D1223766

To Dr. Jem. Milgrim – with respect for his effluvious interest in things orthopedically interesting as well as pragmatic

D. Kelikian

[signature]

[signature]

H. KELIKIAN, M.D.

*Emeritus Professor of Orthopedic Surgery,
Northwestern University Medical School;
Senior Attending Orthopedic Surgeon,
Northwestern Memorial Hospital, Chicago, Illinois;
Consulting Orthopedic Surgeon,
Bethany Methodist, Henrotin, and Augustana Hospitals,
Chicago, Illinois*

CONGENITAL DEFORMITIES *of the* HAND *and* FOREARM

W. B. SAUNDERS COMPANY
Philadelphia, London, Toronto
1974

W. B. Saunders Company: West Washington Square
Philadelphia, Pa.   19105

12 Dyott Street
London, WC1A   1DB

833 Oxford Street
Toronto, Ontario M8Z 5T9, Canada

Congenital Deformities of the Hand and Forearm   ISBN 0-7216-5358-8

Print No.:   9   8   7   6   5   4   3   2   1

To My Children
Armen, Alice and Virginia

PREFACE

Anomalies of the hand and forearm have attracted the attention of surgeons and scientists from the very beginnings of history. An overwhelming mass of writing has been the result. Almost all of it is based on actual experience, but some parts of it are rooted in superstition and others in notions of etiology and classification that spring more from fantasy than from observation.

Surgical management of these difficult handicaps to normal function and normal appearance has been attended at times with indifferent success, and some of the results have been presented with an excess of enthusiasm. There is no consensus on a definition of effective therapy. Confusion also arises from the circumstance that these genetic defects are never exactly alike, and so the surgical attack has always rightly taken individual rather than standardized routes.

This book examines the past and records the author's own experience in a challenging field of surgery. There is no other in which the personal rewards of good planning are as great, but in which the quantitation of results is so unsatisfactory, and moreover in which terminologic confusion is so generalized.

The recording of this experience is in large measure pictorial, and appreciation is due most of all to Irmgard K. Strassburger for drawings that illustrate both the rationale and the detail of surgical technique and to Jack Leblebijian for photographs that illuminate the problems and the results in many individual case histories.

The painstaking search through the literature has involved the help of Georgia Price, of the Northwestern University Medical School library. Also a debt of gratitude is owed to Dr. Hermine Pashayan, who prepared the pedigree chart on symphalangism.

The greatest obligation of all I owe to my family, who quietly supported an endeavor which often seemed endless and who missed—I hope as much as I— the many hours of pleasant companionship I once enjoyed with them.

My publishers, too, had to know patience. Beyond this passive virtue they displayed a sensitive appreciation of my purposes and a thorough technical knowledge of how to secure the results in preparation and in printing that I wanted.

H. KELIKIAN

CONTENTS

Chapter One

DEFINITION AND SCOPE

Our knowledge of congenital anomalies is in a state of flux. What was written about birth defects in the past is at present considered fallacious; what is being written now may well be accorded a similar verdict. Opinions on this subject change from decade to decade, if not from year to year. The pace of this dynamism has been especially accelerated since the establishment of the sciences of genetics and biochemistry, and the advent of radiography and the electron microscope.

When Etienne Geoffroy Saint-Hilaire (1822) conducted his experiments on eggs, the microscope was a crude instrument, hardly in common use; the words biochemistry and microbiology had not yet found their way into dictionaries; Gregor Mendel, founder of the science of genetics, was born in the year Saint-Hilaire published the results of his experiments; and the discoverer of x-ray, Wilhelm Roentgen, 33 years later.

Etienne's son, Isidore Geoffroy Saint-Hilaire (1829, 1832) was a researcher of another sort. In addition to what he had learned from his father, he diligently studied what others had written about structural abnormalities. With a penchant for detail and organization, he catalogued every abnormality he had seen, heard of, or read about; he classified them into groups and assigned to each category an appropriate designation. It was he who introduced the terms *teratology, ectrodactyly, phocomelia,* and numerous others still in use. We may now regard his views on congenital anomalies as obsolete, but we still can learn from him something we seem to have lost sight of, namely, the scholarly method of presenting a subject.

In nineteenth century literature, socially condonable malformations were discussed in connection with gross monstrosities and often became overshadowed by the latter. Deformities of the hand suffered similar submersion. In many modern communications, almost all of the space is allotted to the defects of the skull, the spine, and to the abnormalities of the brain and the heart; discussion of the hand is ignored.

1

CHANGING CONCEPTS OF CONGENITAL ANOMALY

There is considerable disparity of opinion as to what constitutes a congenital abnormality. Vrolik (1849) defined congenital deformities as "deviations of the organism which can be formed only in the early period of gestation, or, at least, previously to the termination of foetal condition." Vrolik was noncommittal as to when, in relation to the moment of birth, congenital malformations became manifest—did they reveal themselves immediately after birth or at some later period?

During the ensuing decades, this question was vehemently debated. The pedantically minded argued that the adjective *congenital* is a compound of the prefix *con* which means with and the word *genital* which is related to genesis, meaning origin. The deformity qualified by the adjective *congenital* must be seen at birth, these purists argued. Those who held a broader view replaced the word *seen* with *present;* they contended that a congenital anomaly can well be present at birth but may not be perceived.

Garrod's (1908, 1923) discovery of inborn errors of metabolism tipped the scale in favor of the more liberal view. Early in the present century, Garrod and his followers established the existence of numerous congenital anomalies which would have remained hidden had they not been revealed with the aid of intricate biochemical studies. In the course of their autopsy examinations of the deeper recesses of the body, pathologists divulged congenital abnormalities which had not been suspected while the person was living. During abdominal explorations, surgeons rediscovered the diverticulum that Meckel (1812) had described a century earlier.

The broad implications of Garrod's discovery do not seem to have been widely appreciated. "Generally when we speak of an error of development, and still more when we use the word 'malformation,' we are not referring to morbid structural development affecting numerous minute tissue elements, but to an obvious anomaly in external form," Lenz (1931) wrote. Murphy (1947) had this to say: "The word congenital . . . denotes present at birth and has no other significance. The term malformation means any gross anatomical deviation from the normal, and is used interchangeably with the terms defect, anomaly, deformity, or abnormality." Murphy conceded that a defect may not be visible at birth and can well be "internal," and that its presence is "disclosed either by operation or necropsy."

The existence of internal structural abnormalities was generally accepted, but the controversy concerning late identification of some anomalies persisted. Under the heading "developmental errors," Fairbank (1948) included a number of skeletal abnormalities which are not suspected at birth but are discovered later when a bone breaks, necessitating roentgenographic survey. McIntosh et al (1954) pointed out that less than half of the congenital anomalies are detected at birth and that diagnosis of the remainder may not be made until long after, if ever.

Writing alone, McIntosh (1959) wondered what should be included in the concept of congenital malformation. "The definition of a malformation would appear to be obvious, almost axiomatic, until one tries to formulate it," he wrote. "A structural deviation from the average norm, if it is rare and unfamiliar and therefore 'unsightly,' and if it is readily recognizable to the naked eye—like a cleft lip or a sixth digit on one hand—patently constitutes a malformation . . . . Shall we admit to the category of congenital malformations only those lesions which can be gauged with the naked eye, or is anything to be gained by including microscopic, even submicroscopic, deviations?"

As if to answer this question, Fraser (1959) wrote: "The term 'congenital malformation' will be used to denote gross structural abnormalities present at birth. Admittedly it can be argued that cellular abnormalities such as spherocytosis and molecular diseases such as sickle cell disease are malformations at the cellular and molecular levels, respectively. However, it is felt that the term, when used at these levels, becomes so all-inclusive that it is no longer meaningful. Certainly, as commonly used, the term refers to anatomic abnormalities as observed at the supercellular level."

During the first international conference on congenital malformations, Tatum (1961), of the Rockefeller Institute and a recent winner of the Nobel prize, considered it necessary to avoid a rigid definition of congenital malformations. He advised including in such a definition "not only anatomic abnormalities present in man at birth but also, and especially, molecular abnormalities detectable in any organism, from virus to man." At the same conference, Ebert (1961) asked: "Are we not agreed that anatomic abnormalities are but an expression of abnormalities of structure, or association, or interaction of molecules?"

It seemed propitious for someone to evoke Garrod's ghost. "Garrod in 1908," Goldberg (1963) wrote, "put forward his theory on inborn errors of metabolism—suggesting that some genetic disorders express themselves through enzyme defects as chemical aberrations of the body. . . .The original concept of Garrod has already proved of decisive importance in medical thought. The future may well show that genetic influences play a much greater part in the etiology of diseases than is at present appreciated." In an article entitled "Studies of molecular basis of congenital malformations," Mackler (1969) spoke of specific submolecular inhibitors which interfere with the activity of electron transport system during the development of the fetus, producing malformations.

A great body of literature has now grown to prove that structural deviations seen by the naked eye often coexist with, or are even caused by, hidden disturbances; there are definite indications that visible and occult deviations may have been caused by the same genetic determinant. There are numerous reported cases of radial ray defect associated with congenital blood dyscrasias, Fanconi's anemia among others. Stiff, contracted fingers are among the many obvious manifestations of disturbed mucopolysaccharide metabolism of bone-forming cartilage cells. Chromosomal aberrations which accompany malformations of the hand or forearm surely belong to the molecular or even submolecular level. There is already a growing body of literature concerning the hand and foot syndrome of sickle cell anemia—the disorder which was classed by Fraser (1959) with molecular diseases. Occasionally in this disease some of the metacarpal bones are short. It is known that subjects with sickle cell anemia have a high incidence of multiple infarction of bone due to plugging of nutrient vessels by emboli. It is possible that shortness of the metacarpals is caused by interference with circulation at the metaphyseo-epiphyseal junction, resulting in hypochondroplasia and premature effacement of growth cartilage line. In another variety of hemolytic disease due to congenital deficiency of pyruvate kinase enzyme, the ulnar metacarpals and fibular metatarsals are dwarfed. Admittedly, in sickle cell anemia and perhaps in pyruvate kinase deficiency, skeletal changes may have developed insidiously during the postnatal period; they may represent somatic consequences and as such are neither genetic nor heritable. The same may be said of malformations which gradually become manifest in the course of congenital analgesia, Ehlers-Danlos syndrome, Marfan's syndrome, multiple enchondromatosis, multiple exostosis, and numerous other complexes. The fact remains that the underlying error of these so-called consequential malformations is congenital (Figs. 1–1 and 1–2).

Too often, the time when a congenital anomaly is recognized is recorded as the time of onset. Recognition depends upon the diagnostic acumen of the clinician. The latter cannot arrive at a diagnosis before he has seen and examined the patient. Doting parents, mothers in particular, are not likely to accept the adverse; they wait, and hope that the deformity in question will in time amend itself. The mother may not even notice that one of her infant's fingers is larger than the corresponding digit on the opposite hand. Even if she does, she is likely to ascribe the enlargement of the finger to a transitory deposit of baby fat. Not until the affected finger grows to grotesque dimensions is the child brought in for examination. In order to avoid the attachment of any stigma to her family or to assuage her own guilt complex, the mother will relate the enlargement of the child's finger to some fortuitous postnatal event – an accident or disease. The examining physician, who has perhaps never seen a macrodactylic digit, may be naive enough to take the mother's word for granted and will record the inception of the digital overgrowth at some later date after birth. Macrodactyly is usually evident at birth, although the affected finger attains its greatest gain in girth and length during the period of accelerated growth in childhood and adolescence. Anomalies of the hand and forearm associated with bone dysplasia often fail to cause symptoms that invite the attention which must precede recognition. What Rubin (1964) said about osteopetrosis applies with equal justification to most skeletal disorders: "The time of recognition is not related to time of onset" (Figs. 1–3 and 1–4).

"In a sense," Mellin (1963) wrote, "life may be described as a continuing genetic potential in a physico-chemical environment . . . . 'Persistence' – not 'presence' – marks the malformation." He gave patent ductus arteriosus as an example. He might have given instead the failure of the mesenchymal precursor of the bones to undergo transverse or longitudinal segmentation. At birth, the carpal bones are still cartilaginous; they ossify between the first and the eleventh years. Roentgenographs taken between these two ages will show the carpal bones as gradually expanding islands of density in a sea of translucency. On viewing roentgenographs taken at maturity, one is often surprised to see two or more carpal bones coalesced. The same is true in some cases of side-to-side fusion of forearm bones (radio-ulnar synostosis) or end-to-end union of phalanges (symphalangism). In these allied anomalies the synostotic tendency persists and bony fusion matures insidiously, progressively (Fig. 1–5).

An epiphysis may be congenitally absent in part or as a whole. The carpal epiphysis of the radius becomes roentgenographically visible as a small ovoid ossicle within cartilaginous growth center around the end of the first year in females and a year later in males. It is now thought that Madelung deformity is due to the absence or underdevelopment of the ulnar half of the distal radial epiphysis, and that the aplasia or the hypoplasia of this sector is genetically determined, since the consequent deformity is known to occur in twins, in several members of the same family, mainly in females, and is bilateral. Gates (1946) categorized this abnormality as a genetic disorder. Most clinicians discuss Madelung deformity in connection with congenital malformations, even though the deformity itself appears around the age of ten. Madelung deformity is just one example of congenital anomalies becoming manifest, hence recognizable, years after birth.

(*Text continued on page 10.*)

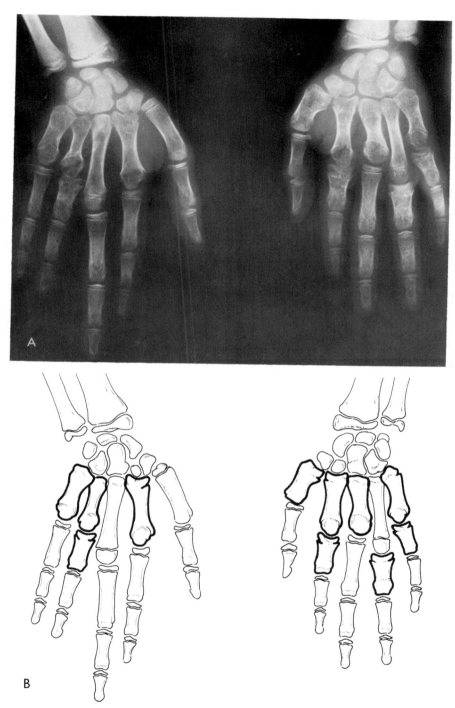

Figure 1–1 Short metacarpals of an 11-year old male with sickle cell disease. *A*, Dorsopalmar roentgenograph of the hands. *B*, Illustrative sketch. In the right hand, the second, fourth, and fifth metacarpals are short. In the left hand, the first, second, third, and fifth are dwarfed. Note the premature closure of the epiphyses of the short metacarpals and short proximal phalanges, also the indentation (remnants of pseudoepiphyses) at the bases of some of the metacarpals.

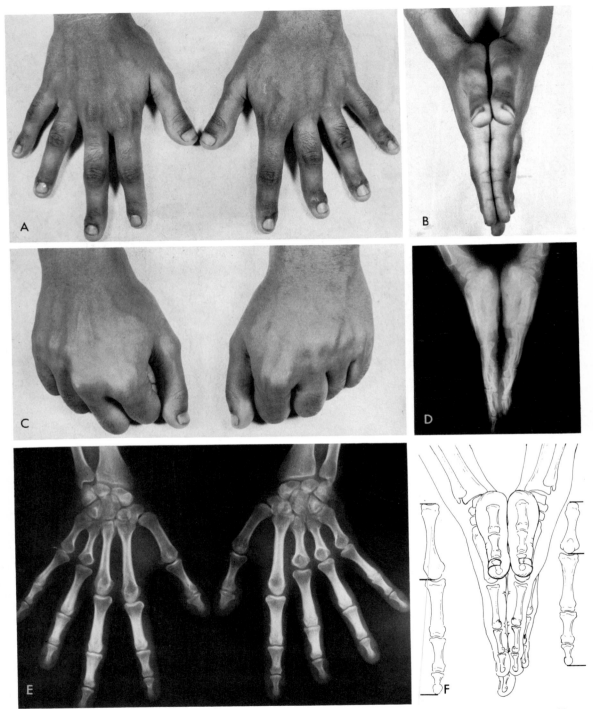

Figure 1–2   Asymmetry and short metacarpals of the hands of a female teenager with congenital pyruvate kinase deficiency. *A*, Dorsal view of the hands: the middle finger of the right hand appears longer than the corresponding digit of the left hand. *B*, Radial view of the same. *C*, Depression of the two ulnar knuckles on the right and three on the left side. *D*, Roentgenograph of the hands in the position shown in *B*. *E*, Dorsopalmar roentgenograph of the hands, showing shortening of the fourth and fifth metacarpals on the right side and shortening of the third, fourth, and fifth on the left side. *F*, Illustrative sketch. This patient also had three short ulnar metacarpals in each foot.

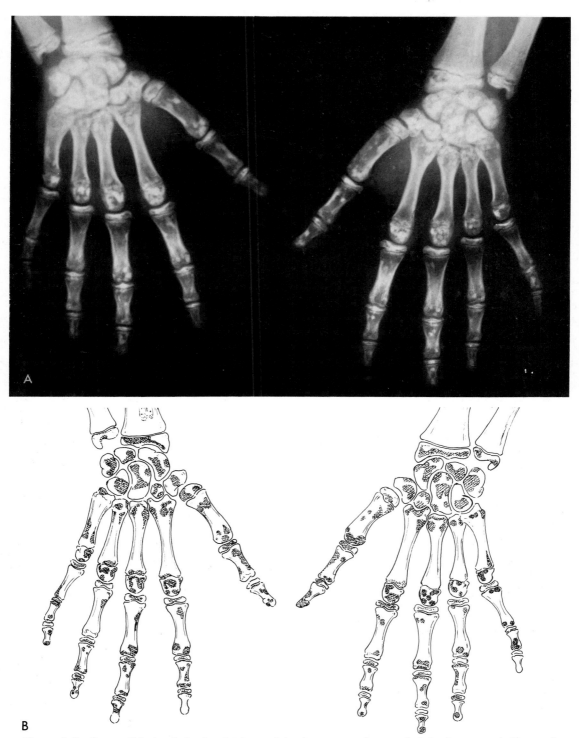

Figure 1–3 Osteopoikilosis of the hands detected in the course of general skeletal survey. *A*, Dorsopalmar roentgenograph of both hands. *B*, Illustrative sketch.

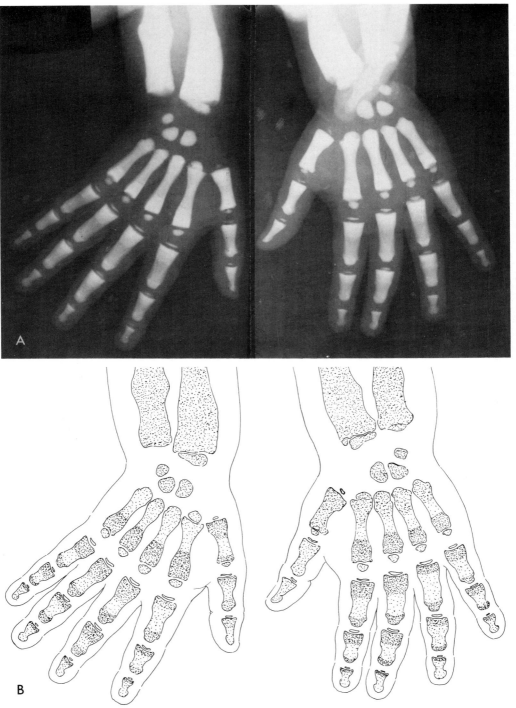

Figure 1–4   Osteopetrosis of the hands of a three-year-old child detected in the course of roentgenographic study necessitated by fracture of the distal radius and ulna of the right forearm. *A*, Dorsopalmar roentgenograph: note the healing fracture of the right distal ulna. *B*, Illustrative sketch.

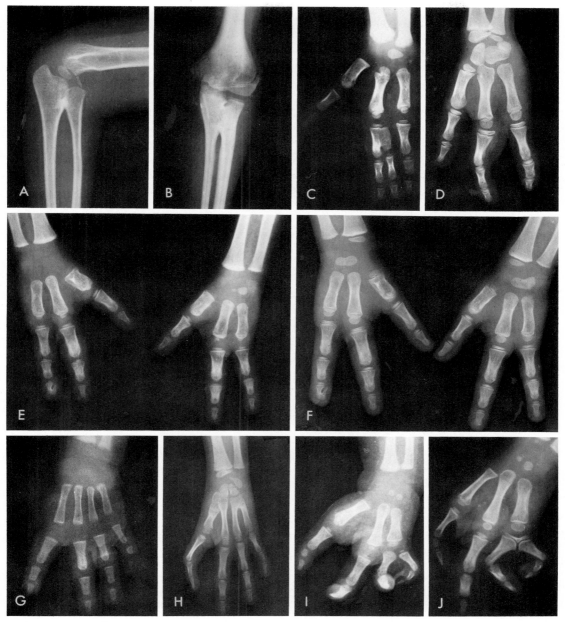

Figure 1-5 Insidious evolution of synostotic states. *A*, Roentgenograph of the right elbow in a three-year-old boy. *B*, The same elbow four years later, showing solid proximal radioulnar synostosis. *C*, Roentgenograph of the left hand of a two-year-old boy with oligosyndactyly. *D*, The same hand five years later, showing fusion of the capitate, hamate, and triquetral bones. *E*, Roentgenograph of the hands of a one-year-old boy with oligodactyly. *F*, The same hands two years later, showing fusion of the capitate and hamate bones. *G*, Roentgenograph of the left hand of a newborn female infant with absent thumb. *H*, The same hand five years later, showing fusion of the last two ulnar metacarpals. The index finger in this child was pollicized. *I*, Roentgenograph of the left hand of a one-year-old female whose index finger was pollicized. *J*, The same hand a year later, showing fusion of the epiphyses of the proximal phalanges of the two ulnar digits.

CONFUSION ABOUT SUNDRY
CONNOTATIONS

Vrolik (1849) distinguished two classes of congenital deformities: (1) those due to "the original deformation of the germ"; and (2) the ones which have resulted from "the subsequent deformation of the embryo by causes operating on its development." Exactly one hundred years later, Birch-Jensen (1949) relabeled Vrolik's two classes with the epithets endogenous and exogenous, respectively. Geneticists have long been teaching that injuries inflicted upon the human embryo by environmental influences would result in malformations which, although congenital, are not hereditary; they have been insisting that these two adjectives should not be used as if they were synonymous. As late as the mid-thirties, when the science of genetics had attained considerable stature, there were still some clinicians who confused the adjective *congenital* with *hereditary*. According to Macklin (1935), this confused coterie felt that in order for a disease to be hereditary it must be congenital or must make its appearance shortly after birth. "Congenital and hereditary are terms which are neither mutually exclusive nor inclusive," Macklin wrote.

The semantic confusion seems to have extended into the sixties. McKusick (1966) introduced the adjective *heritable* "to convey the sense that in a given individual the gene and/or the disease, although transmissible to the offspring, may not have been inherited but rather may have arisen by mutation. The terms *inherited, genetic, hereditary,* and *familial*," McKusick wrote, "are essentially synonymous with *heritable* but have particular shades of meaning. . . . *Congenital* and *hereditary* . . . are not synonymous. . . . A disorder may be congenital and not hereditary, or, conversely, may be hereditary and not congenital. Thalidomide embryopathy is congenital but not hereditary."

Thalidomide taken by the pregnant mother between the thirty-fourth and fiftieth day after her last menstrual period is known to cause malformations in her progeny. Among other parts, the radial component of the forearm and the hand is often involved; the radius, the radial carpal bones, the first metacarpal, and the phalanges of the thumb are absent or hypoplastic. On the whole, except for an occasional occurrence of triphalangeal thumb, the effect of thalidomide is suppressive: elements are subtracted and not added.

CONFUSION CONCERNING THE BORDERS
OF THE HAND AND THE POSTURE OF
THE DIGITS

The adjective *medial* used by some authors—notably by Kanavel (1932) and Entin (1959)— in describing absences of the third digital ray is confusing since this adjective is also utilized in reference to the ulnar or radial border of the hand, depending upon whether the hand is viewed with the palm forward or its back turned towards the inspector. Defects of the third digital ray are best qualified by the adjective *axial*, as the axis of the hand runs through this component. The movements of adduction and abduction of the fingers take place to and away from this axis. The adjectives valgus and varus—employed by Dubreuil-Chambardel (1925) and numerous continental authors—should not be used in descriptions of axial deviations of the digits or the hand; it is best to say that the hand, the finger, or the phalanx is deviated in a radial or ulnar direction. There is no justification for the continuing use of the epithets inner and outer, or medial, or lateral when referring to the borders of the hand; the adjectives *radial* and *ulnar*, or *pre-axial* and *postaxial* are more accurate.

NAMING THE DIGITS

Diemerbroeck (1679) wrote: "The digits, called *daktylos* by the Greeks, are five on each hand, differing in length and thickness. The first, which is thick, because it is equivalent to all the rest in strength is called the thumb. The second, from its use, is called the index and pointer because we are accustomed to using it in pointing out and indicating things. The third, which is the middle finger and the longest, is usually called the impudent, obscene . . . . The fourth is called the ring and medical finger because formerly persons admitted to the doctorate of medicine adorned this digit with a golden ring . . . . The fifth, because of its size, is called little finger and also ear finger since people are wont to clean the dirt out of their ears with it." In Latin we have the ensuing names: pollex, index, medius, annularis, auricularis. Most continental authors employ this nomenclature.

English-speaking authors use the following designations: thumb, index, middle, ring, and little finger. Some authors, mainly in the United States, contend that the hand has a thumb and four fingers and in this group of even number of fingers, therefore, the one next to the index cannot be regarded as being the middle finger; they call this digit the long finger. "It may be better to retain the old established name of middle finger to avoid confusion in cases of congenital or pathological shortening of the middle finger," Kaplan (1965) wrote. Stack (1960) offered the ensuing argument: "The English word 'finger' is considered to have been derived from the pre-Teutonic word 'penge' meaning five, and this means that there is no logical objection to calling the middle digit the middle finger." For reasons already given it would perhaps be less confusing to call this digit the axial finger. In the present book the adjectives *axial* and *middle* are used interchangeably in reference to the third digit of the hand.

NAMING THE BONES OF THE HAND

The metacarpal bones are numbered serially from the radial to the ulnar border of the hand. It is also justifiable to speak of the metacarpal of the thumb, the index, the middle finger, the ring finger, and of the little finger. Some authors number the phalanges in proximodistal sequence: first, second, and third. Others use the adjectives *proximal, middle,* and *distal.* The thumb has only two phalanges: a proximal and a distal. The proximal segment of a digit is also qualified with the adjective *basal,* and the distal phalanx is called terminal or ungual.

NAMING THE BONES OF THE CARPUS

There are two rows of carpal bones. Each row contains four ossicles. The proximal row includes the scaphoid, the lunate, the triquetral, and the pisiform bone. In the distal row are placed the trapezium, the trapezoid, the capitate, and the hamate. All carpal bones have alternate names: the scaphoid is also called navicular; the lunate, semilunar; the triquetral, cuneiform or pyramidal; the pisiform, orbicular; the trapezium, greater multangular; the trapezoid, lesser multangular; the capitate, os magnum; and the hamate, unciform. One may dismiss all these alternate names except navicular which appears as often in the literature as does scaphoid.

THE SCOPE

Topographically, the hand starts at the carpometacarpal junction; it ends at the fingertips. But we cannot conceive of the hand as a functioning organ without a well-positioned wrist and the unimpeded pronation and supination which take place in the forearm. The extrinsic flexors and extensors of the fingers orginate from the distal end of the humerus, from the bones of the forearm, and from the intervening interosseous membrane. Functional boundaries of the hand include the points of origin of these muscles. A few pertinent questions may well be asked: What about the nerves of the hand which orginate from the region of the cervical spine? And why not include the shoulder?

In the wake of cerebral or birth palsy, the hand is often maimed at birth and continues to remain crippled. To be consistent, we should admit these two conditions into the category of congenital abnormalities because they are present at birth. In some cases of cerebral palsy, one could incriminate injury during parturition. In others, as pointed out by McIntosh (1959), one could not place the

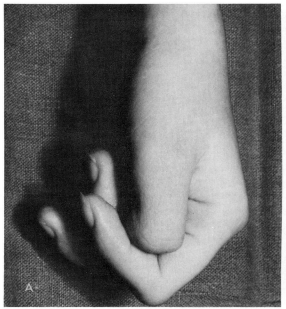
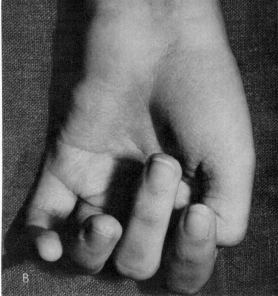

Figure 1–6 "Thumb-clutched hand" or "clasped thumb" of a cerebrospastic young female. This anomaly may be considered as being connatal as well as congenital but is often classed with the former. *A*, Radial view of the left hand. *B*, Palmar view.

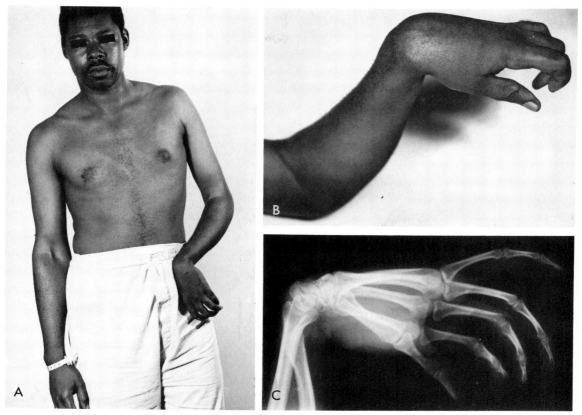

Figure 1–7 Fixed pronation of the forearm and flexion contracture of the wrist and fingers of a man with birth palsy. This deformity is connatal and not congenital. *A*, Frontal view, showing discrepancy between the two upper limbs. *B*, Radial view of the affected right forearm and hand. *C*, Roentgenograph of the same.

onus on injury with any degree of certainty, "and this uncertainty often persists despite intensive clinical observation supplemented by postmorten study of the central nervous system." There should be no uncertainty concerning the crippling of the hand caused by brachial paralysis. In this instance, injury has been inflicted upon an infant who presumably was well formed and equipped with a full quota of functional capacity; the disability resulted from damage incurred during parturition and is, therefore, acquired and not congenital, even though it is present at birth. Not all connatal anomalies are congenital (Figs. 1–6 and 1–7).

As for the shoulder, this author has never understood why Bunnell (1944, 1948, 1956), in the successive editions of his book entitled *Surgery of the Hand*, including those revised by Boyes (1964, 1970), discussed elevation of the scapula, acromioclavicular separation, and tear of the supraspinatus or long head of the biceps. In another book entitled *Hand Surgery*, Aitkin (1966) discussed fractures of the proximal epiphysis of the humerus at length. It may well be asked: What book on the foot mentions slipped capital epiphysis of the femur or tear of the biceps tendon in the thigh?

Most books on the hand suffer from the inclusion of irrelevant items as much as from oversight of more pertinent topics. With the possible exception of Temtamy's (1966) Ph.D. thesis and a treatise by Tridon and Thiriet (1966), almost all books neglect to discuss congenital syndromes implicating the hand. In the present book, an attempt will be made to replenish this deficit.

The scope of the present book has also been amplified by the addition of another chapter which discusses the social and psychological impact of individuals with congenitally malformed hands. Each chapter is accorded as complete a bibliography as it has been possible to secure. In some instances, the list of references is more extensive than the discussion which precedes. This is as it should be. The author considers comprehensive bibliography essential to this book.

SUMMARY

We are beginning to take a breadth and depthwise view of congenital anomalies—a view that goes beyond the arbitrary boundaries in time and space set by earlier authors. At this evolutionary stage in our concept of congenital anomalies, it would seem precarious to formulate an ironclad definition. It is perhaps safe to say that a congenital anomaly is one which has its inception during antenatal development and is present at birth even though it may not be perceived until a later date. A congenital anomaly may be hereditary or nonhereditary, external or internal. In the latter category are included cellular and subcellular disturbances, biochemical disorders, and chromosomal aberrations. These hidden disorders cannot be divorced from the accompanying malformations which are seen by the naked eye. Discussion of congenital anomalies of the hand is extended to include structural and functional deviations of the wrist and forearm as well as syndromes and systemic disorders which implicate the upper limb distal to the elbow proper.

References

Aitkin, A. P.: Fractures of the epiphysis of the upper extremity. *In* Flynn, J. E., (ed.): *Hand Surgery.* Baltimore, Williams & Wilkins Co., pp. 161–183, 1966.

Birch-Jensen, A.: *Congenital Deformities of the Upper Extremities.* Translated from the Danish by E. Aagesen. Copenhagen, Andelsbogtrykkeriet I Odense Det danske Forlag, pp. 9–285, 1949.

Boyes, J. H.: Congenital deformities. Shoulder and elbow. *In* Boyes, J. H., (ed.): *Bunnell's Surgery of the Hand.* Fourth edition. Philadelphia, J. B. Lippincott Co., pp. 55–97, 561–586, 1964. See also fifth edition, pp. 609–647, 1970.

Bunnell, S.: Congenital deformities; shoulder region. *In Surgery of the Hand.* Philadelphia, J. B. Lippincott Co., pp. 609–647; 424–432, 1944. See also second edition, pp. 793–838; 572–584, 1948; third edition, pp. 654–666; 909–962, 1956.

Diemerbroeck, I. de: Digiti. *In Anatome Corporis Humani.* Lugduni, J. A. Huguetan & Soc., pp. 469–470, 1970. See also the French translation by J. Prost. Lyon, Anison and Posuel., Vol. 2, p. 44, 1965.

Dubrueil-Chambardel, L.: Clinodactylies laterales — auriculaire varus, medius valgus, pouce valgus, index varus, etc. *In Le Variation du Corps Humain.* Paris, E. Flammarion, pp. 141–145; figs. 65–70, 1925.

Ebert, J. B.: Antibodies, viruses and embryos. *In First International Conference on Congenital Malformations.* Philadelphia, J. B. Lippincott Co., pp. 291–299, 1961.

Entin, M. A.: Reconstruction of congenital abnormalities of the upper extremities. *J. Bone Joint Surg., 41A*:681–700, 1959.

Fairbank, T.: Abnormalities of the skeleton in children. *Ann. Coll. Surg. Eng., 3*:85–93, 1948.

Fraser, F. C.: Causes of congenital malformations in human beings. *J. Chronic Dis., 10*:97–110, 1959.

Garrod, A. E.: Alkaptonuria. *Lancet, 2*:73–79, 1908.

Garrod, A. E.: *Inborn Errors of Metabolism.* Second edition. London, H. Frowde; Hodder & Stoughton Ltd., pp. 1–16, 1923.

Gates, R. R.: *Human Genetics.* New York, The Macmillan Co., Vol. I, pp. 385–469, 1946.

Goldberg, A.: Inborn errors of metabolism. *Practitioner, 191*:182–191, 1963.

Kanavel, A. B.: Congenital malformations of the hands. *Arch. Surg., 25*:1–53; 282–320, 1932.

Kaplan, E. B.: *Functional and Surgical Anatomy of the Hand.* Second edition. Philadelphia, J. B. Lippincott Co., pp. 23–86, 1965.

Lenz, F.: Anomalies of bodily form. *In* Bour, E., Fischer, E., Lenz, F.: *Human Heredity.* Translated by E. and C. Paul. Third Edition. New York, The Macmillan Co., pp. 285–297, 1931.

Mackler, B.: Studies of the molecular basis of congenital malformations. *Pediatrics, 43*:915–926, 1969.

Macklin, M. T.: The role of heredity in disease. *Medicine, 14*:1–75, 1935.

McKusick, V. A.: *Heritable Disorders of Connective Tissue.* Third edition. Saint Louis, C. V. Mosby Co., pp. 1–3, 1966.

McIntosh, R.: The problem of congenital malformations: general considerations. *J. Chronic Dis., 10*:139–151, 1959.

McIntosh, R., Merritt, K. K., Richard, M. R., Samuels, M. H., and Bellows, M. T.: The incidence of congenital malformations: a study of 5,964 pregnancies. *Pediatrics, 14*:505–521, 1954.

Meckel, J. F.: *Handbuch der pathologischen Anatomie.* Vol. I, pp. 553–597, 1812.

Mellin, G. W.: The frequency of birth defects. *In* Fishbein, M., (ed.): *Birth Defects.* Philadelphia, J. B. Lippincott Co., pp. 1–17, 1963.

Murphy, D. P.: *Congenital Malformations.* Philadelphia, J. B. Lippincott Co., p. 304, 1947.

Rubin, P.: *Dynamic Classification of Bone Dysplasias.* Chicago, Yearbook Medical Publishers, Inc., pp. 258–280, 1964.

Saint-Hilaire, E. G.: *Philosophie Anatomique des Monstruosités Humaines.* Paris, Chez l'Auteur, pp. 473–541, 1822.

Saint-Hilaire, I. G.: *Propositions sur la Monstruosité Considérée chez l'Homme et les Animaux.* Paris, Didot et Le Jeune, pp. 1–74, 1829.

Saint-Hilaire, I. G.: *Histoire Générale et particuliére des Anomalies de l'Organisation chez l'Homme et les Animaux.* Paris, J. B. Balliére, Vol. I, pp. 251–278, 671–702, 1832.

Stack, H. G.: Naming the fingers. *Hand, 1*:146–151, 1969.

Tatum, E. L.: Some molecular aspects of congenital malformation. *In First International Conference on Congenital Malformations.* Philadelphia, J. B. Lippincott Co., pp. 281–288, 1961.

Temtamy, S.: *Genetic Factors in Hand Malformations.* Ph.D. Thesis. Baltimore, Johns Hopkins University, pp. 1–449, 1966.

Tridon, P., and Thiriet, M.: *Malformations Associées de la Téte et des Extrémités.* Paris, Masson et Cie., pp. 1–229, 1966.

Vrolik, W.: Teratology. *In* Todd, R. B., (ed.): *Cyclopaedia of Anatomy and Physiology.* London, Longman, Brown, Green, Longman, & Roberts, *4*:942–976, 1849.

Chapter Two

CAUSAL RELATIONS

The surgeon who undertakes the care of a child born with a malformed hand is often assailed with a barrage of questions: What was the cause of the deformity? Was it "bad blood" on the part of the father or mother? Did it have anything to do with the accident the mother was involved in during her pregnancy? The flu she had? The x-ray which was taken of her? The pills she took? Might the horribly maimed children she saw on television have affected her while she carried her baby? More important, this being her first born, would her next child have the same deformity?

Even the most experienced clinician cannot answer all of these questions. The literature is not of much help because it deals mainly with monstrosities and major malformations. One has to wade through stacks of articles and books to find something specific about hands—it is like looking for a needle in a haystack. There is so much to read to learn so little.

The controversy as to whether the seed or the soil should be blamed for an undesirable crop is very ancient. The familiar parable in the New Testament (Matthew 13:4) about "seeds falling upon stony places where they had not much earth" put the blame upon the soil. Many poets have since identified earth with mother. To some, the warm, loamy earth is like a fertile mother. To others— Swinburne, for one—"chill solemn earth" is a "fatal mother with . . . Niobean womb," meaning a growth-stunting uterus.

Montgomery (1836) considered it a "truth that the seeds of life are often sown adulterated . . . . The germ . . . may have a morbid taint," he wrote and assigned the adjective *innate* to abnormalities resulting from this cause. In the years that followed, this class of congenital anomalies acquired diverse designations: hereditary, familial, inherent, inborn, intrinsic, germinal, genetic, endogenous, genotypic, and biotypic. Malformations caused by external influences acting upon the developing embryo have been variously called amniotic, formative, evolutionary, developmental, environmental, nongenetic, extrinsic, exogenous, and phenocopic.

16

INCIDENCE

Saint-Hilaire (1832) estimated that in Paris 1 out of 3000 newborns was malformed. Following the example set by him almost all teratologists preceded their discussion of congenital anomalies with statistical surveys. According to Murphy (1947), 1 of every 213 infants born in and around Philadelphia was malformed; in families with a previously deformed child, the birth of a subsequent defective offspring was 25 times greater; a child born of an older mother ran a greater risk of being abnormal; and one coming late into a family was more likely to be defective than its predecessors. Carter (1950) pointed out that malformed stillborns and babies with minor malformations were usually left out of reported surveys, and that seemingly unaffected newborns were not followed up sufficiently to see if an undetected anomaly would become manifest. He estimated that if all these cases were included, the incidence of congenital anomalies would rise to 4 or 5 per cent.

None of these authors particularized the malformations of the hand. Birch-Jensen (1949) produced the first statistics of congenital defects of the upper extremity. His survey was confined to one compact country, Denmark. At the time, the population of Denmark was around four million; the total number of defective children was 625. Birch-Jensen estimated that 1 in 6438 newborns suffered from absence of some part of the upper extremity. Birch-Jensen limited his discussion to the deficiencies and made no mention of duplications. Polydactyly, which constitutes one of the most common congenital anomalies of the hand, appears to have escaped Birch-Jensen's attention, perhaps because surplus digits are disposed of soon after birth by the family physician and fail to find their way into official dossiers. Also absent from Birch-Jensen's list are anomalies of segmentation: symphalangism, carpal coalescence, and radioulnar synostosis. One likewise misses discrepancies of digital alignment, Madelung deformity, macrodactylia, and numerous syndromes or systemic disorders which implicate the hand. Canepa and Sanguinetti (1959) studied 40 cases of congenital deformities of the hand. These represented nearly 10 per cent of all skeletal malformations. They considered syndactyly, brachydactyly, and polydactyly as the most common congenital anomalies of the hand. Males seem to be affected more often than females. Conway and Bowe (1956) surveyed the live babies born at the New York Hospital between the years of 1932 and 1954. They placed the incidence of hand anomalies as 1 in 626 live births.

Almost all statistics, including Birch-Jensen's, stress the relative infrequency of congenital malformations. The patient is constantly reminded of his defect, and the awareness of being disadvantageously different from the norm deepens his feeling of alienation. The inevitable psychological turmoil finally compels him or his parents to seek advice. In most instances, the child is brought to a surgeon who is primarily concerned with improving the function and form of the crippled hand.

The surgeon is least interested in defective embryos, monstrosities, and mangled or macerated feti, discussions of which clutter statistical surveys of congenital anomalies. Muench (1953) voiced the sentiment of most practicing surgeons when he said: "To a good many clinicians, a biostatistician is a mechanism devoted mainly to asking embarrassing questions after it is too late to get an answer." Hellman (1953) wrote: "Putting holes in a punched card to record data doesn't impart to that card either a soul or integrity." It is even more difficult to infuse compassion into the computer machines which are now being utilized for statistical surveys.

GENETIC INTERPRETATION

Heredity has long been regarded as a major factor in the causation of congenital anomalies, including those of the hand. Aristotle (384–322 B.C.) had written: "For man is generated from man; and thus it is the possession of certain characters by the parent that determines the development of the characters in the child. . . . A given germ does not give rise to any chance living being, nor spring from any chance one; but each germ springs from a definite parent and gives rise to a definite progeny. And thus it is the germ that is the ruling influence of the offspring."

Heredity is a nebulous subject. It is wrapped in mystery and therefore open to speculation. As often happens in discussions of such topics, rhetoric diverts the attention from reality. Sir Francis Galton (1869–1889), Erasmus Darwin's grandson, extracted the phrase "nature and nurture" from Shakespeare (*The Tempest*: act 3, scene 1, line 188), and dangled it as a decoy before the intellectuals of his time. This bit of Shakespearean euphony reverberated in the writings of numerous authors—Thomson (1908), Reid (1910), Dunn and Dobzhansky (1952), Harris (1959), and many others.

Galton defined nature as "the sum of inborn qualities" and related nurture to environmental influences. He accorded greater importance to the former. Galton's cousin, Charles Darwin (1887), agreed with him on this point. In his turn, Galton (1889) credited Darwin with the idea of "particulate inheritance." Galton also spoke of "heritages that blend." These two concepts—particulate and blended inheritances—are mutually exclusive.

Weismann (1875) brought the concept of heredity down from the speculative stratosphere and tied it to something definite: he allocated the material of heredity within the germ cell, inside the nucleus, and on the chromosomes. Weismann considered the germ cell as the sole conveyor of hereditary qualities and their determinants. It was after the general acceptance of Weismann's views that the word "germinal" appeared in discussions of congenital malformations. Ballantyne (1904) argued that when the same malformation reappears in two or three generations of the same family, one must suspect a teratogenic something in the ovum or the sperm; the occurrence of the same malformation in several members of the same family also required similar explanation.

Ballantyne quoted many authors on heredity but failed to mention Gregor Mendel, the founder of modern genetics. Mendel (1865) had announced his laws of heredity 40 years before the publication of Ballantyne's book. Mendel's principles were entirely overlooked until they were rediscovered by DeVries (1900), Correns (1900), and Tschermak (1900). The interim neglect of Mendel's discoveries has been ascribed to the fact that Mendel was a monk who led a secluded existence, out of contact with other scientists. A more plausible explanation is that during the last four decades of the nineteenth century, intellectuals all over the world were overwhelmingly taken up with the Darwinian theory, and Mendel's "dull and simple ratios, the result of breeding garden peas," passed unnoticed.

Mendel experimented with various kinds of pea plants. When a purebred tall plant was crossed with a purebred dwarf, the hybrids of the first filial generation were all tall. The dwarfs seemed to have slipped out of sight. But this was illusory, because the tall hybrid contained the unseen character of the dwarf. When this tall hybrid was self-pollinated, Mendel obtained a second generation three-quarters of which were tall and one-quarter dwarf, giving a 3:1

ratio. When self-pollinated, all the dwarfs of this second generation bred true, but tall plants manifested varied behavior: one-third produced tall progenies and two-thirds resembled the first generation hybrids. The tall plants of the second generation proved themselves purebred because when pollinated with dwarfs, the progenies were again all tall.

On the basis of such experiments, Mendel formulated his well-known laws of segregation and independent assortment. In effect, Mendel said that in cross-breeding, contrasting characters may seem to have accomplished temporary union, but they are capable of detaching themselves and recombining; in this process of combination, detachment, and recombination, some characters express themselves fairly regularly, while others are suppressed. Mendel gave the epithets *dominant* to the former and *recessive* to the latter.

Mendel was not one to indulge in sweeping generalizations. His interpreters—who are legion—have described Mendelian characters as being durable and discrete: in their passage from generation to generation, dominant and recessive characters lose none of their original attributes; they preserve their prerogative to detach themselves and to return again to their initial state. Mendel's unit character has been dubbed "the dice of destiny," which can be shaken together, separated, recombined, and separated again, eventually achieving "a kind of splendid isolation."

Genetics, deserving the name science, received great impetus after the rediscovery of Mendel's laws in 1900. In the comparatively short span of seven decades, genetics has attained a gigantic scope. Its growth has not ceased; it continues to be dynamic and four dimensional. It now extends in all directions, into every nook and cranny of organic existence, encompassing the entire array of biological sciences and many phases of clinical medicine. That a new and expanding science would require a commensurate vocabulary was foreseen by the earlier exponents of Mendelism.

In due course, geneticists developed a secular argot which now often remains impervious. Geneticists are not likely to condescend and establish a common wavelength with the clinicians. The latter may strike a recalcitrant attitude—as have Barsky and associates (1964)—dismissing the seemingly abstruse terms used by geneticists as "merely convenient pegs on which to hang our hat of ignorance." Geneticists might well ask, Whose ignorance? Refractory remarks do not solve problems. It is time that clinicians make an effort to familiarize themselves with the body of knowledge garnered by geneticists. Knowledge is conveyed by words. Geneticists have concocted their own unique set of words.

Johannsen (1903, 1911) introduced the term "gene" which he considered a very applicable little word, easily combined with others; it stands for the unit-factors in the gametes. Out of one such combination Johannsen derived the designation "genotype," which he defined as the fundamental hereditary constitution of an organism. Johannsen pointed out that the genotype cannot be seen; its presence is surmised by developed, measured realities of qualities and reactions of the organism in question. To this discernible expression of genotype, Johannsen gave the name "phenotype." Johannsen also used the adjectival forms of these terms, evolving the epithets genotypic and phenotypic. Genotype is determined at the time of fertilization, before environmental influences come into play. Phenotype is genotype modified by environment; it is produced by the interreaction of gene and environment. Genes are comparatively stable. Environment varies. In its transmission from one generation to another, the same genotype is often represented by diversified phenotypes.

DeVries (1903) introduced the term *mutation* to indicate a change in genetic constitution. The adjective *mutant* was originally applied to the individual manifesting the nascent trait and, later, to the gene transporting it. "A mutation," Harris (1959) wrote, "presumably alters the structure of a gene in some way and this may be expected to be reflected in its behavior." Seemingly new characteristics, including newly erupting congenital anomalies, may owe their origin to mutant genes and are passed by them to future generations.

Bateson (1906) introduced the terms *allelomorph, homozygote,* and *heterozygote*. Allelomorph is compounded from the Greek roots *allelon* and *morph* which respectively mean alternative and form. Bateson used the term allelomorph for each alternative Mendelian factor. Allele is the abbreviated form of allelomorph. Allelic and allelomorphic are adjectival forms. Zygote denotes a fertilized ovum. When the latter is formed by the union of two gametes carrying analogous alleles, it is called a homozygote; the individual evolving from this union is said to be homozygous. The heterozygote is a hybrid, the product of two gametes of dissimilar genetic constitution. Bateson also introduced the symbols F_1, F_2, F_3, and so forth to represent the successive filial generations. Castle (1931) pointed out that the dominant allele is expressed in the heterozygote, while the recessive is not. It would follow that dominant alleles are regularly expressed in F_1, while the recessives are regularly suppressed in that generation; both variants are expressed in F_2, in which dominants exceed recessives, maintaining the 3:1 ratio. Alleles are now regarded as alternative forms occupying homologous positions or loci on each pair of chromosomes.

Timoféef-Ressovsky (1931) introduced the terms *penetrance* and *expressivity*. Penetrance pertains to the frequency of the phenotypic manifestations in a pedigree group; expressivity denotes the degree to which the effect of the genotype becomes manifest in an individual. A gene is said to have complete penetrance when it produces its full phenotypic effect in every member of a pedigree; when the effect is manifest in only a few members, the gene is said to have low penetrance; when the gene produces diversified effects from one individual to another, it is said to have variable expressivity; when a dominant defect skips a generation in the pedigree, it is considered as lacking penetrance. "Polydactyly is quite uniform in some pedigrees, but in others the extra finger shows all stages of reduction until it is no bigger than a wart in the position where the finger should be," Gates (1952) wrote. He called these muted expressions *formes frustes*.

Goldschmidt (1938) introduced the term *phenocopy* which he regarded as the product of environment only; it is brought about by exogenous influences acting upon the developing embryo by causing alteration of form and function. Phenocopy is an environmentally induced facsimile of phenotype; it is not transmitted from one generation to another; it is not heritable. Malformations of the newborn infant caused by maternal rubella or thalidomide intake are phenocopies of known genetic defects. In phenocopy, only somatic cells suffer alterations; genotype is related to germinal cells as is in part the phenotype.

Montgomery (1906), one of Weismann's disciples, pointed out that the somatic cell reproduces itself, but is incapable of reproducing a whole individual; certain mature germ cells possess this power. At the time, not much was known about the chromosomal content of various cells. It is now definitely established that each human cell contains 23 pairs, or a total of 46 chromosomes. Of these, 22 pairs are alike in both sexes; they are called autosomes. The remaining pair are named sex chromosomes, which vary according to sexes. In the male, an X chromosome is coupled with a Y chromosome; in the female, two X chromosomes constitute the pair.

Karyotype is a term used to distinguish the chromosomal pattern of one individual from that of another. This designation is also employed for the photograph of chromosomes arranged in the standard Denver (1960) classification. Chromosomal pairs are separated into groups. There are seven autosomal groups. Some authors label these groups with capital letters: under A are included autosomal pairs 1 through 3; under B, 4 and 5; under C, 6 through 12; under D, 13 through 15; under E, 16 through 18; under F, 19 and 20; and under G, 21 and 22. The twenty-third pair consists of sex chromosomes. If two or more cells obtained from the tissue of an individual reveal different karyotypes, the tissue or the individual is said to show mosaicism.

Autosomal or somatic cells reproduce themselves within the individual by mitosis; each new cell thus produced contains the exact chromosomal complement of the parent cell: 22 pairs of autosomes and one pair of sex chromosomes, making a total of 46. From a genetic point of view, the chromosomes contained in somatic cells are considered inert; they do not convey inherited characteristics from the individual to the offspring. Transmission of hereditary traits is carried out by the gametes—the sperm and the ovum. These germ cells are produced by a type of division known as meiosis, in which each pair of parental chromosomes loses a partner by a process called disjunction. In the language of the geneticist, during meiosis the diploid cell is converted into a haploid state with half of the chromosomal complement of the parental cell; it now has 22 single autosomes and one sex chromosome. Being haploid, neither the ovum nor the sperm can enter into a reproductive phase unless they first unite and attain a diploid status in the fertilized ovum or the zygote, and the individual regains its full quota of 23 pairs or 46 chromosomes.

In meiosis a chromosome occasionally fails to shed its partner; the failure of a complementary chromosome to separate from its partner is called nondisjunction. In the fertilized ovum, this pair gains another chromosome with the result that, at this particular point, there are now three chromosomes instead of two. Triplication of a numbered pair of chromosomes is called trisomy. The trisomic individual has 47 instead of 46 chromosomes. Alternately, one of the chromosomes may be sluggish in the plane of meiotic division; this is called lagging or anaphase lag. The lingering unit may become attached to another chromosome or get lost; in the latter instance the zygote—and through it the individual— will have 45 chromosomes instead of 46. A particle may break away from a chromosome and disappear; this is called deletion. Occasionally, the portions of the two arms of a chromosome will become detached and the broken ends of the centric segment will rejoin, forming a ring; the detached terminals, having no centromere—the spindly mass of chromatid at the equator as produced in the metaphase of meiosis—are lost. In some cases of deletion, the broken fragment may survive and reattach itself to the same or to another chromosome. If intact, the terminal point of the recipient chromosome is said to repel the invading particle, and it can only give anchorage to the latter when it itself is broken and has given a fragment in exchange; this is called translocation and is often qualified with the adjective "reciprocal." Since exchanged particles are not likely to be of the same size or chromatin content, one chromosome will be different in size and quality from the other. Sex chromatin takes up stain; hence, it is made visible during the resting stage of cell division, providing the cell contains more than one X chromosome, as it does in females; women with paired X chromosomes are chromatin positive, while men with only a single X are chromatin negative.

Homologous chromosomes often exchange particles, and this is considered normal. When the segment acquired by a chromosome has turned upside down, however, the genes on it will be arranged in reverse order; this is called inversion. When a centromere splits crosswise and one chromosome acquires two equal but long arms bearing the same set of genes in reverse sequence, it is called isochromosome. Translocation between homologous chromosomes may result in duplication of the same type of gene in one of the pairs.

Association of chromosomal aberrations with pathologic conditions is now an established fact. There is already a sizeable body of clinically recognizable syndromes connected with chromosomal abnormalities which affect the hand and the forearm. As time goes on, more and more such associations are likely to be established. In discussions of these syndromes by geneticists, such terms as trisomy, triplication, or triploidy, linkage, mosaicism, and many others frequently crop up. The clinician cannot afford to ignore them.

Genes on the same chromosome tend to stay together as they are passed together from parent to child; this is called linkage. Associated abnormalities passed on by the sex chromosome are said to be sex-linked. Most geneticists consider the Y chromosome genetically inactive, and prefer the connotation of X-linked to that of sex-linked. In X-linked disorders, the affected individuals are nearly always male, the mother of the affected male acting as carrier. McKusick (1966) considered the absence of male-to-male or father-to-son transmission as the critical characteristic of X-linked inheritance. "Father-to-son transmission of X-linked traits cannot occur," he wrote.

The term *sex-limited* merely means that the gene concerned expresses itself mainly in males or females. A particular gene may give rise to two or more expressions; in this instance simultaneously appearing phenotypic expressions are associated and not linked. Some traits owe their origin to the concerted action of several biochemical or enzymic processes, each of which may be controlled by a different gene. The inherited trait is then said to be multifactorial.

Genetic disorders transmitted by one of the nonsex chromosomes are called autosomal. In autosomal dominant phenotype, only one parent is affected and the trait can be traced back from one generation to another almost persistently. In autosomal recessive abnormalities, both parents are unaffected, but act as carriers of the responsible gene: the child receives two doses of the mutant gene, one from the mother and one from the father. Parental consanguinity is considered the arena for hidden recessive traits to come into the open.

The literature abounds with numerous reports of genetic disorders of the hand and forearm. The following show distinct autosomal dominant patterns: anonychia, polydactyly, syndactyly, brachydactyly, stub thumb, symphalangism, carpal coalescence, radioulnar synostosis, split hand, and radial ray defect. Most discrepancies of digital posture, especially those due to skeletal abnormalities or aplasia of pollical extensors, are transmitted as autosomal dominant phenotypes. Occasionally one encounters postural misalignments which pursue a recessive mode of inheritance (Figs. 2–1 to 2–6).

The hand and the forearm are also implicated in a number of syndromes, some of which are transmitted as either dominant or recessive phenotypes. The following are considered dominant: achondroplasia, acrocephalosyndactyly, Marfan's arachnodactyly, Holt-Oram syndrome, cleidocranial dysostosis, Klippel-Trenaunay angiodysplastic asymmetry, and most bone dysplasias affecting the hand and forearm. The locus of nail-patella syndrome and that of the ABO blood group are linked. Nail-patella syndrome is considered an autosomally linked trait; it is transmitted as a dominant phenotype. Achondrogenesis, Ellis-van Creveld chondroectodermal dysplasia, congenital analgesia, various

(*Text continued on page 28.*)

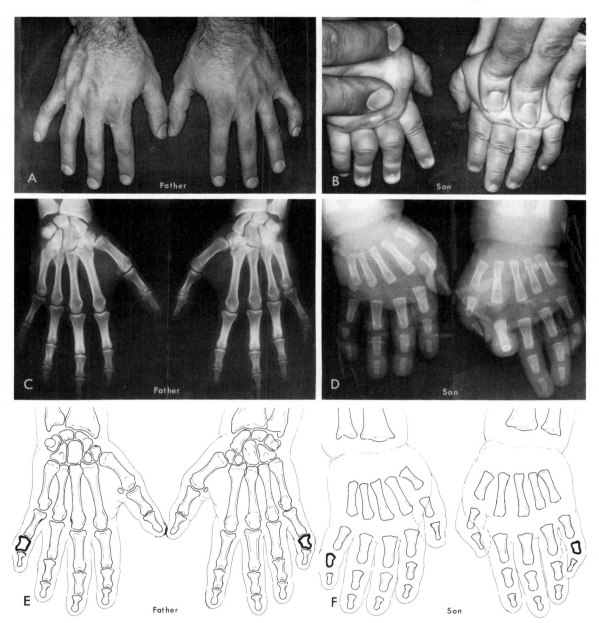

Figure 2–1 Dominant phenotype with unabated expressivity. Bilateral dwarfed middle phalanx (brachymesopha-langy) of the little finger with radial deviation (clinodactyly) of the little finger – more marked in the left side: father-to-son transmission. *A*, Dorsal view of the father's hands. *B*, Dorsal view of the son's hands. *C*, Dorsopalmar roentgenograph of the father's hands. *D*, Dorsopalmar roentgenograph of the son's hands. *E* and *F* illustrate the roentgenographs which appear above each.

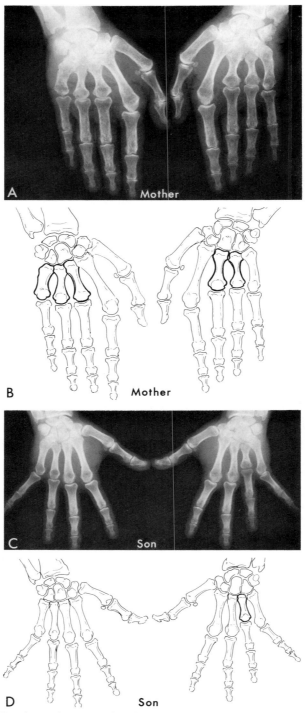

Figure 2–2   Dominant phenotype with abated expressivity. Short metacarpals (brachymetacarpia): mother-to-son transmission. *A*, Dorsopalmar roentgenograph of the mother's hands. *B*, Illustrative sketch of the same. *C*, Dorsopalmar roentgenograph of the son's hands: only the fourth metacarpal of the left hand is short. *D*, Illustrative sketch of the same.

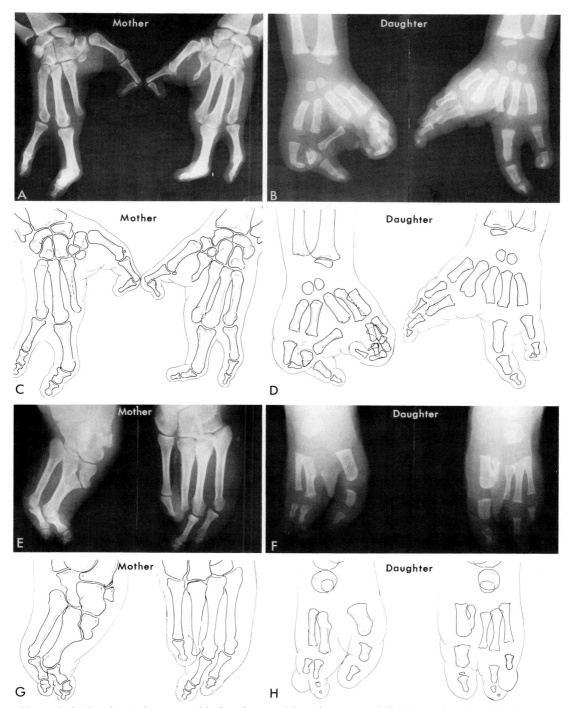

Figure 2–3 Dominant phenotype with abated expressivity. Absent central digits (ectrodactyly; axial adactylia; split hand): mother-to-daughter transmission. *A*, Dorsopalmar roentgenograph of the mother's hands. *B*, Dorsopalmar roentgenograph of the daughter's hands. *C* and *D* illustrate the roentgenographs which appear above each. *E*, Dorsopalmar roentgenograph of the mother's forefeet. *F*, Dorsopalmar roentgenograph of the daughter's forefeet. *G* and *H* illustrate the roentgenographs which appear above each.

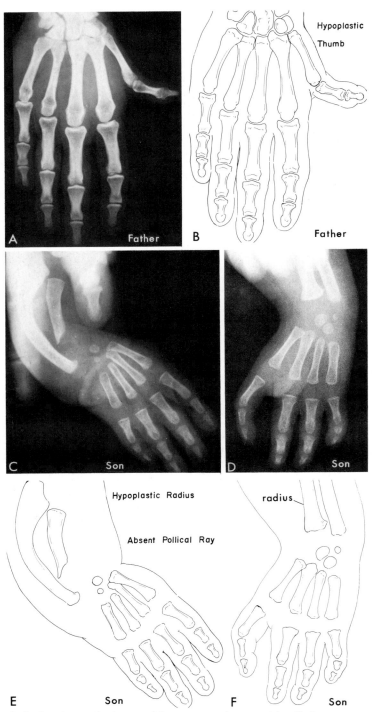

Figure 2–4 Dominant phenotype with accentuated expressivity. Father-to-son transmission. The father had only hypoplasia of the right thumb with thin metacarpal which had been caught in the common bondage of the deep transverse ligament and failed to abduct at the carpometacarpal joint. The son had absence of distal right radius and absence of both pollical rays. *A*, Dorsopalmar roentgenograph of the father's hand. *B*, Illustrative sketch of the same. *C*, Dorsopalmar roentgenograph of the son's right forearm and hand. *D*, Dorsopalmar roentgenograph of the son's left wrist and hand. Note that the more severely affected right upper limb has one carpal bone less than the left wrist. *E* and *F* illustrate the roentgenograph which appears above each.

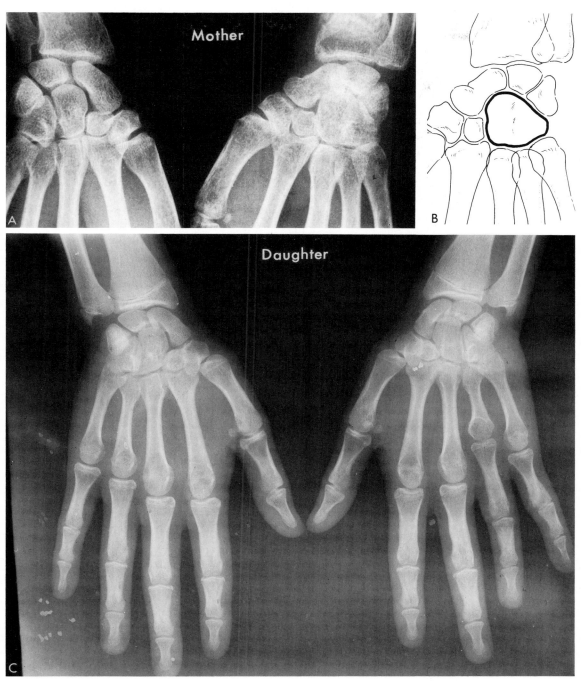

Figure 2–5   Dominant phenotype affecting different elements variously: mother-to-daughter transmission. The mother has coalescence of the capitate and hamate bones of the left wrist. The daughter has a short fourth metacarpal on the left side. The anomalies in both were discovered upon roentgenographic examination for fracture of the left distal radius of the mother and fracture of the proximal phalanx of the daughter's left little finger. *A*, Dorsopalmar roentgenograph of the mother's wrists, showing coalescence of the capitate and hamate bones of the left wrist. *B*, Sketch illustrating the same. *C*, Dorsopalmar roentgenograph of the daughter's hands, showing a short fourth left metacarpal.

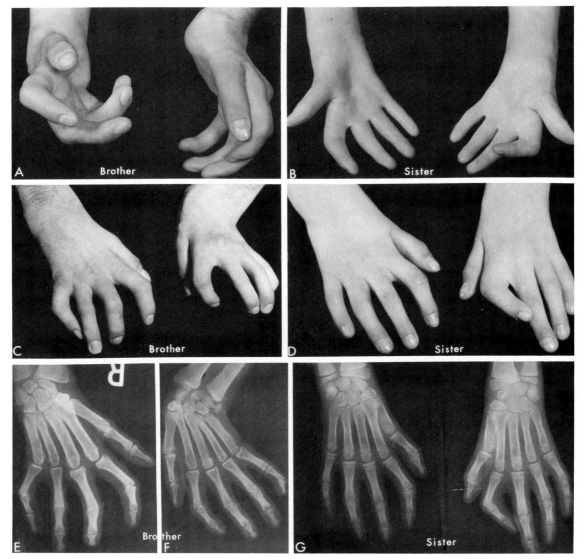

Figure 2–6   Recessive phenotype. Flexion contracture and ulnar drift of the digits (camptoclinodactyly) in a brother and sister born of unaffected parents. *A, C, E,* and *F* represent the brother's hands; *B, D,* and *G* the hands of the younger sister.

forms of mucopolysaccharidosis, and pyknodysostosis are recessive (Figs. 2–7 to 2–11).

There is an erroneous impression that the great majority of congenital hand anomalies are of genetic origin. "A minority of congenital malformations have a major environmental cause. A minority of congenital malformations have a major genetic cause. Most malformations probably result from complicated interactions between genetic predispositions and subtle factors in the intra-uterine environment," Fraser (1959) wrote. Neel (1960) did not think genetic influences would account for more than 20 per cent of congenital anomalies in general.

(*Text continued on page 34.*)

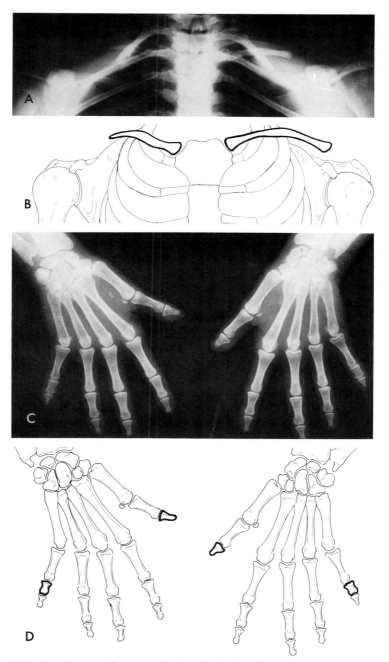

Figure 2–7 Dominant syndrome implicating the hand and showing complete penetrance and slightly variable expressivity. Cleidocranial dysostosis: mother-to-daughter and mother-to-son transmission. In this figure, only the mother's clavicles and hands are shown. She and her other affected children had characteristic skull and pelvic changes, as did the proband shown in Fig. 2–8. *A,* Anteroposterior roentgenograph, showing defective clavicles on both sides. *B,* Interpretative sketch. *C,* Dorsopalmar roentgenograph, showing long second metacarpals, dwarfed middle phalanges of fifth digits, and tuftless terminal phalanges of the thumbs and of the left little finger. *D,* Sketch illustrating the same.

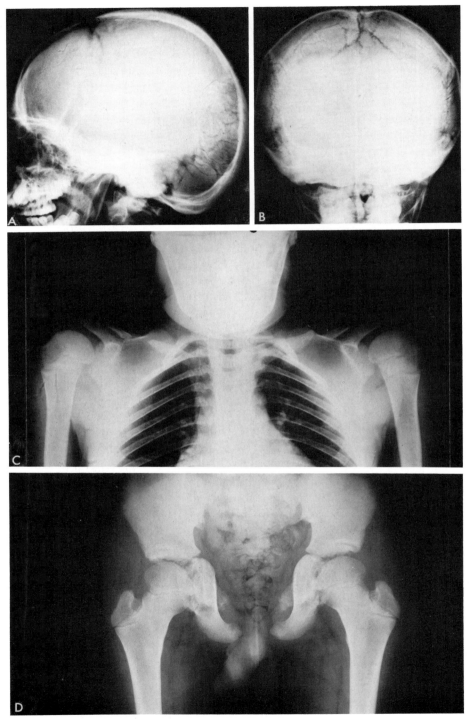

Figure 2–8 The proband was 12 years old when these roentgenographs were taken. *A,* Lateral roentgenograph of the skull, showing a large, open fontanel. *B,* Anteroposterior roentgenograph of the skull, showing as yet open sutures and interposed wormian bones. *C,* Roentgenograph showing central defect of both clavicles. *D,* Roentgenographs showing a wide space between the two pubic bones.

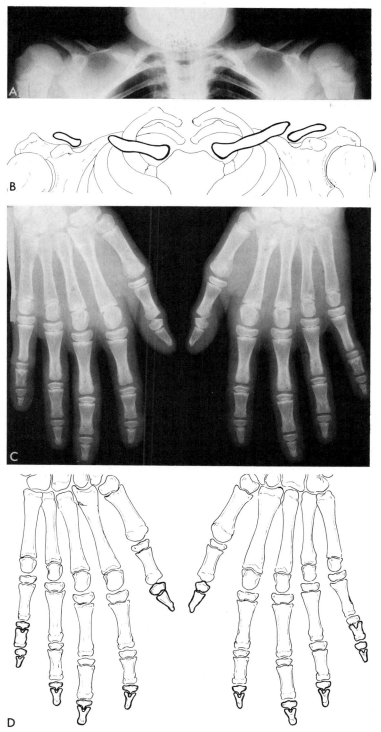

Figure 2–9 Proband's clavicles and hands. *A*, Same as *C* in Fig. 2–8. *B*, Illustrative sketch. *C*, Dorsopalmar roentgenograph of the hands, showing coned ungual epiphyses of the fingers and tuftless terminal phalanges of the thumbs and little fingers. *D*, Illustrative sketch.

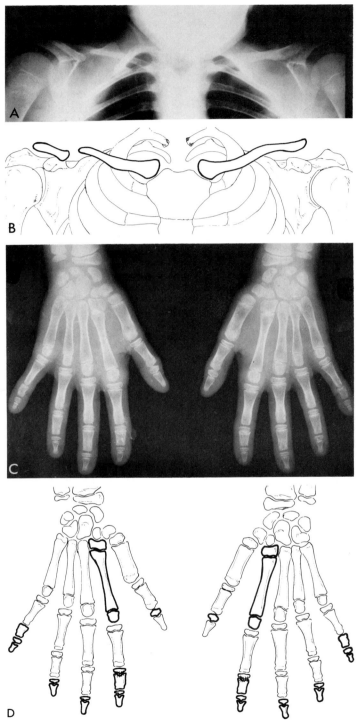

Figure 2–10 Proband's younger sister. *A,* Anteroposterior roentgenograph showing absent midsection of right clavicle and short left clavicle. *B,* Illustrative sketch. *C,* Dorsopalmar roentgenograph of the hands, showing pseudoepiphyses at the proximal end of comparatively long second metacarpals, coned epiphyses of the ungual phalanges of the second to fourth digits and middle phalanges (without epiphyses) of little fingers, and tuftless ungual phalanges. *D,* Interpretative sketch.

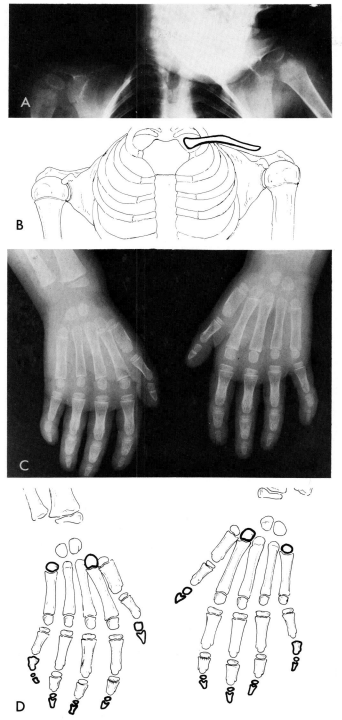

Figure 2–11 Proband's younger brother. *A*, Anteroposterior roentgenograph showing absence of the entire right clavicle and short left clavicle. *B*, Illustrative sketch. *C*, Dorsopalmar roentgenograph of both hands: note the tuftless ungual phalanges of the thumbs, incipient coning of phalangeal epiphyses, pseudoepiphyses at the proximal ends of the second and fifth metacarpals, absence of epiphyses of the short middle phalanges of the little fingers, and radial inclination (clinodactyly) of ungual segments of the same digits. *D*, Illustrative sketch.

There is another lingering half-truth verging on fallacy; it pertains to the presumed symmetry of genetic hand deformities in contrast to environmentally induced defects which are said to be unilateral and asymmetrical. Boorstein (1916) stated that bilateral congenital malformations could generally be traced to heredity, while unilateral ones were due to environmental influences. Danforth (1924) pointed out that hereditary traits do not always find bilateral expression and that the same phenotype may conceivably be produced by a number of different causes. Exogenous malformations produced by thalidomide are often bilateral and, at times, symmetrical. It is also said that endogenous malformations are multiple and generalized, while exogenous defects are confined to one organ or part of the body. Multiplicity of thalidomide-induced defects has also relegated this ever-recurrent adage to the category of half-truths. More than one geneticist has warned against too rigorous application of Mendelian expectation to human beings. Man, especially modern man, is a poor breeder. When married couples produce only one offspring or at most two, the defective child might not have had a chance to be born yet.

EMBRYOLOGIC CORRELATION

Montgomery (1836) pointed out that the human conceptus is most vulnerable during the earlier periods of embryonic development when tissues are undergoing rapid differentiation. During this time many alterations take place: parts fail to form and parts which are already formed are destroyed. Vrolik (1849) listed the following developmental arrests of the upper extremity: (1) absent limbs, (2) absent intermediate segments, (3) truncated limbs, (4) diminished number of fingers, and (5) coalesced fingers or "malformations due to absence of fission." Vrolik was vague about the time of the inception of various anomalies. He stated: "The origin of many malformations of the limbs may be referred to the early period of embryogenesis, but for some of them this is impossible." He probably meant to say that it was difficult to pin down the inception of some deformities to definite days or weeks in early embryonic life.

At the beginning of the present century, Bardeen and Lewis (1901) and Lewis (1901) alone described the embryogenesis of the upper extremity in some detail. They covered the development of the arm and hand from the third to the eighth week after conception. The following is an attempt to cull some pertinent details from their work:

Third week: the arm-bud appears as a slight swelling on the anterior aspect of the Wolffian ridge; the swelling is covered with ectoderm and contains closely packed mesenchymal cells.

Fourth week: the bud enlarges; it extends in the caudal direction; the mesenchyma condenses where future bones are to be deposited; nerves appear at the base of the bud and start connecting with the beginning of the cervicobrachial plexus.

Fifth week: surface lines mark off the upper arm from the forearm and the latter from the hand; the hand is a flat, expanded paddle; its dorsal surface is marked with digital ridges; its free border shows faint indentations, signaling the beginnings of interdigital clefts; the forearm and hand have turned toward the midline of the body. Toward the end of this week, the matrix of the future humerus, ulna, and radius have differentiated into cartilage; nerves reach the hand.

Sixth week: the limb begins to resemble that of an adult; the forearm and the hand are pronated; the indentations on the free border of the hand have deepened; the metacarpals and proximal row of phalanges consist of cartilage; each cartilaginous anlage is surrounded by a thick investment of perichondrium; some carpals and the second row of phalanges are not as yet chondrified; nerves, both sensory and motor, are distributed as in the adult.

Seventh week: muscles are recognizable; all skeletal elements consist of cartilage except the distal row of phalanges of the second to fifth digits; the arm as a whole has migrated caudally.

We are told by Bardeen and Lewis that the structures of the upper arm are differentiated before those of the forearm, and the latter before the hand. During the first two months of embryonic life, the rudiments of muscles, nerves, blood vessels, and skeletal structures are developed. Adult conditions are reached by an increase in size and complexity and by relative shifting of parts.

Writing alone, Bardeen (1910) had this to say: "Agenesis, or failure of skeletal development, may be due either to primary lack of origin of a part or to an affection which destroys the skeletal anlage after it has begun to differentiate."

The earlier limb-bud consists of ectodermal covering and mesodermal content. These elements proliferate and grow simultaneously; the mesoderm condenses and the apical portion of the ectoderm thickens. It is believed that the apical skin ridge acts as an inductor and controls the proximodistal sequence of the development of the limb; the humerus is said to differentiate before the radius and ulna; these in turn chondrify and ossify prior to the differentiation of the metacarpals and phalanges.

Dixey (1881) pointed out that, unlike other tubular bones which acquire their first ring of osseous deposit at about the level of the midshaft, the terminal phalanx obtains a thimble of bone at its tip by direct conversion of condensed mesoderm without the intermediary phase of chondrification. The tip of the terminal phalanx is thus formed by membranous ossification, and growth from this part proceeds proximally toward the shaft. Noback and Robertson (1951) gave the sequence of ossification in the upper extremity as follows: (1) humerus, (2) radius, (3) ulna, (4) distal phalanges, (5) metacarpals, (6) proximal phalanges, and (7) middle phalanges. The ossification in the terminal phalanx is said to commence as early as the seventh postovulatory week—about the same time that the membranous midshaft of the clavicle becomes converted directly to bone. In cleidocranial dysostosis, both the middle portion of the clavicle and the tips of the distal phalanges are defective. The last elements of the hand to become converted into bone are the middle phalanges of the four ulnar digits; in this series the middle phalanx of the little finger ossifies last. Exogenous agents and genetic determinants exercise time and tissue specificity, and the elements which differentiate last tend to be more susceptible to teratogenic influences—the middle phalanx of the little finger is most often misshapen and short (Fig. 2–12).

Streeter (1930) studied 16 fetal specimens with "destroyed parts"; he showed that what had frequently been mistaken for amniotic bands were really macerated sheets of epidermis or strands of hyalinized fibrous tissue overlying areas of focal necrosis. Streeter considered localized deficiencies of the tissue and focal necrosis as causes of congenital deformities. "There is a normal disparity in the quality or vitality of different tissues of the body, and this . . . disparity is inherent in the germ plasm and hereditarily transmitted," Streeter wrote. In his customary role as mentor of basic concepts, Sir Arthur Keith (1940) commented: "Streeter's foetal dysplasia is the source of . . . many congenital malformations . . . . Amniotic adhesions are never formed by a failure in the separation of the

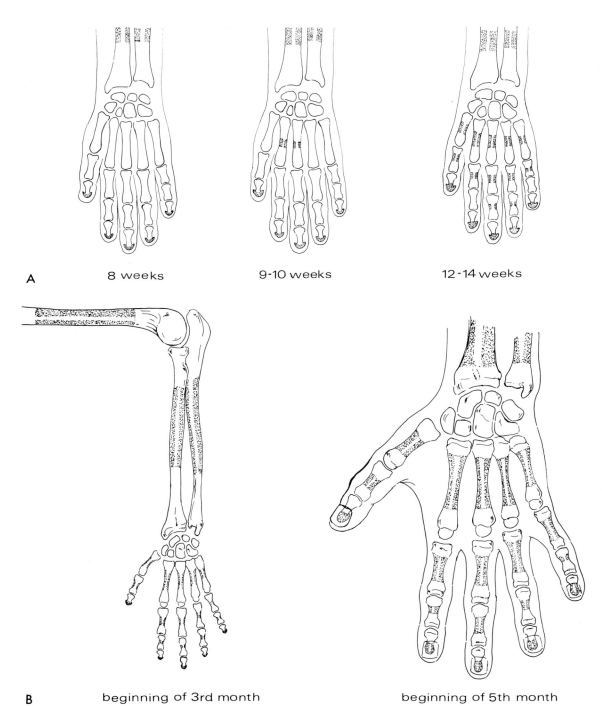

A   8 weeks   9-10 weeks   12-14 weeks

B   beginning of 3rd month   beginning of 5th month

Figure 2–12   Prenatal ossification. *A*, According to Lambertz (1900). *B*, After Bergmann et al (1904).

amnion from the embryo, but are always produced from the foetus — as a result of a dysplasia in foetal tissues. They are the result, not the cause, of foetal malformations."

Harris (1934) featured the hand of a five-week-old human embryo in longitudinal section, showing condensation of the mesenchyma in the precartilaginous skeleton. Another longitudinal section represented the hand of a nine-week-old fetus. It showed the fingers separated from one another; there was some evidence of calcification within the shafts of metacarpals and proximal phalanges; the middle and the terminal phalanges were not shown in this section. Harris advanced the view that vascular bone marrow erupts into and replaces the senescent cartilage in the midshafts of tubular bones; in the hand, this process of invasion and replacement occurs between the ninth and tenth weeks of embryonic life. Prior to this period, the cartilaginous skeleton might have undergone mucoid degeneration and failed to be calcified. Mucoid degenerations might occur within the growth cartilage plate, in which instance the involved bone would remain short; the resulting deformities might range from mild dwarfism to extreme achondroplasia.

These concepts eventually found their way into surgical literature. A number of authors — Bunnell (1944), Ingalls (1954), and Töndury (1965) among others — have correlated the date of inception of various anomalies with the time of the appearance of the involved part during embryonic development. These correlations are based upon the assumption that the embryonic precursor of the affected segment or sector is most likely to undergo focal necrosis before it becomes differentiated. Focal necrosis may be confined to a small area within the limb-bud and cause a circumscribed, limited deficiency, or it may be massive and destroy the entire limb. Depending upon the size and location of the necrotic area, there are various grades of involvement. In some instances, the terminal portion of the limb is affected; in others, the midsegments are involved. In either case, the defect may or may not extend from one border of the limb to the other, and may only affect a small area within these limits.

It may in general be said that when focal necrosis occurs before the third or fourth week of embryonic development — prior to the appearance of the limb-bud — the child may be born without an upper extremity. Necrosis during the fifth week may usher in any of the following anomalies: absence of one or both forearm bones and corresponding digital rays, absence of the central digital rays (split hand) and transverse terminal defect across the wrist. Transverse and longitudinal segmentations of the hand-paddle are initiated around the sixth week; injury during this period is followed by short, webbed, or supernumerary digits. Articular space begins to form around the eighth week. Disturbance at this time may be followed by any of the ensuing synostotic conditions: symphalangism, carpal coalescence, and radioulnar synostosis (Figs. 2–13 and 2–14).

Undifferentiated embryonic tissue is most susceptible to focal necrosis. It is plausible, as suggested by Harris (1934), that the chondrified precursor of one of the bones of the hand or the forearm may undergo mucoid degeneration and pave the way for future dysplastic disturbance. Most skeletal dysplasias involving the hand and the forearm owe their origin to the failure of the chondrified anlagen to become ossified. Chondrodystrophic disorders are said to be initiated around the ninth week of embryonic development.

Bone resists dissolution. Skeletal elements which ossify last, as, for instance, the middle row of phalanges of the fingers, have an extended predifferentiation period and hence a longer span of time to be affected by teratologic influences.

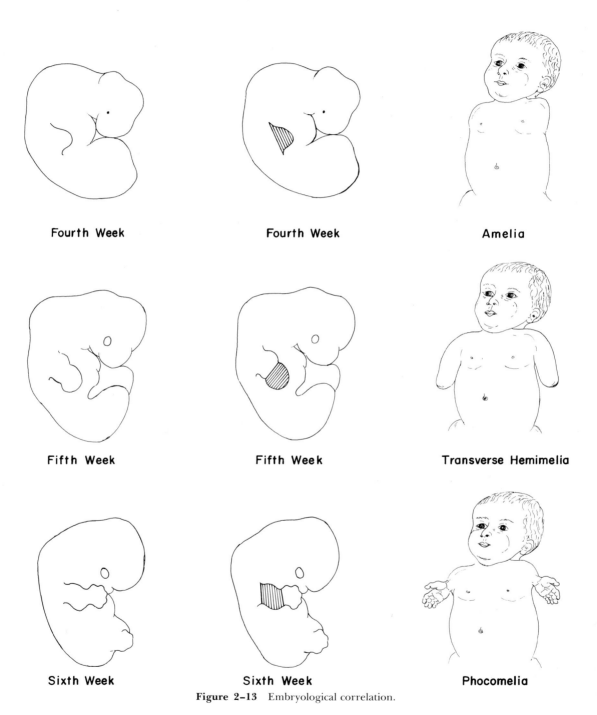

Fourth Week   Fourth Week   Amelia

Fifth Week   Fifth Week   Transverse Hemimelia

Sixth Week   Sixth Week   Phocomelia

Figure 2–13   Embryological correlation.

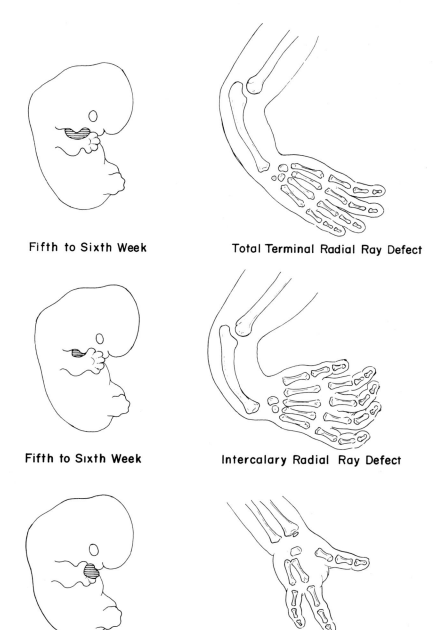

Fifth to Sixth Week

Total Terminal Radial Ray Defect

Fifth to Sixth Week

Intercalary Radial Ray Defect

Sixth Week

Axial Adactylia or Split Hand

Figure 2–14   Embryological correlation.

With the exception of terminal phalanges, each tubular bone of the hand acquires a calcified ring after the ninth postovulatory week; this osseous deposit occurs in the middle of the shaft. It is seldom that the shaft of such a bone is absent while its ends persist. Ossification of the tip of the terminal phalanx precedes that of the shaft; in the anomaly known as acro-osteolysis congenitalis, the ends persist while the shaft is missing. In more severe cases, the entire terminal phalanx is absent.

EXPERIMENTAL DATA

Etienne Geoffroy Saint-Hilaire (1822) and Isidore Geoffroy Saint-Hilaire (1832) conducted some of the earliest teratologic experiments. They shook eggs three days after incubation, pricked them at various points, held them in a vertical position, and insulated them with wax. Various malformations were produced and the Saint-Hilaires drew the inevitable conclusion that the development of the embryo could be modified by external means. These crude experiments were repeated by many others. A notable variation was that introduced by Dareste (1891). He used mercurial vapors and electricity as teratogenic agents and could discern no specificity between cause and effect; the same malformations were produced by different agents.

During earlier decades of the present century, several significant experimental studies were published. Harrison (1918) transplanted the forelimb of an ambystoma and discovered that it possesses self-differentiating potential. That this potential in part depends upon the thickened integument, called ectodermal ridge, extending along the preaxial and postaxial borders of the apical portion of the limb-bud, was proven by Saunders (1948). He first introduced carbon particles into the wing of a chick and followed their fate. As shown by the position of these particles during growth, various segments of the limb seemed to develop spatially in proximodistal sequence. Extirpation of the ectodermal ridge appeared to suppress the growth of the underlying mesenchyma. It seemed reasonable to conclude that apical ectoderm is essential to the highly integrated developmental system made up of ectodermal and mesodermal components of the limb-bud. This conclusion has been confirmed by many. It is now generally agreed that the apical ridge controls the sequential development of the limb. This induction mechanism is regarded as a matter of reciprocal interaction between ectoderm and mesoderm: one discharges stimuli and the other responds. Interference with this exchange—either by genetic determinants or environmental influences—is followed by deleterious consequences. Zwilling (1961) wrote: "Anomalies may result from (1) distortion of the inductive pattern; (2) failure of interactants to make proper contact; (3) loss of inductive capacity, or loss of ability to respond." He attributed polydactyly to "atypical distribution of ridge maintenance."

Stockard (1921) changed the temperature of the environment of the egg and thereby reduced the rate of oxidation. The continuous mode of development of the embryo was thus converted into a discontinuous one. Experimentally induced interruptions of development resulted in more drastic alterations of structure when they occurred during the most active periods of differentiation of the particular part. Stockard called these periods critical. Bagg

(1924) concurred with the view that the experimentally induced abnormality was due to an arrest in the development at the critical period. Based upon his own experiments with irradiation of impregnated mice, Bagg considered focal hemorrhage and formation of a bleb as the precursors of future defects. Bagg (1929) later exposed experimental animals to roentgen rays and produced blebs; these animals eventually developed syndactyly, polydactyly, and other congenital defects.

The list of agents used in experimental teratology is very long. Wilson (1959) counted sixty different agents; these range from physical insults to nutritional deficiencies, growth and metabolic inhibitors, infections, endocrines, and drugs, which had very little in common except their teratogenicity. In many instances, the same effect was produced by withdrawal of a necessary element or by administration of a noxious agent. Despite these experiments, it still remains to be proved that the analogous circumstances will affect human beings in the same way. Nutritional deficiency in experimental animals will cause a variety of congenital malformations. The chief exponent of this method, Warkany (1961), conceded that malformations induced in experimental animals by withdrawal of riboflavin "are not imitated by human circumstances."

Animal experimentations have reaffirmed the fact that the fertilized ovum, which presumably possesses normal genetic endowments, may be damaged by adverse environmental stresses and produce defective individuals. Mall (1917) defined environment as the milieu in which the embryo grows, including influences carried to it "by means of fluids which reach it either before or after the circulation has become established." Many earlier authors identified fetal environment with the uterus and likened the latter to an incubator. This simile scarcely suggests the intimate relationship which exists between the conceptus and its matrix, nor the fact that between these two there is a tissue continuity and uninterrupted exchange of metabolites and electrolytes. More recent authors have expanded the meaning of environment to include enzymes or activators emanating from the chromosomal spiral on which the gene is located, from the neighboring genes, from the ground substance of the nucleus, and from the cytoplasm surrounding the latter. Experience with maternal rubella has definitely confirmed the fact that environmental adversity can induce congenital defects in the human conceptus. Besides infection, as exemplified by maternal rubella, Ingalls (1960) discussed anoxia as a cause of congenital defect. Had he written his article a year later he might have included drugs—thalidomide in particular—among the clinically confirmed exogenous causes of congenital defects. Radiation also belongs to this category.

INFECTION

Syphilis maintained an unchallenged priority as the cause of congenital anomalies until Murphy (1947), after an extensive survey, showed that it had not afflicted the mothers of congenitally malformed offspring more often than those of normal children. Warkany (1961) pointed out that preventive measures and treatment by penicillin had reduced congenital syphilis to a rarity, but congenital malformations continue to flourish.

Warkany singled out two infectious diseases which seem to pass from the

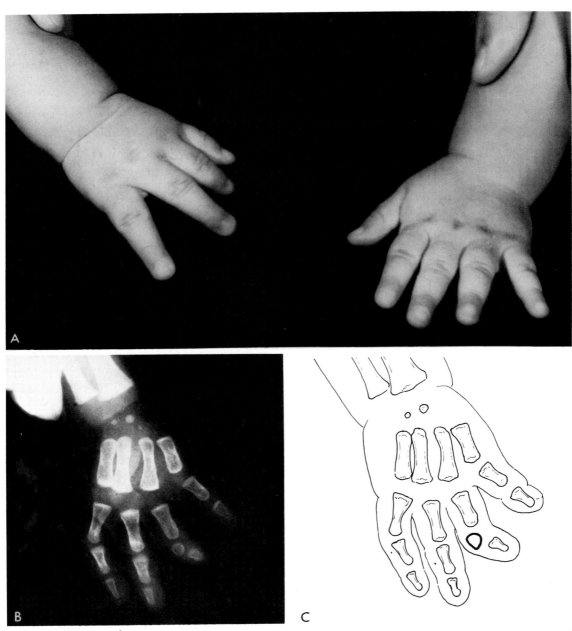

Figure 2–15 Exogenous influence: possible rubella effect. *A*, Dorsal view of hands, showing a smaller right hand with four digits; the thumb is present but is held adducted and does not rotate sufficiently to effect apposition. The next digit – probably the index finger – is bent and radially inclined. *B*, Roentgenograph of the right hand, showing a delta-shaped middle phalanx of the second digit and radial inclination of the distal segment. *C*, Illustrative sketch.

mother to her unborn offspring, causing congenital malformation: toxoplasmosis and rubella. Toxoplasmosis is said to be more destructive to fetal than to embryonic tissue; it causes microthalamus and chorioretinitis; it is not known to produce any specific limb defects. The virus of rubella is embryotoxic. The Australian eye surgeon Gregg (1941, 1945) was first to show that the rubella virus affecting the mother during the first trimester of pregnancy causes a high incidence of cardiac defects, ocular abnormalities, auditory dysfunction, blood dyscrasia, and sundry disturbances of the central nervous system in the child. Gregg's findings have since been confirmed by many others, most of them eye surgeons. In these reports, only rarely are anomalies of the hand incident to the rubella embryopathy mentioned; no specific details or descriptions are given.

The mother of a male infant was exposed to German measles during the second month of pregnancy. She was given an injection of gamma globulin. She did not contract clinically recognizable rubella. Seven months later her son was born with a malformed right hand: the central digit was absent; the metacarpal of the thumb was close to that of the next digit and appeared to be in bondage with the latter; the thumb was unrotated; the middle phalanx of the second digit had triangular configuration (it was shaped like the Greek letter *delta* which made the distal phalanx deviate in a radial direction.)

Admittedly, a single case hardly proves a point and it may be that this is another instance of fortuitous coincidence (Fig. 2–15).

RADIATION

Emil Ries (1926) reported the case of a pregnant woman who had been subjected to three therapeutic irradiations—"at sixty inches skin distance with 0.25 mm. copper filter"—because of bleeding. At approximately near term, she delivered a dead fetus with a malformed forearm and a hand which had only three fingers and no thumb. Goldstein and Murphy (1929) spoke of dead fetuses and microcephalic and mentally and physically subnormal children resulting from pelvic irradiation in the earlier months of pregnancy. They did not mention malformations of the hand. Plummer (1952) and Schull et al (1966) discussed the occurrence of congenital anomalies in infants whose mothers had been exposed during their pregnancy to irradiation from the atomic bomb exploded in Hiroshima and neighboring districts on August 6, 1945. These authors appeared to be primarily concerned with such major malformations as anencephalus and spina bifida. Neel (1958) reported 83 children with simple and 33 with complicated polydactyly.

De Bellefeuille (1962) referred to the mutagenic influence of ionizing radiation on human population; he intimated that the incidence of malformations might increase as a consequence of such exposure. Russell (1963) spoke of "radiation-induced chromosome breakage" and "radiation-induced gene mutations," suggesting that, in both instances, the exposed and successive generations might be affected. He pronounced the majority of diagnostic procedures, with exposures of one roentgen dose or less, harmless to the embryo. Irradiation-induced gene mutation is known to occur in experimental animals. "There is as yet no convincing proof that irradiation produces genetic effects in man," Millen (1963) wrote.

DRUGS

Larsson and Sterky (1960) reported a young mother who had been under continuous tolbutamide treatment for incipient diabetes mellitus; she gave birth to a premature female infant who died 15 minutes after birth. Among other anomalies, this child had only four fingers on each hand, with syndactyly between the second and third digits. In the literature, one finds many scattered reports of congenital anomalies for which a drug or hormone has been incriminated. None of these teratogens seems to possess the time and tissue specificity of thalidomide; nor are they known to result in the distinctive pattern of abnormalities that thalidomide or one of its numerous derivatives produces. Thalidomide shows definite predilection for the extremities, especially for the proximal extremity. Although phocomelia is often reported as the most characteristic abnormality produced by thalidomide, anomalies of the radial component of the forearm and the hand appear to be more common.

Each organ or system has its own specific periods of high sensitivity. These periods coincide with the time of formation of the organ or system and its rapid differentiation. The arm is formed between the third and seventh week of embryonic life and the radial component begins to differentiate during the fifth week. Segmentation of the hand plate and separation of the digits takes place during the ensuing two weeks. As shown in a later chapter, the span between the thirty-fourth and the fiftieth day after the last menstrual day of the pregnant woman is the period during which the embryo is especially susceptible to the teratogenic effect of the thalidomide. A single tablet of thalidomide ingested by the mother during this sensitive period may injure the conceptus. The degree of damage depends upon the time of intake of the drug. Earlier intake causes more drastic damage (Figs. 2–16 and 2–17).

HYPOXIA

Women with severe cyanotic cardiovascular disorders were said by Black-Schaffer (1950) to give birth to babies with "nanosomia and arthropesia." There have been some reports—notably by Alzamora-Castro and coworkers (1953)—of a prevalence of persistent interatrial communications in patients born at altitudes where the oxygen supply is comparatively low. This type of congenital heart disease is often associated with absent thumb or radial ray defect. A schizophrenic woman reported by Wickes (1954) was given insulin-coma treatment from the second month of pregnancy on; her child was born with defective mentality, hypertelorism, and optic atrophy. Wickes ascribed the deleterious effect in this instance to anoxia rather than to an interference with fetal tissue carbohydrate metabolism by insulin. The mother of a child with a missing left hand—reported by Ingalls (1960)—had been under gas-oxygen-ether for an hour during the third month of pregnancy. Ingalls reported another child whose mother "had suffered a severe attack of asthma in early pregnancy for which she had been given morphine"; the child was born with split hand, having only two digits on each hand. Turner (1960) reported a 16-year-old pregnant girl who carried her conceptus under severe emotional stress. Her child was born with a short right shoulder girdle and with only two digits on the left hand. It was surmised that excessive emotional stress in this instance did cause "severe teratogenic effects of a predictable type in the offspring."

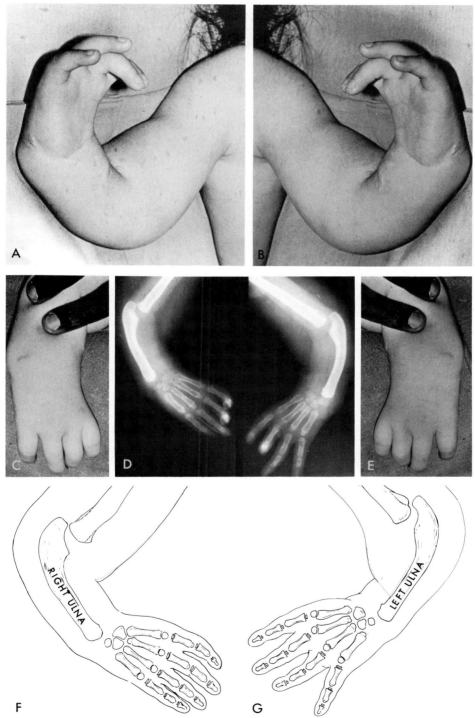

Figure 2-16 Exogenous influence: thalidomide embryopathy, bilateral symmetrical. *A*, Volar view of the right upper limb of a three-year-old female whose mother had taken two tablets of thalidomide while she was in her second month of pregnancy. *B*, Volar view of the left upper extremity. *C*, Dorsal view of the right hand. *D*, Roentgenograph of both upper limbs. *E*, Dorsal view of the left hand. *F*, Illustrative sketch of the right upper limb. *G*, Illustrative sketch of the left upper limb.

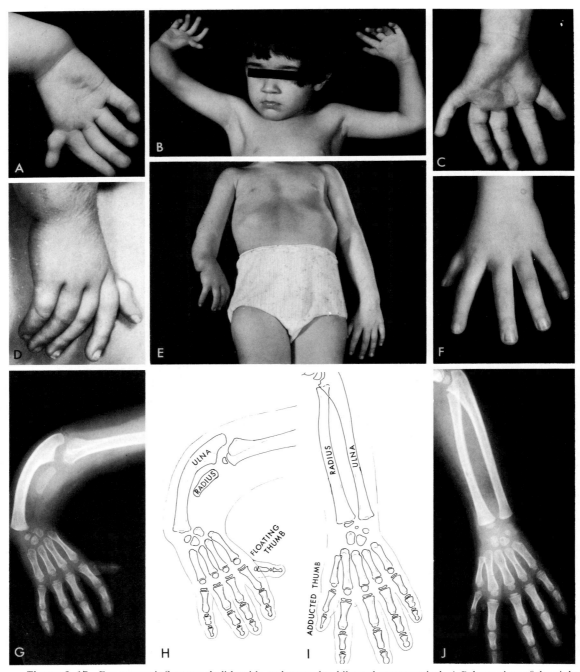

Figure 2–17 Exogenous influence: thalidomide embryopathy, bilateral asymmetrical. *A*, Palmar view of the right hand of a four-year-old female whose pregnant mother had taken a number of thalidomide tablets around the fiftieth day after her last menstrual period. *B*, Frontal view of both upper limbs. *C*, Palmar view of the left hand. *D*, Dorsal view of the right hand. *E*, Dorsal view of both upper limbs. *F*, Dorsal view of the left hand: note that the first webspace is distally placed. *G*, Dorsovolar roentgenograph showing absence of distal half of radius, three carpal ossicles and absent first metacarpal. *H*, Interpretative sketch of *G*. *I*, Interpretative sketch of *J*, showing intact radius, four carpal ossicles, a thin first metacarpal, and attenuated pollical phalanges.

The ancient lore of maternal impression as a cause of congenital abnormalities has been given a newer explanation. It is known that schizophrenic and manic depressive women tend to have frequent abortions and stillbirths and, occasionally, have living offspring with congenital defects; these are now ascribed to the lowered oxygen tension incident to emotional stress. Hypoxia does not seem to produce either a specific or constant pattern of abnormalities, as does thalidomide; its effect is not selectively localized in a set of organs or parts.

SUMMARY

The recognition of a congenital anomaly depends upon the willingness of the parents to seek advice and upon the diagnostic acumen of the consultant; not uncommonly, the clinician is led astray by false inventions emanating from parental guilt complex or memory bias. In some instances the abnormality is not detected at birth; although present, the anomaly is not sufficiently developed to be seen or suspected.

Congenital anomalies of the hand and forearm vary in degree of structural deviation and functional disturbance. They range from crooked little fingers to complete absence of parts, from innocuous spots of osteopoikilosis to the ravaging destruction of bones seen in Maffucci syndrome. In most statistical surveys the less drastic, but by far the majority, of congenital anomalies of the hand are left out. Two main groups of causes for congenital anomalies are recognized and categorized, respectively, as hereditary and environmental. Evidence acquired from studies of pedigrees, twins, contingency, consanguineous marriage, and chromosomes have left no doubt that some malformations are of genetic origin. Observations based upon animal experimentation and experiences with rubella and thalidomide embryopathies support the view that other congenital anomalies are caused by exogenous influences. Genetic determinants and exogenous influences are said to produce maximum degrees of damage during the period of rapid differentiation, which in the human conceptus coincides with the first seven weeks of embryonic development.

Most authors now feel that there are very few purely endogenous or exogenous malformations, and that in many instances the anomaly is the result of both genetic and environmental influences: phenotype is genotype modified by the environment and phenocopy is the replica of phenotype produced by environment. The discernible or detectable abnormality varies from individual to individual because of their diverse genetic constitutions. Radial ray defect and phocomelia are known to have hereditary antecedents and may also be caused by such exogenous influences as thalidomide ingested by the mother during the earlier months of pregnancy.

Heredity features predominantly in the following anomalies: hyperphalangism, brachydactyly, symphalangism, split hand, carpal coalescence, and most skeletal dysplasias implicating the hand and the forearm. Heredity is more often a factor in polydactyly than in syndactyly, and it plays an occasional role in anomalies of digital posture, annular grooves and transverse terminal defects, Madelung deformity, dislocation of radial head, and radioulnar synostosis. Heredity does not seem to play a part in the production of acrosyndactyly, macrodactyly, mirror hand or ulnar dimelia. The concepts of amniogenic malformations and malformations presumably caused by umbilical cord strangulations or arising from atavism will be taken up in pertinent context—in connection with annular grooves and terminal transverse defect and polydactyly.

References

Alzamora-Castro, V., Rotta, A., Battilana, G., Abugattas, R., Rubio, C., Bouroncle, J., Zapata, C., Santa-María, E., Binder, T., Subiría, R., Paredes, D., Pando, B., and Graham, G. G.: On the possible influence of great altitudes on the determination of certain cardiovascular anomalies. *Pediatrics, 12*:259–262, 1953.

Aristotle: De Partibus Animalum (On parts of Animals). Translated by W. Ogle. *In* McKeon, R., (ed.): *The Basic Works of Aristotle.* New York, Random House, pp. 646–649, 1941.

Bagg, H. J.: Etiology of certain congenital structural defects. *Am. J. Obstet. Gynecol., 8*:131–141, 1924.

Bagg, H. J.: Hereditary abnormalities of the limbs, their origin and transmission. *Am. J. Anat., 43*:167–219, 1929.

Ballantyne, J. W.: *Manual of Antenatal Pathology and Hygiene: The Embryo.* Edinburgh, W. Green & Sons, Vol. II, pp. 203–224, 1904.

Bardeen, C. R.: Morphogenesis of the skeletal system. *In* Keibel, F., and Mall, F. P., (eds.): *Manual of Human Embryology.* Philadelphia, J. B. Lippincott Co., pp. 317–443, 1910.

Bardeen, C. R., and Lewis, W. H.: Development of the limbs, bodywall, and back in man. *Am. J. Anat., 1*:1–35, 1901–1902.

Barsky, A. J., Kahn, S., and Siman, B. E.: Congenital anomalies of the hand. *In* Converse, J. M., and Wittler, J. W., (eds.): *Reconstructive Plastic Surgery.* Philadelphia, W. B. Saunders Co., Vol. IV, pp. 1696–1727, 1964.

Bateson, E.: An address on Mendelian heredity and its application to man. *Brain, 29*:157–179, 1906.

Bellefeuille, P. de: A theorem on the genetics of some congenital malformations. *Acta Genet.* (Basel), *12*:129–136, 1962.

Bergman, E. v., Bruns, P. v., and Mikulicz, J. v.: *A System of Practical Surgery.* Translated by W. T. Bull and J. B. Solley. New York, Lea Brothers Co., Vol. III, pp. 270–278, Figs. 174, 175, 179, 1904.

Birch-Jensen, A.: *Congenital Deformities of the Upper Extremities.* Translated from the Danish by E. Aagesen. Copenhagen, Andelsbogtrykkeriet I Odense and Det danske Forlag, pp. 11–14, 1949.

Black-Schaffer, B.: Fetal nanosomia and bone arthropesia in newborn with severe cyanotic cardiovascular anomaly. *Am. J. Obstet. Gynecol., 59*:656–661, 1950.

Boorstein, S. W.: A symmetrical congenital malformation of the extremities. *Ann. Surg., 63*:192–197, 1916.

Bunnell, S.: *Surgery of the Hand.* Philadelphia, J. B. Lippincott Co., pp. 609–647, 1944.

Canepa, G., and Sanguinetti, C.: Deformita congenite della mano. *Arch. Chir. Ortop. Med., 24*:109–146, 1959.

Carter, C. O.: Maternal states in relation to congenital malformations. *J. Obstet. Gynaecol. Br. Emp., 57*:897–911, 1950.

Castle, W. E.: *Genetics and Eugenics.* Cambridge, Harvard University Press, pp. 145–150, 1931.

Conway, G., and Bowe, J.: Congenital deformities of the hands. *Plast. Reconstr. Surg., 18*:286–290, 1956.

Correns, C.: Gregor Mendel's "Versuche über Pflanzenhybriden" und die Bestätigung ihrer Ergebnisse durch die neuesten Untersuchungen. *Bot. Z., 58*:230, 1900.

Danforth, C. H.: The heredity of unilateral variations in man. *Genetics, 9*:199–211, 1924.

Dareste, C.: *Recherches sur la Production Artificielle des Monstruosités ou Essais de Teratogénie Expérimental.* Second Edition. Paris, C. Reinwald et Cie., pp. 73–173, 1891.

Darwin, F., (ed.): *The Life and Letters of Charles Darwin: Including an Autobiographical Chapter.* London, John Murray, pp. 20–25, 1887.

Denver classification of chromosomes. See: Editorial Comment: A proposed standard of nomenclature of human mitotic chromosomes (Denver, Colorado). *Ann. Hum. Genet., 24*:219–325, 1960.

DeVries, H.: Das Spaltungsgesetz der Bastarde. *Ber. Dtsch. Bot. Ges., 18*:83–90, 1900.

DeVries, H.: *Die Mutationstheorie.* Versuche and Beobachtungen über die Entstehung von Arten im Pflanzenreich. Leipzig, Veit & Co., Vol. I, pp. 1–648; Vol. II, 1–752, 1903.

Dixey, F. A.: On the ossification of the terminal phalanges. *Proc. R. Soc. London, 31*:63–71, 1881.

Dunn, L. C., and Dobzhansky, T.: *Heredity, Race and Society.* New York, Mentor Books, pp. 18–39, 1952.

Fraser, F. C.: Causes of congenital malformations in human beings. *J. Chronic Dis., 10*:97–110, 1959.

Galton, F.: *Hereditary Genius: An Inquiry into Its Laws and Consequences.* London, The MacMillan Co., pp. 1–49, 1869.

Galton, F.: *English Men of Science; Their Nature and Nurture.* London, The MacMillan Co., pp. 39–43, 253–260, 1874.

Galton, F.: *Natural Inheritance.* London, The MacMillan Co., pp. 1–17, 192–198, 1889.

Gates, R. R.: *Human Genetics.* New York, The MacMillan Co., Vol. I, pp. 6–49, 1952.

Goldschmidt, R.: The theory of the gene. *Science Monthly, 46*:268–273, 1938.

Goldstein, L., and Murphy, D. P.: Etiology of the ill-health in children born after maternal pelvic irradiation. *Am. J. Roentgenol., 22*:322–331, 1929.

Gregg, N. M.: Congenital cataract following German measles in the mother. *Trans. Ophthal. Soc. Aust., 3*:35–46, 1941.

Gregg, N. M.: Rubella during pregnancy of the mother with its sequelae of congenital defects in the child. *Med. J. Aust.*, *1*:313–320, 1945.

Harris, H. A.: Congenital abnormalities of the skeleton. *In* Blacker, C. P., (ed.): *The Chances of Morbid Inheritance*. London, H. K. Lewis & Co., pp. 378–404, 1934.

Harris, H.: *Human Biochemical Genetics*. Cambridge, Cambridge University Press, pp. 9–34, 1959.

Harrison, R. H.: Experiments on the development of the forelimb of amblystoma, a self-differentiating equipotential system. *J. Exp. Zool.*, *25*:413–459, 1918.

Hellman, L.: Discussions about the statistical approach to the study of congenital malformation. *In* Holt, L. E., Jr., et al., (eds.): *Prematurity, Congenital Malformations and Birth Injury*. New York, Association for the Aid of Crippled Children, pp. 183–191, 1953.

Ingalls, T. H.: Epidemiology of congenital malformations. *In Mechanism of Congenital Malformation. Proceedings of Second Scientific Conference of the Association for the Aid of Crippled Children*. New York, pp. 10–20, 1954.

Ingalls, T. H.: Environmental factors in causation of congenital anomalies. *In Ciba Foundation Symposium on Congenital Malformation*. Boston, Little, Brown & Co., pp. 51–77, 1960.

Johannsen, W.: *Ueber Erblichkeit in Populationen und in reinen Linien*. Jena, G. Fischer, pp. 1–68, 1903.

Johannsen, W.: The genotype conception of heredity. *Am. Nat.*, *45*:129–159, 1911.

Keith, A.: Concerning the origin and nature of certain malformations of face, head, and foot. *Br. J. Surg.*, *28*:173–192, 1940.

Lambertz: Hand und Fuss. *In Die Entwicklung des menschlichen Knochengerüstes während des fötalen Lebens dargestellt an Röntgenibildern*. Hamburg, L. Graff & Sellem, pp. 48–52, 1900.

Larsson, Y., and Sterky, G.: Possible teratogenic effect of tolbutamide in a pregnant prediabetic. *Lancet*, *2*:1424–1425, 1960.

Lewis, W.: The development of the arm in man. *Am. J. Anat.*, *1*:145–183, 1901.

Mall, F. P.: On the frequency of localized anomalies in human embryos and infants at birth. *Am. J. Anat.*, *22*:49–72, 1917.

McKusick, V. A.: *Heritable Disorders of Connective Tissue*. Third edition. St. Louis, C. V. Mosby Co., pp. 1–37, 1966.

Mendel, G.: Experiments in plant hybridization. *In W. Bateson's Mendel's Principles of Heredity*. Cambridge, Cambridge University Press, pp. 335–386, 1913. See also: *J. R. Hort. Soc.*, *26*:1–32, 1901. The original was published in 1865.

Millen, J. W.: Irradiation and congenital malformations. *Practitioner*, *191*:143–151, 1963.

Montgomery, T. H., Jr.: *The Analysis of Racial Descent in Animals*. New York, H. Holt & Co., pp. 42–152, 1906.

Montgomery, W. F.: Foetus, *In* Todd, R. B., (ed.): *The Cyclopaedia of Anatomy and Physiology*. London, Longman, Brown, Green, Longman & Roberts, Vol. II, pp. 316–338, 1836–1839.

Muench, H.: Biostatistics — and why. *Postgrad. Med.*, *13*:334–338, 1953.

Murphy, D. P.: *Congenital Malformations*. Philadelphia, J. B. Lippincott Co., pp. 1–102, 1947.

Neel, J. V.: A study of major congenital defects in Japanese infants. *Am. J. Hum. Genet.*, *10*:398–445, 1958.

Neel, J. V.: Some genetic aspects of congenital defects. *In Congenital Malformations*. Papers and Discussions presented at the First International Conference. Philadelphia, J. B. Lippincott Co., pp. 63–69, 1960.

Noback, C. R. and Robertson, G.: Sequence of appearance of ossification centers in the human skeleton during the first five months of prenatal life. *Am. J. Anat.*, *89*:1–28, 1951.

Plummer, G.: Anomalies occurring in children exposed in utero to the atomic bomb in Hiroshima. *Pediatrics*, *10*:687–693, 1952.

Reid, G. A.: *Laws of Heredity*. New York, MacMillan & Co., pp. 410–435; 514–516, 1910.

Ries, E.: The danger of malformation of fetus in Roentgen-ray treatment during pregnancy. *Am. J. Obstet. Gynecol.*, *11*:261–363, 1926.

Russell, L. E.: Radiation Hazard. *In* Fishbein, M. (ed.): *Birth Defects*. Philadelphia, J. B. Lippincott Co., pp. 156–163, 1963.

Saint-Hilaire, É. G.: *Philosophie Anatomique des Monstruosités Humaines*. Paris, Chez l'Auteur, pp. 473–541, 1822.

Saint-Hilaire, É. G.: *Histoire Générale et Particulière des Anomalies de l'Organisation chez l'Homme et les Animaux*. Paris, J. B. Baillière, pp. 251–278; 670–702, 1832.

Saunders, J. W., Jr.: The proximo-distal sequence of origin of the parts of the check wing and the role of ectoderm. *J. Exp. Zool.*, *108*:363–403, 1948.

Schull, W. J., Neel, J. V., and Hashizume, A.: Some further observations on the sex ratio among infants born to survivors of the atomic bombings of Hiroshima and Nagasaki. *Am. J. Hum. Genet.*, *18*:328–373, 1966.

Stockard, C. R.: Developmental rate and structural expression: an experimental study of twins, "double monsters" and single deformities, and the interaction among embryonic organs during their origin and development. *Am. J. Anat.*, *28*:115–266, 1921.

Streeter, G. L.: Focal deficiencies in fetal tissues and their relation to intra-uterine amputation. *Carnegie Institution of Washington*, Publication #414, *22*:1–44, 1930.

Thomson, J. A.: *Heredity*. New York, G. P. Putnam's Sons, pp. 1–13, 1908.

Timoféef-Ressovsky, H.: Über phänotypische Manifestierung der polytopen (pleitropen) Genovariation Polyphaen von Drosophilia Funebis. *Naturwissenschaften, 19*:765–768, 1931.

Töndury, G.: Etiological factors in human malformation. *Triangle, 7*:90–100, 1965.

Tschermak, E. von: Über kunstliche Kreuzung bei Pisum satirum. *Ber. Dtsch. Bot. Ges., 18*:232–239, 1900.

Turner, E. K.: Teratogenic effects on the human fetus through maternal emotional stress. Report of a case. *Med. J. Aust., 2*:502–503, 1960.

Vrolik, W.: Teratology. *In* Todd, R. B., (ed.): *The Cyclopaedia of Anatomy and Physiology.* London, Longman, Brown, Green, Longman & Roberts. Vol. IV, Part II, pp. 942–976, 1849–1852.

Warkany, J.: Environmental teratogenic factors. *In First International Conference on Congenital Malformations.* Philadelphia, J. B. Lippincott Co., pp. 99–105, 1961.

Weismann, A.: *Studien zur Descendez-Theorie.* Leipzig, W. Engelmann. p. 431, 1875.

Wickes, I. G.: Foetal defect following insulin coma therapy in early pregnancy. *Brit. Med. J., 2*:1029–1030, 1954.

Wilson, J. G.: Experimental studies on congenital malformations. *J. Chronic Dis., 10*:111–130, 1959.

Zwilling, E.: *Congenital Malformations.* Philadelphia, J. B. Lippincott Co., pp. 133–139, 1961.

Chapter Three

CLASSIFICATIONS

Congenital anomalies of the hand do not lend themselves to a comprehensive classification. To classify a subject, one needs a standard terminology. Often enough, diverse names are assigned to one and the same deformity by different authors, and labels which originally were set aside for some malformations have come to be tagged onto others. There is also the intractable confusion about obscure connotations. In a previous communication, the author and a colleague (1957) made a plea in favor of using the English equivalents of complex names derived from Greek or Latin, He conceded that long usage, perhaps also euphony and succinctness, has made such a term as syndactyly acceptable. For analogous reasons one could also retain synostosis, polydactyly, macrodactyly, and some other terms which are easily understood or cause no confusion.

One thinks offhand of the term *camptodactyly* which has been misspelled and misconstrued. This word is derived from the Greek roots *kamptos* and *daktylos* which respectively mean bent and digit. Landouzy (1885, 1906) introduced the term "camptodactyly" to denote flexion deformity of the finger. Cutler (1942) misspelled camptodactylism and evolved comptodactylism which he defined as "congenital distortion of the finger, especially of the distal phalanx, occurring at the interphalangeal joint and resulting in fixed flexion, or less commonly in extension." Bunnell (1944) used the same spelling as Cutler; he surmised that the prefix *compto* stood for the word count and equated comptodactylism with "abnormal number of digits."

In the communication alluded to earlier, this author's main complaint concerned the employment of abstruse names which often necessitate the use of a dictionary. His complaint appears to have gone unheeded. Articles and books published since continue to flaunt such ambiguous designations as peromanus or perodactyly and such a ponderous compounding as streblomicrodactyly. Some of these words are not even recorded in standard medical dictionaries. Notwithstanding the confusion they cause, these terms and many others of the same ilk continue to appear in the literature.

Congenital anomalies of the hand are often too bizarre and complex to be corralled into discrete categories. Cohn (1932) considered any attempt to classify these abnormalities as quixotic—"ridiculous because there are millions of possible combinations of defects." All the same, in the last hundred or more years, numerous such attempts have been made and are still being made. Many recent authors have tried to introduce seemingly novel terms or ascribed newer meanings to old names, thereby augmenting the already existing confusion.

Heretofore published classifications of congenital hand anomalies cannot be said to have followed one another in an orderly time sequence. They seem to have cropped up at irregular intervals. Each successive list has retained part of its predecessor's and appropriated a few points from contemporary tabulations. In consequence, various classifications tend to overlap one another; many even look alike. To use a strained analogy: there is not a single tree; there is a cluster of trees hedged together with their branches touching one another and becoming snarled. But as one can untwine a tangle and trace each twig to its main stem, it is possible to relate sundry classifications to their ancestral source—usually an idea or point of view utilized by an earlier author.

On the basis of the concept they stem from or the trend they pursue, recorded classifications of congenital hand anomalies may be said to belong to one of the following categories: (1) impressionistic gradation of deformities, (2) assessment based upon numerical and dimensional discrepancies, (3) separation of genetic deformities from those caused by environmental influences, (4) tabulations based upon skeletal defects, and (5) all-embracing classifications. In most tabulations, malformations of both upper and lower limbs are included. In our reproductions of published lists, we have deleted lower limb anomalies.

IMPRESSIONISTIC GRADATION

Saint-Hilaire (1829, 1832) characterized congenital anomalies as either slight or severe. If a deformity was appreciably apparent or when it caused functional disturbance, it was considered "a vice of conformation," which was the then currently fashionable substitute for malformation. More than a century later, Kanavel (1932) graded congenital anomalies of the hand as either moderate or severe. An offshoot of this method appeared in Iselin's (1955) book. It was adopted by Benassi and Trabucci (1952) and appeared again in the latest edition of Iselin's (1967) book. Deformities of the hand are classed under two main groups called, respectively, simple and complex. By way of comment upon this method of classification, one can do no better than evoke Bunnell's (1944) verdict—arbitrary (Fig. 3–1).

DISCREPANCIES OF NUMBER AND SIZE

Otto (1831) classified "vices of organization" according to variations of number, size, form, position, connection, color, consistency, continuity, texture, and content. Saint-Hilaire (1836) adopted the first two categories only. Under deficiencies, he discussed ectromelia, hemimelia, and phocomelia—terms he himself coined to denote, respectively, absence of the whole, half, and intermediary segments of the limb. Saint-Hilaire gave polydactyly as an example of numerical augmentation and used ectrodactyly for diminution of digital numbers. Under variations of size, he considered atrophy and hypertrophy of the fingers. This method was adopted and elaborated by many authors, mainly French: Fort (1869), Polaillon (1884), Kirmisson (1898), and Dubreuil-Chambar-

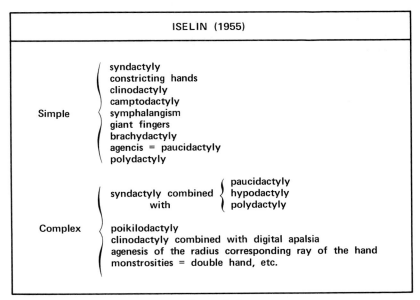

Figure 3-1

del (1925). To the categories of diminution and augmentation, Fort added adhesion, or syndactyly, and axial deviation. Polaillon spoke of developmental arrests and excesses. He considered conjoined, abbreviated, and absent digits as examples of arrested development, and polydactyly and macrodactyly as those of developmental excess. Kirmisson advised that the numerical increase or decrease of the phalanges should also be taken into consideration. Dubreuil-Chambardel included variations from the normal phalangeal formula in his classification (Figs. 3-2 and 3-3).

Young (1894) introduced the designation "perverted development." Thinking perhaps along the same line as Polaillon, Nichols (1902) produced what proved to be the most durable classification of congenital hand anomalies on this side of the Atlantic. To Polaillon's arrested and excessive development, he added Young's coinage—perverted development. Lund (1902) popularized this classification. In his second communication, Nichols (1909) again spoke of perverted development. Some years later, Nichols and Ely (1923) subdivided anomalies due to deficient and excessive development into two subsidiary groups as concerned the number and size of the part. They now described perverted development as being "qualitative or morphological rather than quantitative." They did not explain what they meant. Ahstrom (1965) recently gave a more sophisticated version of Nichols' classification (Figs. 3-4 and 3-5).

Kanavel (1932) used the epithets "hypoplasia" and "hyperplasia" instead of deficient and excessive development and he replaced the designation "perverted development" with "tissue disorientation." "Congenital malformations of the hand," Kanavel wrote, "are due to varying degrees of growth impairment having origin in germ plasm. Moderate growth impairment ends in tissue disorientation. Severe growth impairment ends in aplasia and hypoplasia." Kanavel was equivocal about the nature of hyperplasia. "The orientation of hypertrophy of the fingers with other congenital malformations of the hand presents considerable difficulty," Kanavel confessed. Cutler (1942) attempted to simplify Kanavel's classification. Paletta (1953) revived the original (Fig. 3-6).

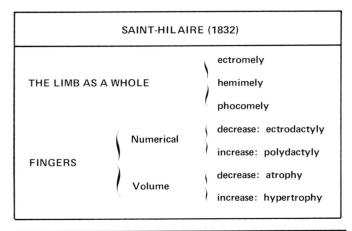

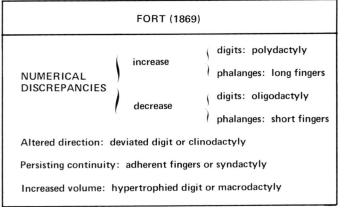

Figure 3–2

SIMPLIFIED CLASSIFICATIONS

Annandale (1866) discussed congenital deformities of the fingers under six headings: (1) hypertrophy, (2) deficiencies, (3) supernumerary fingers, (4) union, (5) contractions, and (6) tumors. With but slight modification, this list reappeared in the writings of Blum (1882), Anderson (1897), and Tubby (1912). Browne (1933) supplied the following list for congenital abnormalities in general: (1) superfluous formation, (2) failure of formation, (3) failure of fusion, (4) failure of atrophy, (5) failure to migrate, and (6) moulding deformities. In applying this classification to the hand, Browne (1939) eliminated failures of fusion and migration and added three new ones. His final list consisted of the following: (1) extra formation as exemplified by polydactyly, (2) failure of atrophy resulting in webbed fingers, (3) hypertrophy—the child having been with "one or more huge and useless fingers," (4) atrophic changes "varying from a slight indentation of the skin to a complete amputation," (5) moulding deformities, "talipes of the hands," and (6) acrocephalosyndactyly, which he considered "mutual deformity" produced by "jamming of the developing limb-buds against the skull in early foetal life." Patterson (1959, 1964) introduced what has come to be

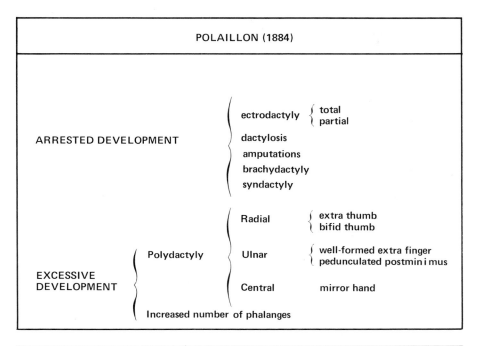

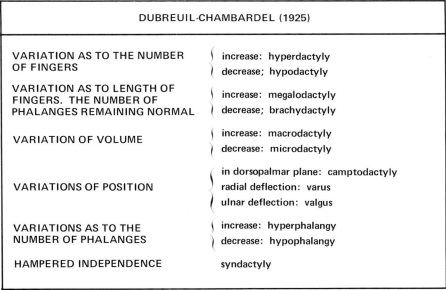

Figure 3-3

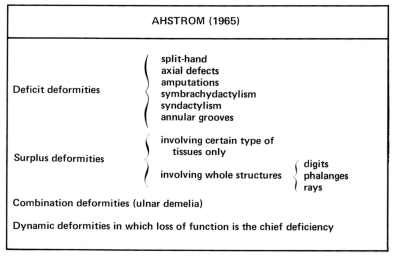

```
┌─────────────────────────────────────────────────────────────────┐
│                        NICHOLS (1902)                           │
├─────────────────────────────────────────────────────────────────┤
│                                                                 │
│                               ⎧                  ⎧ acheiria     │
│   DEFICIENT            ⎧       ⎨ as to the number ⎨ ectrodactylism│
│   DEVELOPMENT          ⎨       ⎩                  ⎩ hypophalangism │
│                        ⎪       ⎧                  ⎧ microcheiria  │
│                        ⎩       ⎨ as to the size   ⎨ microdactylia │
│                                ⎩                  ⎩               │
│                                                  ⎧ polycheiria    │
│   EXCESSIVE           ⎧        ⎧ in numbers       ⎨ polydactylism  │
│   DEVELOPMENT         ⎨        ⎨                  ⎩ polyphalangism  │
│                       ⎪        ⎪                  ⎧ cheiromegaly   │
│                       ⎩        ⎩ in size          ⎨ dactylomegaly  │
│                                                  ⎩                │
│                                ⎧ syndactylism                     │
│                                ⎪ cleft hand                       │
│   PERVERTED           ⎧        ⎪ constrictions    ⎧ of the hand    │
│   DEVELOPMENT         ⎨        ⎨ deflections      ⎨ of the fingers │
│                       ⎩        ⎪ dislocations     ⎩                │
│                                ⎩ tumors                           │
│                                                                 │
└─────────────────────────────────────────────────────────────────┘
```

Figure 3–4

```
┌─────────────────────────────────────────────────────────────────┐
│                        AHSTROM (1965)                           │
├─────────────────────────────────────────────────────────────────┤
│                                                                 │
│                          ⎧ split-hand                           │
│                          ⎪ axial defects                        │
│   Deficit deformities    ⎪ amputations                          │
│                          ⎨ symbrachydactylism                   │
│                          ⎪ syndactylism                         │
│                          ⎩ annular grooves                      │
│                                                                 │
│                          ⎧ involving certain type of            │
│                          ⎪    tissues only                      │
│   Surplus deformities    ⎨                          ⎧ digits     │
│                          ⎪ involving whole structures ⎨ phalanges │
│                          ⎩                          ⎩ rays       │
│                                                                 │
│   Combination deformities (ulnar demelia)                       │
│                                                                 │
│   Dynamic deformities in which loss of function is the chief deficiency │
│                                                                 │
└─────────────────────────────────────────────────────────────────┘
```

Figure 3–5

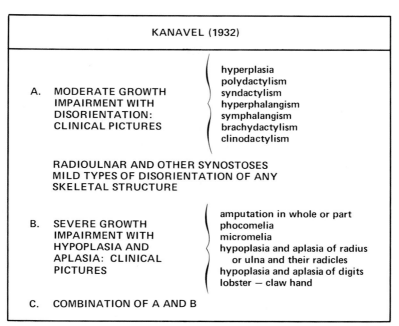

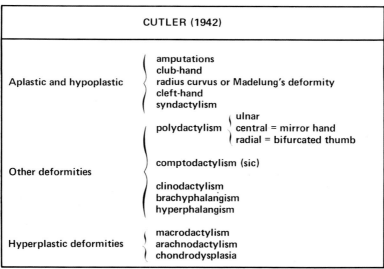

Figure 3–6

known as simplified classification. With very little modification, this list has been reproduced by Clarkson and Pelly (1962), Matthews (1964), and Buchan (1966). Entin (1964) must have had what may well be called the British classification in mind when he spoke of "monotonous enumeration of isolated entities" (Fig. 3–7).

EMBRYOPATHY VERSUS FETOPATHY

Roblot (1906) distinguished congenital anomalies occurring during the formative period from those which presumably had their inception at a later stage

ANNANDALE (1866)
1. Hypertrophy
2. Deficiencies
3. Supernumerary digits
4. Union of adjacent members
5. Contractions
6. Tumors

BROWNE (1939)
Failure of formation: absence of parts
Extra formation: polydactyly
Failure of atrophy: syndactyly
Hypertrophy: "huge useless fingers"
Atrophic changes: ring constrictions
Moulding deformities: talipes of the hands
Acrocephalo - syndactyly

BLUM (1882)

HYPERTROPHY	{	pure: uniform enlargement of all structures
		tumorous: lobules of fat or enlarged vessels
POLYDACTYLY	{	underdeveloped digit held with a pedicle
		developed, but sharing a common metacarpal
		developed, possessing its own metacarpal
		bifid digit, usually the thumb
SYNDACTYLY	{	connected with membrane or web
		ensconced in a common bag of skin
		connected with bone
RETRACTIONS	{	flexion contracture at metacarpophalangeal joints
		flexion contracture at interphalangeal joints

PATTERSON (1964)

1.	WEBBING OF FINGERS	{	(a) with normal digits
			(b) with abnormal digits
2.	ABNORMALTIES OF POSITION	{	(a) a flexion contracture
			(b) lateral displacement
3.	ABSENCE OF PARTS		
4.	RING CONSTRICTIONS		
5.	EXCESS TISSUE		

Figure 3–7

of antenatal development. He then subdivided the former into two smaller groups: (1) anomalies caused by arrested development and (2) the ones resulting from excessive development. He placed absent and short digits under anomalies by arrested development; surplus, long, and large digits were relegated to anomalies by excessive development. Müller (1937) separated anomalies which had their inception in the undifferentiated mesenchymal core of the original hand plate from those that occurred after the transformation of preosseous anlage. Berndorfer (1961) distinguished malformations belonging to the category of embryopathy from those classed as fetopathy on the basis of presumed damage incurred by the conceptus before or after development of the organs. "In general, if we find multiple malformations, we must assume germinal injuries," Berndorfer wrote.

The term *embryopathy* is now used by most authors for defects occurring during the first two months of antenatal life, and *fetopathy* is reserved for anomalies occurring after organogenesis. Toxoplasmosis is said to affect fetal elements, while rubella and thalidomide act on embryonic tissue. Defects caused by the former are classed under fetopathy, and those produced by the latter are categorized as embryopathy. Strictly speaking, all abnormalities—genetic and nongenetic—which have their inception during embryonic development should be considered as embryopathies. But convention has confined the designation embryopathy to anomalies caused by environmental agencies only. Fetopathies are extremely rare (Fig. 3–8).

ROBLOT (1906)

I. **ANOMALIES OCCURRING DURING FORMATIVE (EMBRYONIC) PERIOD**

    A.   **Caused by arrested formation**   { ectrodactyly / brachydactyly / microdactyly

    B.   **Caused by excessive formation**   { polydactyly / macrodactyly

II. **ANOMALIES OCCURRING DURING DEVELOPMENTAL (FETAL) STAGE**

    Syndactyly   { partial / total

    Constricting hands, scars, etc.

    Amputations

    Hypertrophies

    Atrophies

Figure 3–8

ENDOGENOUS AND EXOGENOUS DEFORMITIES

Birch-Jensen (1949) classified congenital deficiencies of the upper limb on the basis of their supposed determination by the gene or subsequent instigation by exogenous agencies. Potter (1952) adopted this distinction and stated that "all bilaterally symmetrical abnormalities and those which consist of excessive numbers of parts are endogenous"—which is not true. We know now that bilaterally symmetrical abnormalities, as well as multiple abnormalities, are often produced by thalidomide, an exogenous agent. We can now say with greater confidence what Nichols (1902) said at the turn of the century: "Identical pathological conditions may result from very different causes." The converse is also ture: identical causes may produce different deformities. Vinke (1956) wrote: "Genetic and environmental factors may lead to the same kind of congenital malformations. Identical malformations may be hereditary in one case and nonhereditary in another." As geneticists would say: phenocopies, which are exogenetically induced, may mimic phenotypes, which are genetically determined. All that can now be said about the Birch-Jensen classification is that it has contributed a pair of useful adjectives (Fig. 3–9).

CLASSIFICATION BASED UPON SKELETAL DEFICIENCIES

Earlier embryologists and anthropologists described primitive carpal bones as being arranged in two transverse series. Leboucq (1884) pointed out that these

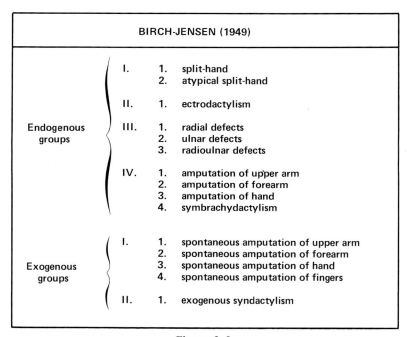

Figure 3–9

ossicles are also arranged along longitudinal lines which stem from the main axis of the limb and pass distally into the fingers. Leboucq mentioned two such rays and called them, respectively, radial and ulnar. Goldmann (1890) added another longitudinal ray and attached to it the epithet "median." Polaillon (1884) used the adjectives "radial," "central," and "ulnar." Klippel and Bouchet (1907) attached the adjective "longitudinal" to radial and ulnar absences. Broca and Mouchet (1912) spoke of total and partial defects. Under the latter, they included longitudinal hemimelia which they defined as absence of the radius or ulna.

Potel (1914) made the distinction between transverse and longitudinal absences. He gave three subgroups of transverse deficiency: (1) total, meaning absence of the entire limb; (2) radicular, representing deformities in which one or both segments between the shoulder and the hand are missing; (3) terminal, as exemplified by the absence of the hand, fingers, or phalanges. Under the heading longitudinal defects, Potel listed: (1) absence of the radius, (2) absence of the radius and corresponding part of the hand, (3) absence of the ulna, and (4) absence of the ulna and one or more fingers on the corresponding side of the hand. Potel attached the epithet "segmental longitudinal" to the absence of the forearm bones alone.

In his book, Jones (1920) included a diagram which showed the axis of the hand passing through the third metacarpal and the middle finger. Structures on the radial side of this axis were named preaxial and those on the ulnar side of this axis postaxial. Kanavel's (1932) diagram showed that the axis of the hand separating the radial from ulnar elements passed through the index finger. Hypoplasia, Kanavel said, may involve "the radial bud and its radicle in whole or in part or . . . the ulnar bud and its radicle in whole or in part." The thumb, he explained, originated directly from the radial bud, while the index finger lay between the two and might be involved in hypoplasia of either ray, although it was more closely associated with the ulnar bud. "Congenital defects of the radius most often involve the thumb," Kanavel wrote. He identified lobster-claw or split hand with hypoplasia of the "median" primordial carpal bud described by Goldmann (1890). His illustrations of this deformity showed absence of the middle finger and part of the third metacarpal.

According to Bunnell (1944), hypoplastic deformities of the hand conform to three distinct patterns named segmental, longitudinal, and annular, respectively. Under segmental defect, Bunnell listed end-to-end synostoses and intercalary deficiencies. Under longitudinal defect, he placed absences of radial and ulnar rays. "There may be," Bunnell wrote, "loss of ulnar or radial digits alone, or instead the defect may be of medial digits and carpal bones." He placed circular soft tissue depressions and transverse terminal deficiencies or amputations under annular defect.

O'Rahilly (1951) reverted to the terminology used by Jones (1920)—for that matter, by most anatomists and anthropologists. What Polaillon (1884) had considered central and Kanavel (1932) median hypoplasia, and Bunnell (1944) medial defect of digits, O'Rahilly (1951) called axial adactylia. This designation appeared in a footnote, and no more was said about it except that it represented "the possible pattern of cleft hand." O'Rahilly was concerned primarily with pre- and postaxial defects, which he collectively called paraxial—parallel to the axis. As had Broca and Mouchet (1912), he assigned the designation "longitudinal hemimelia" to defects of the radial and ulnar rays. O'Rahilly called defects of the radial ray preaxial and those of the ulnar component postaxial.

O'Rahilly considered hemimelia as being transverse or longitudinal (paraxial). He distinguished two types of longitudinal defects, terminal and intercalary. In terminal preaxial hemimelia the following bones are missing: radius, scaphoid, trapezium, first metacarpal, and two phalanges of the thumb. In intercalary preaxial hemimelia one of the following bones may be absent: radius or portions of it, trapezium, and the first metacarpal, in part or as a whole. In terminal postaxial hemimelia, the ulna and the corresponding bones of the wrist and the hand might be missing; in the intercalary postaxial type, the ulna or portions of it, the pisiform, the hamate, triquetrum, or some of the ulnar metacarpals may be absent. O'Rahilly placed what he called "coherence of normally adjacent structures," or synostosis, under fusion hemimelia. O'Rahilly's favorite term for duplications — what earlier authors called numerical augmentation — was polymelia or dimelia.

Frantz and O'Rahilly (1961), Hall et al (1962), and Stelling (1965, 1968) divided skeletal limb defects into two main groups, named, respectively, terminal and intercalary. Each group is further subdivided into transverse and longitudinal, giving two major groups, each with two subgroups or a total of four subdivisions: (1) terminal transverse hemimelia, (2) terminal longitudinal hemimelia, (3) intercalary transverse hemimelia, and (4) intercalary longitudinal hemimelia. Each of these defects is qualified as being partial or complete. Lenz (1969) considered "aplasia of the radius and the thumb" preferable to radial hemimelia. Freire-Maia (1969) retained O'Rahilly's original terminology as did Burtch (1969) except for the use of the ambiguous term *meromelia*, meaning malformed limb (Figs. 3–10 and 3–11).

COMPREHENSIVE CLASSIFICATIONS

Nichols (1902) wrote: "The affections of the hand and fingers include those that are peculiar to or affect this region exclusively; those that may occur elsewhere, but show predilection for, or exhibit special features or modifications in this locality; those conditions affecting the hands equally and indifferently with other parts of the body; and manifestations exhibited by the hand, or general diseases." Nichols shunned the task of classifying congenital hand anomalies upon the broad base he outlined. Where he feared to tread, Potel (1914) rushed in, and produced perhaps the most elaborate classification on record. Steindler (1923) reproduced Potel's classification and, in his turn, attempted to compose one which would be "less complex and applicable to most conditions of the upper limb." Steindler failed. His classification contained such presumptuous connotations as developmental suppression, developmental aberrations, dysplastic conditions, amniotic contractures, and polyglandular dystrophy — as examples of which he gave polydactylia (some cases), macrodactylia, and arachnodactylia (Fig. 3–12).

Another attempt to formulate an all-inclusive classification was made by Entin (1959). He gave the ensuing list: (1) local abnormalities confined to the upper limb, (2) conditions affecting the skeleton as a whole, (3) conditions in which the greatest disturbance is localized in the neuromuscular system, (4) miscellaneous conditions not belonging to the groups mentioned. What O'Rahilly and his followers called transverse terminal defect, Entin considered vertical absence; longitudinal deficiencies in the former classification were renamed by Entin horizontal absences (Fig. 3–13).

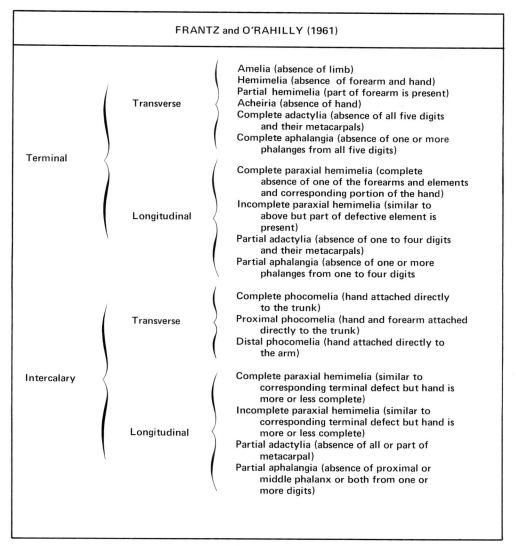

FRANTZ and O'RAHILLY (1961)

Terminal

Transverse

Amelia (absence of limb)
Hemimelia (absence of forearm and hand)
Partial hemimelia (part of forearm is present)
Acheiria (absence of hand)
Complete adactylia (absence of all five digits
and their metacarpals)
Complete aphalangia (absence of one or more
phalanges from all five digits)

Longitudinal

Complete paraxial hemimelia (complete
absence of one of the forearms and elements
and corresponding portion of the hand)
Incomplete paraxial hemimelia (similar to
above but part of defective element is
present)
Partial adactylia (absence of one to four digits
and their metacarpals)
Partial aphalangia (absence of one or more
phalanges from one to four digits

Intercalary

Transverse

Complete phocomelia (hand attached directly
to the trunk)
Proximal phocomelia (hand and forearm attached
directly to the trunk)
Distal phocomelia (hand attached directly to
the arm)

Longitudinal

Complete paraxial hemimelia (similar to
corresponding terminal defect but hand is
more or less complete)
Incomplete paraxial hemimelia (similar to
corresponding terminal defect but hand is
more or less complete)
Partial adactylia (absence of all or part of
metacarpal)
Partial aphalangia (absence of proximal or
middle phalanx or both from one or
more digits)

Figure 3–10

Entin stressed the point that "by emphasizing the derangement of function and structure" his classification crystallized the particular reconstructive procedure needed. Admittedly one needs a plan for sorting out the diversified deformities of the hand. While a classification helps the author to organize his material and present it as best he can, it gives no guidance to the surgeon. The surgeon does not deal with collective categories, but with discrete clinical entities. Syndactyly has been categorized as absence of fission by Vrolik (1849); union of adjacent members by Annandale (1866); developmental arrest by Polaillon (1884); perverted development by Nichols (1902); failure of segmentation by Potel (1914); disorientation of tissue by Kanavel (1932), failure of atrophy by Browne (1939); fusion of adjacent fingers by Cutler (1942), and finally by Bunnell (1944) and Entin (1959) simply as webbed digits. It cannot be said that any of these diversified designations have materially influenced the treatment of syndactylism.

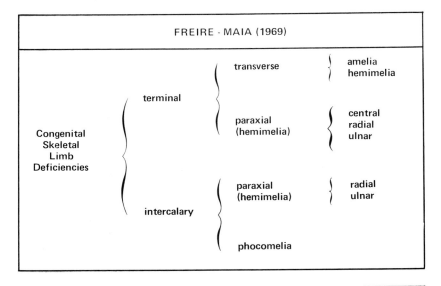

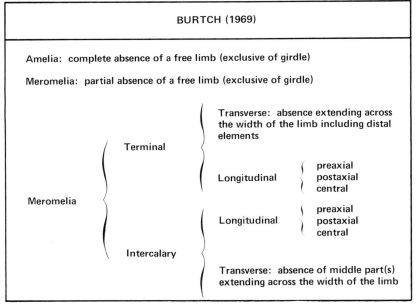

Figure 3–11

In a recent communication, Swanson (1964) gave the following list: (1) failure of separation of parts, (2) duplications, (3) arrest of growth and development, (4) focal deficiency, (5) overgrowth, and (6) general skeletal defects. One may ask, are not failure and arrest of growth and skeletal defects both focal deficiencies? Swanson et al (1968) formulated another classification "on the basis," we are told, "of embryological failure." The following main categories are given: (1) failure of separation of parts, (2) arrest of development of parts, (3) duplications, (4) overgrowth, (5) the congenital circular constriction band syndrome, and (6) generalized skeletal defects. Again one asks, are not "circular constriction band" or annular groove and "arrest of development of parts" produced by the same process, namely focal necrosis in different areas of the embryonic limb?

POTEL (1914)

Absences

transverse
- the entire limb: amelia
- intermediary segments (phocomely)
  - arm and forearm
  - upper arm
  - forearm
- terminal segment
  - hand: ectrocheiry
  - fingers: ectrodactyly

longitudinal
- radius: radial club-hand
- ulna: ulnar club-hand
- radius and corresponding digital rays
- ulna and corresponding digital rays

Hypertrophies

true
- hemihypertrophy involving half of the body
- monomelic hypertrophy
- enlargement of fingers or thumb: macrodactyly

false
- trophic edema, etc.
- neoplasms

Disturbances of Segmentation

defective
- synostoses
  - humerus to forearm bones
  - radioulnar
  - intercarpal
  - intemetarcarpal
  - interphalangeal
- syndactyly of embryonic variety

exaggerated
- transverse: hyperphalangism
- longitudinal : polydactyly

Axial deviation of digits
- forward bending: camptodactyly
- side-to-side deflection: clinodactyly

Heteroplastic aberrations: exostosis, hyperostosis

STEINDLER (1923)

DEVELOPMENTAL SUPPRESSION
- congenital defect of the forearm bones (congenital club-hand)
- the cleft hand (lobster claw-hand)
- extrodactylia (aphalangism)

DEVELOPMENTAL ARREST
- syndactylia
- symphalangism

DEVELOPMENTAL ABERRATIONS
- polydactylia
- hyperphalangism

DYSPLASTIC CONDITIONS
- synostosis
- brachydactylia (some cases)
- fusion of carpal bones

POLYGLANDULAR DYSTROPHY
- polydactylia (some cases)
- macrodactylia (partial gigantism)
- arachnodactylia

CONTRACTURES (NEUROGENIC or AMNIOTIC)
- contracted club-hand
- contracted fingers
- amniotic contractures

Figure 3–12

ENTIN (1959)

Anomaly

A. Absence of parts (agenesis or amputation)

Vertical absence (long axis of the limb)
No arm (abrachius)
No forearm or hand (hemibrachius)
No hand (achirus)
No digits (adactyly)
No phalanges (electrodactylism)

Horizontal absence of parts (forearm and hand)
No forearm (phocomelia)
No radial component (radius and thumb)
No radius or thumb
No radius or its parts
No thumb
No part of thumb (hypoplasia)
No medial component (central digit and carpal bones)
No ulnar component (ulna and three ulnar digits)

B. Deformities or Abnormalties

Shoulder girdle
Upper arm
Forearm
Radio-ulnar fusion
Madelung's deformity
Others (mirror-hand)
Hand and digits
Bone fusion (symphalangism)
Bent digits (clinodactyly)
Short or partially amputated digits (brachydactyly)
Webbed digits (syndactyly)
Others (bifid and supernumerary digits)

Disturbances of Bone Formation or Growth

Chondrodystrophies
Dyschrondroplasia (multiple enchondroma or Ollier's disease)
Achondroplasia (chondrodystrophy foetalis)
Chondro-ectodermal dysplasia (Ellis-van Creveld syndrome)
Metaphyseal and epiphyseal dysplasia
Chondro-osteo dystrophy (gargoylism and Morquio-Brailsford disease)

Osteodystrophies (osteogenesis imperfecta)
Others: arachnodactyly (Marfan's syndrome)
Disturbances of joints and ligaments: multiple dislocations

Neuromuscular Conditions

Arthrogryposis (amyoplasia congenita)
Sprengel's deformity

Cerebral palsy { Spastic hemiplegia and quadriplegia
Athetosis

Others: Mobius' syndrome (facial muscles and upper extremities)

Figure 3-13

RETREAT TOWARD ANATOMICAL CLASSIFICATION

Edwards et al (1964) wrote: "Due to limitation in knowledge of morbid embryology, a system of classifying malformations must be anatomical rather than etiological and should enable syndromes as well as single defects to be both recognized and classified."

O'Rahilly (1969) had this to say: "Although the delineation of limb anomalies may be based, at least in some instances, on clinical, functional, teratogenic, embryological or genetic criteria, the only satisfactory criterion of classification at the present time is anatomic. In relatively few cases can an external agent such as thalidomide be pinpointed, and such disputed causal terms as amputation (which could at best apply to only a small minority) should be rigorously avoided. Moreover, even where a causal agent is known, etiologic classification supplements but does not replace the anatomic . . . . Similarly a genetic basis can be implicated in only some cases, and in those, the genetic data supplement but do not replace the anatomic. Once the anatomic classification be established . . . the additional information can be superimposed." O'Rahilly advised that, for each anatomic category, a distinction be made according to whether the anomaly is isolated, is confined to the limbs, or has occurred as part of a syndrome with other systems or regions involved.

The anatomical classification originally suggested by O'Rahilly (1951) and later elaborated by many of his followers comes as near to being rational as can be expected at this stage of our knowledge. Somewhere along the way, duplications and fusion hemimelias that O'Rahilly had discussed seem to have been overlooked by his followers. Also missing in subsequent tabulations are intercalary inclusions. In the classification proposed by O'Rahilly and his followers, ab-

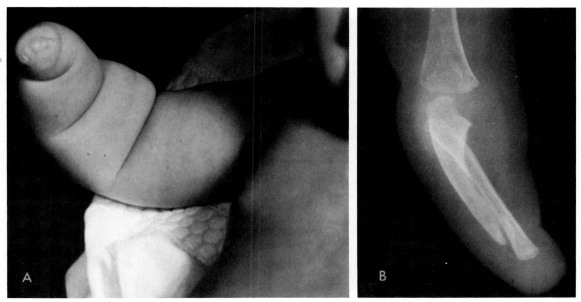

Figure 3–14 Transverse terminal (peripheral) defect: transantebrachial agenesis of the right upper limb. *A,* Frontal view of the right upper limb of a 12-month-old infant. *B,* Lateral roentgenograph of the same.

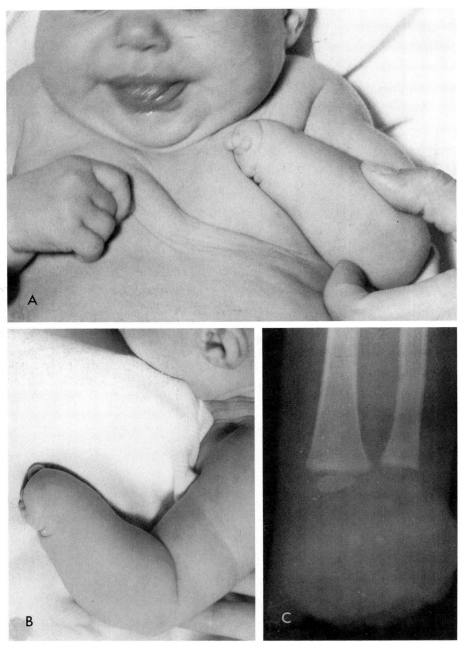

Figure 3–15 Transcarpal agenesis of the left upper limb resulting in absence of a hand or acheiria. *A*, Frontal photograph of a 13-month-old infant. *B*, Dorsal view of the left arm. *C*, Dorsovolar roentgenograph of the defective limb.

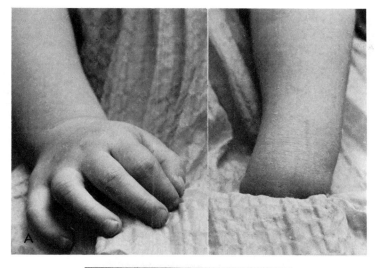

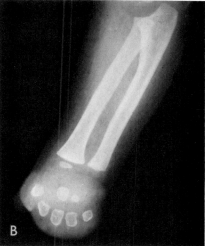

Figure 3–16 Transmetacarpal agenesis (adactylia). *A*, Frontal view of the upper limbs of a two-year-old female. *B*, Dorsvolar roentgenograph of the left limb.

sence of the radius alone is assigned to the category of intercalary defects. Smith (1964) described a number of cases of aplasia of the radius of which he wrote: "Radial paraxial intercalary hemimelia is neither paraxial intercalary nor hemimelic. It represents a variable but diffuse series of congenital abnormalities affecting the entire upper limb." One could level the same criticism against any designation denoting a particular hand defect. For a missing radius, Smith used the term radial club hand, which is nowhere as specific as intercalary radial hemimelia of O'Rahilly's classification. No less an authority than Lenz (1969) considered the terminology proposed by O'Rahilly and his followers as "one of the main descriptive systems . . . . Its main use is to serve as a standard nomenclature which may facilitate mutual understanding in the field in which a wide variety of difficult jargon is used. Unfortunately, as has been said, some authors would sooner use somebody else's toothbrush than his terminology." (See Figs. 3–14 to 3–34.)

(*Text continued on page 86.*)

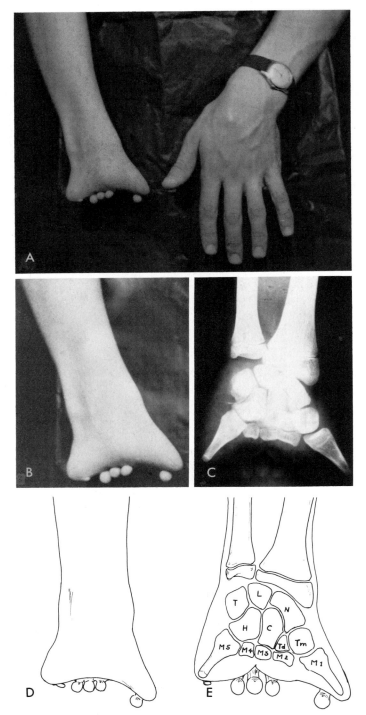

Figure 3–17 Transmetacarpal defect of skeletal elements with bubble-like soft tissue vestiges of ungual phalangeal pulps. *A*, Dorsal view of the hands of a 10-year-old boy. *B*, Photograph of the right hand—enlarged. *C*, Dorsopalmar roentgenograph of right hand. *D* and *E* illustrate *B* and *C*, respectively.

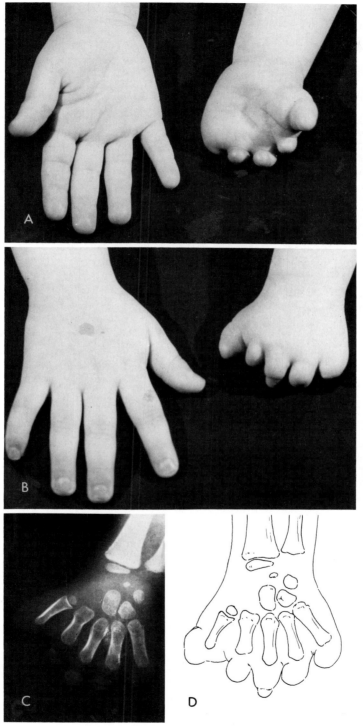

Figure 3–18 Absence of all phalanges. *A*, Palmar view of the hands of a four-year-old female. *B*, Dorsal view of the same. *C*, Dorsopalmar roentgenograph of the left hand. *D*, Illustrative sketch.

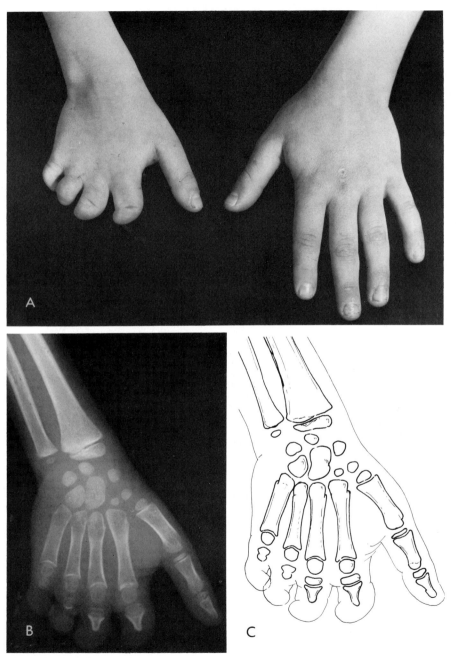

Figure 3–19   Absence of most phalanges of the lesser digits. *A,* Dorsal view of both hands. *B,* Dorsopalmar roentgenograph of the right hand. *C,* Illustrative sketch.

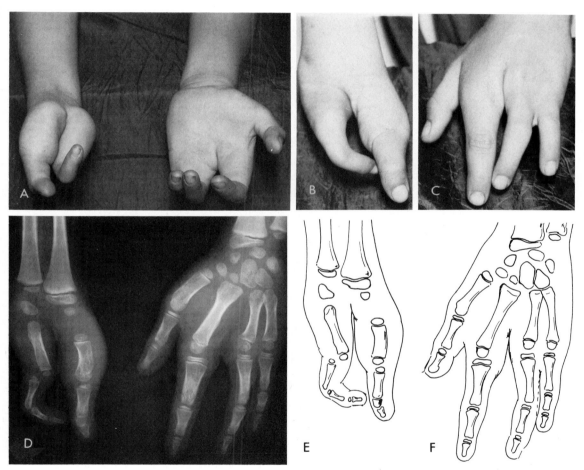

Figure 3–20 Terminal longitudinal defect of the central digital rays (axial adactylia; split hand) of an eight-year-old boy. *A*, Palmar view of the hands. *B*, Dorsal view of the right hand. *C*, Dorsal view of the left hand. *D*, Dorsopalmar roentgenograph of both hands. *E* and *F* illustrate *D*.

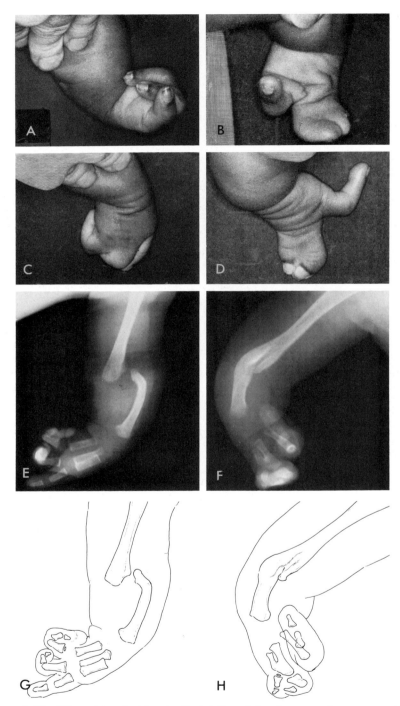

Figure 3–21 Bilateral terminal longitudinal defect of the ulnar ray of a one-year-old boy. *A*, Palmar view of the right hand. *B*, Palmar view of the left hand. *C*, Dorsal view of the right hand. *D*, Dorsal view of the left hand. *E*, Roentgenograph showing absence of the right ulna. *F*, Roentgenograph showing absence of the left ulna and fusion of the radius with the humerus as well as fusion of two radial metacarpals with syndactyly of the corresponding digits. *G* and *H* illustrate the roentgenograph above each.

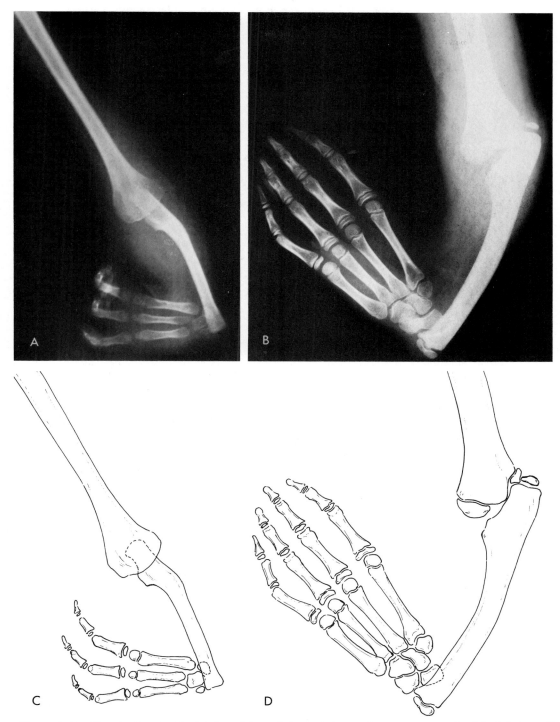

Figure 3–22   Terminal longitudinal defect of the radial ray. *A*, Dorsovolar roentgenograph of the left upper limb of a two-year-old female, showing absence of the radius and the two radial digits. *B*, Dorsovolar roentgenograph of a seven-year-old male, showing absence of the pollical ray. *C* and *D* illustrate the roentgenograph above each.

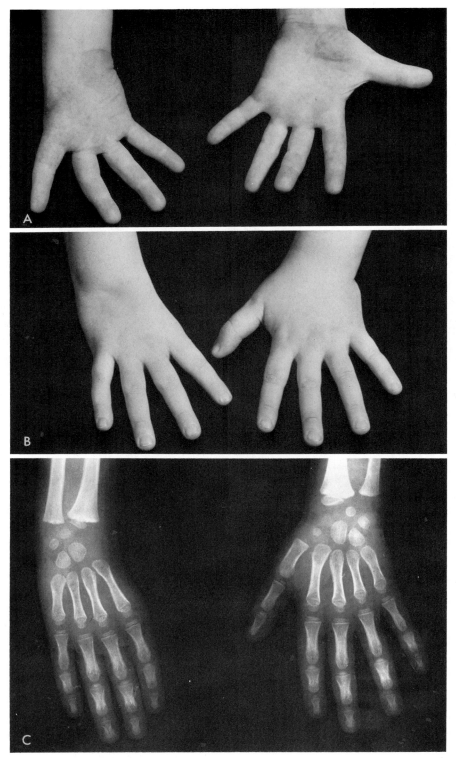

Figure 3–23 Terminal longitudinal defect of the pollical component of the right hand of a five-year-old child. *A*, Palmar view of the hands. *B*, Dorsal view of the same. *C*, Dorsopalmar roentgenograph of the hands.

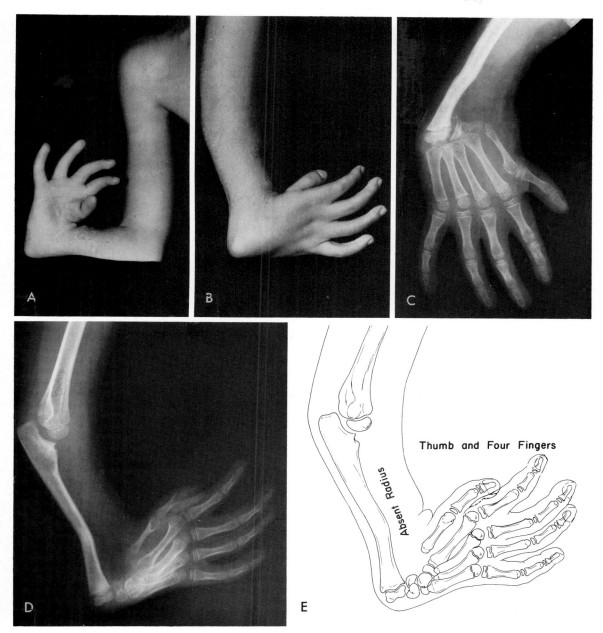

Figure 3-24 Intercalary defect involving the right radius of an 11-year-old boy who had been subjected to osteotomy of the ulna to correct its curvature. *A*, Volar view of the right upper limb. *B*, Dorsal view of the same. *C*, Dorsopalmar roentgenograph of the right hand—enlarged. *D*, Dorsopalmar roentgenograph of the forearm and the hand. *E*, Interpretative sketch.

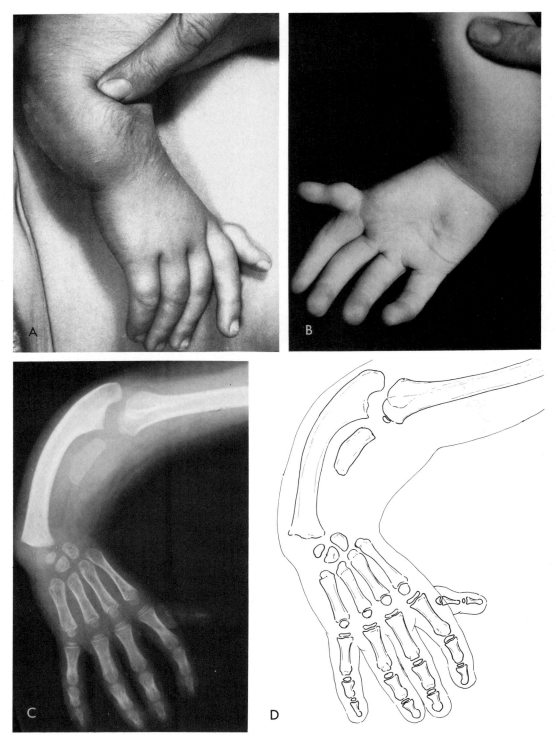

Figure 3–25   Intercalary defect involving the distal half of the right radius and the first metacarpal of a five-year-old female. *A*, Dorsal view of the hand and forearm. *B*, Palmar view. *C*, Dorsopalmar roentgenograph. *D*, Illustrative sketch.

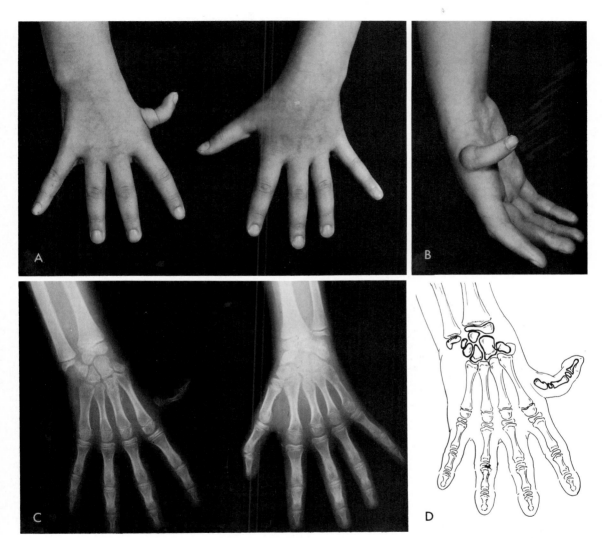

Figure 3–26 Intercalary radial ray defect involving the carpal scaphoid and the proximal part of the first metacarpal. *A*, Dorsal view of the hands of a 10-year-old female. *B*, Radial view of the affected right hand. *C*, Dorsopalmar roentgenograph of both hands. *D*, Sketch of the roentgenograph of the right hand.

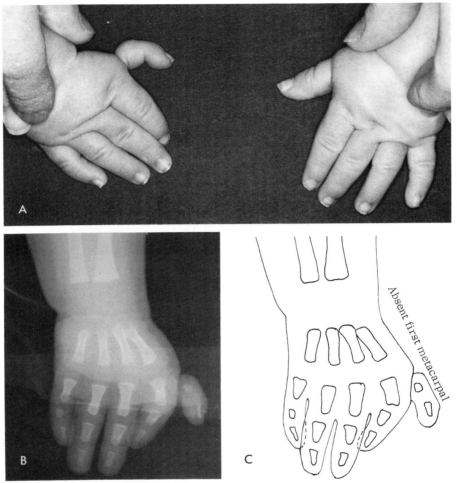

Figure 3–27   Intercalary defect of the right hand of a three-month-old infant involving the first metacarpal bone. *A*, Dorsal view of the hands. *B*, Dorsopalmar roentgenograph of the right hand. *C*, Illustrative sketch.

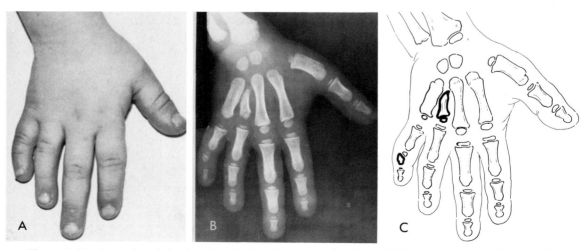

Figure 3–28   Intercalary defect involving the fourth metacarpal and the middle phalanx of the right hand of a two-year-old boy. *A*, Dorsal view of the right hand showing a short ring finger. *B*, Dorsopalmar roentgenograph showing absence of the proximal extremity of the fourth metacarpal and an irregularly shaped fifth metacarpal as well as a squat middle phalanx of the little finger. *C*, Sketch illustrating the same.

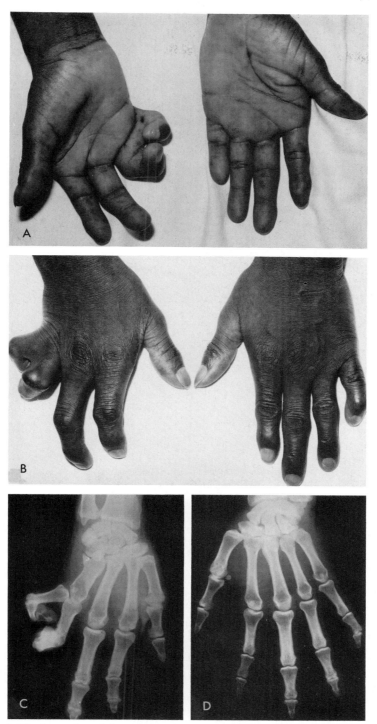

Figure 3–29 Intercalary defect of the ulnar ray involving the fifth metacarpal of an adult male. In this case a short ulnar metacarpal bone supports two crooked, partly webbed ulnar digits. *A*, Palmar view of both hands. *B*, Dorsal view. *C*, Dorsopalmar roentgenograph of the right hand, with missing metacarpal. *D*, Dorsopalmar roentgenograph of the left hand.

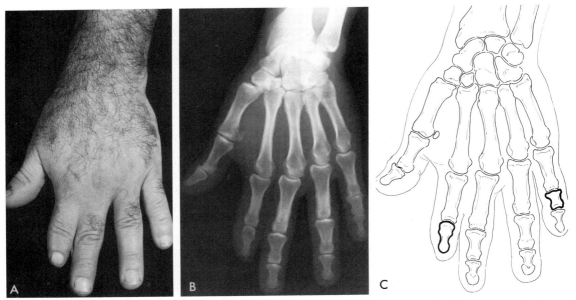

Figure 3-30 Intercalary defect of the left hand of an adult male, involving the second phalanges of the index and little fingers. *A*, Dorsal view of the left hand, showing cutaneous syndactyly of the dwarfed index finger with its ulnar neighbor. *B*, Roentgenograph of the same, showing that the index finger lacks a middle phalanx and the middle phalanx of the little finger is short. *C*, Sketch illustrating the same.

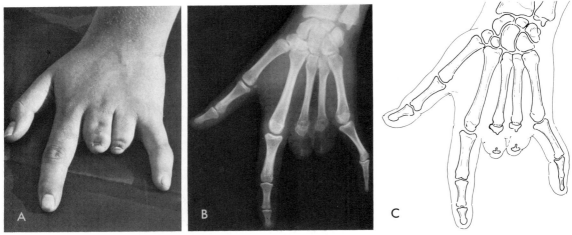

Figure 3-31 Intercalary defect of the middle and ring fingers. *A*, Dorsal view of the right hand; both affected digits bear rudimentary nails. *B*, Dorsopalmar roentgenograph: ungual phalanges of the affected digits are shown as small slivers with flared-out tufts. Bases of proximal phalanges are also present; the shafts are missing. *C*, Sketch illustrating the same.

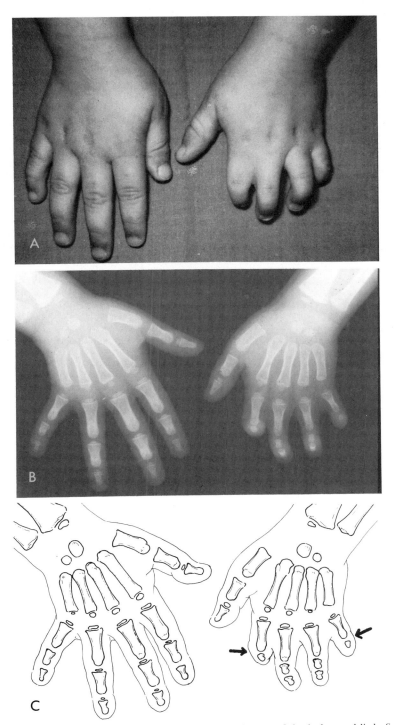

Figure 3-32 Intercalary absence of the middle phalanges of the index and little fingers in a two-year-old boy with short, webbed fingers of the left hand. *B*, Dorsopalmar roentgenograph: left index and little fingers lack a middle phalanx. *C*, Sketch illustrating the same.

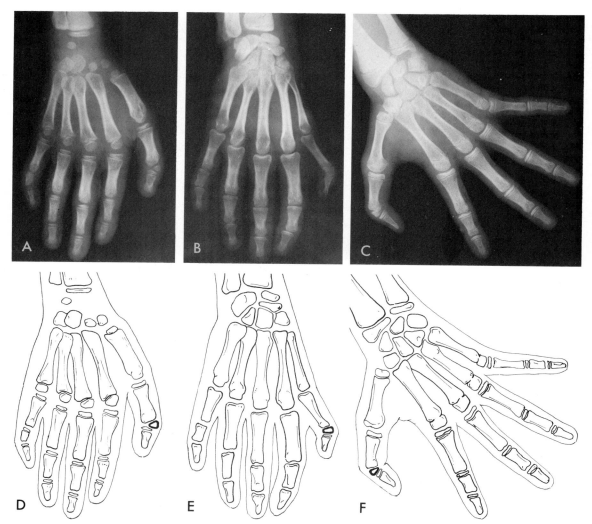

Figure 3–33 Intercalary inclusions. *A*, Dorsopalmar roentgenograph showing a triangular piece of bone interposed between the proximal and distal phalanges of the right thumb. *B*, Roentgenograph of a similar case in which the interposed bone is rhomboid in shape. *C*, Roentgenograph of the left hand of another patient—here again the interposed bone is triangular in shape. *D*, *E*, and *F* illustrate the roentgenograph above each.

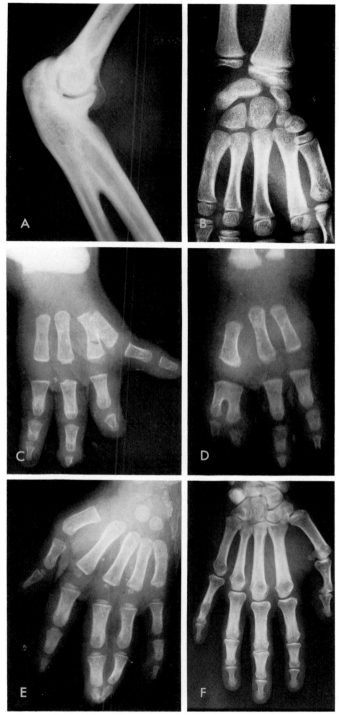

Figure 3–34 Fusion anomalies. *A*, Radioulnar synostosis. *B*, Lunotriquetral coalescence. *C*, Side-to-side fusion of two radial metacarpals. *D*, Side-to-side fusion of phalanges. *E*, Confluence of the tips of the ungual phalanges of the middle and ring fingers. *F*, End-to-end fusion of the proximal and middle phalanges of the little finger.

SUMMARY

We have not as yet attained enough latitude of knowledge about congenital hand anomalies to formulate a comprehensive classification. Numerous attempts in this direction can be credited with one positive contribution: they have bequeathed a number of more sophisticated and perhaps more accurate designations. The adjective exogenous is more specific than environmental. Heretofore, the uterus of the mother was considered the main environment of the zygote, but many recent authors speak of internal or microenvironment, meaning all that exists outside of the particular gene on the chromosomal spiral. The phrase "peripheral agenesis" says more and does not convey the unwarranted implication that "spontaneous amputation" does. The classification of skeletal defects—originally proposed by O'Rahilly (1951) and elaborated by many others—has much to commend it, but it is at best confining: it leaves out anomalies of augmentation of size (macrodactyly, angiodysplastic enlargements, monomelic and hemihypertrophies); synostotic states (symphalangism, side-to-side coalescence of metacarpals and phalanges, carpal coalescence, and radioulnar synostosis); intercalary inclusions (triphalangeal thumb); longitudinal inclusions (supernumerary metacarpals and phalanges); and many other abnormalities.

References

Ahstrom, J. P., Jr.: Classification of congenital deformities of the hand. *J. Bone Joint Surg.*, *47A*:643, 1965.

Anderson, W.: *The Malformations of the Fingers and Toes.* London, J. & A. Churchill, pp. 129–149, 1897.

Annandale, T.: *The Malformations, Diseases and Injuries of the Fingers and Toes and their Surgical Treatment.* Philadelphia: J. B. Lippincott Co., pp. 1–72, 1866.

Benassi, V., and Trabucci, L.: Terapia chirurgica delle deformita congenite della mano. *Chir. Organi Mov.*, *51*:177–197, 1952.

Berndorfer, A.: Some problems in connection with congenital malformations of the hands. *Acta Chir. Plast.* *3*:219–228, 1961.

Birch-Jensen, A.: *Congenital Deformities of the Upper Extremities.* Translated by E. Aagesen. Copenhagen, Andelsbogtrykkeriet I Odense and Det danske Forlag, pp. 15–26, 1949.

Blum, A.: *Chirurgie de la Main.* Paris, Asselin et Cie, pp. 1–16, 1882.

Broca, A., and Mouchet, A.: *Difformités Congénitales des Membres.* Paris, G. Steinheil, pp. 1–158, 1912.

Browne, D.: Congenital malformation. *Practitioner*, *131*:20–32, 1933.

Browne, D.: Congenital anomalies of the extremities. *Practitioner*, *142*:270–277, 1939.

Buchan, A. C.: Congenital malformations of the hand. *In* Pulvertaft, R. G., (ed.): *The Hand.* London, Butterworths, pp. 32–64, 1966.

Bunnell, S.: *Surgery of the Hand.* Philadelphia, J. B. Lippincott Co., pp. 609–647, in particular p. 621, 1944.

Burtch, R. L.: Classification nomenclature for congenital skeletal limb deficiencies. *In* Swinyard, S. J., (ed.): *Limb Development and Deformity: Problems of Evaluation and Rehabilitation.* Springfield, Ill., Charles C Thomas, pp. 505–538, 1969.

Clarkson, P., and Pelly, A.: *The General and Plastic Surgery of the Hand.* Philadelphia, F. A. Davis Co., pp. 396–419, 1962.

Cohn, I.: Skeletal disturbances and anomalies. A clinical report and a review of the literature. *Trans. South Surg. Assoc.*, *44*:485–521, 1932.

Cutler, C. W.: *The Hand, Its Disabilities and Diseases.* Philadelphia, W. B. Saunders Co., pp. 401–444, 1942.

Dubreuil-Chambardel, L.: *Les Variations du Corps Humain.* Paris, Flammarion, pp. 99–100, 1925.

Edwards, J. H., Leck, I., and Record, R. G.: A classification of malformations. *Acta Genet. (Basel)*, *14*:76–90, 1964.

Entin, M. A.: Reconstruction of congenital abnormalities of the upper extremities. *J. Bone Joint Surg.*, *41A*:681–700, 1959.

Entin, M. A.: Reconstruction of congenital aplasia of the radial component. *Surg. Clin. North Am.*, *44*:1091–1105, 1964.

Fort, J. A.: *Des Difformités Congénitales et Acquisés des Doigts.* Thèse. Paris, A. Delahaye, pp. 8–11, 1869.

Frantz, C. H., and O'Rahilly, R.: Congenital skeletal limb deficiencies. *J. Bone Joint Surg.*, *43A*:1202–1224, 1961.

Freire-Maia, N.: Congenital skeletal limb deficiencies. *In* Bergsma, D., (ed.): *Birth Defects. Original Article Series.* New York, National Foundation—March of Dimes. Vol. V, No. 3:7–13, 1969.

Goldmann, E. E.: Beitrag zur Lehre von den Missbildungen der Extremitäten. *Beitr. Klin. Chir.*, *7*:239–256, 1890.

Hall, C. B., Brooks, M. B., and Dennis, J. F.: Congenital skeletal deficiencies of the extremities. *J.A.M.A.*, *180*:590–599, 1962.

Iselin, M.: *Chirurgie de la Main.* Paris, Masson et Cie., pp. 585–616, 1955.

Iselin, M., and Iselin, F.: *Traité de Chirurgie de la Main.* Paris, Flammarion, pp. 773–817, 1967.

Jones, F. W.: *The Principles of Anatomy as Seen in the Hand.* London, J. & A. Churchill, pp. 7–19; 46–56; fig. 24, 1920.

Kanavel, A. B.: Congenital malformations of the hands. *Arch. Surg.*, *25*:1–53; 282–320, 1932.

Kelikian, H., and Doumanian, A.: Congenital anomalies of the hand. *J. Bone Joint Surg.*, *39A*:1002–1019; 1249–1366, 1957.

Kirmisson, E.: *Traité des Maladies Chirurgicales d'Origine Congénitale.* Paris, Masson et Cie., pp. 417–484; 732–747, 1898.

Klippel, M., and Bouchet, P.: Hémimélie avec atrophie numérique des cas. *Nouv. Iconog. Salp.*, *20*:290–334; 396–417, 1907.

Landouzy, L.: Sur une déformation particulière des doigts propre á l'arthritisme. *J. Med. Chir. Pratique* (3 s.) *56*:485–489, 1885.

Landouzy, L.: Camptodactylie. Stigmate organique précoce du neuro-arthritisme. *Presse Méd.*, *14*:250–253, 1906.

Leboucq, J.: Recherches sur la morphologie du carpe chez les mamifères. *Arch. Biol.*, *5*:35–102, 1884.

Lenz, W. A.: Bone defects of the limbs—an overview. *In* Bergsma, D., (ed.): *Birth Defects. Original Article Series.* New York, National Foundation—March of Dimes. Vol. V, No. 3:1–6, 1969.

Longhi, L.: Malformazioni congenite dell mani (tentative di classificazione e contributo casistico). *Arch. di Ortop.*, *55*:183–212, 1939.

Lund, F. B.: Congenital anomalies of the phalanges with report of cases studied by skiagraphy. *Med. Surg. Rep. Boston City Hosp.*, (13 s.) pp. 1–21, 1902.

Matthews, D.: The congenitally deformed hand. *Br. J. Plast. Surg.*, 17:366–375, 1964.

Müller, W.: *Die angeborenen Fehlbildungen der menschlichen Hand.* Leipzig, G. Thieme, pp. 11–20, 1937.

Nichols, J. B.: Hand. *In* Buck, A., (ed.): *Reference Handbook of the Medical Sciences.* New York, William Wood & Co., Vol. IV, pp. 479–533, 1902.

Nichols, J. B.: *W. W. Keen's Surgery.* Philadelphia, W. B. Saunders Co., Vol. II, pp. 21–25, 1909.

Nichols, J. B., and Ely, L. W.: *A Reference Handbook of the Medical Sciences.* New York, William Wood & Co., Vol. IV, pp. 855–901, 1923.

O'Rahilly, R.: Morphological patterns in limb deficiencies and duplications. *Am. J. Anat.*, 89:135–194, 1951.

O'Rahilly, R.: The nomenclature and classification of limb anomalies. *In* Bergsma, D., (ed.): *Birth Defects. Original Article Series.* New York, National Foundation — March of Dimes. Vol. V, No. 3:14–17, 1969.

Otto, A. W.: *A Compounding of Human Comparative Pathological Anatomy.* Translated from German with additional notes and references by I. F. Souk. London, B. Fellows, pp. 1–41; 216–220, 1831.

Paletta, F. X.: Congenital deformities of the hands and feet. *Missouri Med.*, 50:19–23, 1953.

Patterson, T. J. S.: Congenital deformities of the hand. *Ann. R. Coll. Surg. Eng.* 25:306–330, 1959.

Patterson, T. J. S.: Classification of the congenitally deformed hand. *Br. J. Plast. Surg.*, 17:142–144, 1964.

Polaillon: Doigt. *In* Dechambre, K., (ed.): *Dictionnaire Encyclopédique des Sciences Médicales.* Pairs, G. Masson et P. Asselin et Cie., 30:115–353, 1884.

Potel, G.: Essai sur les malformations congénitales des membres. Leur classification pathogénique. *Rev. Chir.* 49:293–326; 625–648; 822–858; 50:84–114, 1914.

Potter, E.: *Pathology of the Fetus and the Newborn.* Chicago: Year Book Medical Publishers, Inc., pp. 483–498, 1952.

Potter, E.: Classification and pathology of congenital anomalies. *Am. J. Obstet. Gynecol.* 90:985–993, 1964.

Roblot, G.: *La Syndactylie Congénitale.* Paris, Imprimerie Maulds, Doumeng & Cie., pp. 11–21, 1906.

Saint-Hilaire, I. G.: *Propositions sur la Monstruosité.* Paris, Imp. Didot le Jeune, pp. 18–19, 1829.

Saint-Hilaire, I. G.: *Histoire Générale et Particulière des Anomalies de l'Organisation chez l'Homme et les Animaux.* Paris, J. B. Baillière, pp. 257–278; 670–702, 1832.

Saint-Hilaire, I. G.: *Histoire Générale et Particulière des Anomalies de l'Organisation chez l'Homme et les Animaux.* Paris, J. B. Bailière, Tome II, pp. 206–237, 1836.

Smith, R. J.: Radial club hand. *Bull. Hosp. Joint Dis.*, 25:85–93, 1964.

Steindler, A.: *Reconstructive Surgery of the Upper Extremities.* New York, Appleton & Co., pp. 210–249, 1923.

Stelling, F.: Congenital anomalies of the upper extremity. *J. Med. Assoc. Ga.*, pp. 402–409, 1965.

Stelling, F.: The upper extremity: congenital anomalies. *In* Ferguson, A. B., Jr., (ed.): *Orthopedic Surgery in Infancy and Childhood.* Third edition. Baltimore, Williams & Wilkins Co., pp. 293–339, 1968.

Swanson, A. B.: A classification for congenital malformations of the hand. *Acad. Med. Bull. New Jersey*, 10:166–169, 1964.

Swanson, A. B.: Classification of limb malformations on the basis of embryological failures. *Inter-Clinic Inf. Bull.*, 6:1–22, 1966.

Swanson, A. B., Barsky, A. J., and Entin, M. A.: Classification of limb malformation on the basis of embryological failure. *Surg. Clin. North Am.*, 48:1169–1179, 1968.

Tubby, A. H.: *Deformities Including Diseases of the Bones and Joints.* Second edition. London, MacMillan & Co., Vol. I, pp. 76–108, 1912.

Vinke, T. H.: Re-evaluation of etiologic factors in congenital anomalies of the skeleton. *Clin. Orthop.*, 8:7–19, 1956.

Vrolik, W.: Teratology. *In* Todd, R. B., (ed.): *The Cyclopaedia of Anatomy and Physiology.* London, Longman, Brown, Green, Longman & Roberts, Vol. IV, Part II, pp. 942–976, 1849–1852.

Young, J. K.: *A Practical Treatise on Orthopedic Surgery.* Philadelphia, Lea Brothers & Co., pp. 420–431, 1894.

Chapter Four

SYNDROMES IMPLICATING THE HAND AND THE FOREARM

Dictionaries are equivocal as to what constitutes a syndrome. They seem content with so glib a definition as the following: an aggregate of symptoms which, associated together, conjure up the picture of a disease. One lexicon is more circumspect; it has replaced the word "disease" with the phrase "clinical picture."

The word "disease" denotes an active morbid process which is not present in every syndrome. A congenital syndrome may have been initiated by a dynamic disturbance during embryonic development; when seen at birth or soon after, in most instances, it represents the aftermath of an activity already abated.

It is an ancient truism that when there is one congenital anomaly there are usually two or more. Perhaps all isolated congenital anomalies are constituents of as yet unidentified syndromes. Individual components of a syndrome may each involve separate organs, systems, or tissues derived from diverse embryonic layers. The fact that they occur together in unrelated individuals or in members of the same family suggests a common bondage. In all likelihood this association is determined by genes which share the same chromosome but, individually, are responsible for different symptoms, or by a single gene with multiple effects. Concurrence in time when the affected organs are beginning to develop also plays a part in establishing an association between various symptoms.

Genes as well as exogenous influences have time and tissue specificity. The nature of the particular defect is determined not only by the inherent properties of the affected tissue but also by the time when the original insult is inflicted. During their period of rapid differentiation, tissues belonging to various embryonic layers become teratogenically susceptible to the same genetic determinant or exogenous agent; simultaneously developing organs and systems are affected at the same time. Concurrence of multiple symptoms constitutes a syndrome.

Organs with widespread effects, such as the heart, brain, endocrine glands, or the kidneys, which have undergone defective development during embryonic life may, in their turn, induce disturbances in distant parts. Propinquity of developing parts also plays a role in the production of associated defects; the developmental disturbance of one embryonic layer is likely to affect the cells of the contiguous strata; it is not uncommon for tissues or organs derived from various embryonic layers to be affected simultaneously.

The distinction between syndromes and systemic disorders seems arbitrary. Some syndromes have sufficiently extensive ramifications to be regarded as systemic disorders. In many instances, one cannot categorically state whether a set of associated symptoms constitutes a syndrome or a systemic disorder. Traditionally, syndromes have been segregated from systemic disorders, sorted into separate categories, and tagged with distinctive labels. Even if ascertained — as has happened often in the past — that a syndrome, which was originally considered confined to a limited number of organs, involves every system of the body, it will continue to be recognized by its baptismal name. It may someday be proved that what we now consider syndromes are all systemic disorders, but the traditional way of naming them is likely to persist. Traditions resist change, reject innovations.

Over one hundred years ago, Down (1886) wrote a highly speculative article about a congenital idiocy which has since become identified with his name. Down advanced the view that in this particular brand of imbecility, the affected child departed from its stock and assumed the characteristics of another ethnic group: the European infant resembled a Mongol child born in Asia, both in appearance and "mental power." Down coined the designation mongolism and indicated that the assumption of mongoloid features by a Caucasian child was a sign of degeneracy.

There have been a number of attempts to dispose of such incriminatory designations as mongolism or mongol child. The term acromicria relates to the type of developmental deficiency characterized by the smallness of the acral parts, in opposition to acromegaly, in which these parts are overdeveloped. Clift (1922) and Benda (1946) used the term acromicria as a substitute for mongolism. Goldstein (1956) suggested the name congenital acromicria syndrome for children who are "immature in body build, in most of their organ and brain development, and in their bodily and mental functions and/or responses." Not long after, Lejeune et al (1959) ascertained that the type of imbecility described by Down is associated with an abnormality of chromosomes, and justifiably called the syndrome trisomy 21. With 18 other signatories, Allen (1961) penned a protest letter urging the elimination of the expressions mongolian idiocy and mongolism, regarding them as unjustifiable and erroneous. "The occurrence of this anomaly in Europeans and their descendants is not related to the segregation of genes derived from Asians," Allen and his colleagues wrote. Lennox (1961) considered trisomy 21 as a highly specific designation and hoped that such hackneyed terms as Down's mongolism and its ilk would be kept out of scientific communications. Notwithstanding, these terms continue to appear in the most modern, most sophisticated scientific publications.

CHROMOSOMAL ABERRATIONS

Trisomy 21, just mentioned, is one of several chromosomal aberrations which implicate the hand. In about half the subjects with this complex, the palm possesses a four-finger line or simian crease, the middle phalanx of the fifth digit is short and rhomboidal in shape, and its distal segment inclines in a radial direction; less commonly, the thumb is clasped in the palm. In trisomy 13–15, the fingernails are hyperconvex, and there is usually an extra digit. In trisomy 18, the fingers are contracted and overlap, and the radius may be missing (Figs. 4–1 to 4–3).

Congenital anomalies associated with autosomal chromosomal aberrations are frequently fatal and are usually more severe than those of sex chromosomes X and Y. In XO complex or Turner's syndrome, the carrying angle of the elbow is exaggerated and the fourth metacarpal may be short. In XXY, XXXY, XXXXY, or Klinefelter's syndrome, and in XYY constitution, there may be radioulnar synostosis. There are some other anomalies of the hand and forearm seen in connection with chromosomal aberrations. As noted elsewhere, these complexes are described by geneticists whose jargon is not always clear—not for the general clinician (Figs. 4–1 to 4–4).

SKELETAL DISORDERS

If the secular verbiage of geneticists appears opaque, that used by authors describing skeletal disorders is confounding for another reason. Geneticists are at least consistent in the terms they use. Authors describing skeletal disorders often employ different designations for the same entity or the same designation for different entities. Dystrophy denotes a weakened condition of tissue caused by faulty nutrition; dysplasia signifies abnormal tissue development; dysostosis has a vague connotation—some dictionaries define it as defective formation of bone. These three terms are often employed interchangeably in classifications of developmental abnormalities of the skeleton.

Sear (1953) used the term dystrophy in the heading of his classification of congenital disorders of bone. He drew attention to the fact that seemingly discrete dystrophies often present several features in common. To illustrate his point, Sear referred to the description of the terminal phalanges in cleidocranial dysostosis given by Jansen (1919) and quoted the case of osteopetrosis reported by Seigman and Kilby (1950). In the article referred to by Sear, Jansen pointed out that in cleidocranial dysostosis the terminal phalanges lack ungual tufts which are formed in membrane: terminal phalanges appear tapered—they "look as though they had been nibbled off." The case diagnosed as osteopetrosis reported by Seigman and Kilby showed absence of development of the distal portions of the ungual phalanges. This case has since been reclassified by McKusick (1968) as pycnodysostosis.

Structurally and genetically the two disorders—cleidocranial dysostosis and pycnodysostosis—differ greatly from each other. In pycnodysostosis, dwarfism is disproportionate and pronounced; the bones are dense and brittle; the ungual phalanges are short and squat and often shaftless, and inheritance is autosomal recessive. In cleidocranial dysostosis, dwarfism is proportionate and moderate; the bones have normal texture and the inheritance is autosomal dominant; the tufts of the terminal phalanx are often missing and, in consequence, this bone appears spiked, spear-shaped; periosteal deposition of bone is also interfered with, causing attenuation of phalangeal and metacarpal shafts; the middle phalanges of the index and little fingers are dwarfed, and the second metacarpal is comparatively long (in the young, this bone bears an additional epiphysis at its

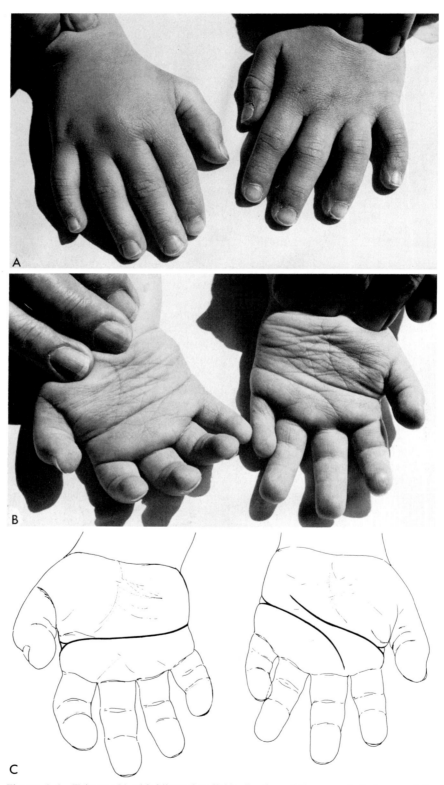

Figure 4–1   Trisomy 21 with bilateral radial inclination of the ungual phalanges of the little fingers (clinodactyly) and unilateral simian crease. *A*, Dorsal view of the hands. *B*, Palmar view. *C*, Sketch illustrating the same.

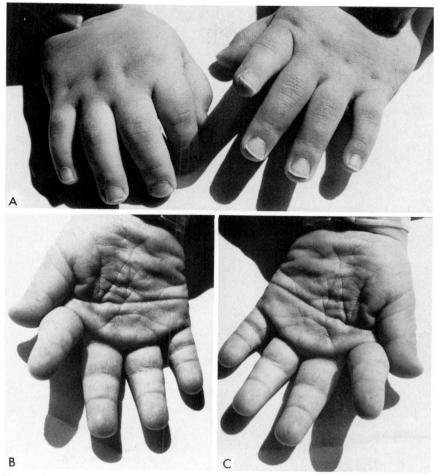

Figure 4-2 Trisomy 21 with simian crease of the palms. *A,* Dorsal view of the hands. *B* and *C,* Palmar views.

proximal extremity; in the young also some of the phalanges possess cone-shaped epiphyses). (See Fig. 4-5.)

Sear stressed the point that different bone disorders often produce analogous changes which doom any attempt at classification of clinical manifestations. He also expostulated about the difficulty of segregating skeletal dystrophies into discrete groups. After this warning, one would think that he would have avoided classifying bone dystrophies. But, as many others before him—and some since—he apparently could not resist the temptation. Sear classified congenital bone dystrophies according to the nature of the ossification of the involved elements—as to whether the affected bones are formed by membranous, cartilaginous, or periosteal ossification. The distinction between the first and last categories appears unjustifiable; most authors consider that bone laid down by the periosteum is of membranous origin. In Sear's classification there is, moreover, considerable overlapping; several dystrophies appear in two and even in three main groups.

Rubin (1964) chose the term dysplasia, defining this designation as "a disturbance in the bone form or modeling which assumes a disturbance in growth, in-

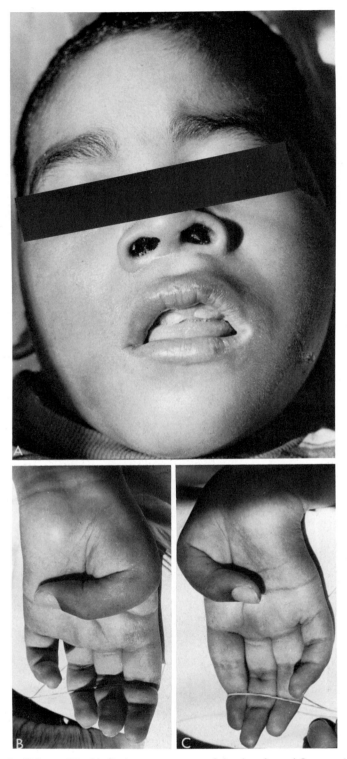

Figure 4–3   Trisomy 21 with flexion contractures of the thumbs and fingers. *A*, Frontal photograph of a nine-year-old boy's face. *B*, Palmar view of the hands.

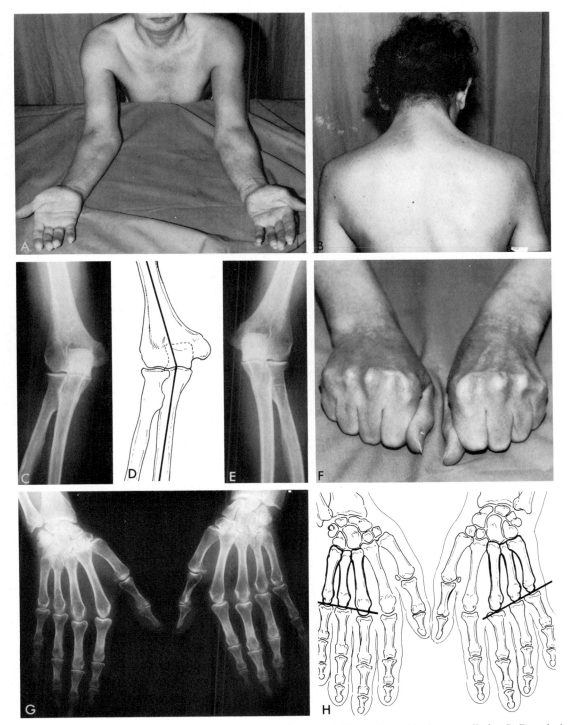

Figure 4–4 Female with XO complex (Turner's syndrome). *A*, Volar view of both upper limbs. *B*, Dorsal view showing the webbing of the neck. *C*, Anteroposterior roentgenograph of right elbow. *D*, Sketch of the same showing exaggeration of carrying angle. *E*, Anteroposterior roentgenograph of left elbow. *F*, Fisted hands — note that the fourth knuckle of the left fist is less prominent. *G*, Dorsopalmar roentgenograph of both hands. *H*, Sketch showing the shortness of the right fourth metacarpal.

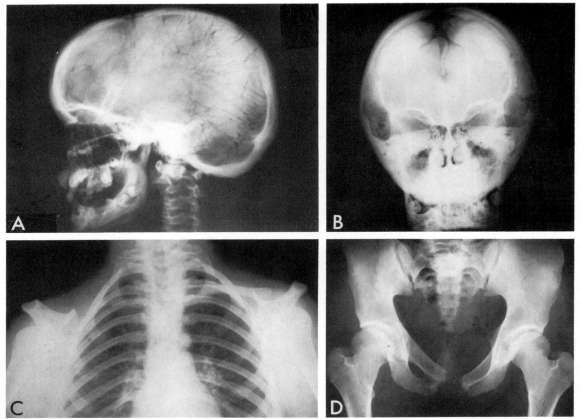

Figure 4–5   Cleidocranial dysostosis in an adult female. *A*, Lateral roentgenograph of the skull showing open fontanels and delayed closure of sutures. *B*, Anteroposterior view of the same. *C*, Anteroposterior roentgenograph showing absence of the right clavicle and short left clavicle. *D*, Anteroposterior view of the pelvis, showing a wide space in the region of the symphysis pubis.

trinsic to bone." Rubin classified dysplasias of the growing bone according to the location of the modeling error in the epiphysis, physis, metaphysis, or diaphysis. Each class of dysplasia—named, respectively, epiphyseal, physeal, metaphyseal, and diaphyseal—was further divided into two subclasses: hypoplastic and hyperplastic types, and under these were listed sundry clinical entities. This classification has some attractive features, not the least of which is its simplicity.

Aegerter and Kirkpatrick (1968) considered Rubin's classification as being "difficult to put . . . into practical usage." Rubin had classed Morquio's disease with epiphyseal dysplasia. Aegerter and Kirkpatrick pointed out that Morquio's disease is a disturbance of mucopolysaccharide metabolism of all bone-forming cartilage cells and not just those of one zone. In their turn, Aegerter and Kirkpatrick offered a classification of bone dysplasias which swung to the opposite extreme from the simple one proposed by Rubin; it became too cluttered with what they called "a confoundingly heterogenous group of disorders" to be put into any "practical usage."

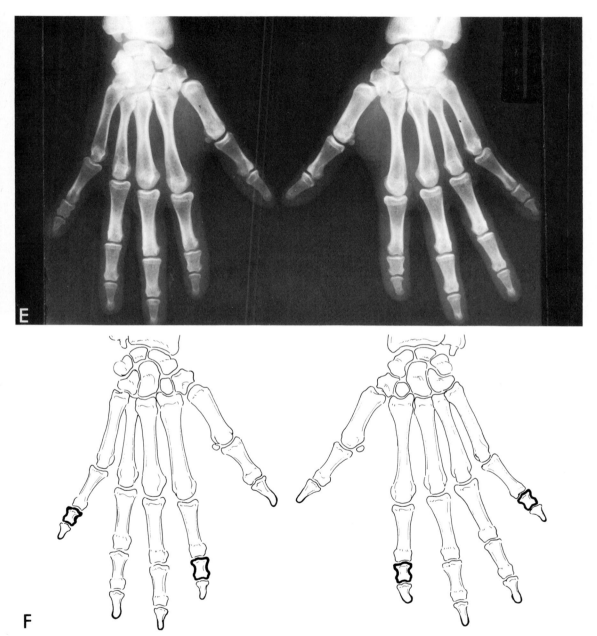

Figure 4–5 *Continued. E*, Dorsopalmar roentgenograph of both hands—note the absence of ungual tufts in some of the digits (particularly of the thumbs and little fingers) and dwarfed middle phalanges of the second and fifth digits. *F*, Sketch illustrating the same.

Classifications of bone dysplasias oscillate between two extremes: oversimplification and involuted redundancy. In both instances one notes overlapping of entities. Our knowledge of these conditions is changing from day to day. As in the case of mucopolysaccharidoses, we are beginning to discern common denominators among a few bone dysplasias. The majority of these skeletal disorders continue to constitute "a confoundingly heterogenous group." Until we can establish a valid basis of classification, we should consider most bone dysplasias as separate entities. It needs to be pointed out that in almost all congenital anomalies of the hand and forearm—polydactyly, syndactyly, brachydactyly, split hand, radial and ulnar ray defects, dislocations, and synostoses—one finds variable degrees of osseous dysplasia. Conversely, the anomalies mentioned also occur as components of syndromes of which bone dysplasia is but another constituent. Aegerter and Kirkpatrick spoke of Morquio's disease. One may also mention acrocephalosyndactyly, arachnodactyly, chondroectodermal dysplasia, and numerous other complexes which present several salient features besides skeletal disturbances.

METABOLIC AND ENDOCRINE DISORDERS

Morquio's disease, mentioned in the preceding section, is one of the better known mucopolysaccharide storage disorders of bones formed from cartilage. There are now about a half dozen distinct skeletal disorders which are ascribed to, or associated with, deranged mucopolysaccharide metabolism. The basic disturbance is a failure of the overloaded cells of the growth cartilage plate to proliferate and become converted into shapely bones. Among other skeletal elements, the bones of the hand, wrist, and forearm are implicated. The affected individual is a dwarf and has short limbs and short digits and usually stiff, contracted metacarpophalangeal and interphalangeal joints.

Delayed appearance of carpal ossicles is a feature of mucopolysaccharidoses and also of congenital hypothyroidism. Homocystinuria is a metabolic disorder occurring in sibs with unaffected parents. The urine of the affected child contains elevated amounts of homocystine as well as methionine. In two-thirds of the reported cases there has been mental retardation. At about the age of 10, the child develops ectopia lentis. The skeletal features suggest Marfan's (1896) arachnodactyly which, unlike homocystinuria, is inherited as an autosomal dominant trait. Congenital hypophosphatasia is another metabolic disorder, also inherited as an autosomal recessive phenotype, in which the long bones, including those of the hand, manifest varying degrees of diffuse and localized rarefaction; if the child survives, it evolves as a dwarf and has short stubby fingers. To the list of metabolic and/or endocrine disorders affecting the hand and the forearm should be added the following: Albright's hereditary osteodystrophy, which comprises pseudohypoparathyroidism and pseudopseudohypoparathyroidism, with characteristic dwarfing of ulnar metacarpals; essential familial hypercholesterolemia which is often accompanied by nodular thickening of the digits and xanthoma tuberosum and tendinosum; and perhaps leprechaunism in which the affected child is a mentally retarded dwarf with disproportionately large hands and feet and gnomelike features (Figs. 4–6 to 4–12).

(*Text continued on page 106.*)

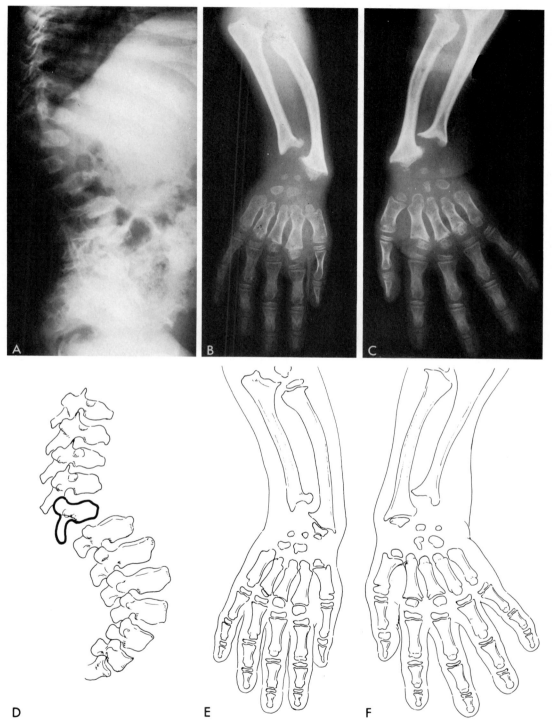

Figure 4–6 Morquio's mucopolysaccharidosis. *A*, Lateral roentgenograph of the spine of a seven-year-old child, showing beaked vertebrae. *B*, Dorsovolar roentgenograph of the right forearm and hand: trapezium, trapezoid, and scaphoid bones have not yet appeared. *C*, Roentgenograph of the left forearm and hand. *D*, *E*, and *F* illustrate the roentgenograph above each.

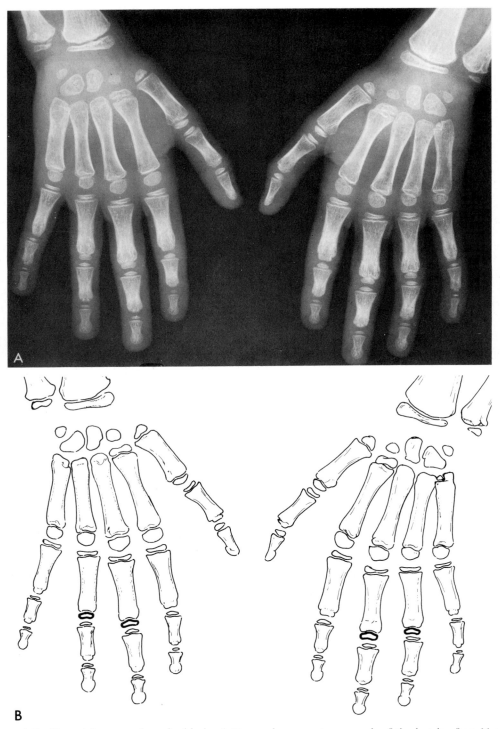

Figure 4–7 Morquio's mucopolysaccharidosis. *A*, Dorsopalmar roentgenograph of the hands of an 11-year-old boy, showing absence of the proximal row of carpal bones, accessory epiphyses at the proximal ends of the second metacarpals and distal ends of the first metacarpal and at the distal ends of the proximal phalanges of the middle and ring fingers. *B*, Sketch illustrating the same.

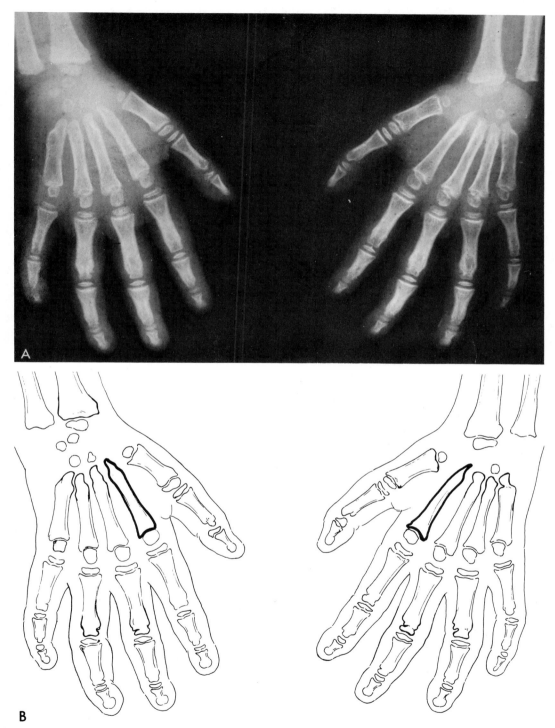

Figure 4–8 Hurler's mucopolysaccharidosis—milder form. *A*, Dorsopalmar roentgenograph of the hands of a seven-year-old child. *B*, Sketch showing vagrancy in the appearance of carpal ossicles in the right and left wrists and spiking of the proximal ends of four ulnar metacarpals.

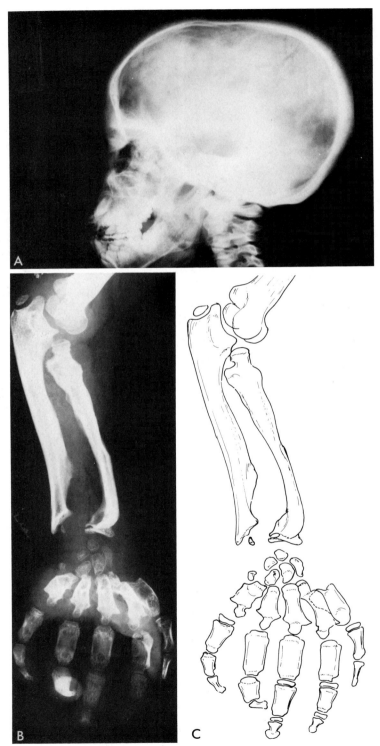

Figure 4–9 Hurler's mucopolysaccharidosis—severe form. *A*, Lateral roentgenograph of the skull of a teenager showing brachycephaly. *B*, Dorsopalmar roentgenograph of the right forearm and hand showing irregularity in the shape of the bones. *C*, Sketch illustrating the same.

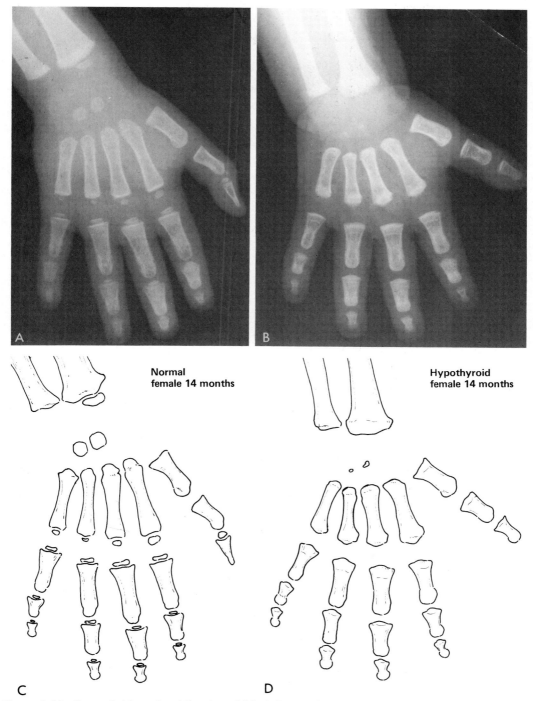

Figure 4-10 Congenital hypothyroidism in a child. *A*, Dorsopalmar roentgenograph of the right hand of a 14-month-old female showing timely appearance of the following bones: carpal epiphysis of the radius, capitate and hamate bones of the wrist, epiphysis of second to fifth metacarpals and of corresponding proximal phalanges, and epiphysis of the ungual phalanx of the thumb. *B*, Dorsopalmar roentgenograph of the right hand of a child with congenital hypothyroidism. *C* and *D* illustrate the roentgenograph above each.

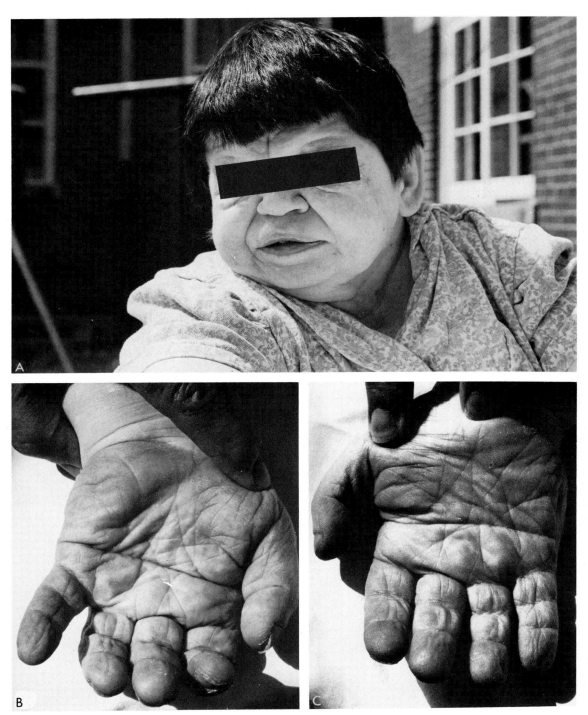

Figure 4–11   Congenital hypothyroidism in an adult dwarf. *A,* Photograph of the face showing thick, pudgy features. *B* and *C,* Palmar photographs of the hands showing simian creases and short isometric fingers.

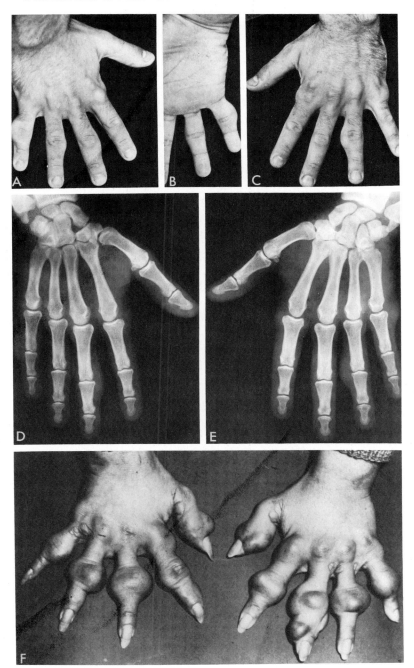

Figure 4–12   Essential hypercholesteremia. *A*, Dorsal view of the right hand of an 18-year-old male whose blood cholesterol has ranged between 350 and 400 mg. per 100 ml. since early childhood: note the swelling on the ulnar aspect of the little finger and on the dorsum of second metacarpophalangeal joint. *B*, Palmar view of the right little finger. *C*, Dorsal view of the left hand. *D* and *E* are the roentgenographs of the right and left hands, respectively, showing that the swellings of the fingers are extraskeletal. *F*, Dorsal view of the hands of another case (Dr. A. K. Kachadourian's patient). This patient, a 30-year-old female, is reported as belonging to a family with several sibs affected similarly. Her blood cholesteral has ranged between 700 and 800 mg. per 100 ml. since childhood.

DWARFISM AND DIGITAL DEFORMITIES

Almost all metabolic or endocrine disorders mentioned in the preceding section and most congenital bone dysplasias are associated with shortness of stature, short upper extremities, and short fingers. Dwarfism is described as being total or partial. In the former, the vertebral column is affected as well as the limbs. Dwarfism due to the shortening of the limbs alone is characterized as being rhizomelic, mesomelic, or acromelic. In the rhizomelic form, the root segments of the limbs — the humerus in the upper and the femur in the lower extremities — are primarily affected. In the mesomelic type, the midsegments of the limbs are mainly short. In acromelic dwarfism, stunting chiefly involves the bones of the peripheral portion of the limb. It should be understood that these designations — rhizomelic, mesomelic, and acromelic — are relative; they merely particularize the segment which seems to have suffered the greatest degree of abbreviation in length; in no instance is one segment of the limb affected to the exclusion of the others. In the mesomelic variety, when one of the two parallel bones of the midsegment is primarily hypoplastic, the dwarfism is qualified with the adjective hemimelic, and, in unilateral cases, the other bone is usually shorter than the corresponding element of the opposite limb.

The compendium of dwarfism and digital anomalies should include the following disorders: achondrogenesis, achondroplasia, Albright's hereditary osteodystrophy, bird-headed dwarfism, cartilage-hair hypoplasia, chondrodysplasia punctata, cleidocranial dysostosis, de Lange degeneration, deafness and synostotic states (Vessel-Forney syndrome), dyschondrosteosis, Ellis-van Creveld chondroectodermal dysplasia, focal dermal hypoplasia, hypochondroplasia, hypophosphatasia, infantile thoracic dystrophy, Maffucci's angiodysplastic enchondromatosis, metaphyseal dysostosis of Jansen or Schmid, mesomelic dwarfism of hypoplastic ulna-fibula-mandible, mucopolysaccharidoses, multiple epiphyseal dysplasia, multiple exostosis, Nievergelt's syndrome, Ollier's enchondromatosis, pyknodysostosis, Russell-Silver dwarfism, trisomies, Weill-Marchesani spherophakiabrachymorphia, XO complex, and several other heterogeneous constellations.

HEAD AND HAND COMPLEX

More than half of the syndromes mentioned in the preceding section should reappear in the compendium dealing with head and hand complexes which, in addition, would contain the following: acrocephalosyndactyly, acrofacial dysostosis, acro-osteolysis, craniocarpotarsal dysplasia, craniometaphyseal dysplasia, craniofacial dysostosis of Crouzon, craniosynostosis and radial ray defect, Hanhart's micrognathia-peromelia, Weyers' oligodactyly syndrome, and various other heterogeneous entities. It should be pointed out that the eye, ear, and mouth constitute integral parts of the head, and each of these sense organs has its own cluster of associated anomalies (Fig. 4–13).

OCULOMELIC COMPLEXES

"Probably more abnormalities are known of the hands than any other part of the body except the eye," Gates (1946) wrote. It is not surprising that

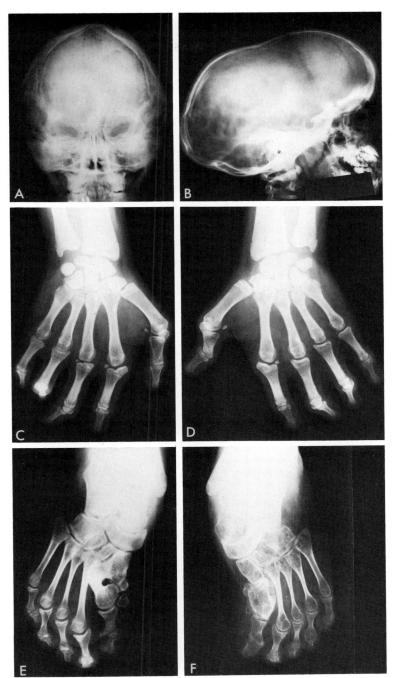

Figure 4–13 Cranioacral malformation. *A,* Anteroposterior roentgenograph of the skull of an adult, showing diminished side-to-side but increased vertical diameter. *B,* Lateral view showing increased anteroposterior diameter. *C,* Dorsopalmar roentgenograph of the right hand: the fingers are inclined in ulnar direction and each one lacks a phalanx. *D,* Dorsopalmar roentgenograph of the left hand, showing similar defects and deviations: the proximal phalanx of the thumb is short on the radial side, causing deviation of the ungual segment in radial direction. *E,* Dorsopalmar roentgenograph of the right foot: the cuboid bone has coalesced with the short, curved first metatarsal. *F,* Dorsoplantar roentgenograph of the left foot: the first metatarsal is short and there is hallux varus interphalangeus. The configuration of the skull of this patient is typical of acro-osteolysis congenita.

anomalies of the hand and eye often are associated. In acrocephalosyndactyly, the fingers are confluent, and there is often atrophy of the optic nerve. In Ehlers-Danlos syndrome, the fingers are hyperextensible, and accompanying anomalies of the eye range from microcornea to keratoconus. In the facial diplegia named after Möbius, symbrachydactyly may coexist with ptosis or proptosis. Polydactyly and retinitis pigmentosa constitute the two main components of Laurence-Moon-Bardet-Biedl syndrome. Marfan's arachnodactyly is associated with subluxation of the lens. In most mucopolysaccharidoses—Hurler, Morquio, Scheie, and Maroteaux-Lamy types—the fingers are contracted and the cornea is cloudy. Oculodentoosseous—also called oculodentodigital—dysplasia consists of microcornea, enamel hypoplasia, and soft tissue syndactyly of ring and little fingers; the involved digits are deviated in ulnar direction and, upon roentgenographic examination, may show lack of modeling and cube-shaped middle phalanges and bony union of ungual segments. Sorsby syndrome consists of apical dystrophy of the digits and macular coloboma. In trisomy 13–15, polydactyly coexists with microphthalmia. In trisomy 18, the fingers overlap, the cornea is opaque, and the eyelids droop. In trisomy 21, there is only a single transverse palmar crease, the little finger is curved radialward, and myopia is frequent. In Weill-Marchesani complex, the fingers are short and the lens is round.

One could run through the entire gamut of syndromes with multiple manifestations and ferret out associated anomalies of the hand and eye. These complexes have been described mainly by ophthalmologists; the major portion of their discussion is devoted to the abnormalities of the eye. Anomalies of the hand are merely mentioned in passing and are rarely described in detail. Such obvious abnormalities as syndactyly and polydactyly are often noted; however, it is not stated whether the webbed or surplus digits belong to the hand or the foot. Only occasionally is a hint given in the titles of these articles about the accompanying digital defect.

Ophthalmologists use the terms anophthalmia and microphthalmia interchangeably. In a literal sense the former means absent eyeball and the latter, small eyeball. The real distinction depends upon the presence or absence of the nervous mechanism necessary for vision.

The development of this mechanism coincides with that of the digits. The condensation of the mesenchyme, which is to form the sheath of the optic nerve, appears around the fifth week of embryonic life; the axis cylinders of the nerve itself are not seen until the middle of the sixth week, when segmentation of the handplate and the separation of the digits is in process. Polydactyly and syndactyly are known to occur in association with anophthalmia or microphthalmia. Split hand has been reported in connection with congenital cataract.

OROMELIC COMPLEXES

In the embryo, the development of the oral cavity, its contents, and surrounding structures coincides with that of the upper extremity. In both instances, organogenesis is initiated around the fourth postovulatory week, and structures attain definitive shapes by the end of the seventh week. The upper limb, the hand in particular, develops by a process of fission of a solid mass of tissue. The mouth attains its final form by fusion of the following separate parts: the mesial and lateral nasal buds, paired maxillary processes, and the rami of the mandibular arch. Congenital anomalies of the hand and forearm may be due to absent or excessive segmentation, while those of the mouth result from failure of initially discrete anlagen to coalesce. In most malformations of the mouth, one single structure (for instance, the tongue) is rarely affected alone. There are often associated anomalies of the teeth, mandible, and maxilla. It is to be remembered that the mouth constitutes an integral part of the face as well as of the alimentary canal.

Cleft lip-palate is classed with anomalies of both the face and the oral cavity; it provides a salient example of the principle that anomalies of the mouth are due to the failure of fusion of disparate parts. Cleft lip-palate is known to be accompanied by excessive longitudinal segmentation of the embryonic handplate, as exemplified by polydactyly, or failure of longitudinal fission, which results in syndactyly.

The same principle is illustrated again by the associated anomalies of the tongue and the hand. At about the fourth week of embryonic life, simultaneous with the appearance of the limb buds, a swelling appears on the floor of the pharynx. The smaller posterior portion of the tongue is developed from this swelling; the larger anterior part is formed by the fusion of two lateral buds arising from the inner aspects of the right and left rami of the mandibular arch. The fusion of the lateral halves of the tongue is completed after the seventh week of embryonic life, as at this time its tip is still split. The period of development of the tongue corresponds with that of the fingers: the absence or underdevelopment of the tongue is often associated with digital anomalies, in particular, with short webbed digits or symbrachydactyly due to defective longitudinal as well as transverse segmentation of the handplate.

OTOMELIC COMPLEXES

In the embryo, the auditory pit makes its appearance about a week earlier than the limb bud. While the canonical elements of the hand and arm attain definitive configuration by the end of the seventh week, the receiving and transmitting mechanisms of the ear do not become established until after the third month of intrauterine development. The development of perceiving elements of the ear coincides with that of the hand.

Congenital deafness may be due to defective nerve connections or to imperfect development of the conductive system. Perceptive elements of the ear, as of other sense organs, are derived from ectoderm. Congenital sensorineural deafness is usually accompanied by anomalies of the nails, the pilosebaceous apparatus, and the teeth—elements derived from ectoderm. The receiving apparatus of the ear has a mixed origin; the skin of the external ear originates from ectoderm, while its cartilaginous and bony elements are derived from mesoderm. Anomalies of the receiving apparatus are likely to be accompanied by skin and osteocartilaginous changes elsewhere.

The middle ear contains three bony elements called, respectively, malleus, incus, and stapes. They are derived from mesoderm and constitute parts of the conductive mechanism. There is a joint between the stapes and the vestibular apparatus. Ankylosis of this articulation has come to be known as otosclerosis, which is clinically manifest as conductive deafness. The failure of formation of a joint between two consecutive phalanges has its inception around the eighth or ninth week of embryonic development, but osteosynthesis culminating in symphalangism may not become established until many years after birth. Otosclerosis, which is seldom detected in childhood, is not an uncommon accompaniment of symphalangism. Conductive deafness is also known to occur in such other synostotic states as carpal coalescence, Klippel-Feil syndrome, and radioulnar synostosis. Conductive hearing loss has been noted in cases with Madelung deformity.

In the syndrome known as auriculo-osteodysplasia, the lobule of the external ear is posteriorly displaced and elongated; there is dysplasia of the radiocapitular articulation, and the head of the radius is dislocated. Sensorineural deafness at times accompanies ectodermal dysplasia with polydactyly or syndactyly. In keratopachyderma there is deafness, thickening of the skin of the palms and soles, and annular grooves around the digits. Sensorineural deafness has also been reported in association with leukonychia, onychodystrophy, and split hand. In otopalatodigital (OPD) syndrome, there is deafness, dwarfism, cleft palate, dislocation of the radial head, and clinodactyly of the little finger.

HEMATOMELIC DEFICIENCIES

Primitive blood cells begin to form in the yolk sac during the fourth week of embryonic development—at about the time of the appearance of the limb bud. Hematopoiesis starts within the body mesenchyma and the liver during the fifth or sixth week—around the time of the critical differentiation of the radial ray. The most common hand and forearm anomaly seen in association with congenital blood dyscrasia is radial ray defect. As will be pointed out in the next section, the components of the radial ray also are preferentially affected in heart and hand complexes. These three anomalies—congenital heart disease, blood dyscrasia, and radial ray defect—are known to coexist, in which instance the infant usually dies soon after birth. Survival is not uncommon when only two defects occur or when the three abnormalities are not severe.

Radial ray deficiency is most commonly seen in panmyelopathy and in connection with platelet hypoplasia. Triphalangeal thumb is occasionally seen in infants with hypoplastic anemia. In the hand and foot syndrome of sickle cell anemia, the digits are swollen and painful owing to punctate areas of bone destruction and, at times, avascular necrosis of epiphyseal centers; the affected metacarpals and phalanges may remain short. Female subjects with sickle cell anemia will occasionally possess thin, long, hypermobile fingers, not unlike those seen in Marfan's arachnodactyly. As noted in Chapter 1, in congenital pyruvate kinase (PK) deficiency, the ulnar metacarpals and fibular metatarsals are dwarfed (Fig. 4–14).

CARDIOMELIC COMPLEXES

The limb buds and the primitive heart tube appear about the same time in the embryo and develop simultaneously. The upper extremity differentiates earlier than the lower and its development follows more closely that of the heart; hence the preferential association of heart and upper limb anomalies. In the

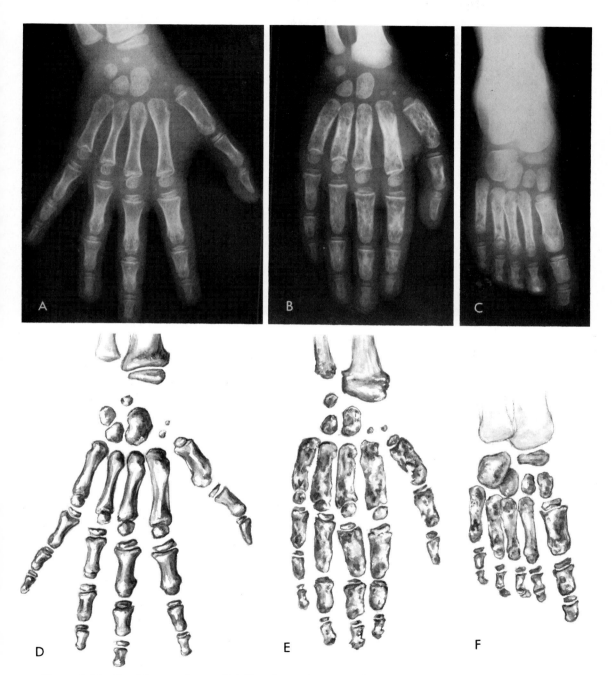

Figure 4–14   Hand-foot syndrome of sickle cell anemia. *A*, Dorsopalmar roentgenograph of the right hand of a normal six-year-old child with normal texture and configuration of the bones. *B*, The right hand of a child of the same age with sickle cell disease: note the expansion of the cortices and disseminated erosion of the tubular bones. *C*, Roentgenograph of the right foot of the same subject showing similar changes. *D, E,* and *F* illustrate the roentgenograph above each.

resulting complex, the most common cardiac anomaly is atrial septal defect; the most frequent skeletal abnormality is defect of the radial ray. Individuals with more pronounced radial ray defect ran a greater risk of having defective hearts.

Concurrent deficiencies of the radial ray and heart are said to start around the fifth postovulational week. During the sixth week, longitudinal and transverse segmentations are taking place in the handplate. Occasionally, polydactyly and syndactyly are seen in connection with congenital heart disease. In some instances there are also chondrodystrophic changes involving the metacarpal and phalangeal bones. Mesenchymal condensation of the skeletal elements of the hand and forearm occurs between the fifth and sixth weeks of embryonic life; chondrification takes place a week later; ossification appears in the tuft portion of the terminal phalanges between the seventh and eighth week; and in metacarpals and proximal phalanges around the ninth week. In some heart and hand complexes, chondrodystrophic changes of the bones of the hand are seen in association with interatrial septal defect. To explain this occurrence, it is contended that the teratogenic effect might start earlier but continues to exert its influence during later months when the skeletal anlagen begin to ossify and the interatrial septum becomes established.

Atrial septal defect and nonopposable triphalangeal thumb are the main features of the Holt-Oram syndrome. In the upper limb–cardiovascular complex named after Lewis, the involvement of the proximal extremity is more extensive and varied; there may be partial or complete absence of the radial ray. Tabatznik syndrome is characterized by cardiac arrhythmia and stub thumb. In an article entitled "The hand and the heart," Silverman and Hurst (1968) noted the following additional associations: in Hurler's mucopolysaccharidosis, the hand is broad and has short, stubby digits and there is often incipient coronary arteriosclerosis; in trisomy 13–15, postaxial polydactyly is associated with ventricular septal defect; in Marfan syndrome, the fingers are long, thin, and tapered and at times there is aortic regurgitation; in Rubinstein-Taybi broad thumb big toe complex, there may be pulmonic stenosis; in de Lange degeneration, proximally positioned thumb or "chicken-wing" appendage of a monodactylic hand is associated with ventricular septal defect; and in trisomy 21, the palm is marked by a simian crease, the terminal phalanx of the little finger inclines in radial direction, and there is a defect of the atrioventricular canal. Associated anomalies of the hand and heart are also known to occur in Ellis-van Creveld chondroectodermal dysplasia, Ehlers-Danlos syndrome, Laurence-Moon-Bardet-Biedl syndrome, thalidomide embryopathy, trisomies 13–15 and 18, and in XO complex.

RENAL-ACRAL COMPLEXES

Like the tongue, the urogenital system is formed by fusion of separate parts; these parts begin to coalesce during the fifth and sixth weeks of embryonic life—at the same time that the transverse and longitudinal segmentation of the limb bud is delineated. Concurrent defects of the limbs and urogenital system follow the general rule which holds that simultaneously developing parts are likely to become teratogenically affected at the same time and to develop associated defects. The critical period of development of the upper limb coincides more closely with the organogenesis of the heart than of the kidney. The development of the lower limb lags behind that of the upper extremity and coincides with the formation of the kidney.

It is not surprising that more cases of upper limb abnormalities are recorded in connection with congenital heart disease, while lower limb defects seem to occur more often in association with renal agenesis and dysgenesis. In their review of 364 cases of congenital renal defects, Ashley and Mostofi (1960) recorded five instances of upper limb involvement and 31 cases in which the lower extremity was affected. The exact nature of the upper limb defect was not specified. Dieker and Opitz (1969) reported two cases with associated anomalies of the urogenital system and the hand: the first case had short webbed fingers and rudimentary postaxial polydactyly of the right hand; the second patient lacked a middle finger on the left hand. Ectrodactyly of the middle finger of the left hand was a feature of the case described by Curran and Curran (1972). This patient also had short middle phalanges of both little fingers, with radial inclination of the distal segment. A short tuftless ungual phalanx is perhaps the most common hand anomaly seen in connection with congenital renal defects; occasionally, the phalangeal epiphyses are coned. In renal-acral complexes, there are usually other associated anomalies, such as Klippel-Feil deformity and conductive deafness. Renal insufficiency is also known to occur in subjects with the nail-patella syndrome. One need also mention the so-called renal rickets which often becomes manifest in infancy and early childhood (Figs. 4–15 and 4–16).

TEGUMENTARY COMPLEXES

It used to be thought that certain genes could selectively affect one of the three primary body layers to the exclusion of the other two. It is perhaps more correct to say that some genes exert greater influence on a particular primary layer, but they also involve the layer next to it. Defective mesodermal elements — bone, joints, muscles, and blood vessels — often accompany abnormalities of ectodermal structures — the epidermis and its appendages. Clinically manifest associated anomalies of ectodermal and mesodermal derivatives are numerous. The following must be mentioned, as they often implicate the hand: anonychia-ectrodactyly syndrome; cartilage-hair hypoplasia; associated defects of the skull, scalp, and limbs; dyskeratosis congenita; ectodermal dysplasia; focal dermal hypoplasia syndrome; pachyonychia congenita; Puretic syndrome; Rothmund-Thomson poikiloderma, tuberous sclerosis, and tylosis (Fig. 4–17).

THALIDOMIDE EMBRYOPATHY

It is now definitely established that thalidomide intake by the mother during her earlier months of pregnancy will cause malformations in the child. No correlation has yet been established between the dosage of the drug and the degree of the damage. The drug exerts its embryotoxic effect during the sensitive period of organogenesis — during the interval between the thirty-fourth and fiftieth day after the last menstruation, rarely a few days later. Within this period there appears to be close correspondence between the time of intake and the severity of the malformation. When ingested early — between the thirty-fourth and thirty-ninth day — the ears and cranial nerves might be affected. Intake between the thirty-ninth and forty-third day would result in severe defects of the arms: amelia, abrachia, and phocomelia.

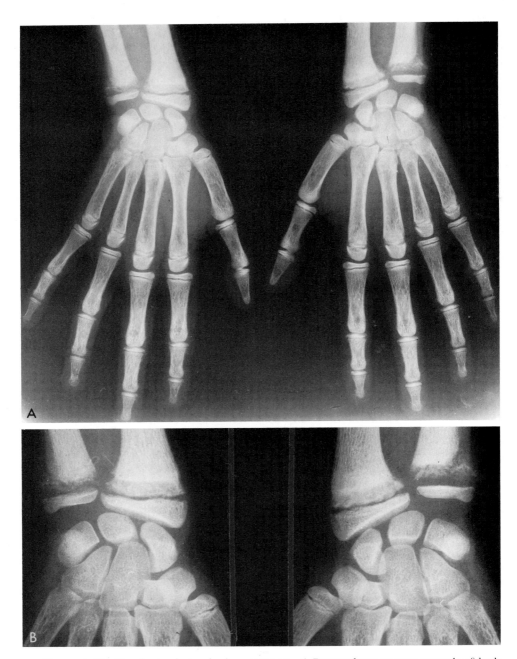

Figure 4–15 Renal osteodystrophy in a teenager. *A*, Dorsopalmar roentgenograph of both hands: note the disturbance of the metaphyseo-epiphyseal junction of the forearm bones, generalized osteoporosis producing attenuated shafts of the tubular bones, and tuftless terminal phalanges, especially of the thumbs. *B*, Enlarged roentgenograph of the wrists.

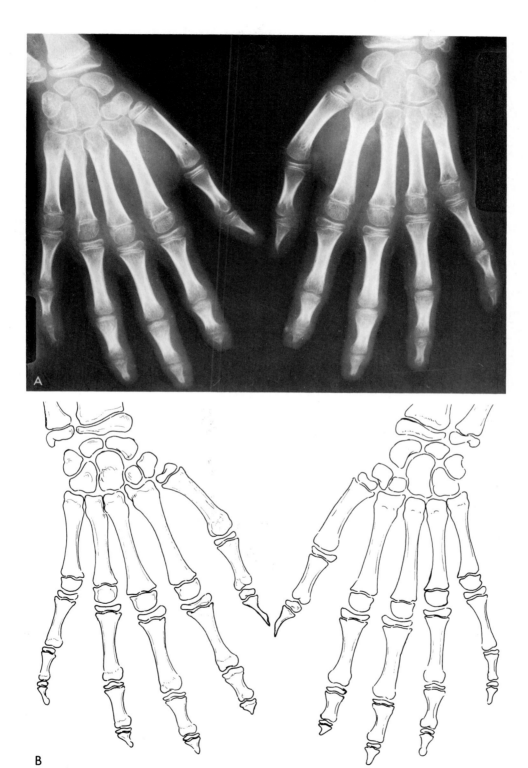

Figure 4–16 Spear-shaped ungual phalanges in a case of congenital renal insufficiency. *A*, Dorsopalmar roentgenograph of both hands. *B*, Sketch illustrating the same.

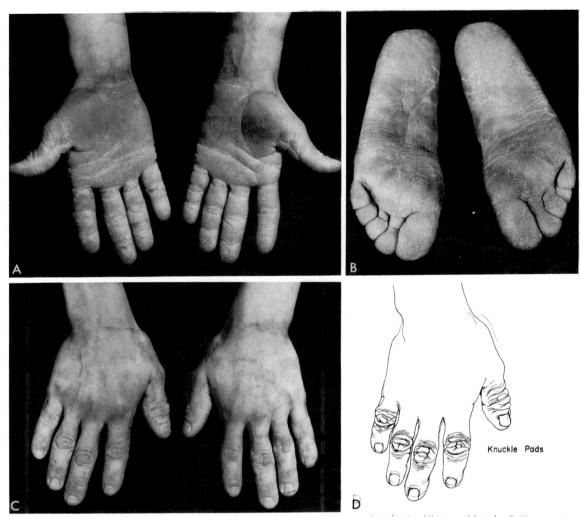

Figure 4–17   Tylosis (keratosis palmoplantaris). *A*, Palmar view of the hands of a 19-year-old male. *B*, Plantar view of the feet. *C*, Dorsal view of the hands. *D*, Sketch illustrating the dorsal aspect of the right hand, showing precocious knuckle pads.

Thalidomide embryopathy shows distinct predilection for the radial component. Ingestion of the drug between the forty-fourth and forty-eighth day might
cause total or partial radial ray defect. When taken around the fiftieth day after
the last menstrual period, or a few days later, one might expect such minor abnormalities as floating thumb, triphalangeal thumb, or hypoplasia of the thenar
eminence. Thalidomide embryopathy, which is an exogenous disorder, often
mimics endogenous anomalies of the hand and forearm seen in association with
congenital heart disease. Thalidomide embryopathy which is a phenocopy is
often strikingly similar to the phenotypic expressions of Holt-Oram syndrome,
which is a heritable disorder. Thalidomide embryopathy also simulates upper
limb abnormalities seen in connection with three other genetic disorders: throm-
bocytopenia-radius aplasia syndrome; Fanconi's panmyelopathy; and the syndrome of deletion of the long arm of D chromosome, also known as 13q or 13r
syndrome (Fig. 4–18).

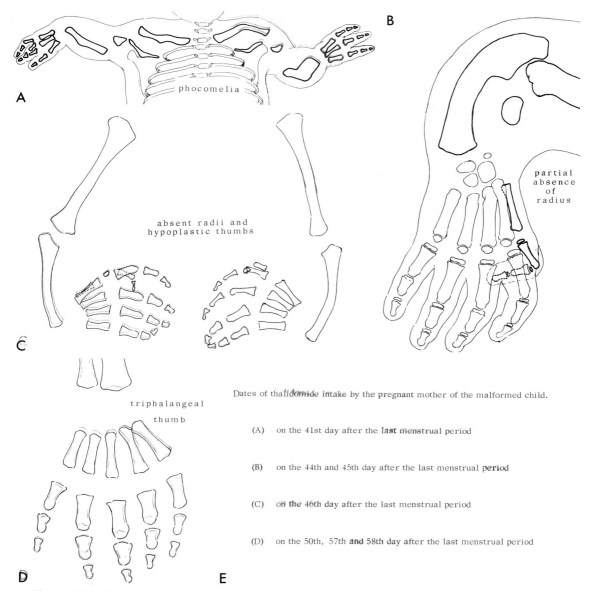

phocomelia

absent radii and
hypoplastic thumbs

partial
absence
of
radius

triphalangeal
thumb

Dates of thalidomide intake by the pregnant mother of the malformed child.

(A)   on the 41st day after the last menstrual period

(B)   on the 44th and 45th day after the last menstrual period

(C)   on the 46th day after the last menstrual period

(D)   on the 50th, 57th and 58th day after the last menstrual period

Figure 4-18   Correspondence between the time of ingestion of thalidomide by the pregnant mother and the type of upper limb malformation inflicted upon the offspring. The sketches in this figure were taken from roentgenographs provided by the courtesy of Professor W. Lenz of Munster, West Germany.

SYNDROMES WHICH TEND TO PRODUCE ANALOGOUS LOCAL DEFECTS IN THE HAND OR FOREARM

The same localized dysmorphic effect may occur in different syndromes. Arachnodactyly, heretofore regarded as being characteristic of Marfan's syndrome, is also seen in homocystinuria and in some female subjects with sickle cell anemia. Dislocation of the radial head is known to occur in auriculo-osteodyspla-

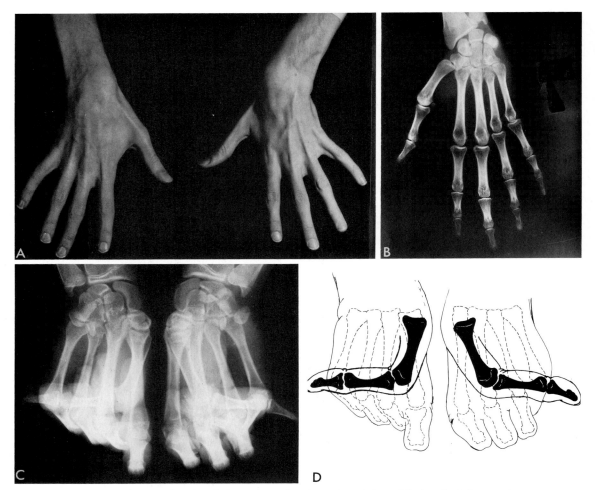

Figure 4–19   Marfan's arachnodactyly in a teenage female. *A,* Dorsal view of the hands. *B,* Dorsopalmar roentgeno-graph of the left hand. *C,* Roentgenograph of clenched fists with the tips of the thumbs extruding beyond the ulnar border of the hand. *D,* Sketch illustrating *C.* Compare this figure with Figure 4–20.

sia, bird-headed dwarfism, craniosynostosis, de Lange degeneration, Klippel-Trennaunay syndrome, Larsen's syndrome, Morquio's mucopolysaccharidoses, multiple enchondromatoses with or without hemangioma, multiple exostosis, nail-patella syndrome, ophthalmo-mandibulo-melic dysplasia, otopalato digital syndrome, pterygium anticubiti, and in many more complexes. There must be at least two dozen syndromes associated with short metacarpals and twice as many complexes which are accompanied by short middle phalanx of the little finger and radial inclination of the ungual segment (Figs. 4–19 and 4–20).

SYNDROMES WITH DIVERSIFIED PHENOTYPIC EFFECTS IN THE HAND OR FOREARM

These are numerous. Multiple exostoses or diaphyseal aclasis is perhaps the most common ubiquitous complex; besides causing bizarre malformations else-where, it affects the skeletal elements of the hand and forearm variously. It may

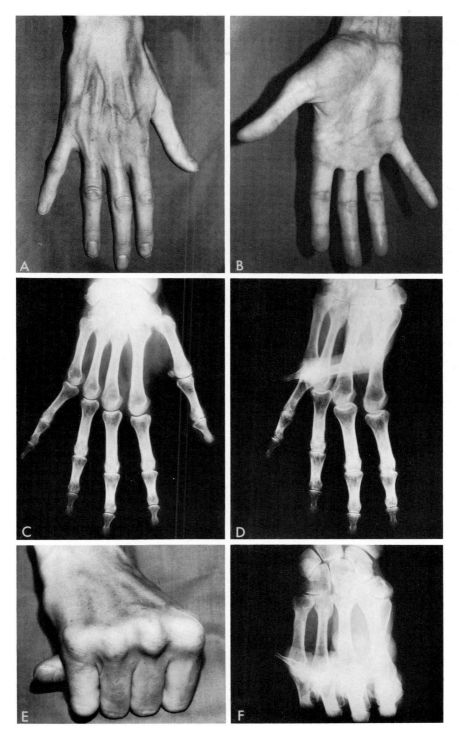

Figure 4–20 Arachnodactyly in a female teenager with sickle cell anemia. She had no ectopia lentis characteristic of Marfan's arachnodactyly nor any sign of homocystinuria. *A*, Dorsal view of the right hand showing thin, long, tapered fingers. *B*, Palmar view. *C*, Roentgenograph of the same. *D*, Roentgenograph of the hand with extended fingers showing protrusion of the thumb beyond the ulnar border of the hand. *E*, Protrusion of the thumb beyond the ulnar border. *F*, Roentgenograph of the same.

be accompanied by any or several of the following malformations: massive tumors, dislocation of the radial head, short ulna, interlocked forearm bones, Madelung deformity, short metacarpals, and axially deviated ungual phalanges (Figs. 4–21 to 4–25).

(*Text continued on page 125.*)

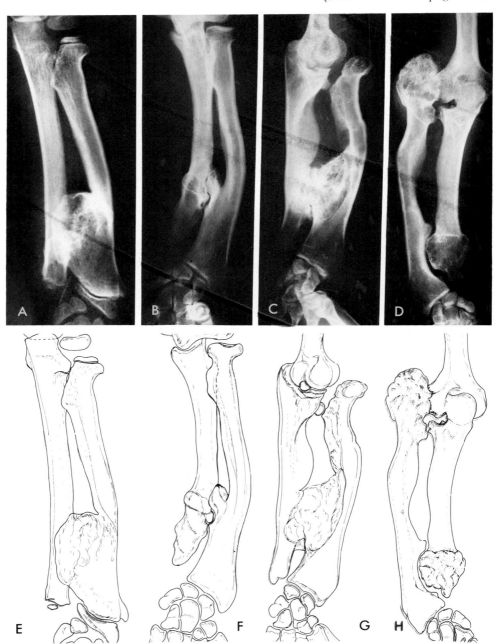

Figure 4–21   Multiple exostoses associated with sundry malformations of the forearm bones. *A,* Exostosis emanating from the ulnar aspect of the right radius, causing shortening of this border and pseudo-Madelung deformity of the wrist. *B,* In this figure radius and ulna are interlocked, preventing pronation and supination of the hand. *C,* Interlocking is also seen in this roentgenograph; in addition, the head of the radius is dislocated. *D,* The heads of both radius and ulna are bulbous in this roentgenograph; the head of the radius is dislocated; the head of the ulna fails to reach the carpus. *E, F, G,* and *H* illustrate the roentgenograph above each.

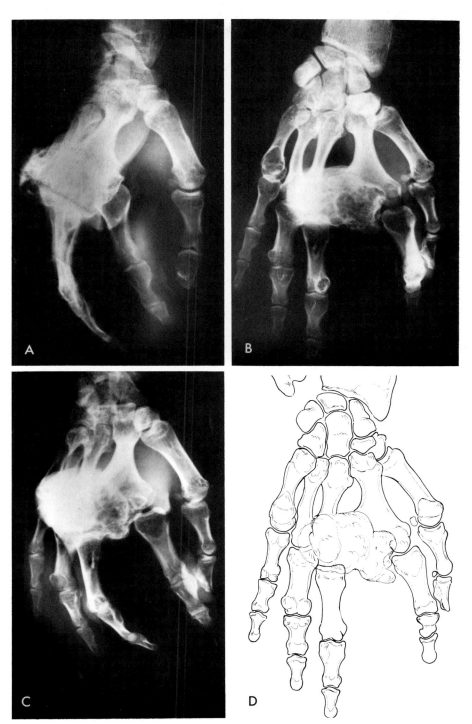

Figure 4–22 Multiple exostoses: massive tumor of metacarpal bone. *A,* Lateral roentgenograph of the left hand, showing a large tumor emanating from the distal end of the second metacarpal. *B,* Dorsopalmar view. *C,* Oblique view. *D,* Illustrative sketch.

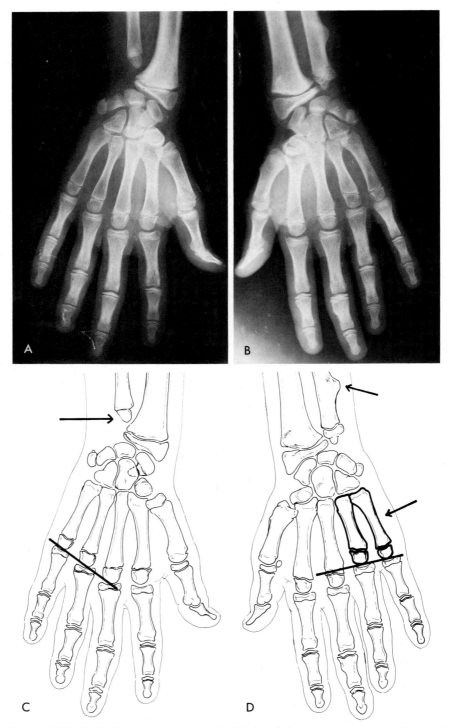

Figure 4–23 Multiple exostoses associated with dwarfed ulnar metacarpals. *A*, Dorsopalmar roentgenograph of the right hand and distal forearm: the ulna on this side is short and tapered. *B*, Dorsopalmar roentgenograph of the left hand of the same patient: the ulna on this side bears an exostosis; the last ulnar two metacarpals are dwarfed. *C* and *D* illustrate the roentgenograph above each.

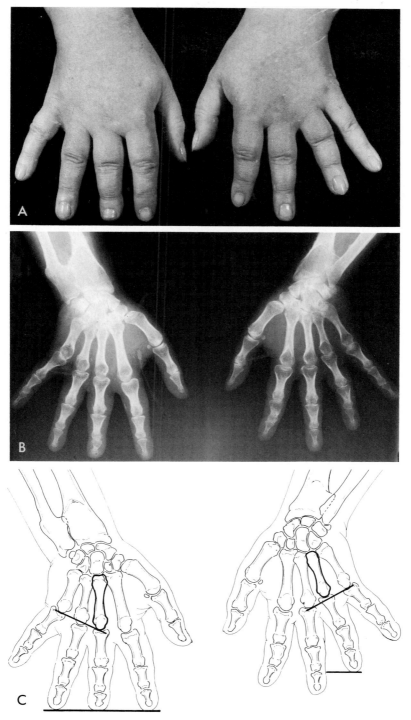

Figure 4–24 Multiple exostoses: isometric central digits and short metacarpal. *A*, Dorsopalmar roentgenograph of both hands: the three central digits of the right hand are equal in length; the left little finger is almost as long as the ring finger next to it. *B*, Dorsoplantar roentgenograph of the same, showing a dwarfed right third and left fourth metacarpal. *C*, Sketch illustrating the same.

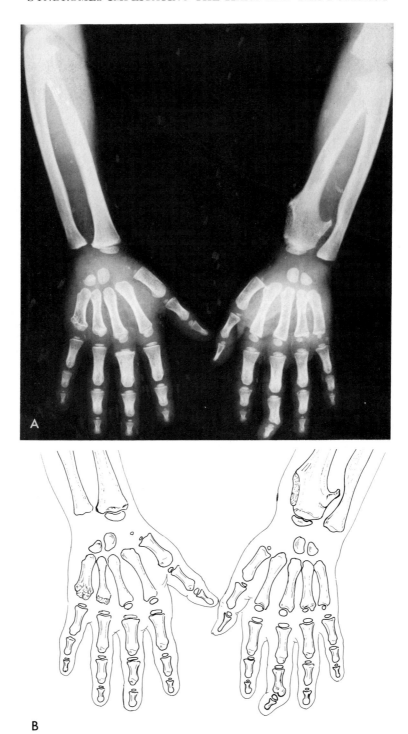

Figure 4–25 Multiple exostoses associated with misshapened metacarpals and axially deviated phalanx. *A*, Dorsopalmar roentgenograph of a 22-month-old female: the fourth and fifth metacarpals of the right hand bear no epiphyses and the ungual phalanx of the left middle finger is deviated in radial direction. *B*, Illustrative sketch.

CONGENITAL SYNDROMES WITH CONSEQUENTIAL POSTNATAL MALFORMATIONS

There are a number of syndromes with underlying defects which are congenital as well as heritable and which, during the postnatal period, surreptitiously engender devious somatic effects. In the syndrome known as congenital analgesia, the child is born without any detectable defect. The primary lesion is thought to reside in the dorsal root ganglia and to consist of degeneration of

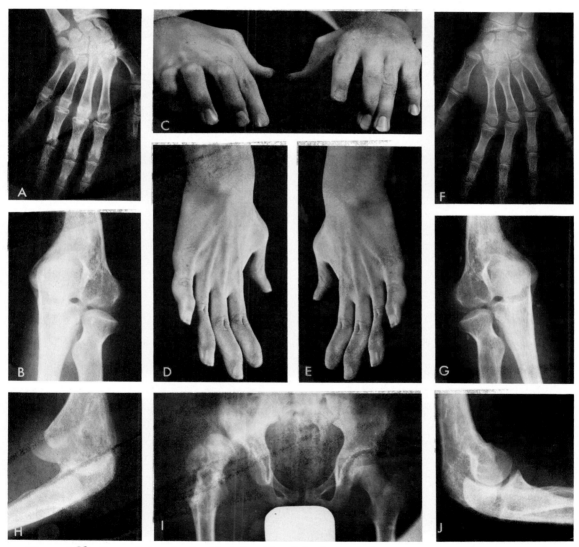

Figure 4=26   Congenital analgesia with deformities of the fingers and sundry subluxations in a 14-year-old boy whose parents were first cousins. Another brother was similarly affected. A female sibling was unaffected. *A,* Roentgenograph of the right hand, showing ulnar drift of the fingers. *B,* Anteroposterior roentgenograph of the right elbow, showing radiocapitellar dysplasia. *C,* Dorsal view of the hands, showing facultative camptodactyly. *D* and *E* show swan-neck deformity of extended fingers. *F* shows radially inclined three central digits of the left hand. *G,* Radiocapitellar dysplasia of the left elbow. *H,* Posterior dislocation of the right radial head. *I,* Dislocation of the right femoral head. *J,* Minimal posterior subluxation of the left radial head.

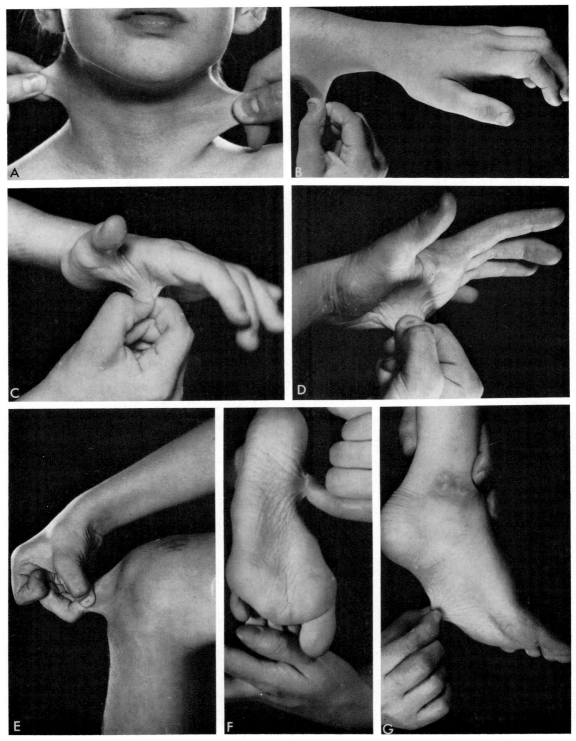

Figure 4–27 Ehlers-Danlos syndrome: hyperelasticity of the skin. Photographs showing hyperelasticity of the skin of the neck *(A); B, C* and *D,* palm; *E,* extensor surface of the knee; *F* and *G,* sole of the foot.

ganglion cells; biopsy has shown complete demyelinization of sensory nerves. Gradually, neuropathies develop: joints are dislocated, the fingers are clubbed and assume bizarre postures. Ehlers-Danlos syndrome provides another example. This complex consists of hyperelasticity of the skin, hypermobility of the joints, and fragility of small vessels. Post-traumatic parchment-thin scars and insidiously developing deformities, such as those of the spine, hands, and feet, are consequential (Figs. 4–26 to 4–30).

(*Text continued on page 131.*)

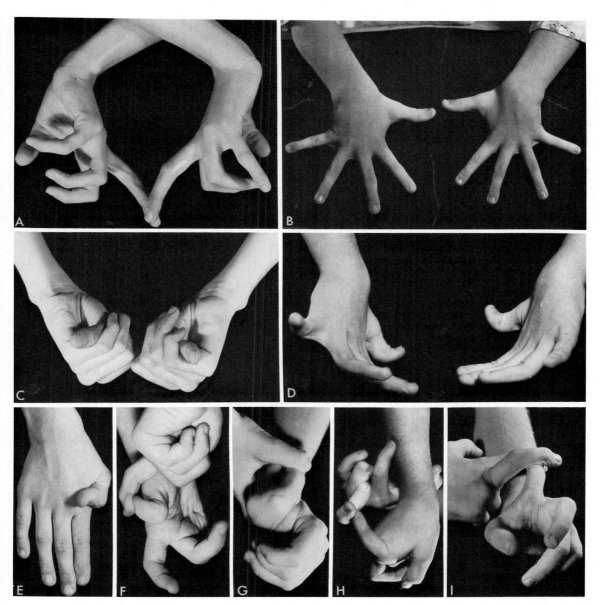

Figure 4–28   Ehlers-Danlos syndrome: hypermobility of the digits. *A*, Ulnar photograph of both hands. *B*, Dorsal view showing the extent of abduction of the non-axial digits. *C*, Ulnar view showing protrusion of the thumbs beyond the ulnar border of the hands. *D*, Ulnar view showing active extension of the digits. *E*, Active clockwise rotation of the right thumb. *F*, *G*, *H*, and *I* demonstrate passive extensibility of the thumbs and index fingers.

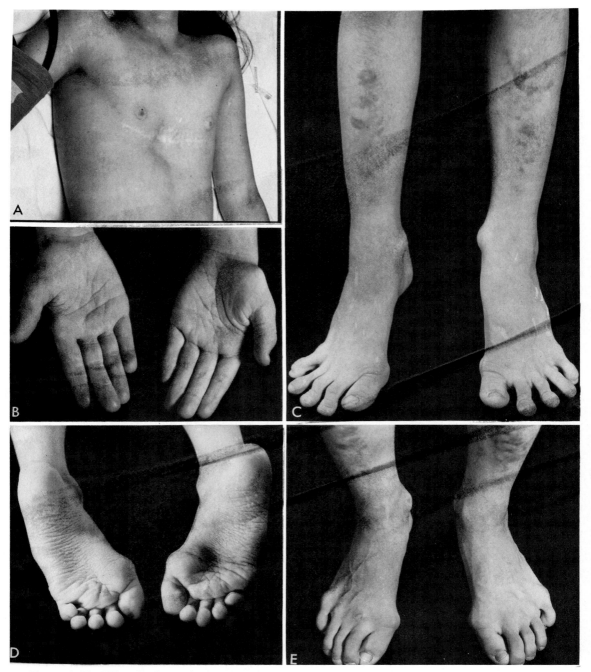

Figure 4–29   Ehlers-Danlos syndrome: objectively observed stigmata. *A*, Frontal view of the chest, which had been operated on for pectus excavatum which was followed by recurrence. *B*, Palmar view of the hands: note corrugation of the skin. *C*, Frontal view of the legs and feet: note the parchment-thin scars of the shins and splaying of the forefeet on weight bearing. *D*, Plantar view of the feet, showing extensive corrugation of the skin. *E*, Dorsal view of the feet, showing bilateral hallux valgus and bunions on the side of the first and fifth metacarpophalangeal joints.

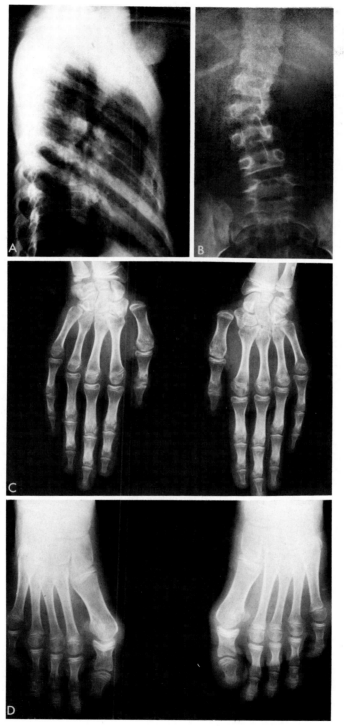

Figure 4–30 Ehlers-Danlos syndrome: roentgenographically detectable skeletal changes. *A*, Lateral view of the chest, showing diminished anteroposterior diameter. *B*, Lumbar scoliosis. *C*, Dorsopalmar view of the hands, showing bilateral dislocation of the first metacarpal at the carpometacarpal joint. *D*, Dorsoplantar view of the feet, showing bilateral metatarsus primus varus and hallux valgus.

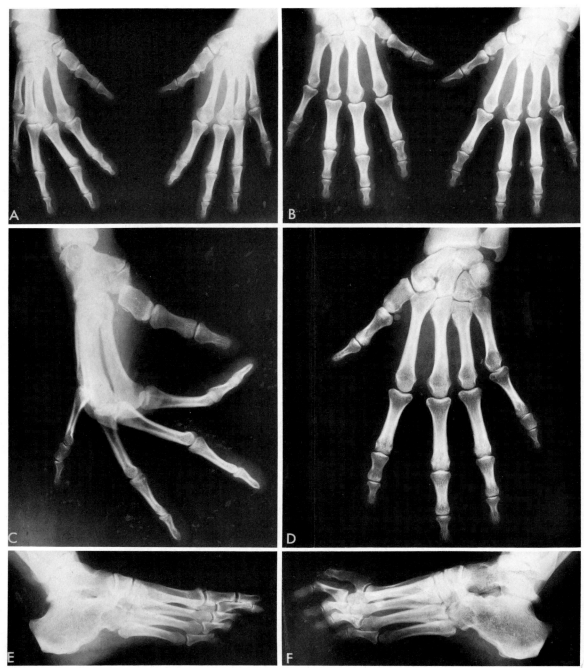

Figure 4–31   Hand-foot-uterus (?) syndrome. *A*, Oblique roentgenograph of the hands of a female adult whose genital organs were not examined to determine the status of her uterus. *B*, Dorsopalmar roentgenograph of the hands. *C*, Enlarged oblique view of the right hand, showing dwarfed first metacarpal. *D*, Enlarged dorsopalmar roentgenograph of the left hand: note the coalescence of the scaphoid with the trapezium and also the shortness of the middle phalanx of the little finger and of the first metacarpal. *E*, Lateral roentgenograph of the right foot, showing fusion of the os calcis with the cuboid bone. *F*, Lateral roentgenograph of the left foot, showing, in addition to calcaneocuboid coalescence, symphalangism of the great toe and absence of a phalanx (probably due to distal symphalangism) in each lesser toe.

HAND AND FOOT COMPLEXES

Serial homology is often seen in polydactyly and syndactyly. In almost all cases of split hand the feet are cloven, manifesting more typically lobster-claw deformity. Comparable malformations of the hands and feet are also seen in many cases of brachydactyly, symphalangism, and congenital clubbing of the digits. Coalescence of carpal ossicles is often associated with fusion of the tarsal bones. In the hand-foot-uterus syndrome described by Stern et al (1970) and Poznanski and associates (1970) there is coalescence of the carpal scaphoid with the trapezium; the first metacarpal is dwarfed, the hallux is short and has a spiked terminal phalanx, and the os calcis is fused with the cuboid bone. Hand-foot syndrome sickle cell anemia is characterized by painful swelling of the hands and feet of infants. The hands and the feet are analogously affected in numerous better known syndromes: arthrogryposis multiplex congenita, craniosynostosis, Ellis-van Creveld chondroectodermal dysplasia, Larsen's syndrome, Laurence-Moon-Bardet-Biedl syndrome, and tylosis, among others (Fig. 4–31).

SUMMARY

A congenital syndrome is defined as a constellation of anomalies which concur with sufficient constancy as to suggest prenatally determined association. Not all—in fact, comparatively very few—syndromes implicating the hand and the forearm can be fitted into coherent, meaningful compendia. Most of these overlap and some of them tend to become too diffuse and overextended to drive home a durable meaning. The names given to syndromes are either eponymic or descriptive. Preference is accorded to descriptive names, and eponyms are used only when the former seem confusing or presumptive. A number of syndromes are associated with more than one morphological variant of the hand and forearm abnormality. Reference to each one of these deformities will be made in the proper context.

References

Aegerter, E., and Kirkpatrick, J. A.: *Orthopedic Diseases*. Third edition. Philadelphia, W. B. Saunders Co., pp. 95–98, 1968.

Allen, G., Genda, C. E., Book, J. A., Carter, C. O., Ford, C. E., Chu, E. H. Y., Hanhart, E., Jervis, G., Langdon-Down, W. (original Langdon Down's grandson), Lejeune, J., Nishimura, H., Oster, J., Penrose, L. S., Polani, P. E., Potter, E. L., Stern, C., Turpin, R., Warkany, J., and Yannet, H.: "Mongolism." *Lancet*, *1*:775, 1961.

Ashley, D. J. B., and Mostofi, F. K.: Renal agenesis and dysgenesis. *J. Urol.*, *83*:211–230, 1960.

Benda, C. E.: *Mongolism and Cretinism*. New York. Grune and Stratton, pp. 5–6, 1946.

Clift, W.: Roentgenological findings in mongolism. *Am. J. Roentgenol.* 9:429–432, 1922.

Curran, A. S., and Curran, J. P.: Associated acral and renal malformations. A new syndrome? *Pediatrics*, *49*:276–725, 1972.

Dieker, H., and Opitz, J. M.: Associated acral and renal malformations. *In* Bergsma, D., (ed.): *Birth Defects. Original Article Series*. New York, National Foundation—March of Dimes, *3*:68–77, 1969.

Down, J. L. H.: Observations on an ethnic classification of idiots. Clinical Lectures and Reports by the Medical and Surgical Staff of the London Hospital. *3*:259–262, 1866.

Gates, R. R.: *Human Genetics*. New York, The MacMillan Co., pp. 156–244; 385–469, 1946.

Goldstein, H.: Congenital acromicria syndrome. *Arch. Pediatr.*, *73*:115–124, 1956.

Jansen, M.: La dysostosi cleidocranica. *Arch. Ortop.*, *35*:270, 1919.

Lejeune, J., Gautier, M., and Turpin, R.: Etude des chromosomes somatiques de neuf enfants mongoliens. *C. R. Acad. Sci., 248*:1721–1722, 1959.

Lennox, B.: Down's syndrome (mongolism). *Lancet, 2*:1093, 1961.

Marfan, A. B.: Un cas de déformation congénital des quatre membres plus prononcée aux extremités, characterisée par l'allongement des os avec un certain degré d'amincissement. *Bull. Soc. Méd. Hôp.* (Paris), *13*:220–226, 1896.

McKusick, V. A.: *Mendelian Inheritance in Man.* Second edition. Baltimore, Johns Hopkins Press. Entry 2525; p. 253, 1968.

Opitz, J. M., Johnson, R. C., McCreadie, S. R., and Smith, D. W.: The C syndrome of multiple congenital anomalies. *In Birth Defects: Original Article Series.* Vol. V, No. 2, pp. 161–166, 1969.

Poznanski, A. K., Stern, A. M., and Gall, J. C., Jr.: Radiographic findings in hand-foot-uterus syndrome (HFUS). *Radiology, 96*:129–134, 1970.

Rubin, P.: *Dynamic Classification of Bone Dysplasias.* Chicago, Year Book Medical Publishers, Inc., pp. 76–84; 258–280, 1964.

Sear, H. R.: The congenital bone dystrophies and their correlation. *J. Faculty of Radiologists, 4*:221–234, 1953.

Seigman, E. L., and Kilby, W. L.: Osteopetrosis. Report of a case and review of recent literature. *Am. J. Roentgenol., 63*:865–874, 1950.

Silverman, M. E., and Hurst, J. W.: The hand and the heart. *Am. J. Cardiol., 22*:718–728, 1968.

Stern, A. M., Gall, J. C., Jr., Perry, B. L., et al.: The hand-foot-uterus syndrome. *J. Pediatr., 77*:109–116, 1970.

Chapter Five

ANCILLARY
CONSIDERATIONS

The care of a congenitally malformed child often requires the concerted efforts of a geneticist, pediatrician, and surgeon. Before he undertakes an operation on a crippled hand, the surgeon should find out if the condition is hereditary and whether it is associated with anomalies of other parts — in particular the nervous, cardiovascular, and hemic systems: the surgeon must be assured that the child is on par mentally and has no congenital heart disease or blood dyscrasia. The surgeon should be familiar with what has been done for similar deformities in the past. He need not, however, feel tradition-bound. Perplexingly diverse congenital malformations of the hand do not always lend themselves to set surgical procedures. The surgeon should modify the method of his choosing to meet the exigencies of the case. Diversified structural deviations can only be coped with by flexibility of mind and an imaginative approach.

QUALIFICATIONS OF THE HAND
SURGEON

The question is often raised as to who should undertake the surgical treatment of maimed hands. Bunnell (1944) considered the problem of the crippled hand to be composite, "requiring correlation of the various specialities — orthopedic, plastic and neurologic surgery. As the problem is composite, the surgeon must also be. It is impractical for three specialists to work together or in series. There is no shortcut. The surgeon must face the situation and equip himself to handle any and all tissues in a limb." Lipscomb (1961) also stressed the necessity of training in orthopedic, plastic, and neurosurgery. Littler (1964) regarded hand surgery as a "regional endeavor," which "represents only a segmental interest in the broad field of reconstructive surgery."

It is unfortunate that the field of hand surgery has been converted into an arena of contention among various surgical specialists—orthopedic and plastic surgeons in particular. Curiously, neither of these contending groups can claim historical precedence for some of the procedures which they insist belong to their respective domains. Almost all orthopedic procedures utilized in hand surgery—osteotomy, bone resection, arthroplasty, and arthrodesis—were developed by general surgeons, as were many of the methods of plastic surgery.

Littler likened hand surgery to ophthalmology in that both required "a particular and refined attitude" for the best management of their complex structures. There is more to be said. Some of the most delicate techniques used in hand surgery—advancement or recession of tendons, for example—were suggested by similar procedures long in practice in ophthalmology. Eye surgeons developed many of the skinplasty techniques now commonly used in hand surgery: the Z-plasty, the full thickness free skin graft, the island graft, and bipedicled tube, all of which will be discussed in Chapter Six. As was indicated in Chapter Two, the embryotoxic effect of the rubella virus was demonstrated by eye surgeons who settled, once and for all, the vexing question of exogenous agents causing congenital anomalies. The most exhaustive documentation of hand deformities—as components of congenital syndromes—is found between the covers of two massive volumes entitled *Genetics and Ophthalmology*, authored by Waardenburg, Francheschetti, and Klein (1961) and again by Waardenburg (1963). Almost all oculomelic syndromes were described by eye surgeons.

Hand surgery is nobody's secular domain. Men from many surgical specialties have contributed to its development. The question as to who should undertake the treatment of a crippled hand can be answered simply and succinctly: he who can improve its function and better its appearance.

FUNCTIONAL IMPROVEMENT IS THE PRIMARY AIM OF SURGICAL INTERVENTION

"Congenital deformities of the forearm and hand are susceptible to great relief by plastic operations," Roberts (1919) wrote. He meant relief from disability. Roberts insisted that the primary aim of reconstructive surgery of the hand is improvement of function. The patient's "mental attitude toward deformity," Roberts wrote, "must be modified by insistence that good looks are less valuable than good works. Sentimental timidity of the patient has no place in reconstructive surgery of the hand. After the surgeon has rebuilt the crippled hand, making it capable of improved function, the patient must be urged and driven. . . to develop manual facility."

It is tempting to wax rhetorical about the munificence of the hand. From Quintilian (A.D. 35–97) to Khaldun (1394), Mateos Djughaetsi (1470?), and Montaigne (1580); from Bell (1835) to Nichols and Ely (1923), Wessel (1935), Bunnell (1944), Kaplan (1965), and Sorrel (1967)—many an author has succumbed to the temptation. We are told that hands "speak themselves," "emulate speech," defend "against aggression" and serve as "instruments of thought and creation"; that the word *chirurgie* is derived from the Greek roots *cheir* and *ergon* meaning, respectively, *hand* and *work* and from "the Latin *manus* are derived *manage, management, mandate, manipulate, maintain, manner, manuscript, manufac-*

ture"; that "the hand grasps. . . the world it creates. In serving its master it reflects his being, as if through a mirror, in a thousand ways"; and finally—there is actually no end to the hyperbolic incantations—"the hand is the outside brain of man."

Wood Jones (1944) advised transferring our admiration from the human hand to the human brain, which composes action patterns for the hand. "It is useless," he said, "to praise the human hand for the wonderful things the brain can find for it to do. . . ." Jones called attention to the fact that the central nervous system is merely the inturned portion of the great surface of the embryogenic body; it is similar in derivation to the skin, which he regarded as an exteriorized nervous system, with the hand serving as its main testing organ. He pointed out that in the process of hand-testing, the fingers—which receive their volar sensory supply from the median nerve—especially the index, play a prominent role. "The median nerve is the channel by which the large bulk of our informative sensory stimuli is carried to the brain," Jones concluded.

It is now generally appreciated that the hand subserves the brain in more than one way. The hand harvests information concerning the size, form, and number of objects, their position in space, and the sense of pain or pleasure they impart. The data thus gleaned are conveyed to the brain which, in turn, coordinates action patterns which have been categorized as pinch, grasp, and grip.

The action pattern in which the palm serves as a platform on which the thumb and fingers close is variously called grasp or grip. The former is said to require the services of the extrinsic muscles of the hand with little aid from the intrinsic group. Grip is stronger; it requires the full force of both groups of muscles and its power depends upon the amplitude of the palm—the broader the palm, the stronger the grip. Two types of pinch are distinguished: pulp-to-pulp, as enacted by the thumb and one of the fingers, and side-to-side pinch, as performed between two neighboring fingers. Side-to-side pinch is no more than a pincer action; it is weaker and far less effective than the pulp-to-pulp pinch. Two varieties of the latter are recognized and called, respectively, power pinch—as exemplified by the act of holding fast to a coin with the thumb and the index finger—and precision pinch, in which the opposing digits hold an object, a pencil for instance, without exerting a great deal of pressure upon it. In the act of picking up a fine object such as a pin or needle, the nail of the thumb and the tip of the opposing digit, usually the index finger, are used. The thumb is essential for effective grip and for precision and power pinch (Figs. 5–1 and 5–2).

The ultimate aim of reconstructive surgery of the hand is to enhance the efficacy of these action patterns and preserve whatever sensibility the maimed parts possess. One aims for the optimum, which is a hand with effective pulp-to-pulp apposition, strong grip, and discriminating touch. But in some instances, one learns to settle for less. Not infrequently, the surgeon is forced to remain content with having obtained a hand which merely serves as a pincer, hook, paddle, or reshaped stump to be fitted with a prosthesis. If the child is born with only a thumb, the surgeon is justified in building an apposition strut with the aid of a composite skin and bone graft. The post thus formed is to be regarded as an improvement, even if it remains devoid of perception or at best conveys a dull sensation. Improvement in appearance is also relative. Except in some forms of polydactyly, the reconstructed hand rarely appears as attractive as its opposite, unaffected mate. The surgeon may again have to settle for a hand which looks only a little less repulsive than before surgery.

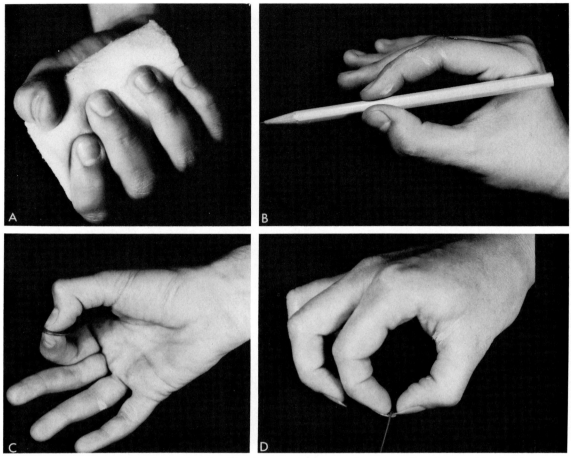

Figure 5-1 Grip and pinch. *A,* Here the object is pressed energetically against a broad palm with a bulging thenar eminence. *B,* Precision pinch. *C,* Pinching a coin with overt power. *D,* Holding a pin between the thumbnail and the tip of the index finger.

CONTRAINDICATIONS TO SURGERY

Since the hand is under the control of the cerebral cortex, surgery upon it should not be contemplated if its possessor is mentally defective or lacks coordination. One also hesitates to operate upon a hand with weak motor power and diminished sensibility. The arm and the forearm together serve as a segmented bridge between the brain and the hand. In the absence of these segments, as in classic phocomelia, one avoids surgery. Surgical interference is contraindicated in the treatment of radial ray defect associated with extensive congenital heart disease and with uncontrolled blood dyscrasias — Fanconi's anemia in particular. One also hesitates to separate the fingers in children with acrocephalosyndactyly when there is already an established atrophy of the optic nerve or when vision is irretrievably lost. Older children who are psychologically adjusted to their deformity and have developed considerable dexterity with their deformed hands are better left alone (Figs. 5-3 to 5-8).

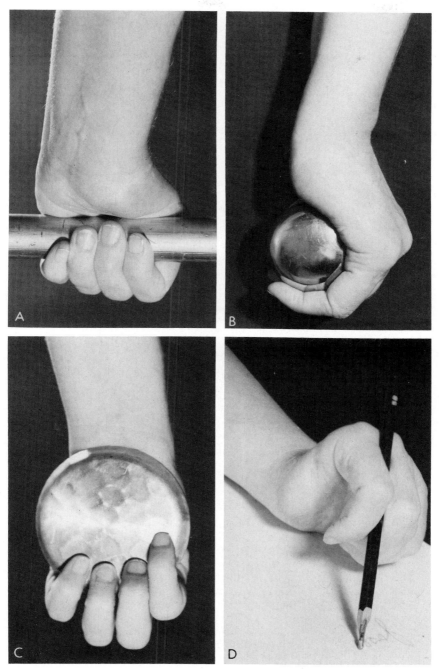

Figure 5–2 The functions of a thumbless hand. *A*, A thumbless hand presses a bar against the palm which is narrow and has no thenar eminence. *B*, Side view of the same. *C*, The four fingers curl around a round object, such as a doorknob, and fail to rotate it effectively. *D*, Side-to-side pinch.

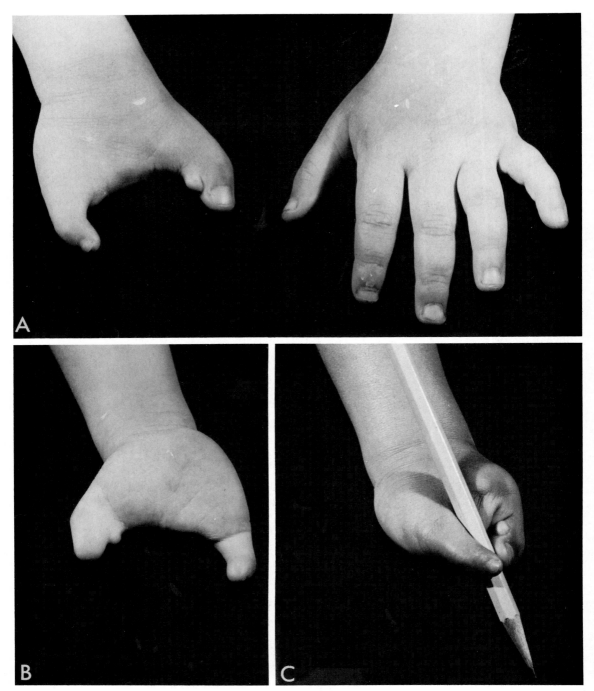

Figure 5–3 Child with absent central digits. *A*, Dorsal view of both hands. *B*, Palmar view of the right hand. *C*, Showing excellent pulp-to-pulp pinch.

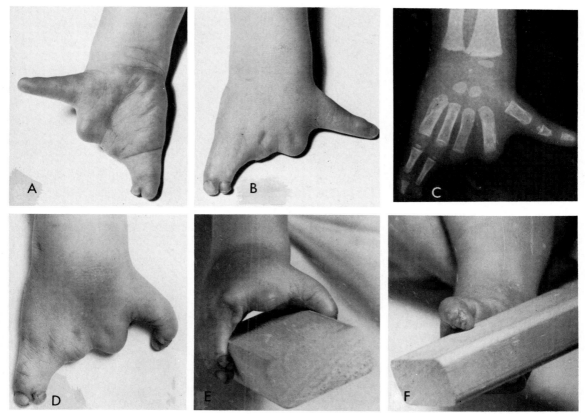

Figure 5–4 Child with agenesis of the index and middle fingers and syndactyly of the ring and little fingers. *A*, Palmar view of the right hand. *B*, Dorsal view of the same. *C*, Dorsopalmar roentgenograph. *D*, Dorsal view, showing flexion of the thumb. *E* and *F* demonstrate an effective grip.

PROPITIOUS TIME FOR SURGICAL
INTERFERENCE

A persistent fallacy in the literature pertains to the postponement of surgical interference until the child is four or five years old. One of the spurious reasons given is that prior to this age, the hand is too small to be splinted or immobilized postoperatively. One wonders if the authors who commit such statements to print have ever learned to apply properly a pressure dressing on the hand or have ever thought of utilizing a percutaneous Kirschner wire for internal splintage—procedures which will be taken up in Chapter Six.

Functional use is the greatest stimulus to growth. It also helps the child to develop coordination. Fingers will grow and become useful if they are freed from restraint and placed in position to perform. The thumb may be regarded as the functional terminus of the rotational ray of the forearm and the hand. In the absence of the thumb, the radius does not develop and often establishes a fibrous or even osseous union proximally with the ulna; pronation and supination, essential to a well-functioning hand, are then completely lost. These haz-

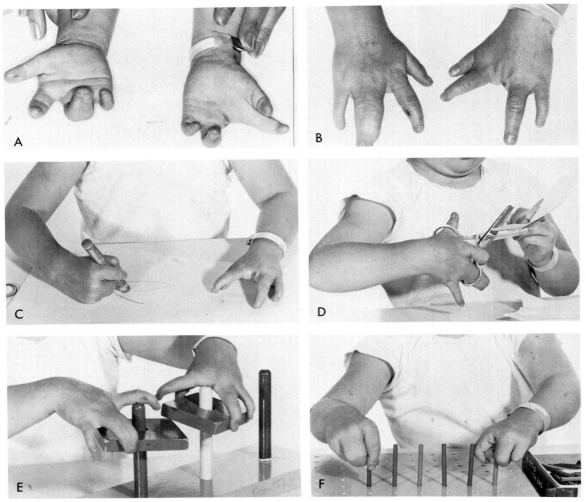

Figure 5–5   Child with syndactyly of the right middle and ring fingers and agenesis of the left middle finger. *A*, Palmar view of the hands. *B*, Dorsal view. *C*, Wielding a crayon. *D*, Wielding scissors. *E* and *F* demonstrate fairly intricate performances.

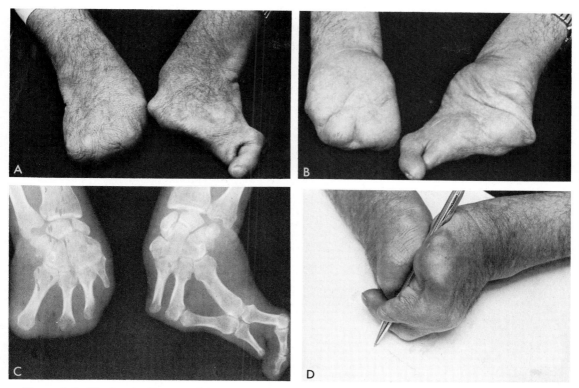

Figure 5–6 The hands of a successful attorney-at-law with split hand complex. *A*, Dorsal view of the hands. *B*, Palmar view. *C*, Dorsopalmar roentgenograph of the hands. *D*, Wielding a pen with the hands.

ards are obviated when the index finger is pollicized early in infancy, thus supplying the radius with a functional stimulus for growth and permitting it to move around the ulna and avoid becoming fused with it. Conversely, in clubhand due to a defective radius, unless the carpus is brought in line with the ulna early in infancy, the distal ulnar epiphysis does not develop and cannot provide a broad, stable support for the hand.

There are some procedures, however, which should not be attempted in early life. A growing child should not be subjected to such operations as arthrodesis, arthroplasty, or joint resection—measures which may damage the epiphyseal disc and stunt the growth of the involved bone. Other procedures, such as separation of confluent fingers, osteotomy of the metacarpal shaft, tendon transfers, and digital shift, can safely be carried out early in life, even during infancy.

The psychological orientation of the child must also be taken into consideration. Children before the age of four are not self-conscious about their deformity, and we must presume that they do not as yet feel branded with the stigma which sets them off from their fellows. A child who has been operated on prior to this age does not usually remember the operation—which must have caused considerable pain and suffering. Reconstructive surgery should, if possible, be completed during preschool years, so that by the time the child enters school he has become used to the form in which his hand will remain.

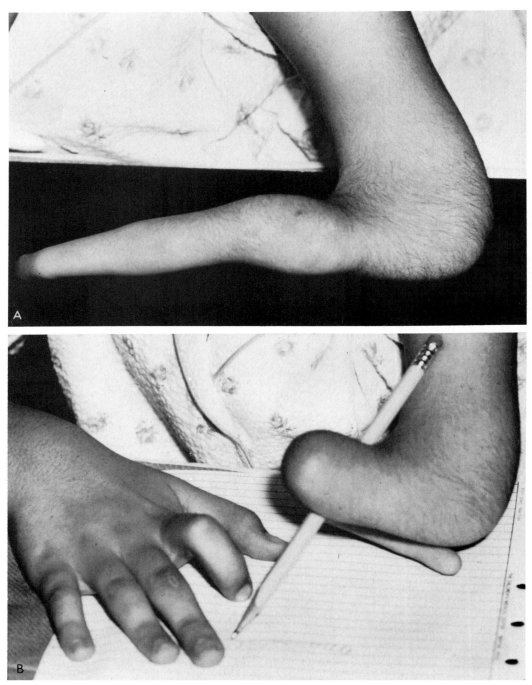

Figure 5–7   The left upper limb of a left-handed monodactylous teenage female. *A*, Radial view of the limb. *B*, Wielding a pencil which is held at the wrist.

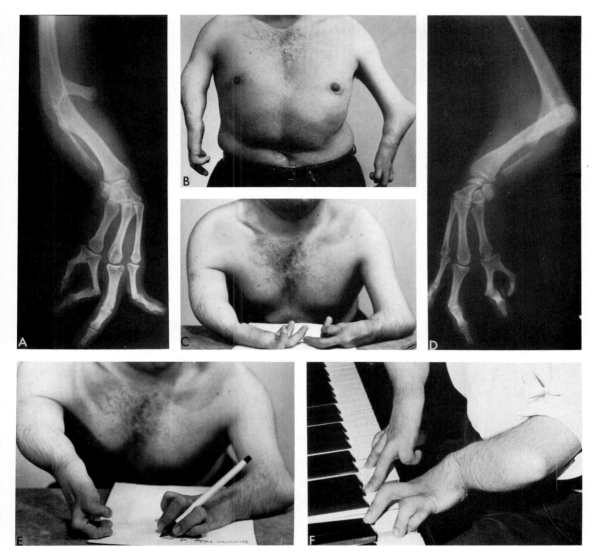

Figure 5–8 Young man with bizarre (phocomeloid with defective ulnar ray) malformations of both upper limbs. *A,* Roentgenograph of right upper limb. *B,* Frontal view, showing the range of extension at the left elbow. *C,* Showing the range of flexion. *D,* Roentgenograph of left upper limb. *E,* Writing with the left hand, which can be pronated. *F,* Playing the piano. This young man drives a car and has learned to use his right shoulder to compensate for lack of flexion and rotary movements at the elbow.

SUMMARY

Operative methods are transposable from one surgical specialty to another. Procedures and technical refinements that have been developed by other surgical specialists—ophthalmic and general surgeons in particular—have been adopted by plastic and orthopedic surgeons who have converted hand surgery into an arena of contention. Hand surgery is not the secular domain of any one coterie of surgeons. Any surgical specialist who can improve the function of the crippled hand and better its appearance is qualified to undertake its treatment.

In consideration of corrective measures, function takes precedence over cosmetic appearance. Functional use is the greatest stimulus to growth. The earlier a congenitally malformed hand is operated upon and put to use the better. If possible, the child with a congenitally malformed hand should have corrective surgery prior to school age, preferably before the age of four.

References

Bell, C.: *The Hand: Its Mechanism and Vital Endowments, as Evincing Design.* Philadelphia, Carey, Lea & Blanchard, pp. 130–168, 1835.

Bunnell, S.: *Surgery of the Hand.* Philadelphia, J. B. Lippincott Co., Preface and p. 31, 1944.

Djughaetsi, M.: 15th century scientist quoted by Emin, K. *In Seven Songs of Armenia.* Yerevan, Government Publishing Co., p. 63, 1970.

Jones, F. W.: *The Principles of Anatomy as Seen in the Hand and Brain, etc.* Second edition. London, Baillière, Tindall & Cox, pp. 298–348, 1944.

Kaplan, E. B.: *Functional and Surgical Anatomy of the Hand.* Second edition. Philadelphia, J. B. Lippincott Co., pp. 3–19, 1965.

Khaldun, Ibn: *The Muguaddimah.* An Introduction to History. (Translated from the Arabic by F. Rosenthal.) London, Routledge & Kegan Paul Ltd., Vol. I, p. 90, 1958. The original is said to have been published in 1394.

Lipscomb, P. R.: Who should do surgery of the hand? *Surg. Gynecol. Obstet., 113*:233, 1961.

Littler, J. W.: Principles of reconstructive surgery of the hand. *In* Converse, J. M., (ed.): *Reconstructive Plastic Surgery.* Philadelphia, W. B. Saunders Co., Vol. IV, pp. 1612–1673, 1964.

Montaigne, M. de: *Essays of Michel de Montaigne.* (Translated by C. Cotton.) Selected and illustrated by Salvadore Dali. New York, Doubleday & Co., Inc., pp. 161–162, 1947. The original is said to have been published in 1580.

Nichols, J. B., and Ely, L. W.: *A Reference Handbook of the Medical Sciences.* New York, William Wood & Co., Vol. IV, pp. 855–901, 1923.

Quintilian, M. F.: His writings appeared in a volume called: *Institute of Elegance,* published in London, 1805. See also: *Quintilian on Education.* (Translated by W. M. Smail.) New York, Teachers College Press, 1938. And: Radermacher, L., (ed.): *M. Fabi Quintiliani Institutionis Oratoriae,* Libri XII, Vols. I & II. Tuebneri, Lipsiae in Aedibus B. G., 1965. The quotation in the present book is from Sir Charles Bell's treatise: *The Hand: Its Mechanism and Vital Endowments as Evincing Design.* London, Bell & Baldy, pp. 166–167, 1865.

Roberts, J. B.: Salvage of the hand by timely reparative surgery. *Ann. Surg., 70*:627–632, 1919.

Sorrel, W.: *The Story of the Human Hand.* Indianapolis, Bobbs-Merrill Co., p. xvii, 1967.

Waardenburg, P. J., Francheschetti, A., and Klein, D.: *Genetics and Ophthalmology.* Netherlands, Royal Van Gorcum Publishers Assn., Vol. I, pp. 1–992, 1961.

Waardenburg, P. J.: *Genetics and Ophthalmology.* Netherlands, Royal Van Gorcum Publishers Assn., Vol. II, pp. 993–1914, 1963.

Wessel, N. Y.: Judgment of manual expression. *Psychol. Bull., 32*:571–572, 1935.

Chapter Six

USABLE TENETS OF TREATMENT

It is often stated that surgery of the congenitally maimed hand is quite different from that utilized in the treatment of the injured hand. Except for its size, the hand of a child is no different from that of an adult. An injured hand is more likely to be infected or scarred. Not infrequently, a congenitally malformed hand has been surgically scarred or infected before the patient seeks further consultation. Too often congenital hemangiomas and moles have been overtreated by radium or x-ray with disastrous consequences, necessitating an array of surgical procedures employed to reconstruct extensively traumatized limbs (Fig. 6–1).

A crippled hand is a crippled hand, whether caused by events antedating the birth of its possessor or by injury or infection in later life. Surgical techniques are transposable from one lesion to another. Frequently, congenitally malformed hands simulate acquired deformities. Surgical procedures originally performed on hands distorted during postnatal life are advantageously utilized to amend analogous deformities having their inception in the antenatal period. Splints, skinplasty, tendon surgery, nerve suture, bone and joint work, and digital transfer and amputation, commonly practiced in the treatment of injured hands, are also employed in attempts to improve the function and, if possible, the appearance of congenitally malformed hands.

EXTERNAL APPLIANCES

One of the marks of sound reconstructive surgery of the hand is the sparse use of external appliances. The hand is not like the foot. Clubhand is not like clubfoot. The foot can be manipulated, wrenched, and casted. The cast can be wedged and rewedged, and immobilization may be carried on for weeks and months, even years, without jeopardizing the usefulness of the foot. The essential function of the foot is stability. Movement is paramount in the hand; protracted immobilization of the fingers is certain to cause stiffness. Rigid external appliances, which may at times become expedient, are rarely extended past the distal palmar crease. As a rule, the fingers are left free to flex and extend.

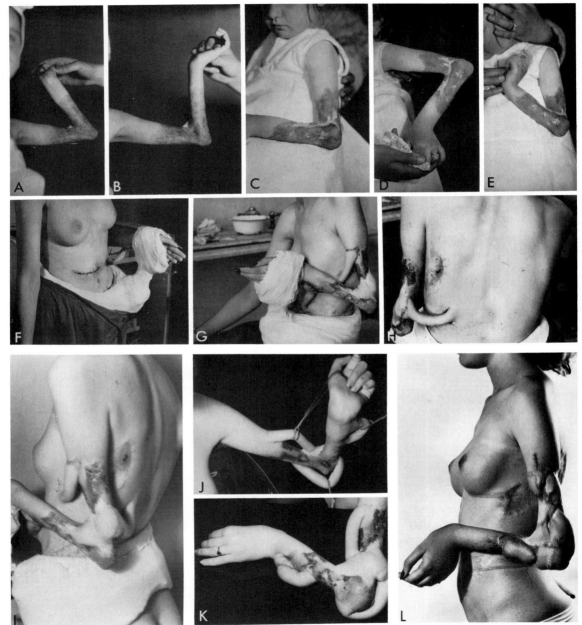

Figure 6–1   *A, B, C, D,* and *E:* various views of the left arm of a three-year-old female who was born with a hairy mole around the elbow. The mole was treated by radium which resulted in atrophy of the underlying muscles, fibrous ankylosis of the elbow joint, and wrist drop. The functional restoration of this limb necessitated the employment of numerous surgical procedures used for reconstruction of a severely injured limb. In this figure are shown only some of the preliminary steps used for the replacement of bone-bound hirsute scar. *F* and *G* show the plaster apparatus used to hold the hand in dorsiflexion and procure a measure of immobilization while three tubed grafts are being transferred from the torso to the arm. *H* shows one of the tubed grafts. *I,* Hirsute scar has been partly replaced by pliable skin. *J* and *K* show the transferred tubes. *L* shows flattened tubes.

External appliances are used to prevent deformity and procure rest for traumatized tissue. The deformities due to absence of the radius and arthrogryposis are progressive. In both of these conditions, one is justified to manipulate the hand and hold it in functional position—20-degree extension at the wrist and neutral as to ulnar or radial deviation—with a circular cast. After four weeks, the

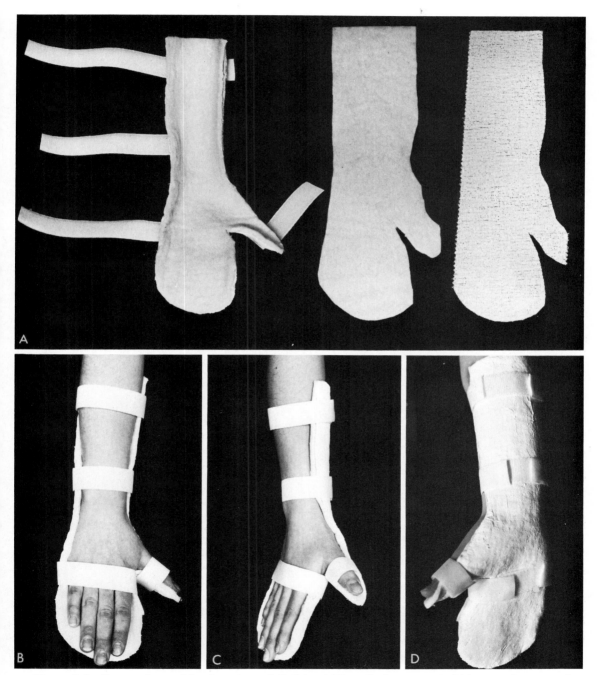

Figure 6–2   Gutter splint used for the wrists and all digits. *A*, The splint is composed of felt pad and plaster, which are shown next to it. It is held in place by porous adhesive straps. *B*, *C*, and *D*, Various views of the splint holding the hand in position.

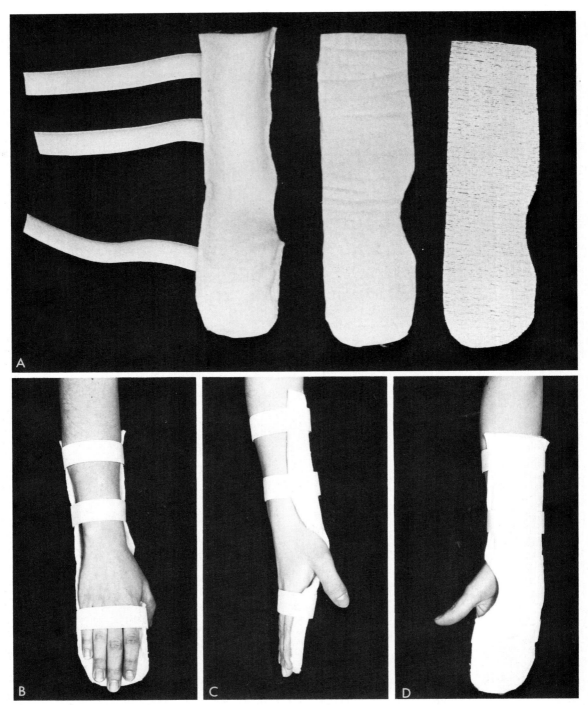

Figure 6–3   Gutter splint which leaves the thumb free. *A*, The splint and component materials. *B, C,* and *D,* Various views of the splint holding the hand in position.

cast is replaced by a volar gutter splint which is worn at night, leaving the hand free during the day to allow muscular contractions and mobility of the joints. Improvised functional splints are also used after surgical procedures for correction of the flexion contractures of the digits or camptodactyly (Figs. 6–2 to 6–7).

Refined surgical technique and respectful tissue touch on the part of the surgeon do make a difference. Nonetheless, surgery is injury. Following surgical intervention, attempts should be made to prevent swelling of the hand. Postoperatively, pressure dressing is applied and the hand is elevated—better still,

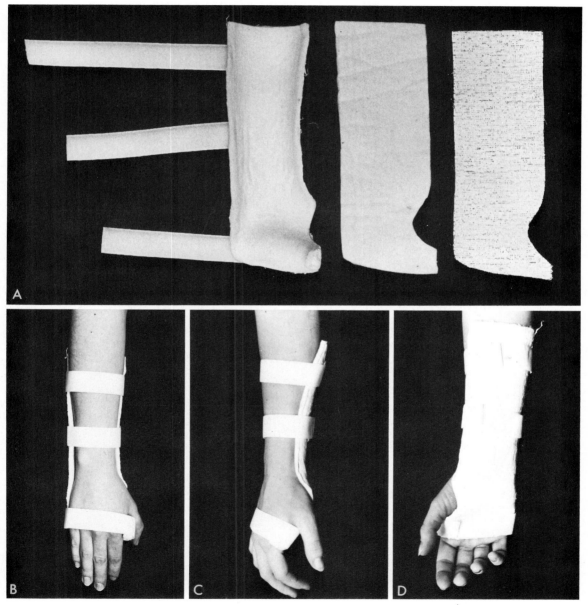

Figure 6–4   Gutter splint supporting only the wrist. *A*, The splint and its components. *B*, *C*, and *D*, Various positions of the splint supporting the wrist.

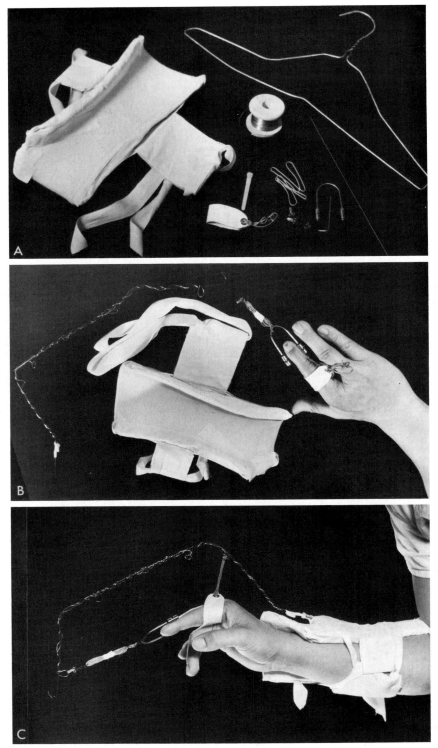

Figure 6–5 Improvised splint for functional exercises of the finger after arthroplasty. *A*, Gutter splints and material used for traction and exercises under tension. *B*, Splint and the hand. *C*, Hand in the splint.

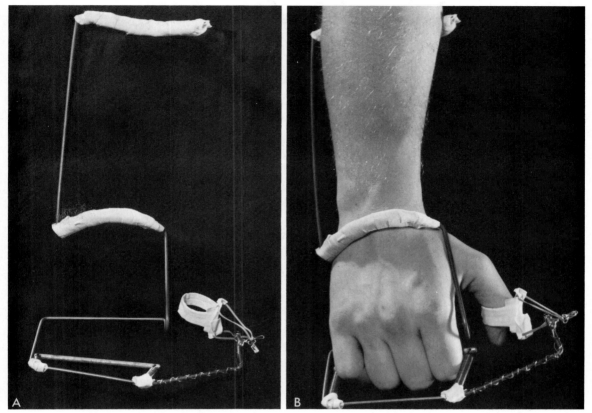

Figure 6–6 Improvised splint for supporting the wrist and exercising the thumb. *A,* The splint and its adjuncts. *B,* Hand in the splint.

suspended. After tendon and nerve sutures and corrective osteotomy, immobilization for at least four weeks is requisite. After cross skin grafts from abdomen to hand, a Velpeau bandage is used (Figs. 6–8 and 6–9).

PRELIMINARY STEPS

The child is put under general anesthesia; the part to be operated on is scrubbed with soap and water. Children have hairless, smooth skin; the hand and the forearm can be rendered clean in half the time it would require to prepare the same parts in adults. Children, moreover, have delicate, bruisable integument. The standard 10-minute scrubbing with even the mildest detergent is likely to cause excoriation of the skin; five minutes of scrubbing with soap and water will suffice. The parts are then rinsed with alcohol. Not much more need be done in the way of sterilization. If felt necessary, the parts may be swabbed with one of the nonstaining antiseptics—aqueous Zephiran, for instance. Antiseptics that color the skin make it difficult for the surgeon to check the circulation of the fingers at intervals during surgery.

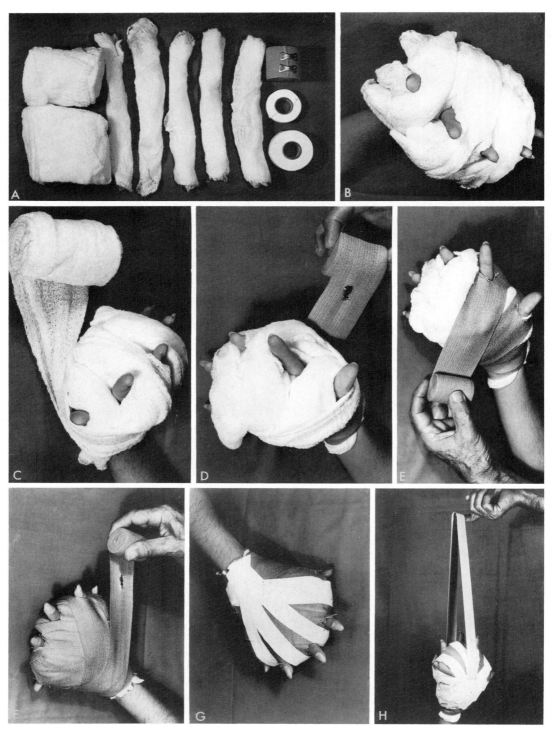

Figure 6–7 Material and method of postoperative pressure dressing and suspension. *A*, Fluffed gauze, bandage gauze strips, hernia tape, adhesive tape, and stretchable bandage. *B*, Packing of the interdigital spaces. *C*, Application of fluffed gauze bandage. *D, E, F,* and *G*, Application of stretchable bandage and adhesive tape. *H*, The hernia tape used for suspension of the operated hand.

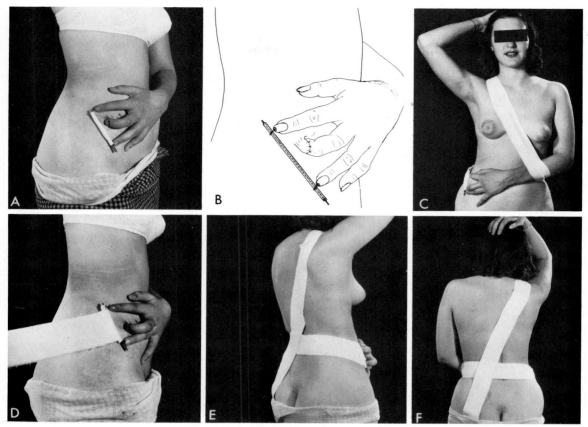

Figure 6–8 Adhesive Velpeau strap attached to a spreader bar. *A,* Spreader bar sutured to the fingernails. *B,* Sketch of the same. *C, D, E,* and *F,* Various steps of applying the adhesive strap.

The arm is draped in the usual manner. The hand is rendered bloodless: in children we prefer a sterile rubber catheter for a tourniquet, and apply it at a point proximal to the wrist or elbow. During surgery, the tourniquet is loosened at intervals; the bleeders are ligated; the circulation of the fingers is checked. Preliminary to incision, the fingers are held in extension with the aid of tension sutures passing through their tips (Fig. 6–10).

INCISIONS

It would be repeating a time-honored axiom to say that incisions on the hand should not cross the flexion creases of the palm and fingers, nor should they overlie tendons and run in the same direction. Skin cuts which cross the flexion creases inevitably heal with thick contracting scars; longitudinal incisions over tendons produce adhesions. When the lines of closure lie directly over the tendons, the tendons will gradually become bound down by dense adhesions and fail to function. The usual lateral longitudinal incision along the fingers must not

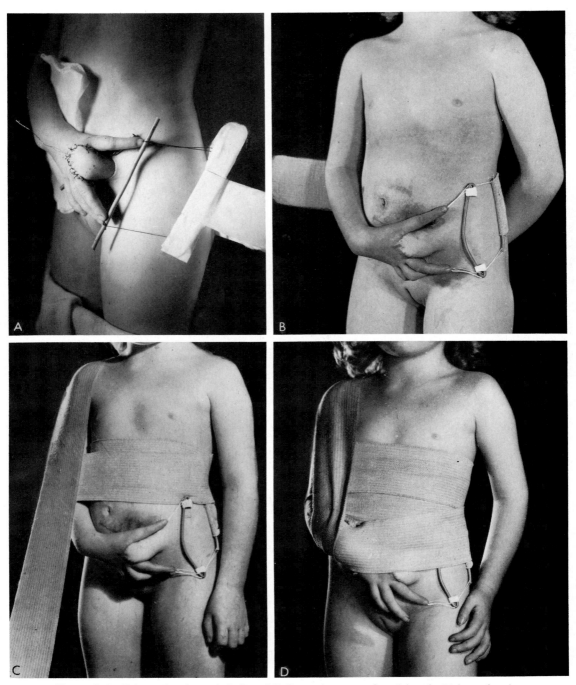

Figure 6–9 Velpeau bandage. *A, B, C,* and *D,* Successive steps of applying the Velpeau bandage.

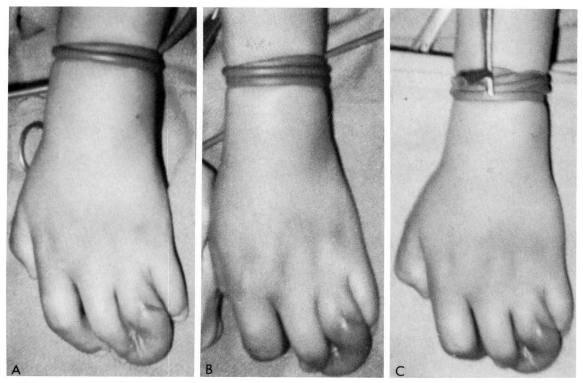

Figure 6–10 The use of a rubber catheter as a tourniquet. *A*, Two coils of the rubber catheter, one locking the other. *B*, Another coil has been added, making certain that the coils are snug against each other. *C*, The ends of the catheter are held with a hemostat.

overlie the neurovascular bundle, but should be placed on a more dorsal plane; it is better for this incision to undulate instead of tracing a straight line. The edges of the skin are retracted by a suture (Fig. 6–11).

At the conclusion of the main reconstructive work, the tourniquet is again released and hemostasis secured, using very fine 6–0 plain catgut for ligature. Approximation of subcutaneous tissue is not necessary in children, except in cases in which there is a dead space which needs to be obliterated. At points of tension the skin edges are brought together with a few interrupted sutures, using 34 nonfilament stainless steel. The intervening gaps are closed with 5–0 absorbable (polyglycolic acid or Dexon) suture.

In the closure of the surgical wound, the margins of the skin are brought back to their original line and sutured together. When the edges of the skin are mobilized, made to extend beyond the original line of incision and anchored at some distance from it, the procedure ceases to be simple closure and evolves into plastic repair. Skinplasty is also necessitated when the gap between the margins of the incision is too wide to be spanned without great tension, or when more skin is needed in anticipation of future reconstructive work. In both of these circumstances, skin for coverage is transferred from a more remote region of the body as a completely detached piece (free graft) or as a flap which remains temporarily connected to the donor area (pedicled graft).

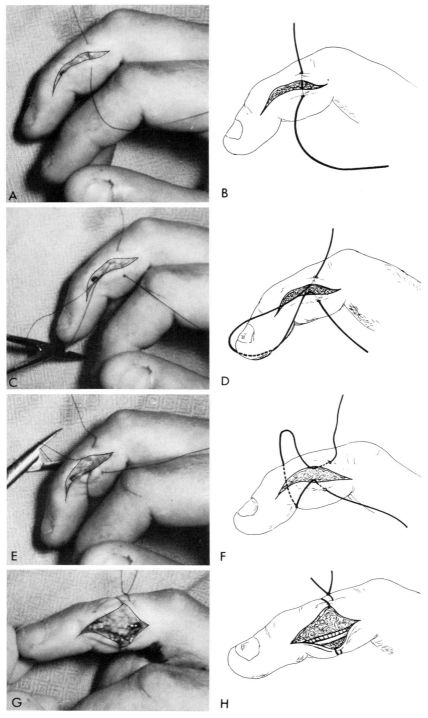

Figure 6–11   *A*, Dorsolateral undulating incision on the radial aspect of the middle finger. The skin edges are undermined and a suture is passed from one edge to the other. *B*, Sketch illustrating the same. In *C* and *D* is seen the central loop of the suture passing over the tip of the finger. *E* and *F* show the loop well on the ulnar aspect of the finger. The ends of the suture are now tied together, as shown in *G* and *H*, procuring adequate, atraumatic retraction.

FREE SKIN GRAFT

Historians of skinplasty—Davis (1919), Gnudi and Webster (1950), Rogers (1959) and Gibson (1961), to mention a few—have aired the sensational lore of what is called the ancient Indian method, also known as flagellation and free skin grafting. This story began to spread in European professional circles soon after the appearance of a letter by Dutrochet (1817) in *Gazette de Santé*. This letter reveals that in order to cover a defective area elsewhere on the body, Indians beat the donor site with a shoe "blow after blow" until it became congested; an appropriate piece of "skin and subcutaneous tissue" was then fashioned and fixed on the recipient site "with agglutinative plasters." Historians have also propagated the story about a female charlatan named Gambarcurta. Early in the eighteenth century, this woman is said to have peddled a wound-healing balsam in Florence. To dramatize her commodity, she would cut a piece of skin from her thigh and stick it back in place with her balsam. The skin thus glued is said to have "taken" the following evening.

Fascinating as these reports are, they lack detailed description of technique and trustworthy records of long-term results. They must be dismissed with an aphorism of Virginia Woolf, quoted by her biographer, Aileen Pippett (1953): "Nothing can exist unless it is properly described."

The first comprehensive description of free skin grafting was recorded by Reverdin (1870). "With the point of a lancet," he wrote, "I raised two little flaps from the right arm, taking care not to cut the dermis." He applied these pieces to the granulating surface. Ollier (1872) and, following him, Thiersch (1886), lifted larger and thicker shavings of skin. Wolfe (1875), an eye surgeon, used full-thickness skin; this method was elaborated by Krause (1893). Davis (1919) hyphenated the name of Ollier with that of Thiersch and the name of Wolfe with Krause. Blair and Brown (1929) replaced these eponymic titles with the more descriptive adjectives *split* or *thin* (Reverdin), *intermediate* (Ollier-Thiersch), and *thick* (Wolfe-Krause).

It was inevitable that someone should think of covering with free graft the raw surfaces left after the separation of webbed fingers. Lennander (1891) was probably the first to practice this method. He used Thiersch graft. Thinner grafts are more certain to take but tend to contract, and the color and appearance of the healed surface are conspicuously unsightly as compared to the color and appearance which follow successful full-thickness graft. In restorative surgery of congenitally malformed hands, thin and intermediate free grafts are seldom utilized. The choice remains with full-thickness free skin or transferred flaps (Figs. 6–12 and 6–13).

LOCAL FLAPS

By definition, an attached flap includes skin and subcutaneous tissue sufficient to afford passage for nourishing vessels. These vessels penetrate the flap at its attached end and pass on toward its free border. The attached end of the flap is called the pedicle. When a flap is procured from the skin bordering the wound, it is qualified as being local. Celsus (circa 25 B.C.) described an ingenious method of spanning a skin defect with local flaps. He outlined two quadrilateral flaps on the opposite sides of the skin defect, mobilized the edges of the flaps nearer to the defect, drew them together, and sutured them over the wound. If

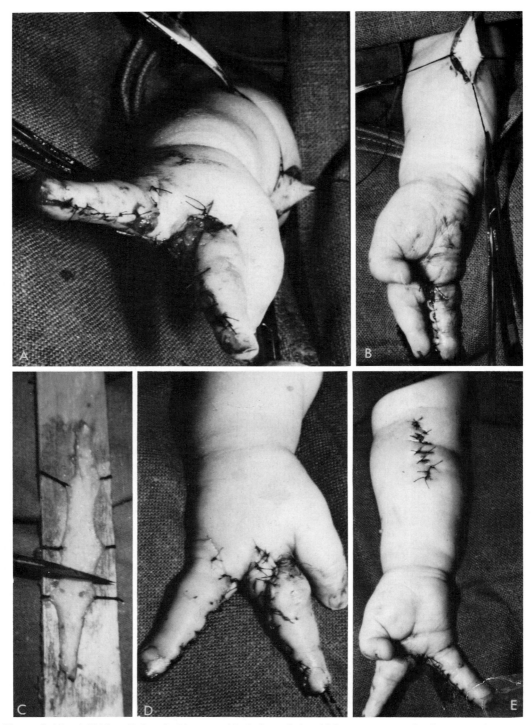

Figure 6–12   *A,* Tridactylic hand with two webbed ulnar digits which were separated. The raw surfaces were covered with the aid of local flaps, leaving small, denuded areas near the base of each digit. *B,* Elevation of an elliptical piece of free skin from the flexor aspect of the proximal forearm. *C,* The graft was placed on a tongue depressor with its raw surface up and tied under tension; fatty and areolar tissue was scraped and the graft was bisected, yielding two triangular pieces. *D,* Each piece was utilized to cover the raw surfaces of the separated digits. *E,* Closure of the forearm defect by Z-plasty.

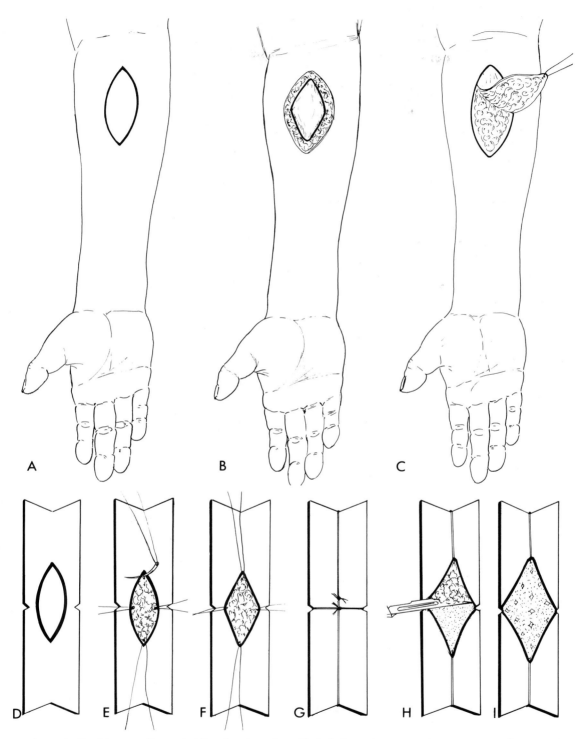

Figure 6–13 Diagrams illustrating the elevation of an elliptical piece of skin from the proximal volar surface of the forearm and its conversion to a full-thickness graft. *A, B,* and *C* show the elevation of an elliptical piece of skin which is laid (*D*) on a notched tongue depressor with its raw surface up. *E* and *F* show suturing and tying the piece of skin to the underlying tongue depressor. *G* shows the reverse side of the tongue depressor. *H,* The areolar tissue is being scraped from the graft, and punctate stab apertures are seen in *I.*

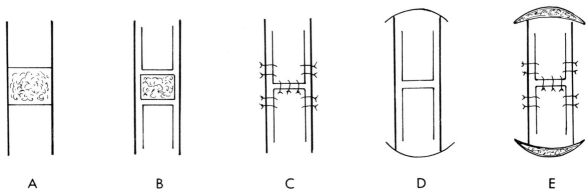

Figure 6–14 Celsus method of advancing local flaps for surfacing a defect. *A*, Dotted area represents the defect, on either side of which quadrilateral incisions are made. *B*, Advancement of quadrilateral flaps. *C*, Closure. *D*, Semilunar incision at the base of each quadrilateral flap to relieve tension. *E*, Relaxed flaps are drawn together and sutured.

the flaps could not be approximated, Celsus resorted to relaxing incisions. He insisted that these cuts should go deeper than the skin. He also advised against suturing the skin flaps under undue tension. Historians of skinplasty seem to have overlooked Celsus: they credit Serre (1842) of Montpellier, who merely popularized the procedure. It is perhaps because of this that the operation has come to be known as the French method (Fig. 6–14).

Zeller (1810) was first to apply the principle of local skin flap in hand surgery. He made a V-shaped incision on the dorsal aspect of the hand between the bases of the syndactylized fingers. The triangular flap, thus fashioned, had a broad proximal base and pointed distal apex. After separating the conjoined fingers from each other, Zeller advanced the triangular flap over the newly formed commissure and anchored its apex to the skin of the palm. Dieffenbach (1834) blunted the tip of Zeller's flap and gave it the configuration of a horseshoe. More than a century later, Iselin (1960) described a flap not unlike Dieffenbach's and called it "procede de M. Iselin" (Fig. 6–15).

To diminish the side-to-side span of the upper lip, Teale (1858) developed two transversely disposed triangular flaps, pulled them side by side, and sutured them together. Norton (1881) applied this principle in establishing a commissure between webbed fingers. The Teale-Norton procedure was revived more recently by MacCollum (1940). After separating the webbed fingers, MacCollum developed two triangular flaps, a palmar and a dorsal; these flaps were raised from the corresponding surfaces of the hand between the bases of the webbed digits. MacCollum pulled the dorsal and palmar flaps across the webspace, suturing the side bar of the one to the corresponding limb of the other, and used free skin grafts for surfacing the sides of the separated digits. He described his method of suturing the triangular flaps as having the form of a "Z". He did not mention the originator of this design (Fig. 6–16).

Denonvilliers (1856), a French eye surgeon, devised the Z-plasty technique in an attempt to correct the contracture of the lower eyelid. Morestin (1914) applied this procedure to the hand. Pieri (1920) included in his articles drawings showing Z-cuts on the volar aspect of a contracted finger. In Steindler's (1925) article, another set of drawings appeared, illustrating what he called "Pieri's method of thumb web plasty." Pieri, we are told, used a Z-shaped incision to widen the webspace between the thumb and index finger. In addition to its use for correction of flexion deformity of fingers and adduction contracture of the

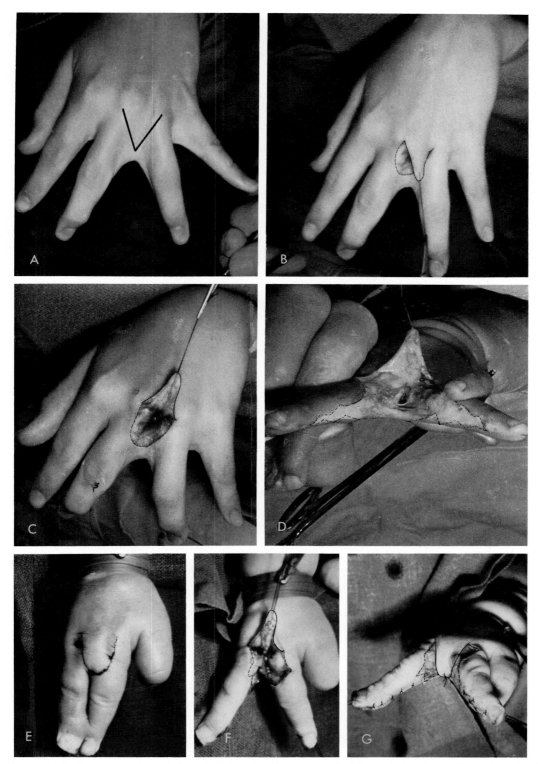

Figure 6–15 Dorsal commissural flaps. *A, B, C,* and *D* demonstrate incision and elevation, Zeller's triangular flap. In *E, F,* and *G* is seen Dieffenbach's flap.

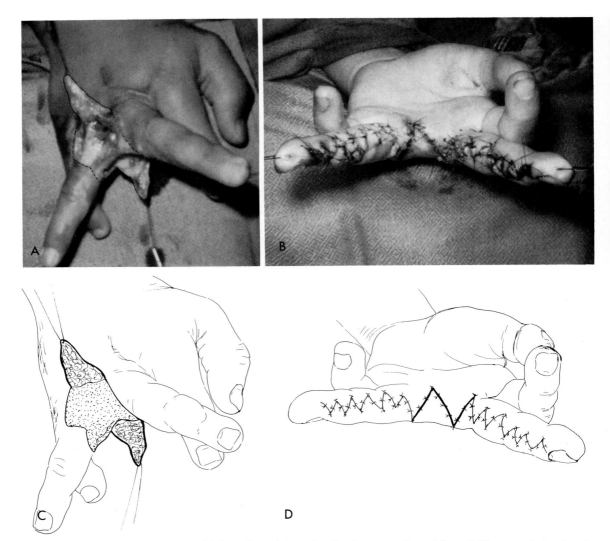

Figure 6–16 Teale-Norton-MacCollum flaps. *A,* Dorsal and palmar commissural flaps. *B,* Photograph showing the two commissural flaps used in connection with small Z-plasty cuts to cover the raw surfaces of the webbed third and fourth digits which had been separated. *C* and *D* illustrate photograph above each.

thumb—both of which may be of congenital origin—Z-plasty is advantageously utilized in repair of annular grooves and in release of contracture around the wrist.

Szymanowski (1870) illustrated the design of the Z-incision and Limberg (1964) discussed the theory behind this method, giving its practice mathematic precision. In single Z-plasty, the triangular flap on one side is transposed to cover the defect produced by the elevation of the other and vice versa. To repair longer contractures, multiple Z-incisions are used. The main line of incision runs lengthwise along the course of the contracting band. The skin edges are undermined to bring into view the underlying contracted band. The latter is dissected out. The cut margins of skin are split with slanting small incisions. Side incisions are set at about 60 degrees to the longitudinal cut. The side V-flaps raised are mobilized and made to exchange places across the main line of the surgical wound (Figs. 6–17 to 6–19).

(Text continued on page 166.)

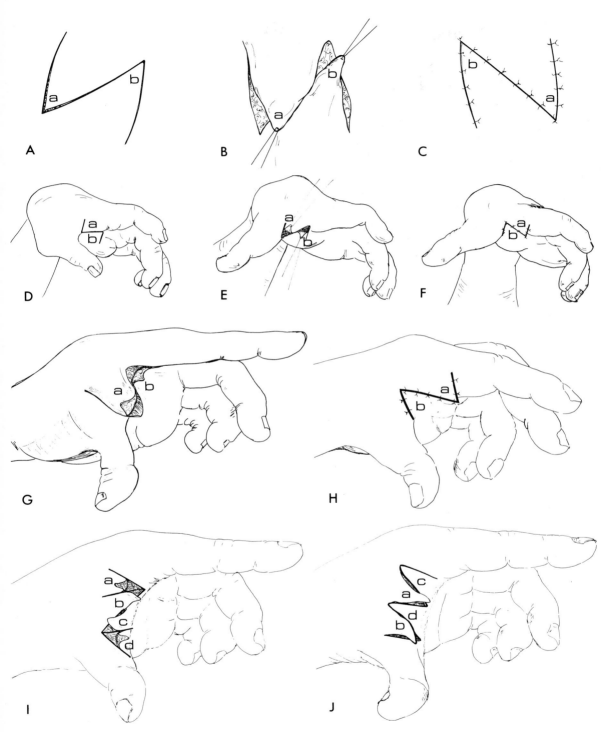

Figure 6–17 *A*, Incision for two-flap Z-plasty. *B*, Elevation of flaps. *C*, Reversal of loci. *D*, *E*, *F*, *G*, and *H* illustrate application of two-flap Z-plasty for widening the first webspace. *I* and *J* show that the space may also be widened by bisecting each flap and producing four shorter flaps.

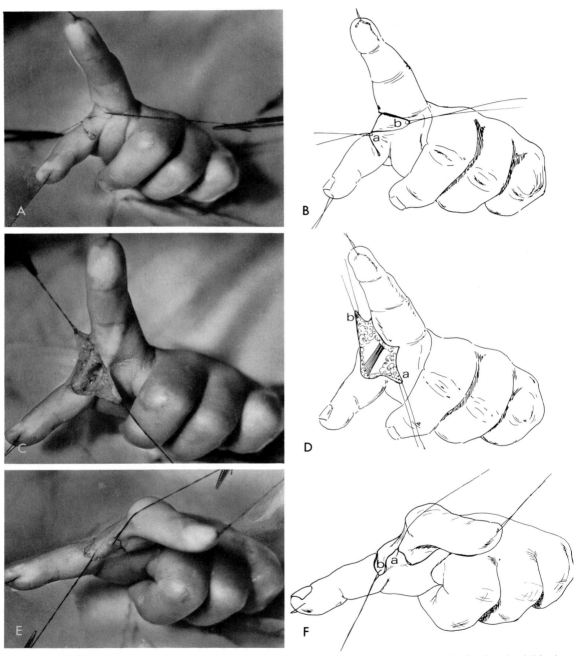

Figure 6–18 Application of Z-plasty for widening the first webspace. The right hand of a female child whose thumb was distally placed and appeared to have been caught in the common bondage of deep transverse metacarpal ligament; the first webspace was narrow. *A* and *B* show the initial incision. *C* and *D* demonstrate the elevation of the triangular flap and the exposure of the anomalous band of the deep transverse ligament which anchored the proximal phalanx of the thumb; this band was excised. *E* and *F* show that each triangular flap has been shifted to cover the area from which the other was lifted.

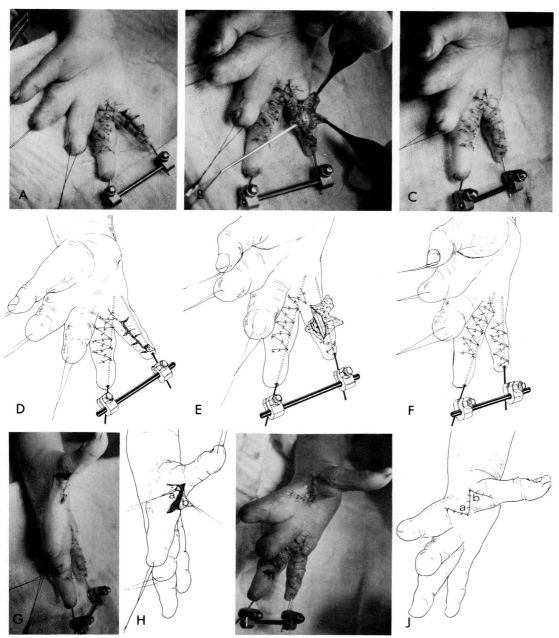

Figure 6–19 Multiple Z-plasty. The hand of a 3-year-old female who was born with an adduction contracture of the thumb, absent terminal phalanges of the index and middle fingers, and flexion contracture of the fourth and fifth digits. *A* shows Z-plasty of the ring and little fingers—the flaps on the former were sutured; multiple cuts were made at an angle of 60 degrees to the contracted scar of the little finger; percutaneous K-wires (Kirschner wires) have been inserted to hold the fingers in extension so that the triangular flaps may be sutured under tension. *B* shows that the flaps on the little finger have been lifted, a bistuary was passed behind the flexor tendons, and anterior capsulotomy of the first interphalangeal joint was performed. *C*, Closure of the triangular flaps of the little finger. *D*, *E*, and *F* illustrate the photograph above each. *G* and *H* show Z-incision in the first webspace, and *I* and *J* demonstrate alternation of the triangular flaps of the first webspace.

Szymanowski (1870) described numerous variations of flaps raised from the immediate vicinity of the skin defect; his designs have been reproduced in many books and articles dealing with skinplasty. Besides advancing or sliding flaps, Szymanowski also described others which were made to rotate or twist on their attached bases. Lewin's (1951) rotation finger flap, the cocked-hat flap of Gillies and Millard (1957), and numerous other named flaps may be traced to Szymanowski's models. In these later modifications, the defect left by the displaced flap is covered by free skin graft, descriptions of which had just begun to appear in Szymanowski's day.

REGIONAL FLAPS

When the flap is raised from the same area as the defect and an intervening zone of intact skin separates the two, the surfacing is said to have been accomplished by the Indian method. We learn from Fayrer (1866) that members of the Kimar tribe in India devised this method. According to Davis (1919), members of the tilemaker caste perfected the technique of elevation and transfer of regional flaps.

To the category of regional flaps belong the palmar or thenar grafts of some years back and the transdigital or cross-finger grafts of more recent vintage. Thenar or palmar flaps entail sacrifice of valuable skin from the volar aspect of the hand and necessitate acute flexion of the finger for several weeks; not infrequently, the grafted finger fails to extend fully after it has been weaned from the donor site. The discomfort accompanying cross-finger flaps is minimal, and postoperative disability of the donor digit is practically nil. The dorsal skin of one of its neighboring digits provides the best coverage for small defects on the volar aspect of the finger. The defect of the donor site is surfaced by full-thickness free skin. The flap is detached from the donor site after five weeks (Fig. 6–20).

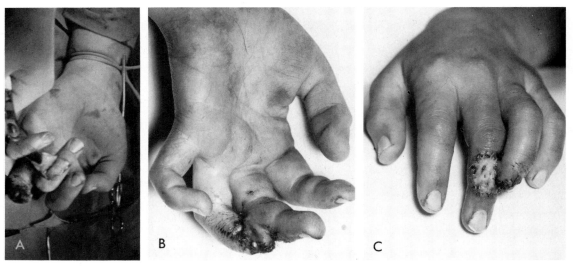

Figure 6–20   Cross-finger flap. *A* shows a rectangular flap lifted from the dorsal aspect of the middle finger to be transferred to the volar surface of the ring finger. *B*, Palmar view of the transferred flap. *C* shows that the back of the donor finger has been covered by full-thickness graft.

To the class of regional flaps also belongs the recently revived and popularized neurovascular island graft. This method owes its origin to Gersuny (1887), who covered a defect in the lower face by a rotation flap from the neck. Dunham (1893) split the bridge of skin between the donor and recipient areas, and buried the nourishing stalk of the flap. The principle of passing the island graft through a tunnel under the skin was introduced by Monks (1898), another eye surgeon. Somehow this operation came to be identified with Esser's name. The only contribution Esser made is the coinage of the term *island flap*. According to Peacock (1960), Esser reported 14 cases in which the principles of island transfer had been applied to the hand. In Esser's (1917) article referred to, no mention of any work on the hand is found.

The stalk of the island flap, described by Dunham (1893) and Monks (1898), consisted of nourishing vessels, mainly an artery. Littler (1960) incorporated into the stalk a sensory nerve as well. He stressed the importance of sensation in the hand. "Anaesthetic hand," he wrote, "is a blind hand." Such a hand is in constant jeopardy, since it cannot perceive and ward off injuries. Without sensation, moreover, the prehension of the hand is impaired. Littler advised expending every effort to restore sensation at the opposing areas of the digits—in particular, the volar aspect of the thumb and the radiovolar surface of the index finger.

To replenish critical pulp sensitivity in the above areas, an island of skin and subcutaneous tissue is raised from the ulnar pulp of the middle or ring finger. The nerve and vessels leading to this island are dissected out from the distal palmar crease onward. To gain unfettered mobility for the neurovascular pedicle, the artery forking out from the common volar vessel and going to the adjacent finger is doubly ligated and severed between the two ligatures; for analogous reasons the dorsal branch of the digital nerve is sacrificed. The island of skin, with its neurovascular stalk, is now led through a subfacial tunnel to the base of the insensitive digit. The bridge of skin on the digit is slit, and a groove is developed to comfortably contain the stalk of the island flap. An appropriate patch of skin and subcutaneous tissue is removed from the recipient digit, and the island flap is sutured in its place. The neurovascular stalk is buried in the previously prepared groove on the side of the insensitive digit. The defect on the donor finger is surfaced with free full-thickness skin (Fig. 6–21).

REMOTE FLAPS

The operation of replenishing skin and subcutaneous tissue with the aid of pedicled grafts obtained from distant areas has come to be called the Italian method, since it was originally described by Tagliacozzi (1597), the Italian surgeon. This method was applied to the hand by Kummer (1891), who raised a flap of skin from the chest to line the raw surface of webbed fingers which had been surgically separated. Not long after, Stone (1908) wrote: "In plastic restoration of the hand the most valuable procedure, one seldom used, is the adaptation of the Italian method of fixing the part of the skin of another portion of the body, and, after an interval, severing the flap. This method is . . . easily applied . . . to the hand. . . ."

Pedicled flaps transposed from distant areas are qualified as being tubed or untubed. Tubulation of the skin was described by Prince (1868), who recorded a "triumphant example" of its application. Prince distinguished two types of tubes: those formed by inversion and the ones fashioned by eversion. Nicoladini (1897)

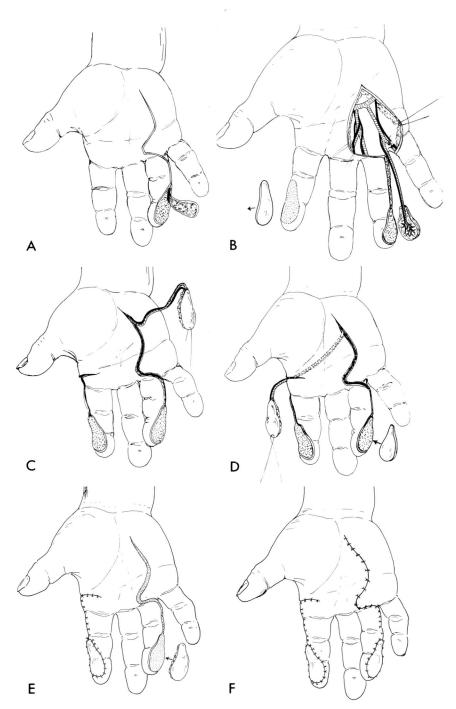

Figure 6–21   Sketches illustrating the technique of neurovascular island graft. *A,* Incision for elevation of the island graft from the ulnar aspect of the ring finger pulp. *B,* Isolation of the neurovascular stalk. *C,* Incision for the removal of insensitive skin on the radial side of the index pulp and for the groove into which the stalk of the island graft is to be buried. *D,* Passing the graft through a tunnel in the palm and free full-thickness graft to surface the denuded area on the ulnar aspect of the ring finger pulp. *E,* Suturing the island graft to the index finger. *F,* Closure.

discussed the use of a closed tube in reconstructing the thumb. He spoke of raising a flap from under the breast, converting it into a tube, and inserting the raw stump of the thumb into it. Nicoladini also suggested incorporating a piece of bone inside the tube as a method of reconstructing the thumb, thus foreshadowing the composite grafts of more recent surgeons. *Marsupialization* is a modern term for tubes formed by eversion.

Webster (1959), who otherwise produced an excellent review of the early history of the tubed flap, overlooked the contributions of Prince and Nicoladini. Webster devoted considerable space to the controversy as to who originated the bipedicled tube — Filatov or Gillies. Filatov (1917), the Russian eye surgeon, described a tube he had raised in September, 1916. Gillies (1920), who is widely credited for this method, performed his operation in October, 1917, and published his first paper on the subject three years later.

The elevation and transfer of pedicled flaps is now well standardized. It is important that the area selected for the donor site have very little subcutaneous fat and possess no hair, nor latent potentiality to grow hair. In adults, one can see if the donor site is hairy or not. In children, it is often difficult to ascertain if the area selected will or will not sprout hair in the future. The sex of the child and its ancestry may provide clues: hairy parents, especially those of southern European and Mediterranean extraction, beget hairy offspring; in females, the skin over the lower ribs and upper abdomen is not likely to sprout hair. For comfort, the side of the torso opposite the hand to which the flap is to be attached is selected.

When the mobility of the skin of the donor site is tested, it will be found that the fold, which is easily plucked, will slant in the direction of the cleavage lines of the area: in the upper abdomen it will incline from the lateral border down and medially toward the umbilicus. This portion of the abdominal wall receives its main nutrient supply from the lower intercostal and the lateral lumbar arteries. These vessels are segmentally arranged and pierce the deep fascia along the outer border of the abdomen; they then run downward parallel with the tension lines, or in the same direction as the pluckable fold of skin. For better nourishment, the flap should also have a wide base which falls in the path of the segmental vessels mentioned. If the incisions are made parallel with the tension lines, more pliable skin will be obtained.

For elevation of a bipedicled tube, two parallel incisions are made in the selected donor area. The length of these incisions may vary from 8 to 12 cm., depending on the amount of skin needed; the interval between them should not be less than one-third of their length. In the upper quadrant of the abdomen and the adjoining area of the lower chest, the proximal incision starts at a point 2 or 3 cm. medial to the inception of the distal incision and ends that much closer to the midline of the abdomen. If one visualizes imaginary lines connecting the beginnings and the ends of the two incisions, the results would be a parallelogram. This pattern provides a broad base to each pedicle and makes it available for a greater number of segmental vessels than if the pattern simulates a rectangle.

The skin incisions are developed down to, but not through, the deep fascia; the interval between the two parallel incisions is undermined; the flap thus procured is lifted. The underlying raw surface is covered by subjecting the margins of the abdominal incision to Z-plasty and approximating them. The cut margins of the lifted flap are now defatted and sutured together, closing its areolar interior.

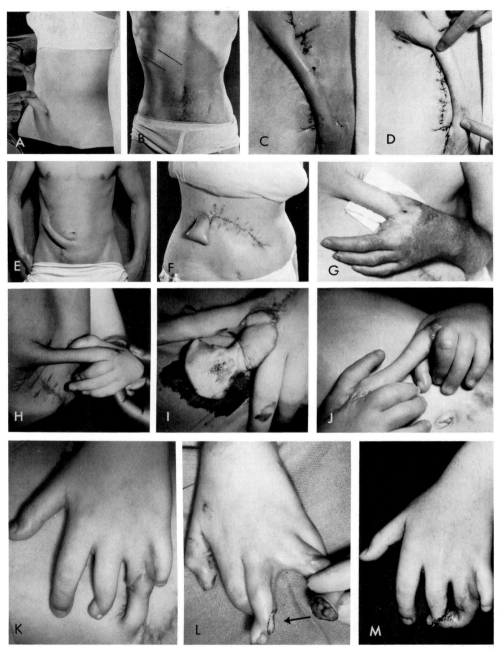

Figure 6–22   Tubes. *A,* Selection of the skin to be tubed from a pluckable hairless area. *B,* Design and spacing of the incisions. *C,* Closure of the superior corner of the donor area by Z-plasty. *D,* Closure of the inferior corner of the donor area. *E,* The tube after the incisions have healed. *F,* The tube whose detached end has been closed upon itself. *G,* Attachment of the tube to a hand without a thumb and index finger: later, on a bone peg was inserted into it for procuring an oppositional post. *H,* Attachment of the tube to the widened webspace between the index and middle fingers. *I,* The other end of the tube is detached from the abdomen and (*J*) connected to the deepened webspace between the index and middle fingers of the opposite thumbless hand. *K,* Attachment of the tube to a congenitally stunted ring finger. *L,* Weaning of the tube. *M,* Attachment of the weaned end to the scarred distal phalanx of the middle finger to provide pliable skin preliminary to corrective osteotomy of the angulated bone.

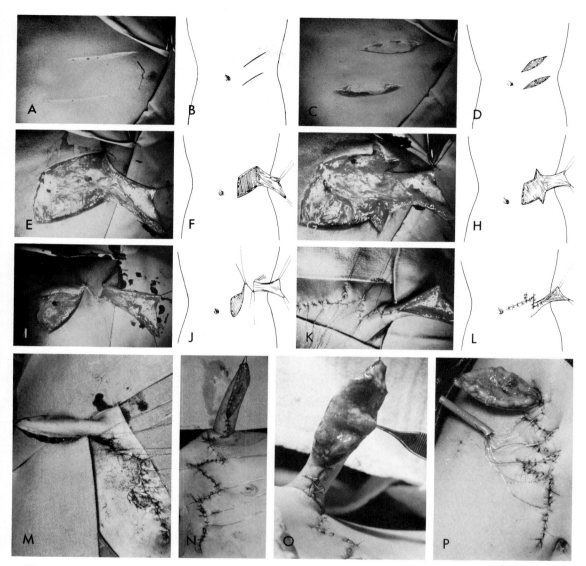

Figure 6–23 Elevation of partially tubed (petal) flap. *A* and *B* demonstrate parallelogram design for incisions in the left upper quadrant of the abdomen. *C* and *D* show deepening of the incision down to the deep fascia. In *E* and *F* is seen the lifted flap, and in *G* and *H* are shown the side cuts in the donor area in preparation for Z-plasty. *I* and *J* show the beginning of Z-plasty, and the completion of closure of the abdominal wound and tubing of the stem of the flap are seen in *K* and *L*. Depending upon the direction of the first triangular flap at the base of the pedicle, the flap graft may be made to turn toward the right *M*, face forward, as in *N* and *O*, or turn toward the left *P*.

For attachment to the hand, the pedicle nearer the midline is disconnected from the abdomen—usually in two or three weeks—by an oval incision. The end petal of skin thus raised should be about 4 cm. in diameter. The oval area of defect on the abdomen is closed by undermining the skin edges and drawing them together with interrupted sutures. Near the midline there will be some puckering, which is done away with by running a small slit from the dome of the oval cut toward the midline and trimming the sharp corners ("dog ears") thus created. If the circulation of the detached end appears precarious, it may be wise to postpone the attachment of the graft to the hand; the end flap of the graft is

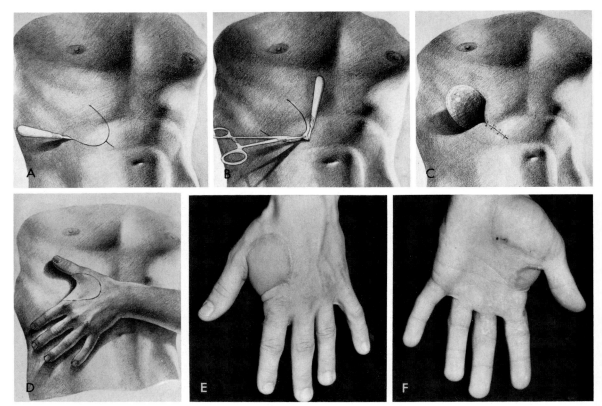

Figure 6-24   Petal flap. *A,* Incision in the right upper quadrant of the abdomen. *B,* The "dog-ears" of donor-site skin are being cut. *C,* Closure of the donor site. *D,* Design for application of the petal to the widened first webspace of the left hand. *E,* Dorsal view of the grafted left hand. *F,* Palmar view.

temporarily closed on itself to see how much of it will slough. Avascular skin will turn purplish or black in a week; the necrotic skin is trimmed down to a bleeding point, and then the tube is connected to the hand. Six weeks after connecting the tube to the hand, the nourishing pedicle of the tube is weaned from the abdomen. In some cases, the opposite hand also requires reconstructive work. The weaned end of the tube is connected to this hand. After seven weeks, the tube is divided in the middle and portioned between the two hands. The technique of elevating and transferring untubed (petal), partly tubed (stemmed petal), or folded (pillow-case) flaps with a single pedicle is not unlike that employed for bipedicled tubes. The petal or stemmed petal flap with a single pedicle has an advantage in that it need not be delayed for three weeks after it is raised but can be attached to the hand at the same sitting (Figs. 6–22 to 6–26).

    Tubes provide thick, unwieldy skin. When thinner skin is needed, as over the fingers and the dorsum of the hand, especially when one hand is involved, flaps are preferred. Tubes, as well as flaps, transferred from distant areas tend to become pigmented and they get fatter if the donor site—from which they have been detached—becomes fatter. Disregarding this latent potentiality and in anticipation of future reconstructive work, it is judicious to pile up on the hand more skin than is needed, making allowance for wastage and refinement; bulky grafts may be defatted and readjusted at a future time.

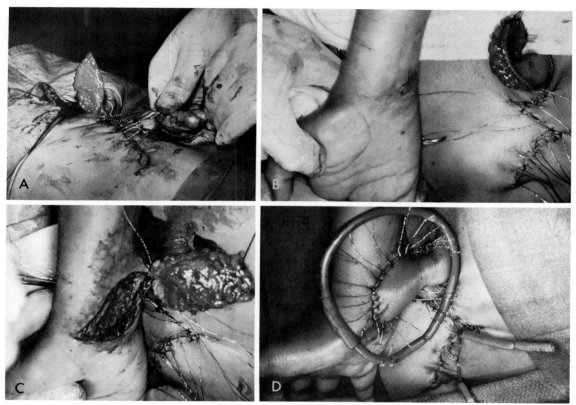

Figure 6-25   *A*, Petal flap raised from the abdomen. In *B*, the same flap facing the volar surface of the right wrist is shown: this area had been subjected to Z-plasty which resulted in an ulcer surrounded by scar tissue adhering to the underlying tendons. *C*, The ulcer and the scar of the wrist have been resected and the petal flap is approximated to it. *D*, Closure with wire sutures which are tied to a catheter to prevent the ends from sticking the patient.

Skin grafting is just one link in the chain of procedures used to improve the function and appearance of congenitally maimed hands. In some malformations, timely skin grafting makes corrective operations of the bones and joints unnecessary. Syndactylism of two fingers of unequal length provides a pertinent example. When fingers are bound together up to their tips, the longer of the two tends to incline towards its shorter mate; the joints of the one digit are splinted by the bones of the other and lose their mobility. Timely separation of such fingers and the insulation of each with skin will do away with the necessity of performing angulation osteotomy of the deviating digit or arthroplasty of the stiff joint.

DIGITAL DISENGAGEMENT

Separation of webbed fingers also serves as a salient example of what the author has chosen to call digital disengagement. In the treatment of syndactylism, in addition to splitting the cutaneous web between the conjoined digits, the author severs the deep transverse ligament proximally in order to establish a sufficiently deep commissure and obviate future recurrence. In pollicization of the

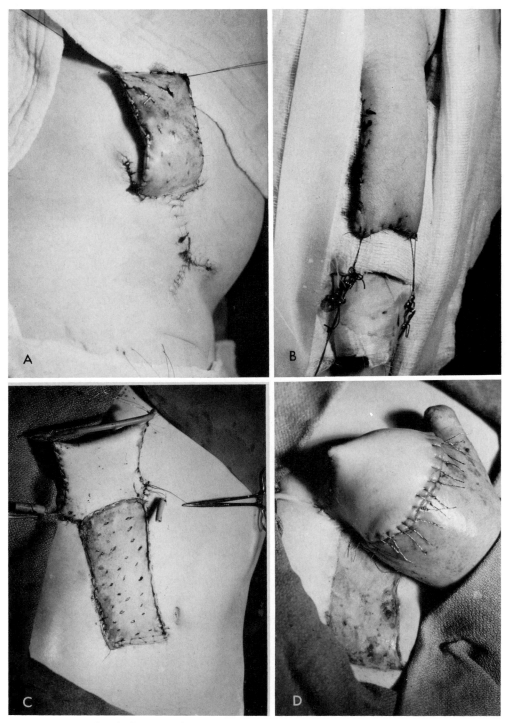

Figure 6–26   Seamed and pillow-case flaps. *A,* The undersurface of a flap—note that the raw surface is covered with split-thickness free graft. *B,* The graft is turned over a fine mesh gauze and held under tension by sutured eyes and hooks. *C,* The donor site is surfaced by free graft and the half of the flap is made to cover the other half. The denuded remnants of metacarpals of the left hand were later inserted into this pillow-case, as shown in *D.*

index finger, the following binding elements are cut: the juncture tendinum, which connects the extensor tendons of the index and long fingers; the deep transverse ligament between the metacarpals of the two digits and the interosseous ligament binding these bones proximally; the digital artery of the middle finger and the overlying transverse strands of palmar apaneurosis. In some cases of radial ray defect, the thumb is hypoplastic — it can be flexed and extended, but cannot be abducted and turned into opposition. In this condition and in the nonopposable variety of triphalangeal thumb, the first metacarpal is caught in the common bondage of the deep transverse ligament, which needs to be severed (Figs. 6–27 and 6–28).

SURGERY ON MUSCLES AND TENDONS

In 1852, Huguier (1874) operated on a patient with missing phalanges of the thumb. In order to deepen the first intermetacarpal space, he stripped the insertion of the thumb adductor. This was the first operation involving one of the muscles of the hand.

In earlier operations for correction of deformity of the hand due to an absent radius, the flexor tendons at the wrist were severed or subjected to Z-plasty. For some years now the author has been stripping the origin of contracted flexors from the medial epicondyle of the humerus. In connection with his swivel operation for proximal radioulnar synostosis, the author transfers the extensor carpi ulnaris and connects it to the tendon of the brachioradialis. In cases with congenital absence of the extensor pollicis longus, the author again uses the extensor carpi ulnaris as a motor and connects it, with the aid of an intermediary free tendon graft, to the terminal phalanx of the thumb. In congenital absence of lumbricals, the sublimis of the affected digit is transferred to its extensor expansion.

Occasionally, a child is born with two vestigial digits without flexors to pull them together and effect a pinch. In such a case, the author has obtained a free tendon graft from the extensor of the fourth toe, converted it into a "V," hooked the flexor carpi radialis to the apex of the "V," and connected the ends of the tendon graft to the terminal bones of each digit.

NERVE SUTURE

This is rarely indicated in congenital hand defects. In one variety of macrodactyly, the digital nerve is almost twice as long as the finger it supplies. The width of the macrodactylic digit cannot be reduced unless the redundant segment of the nerve is resected. The remaining ends are then sutured together.

SURGERY ON BONES AND JOINTS

Rather than amputate a macrodactylic digit, Massonnaud (1874) recommended surgical destruction of the growth cartilage plate. In some cases of

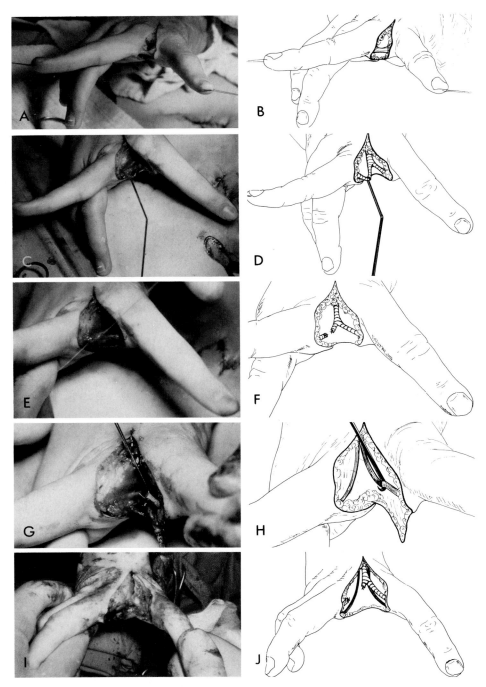

Figure 6–27 Digital disengagement. *A* and *B* show the incision across the web between the index and middle fingers to expose the deep transverse ligament which is cut. *C* and *D* demonstrate isolation of the digital artery running along the radial aspect of the middle finger; this artery is doubly ligated and severed between the ligatures, as shown in *E* and *F*. In *G* and *H* is seen the isolation of the digital nerve passing along the ulnar aspect of the index finger. As shown in *I* and *J*, the interdigital cleft is deepened proximally between the digital nerves supplying the contiguous sides of the index and middle fingers.

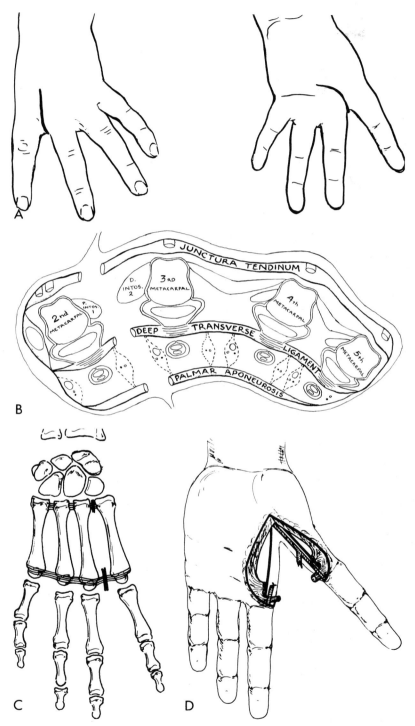

Figure 6–28 *A* shows the incisions for pollicization of the index finger. *B*, Fascial structures which need to be severed. *C*, Severance of deep transverse intermetacarpal ligament. *D*, Severance of the artery going to the middle finger.

macrodactyly, the ligaments around one of the joints are lax or the articular ends of the bones are interlocked. Nineteenth century authors recommended resection of incongruous bones and fusion of the joints for these cases. Both of these operations—epiphysiodesis and arthrodesis—have been revived recently.

Guermonprez (1887) ran through the entire gamut of joint resections and excision of bones to improve the function of the crippled hand. One of his favored operations was clefting of digitless hands or creation of lobster-claw deformity for a hand in which the digitless central three metacarpals prevented the two marginal digits from effecting a pinch: he removed the central three metacarpals. Guermonprez was also the first to pollicize one of the lesser digits, in particular the index and middle fingers. Lauenstein (1888) osteotomized the sec-

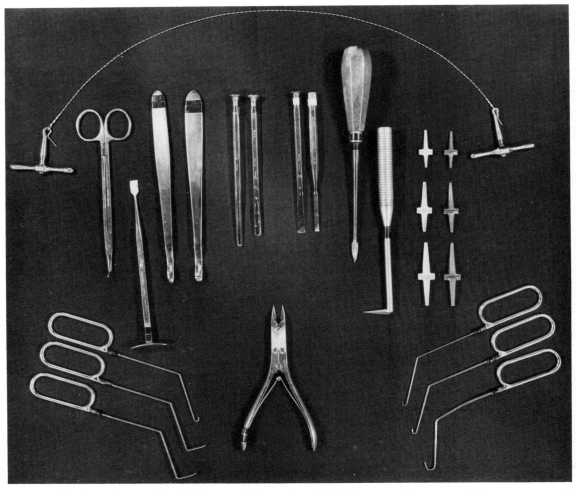

Figure 6–29 Armamentarium for bone and joint surgery. In this figure are shown some of the more commonly used retractors, curved and straight chisels, angular and straight ice-pick, and bone cutter. On the right, in the middle, are shown silicone rubber prostheses. Missing from this figure are the following: hand-drill, power-driven saw, and burr.

ond and fifth metacarpals of a thumbless hand, and rotated the index and little fingers into apposition. Herzog (1892) undertook two procedures to correct the angular deformity of the thumb: excision of the distal articular end of the proximal phalanx and cuneiform osteotomy through the shaft of this bone (Figs. 6–29 to 6–33).

Comparatively inert implants composed of vitallium, stainless steel, or silicone rubber are only occasionally used in the treatment of congenital anomalies of the hand and the forearm. In proximal radioulnar synostosis, the author utilizes a stainless steel swivel which will be described in Chapter Twenty-eight. In an occasional case of a stiff or interlocked proximal interphalangeal joint, oc-

(Text continued on page 183.)

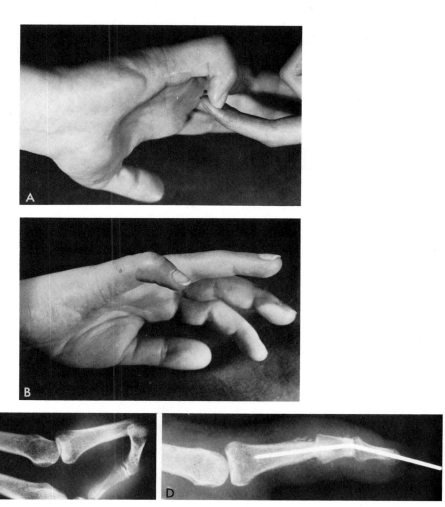

Figure 6–30 Interphalangeal fusion is occasionally indicated in congenital flexion contracture (camptodactyly) which affects the little finger most commonly. *A*, Ulnar view of the little finger which had been subjected to multiple operations, each aggravating the flexion deformity. *B*, Postoperative photograph. *C*, Preoperative roentgenograph. *D*, Postoperative roentgenograph; the K-wire was removed seven weeks after surgery.

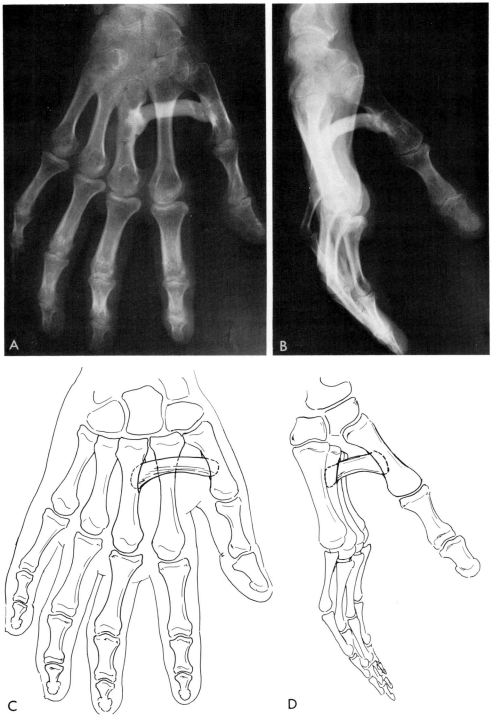

Figure 6–31   Intermetacarpal bone graft. *A*, Dorsopalmar roentgenograph of the right hand showing bone graft between the first and third metacarpals. *B*, Lateral view of the same. *C* and *D* are illustrative sketches of *A* and *B*, respectively. This operation is indicated in old cases of absent extensors and abductors of the thumb and in arthrogryposis.

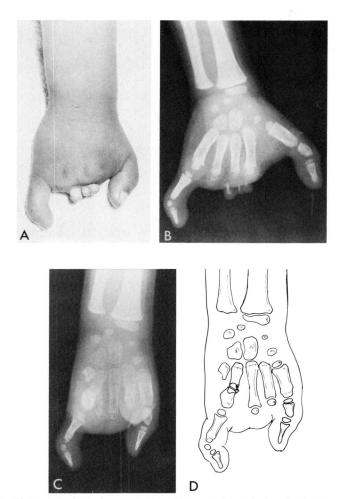

Figure 6–32   Shift of the little finger. *A*, Dorsal view of the right hand of a five-year-old female with agenesis of the central digits. She could not oppose the two remaining digits. Two alternative procedures were considered: (1), removal of portions of the central metacarpal in order to create a cleft with its apex pointing proximally, which would result in a lobster-claw deformity; (2), bringing the little finger closer to the thumb. The last procedure was chosen from both cosmetic and functional points of view — functional because it would procure a comparatively broader palm. *B*, Preoperative dorsopalmar roentgenograph of the hand. *C*, Postoperative roentgenograph. *D*, Sketch illustrating the surgical procedure.

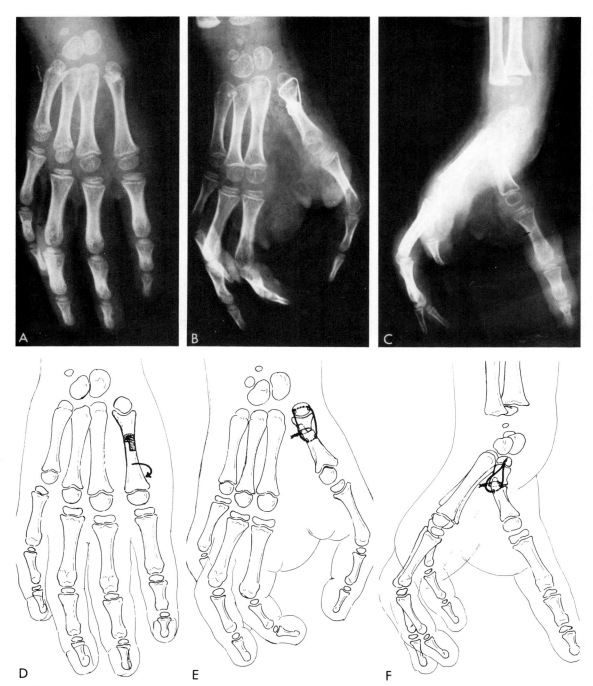

Figure 6–33 Shortening and rotation-angulation osteotomy of the index metacarpal and arrest of growth from accessory epiphysis. *A*, Roentgenograph of the hand of a three-year-old female with absent pollical ray — note that the metacarpal of the index bears an accessory epiphysis at its proximal end. *B*, The shortened metacarpal of the index finger has been moved away from its ulnar neighbor; a loop of wire is used to arrest the growth from the accessory epiphysis. *C*, The distal fragment of the osteotomized metacarpal is angulated in the palmar direction. *D*, *E*, and *F* illustrate some of the procedures mentioned.

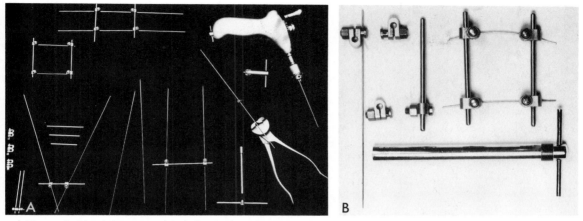

Figure 6–34 *A,* Armamentarium for the insertion of Kirschner wire (K-wire). *B,* Armamentarium for external fixation.

curring in late stages of macrodactyly, the affected articulation is mobilized with the aid of a silicone rubber insert.

USES OF THE KIRSCHNER WIRE

Lambotte (1928) appears to have been the first to attempt intramedullary fixation of the bones in the hand. In time, the Lambotte pin was replaced by Kirschner wire, K-wire for short, which has proved itself indispensable in

(Text continued on page 189.)

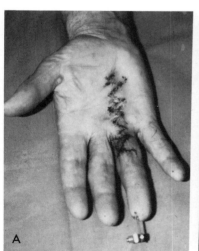
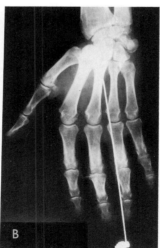
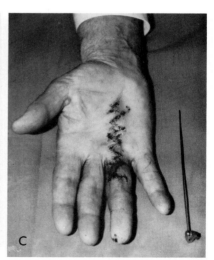

Figure 6–35 Percutaneous K-wire for internal splintage. *A,* Palmar view of the right hand which has been subjected to Z-plasty for contracture of the ring finger. *B,* Roentgenograph showing that the K-wire passes through soft tissues and thus acts as an internal splint during the postoperative period. *C,* The K-wire and its terminal nut after it has been extracted from the hand.

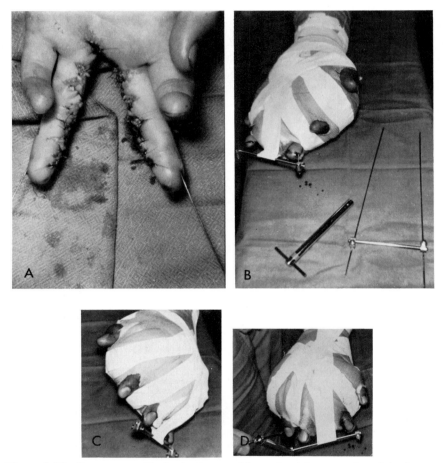

Figure 6–36   Percutaneous K-wire is often used for maintaining extension of the fingers after Z-plasty for flexion contracture of the fingers and after separation and surfacing of webbed fingers. *A*, K-wire is passed through the soft tissue on the radial aspect of the middle finger which had been separated from its ulnar neighbor and surfaced. *B*, Palmar view of the bandaged hand showing that K-wire has also passed through the ulnar aspect of the ring finger; the two digits thus splinted internally are held apart by a spreader bar. *C*, Dorsal view of the bandaged hand. *D* shows the use of a small wrench to tighten the nut over the spreader bar.

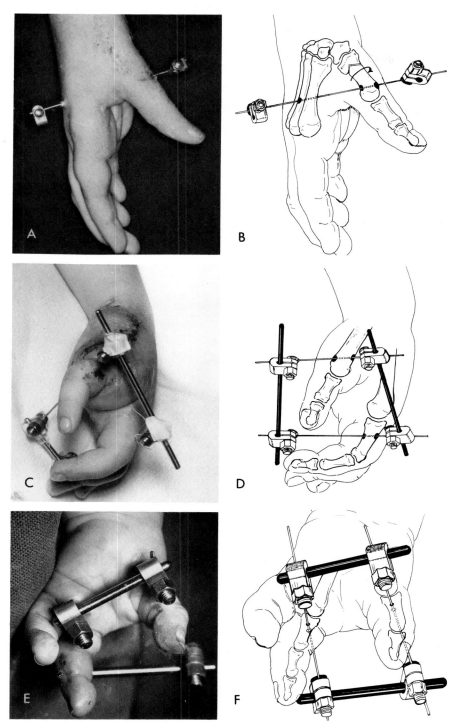

Figure 6–37 *A* and *B* show transfixation of the rotated distal fragment of the osteotomized first metacarpal to the metacarpal of the middle finger. In *C* and *D*, the metacarpal of the pollicized index finger is transfixed to the proximal phalanx of the middle finger. *E* and *F* show transfixation of the proximal phalanx of the thumb to the proximal phalanx of the neighboring digit in a tridactylic hand.

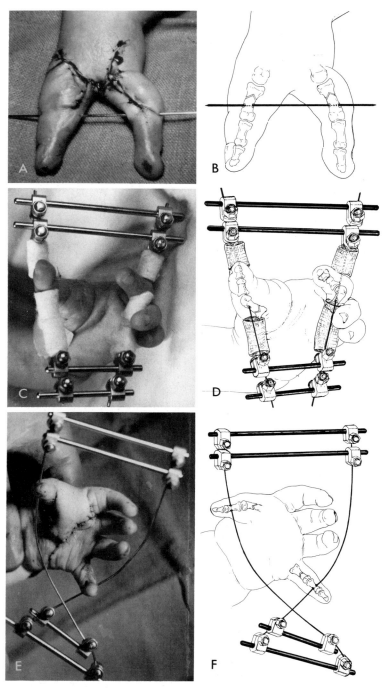

Figure 6–38 *A,* Transfixation after rotary osteotomy of the proximal phalanges of a child with two digits whose nails were in the same plane and failed to effect opposition. *B,* Illustrative sketch of the same. *C,* Transfixation after pollicization of the index finger. *D,* Illustrative sketch of same. *E* represents a hand with adduction contracture of the thumb, short fingers, and partly webbed fourth and fifth digits; the origin of the adductors transversus was released, the first metacarpal and proximal phalanx of the little finger were osteotomized, placed in opposition, and held with external fixation as shown in *F.*

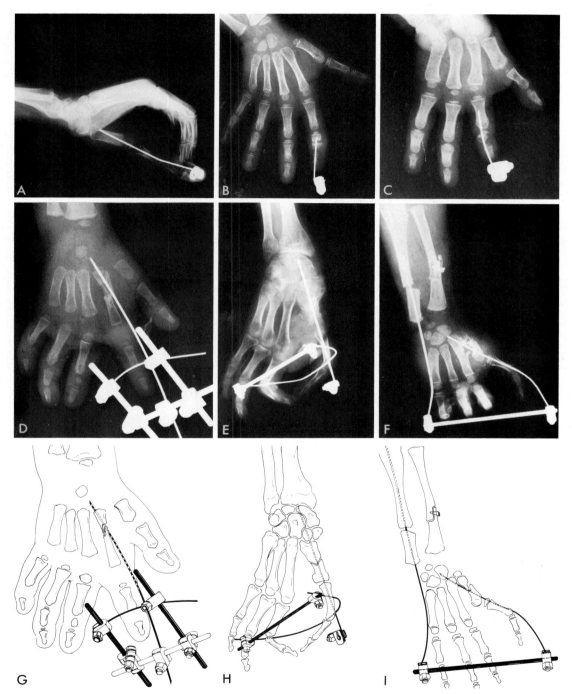

Figure 6–39 Axial intra-osseous insertion of K-wire. *A*, K-wire inserted through the phalanges of the thumb into the first metacarpal for fusion of the metacarpophalangeal joint. *B*, Inadequate transfixation of a fragment in a patient in whom osteotomy of the middle phalanx of the index finger has been performed for angular deformity at the second interphalangeal joint. *C*, Adequate transfixation after osteotomy through the delta-shaped middle phalanx. *D*, Transfixation after elongation osteotomy of the index metacarpal. *E*, Transfixation after pollicization of the index finger. *F*, shows the hand and forearm of a five-year-old boy who had a short radius, absent radial epiphysis, and curved ulna and absent pollical ray; in this case both the pollicized index finger and osteotomized ulna were transfixed by axially directed intra-osseous K-wires. *G*, *H*, and *I* are illustrative sketches of the roentgenograph above each.

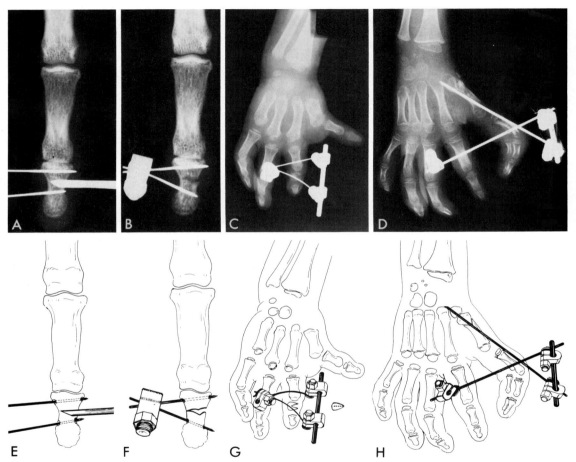

Figure 6–40 *A* shows two K-wires inserted into the ungual phalanx which deviated radially upon flexion at the distal interphalangeal joint. *B*, External transfixation after corrective osteotomy. *C*, External fixation after osteotomy for axial deviation of the index finger. *D*, Transfixation after rotary osteotomy of the first metacarpal in a patient in whom the first digital ray had two sets of three phalanges which failed to oppose the lesser digits. *E*, *F*, *G*, and *H* illustrate roentgenograph above each.

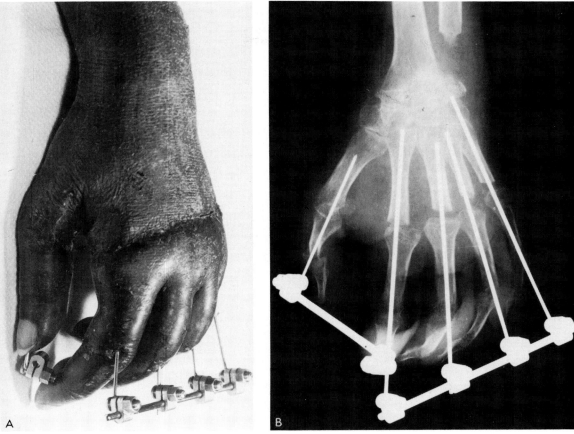

Figure 6–41 *A* and *B*, The use of K-wire after fusion of the metacarpophalangeal joint of the thumb and excision of the lesser metacarpal heads for the so-called wind-blown deformity of the digits.

surgery of the hand. In work on bone, K-wire is inserted either axially through the medullary cavity or transversely across the shaft of the bone. When only soft tissue work is done, the wire is made to pass under the skin, along the side of the skeletal elements. The protruding ends of the wires are transfixed externally (Figs. 6–34 to 6–41).

SUMMARY

Surgical techniques are transposable from one lesion to another, from one region of the body to another. Almost all procedures used in attempts at redressing acquired deformities are also utilized in the treatment of congenitally malformed hands. The most commonly employed methods are skinplasty, corrective osteotomy of bones, and digital transfer operations. Kirschner wire is considered an indispensable addition to the armamentarium of the hand surgeon.

References

Blair, V. P.: The full thickness skin graft. *Ann. Surg., 80*:298–314, 1924.

Blair, V. P., and Brown, J. B.: The use of large split skin grafts of intermediate thickness. *Surg. Gynecol. Obstet., 49*:87–96, 1929.

Celsus, A. C.: *De Medicina.* (With English translation by W. G. Spencer.) Cambridge, Massachusetts, Harvard University Press, Vol. 3, Book 7, pp. 362–364, 1935–1938. Original appeared around 25 B.C.

Davis, J. S.: *Plastic Surgery: Its Principles and Practice.* Philadelphia, P. Blakiston's Son & Co., pp. 1–35, 1919.

Denonvilliers: Blépharoplastie. *Bull. Soc. Chir., 7*:243, 1856–1857.

Dieffenbach, J. F.: *Chirurgische Erfahrungen besonders über Wiederherstellung zerstörter Teile des menschlichen Körpers nach neuen Methoden.* Berlin, T. C. F. Enslin, 1834.

Dunham, T.: A new method for obtaining a skin flap from the scalp and a permanent buried vascular pedicle for covering the face. *Ann. Surg., 17*:677–679, 1893.

Dutrochet, H.: Examples of reunion of parts completely separated from the body. *Gaz. de Santé.* Mar. 21, 1817. English translation in Gibson's (1961) article.

Esser, J. F. S.: Island flaps. *New York Med. J., 106*:264–265, 1917.

Fayrer, J.: *Clinical Surgery in India.* London, Churchill & Sons, pp. 595–601, 688–706, 1866.

Filatov, V. P.: Plastic procedure using a round pedicle. *Vestn. Oftalmol., 34*:149–153, 1917. See translation in *Surg. Clin. North Am., 39*:277–287, 1959.

Gersuny, R.: Plastischer Ersatz der Wangenschleimhaut. *Cbl. Cirs., 14*:706–708, 1887.

Gibson, T.: Flagellation and free grafting. *Br. J. Plast. Surg., 13*:195–203, 1961.

Gillies, H. D.: The tubed pedicle in plastic surgery. *New York Med. J., 111*:1–12, 1920.

Gillies, H. D., and Millard, D. R., Jr.: *The Principles and Art of Plastic Surgery.* Boston, Little, Brown & Co., Vol. 7, pp. 481–495, 1957.

Gnudi, M. T., and Webster, J. P.: *The Life and Times of Gaspare Tagliacozzi.* New York, H. Reichner, pp. 183–216; 305–332, 1950.

Guermonprez, F.: *Notes sur quelques Resections et Restaurations du Pouce.* Paris, P. Aselin, pp. 5–52, 1887.

Herzog, W.: Über angeborene Deviation der Fingerphalangen. *Münch. Med. Wochenschr., 39*:344–345, 1892.

Huguier, P. C.: Considérations anatomiques et physiologiques sur le rôle du pouce et sur la chirurgie de cette organ. *Arch. Gén. Méd., 2*:404–421; 567–580; 692–707, 1873, and *1*:54–82, 1874.

Iselin, F.: Traitement chirurgical des syndactylies congénitales. *Rev. Prat., 10*:2511–2620, 1960.

Krause, F.: Über die Transplantation grosser, ungestielter Hautlappen. *Arch. Klin. Chir., 46*:177–182, 1893.

Kummer, E.: Syndactylie congénitale anaplastie d'après la methode Italienne. *Rev. d'Orthop., 2*:129–133, 1891.

Lambotte, A.: Contribution à la chirurgie conservatrice de la main dans les traumatismes. *Arch. Franco-Belges. Chir., 31*:759–764, 1928.

Lauenstein, C.: Ein neuer Vorschlag auf operativem Weg die Brauchbarkeit der daumenlosen Hand zu verbessern. *Dtsch. Med. Wochenschr., 14*:612–613, 1888.

Lennander, K. B.: Fall af kongenital syndaktyli, opereradt med hjelp af Thiersch's hudtransplantationsmetod. *Upsala Lak. Forhandlingar., 26*:151–152, 1891.

Lewin, M. L.: Digital flaps. *Plast. Reconstr. Surg., 7*:46–49, 1951.

Limberg, A. A.: *Collection of Scientific Works in Memory of 50th Anniversary of the Medical Postgraduate Institute.* Leningrad, pp. 461–489, 1964. Original said to have been published 1929. See: *Planning of Local Plastic Operations of Body's Surface.* (In Russian.) Leningrad, Medgiz, pp. 145–593, 1963. Also: Design of local flaps. *In* Gibson, T., (ed.): *Modern Trends in Plastic Surgery.* Second series. London, Butterworth, p. 38, 1966.

Littler, J. W.: Neurovascular skin island transfer in reconstructive surgery of the hand. *Tr. Int. Soc. Plast. Surgeons.* London, E. & S. Livingstone Ltd., pp. 175–178, 1960.

MacCollum, D. W.: Webbed fingers. *Surg. Gynecol. Obstet., 71*:782–789, 1940.

Massonnaud, A.: *Essai sur la Pathogénie de l'Hypertrophie Unilatérale.* Thèse. Paris, A. Parent, pp. 5–34, 1874.

Monks, G. H.: The restoration of a lower eyelid by a new method. *Boston Med. Surg. J., 139*:385–387, 1898.

Morestin, H.: De la correction des flexions permanentes des doigts consécutives aux panaris et aux phlegmons de la paume de la main. *Rev. Chir., 50*:1–27, 1914.

Nicoladini, C.: Daumenplastik. *Wien. Klin. Wochenschr., 10*:663–665, 1897.

Norton, A. T.: A new reliable operation for the cure of webbed fingers. *Br. Med. J., 2*:931–932, 1881.

Ollier, L.: Greffe cutanée ou autoplastique. *Bull. Acad. Med., 1*:243–250, 1872.

Peacock, E. E., Jr.: Reconstruction of the hand by the local transfer of composite tissue island flaps. *Plast. Reconstr. Surg., 25*:298–322, 1960.

Pieri, G.: Plastica cutanea per le retrazioni cicatriziali delle dita. *Chir. Org. Mov., 4*:303–306, 1920.

Pippett, A.: *The Moth and the Star: A Biography of Virginia Woolf.* Boston, Little, Brown & Co., p. 64, 1953.

Prince, D.: *Plastics: A New Classification and Brief Exposition of Plastic Surgery.* Philadelphia, Lindsay and Blakiston, pp. 31–32, 1868.

Reverdin, J.: Greffe épidermique. *Bull. Soc. Imp. Chir., 10*:511–515, 1870.

Rogers, B. O.: Historical development of free skin grafting. *Surg. Clin. North Am., 39*:290–309, 1959.

Serre: *Traite sur l'Art de Restaurer les Difformités de la Face.* Montpellier, L. Castel, Paris, J. B. Baillière, pp. 1–468, 1842.

Steindler, A.: Skin flap methods in the upper extremity. *J. Bone Joint Surg., 7*:512–527, 1925.

Stone, J. S.: Plastic surgery. *In* Bryant, J. D., and Buck, A. H., (eds.): *American Practice of Surgery.* New York, William Wood & Co., *4*:610–636, 1908.

Szymanowski, J. V.: *Handbuch der operativen Chirurgie.* Braunschweig, Druck. Verlag von Friedrich Vieweg und Sohn, pp. 167–205, 1870.

Tagliacozzi, G.: *De Curtorum Chirurgia.* See Gnudi, M. T., and Webster, J. P.: *The Life and Times of Gaspare Tagliacozzi.* New York, H. Reichner, pp. 183–208, 1950. Original published in 1597.

Teale: On plastic operations upon the face and neck. *The Half Yearly Abstract of the Medical Sciences, 26*:152–154, 1858.

Thiersch, C.: Über Hautverpflanzung. *Verh. Dtsch. Ges. Chir., 15*:18–19, 1886.

Webster, J. P.: The early history of the tubed pedicle flap. *Surg. Clin. North Am., 39*:261–275, 1959.

Wolfe, J. R.: A new method of performing plastic operations. *Br. Med. J., 2*:360–361, 1875.

Zeller, S. J.: *Über die ersten Erscheinungen venerischer Localkrankheit.* Vienna, J. G. Bibz. pp. 107–112, 1810.

Chapter Seven

ANOMALIES OF THE NAILS

The nails are epidermal appendages. Like the superficial layer of the skin, pilosebaceous apparatus, the teeth, mammary glands, the linings of bodily apertures, nerves, and many elements of the eye, including the lens, they are derived from ectoderm. Most congenital anomalies of the nails are components of syndromes in which a varying number of ectodermal derivatives are affected. The nails also reflect abnormalities in size and shape of the underlying phalanges, which are mesodermal derivatives.

DEVELOPMENT AND GROWTH OF THE NAIL

The nails are the last elements of the embryonic hand to develop. By the tenth week of intrauterine life, the three layers of the epidermis—periderm (epitrichium), stratum intermedium, and stratum germinativum—have become differentiated. The fetal periderm and stratum intermedium represent, respectively, the stratum corneum and stratum lucidum of the mature epidermis.

During the tenth week of intrauterine life, a depression becomes delineated over the dorsal tip of the fetal finger. This area marks the site of the nail field. The future nail plate is formed within the stratum intermedium; it is covered on the top by a continuation of the periderm and rests on the deeper stratum germinativum.

From the tenth to the twentieth weeks of intrauterine life, the nail field undergoes a number of changes. It sinks deeper below the general surface of the skin covering the dorsum of the terminal phalanx, and expands sideways, backward, and forward, establishing distinct boundaries. Proximally, the nail field is bounded by an epidermal infolding, which is to become the future nail fold. Two shallow grooves mark the sides of the nail field, and in front there is a distinct flat depression called the distal groove.

The buried strip of stratum intermedium undergoes a process of hardening, which is not well understood but is considered akin to keratinization. The keratinized nail plate erupts, as do teeth, through the overlying periderm. The periderm gradually disappears from all areas except from a small section just in front of the nail fold. This remnant periderm is called eponychium. Simultaneous with the shedding of its surface covering, the nail plate pushes its way backward and becomes firmly rooted beneath the eponychium. At the same time, the nail plate grows forward until its free margin forms an eave atop the fingertip. The remnant of the periderm beneath the free border of the nail is called hyponychium. At full term, the cornified content of stratum intermedium, now resembling an adult nail in miniature, juts forward and may need trimming. The mature nail consists of a visible part and a root which lies hidden under the nail fold.

The nail as a whole is provided with a bed which is lined with stratum germinativum. The proximal part of the nail bed is called the germinal matrix because it is concerned with the formation and growth of the nail. The part of the visible nail overlying the germinal matrix is called the lunula; this is a grayish, opaque crescent which occasionally — most commonly in the young — is seen distal to the eponychium. The germinal matrix lies under the lunula, extending from the distal margin of the lunula backward under the nail root to where the nail fold is reflected as the roof of the nail root. Some authors think the reflected portion of the nail fold contributes to the formation of the superficial lamina of the nail, while the matrix below generates the deeper layers. The germinal matrix progressively contributes to the thickness of the nail. As a result, the nail is thicker at the distal lunula than near the nail fold. From the distal border of the lunula forward, the nail is uniform in thickness. The cuticle trimmed by the manicurist is the cornified edge of the eponychium.

The part of the nail bed distal to the germinal matrix is called the sterile matrix, since it does not contribute to the growth of the nail but merely provides a smooth surface over which the growing nail glides forward. The nonfecund matrix extends from under the distal border of the lunula to a line which separates the anterior margin of the nail from the underlying skin of the fingertip. Boas (1894) advanced the view — which many authors have since supported — that the terminal strip of the nail bed, the "sole horn," is capable of proliferative activity and contributes to the horny substance of the nail. It is presumed that overactivity of this distal germinal matrix might bring about hyperkeratotic conditions. The nail bed controls the longitudinal striation and smoothness of the overlying plate, and its irregularities lead to distortion of the latter (Fig. 7–1).

The nail grows constantly. It grows forward instead of backward owing to the pressure exerted by the posterior reflected wall of the nail fold. The growth of the nail is accelerated in childhood; it becomes sluggish with advancing age. The nail grows more rapidly in boys than in girls; it grows faster in nail-biters; it grows less rapidly in poorly nourished than in well-nourished children. The growth of the nail is most rapid in the middle or axial digit; it is slowest in the little finger. The growth of the fingernail is said to vary between 0.5 and 1.2 mm. per week. On the average, the fingernail grows at the rate of 119 microns per day or 3 mm. a month. It takes about 180 days for an avulsed nail to renew itself, providing that the underlying matrix remains undamaged and in situ.

TERMINOLOGY

Nineteenth century authors distinguished three classes of congenital anomalies of the nail: (1) absences; (2) anomalies of augmentation; and (3) abnor-

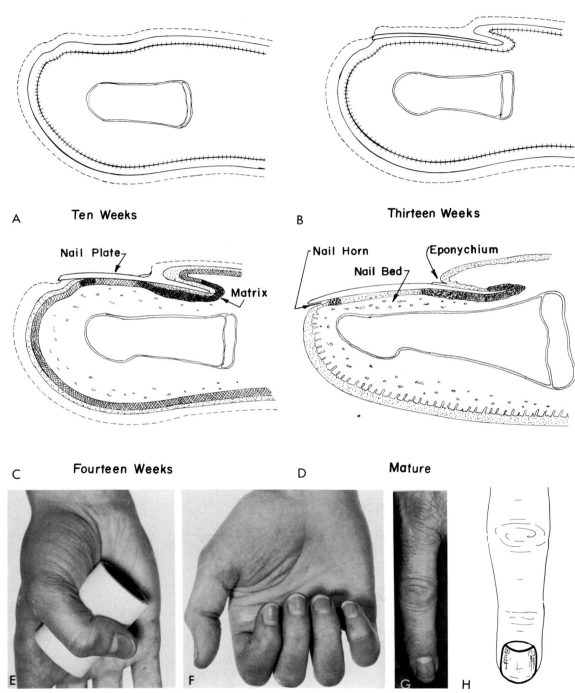

Figure 7–1   The development and maturity of the nail. Sketches *A, B, C,* and *D* illustrate various stages of the development of the nail. In *E, F,* and *G* are seen mature thumb and fingernails. *H,* Sketch illustrating the lunula seen in *G.*

malities of implantation. The last group includes nail formation in ectopic areas (for example, in the palmar aspect of the finger). Heterotopic nails are extremely rare. Under the second group are considered augmentation of number seen in polydactyly and increase in size occurring in syndactyly, when two or more confluent digits share one large nail, and in macrodactyly. Abnormally developing nails assume bizarre configurations, consistency, and coloring or lack of coloring. Occasionally, nails fail to develop altogether or are represented by atrophic rudiments.

Total or partial absence of a nail has come to be known as anonychia. There are clinical gradations of this condition, ranging from total, through partial absence, to stunting of the nail. Nails which have been reduced to rudiments are said to be atrophic, and the condition is onychatrophy. Vestigial nails approach normalcy as one passes from the radial to the ulnar border of the hand. In most cases of onychatrophy, the thumb or the index finger or both may be without any nail, while the nail of the little finger is normal. Anonychia and onychatrophy are considered variations of the same disorder and are often discussed together. In both anonychia and onychatrophy, comparable changes affect the toenails. Similarly, in the foot, the nails on the preaxial digits—on the big toe in particular—are more extensively affected.

Onychodystrophy is a generic term which is sometimes employed synonymously with anonychia or onychatrophy, but it is more often used in referring to the following disorders: koilonychia, leukonychia, onychogryposis, and pachyonychia. Koilonychia means spoon-shaped nail, and leukonychia, white nail. Onychogryposis refers to the hypertrophy and thickening of the nail. In pachyonychia, the nail plate is thick but not elongated; in addition, the space under the free margin of the nail is packed with a dark, friable, horny mass. Because of its resemblance to a miniature tennis racket, DuBois (1926) applied the designation racket nail—*ongle en raquette*—to the short, oblong nail overlying stub thumb. Prado-Castello and Prado (1960) preferred the term micronychia for such nails and referred to nails seen on oversized digits as macronychia (Fig. 7–2).

HYPERKERATOSIS OF THE NAIL BED

Wilson (1905) described a pedigree in which eight members in three generations were affected with uncomplicated hyperkeratosis of the nail beds. The proband was a 10-month-old male infant. He had normal appearing skin, hair, and teeth, and did not seem to have any other congenital defects. The surface of the nail was smooth. The nail itself appeared normal at its base, but toward the free extremity it was lifted from its matrix by a dark, friable, horny mass. The nail seemed to grow faster than the horny tissue underneath; the latter sloped down and backward from the free border of the nail.

Murray's (1921) case was a 12-year-old female whose fingernails were raised at their free ends by dark, yellowish, horny masses which projected at an angle from the nail beds. This girl's grandfather, her own mother, and two other children in the same family were similarly affected; all of them also had erupted teeth at birth. Thomson's (1928) patient was a five-year-old female with brittle nails which became thicker toward the distal ends. Thomson referred to this anomaly as hereditary dystrophy of the nails and traced its transmission through four generations.

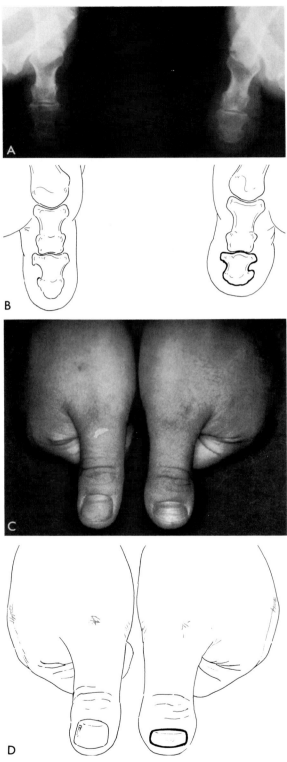

Figure 7–2   Racket nail. *A*, Dorsovolar roentgenograph of right and left thumbs; the latter has a squat ungual phalanx. *B*, Sketch illustrating the same. *C*, Dorsal view of the thumbs of a patient with left racket nail. *D*, Sketch illustrating the same.

ONYCHOGRYPOSIS

This designation refers to nails which are thick, long, and curved. As a congenital anomaly, onychogryposis most often occurs in the big toe. Vidal (1865) reported a case of pre-axial polydactyly. The first radial digit in this hexadactylic hand had a nail which was very thick and curved, and looked like the claw of a carnivorous animal. Sympson's (1888) case with claw-shaped nails was an 11-year-old girl whose mother stated that "the malformation . . . was present at birth." Clement (1928) described a family in which six members in two generations—four men and two women—showed claw fingers, meaning fingers with onychogryptotic nails. Hereditary onychogryposis is transmitted as an autosomal dominant trait.

LEUKONYCHIA

Total, partial, or striated white nails in newborns have been reported by the following authors: Furst (1884), Hedderich (1910), Sibley (1922), DuBois (1926), Becker (1930), Costa (1947), Lingamfelter and Whitmore (1954), and Harrington (1964). Harrington's patient had "porcelain white and lusterless" nails which he considered as belonging to the category of congenital leukonychia totalis. Harrington estimated that up to 1960 a total of about 60 cases of inherited leukonychia totalis has been reported. Congenital leukonychia appears to be about one-tenth as common. In hereditary cases, the trait of leukonychia is transmitted as an autosomal dominant trait. In the pedigree described by Bauer (1920), all but two individuals with leukonychia had multiple sebaceous cysts. Cockayne (1933) explained this association on the basis of a linkage of two independent genes. Graciansky and Boulle (1961) are among many who have noted the concomitant occurrence of leukonychia and koilonychia or spoon nails (Figs. 7–3 and 7–4).

KOILONYCHIA

Children are born with comparatively flat nails. This condition is called platonychia. As children grow, the nail gradually becomes convex. In some instances, the nail is concave at birth, and this condition persists for the rest of the person's life. Ormsby (1917) presented a 14-year-old girl whose nails were so deeply hollowed out that some of them could hold ten drops of water. Cipollaro (1930) described a 31-year-old female who had spoon-shaped nails since birth. The nails of both hands were affected. The anomaly was most marked in the thumbnails. It became progressively less conspicuous toward the ulnar border of the hand. The affected nails were painful at the points of greatest depression. The right thumbnail possessed the greatest depression and had a capacity of 0.25 cc. of water. Halperin (1967) reported a case of congenital koilonychia in a six-year-old child. Inherited koilonychia is comparatively rare and is transmitted as an autosomal dominant trait.

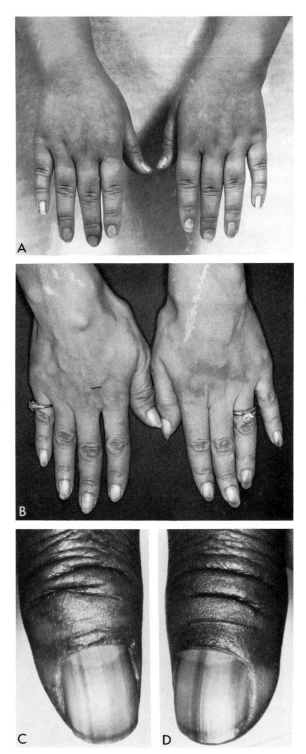

Figure 7–3   *A*, Total leukonychia of the fingernails of the little fingers, and punctate and patchy involvement of some other nails. *B*, Partial leukonychia of the nails. *C* and *D*, Thumbnails with striated leukonychia.

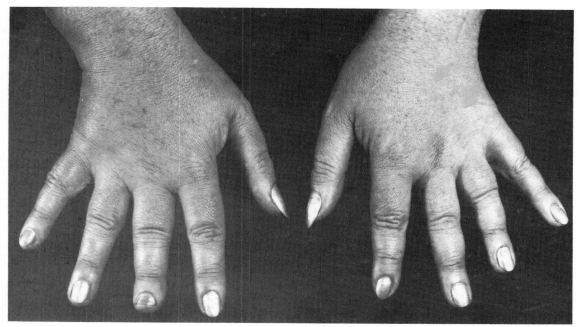

Figure 7–4   Total leukonychia of three nails in each hand and partial involvement of the others.

ABSENCE OF THE NAIL FOLD

Jamieson (1893) presented a 22-year-old female whose nail seemed "to grow directly from the epidermis covering the dorsum of the finger—the nail fold which covers and protects the nail-plate being absent." The nail plate was thin at its posterior part; it gradually became denser and harder, and tended to split longitudinally. The propositus could not remember her "nails in any other state." Jamieson considered her condition as one of congenital origin. An elder sister also had nails like the patient, but "recovered."

NEVUS STRIATICUS SYMMETRICUS UNGUIS

Oppenheim and Cohen (1942) reported a 38-year-old woman with a malformation of the thumbnails. The condition has been present since birth. In the center of each thumbnail there was a linear area measuring 3 mm. in width and 13 mm. in length. This area was marked by parallel dark lines which extended from the posterior nail fold to the free border of the nail. Oliver and Bluefarb (1944) presented a 12-year-old girl with a similar anomaly which also affected the nails of her little fingers (Fig. 7–5).

ANONYCHIA AND ONYCHATROPHY

Sporadic cases of absent or atrophic nails have been reported by the following authors: Eichhorst (1893), Bergé and Weisenbach (1912), Sibley (1919–

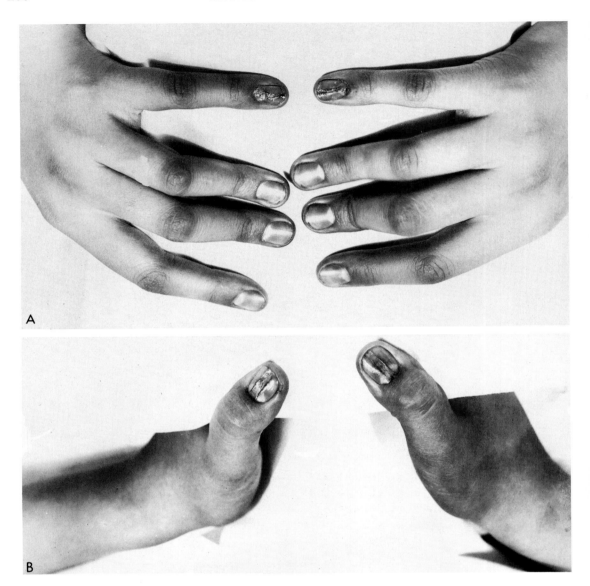

Figure 7–5 Nevus striaticus symmetricus unguis. *A*, Dorsal view showing longitudinal grooving of the fifth digital nails. *B*, Thumbnails showing an analogous defect. (Courtesy of Dr. S. M. Blufarb.)

1920), and Lutembacher (1920). Cockayne (1933) distinguished four varieties of hereditary absence or atrophy of the nails: (1) recessive variant; (2) dominant type; (3) anonychia pollicum; and (4) onychatrophy associated with rudimentary patella. Exemplary cases of recessive anonychia have been reported by Heid-ingsfeld (1913), O'Neill (1916), Cutore (1927), Listengarten (1931), Littman and Levin (1964), and by Timmer and Wildervanck (1969). Some of these authors used the designation "anonychia totalis congenita." Several pointed out that the anomaly had been present since birth. All attested to the recessive mode of in-heritance of the trait.

Isolated cases of dominant anonychia or onychatrophy affecting more than one digit in each hand have been reported by Charteris (1918), Pires de Lima (1924), Hobbs (1935), Vogel and Horn (1964)—who used the title "anonychia congenita"—and by Timmerman et al (1969). Cases belonging to Cockayne's third class, anonychia pollicum or absent thumbnails, were described by Tridon (1912), Ebstein (1919), Strandskov (1939), and by Levan (1961). This trait is also classed with autosomal dominant phenotypes. Cockayne's fourth class, nail-patella syndrome, constitutes the most common variety of congenital anonychia or onychatrophy. Nail-patella syndrome deserves a separate section, as do some other well-defined symptom complexes implicating the nails. These syndromes will be taken up in alphabetical order.

REGIONAL ASSOCIATIONS

One cannot conceive of a normal nail atop an anomalous ungual phalanx. The nails are absent in transverse terminal defects of the digits with missing ungual phalanges. Baisch (1931) described an 18-month-old female with supernumerary webbed digits and almost complete absence of the nails. The nails are expanded and thick in macrodactyly. They are absent in the variety of brachydactyly known as apical dystrophy, in which the ungual phalanges of the four ulnar digits are missing. The terminal phalanges which are implicated by some locally confined disorders, a number of regional abnormalities, and some syndromes, in their turn, implicate the overlying nails (Fig. 7–6).

REMOTE ASSOCIATIONS

The nails are affected in almost all ectodermal dysplasias, in chondroectodermal dysplasias (cartilage-hair hypoplasia and Ellis-van Creveld syndrome), and in tegumentary complexes (focal dermal hypoplasia, plantar and palmar keratosis, and epidermolysis bullosa).

ABSENT MIDDLE PHALANGES AND HYPOPLASTIC NAILS

Under this heading, described in greater detail in Chapter Nine, a symptom complex has been identified characterized by brachydactyly due to the absence of the middle row of phalanges of the fingers, duplication of the ungual phalanges of the thumb, hypoplasia of the auricular cartilage, and hypoplasia of both finger- and toenails.

ANONYCHIA-ECTRODACTYLY SYNDROME

Lees et al (1957) described a condition in which the nail beds, as well as the nails, were absent and, in some instances, one or two digital rays were missing. The feet were likewise affected. The gene responsible for this syndrome was said to manifest its effect in the heterozygous state; it was suggested that the nest of this gene might be linked with the Lutheran blood group locus.

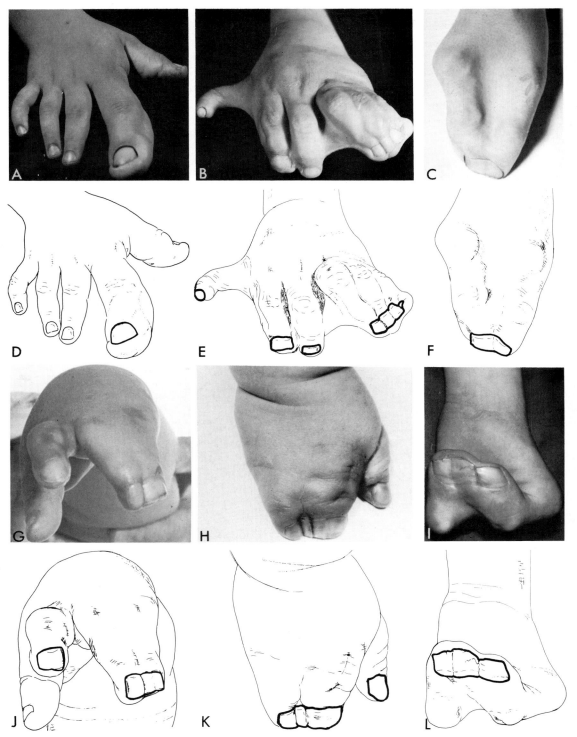

Figure 7–6 Macronychia and confluent nails. *A*, Macronychia in a case of macrodactyly. *B*, Fused fingers and nails in a case of polydactyly and syndactyly. *C*, *G*, *H*, and *I* represent cases of oligosyndactyly. *D*, *E*, *F*, *J*, *K*, and *L* illustrate photograph above each.

CONGENITAL ERYTHROPOIETIC PORPHYRIA (Günther Syndrome)

This is a metabolic disorder, the first sign of which is a red stain on the diaper due to porphyrinuria. The second sign is photosensitivity: when the infant is exposed to sunlight, the acral parts—external ears, the nose, and fingertips—undergo bulbous eruption. Chaudhuri et al (1958) presented a congenital case with hyperpigmentation, ulceration, and scarring on the dorsum of the hand. The fingers were thick; the ungual phalanges were defective at their tips, having lost considerable tissue; the nails were broken.

DEFECT OF THE SCALP AND DYSTROPHY OF THE NAIL

Swart and Calvert (1970) presented an eight-year-old female who had, at birth, an ulcerating lesion over the vertex of the scalp, dystrophy of the finger- and toenails, and a short right index finger. Later, she developed convergent squint and dental caries.

DIFFUSE GASTROINTESTINAL POLYPOSIS AND ECTODERMAL DYSPLASIA (Cronkheite-Canada Syndrome)

This complex consists of generalized gastrointestinal polyposis, alopecia, atrophy of the nails and hyperpigmentation of the skin. Exemplary cases have been reported by Cronkheite and Canada (1955), Johnston et al (1962), Jarnum and Jenson (1966), Manousos and Webster (1966), and Dacruz (1967). All reported cases have been sporadic. The ectodermal changes, including the dystrophy of the nails, is considered to be an inherent component of the syndrome and not secondary to malabsorption which accompanies the intestinal polyposis.

DYSKERATOSIS CONGENITA (Zinsser-Engman-Cole Syndrome; Cole-Rauschkolb-Tommey Syndrome)

This complex presents the following features: dyskeratosis, pigmentation of the skin, leukoplakia of the tongue and of the hard palate, hypersplenism, thrombocytopenia, hyperhidrosis of the palms, and dystrophy of the nails. With the possible exception of the patients presented by Moon-Adams and Slatkin (1954), all reported cases have been males. The trait is considered to be an X-linked recessive.

ELLIS-VAN CREVELD CHONDROECTODERMAL DYSPLASIA

This syndrome, to be discussed in greater detail in Chapter Thirteen, is characterized by (1) dwarfism of acromelic variety; (2) congenital heart disease, usually septal defect and single atrium; (3) coalescence of the carpal hamate and capitate bones; (4) polydactyly; (5) dystrophy of the nails; and (6) autosomal recessive mode of inheritance.

EPIDERMOLYSIS BULLOSA CONGENITA

Constant eruption and bullae formation is known to occur over the bodies of newborn infants, in particular on the feet and the hands. Gedde-Dahl (1971) described a number of congenital cases of epidermolysis bullosa with destruction of fingernails and terminal phalanges.

FIBROMATOSIS-ANONYCHIA COMPLEX
(Gingival Fibromatosis with Abnormal Fingers and Fingernails)

Jacoby et al (1940–41) presented a little girl with massive hypertrophy of the gums, delayed eruption of the teeth, precocious ossification of the bones, including those of the hand, and absence of some of the phalanges and fingernails. The trait was transmitted as an autosomal recessive. Alvandar (1965) described two Asiatic Indian families in which gingival fibromatosis occurred in association with "whittling" of the terminal phalanges and anonychia or dysplasia of the fingernails. In these families, the trait was transmitted as an autosomal dominant.

INFANTILE HYPOPARATHYROIDISM

Hypoparathyroidism is known to occur in very young children, and occasionally it becomes manifest very soon after birth. In the idiopathic variety of hypoparathyroidism, as noted by Klein (1969), the fingernails and toenails are brittle and transversely ridged. Emerson et al (1941) presented a young boy with idiopathic hypoparathyroidism which "may have been of congenital origin." The Chvostek sign was strongly positive. Trousseau's sign was positive after the tourniquet had been applied for 90 seconds. Serum calcium was 5.0 mg. per 100 ml. and inorganic phosphate was 12.1 mg. per 100 ml. The boy had rough, short, thick fingernails "largely overgrown by skin." His toenails were similarly affected.

NAIL-PATELLA SYNDROME (Österreicher Syndrome; Turner-Kieser Syndrome; Familial Dyschondroplasia Associated with Anonychia; Hereditary Arthrodysplasia Osteo-Unguiae)

Pye-Smith (1883) reported a man with the following symptoms: prominent ulnar condyle of the humerus, limited supination of the forearm, recurrently dislocating patella, and "contracted" feet. This man had 11 children. With the exception of one child who was normal and another who died in infancy, all the others presented deformities resembling those of their father. In addition, the children had "ill developed," "poorly formed," "imperfect" nails. Most members of the second generation had limited extension of the elbow; they could pronate their forearms and hands freely, but were unable to supinate these parts fully. The footnote at the end of Pye-Smith's communication states that when the fourth child, a boy, died and his elbow was dissected, the head of the radius was found dislocated posteriorly. One of the daughters married and had three well-formed children; a fourth child had a contracted foot and "ill-formed thumb nails." Stocks (1925) supplied the additional information that a female member of this same family was presented to the Sheffield Medico-Chirurgical Society and showed "backward displacement of left radius"; one of her brothers also had posterior dislocation of the right radial head. In later years, such other components as bilateral absence of the patella, iliac horns, and nephropathy were added to the complex described by Pye-Smith.

In the numerous cases that have since been reported, heredity has featured prominently, the trait being transmitted as an autosomal dominant. Renwick and Lawler (1955) established linkage between the gene responsible for the nail-patella syndrome and that for the ABO blood group. This was considered to be one of the few examples of autosomal linkage established in man. More recently, Schleutermann and colleagues (1969) and Sobel et al (1971) have reported families demonstrating linkage between adenylate kinase and nail-patella foci; coupling of the respective alleles is now regarded as being responsible for the nail-patella syndrome (Figs. 7–7 and 7–8).

OCULO-UNGUAL COMPLEXES

The lens is derived from the ectoderm, as are the epidermis and the nails. Congenital cataract is known to be associated with dyskeratosis palmoplantaris and with ectodermal dysplasia. Papastigakis (1922) reported a patient with total alopecia, congenital cataract, and dystrophic nails. Heidensleben's (1969) patient had congenital koilonychia and cataract.

ONYCHODYSTROPHY-LYMPHEDEMA COMPLEX

Everly Jones (1960) reported a series of seven children with edema of the ankles and feet and, in some, of the hands as well. The edema was said to have

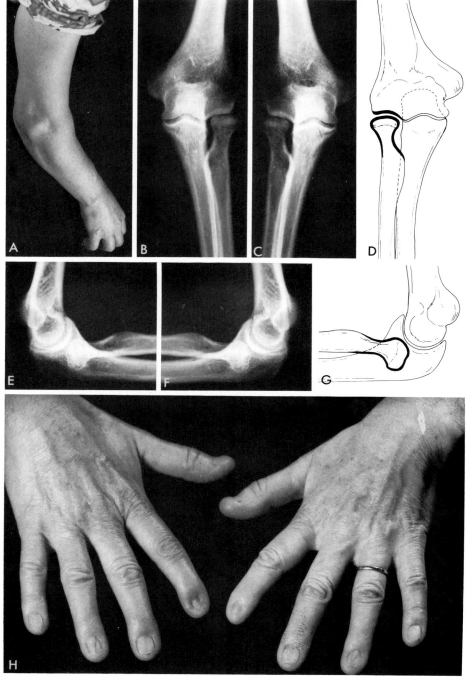

Figure 7-7   Nail-patella syndrome. *A*, The right elbow of a 32-year-old female whose father had absent patellas and dystrophic nails. *B*, Dorsovolar roentgenograph of the right elbow. *C*, Dorsovolar roentgenograph of the left elbow. *D*, Sketch illustrating hypoplastic dome-shaped left radial head and dysplasia of the corresponding capitulum. *E* and *F*, Lateral roentgenographs of the right and left elbows, respectively, showing posterior dislocation of both radial heads. *G*, Sketch illustrating *F*. *H*, Dorsal view of hands showing dystrophy of all nails except the nails of the middle and little fingers.

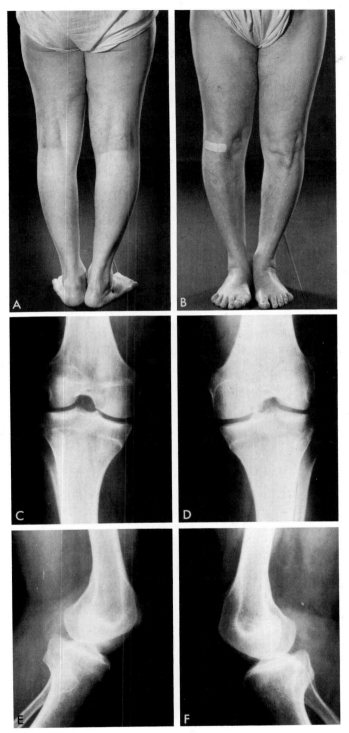

Figure 7–8 *A,* Dorsal view of the lower limbs of the same patient shown in Figure 7–7—note the bowing of the legs. *B,* Frontal view of the same. *C* and *D,* Roentgenographs of the right and left knees, showing bilateral tibia vara. *E* and *F,* Lateral roentgenographs of the same, showing bilateral absence of the patella.

been present since birth and tended to disappear gradually. In five of the seven cases, the toenails were dystrophic. Dystrophy of the nails persisted after the edema cleared. It was suggested that these children were affected by Turner's syndrome. Maisels (1966) described a woman who had been born with complete absence of all toenails and partial anonychia of the hands. At about age 20, she developed edema of the lower extremities. None of her 42 relatives had lymphedema or abnormalities of the nails.

OSTEOGENESIS IMPERFECTA

Atrophy of the fingernails is not an uncommon occurrence in blue sclerotics with brittle bones. This trait is transmitted as an autosomal dominant (Fig. 7–9).

OTO-UNGUAL COMPLEXES

As will be shown in subsequent chapters, there are two main classes of ectodermal dysplasia called, respectively, hidrotic and unhidrotic. The hidrotic variety is inherited as an autosomal dominant phenotype and is characterized by hyperactive sweat and sebaceous gland function, alopecia, absent or malformed teeth, and dystrophy of the nails. In the pedigree described by Robinson et al (1962) several members had sensorineural deafness, "dystrophic nails with furrows and cracks," dental defects ranging from delayed eruption of permanent teeth to partial anodontia, and elevation of the chloride concentration in sweat. "The association of hereditary ectodermal dysplasia and involvement of other ectodermal derivatives, namely, the otocyst and in turn the cochlea, is perhaps not a suprising finding," Robinson and his colleagues wrote.

Feinmesser and Zelig (1961) described two siblings, both females, with bilateral nerve deafness and dystrophy of the nails. Their parents were unaffected, although they were first cousins on the maternal and second cousins on the paternal side. Since auditory nerves and nails are both derived from ectoderm, Feinmesser and Zelig attributed this syndrome to an ectodermal defect of recessive nature. Goodman et al (1969) described a mother with sensorineural deafness, hypoplastic nails and bulbous tumefaction of the ungual segments of the thumbs and the little fingers.

Schwann (1963) presented a child who had been deaf since birth and had leukonychia. Schwann thought this trait was transmitted as an autosomal dominant. Bart and Pumphrey (1967) described a kindred in which many members had sensorineural deafness, palmar and plantar keratosis, leukonychia, and knuckle pads.

PACHYONYCHIA CONGENITA (Jadassohn-Lewandowski Syndrome)

Jadassohn and Lewandowski (1906) coined this term. The symptom complex it represents consists of thick, twisted nails, hyperkeratosis of the palms and soles, and leukoplakia of the oral mucous membrane. An infant reported by Andrews and Stumwasser (1929) began to show characteristic changes of the

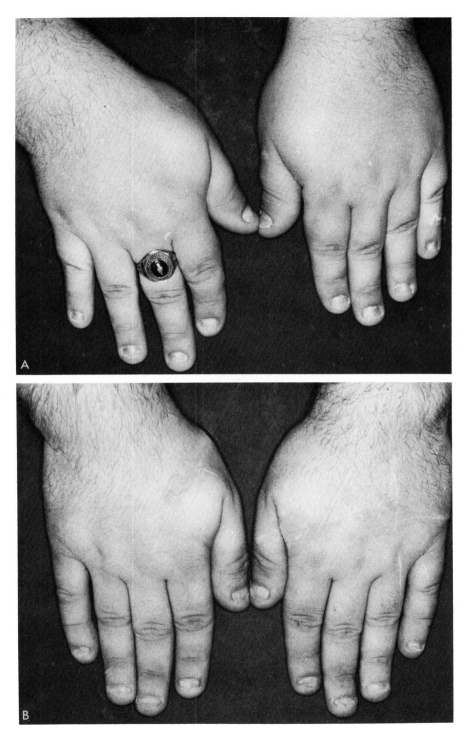

Figure 7–9 *A*, Dorsal view of the hands of a girl with osteogenesis imperfecta; her mother, two brothers, and an older sister all had multiple fractures of the long bones. *B*, Dorsal view of the hands of an older sister; dystrophy of the nails is more marked in this instance.

nails two weeks after birth. Pachyonychia congenita affects males chiefly, and appears to be most prevalent among Slavs and Jews of Slavonic origin. Jackson and Lawler (1951–1952) described six affected members in three generations. The trait is listed among autosomal dominant phenotypes.

TRISOMY 13–15 OR B

Smith (1969) gave "hyperconvex narrow fingernails" as one of the main features of trisomy 13–15.

TREATMENT OF ABSENT OR ATROPHIC NAILS

It is now definitely established that absent nails can be replenished by free-nail graft or camouflaged by plastic substitution. When the nail is lifted up surgically, the matrix remains attached to the nail plate. The nail plate with its matrix makes an ideal free graft, analogous to the full-thickness graft of the skin. Detached nail plate is like split-thickness skin graft. It is well known that split-thickness skin grafts have a greater chance of survival than thicker grafts. The same principle applies to nail grafts.

With varying degrees of success, split- or full-thickness nail grafts have been carried out on traumatic cases by the following authors: Sheehan (1929), Swanker (1947), Berson (1950), McCash (1956), Massè (1967), and Papavassiliou (1969). In these operations, the nail of another digit of the hand or the great toe is used as a graft. In most cases of anonychia, except in the very rare anonychia pollicum, almost all the nails are defective, particularly the nails of the great toes. Buncke and Gonzales (1962) devised an ingenious method of reconstructing a nail bed, nail fold, and a skin-lined nail pouch which would hold a prosthetic nail plate. Langhof and Metzner (1965) utilized "plastic fibric" substitutes in the treatment of onychodystrophy.

Shoemaker (1890) considered the nails as "ornamental, useful appendages of the skin." The nail serves a number of purposes. It provides a protective shield for the most sensitive, perceptive, and vulnerable part of the digit, and helps the latter in picking up finer objects—a needle, for instance. A hand without nails is at a disadvantage. Notwithstanding, the main reason for replenishing absent nails is cosmetic.

SUMMARY

The nails are epidermal appendages and are derived from the ectoderm, the outermost primary layer of the body. Congenital anomalies of the nails are more often seen in connection with such complexes as nail-patella syndrome and syndromes which implicate other ectodermal derivatives than in connection with isolated entities. The nail is supported by the terminal phalanx of each digit, and it reflects the deviation in size and contour of the underlying bone. The main justification for surgical interference in cases of absent or dystrophic nails is cosmetic.

References

Alvandar, G.: Elephantiasis gingivae. Report of an affected family with associated hepatomegaly, soft tissue and skeletal abnormalities. *J. All India Dent. Assn.*, *37*:349–353, 1965.

Andrews, G. C., and Strumwasser, S.: Pachyonychia congenita. *N.Y. State J. Med.*, *29*:747–749, 1929.

Baisch, A.: Anonychia congenita, kombiniert mit Polydaktylie und verzögertem abnormen Zahndurchbruch. *Dtsch. Z. Chir.*, *232*:450–457, Abb. 1, 1931.

Bart, R. S., and Pumphrey, R. E.: Knuckle pads, leuconychia and deafness—a dominantly inherited syndrome. *N. Eng. J. Med.*, *276*:202–207, 1967.

Bauer, A. W.: Beiträge zur klinischen Konstitutionspathologie. V. Heredo-familiare Leukonychie und multiple Atherombildung der'Kopfhaut. *Z. Angew. Anat. Konstitutionsl.*, *5*:44–58, 1920.

Becker, S. W.: Leukonychia striata. *Arch. Derm. Syph.*, *21*:957–960, 1930.

Bergé, A., and Weisenbach, R. J.: Absence congénitale complète des ongles de tous les doigts—biopsie. *Ann. Derm. Syph.*, (5 s.) *3*:244–249, 1912.

Berson, M. J.: Reconstruction of the index finger with nail transplantations. *Surgery*, *27*:594–599, 1950.

Boas, I. E. V.: Zur Morphologie der Wirbeltierkralle. *Morph. Jb.*, *21*:161–311, 1894.

Buncke, H. J., and Gonzalez, R.: Fingernail reconstruction. *Plast. Reconstr. Surg.*, *30*:452–461, 1962.

Charteris, F.: Case of partial hereditary anonychia. *Glasgow Med. J.*, *89*:207–209, 1918.

Chaudhuri, A., Chaudhuri, J. W., and Chaudhuri, K. C.: Congenital porphyria in siblings. *Indian J. Pediat.*, *25*:157–171; Fig. 4, 1958.

Cipollaro, A. C.: Koilonychia, report of a case and review of literature. *N.Y. State Med. J.*, *30*:380–385, 1930.

Clement, L. S.: A claw-fingered family. The inheritance of nail mutation in man. *J. Hered.*, *19*:529–536, 1928.

Cockayne, E. A.: *Inherited Abnormalities of the Skin and Appendages.* London, Oxford University Press, pp. 265–273, 1933.

Costa, O. G.: Leuconychia total congenita. *An Bras. Dermatol.*, *22*:147–149, 1947.

Cronkheite, L. W., Jr., and Canada, W. J.: Generalized gastrointestinal polyposis; an unusual syndrome of polyposis, pigmentation, alopecia and onychotropia. *N. Eng. J. Med.*, *252*:1011–1015, 1955.

Cutore, G.: Sterethonichia (macanza di ununghie) ereditaria. *Riv. Biol.*, *9*:1–10, 1927.

Dacruz, G. M. C.: Generalized gastrointestinal polyposis. An unusual syndrome of adenomatous polyposis, alopecia onychotrophia. *Am. J. Gastroenterol.*, *47*:504–510, 1967.

DuBois, C.: Quelques dystrophies localisés de l'heredo-syphilis. *Ann. Derm. Syph.*, *7*:415–425; Fig. 3, 4, 1926.

Ebstein, E.: Angeborene familiäre Erkrankumg an den Nageln. *Derm. Wochenschr.*, *68*:113–118, 1919.

Eichhorst, H.: Angeborene Nagelmangel. *Cbl. Klin. Med.*, *14*:289–291, 1893.

Emerson, K., Jr., Walsh, F. B., and Howard, J. E.: Idiopathic hypoparathyroidism. A report of two cases. *Ann. Intern. Med.*, *14*:1256–1270; Fig. 3, 1941.

Feinmesser, M., and Zelig, S.: Congenital deafness associated with onychodystrophy. *Arch. Otolaryngol.*, *74*:507–508, 1961.

Furst, L.: Allgemeiner Fingernagel-Wechsel bei einem ½ jahrige Kinde. *Arch. Path. Anat. Physiol.*, *96*:355–357, 1884.

Gedde-Dahl, T., Jr.: *Epidermolysis Bullosa.* Baltimore, Johns Hopkins Press, pp. 66–98; Figs. 13–15, 19, 23, and 35, 1971.

Goodman, R. M., Lockareff, S., and Gwinup, G.: Hereditary congenital deafness with onychodystrophy. *Arch. Otolaryngol.*, *90*:474–477, 1969.

Graciansky, P.de, and Boulle, S.: Association de koilinychie et de leukonychie transmisés en dominance. *Bull. Soc. Fr. Derm. Syph.*, *68*:15–17, 1961.

Günther, H.: Die Hämatoporphurine. *Dtsch. Arch. Klin. Med.*, *105*:88–146; Figs. 1–3, 1912.

Halperin, K. M.: Afflictions of vestigial appendages. I. Congenital defects of the human nail and systemic influences. *J.A.M.A.*, *202*:645; Fig. 4, 1967.

Harrington, J. F.: White fingernails. *Arch. Int. Med.*, *114*:301–306, 1964.

Hedderich: Über Leakonychia totalis. *Derm. Cbl.*, *13*:264, 1910.

Heidensleben, E.: Hereditary congenital koilonychia associated with syndermatotic cataract. *Acta Ophthalmol.*, *38*:1–4, 1969.

Heidingsfeld, M. L.: Congenital absence of finger and toe nails (Anonychia congenitalis totalis). *In Tr. 17th Internat. Congress Med. London.* London, Oxford Press, Section XIII, pp. 93–96, 1913.

Hobbs, M. E.: Hereditary onychial dysplasia. *Am. J. Med. Sci.*, *190*:200–206, 1935.

Jackson, A. C., and Lawler, S. D.: Pachyonychia congenita. A report of six cases in one family, with a note on linkage data. *Ann. Eugen.*, *16*:142–146, 1951–1952.

Jacoby, N. M., Ripman, H. A., and Munden, J. M.: Partial anonychia (recessive) with hypertrophy of the gums and multiple abnormalities of the osseous system. *Guy's Hosp. Rep.*, *90*:34–40, 1940–1941.

Jadassohn, J., and Lewandowski, F.: Pachonychia congenita. Keratosis disseminata circumscripta (follicularis). Tylomata. Leukokeratosis lingae. *In Neisser, A., and Jacob, E., (eds.): Iknographia Dermatologica.* Berlin, Uber und Schwarzenber, pp. 29–31, 1906.

Jamieson, A.: Congenital malformation of nails. *Tr. Med. Chir. Soc.*, Edinburgh, *12* :191–192, 1893.

Jarnum, S., and Jenson, H.: Diffuse gastrointestinal polyposis with ectodermal changes. *Gastroenterology*, 50:107–118; Fig. 2, 1966.

Johnston, M. M., Vosburgh, J. W., Weems, A. T., and Walsh, G. C.: Gastrointestinal polyposis associated with alopecia, pigmentation, and atrophy of the fingernails and toenails. *Ann. Intern. Med.*, 56:935–940, 1962.

Jones, H. E.: Symmetrical peripheral edema of infants. *Arch. Dis. Child.*, 35:192–196, 1960.

Klein, R.: Hypoparathyroidism. *In* Gardner, L. I., (ed.): *Endocrine and Genetic Diseases of Childhood*. Philadelphia, W. B. Saunders Co., pp. 376–391; Fig. 4–12, 1969.

Langhof, H., and Metzner, H.: Kunstoffingernagelersatz bei onychodystrophie. *Aesthet. Med.* (Berl.), 9:150–152, 1965.

Lees, D. H., Lawler, S. D., Renwick, J. H., and Thoday, J. M.: Anonychia with ectrodactyly. Clinical and linkage study. *Ann. Hum. Genet.*, 22:69–79, 1957.

Levan, N. E.: Congenital defect of thumb nails. *Arch. Dermatol.*, 83:938–940, 1961.

Lingamfelter, C. S., and Whitmore, C. W.: Leuconychia totalis. *Va. Med. Mon.*, 81:68, 1954.

Listengarten, A.: Ein Fall von Anonychia totalis congenita. *Derm. Wochenschr.*, 92:691–695, 1931.

Littman, A., and Levin, S.: Anonychia as a recessive autosomal trait in man. *J. Invest. Dermatol.*, 42:175–178, 1964.

Lutembacher, R.: Atrophie ungueale congénitale. *Ann. Derm. Syph.* (6 s.) *1*:461–462, 1920. Review in: *Arch. Derm. Syph.*, *3*:437, 1921.

Maisels, D. O.: Anonychia in association with lymphoedema. *Br. J. Plast. Surg.*, 19:37–42, 1966.

Manousos, O., and Webster, C. U.: Diffuse gastrointestinal polyposis and ectodermal changes. *Gut*, 7:375–379; Fig. 1, 1966.

Massè, G.: La riparazione dell'apparato ungueale nell lesioni traumatiche delle dita. *Minerva Ortop.*, 18:919–922, 1967.

McCash, C. R.: Free nail grafting. *Br. Plast. Surg.*, 8:19–33, 1956.

Moon-Adams, D., and Slatkin, M. H.: Familial pigmentation with dystrophy of the nails. *Arch. Dermatol.*, 71:591–598, 1954.

Murray, F. A.: Congenital anomalies of the nails, four cases of hereditary hypertrophy of the nail bed associated with a history of erupted teeth at birth. *Br. J. Derm. Syph.*, 33:409–411, 1921.

Oliver, E. A., and Bluefarb, S. M.: Nevus striations symmetricus unguis: report of a case with involvement of thumbs and little fingers. *Arch. Derm. Syph.*, 49:190, 1944.

O'Neill, B.: A case of congenital absence of nails. *Lancet*, 12:979–980, 1916.

Oppenheim, M., and Cohen, D.: Nevus symmetricus of the thumbs. *Arch. Derm. Syph.*, 45:253, 1942.

Ormsby: Koilonychia. Congenital alopecia. Deformed teeth. *J. Cutan. Dis.*, 35:856, 1917.

Papastigakis: Un nouveau syndrome dystrophique juvénale, alopécia totale associé à la cataract et altérations ungueales. *Paris Med.*, 45:475, 1922.

Papavassiliou, N. P.: Transplantation of the nail. *Br. J. Plast. Surg.*, 22:274–280, 1969.

Pires de Lima, J. A.: Onychatrophie familiale congenitale. *Ann. Derm. Syph.*, (6 s.), 5:266–271, 1924.

Prado-Castello, V., and Prado, O. A.: *Diseases of the Nails*. Third edition. Springfield, Illinois, Charles C Thomas, pp. 3–16; 220–237, 1960.

Pye-Smith, R. J.: Notes on a family presenting in most of its members certain deformities of the joints of both limbs. *Med. Press Circular*, 34:504–505, 1883.

Renwick, J. R., and Lawler, S. D.: Genetical linkage between the ABO and patella loci. *Ann. Hum. Genet.*, 19:312–331, 1955.

Robinson, G. C., Miller, J. R., and Bensimon, J. R.: Familial ectodermal dysplasia with sensorineural deafness and other anomalies. *Pediatrics*, 30:797–802, 1962.

Ronchese, F.: Peculiar nail anomalies. *Arch. Derm. Syph.*, 63:565–580, 1951.

Schleutermann, D., Bias, W. B., Murdock, J. L., et al: Linkage of loci for nail-patella syndrome and adenylate kinase. *Am. J. Hum. Genet.*, 21:606–630, 1969.

Schwann, J.: Keratosis palmaris et plantaris cum surditate congenita et leuconychia totali umgium. *Dermatologica*, 125:335–353, 1963.

Sheehan, J. E.: Replacement of the thumb nail. *J.A.M.A.*, 92:1253–1255, 1929.

Shoemaker, J. V.: Diseases of the nails. *J. Cut. Genitourin. Dis.*, 8:334–344; 388–393; 419–425; 476–482, 1890.

Shoemaker, J. V.: Some notes on the nails. *J.A.M.A.*, 15:427–428, 1890.

Sibley, W. K.: Case of onychatrophia. *Proc. R. Soc. Med.* London 13 (Section of Derm.), 8:1919–1920.

Sibley, W. K.: Leukonychia striata. *Br. J. Derm.*, 34:238–239, 1922.

Smith, D. W.: The 18 trisomy and D1 trisomy syndromes. *In* Gardner, L. I., (ed.): *Endocrine and Genetic Diseases of Childhood*. Philadelphia, W. B. Saunders Co., pp. 638–652, 1969.

Sobel, R. C., Tiger, A., and Gerald, P. S.: A second family with the nail-patella allele and adenylate kinase allel in grouping. *Am. J. Hum. Genet.*, 23:146–149, 1971.

Stocks, P.: Hereditary disorders of bone development. *In* Pearson, K., (ed.): *The Treasury of Human Inheritance*. London, Cambridge University Press, Vol. III, pp. 7–48, 141–167, 1925.

Strandskov, H. H.: Inheritance of absence of thumb nails. *J. Hered.*, 30:53–54, 1939.

Swanker, W. A.: Reconstructive surgery of the injured nail. *Am. J. Surg.*, 74:341–345, 1947.

Swart, E., and Calvert, H. T.: Congenital ectodermal defect with nail dystrophy and resorption of terminal phalanges. *Br. J. Dermatol.*, 82:93, 1970.

Sympson: Congenital deformity of the nails (onychogryposis). *Lancet*, *1*:722–723, 1888.

Thomson, H. B.: Hereditary dystrophy of the nails. *J.A.M.A.*, *91*:1574, 1928.

Timmer, J., and Wildervanck, L. S.: Anonychia congenita totalis van vingers en tenen. *Nederl. T. Geneesk.*, *113*(1):395–397, 1969.

Timmerman, I., Museteanu, C., and Simionscu, N. N.: Dominant anonychia and onychodystrophy. *J. Med. Genet.*, *6*:105–106, 1969.

Tridon, P.: Absence congénitale des ongles des pouces. *Rev. d'Orthop.*, (3 s.), *3*:192, 1912.

Vidal, J. P. S.: Note explicative sur un pouce double d'annamite. *Rec. Mem. Med. Chir. Pharm. Milit.*, (3 s.), *13*:71–74, 1865.

Vogel, F., and Horn, H.: Anonychia congenita. *In* Becker, P. E., (ed.): *Humangenetik*. Stuttgart, G. Thieme, Vol. 4, pp. 489–490, 1964.

Wilson, A. G.: Three cases of hereditary hyperkeratosis of the nail-bed. *Br. J. Dermatol.*, *17*:13–14, 1905.

Chapter Eight

ANOMALIES OF THE
UNGUAL PHALANGES

It was noted in Chapter Seven that nails reflect the abnormalities in size and shape of the underlying phalanges and that, in their turn, the ungual phalanges are implicated by a few locally confined disorders, a number of regional anomalies, and some syndromes. As in the case of the nails, most congenital anomalies of the ungual phalanges are syndromic. The few exceptions are stub thumb, congenital clubbing of the fingers, and Kirner's deformity of the little finger. Stub thumb has been classified with brachydactyly but seems to affect the ungual phalanx of the thumb selectively. Ungual phalanges are also deferentially affected in congenital clubbing of the fingers and in Kirner's deformity.

ANATOMY

The ungual phalanges of the thumb and fingers are peculiar in that each one possesses three centers of ossification—one at the distal end, another inside the midshaft, and a third at the proximal extremity or the base. The anlage of the distal tip is membranous. The precursors of the two other centers are cartilaginous. The ungual phalanges are the first skeletal elements of the embryonic hand to begin ossifying. Bone begins to be deposited within the distal membranous center as early as the seventh week of intrauterine life and gradually expands to form a crescent-shaped cap for the ungual tuft. The basal epiphyses of all phalanges are cartilaginous at birth. The appearance of the epiphysis of the terminal phalanx of the thumb is variable: it is known to appear as early as 12 months after birth but may not become roentgenographically manifest until the end of the second year. The corresponding centers of the middle and ring fingers receive their osseous cores soon after. These epiphyses unite with their respective shafts at about the age of 13 or 14 in girls and a year later in boys. The last phalanx of the thumb is the earliest to acquire an ossific epiphysis and the earliest to become consolidated as a homogeneous bone. The epiphyses of the terminal phalanges of the brachydactyly-prone and angulation-prone index and little fingers are last to appear (Figs. 8–1 to 8–3).

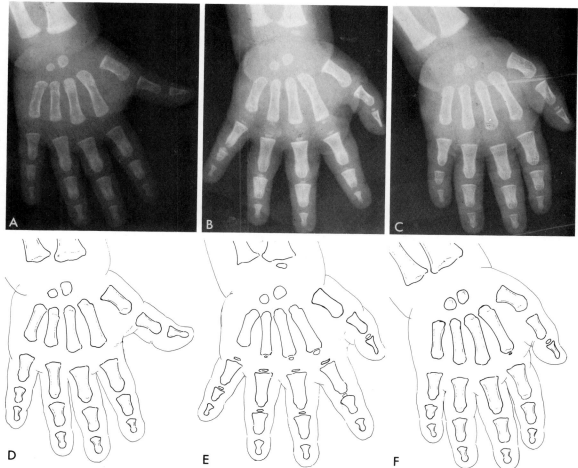

Figure 8–1 The appearance of epiphyses of the ungual phalanges. *A*, Dorsopalmar roentgenograph of a 10-month-old male: none of the epiphyses of the metacarpals and phalanges are roentgenographically manifest. *B*, Roentgenograph of an 11-month-old female, showing the first appearance of the ungual phalangeal epiphysis of the thumb. *C*, Roentgenograph of a 12-month-old male, again showing the first appearance of the epiphysis of the ungual phalanx of the thumb. In both *B* and *C* one notes the absence of corresponding epiphyses of the lesser digits. *D*, *E*, and *F* illustrate the roentgenograph above each.

Each mature ungual phalanx has a spongy expansion at its tip called a tuft, a constricted tubular shaft, and a broad cancellous base. The shaft is thicker on the palmar than on the dorsal aspect. The wide palmar surface is roughened to provide anchorage for the fibro-fatty pad of the terminal pulp, which contains the perceptive elements of tactile sensibility. The base of the distal phalanx of each finger gives attachment to the deep flexor tendon on its palmar aspect and to the extensor expansion on its dorsal side. The base of the last phalanx of the thumb provides anchorage for the extensor pollicis longus on its dorsal aspect and the flexor pollicis longus on its volar side. In some congenital anomalies, the stronger flexor tendons tend to hold the ungual phalanges partly flexed and turned sideways. The ungual phalanges are farthest away from the central circulation and are subject to greater circulatory derangements. They are also at a disadvantage because of their acral position which makes them liable to injury, either *in utero* or outside.

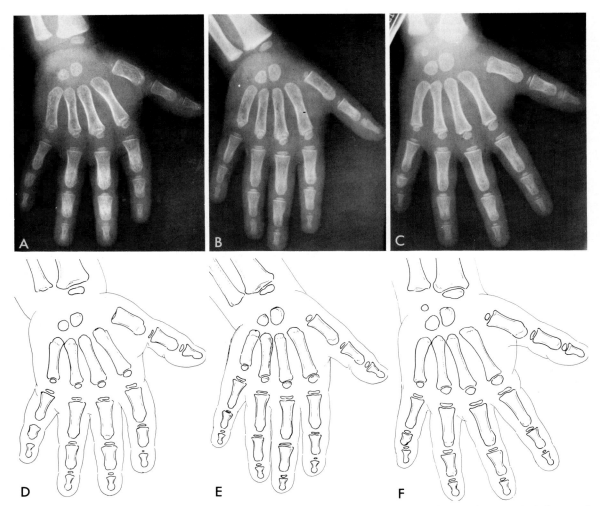

Figure 8–2   *A*, Dorsopalmar roentgenograph of the right hand of an 18-month-old male: the ungual phalanges of the thumb, middle, and ring fingers have fairly large epiphyses; the ungual phalanx of the index finger has a barely discernible epiphyseal seed; the epiphysis of the ungual phalanx of the little finger has not become roentgenographically manifest as yet. *B*, Roentgenograph of a 19-month-old female and *C*, roentgenograph of a 22-month-old male, showing the first appearance of the ungual phalangeal epiphyses in female and male, respectively. *D, E,* and *F* illustrate the roentgenograph above each.

STUB THUMB (Brachydactyly Type D; Brachymegalodactylism; Brachytelephalangy of the Thumb; *Kolbendaumen;* Potter's Thumb; Murderer's Thumb)

In this anomaly, the terminal phalanx of the thumb is short and broad. Thomsen (1928) pointed out that in unilateral cases of stub thumb the growth cartilage plate of the anomalous phalanx is obliterated while the corresponding line on the unaffected side is still intact. Burrows (1938) related the anomaly of stub thumb to the tendency of the growth cartilage line of its terminal phalanx to

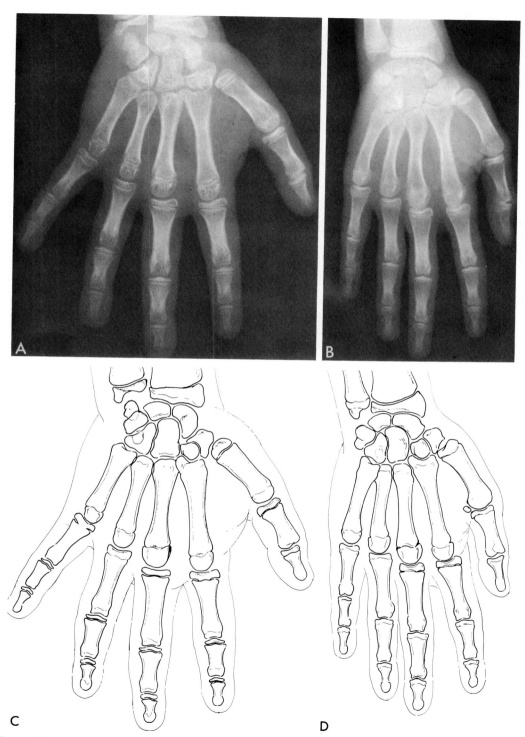

Figure 8–3   *A,* Dorsopalmar roentgenograph of the right hand of a 13-year-old female. The epiphysis of the pollical ungual phalanx has united with the shaft, while the corresponding physes of lesser digits are still open. *B,* Dorsopalmar roentgenograph of a male, 14 years and three months old, showing closure of the physes of all ungual phalanges. *C* and *D* illustrate roentgenograph above each.

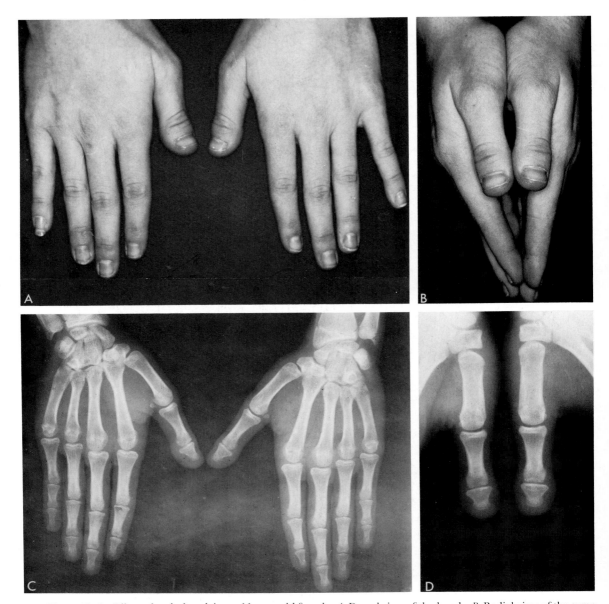

Figure 8–4   Bilateral stub thumb in an 11-year-old female. *A*, Dorsal view of the hands. *B*, Radial view of the same. *C*, Dorsopalmar roentgenograph of both hands. *D*, The same of the thumbs.

close earlier. According to Stecher (1957) the anomaly of short pollex is called potter's or murderer's thumb. Potter's thumb is an acquired deformity. There is no justification for tagging the stigma of criminality to individuals with stub thumbs. Stub thumb is usually an isolated anomaly and is preeminently a genetic disorder, being transmitted as an autosomal dominant trait. The anomaly is also known to occur in connection with a number of syndromes which will be discussed in the ensuing pages (Figs. 8–4 and 8–5).

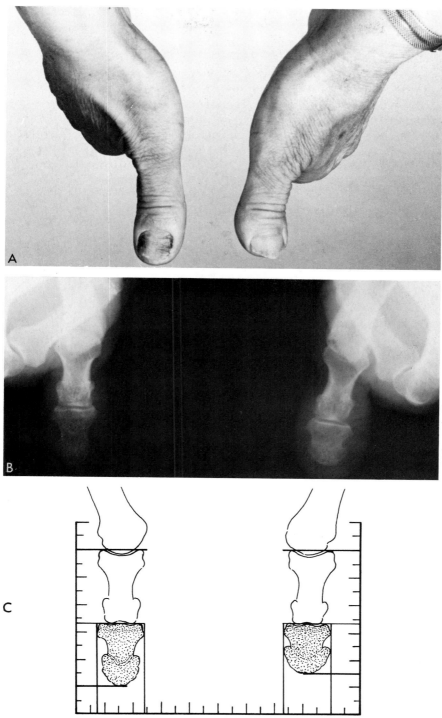

Figure 8–5   Unilateral stub thumb. *A*, Dorsal view of both thumbs. *B*, Dorsopalmar roentgenograph of the same: the ungual phalanx of the left thumb is broader and shorter. *C*, Sketch illustrating the same.

CONGENITAL CLUBBING OF UNGUAL PHALANGES

In clubbing, the ungual segment of the digit appears bulbous and the nail is curved longitudinally. This so-called Hippocratic finger is often seen in individuals who suffer from chronic cardiac or pulmonary diseases. The deformity of the finger in these cases is acquired and not congenital. One finds a number of articles in the literature under the heading of "Congenital clubbing of the fingers and toes." In almost all of them, the congenital origin of the anomaly is emphasized and mention is made of the absence of any heart or lung diseases. Exemplary cases have been reported by Eiselsberg (1911), Weber (1919), Ebstein (1919), Kayne (1933), Witherspoon (1935), Horsfall (1936), and Seaton (1938). Congenital clubbing of the fingers is more frequent in males; it is transmitted as an autosomal dominant trait. The anomaly is almost invariably seen in association with clubbing of the toes. It is simulated by a number of syndromes.

KIRNER'S DEFORMITY (Dystelephalangy)

In this anomaly, named after Kirner (1927), the interphalangeal joint and the basal epiphysis of the terminal phalanx of the little finger are intact but the shaft of the bone is bowed and its tip points toward the radial border of the hand. Thomas (1936), wrote an article bearing the title "A new dystrophy of the little finger," in which he described the curved shaft of the terminal phalanx in three unrelated young females. "The phalanx," he wrote, "takes on the curved 'taloned' effect." Wilson (1952) reported four analogous cases, three females and one male. In one of the young girls, the deformity became manifest at the age of five years and there was "a family history of a similar deformity in her father, her father's mother, and her younger brother." Blank and Girdany (1965) gave the pedigree of a family in which seven members, four males and three females, in three generations were affected. They described the deformity as "symmetrical bowing of the terminal phalanges of the fifth fingers" and considered the trait as simple autosomal dominant. Unlike congenital clubbing of the finger, Kirner's deformity is more common in females. At times, it is seen in subjects with split hand deformity (Fig. 8–6).

ASSOCIATIONS

Ungual phalanges are variously affected in some forms of syndactyly (symbrachydactyly, acrosyndactyly, and acrocephalosyndactyly), in the variety of brachydactyly known as apical dystrophy; in distal type symphalangism, in terminal transverse defects, and in macrodactyly. The ungual phalanges are short in most syndromic disorders which cause dwarfing (for instance, acrodysostosis, Ellis-van Creveld chondroectodermal dysplasia, and peripheral dysostosis). The following sections will be devoted to syndromes which deferentially affect the ungual phalanges.

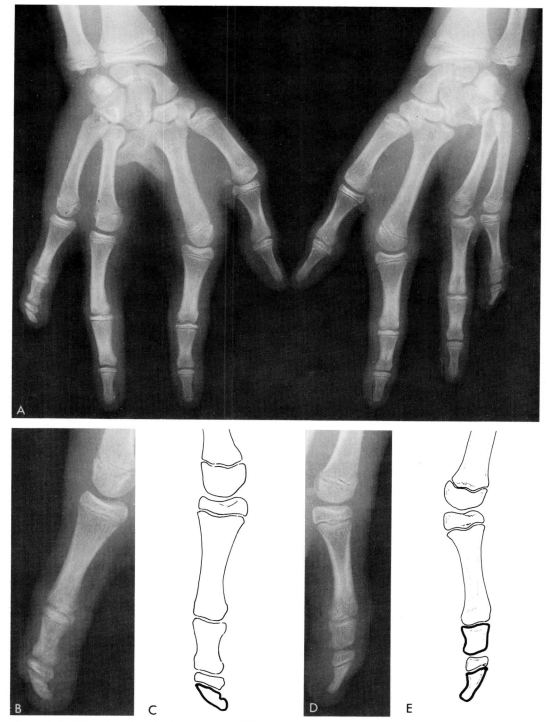

Figure 8–6 Kirner's deformity in an 11-year-old boy with an absence of middle fingers (split hand). *A*, Dorsopalmar roentgenograph of both hands showing curved shafts of the ungual phalanges of the little fingers. *B*, Enlarged roentgenograph of the right little finger. *C*, Sketch illustrating the same. *D*, Enlarged roentgenograph of the left little finger. *E*, Sketch illustrating the same.

ACRO-OSTEOLYSIS CONGENITA (Cheyney Syndrome)

The designation acro-osteolysis was introduced by Harnash (1950). The word osteolysis conveys the impression that there was a preexisting, well-formed bone which subsequently underwent lytic change. There are a number of metabolic, neuropathic, and sclerodermic disorders in which fully developed terminal phalanges undergo secondary dissolution. It is suggested that the adjective *congenital* be used to distinguish what appears to be a developmental disorder which probably had its inception before birth.

Hajdu and Kauntze (1948) described a middle-aged man with foreshortened, broad distal phalanges associated with marked increase of the bitemporal diameter of the skull and flattening of the vertex; the calvarium had the appearance of having been pressed from above, pushing the occiput posteriorly until it formed an overhanging cliff above the nape; and the metopic suture persisted. The ungual phalanges of the hand were short and bulbous; the terminal segments of the fingers felt as if they contained no bones. Upon roentgenographic examination, each ungual phalanx was found to consist of two ossicles which were separated from each other by a radiolucent gap: the proximal piece, representing the epiphyseal element, had the shape of a blunt, conical stump; the distal fragment consisted of a squat little cap of cortical bone overlying a rudimentary cancellous tuft. Comparable changes also occurred in the feet, and the head of the radius on one side was dislocated. A photograph of the patient at four years of age already showed an abnormal configuration of the skull. Hajdu and Kauntze considered the deformity of the calvarium and the peculiar configuration at the occipito-cervical junction to be *prima facie* evidence of an early developmental defect and placed the basic "fault in the mesodermal tissue," which is another way of saying that the disorder had its inception during embryonic development. Papavasiliou et al (1960) categorized this condition as a "generalized congenital osseous dysplasia." Chawla's (1964) patient, a female, "had been aware of the bulbousness of the fingers since childhood." Cheyney (1965) emphasized the congenital aspect of the shaftless terminal phalanges associated with an anteroposteriorly elongated skull, osteoporosis of the mandible, and other skeletal changes. Most reported cases of congenital acro-osteolysis have been sporadic. The trait is listed with autosomal dominant phenotypes (Fig. 8-7).

BERK-TABATZNIK SYNDROME

Berk and Tabatznik (1961) reported a case of a South African Bantu girl who had the following congenital abnormalities: bilateral optic atrophy, localized cervical kyphosis, stub thumb, and short terminal phalanges of all fingers except the little finger. Brachytelephalangy imparted to the affected digit the appearance of a drumstick.

CARTILAGE-HAIR HYPOPLASIA

McKusick (1966) described a form of short-limbed dwarfism prevalent among the Old Amish, a religious isolate. The affected individual is short in

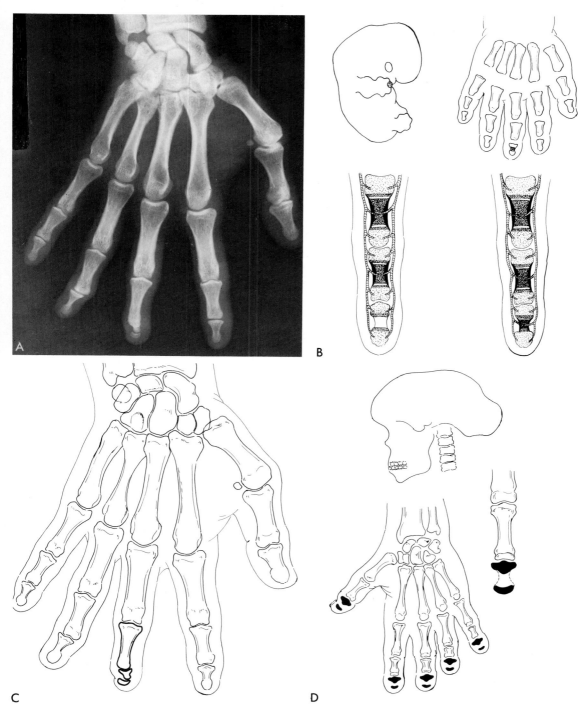

Figure 8–7 *A*, Dorsopalmar roentgenograph of the right hand of an adult male who has had a short middle finger since birth. The tuft of the ungual phalanx has established no osseous continuity with the basal epiphysis. *B*, Sketches illustrating possible causes of this shaftless ungual phalanx; namely, that it is caused by (a) focal necrosis, or (b) absence of nutrient vessel. *C*, Illustrates *A. D*, Sketches illustrating the cranial and digital abnormalities of classic congenital acro-osteolysis.

stature and has thin, sparse hair. The hands are pudgy. The fingers are short, the shortness being most pronounced in the terminal phalanges. The fingernails are broad. The carpal bones are tardy in development. The skeletal changes are ascribed to hypoplasia of the cartilage or to hypochondroplasia. The trait is an autosomal recessive.

CLEIDOCRANIAL DYSOSTOSIS

This well-known, dominantly inherited congenital syndrome has been repeatedly referred to in previous chapters. It affects primarily membranous tissue which is found between the two cartilaginous anlagen of the clavicles and in the midline of the body where two paired bones meet—as do the bones of the cranial vault, the mandibular rami, the neural arches, and the bones on either side of the symphysis pubis. The disorder is ascribed to the failure of the junctional zone between two bony elements to become ossified. Bone is deposited in the membranous midportion of the clavicle at the sixth postovulatory week—about one week before it appears at the tips of the terminal phalanges. The ossification of the tip of the ungual phalanx precedes the deposition of bone by endochondral ossification in its proximal shaft. A strip of mesenchyma separates the two bony nuclei. In some cases of cleidocranial dysostosis, the two nuclei fail to establish a continuity; in others, the ungual tufts fail to develop. The ungual phalanges remain tuftless and upon roentgenographic study give the impression of having assumed the shape of a miniature spear. Usually there are some other hand anomalies (Fig. 8–8).

LARSEN'S SYNDROME

This syndrome has also been mentioned previously. It will be referred to again in Chapter Twenty-one and described in greater detail in Chapter Twenty-seven. Briefly, it consists of peculiar facies (prominent forehead, depressed nasal bridge, and wide-spaced eyes), multiple dislocations (of knees and elbows, in particular), short metacarpals, cylindrical fingers, and stub thumbs (Fig. 8–9).

OTOPALATODIGITAL SYNDROME (Taybi Syndrome; OPD)

Smith (1970) stated that three siblings with this complex were described by Taybi and a fourth case was reported by Dudding et al (1967). It is the other way around. Taybi (1962) reported a 10-year-old boy; Dudding et al (1967) described three male siblings; and Langer (1967) detailed the roentgenographic features of the same three brothers. It is not decided as to whether the trait is transmitted as an autosomal or X-linked recessive. The affected child is moderately retarded mentally and physically. The occiput is prominent and the frontal

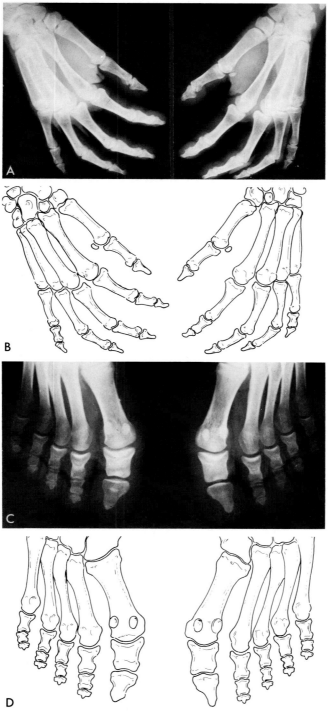

Figure 8–8 Spear-shaped ungual phalanges in cleidocranial dysostosis. *A*, Oblique roentgenograph of an adult female with cleidocranial dysostosis: almost all ungual phalanges are tuftless. *B*, Sketch of the same. *C*, Dorsoplantar roentgenograph of the forefeet of an adult male with cleidocranial dysostosis, showing short proximal phalanges of the great toes and dwarfed and spiked ungal phalanges of the lesser toes. *D*, Sketch illustrating the same.

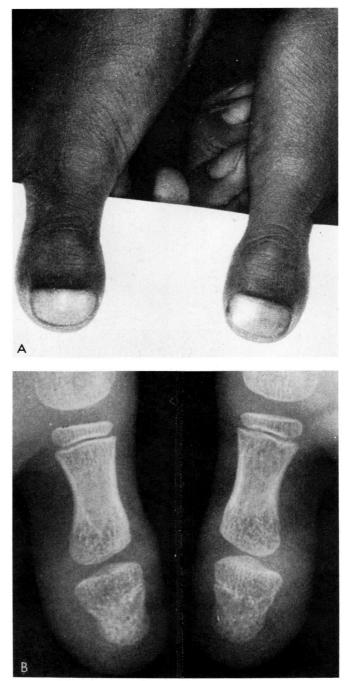

Figure 8–9 Stub thumb in a four-year-old boy with Larsen's syndrome. *A*, Dorsal view of the thumbs. *B*, Dorsopalmar roentgenograph of pollical phalanges, showing precocious effacement of physes of the ungual phalanges.

bone is thick; the facial bones are hypoplastic; the nose has a broad root and there is hypertelorism. The mouth is small and the palate cloven. There is conductive deafness. The hamate and the capitate bones of the wrist are fused and there is a pseudoepiphysis at the base of the second metacarpal. The ungual phalanges of the thumbs and toes and, to a lesser extent, of the other digits are broad and short.

PACHYDERMOPERIOSTITIS (Primary or Idiopathic Hypertrophic Osteoarthropathy)

This condition is considered akin to congenital clubbing of the fingers. It presents the following additional features: thickening of the skin and periosteum of the acral parts of the limb; thickening and seborrhea of the skin of the face and forehead and excessive sweating. Thomas (1942) entitled his article "Agnogenic congenital clubbing of the fingers and toes." He gave the name acropachy to the combination of clubbing of the fingers and painful thickening in the bones. Later authors—Vogl and Goldfischer (1962), Fischer et al (1964), and Rimoin (1965)—renamed this combination pachydermoperiostitis. The trait is considered hereditary. It is transmitted as an autosomal dominant phenotype.

PURETIC SYNDROME

Under the heading "mesenchymal dysplasia," Puretic et al (1962) described a boy with contracture of the joints, stunted growth, osteolysis of terminal phalanges, and multiple subcutaneous nodes—involvement of elements derived from mesoderm. In addition, the boy had "dysseborrhoeic sclerodermiform and atrophic changes of the skin." The proband had a brother and sister who are said to have been similarly affected and who died in infancy with painful flexion contractures of the elbows. The trait in this family is regarded as an autosomal recessive.

PYCNODYSOSTOSIS (Pyknodisostosis)

In compounding this designation, Maroteaux and Lamy (1962) utilized the Greek word *pykos* which means dense. These authors described a variety of dwarfism characterized by sclerotic and moderately brittle bones, protruding temporal ridges, obtuse mandibular angles, stubby digits simulating clubbing of the fingers, and a recessive mode of inheritance. The ungual phalanges are squat—they are tuftless and shaftless. The nails are short and brittle—dystrophic. The trait is transmitted as an autosomal recessive (Fig. 8–10).

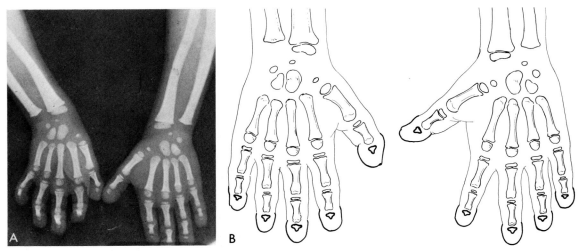

Figure 8–10 Pycnodysostosis. *A*, Dorsovolar roentgenograph of the distal forearms and hands of a five-year-old child with pycnodysostosis, showing miniature ungual phalanges. *B*, Enlarged sketch of the skeletal components of the hands.

RENAL-ACRAL   SYNDROME

A patient who came under the author's care had tuftless "spear point" terminal phalanges. He had a horseshoe kidney from which he eventually died (Fig. 8–11).

ROTHMUND   POIKILODERMIA

This is a hereditary syndrome, probably transmitted as a recessive phenotype. Its main features are atrophy, pigmentation and telangiectasia of the skin, and, at times, juvenile cataract. The subjects are small in stature and have short terminal phalanges—brachytelephalangy. Dwarfism is proportionate.

RUBINSTEIN-TAYBI   SYNDROME

Carpenter (1909) reported a male infant who, since birth, had broad thumbs which were flat at their free ends. The great toes were narrow at their bases and broad at their free ends. The palate was high and narrow. Almost half a century later, Rubinstein and Taybi (1963), whose hyphenated names this syndrome bears, identified the following features: high arched palate, short stature, mental retardation, peculiar facies with prominent forehead, elevated eyebrows, antimongoloid slant of the palpebral fissures, beaked nose with flat bridge and downward projection of the septum, and thumbs and great toes with broad terminal segments. Not infrequently, the ungual phalanx of the thumb turns in radial direction owing to abnormal configuration of the proximal phalanx; the ungual phalanx of the thumb is broad and short. The trait is regarded as an au-

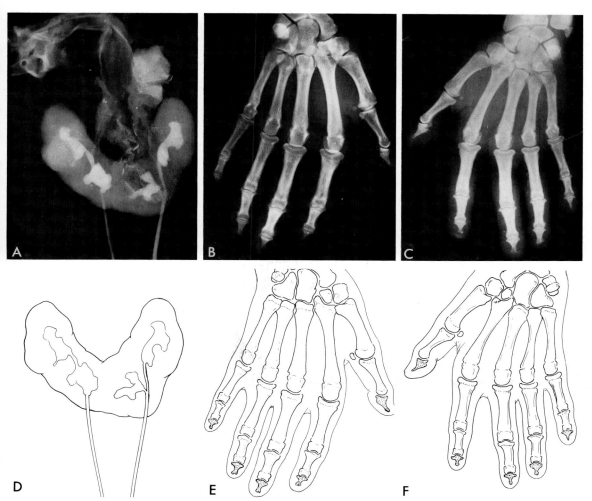

Figure 8–11   Renal osteodystrophy in an adult with horseshoe kidney. *A*, Pyelogram of a horseshoe kidney. *B* and *C* represent right and left hands respectively and show tuftless spear-shaped terminal phalanges. *D*, *E*, and *F* illustrate roentgenographs above each.

tosomal dominant. Marshall and Smith (1970) described a boy with broad thumbs and great toes and normal intelligence. The trait in this instance appeared to be dominant with variable expression.

TABATZNIK HEART AND HAND COMPLEX

McKusick (1968) mentioned a variant of the heart and hand syndrome to which he assigned the eponym Tabatznik, and gave the following as cardinal features: "cardiac arrhythmia and malformation of the upper extremities, particularly 'stub thumb' (brachydactyly, type D)." McKusick catalogued this syndrome with the autosomal dominant phenotypes.

SUMMARY

Stub thumb, congenital clubbing, and Kirner's deformity constitute a triad of anomalies which selectively affect the terminal phalanges. Stub thumb is preeminently a genetic disorder and is encountered quite often. Congenital clubbing of the fingers is comparatively rare; it is a hereditary trait transmitted as an autosomal dominant and is more common in males. Kirner's deformity is characterized by bilateral radial curvature of the attenuated shaft of the ungual phalanx of the little finger; it is also transmitted as an autosomal dominant phenotype but is more common in females. Most abnormalities of the ungual phalanx are syndromic. Stub thumb is known to occur in connection with Berk-Tabatznik syndrome, Larsen's syndrome, otopalatodigital syndrome, and the Tabatznik heart and hand constellation. Congenital clubbing of the fingers is simulated by the following complexes: congenital acro-osteolysis, cartilage-hair hypoplasia, pachydermoperiostitis, peripheral dysostosis, palmar and plantar keratosis, and pycnodysostosis. In cleidocranial dysostosis and in renal-acral syndrome, the ungual phalanx is tuftless; in acroosteolysis, its shaft is absent; and in pycnodysostosis, both tuft and shaft are missing and only the basal epiphysis remains. In pachydermoperiostitis, the phalanx as a whole is thick. None of the congenital anomalies of the ungual phalanx require surgical interference.

References

Berk, M. E., and Tabatznik, B.: Cervical dyphosis from posterior hemivertebrae with brachyphalangy and congenital optic atrophy. *J. Bone Joint Surg., 43B*:77–86, 1961.

Blank, E., and Girdany, B. R.: Symmetric bowing of the terminal phalanges of the fifth fingers in a family (Kirner's deformity). *Am. J. Roentgenol., 93*:367–373, 1965.

Burrows, H.: Developmental abbreviation of terminal phalanges. *Br. J. Radiol., 11*:165–176, 1938.

Carpenter, G.: An infant with malformations of thumbs and toes. *Proc. R. Soc. Med., 2*:59–60, 1909.

Chawla, S.: Cranio-skeletal dysplasia with acro-osteolysis. *Br. J. Radiol., 37*:702–705, 1964.

Cheyney, W. G.: Acro-osteolysis. *Am. J. Roentgenol., 94*:595–607, 1965.

Dudding, B. A., Gorlin, R. J., and Langer, L. O.: The oto-palato-digital syndrome. A symptom complex consisting of dwarfism, cleft palate, characteristic facies and a generalized bone dysplasia. *Am. J. Dis. Child., 113*:214–221; Fig. 8, 1967.

Ebstein, E.: Vererbung der hippokratischen Nagelkrümmung bzw. der Trommelschlegelfinger. *In* Angeborene, familiäre Erkrankungen an den Nageln. *Derm. Wschr., 68*:113–124, 1919.

Eiselsberg, V.: Besprechung eines Falles von multiplem, unter dem Bilde von Trommelschlägelfingern Einhergehendem Lumphangiom der Endphalangen. *Münch. Med. Wschr., 58*:1591, 1911.

Fischer, D. S., Singer, D. H., and Feldman, S.: Clubbing, a review, with emphasis on hereditary acropachy. *Medicine, 43*:459–479, 1964.

Hajdu, N., and Kauntze, R.: Cranio-skeletal dysplasia. *Br. J. Radiol., 21*:42–48, 1948.

Harnash, H.: Die Akroosteolysis, ein neues Krankheitsbild. *Fortschr. Röntgenstr., 72*:352–359, 1950.

Horsfall, F. L., Jr.: Congenital familial clubbing of the fingers and toes. *Canad. Med. Assn. J., 34*:145–149, 1936.

Kayne, G. G.: Familial clubbing of the fingers and toes. *Proc. R. Soc. Med., 26*:270–271, 1933.

Kirner, J.: Doppelseitige Verkrümmungen des Kleinfingerendgliedes als selbständiges Krankheitsbild. *Fortschr. Röntgenstr., 36*:804–806, 1927.

Langer, L. O., Jr.: The roentgenographic features of the oto-palato-digital syndrome. *Am. J. Roentgenol., 100*:63–70, 1967.

Maroteaux, P., and Lamy, M.: La pycnodysostose. *Presse Méd., 70*:999–1002, 1962.

Marshall, R. E., and Smith, D. W.: Frontodigital syndrome: a dominantly inherited disorder with normal intelligence. *J. Pediatr., 71*:129–136, 1970.

McKusick, V. A.: *Heritable Disorders of Connective Tissue.* Third edition. St. Louis, C. V. Mosby Co., pp. 441–442; 463–469, 1966.

McKusick, V. A.: *Mendelian Inheritance in Man.* Third edition. Baltimore, Johns Hopkins Press. Entry 1733; p. 199, 1968. Also in Third edition Entry 18680, p. 274, 1971.

Papavasiliou, C. G., Gargano, F. P., and Walls, W. L.: Idiopathic non-familial acro-osteolysis associated with other bone abnormalities. *Am. J. Roentgenol., 83*:687–691, 1960.

Puretic, S., Puretic, B., Fiser-Herman, M., and Adamcic, M.: A unique form of mesenchymal dysplasia. *Br. J. Dermatol., 74*:8–19, 1962.

Rimoin, D. L.: Pachydermoperiostosis (idiopathic clubbing and periostosis). Genetic and physiologic considerations. *N. Engl. J. Med., 272*:923–931, 1965.

Rubinstein, J. H., and Taybi, H.: Broad thumbs and toes and facial abnormalities. *Am. J. Dis. Child., 105*:588–608, 1963.

Seaton, D. R.: Familial clubbing of fingers and toes. *Br. Med. J. 1*:614–615, 1938.

Smith, D. W.: *Recognizable Patterns of Human Malformation.* Philadelphia, W. B. Saunders Co., Entry 48; pp. 128–129, 1970.

Stecher, R. M.: The physical characteristics and heredity of short thumbs. *Acta Genet., 7*:217–222, 1957.

Taybi, H.: Generalized skeletal dysplasia with multiple anomalies. A note on Pyle's disease. *Am. J. Roentgenol., 88*:450–457, figs. 2 and 7B, 1962.

Thomas, A. R.: A new dystrophy of the fifth finger. *Lancet, 1*:1412–1413, 1936.

Thomas, H. B.: Agnogenic congenital clubbing of the fingers and toes. *Am. J. Med. Sci., 203*:241–246, 1942.

Thomsen, O.: Hereditary growth anomaly of the thumb. *Hereditas, 10*:261–273, 1928.

Villaverde, M.: Systema endocrina y anomalias congenitas (estudio de la braquifalangia terminal del pulgar). *Vida Nueva, 51*:228–254, 1943.

Vogl, A., and Goldfischer, S.: Pachydermoperiostosis. Primary idiopathic hypertrophic osteoarthropathy. *Am. J. Med., 33*:166–187, 1962.

Weber, F. P.: The occurrence of clubbed fingers in healthy persons as a familial peculiarity. *Br. Med. J., 2*:379, 1919.

Wilson, J. N.: Dystrophy of the fifth finger. Report of four cases. *J. Bone Joint Surg., 34B*:236–239, 1952.

Witherspoon, J. T.: Clubbing of the fingers inherited. First incidence reported in Negro race. *J. Hered., 26*:15–16, 1935.

Chapter Nine

BRACHYDACTYLY

The anomaly of short digits has several claims for distinction. It is the most thoroughly studied congenital abnormality of the hand and has evoked a number of communications which vie with one another in excellence. The skeletal defect underlying short digits was one of the first anomalies to be demonstrated by what was called the "roentgen process": the reproduction of a roentgenograph which appeared in the February, 1896 issue of the *Boston Medical and Surgical Journal* showed the middle phalanx of the forefinger wanting and the middle phalanx of the little finger stunted. It was during this year again that Smith (1896) studied the hands of a child with Down's syndrome; he found that the middle phalanx of the little finger was short and the distal segment deviated in radial direction. A short middle phalanx and a radially inclining ungual segment of the little finger are now considered as common features of trisomy 21.

Digital dwarfing was the first physical abnormality in man to be accorded Mendelian interpretation and assessed as a dominant trait. As will be discussed in Chapter Twenty-nine, short digits can also claim priority in that they have been used as evidence to prove the paternity of a man who denied he had fathered an illegitimate child. Digital dwarfing, moreover, is the most common hand anomaly seen in connection with syndromes and systemic disorders.

Most authors writing about dwarfed digits of the hand also include short toes in their discussions. Even though, in the majority of cases, the digits of both the hand and the foot are affected, this discussion shall be limited to the former. Short toes are not disabling and remain hidden in shoes most of the time. Short fingers cannot be concealed indefinitely and invite attention. In some instances, dwarfed digits of the hand are also stiff or misaligned; they cannot be expected to perform as efficiently as fingers with normal posture, normal length, and three flexible joints.

TERMINOLOGY

Leboucq (1896) took into consideration the general reduction of digital length and used the term *brachydactyly*. Drinkwater (1908–1916) adopted the same nomenclature, but distinguished two subgroups: (1) minor brachydactyly, in which the middle phalanges of the four ulnar digits are short, but reduction of digital length as a whole is moderate; (2) brachydactyly proper, in which the middle phalanges are either rudimentary or fused with the ungual segments, causing drastic reduction in digital length. Farabee (1905) described the latter variety and called it hypophalangia. He supposed that the middle phalanx had completely disappeared. Haws and McKusick (1963) visited the clan Farabee had described. They examined the hands of the living descendants and concluded that the main change was not absence, but hypoplasia of the middle phalanges which often became fused with the distal bones. Haws and McKusick retained Leboucq's terminology.

Pfitzner (1898) wrote about this subject only two years after Leboucq. He pointed out that in most instances the short phalanx was responsible for the reduced digital length. Pfitzner considered brachyphalangy as a more appropriate designation. Mohr and Wriedt (1919) contended that "not the finger . . . as a whole, but . . . phalanges are shortened." They also preferred the term brachyphalangy. Most German authors—Pol (1914) among others—considered the term brachyphalangy more precise. MacArthur and McCullough (1932) also adopted this; they argued that the disturbance causing short digits was restricted to certain bones, most commonly to the metacarpals or middle phalanges of the fingers, or to the terminal phalanx of the thumb. The inclusion of metacarpals refutes the contention that the reduced length of the digit is invariably due to a shortened phalanx or brachyphalangy. MacArthur and McCullough described a comparatively uncommon variety of short digits and used the designation apical dystrophy.

In discussions about digital dwarfing, terms with specific reference to various segments are often employed. Brachymegalodactylism denotes a stub thumb. Brachybasophalangy, brachymesophalangy, and brachytelephalangy, respectively, incriminate the basal, middle, and terminal phalanges. Brachymetacarpia refers to reduced digital length due to short metacarpals. Brachyhypophalangy refers to reduction in the number of phalanges. In brachyclinodactyly, the dwarfed digit is deviated sideways; in brachycamptodactyly, it is bent forward; and in brachyclinocamptodactyly, it inclines in both directions. Brachysymphalangy denotes end-to-end fusion of short phalanges. Symbrachydactyly refers to short, webbed digits.

CLASSIFICATION

MacArthur and McCullough (1932) differentiated two main groups of short digits: (1) those which are apparent at birth; and (2) the ones that become conspicuous as the child grows, usually before the age of 10 years. In the first class, MacArthur and McCullough placed the apical dystrophy they described. In the second group were included short digits due to precocious ossification or absent epiphyses of metacarpals and phalanges. Bell (1951) distinguished five main types of brachydactyly and labeled them respectively with letters A, B, C, D, and E. Bell's classification is reproduced here with a few modifications:

A. *Brachymesophalangy*
    1. Farabee (1905) type involves all five digits: the index and little fingers tend to be more severely affected; the middle phalanges of the second to fifth

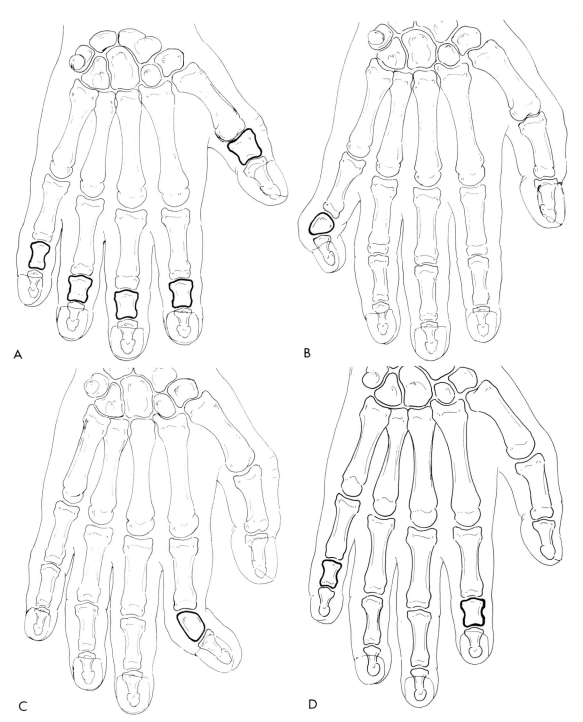

Figure 9–1   Sketches illustrating variants of brachymesophalangy. *A*, Farabee type. *B*, Brachydactyly of the little finger. *C*, Mohr-Wriedt type. *D*, Brachymesophalangy of the index and little fingers.

digits are rudimentary or fused with the terminal segments; the proximal phalanx of the thumb is short.

2. Mohr-Wriedt (1919) type affects the index finger alone; the middle phalanx is rhomboid or triangular in shape, with a broad ulnar border which causes the terminal segment to tilt toward the thumb.

3. Brachymesophalangy of the little finger: shortening is limited to the middle phalanx of the fifth digit; the affected bone is rhomboid or triangular in shape, with a broad ulnar base which causes the distal segment to incline in the radial direction.

B. *Apical dystrophy* of MacArthur and McCullough (1932), or banana fingers: in this variant the four ulnar digits barely project beyond the thumb and resemble stumps left after amputation; the fingers have no nails; the thumb retains its length, but is broad; it is at times bifid and bears a split or double nail; in some cases, the third and fourth digits are webbed.

C. *Drinkwater type*: dwarfing involves mainly the index and middle fingers, and is ascribed to the shortness of the proximal and middle phalanges of these digits; in comparison, the ring finger appears long; the index finger inclines toward the ulnar border of the hand.

D. *Brachymegalodactyly* or stub thumb: the terminal phalanx of the thumb is broad and squat.

E. *Brachymetacarpia:* shortening is confined to the metacarpal bones, more commonly of the fourth and the fifth digital rays.

One wishes that the types outlined in the preceding paragraphs were as clear-cut as they have been made to appear in the literature. In many cases, two or even three types co-exist. One often sees short middle phalanges with short ungual segments and dwarfed metacarpals and short phalanges in the same or opposite hand (Figs. 9–1 to 9–7).

In Bell's classification, one also notes the absence of any mention of brachybasophalangy, which seems to favor the index and ring fingers, usually the former. Vidal (1909), and after him Cohn and Raven (1941), described a type of brachydactyly in which the index finger is drastically reduced in length and deviated toward the ulnar border of the hand. Upon roentgenographic examination, one sees in children a triangular piece of bone which is lodged between the base of the proximal phalanx and the second metacarpal. The triangular ossicle has a broad radial base which causes the index finger to tilt away from the thumb. The index finger has a normal terminal phalanx and a very short middle phalanx. The wedge-shaped piece of bone at the base of the proximal phalanx may eventually fuse with the latter or remain discrete. In either case, the index finger is short and deflected toward the ulnar border of the hand. It often rides astride the middle finger. The anomaly is bilateral and symmetrical (Fig. 9–8).

Not long after the inception of diagnostic roentgenography around 1896, Friedrich et al (1901) included in their book a roentgenograph of a hand with short fingers. The middle phalanx of the index finger was replaced by a triangular piece of bone with a broad ulnar base, causing the ungual segment to tilt toward the thumb. Mohr and Wriedt (1919) described this variety in great detail, and the anomaly is often called Mohr-Wriedt type of brachydactyly. Blondell Jones (1964) assigned the epithet *delta* to the triangular ossicle. The anomaly is often seen in tetradactylic hands and it is at times associated with syndactyly of either the same or opposite hands (Fig. 9–9).

The most common type of brachymesophalangy is that which affects the

(Text continued on page 244.)

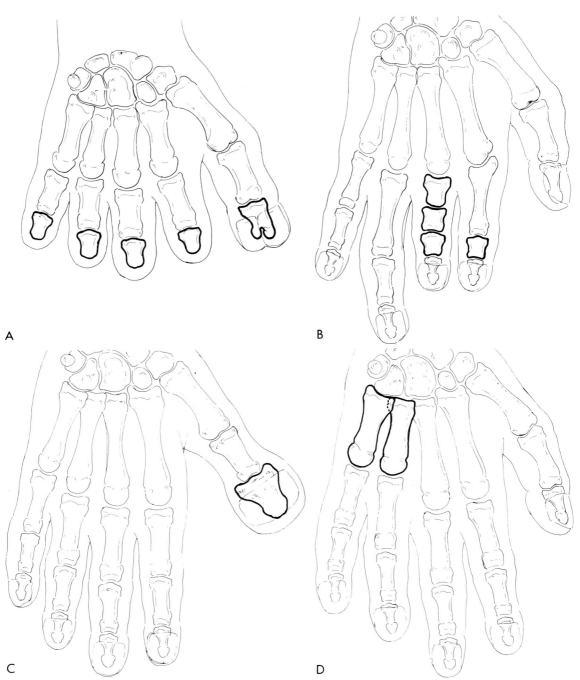

Figure 9–2 *A,* Sketch illustrating apical dystrophy of MacArthur and McCullough. *B,* Drawing illustrating Drinkwater type of brachydactyly. *C,* Drawing showing brachymegalodactyly or stub thumb. *D,* Sketch illustrating brachymetacarpia.

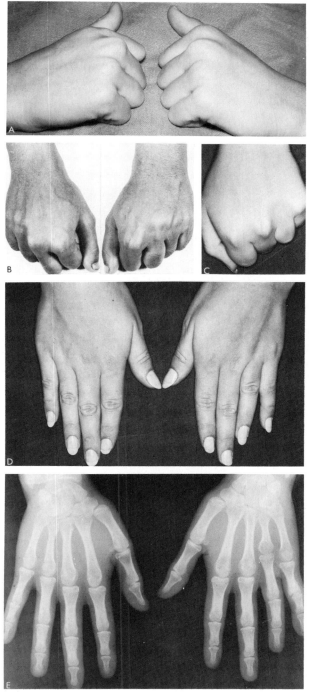

Figure 9–3 Brachymetacarpia. *A,* Test indicating shortened right second metacarpal. *B,* Test denoting dwarfed fourth and fifth metacarpals of the right hand and third, fourth, and fifth metacarpals of the left hand of the same patient. *C,* Sunken knuckle of the left ring finger auguring the most common type of brachymetacarpia—that of the fourth metacarpal. *D,* Dorsal view of the hands of the same patient: note that the left ring finger is shorter than the right ring finger. *E,* Dorsopalmar roentgenograph of the same, showing a dwarfed left fourth metacarpal; the fracture of the proximal phalanx of the little finger was an incidental finding—it was, in fact, the main reason for taking this roentgenograph.

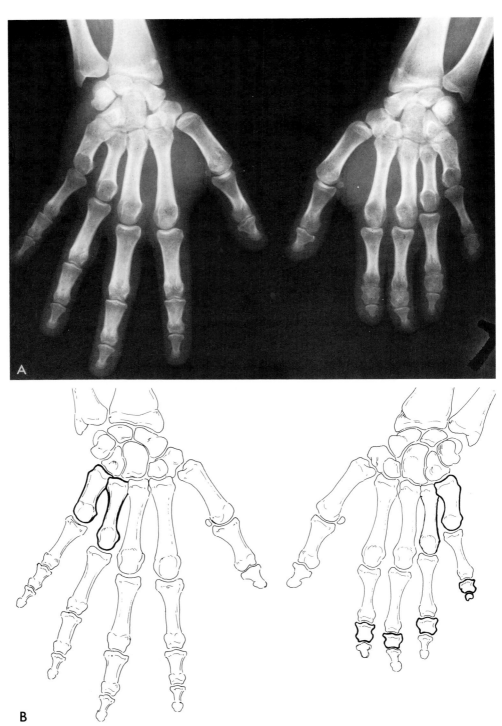

Figure 9–4   Bilateral brachymetacarpia of the fourth and fifth digital rays of both hands associated with brachyme-sophalangy of digits two to five and brachytelephalangy of the index and little fingers of the left hand. *A*, Dorsopalmar roentgenograph of the hands. *B*, Sketch illustrating the same.

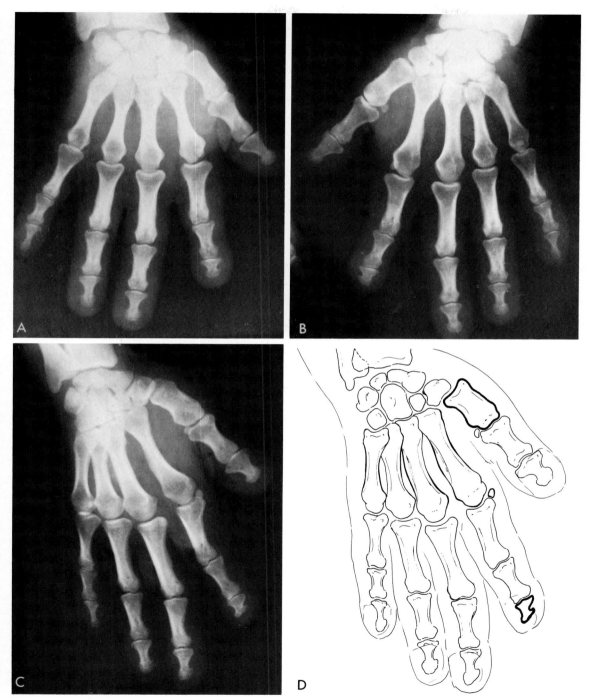

Figure 9–5 Short first metacarpal associated with brachytelephalangy of the index finger. *A* and *B*, Dorsopalmar roentgenograph of the right and left hands. *C*, Oblique view of the right hand. *D*, Sketch illustrating the same.

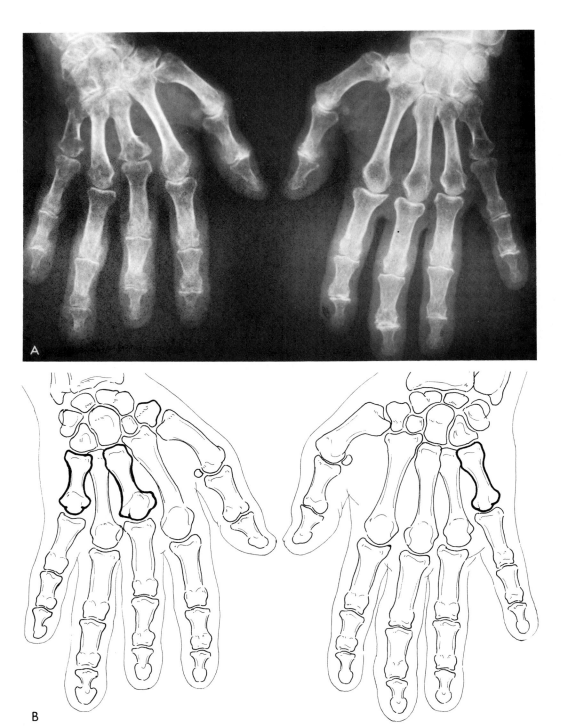

Figure 9–6 Short metacarpals. *A*, Dorsopalmar roentgenograph of the hands of an adult female with short third and fifth metacarpals of the right hand and short fifth metacarpal of the left hand. *B*, Sketch illustrating the same.

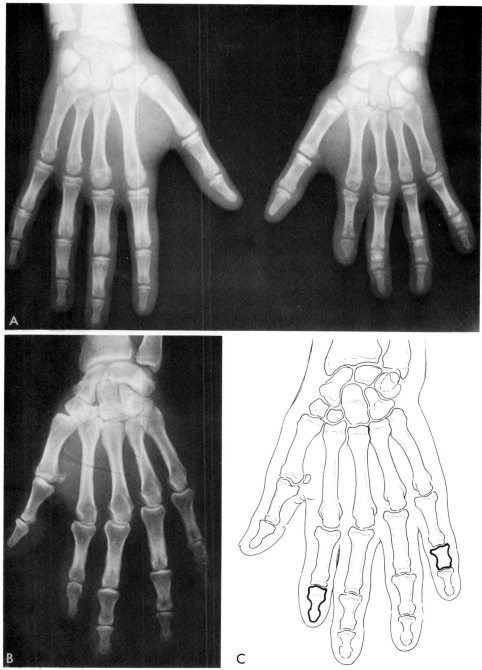

Figure 9–7   Absent middle phalanx of the index finger associated with brachymesophalangy of the little finger. *A*, Dorsopalmar roentgenograph of the hands of a 10-year-old male, showing absence of a phalanx in the left index finger and squat middle phalanx of the little finger: note the absence of an epiphysis at the base of the last phalanx of the index finger and middle phalanx of the little finger. *B*, Dorsopalmar roentgenograph of the left hand six years later or after the closure of the epiphyses. This young man has a nail on the index finger and it must be presumed that the ungual phalanx has in part survived; this last bone which had no epiphysis and appeared spiked in the earlier roentgenograph has acquired a tuft (probably by deposition of bone by its membrane tip) and gained in stature (possibly by fusion of the remnants of the middle phalanx and ungual tuft); it is in fact longer than the ungual phalanges of the other digits. The middle phalanx of the little finger is short. *C*, Sketch illustrating the same.

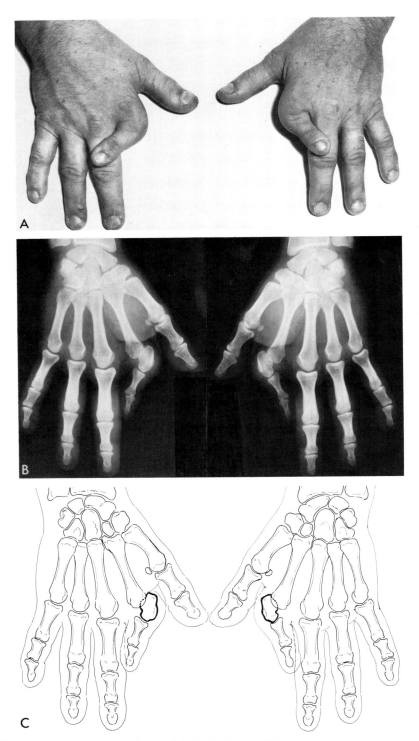

Figure 9–8 Brachybasophalangy of the index finger (Vidal type) *A*, Dorsal view of the hands of an adult male with anomalous basal phalanges of both index fingers with ulnar deviation of the distal segments. This man's son was similarly affected (see Fig. 9–18). *B*, Dorsopalmar roentgenograph of both hands. *C*, Sketch illustrating the same.

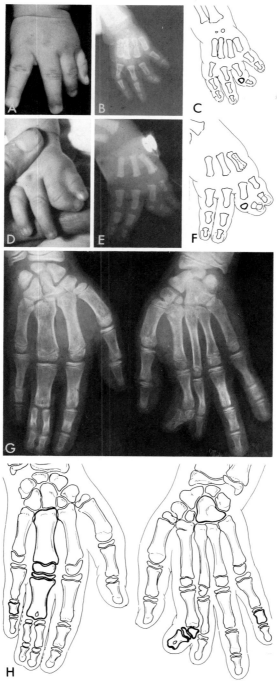

Figure 9–9 Brachymesophalangy of the index finger. *A*, Dorsal view of the tetradactylic right hand of a five-month old boy. *B*, Dorsopalmar roentgenograph of the same, showing a small, almost triangular middle phalanx, causing the ungual segment to tilt toward the thumb. *C*, Sketch illustrating the same. *D*, Dorsal view of the right hand of a younger tetradactylic infant with syndactyly of the two radial digits. *E*, Roentgenograph of the same, showing a dwarfed triangular middle phalanx. *F*, Sketch of the same. *G*, Dorsopalmar roentgenograph of the hands of a teenager: in the right hand, the metacarpals and the proximal phalanges of the third and fourth digits seem to have effected osseous union, while the middle and ungual phalangeal bones remain separated but are enclosed in the same sleeve of skin; in the left hand, the middle phalanx of the index finger is triangular in shape, while the ungual bone is thick, squat, and fenestrated. *H*, Sketch illustrating the same.

fifth digit of the hand. The middle phalanx of the little finger may be missing altogether. It is usually dwarfed, and it is shorter on its radial border than on its ulnar aspect. In consequence, the terminal phalanx inclines toward the thumb. In other words, there is clinodactyly in addition to brachydactyly. Hersh et al (1953) estimated the incidence of this anomaly in the population to be about one in a thousand. This type of brachymesophalangy is the most common hand anomaly seen in connection with dysmorphic syndromes or syndromes with multiple primary defects. In more severe cases, besides being tilted toward the thumb, the ungual segment of the little finger is flexed, producing the deformity of brachyclinocamptodactyly (Figs. 9–10 to 9–13).

ABNORMALITY OF TRANSVERSE SEGMENTATION AS A BASIS OF DIGITAL DWARFING

Drinkwater (1916) related the reduction of digital length to an abnormality of transverse segmentation involving the tubular bones of the hand. These bones are either absent, prematurely ossified, or fused together. In the embryonic handplate, the metacarpals and the phalanges are first represented by rods of condensed mesenchymal tissue. These rods are axially disposed and are intercepted at intervals by transverse zones. These interzones mark the sites of future metacarpophalangeal and interphalangeal joints. Condensed mesenchymal rods become converted into cartilage.

The condensation and chondrification of embryonic tissue starts in the proximal row of phalanges and proceeds distally. Except for the fact that it skips the middle phalanges, ossification proceeds in the opposite direction. It starts at the tips of the terminal phalanges and proceeds proximally. The first bone of the hand to ossify is the terminal phalanx of the thumb. Mall (1906) found bone at the tip of the phalanx in the embryo at the fifty-sixth day. At about the ninth week of embryonic existence, the primary centers of ossification of the metacarpal bones and the proximal row of phalanges appear. The metacarpals of the index and middle fingers ossify earlier and are less likely to remain short. Brachymetacarpia seems to favor metacarpals with delayed ossification—in particular, the metacarpals of the ring and little fingers (Fig. 9–14).

The last bones of the hand to ossify are the middle row of phalanges; ossification occurs in these segments around the eleventh or twelfth week. The last bones to ossify in this row are the middle phalanges of the index and the little fingers, and brachymesophalangy affects these digits most often. Mall (1906) pointed out that, for a protracted period during embryonic development, the ulnar border of the middle phalanx of the little finger is longer than its radial side. This discrepancy persists and reveals itself in brachyclinodactyly of the little finger.

At birth, all the primary centers located in the shafts of the metacarpals and phalanges are ossified, but the epiphyses are still cartilaginous. The phalanges which are most prone to remain short are those of the second row. In the third row, the epiphyses of the bones belonging to the middle and ring fingers appear earlier than those of the index and little fingers. The middle and ring fingers—especially the latter—usually retain their length in most cases of brachydactyly (Fig. 9–15).   (Text continued on page 250.)

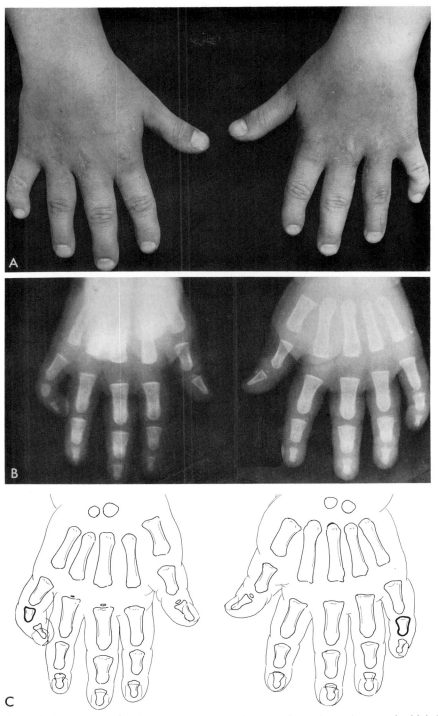

Figure 9–10 Bilateral brachymesophalangy of the little finger in a nine-month-old infant, showing radially inclined flexed distal segments of the little fingers. *A*, Dorsal view of the hands. *B*, Dorsopalmar roentgenograph of the hands: the middle phalanx of each little finger is longer on the ulnar than on the radial side. *C*, Sketch illustrating the same.

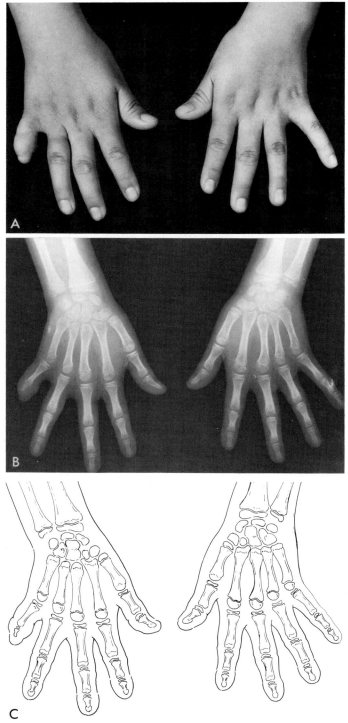

Figure 9–11   Absent middle phalanx of the little finger. *A*, Dorsal view of the hands of an eight-year-old female: note that the right little finger bears a small nail. *B*, Dorsopalmar roentgeno-graph of the hands, showing absence of a middle phalanx in the right little finger and dwarfed ungual segment. *C*, Sketch illustrating the same.

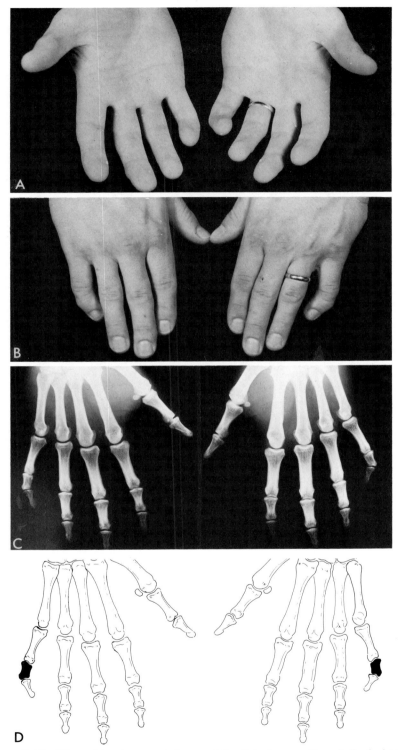

Figure 9–12 Bilateral brachymesophalangy of the little finger with radially deviated flexed ungual segment. *A*, Palmar view of the hands. *B*, Dorsal view. *C*, Roentgenograph of the hands. *D*, Sketch illustrating the same.

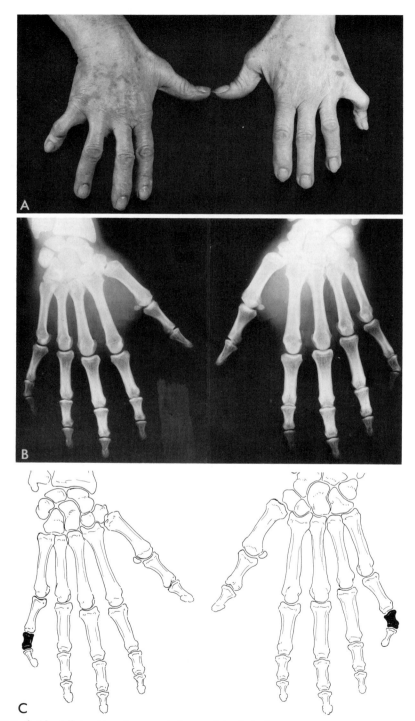

Figure 9–13 Bilateral brachymesophalangy of the little finger with flexed middle and radially deviated distal segments (brachyclinocamptodactyly). *A*, Dorsal view of the hands. *B*, Dorsopalmar roentgenograph of the same: not only is the middle phalanx of each little finger dwarfed as a whole but also its radial border is shorter than its ulnar margin. *C*, Sketch illustrating the same.

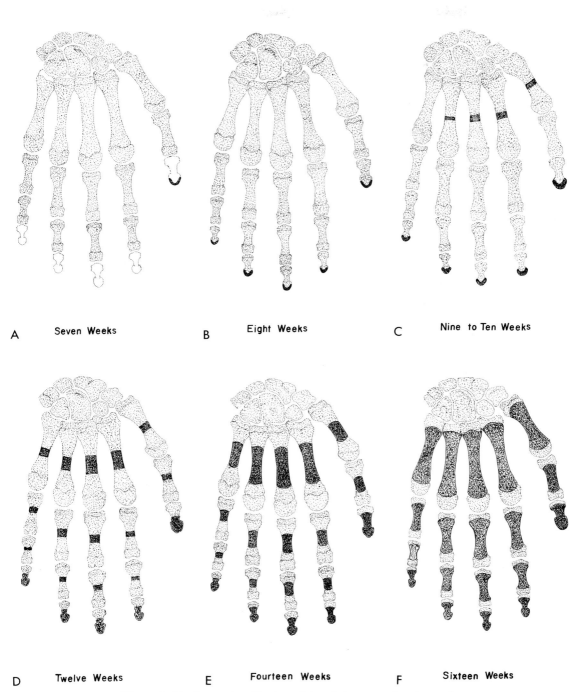

A   Seven Weeks   B   Eight Weeks   C   Nine to Ten Weeks

D   Twelve Weeks   E   Fourteen Weeks   F   Sixteen Weeks

Figure 9–14 Prenatal ossification of the phalanges and metacarpals.

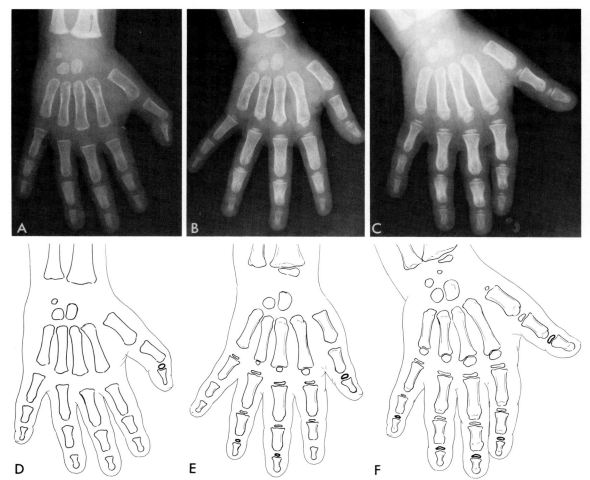

Figure 9–15 As with other secondary growth centers, there is considerable variation and vagrancy in the appearance of epiphyses of the tubular bones of the hands. These centers appear earlier in girls than in boys, and earlier in northern Europeans than in Mediterranian races. For this figure the right hands of three boys belonging to the latter group were roentgenographed. *A,* The right hand of a 21-month-old male: the distal epiphysis of the radius is not yet visible; there are three carpal ossicles and, of the tubular bones of the hand, only the ungual phalanx of the thumb possesses an epiphysis. *B,* The hand of a 28-month-old boy: the epiphyses of the proximal phalanx of the thumb, of the middle and ungual phalanges of the little finger, and of the fifth metacarpal bone are not visible; there are only two carpal bones and a sizable radial epiphysis. *C,* The hand of a 33-month-old boy of the same ethnic origin: all tubular bones of the hand have acquired secondary growth centers; there are four carpal bones and the radius possesses a small distal epiphysis — much smaller than the corresponding center of the five-months-younger boy whose hand is shown in *B.* Sketches *D, E,* and *F* illustrate the roentgenograph above each.

Nissen (1933) considered delayed appearance of the secondary centers of the terminal phalanges of the index and little fingers to be significant. In the series of short digits which he reported, the epiphyses were frequently absent from the terminal phalanges, especially in the index and little fingers, though they were always present in the thumb. Epiphyses were consistently absent in the middle phalanges, thus providing another reason for their shortness. "Where epiphyses are absent from both middle and terminal phalanges," Nissen wrote, "it may be assumed that bony union is facilitated between the ossifying middle phalanx and the phalanges proximal and distal to it."

   Prior to the establishment of bony union between epiphyses and the shaft, a
plate of growth cartilage intervenes between them. In the metacarpals and phalanges, this plate is disposed transversely. The longitudinal growth of each metacarpal or phalanx depends primarily upon the new bone laid down by the
growth cartilage plate. Occasionally, a strip of fibrous tissue or cartilage intervenes between the bone deposited by the growth cartilage plate and the already
ossified shaft, leading to what is known as hypersegmentation. These interposed
strips temporarily impede longitudinal growth. They may eventually vanish or
persist. In either case, the affected digital ray remains short (Fig. 9–16).

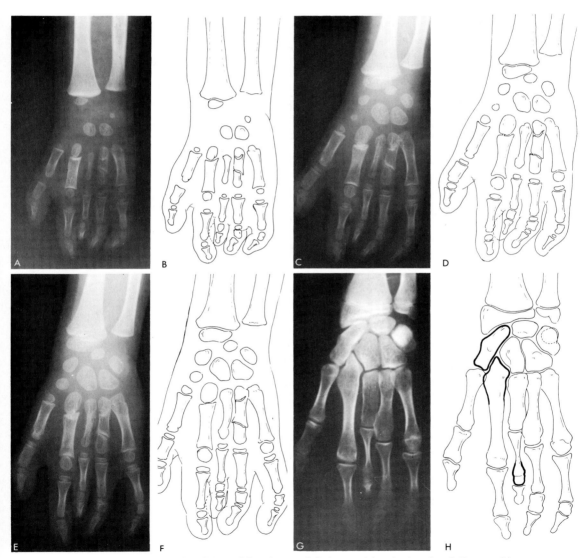

Figure 9–16 Hypersegmentation followed by abnormal fusion and brachydactyly. *A*, Dorsopalmar roentgenograph of the left hand of a three-year-old female. *B*, Sketch of the same. *C*, Roentgenograph of the hand two years later.
D, Sketch of the same. *E*, Roentgenograph of the hand at the age of six years. *F*, Sketch illustrating the same. *G*, Roentgenograph at the age of 13, showing coalescence of scaphoid with trapezium and trapezoid with second metacarpal,
absence of middle phalanges of the second and third digits, squat middle phalanges of the ring and little fingers, and a
dwarfed third metacarpal. *H*, Sketch illustrating the same.

Abnormality of transverse segmentation may involve various elements—joints, growth plates, and shafts of bones. Parts are absent, or have grown together where they should not, or failed to unite when they should. Absences are either terminal or intercalary. In terminal transverse absence, the dwarfed digits have lost varying portions of their ungual and, at times, their middle phalanges. What remains resembles the stumps left after amputation. This defect is easily recognizable at birth. The category of transverse intercalary abnormalities includes precocious closure of growth plates, fusion of two consecutive bones, and hypersegmentation of the shafts. Precocious closure of growth plates leaves the involved bone short. In end-to-end union of two consecutive phalanges, the single segment produced is shorter than the added length of the two separate bones. In hypersegmentation, the combined length of four or more small ossicles is less than that of three normal phalanges. Digital dwarfing caused by intercalary abnormalities is insidious: its development may not become manifest until years after birth. MacArthur and McCullough (1932) must have had these intercalary abnormalities in mind when they said, "Short digits, like stature, are not always detectable until a certain age is reached."

HEREDITY

Nineteenth century authors—Kellie (1808), MacKinder (1857), and many others—reported cases of dwarfed digits reappearing in successive generations of the same family. In 1903—three years after the rediscovery of Mendel's principle of heredity—Farabee submitted his doctoral thesis. The subjects of Farabee's study belonged to a family in Pennsylvania. More than half of the members of this clan had short digits. Farabee concluded that the anomaly was inherited "in conformity with Mendel's law for five generations," meaning it was strictly a dominant trait. This verdict has not been changed and has been applied to other forms of short digits: apical dystrophy, stub thumb, brachymetacarpia, and brachydactyly due to hypersegmentation. In the pedigree described by Mohr and Wriedt (1919), the affected members were heterozygous with one exception. "This individual," Mohr and Wriedt wrote, "resulted from an intermarriage with the affected lines, and therefore may have been homozygous for the factor. . . . She was a cripple without fingers. . . . She died at the age of one year." To be lethal in the homozygous state, a gene must be very potent—in MacKinder's (1857) language, it must have a "rigorous root." Hersh et al (1953) described a pedigree of brachymesophalangy of the little finger with radial inclination of the distal phalanx; they considered the trait to be an autosomal dominant with a slight variation of penetrance. Brachybasophalangy of the index finger is also transmitted as an autosomal dominant trait (Figs. 9–17 and 9–18).

ASSOCIATIONS

In Farabee's (1905) pedigree, every brachydactylous man was shorter and stouter than his normal brother, and the affected woman was shorter than her unaffected sister. Haws and McKusick (1963) examined the descendants of this family and found evidence of epiphyseal disturbance in other parts of the skeleton—particularly in the appendicular skeleton. The affected individuals

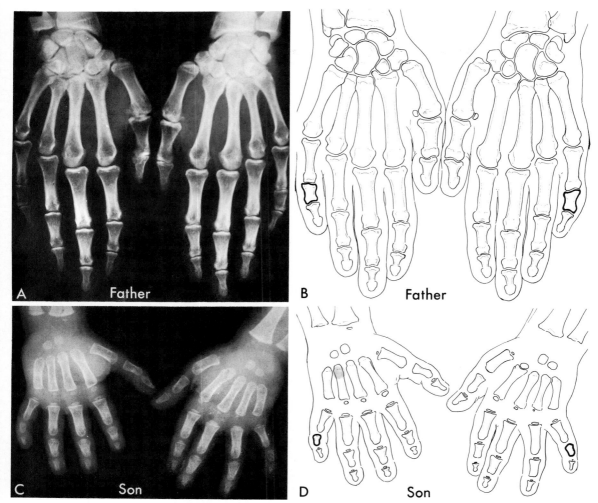

Figure 9–17 Father-to-son transmission of bilateral brachyclinodactyly of the little finger. *A*, Dorsopalmar roentgenograph of the father's hands. *B*, Sketch illustrating the same. *C*, Dorsopalmar roentgenograph of the son's hands. *D*, Sketch illustrating the same.

had short arms and short legs, but their sitting height was nearly normal; they also had short toes. Nissen (1933) noted the presence of accessory bones in the wrists and ankles in many of the members of the pedigree he described. End-to-end fusion of the phalanges or symphalangism is a common finding in brachydactyly. Roederer (1914) noted the association of a short third metacarpal with scoliosis. In a brachydactylous family reported by Brailsford (1946), affected members developed precocious bilateral osteoarthritis of the hip. Shafar (1941) traced a variety of hereditary chondro-osteodystrophy through these generations. The affected individuals had small hands with short digits, owing to irregular involvement of the metacarpals and the middle and distal phalanges. The 18-month-old child with brachybasophalangy and ulnar deviation of the index finger reported by Cohn and Raven (1941) had hallux valgus interphalangeus. In symbrachydactyly, the digits are short and webbed. Brachymetacarpia of the first metacarpal is at times seen with a short ulna (Figs. 9–19 and 9–20).

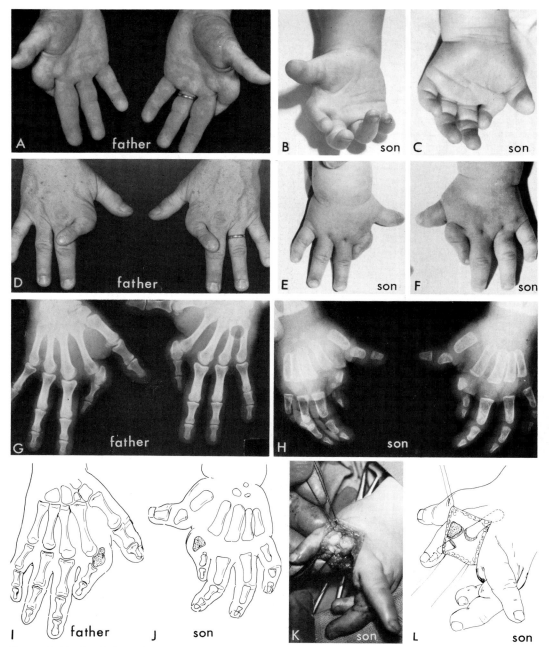

Figure 9–18 Brachybasophalangy of the index fingers with ulnar deviation of distal segments. Father-to-son transmission. *A,* Palmar view of the father's hands. *B* and *C,* Palmar view of the son's hands. *D,* Dorsal view of the father's hands. *E* and *F,* Dorsal view of the son's hands. *G,* Dorsopalmar roentgenograph of the father's hands. *H,* Dorsopalmar roentgenograph of the son's hands. *I,* Sketch illustrating the roentgenograph of the son's hands. *J,* Sketch illustrating the roentgenograph of the son's left hand. *K,* This hand was surgically explored: the triangular proximal phalanx of the index finger was found in an eccentric position, as shown in sketch *L.*

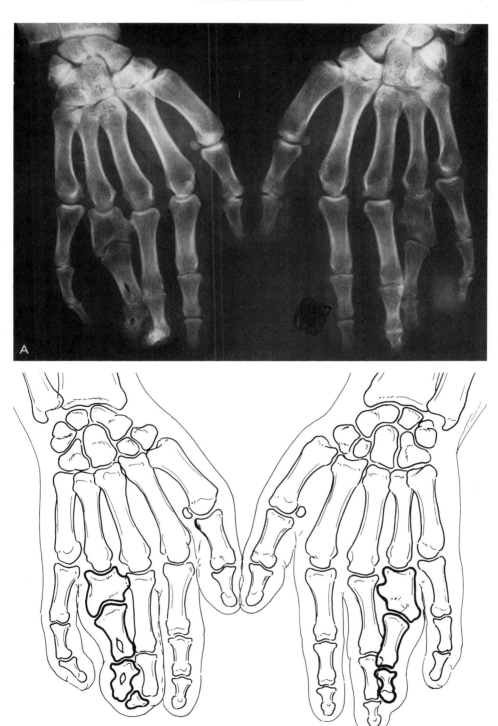

Figure 9–19 Bilateral brachybasophalangy of the ring finger in a patient with syndactyly of the third and fourth digits. *A,* Dorsopalmar roentgenograph of the right and left hands. *B,* Sketch illustrating the same.

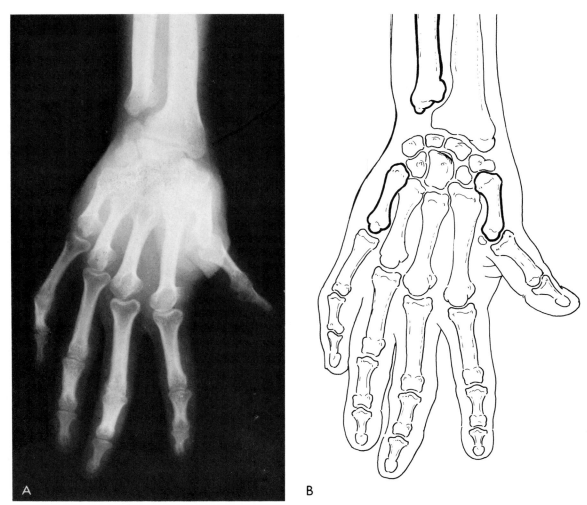

Figure 9-20   Short first and fifth metacarpals associated with a short right ulna. *A*, Dorsopalmar roentgenograph of the right hand. *B*, Sketch illustrating the same.

All dwarfs have short digits. As indicated in Chapter Four, the compendium of dwarfism contains more than 40 generalized disorders. The fingers are short in all forms of mucopolysaccharidosis and in such metabolic and endocrine disorders as congenital hypothyroidism and hypophosphatasia. It would take several hundred pages to discuss all of these, and their discussion would lead us too far afield. We shall also eschew innumerable syndromes which are accompanied by short middle phalanx of the little finger with radial deviation of the distal segment. The complexes paraphrased in the ensuing sections represent a selected group. They may give an idea concerning the catholicity of syndromic brachydactyly.

ABSENT MIDDLE PHALANGES AND HYPOPLASTIC NAILS

Bass (1968) described a family in which 13 members in four generations had hypoplastic finger- and toenails, absent middle phalanges in the four ulnar and four fibular digits, duplicated distal phalanges of the thumbs, and possible hypoplasia of the auricular cartilage. In the pedigree traced by Cueva-Sosa and Garcia-Segur (1971), an analogous cluster of anomalies ran through seven generations. Some members of this clan presented variable degrees of hypoplasia of the terminal phalanges of the fingers.

ACHONDROGENESIS

This is a severe form of micromelic dwarfism. Affected infants have rudimentary, short digits, each digit being composed of a single segment. Two varieties now recognized: lethal and nonlethal. Lethal cases were reported by Parenti (1936) and Fraccaro (1952); Grebe (1952) and Quelce-Salgado (1964) described living subjects. The trait is regarded as an autosomal recessive (Fig. 9–21).

ACHONDROPLASIA

Parrot (1878) introduced the designation achondroplasia, which many authors consider a misnomer. Notwithstanding, this name has become deeply etched in the literature and has not been dislodged by any suggested substitute. Achondroplasia is regarded as the prototype of short-limbed dwarfism. It is classed under the rhizomelic variety, since the bones close to the roots of the limbs are more extensively affected than those of the midsegment and these, in turn, more than the terminal segments. The basic disturbance is faulty endochondral ossification. In long bones, the growth from the epiphyseal area is kept in abeyance, while deposition of bone around the shaft by the periosteum continues. In consequence, the involved bones have bulbous ends and short, thick shafts. Soft tissues overlying the affected bones are bulky. The hand is fleshy, plump, and spatulate. The pudginess of the digits does not extend beyond the proximal phalanges; when fingers are extended and proximal phalanges touch one another, the terminal segments remain separated. The hand is then said to be trident. The four ulnar digits are also described as being isometric, or equal in length. It would be more accurate to say that these fingers are nearer the same length than is normal.

A number of atypical forms of achondroplasia have been described in the literature. In some of these the trident arrangement of the fingers is missing, but the digits are short. Advanced paternal age is said to play a definite role in the causation of achondroplasia; this is in contrast to trisomy 21, in which advanced maternal age is considered a factor. Achondroplasia is transmitted as an autosomal dominant trait (Figs. 9–22 and 9–23).

ACRODYSOSTOSIS

This designation was introduced by Maroteaux and Malamut (1968). Robinow et al (1971) reported 11 cases and gave the following as the major features: peripheral dysostosis, nasal hypoplasia, mental defect, and premature

(Text continued on page 261.)

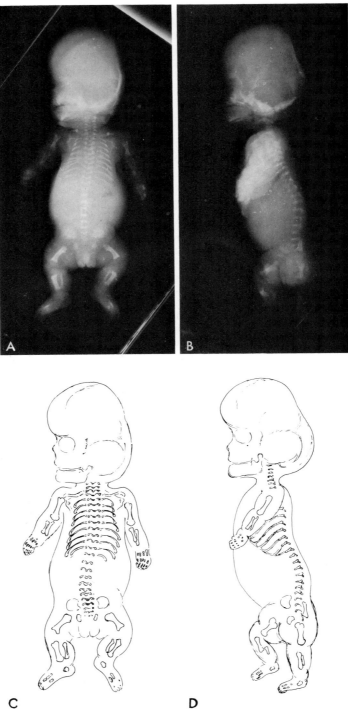

Figure 9–21 The skeleton of a mesomelic stillborn dwarf: probably a case of achondrogenesis. *A*, Anteroposterior roentgenograph. *B*, Lateral roentgenograph. *C* and *D* illustrate roentgenograph above each.

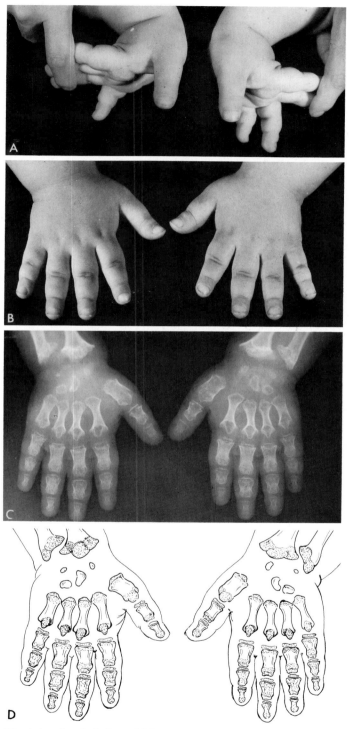

Figure 9–22   Achondroplasia in a child. *A*, Radial view of the hands, showing hyperextensibility of the fingers. *B*, Dorsal view, showing trident fingers. *C*, Dorsopalmar roentgenograph of the hands. *D*, Sketch illustrating the same.

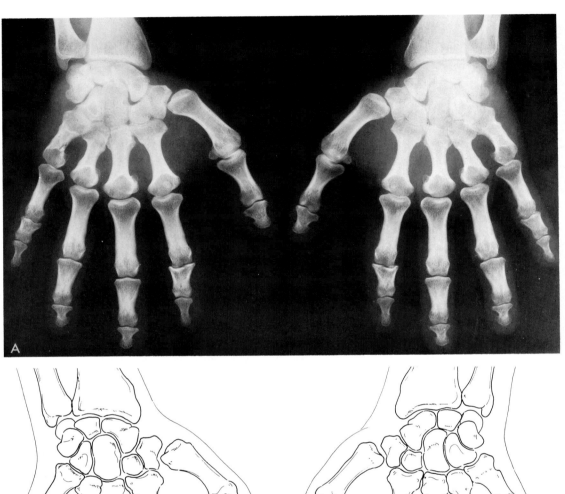

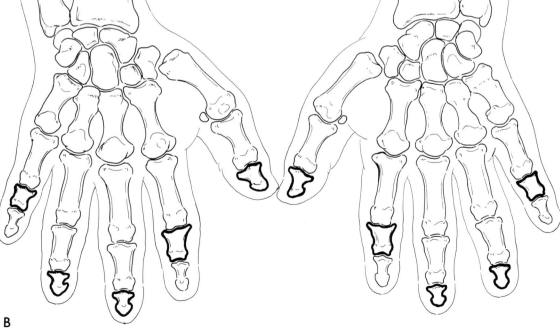

Figure 9–23 Adult achondroplastic dwarf. *A*, Dorsopalmar roentgenograph of the hands, showing that the four ulnar metacarpals are shorter than the corresponding proximal phalanges; the middle phalanges of the index and little fingers are dwarfed as are the ungual phalanges of the thumbs and middle and ring fingers. *B*, Sketch illustrating the same.

skeletal maturation. The phalanges have cone-shaped epiphyses and are short, as are the metacarpals. Brachydactyly becomes progressively manifest during the growth period. No familial incidence has been recorded.

ALBRIGHT'S HEREDITARY OSTEODYSTROPHY (AHO)

This is a genetic disorder characterized by a round face, short stature, obesity, dwarfed metacarpals, and insensitivity on the part of the end-organs (renal tubules) to parathyroid hormone; administration of large doses of parathyroid hormone to these patients has little or no effect on serum calcium or phosphorus or on urinary phosphate excretion. Two subgroups of AHO are recognized and called, respectively, pseudohypoparathyroidism (PHP) and pseudopseudohypoparathyroidism (PPHP). Subjects with PHP have normal serum phosphatase activity and low calcium; hence, they present with tetany, positive Chvostek and Trousseau signs, and ectopic calcification. In PPHP, the serum calcium is normal, and the symptomatology related to hypocalcemia is lacking. Most authors consider PPHP as the incomplete expression of PHP, since they are known to co-exist in the same kinship. PPHP is said to be associated with dwarfed metacarpals more often than PHP. In young patients, the affected metacarpal—the third, fourth, or fifth, or, rarely, the second—has a narrow growth cartilage plate which is often effaced prematurely. The trait of PHP or PPHP is transmitted as an autosomal dominant with incomplete penetrance and variable expressivity; females are affected more often than males (Fig. 9–24).

BANKI SYNDROME

Banki (1965) described a family in which several members in three generations showed the following anomalies: synostosis of lunate and triquetral bones, clinodactyly, and short metacarpals with thin shafts. This syndrome is catalogued with the autosomal dominant phenotypes.

BASAL CELL NEVUS SYNDROME

Glendenning et al (1963), Block and Glendenning (1963), Gorlin and associates (1963, 1965), and Ferrier and Hindrichs (1967) have described a symptom complex consisting of carcinoma-prone basal cell nevi, odontogenic cyst of the mandibles, and some other skeletal anomalies. Among the latter is included dwarfing of the fourth metacarpals. Patients with this syndrome often manifest hyporesponsiveness to parathormone and tend to have ectopic calcifications, which has led some authors to lean towards the view that this complex might be related to pseudohypoparathyroidism.

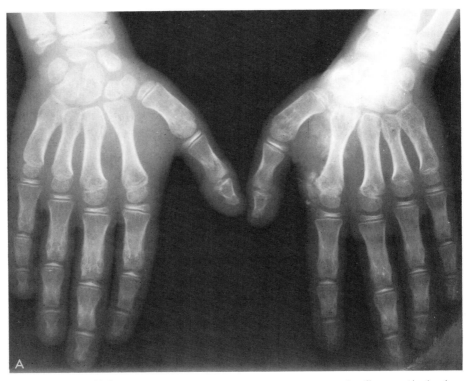

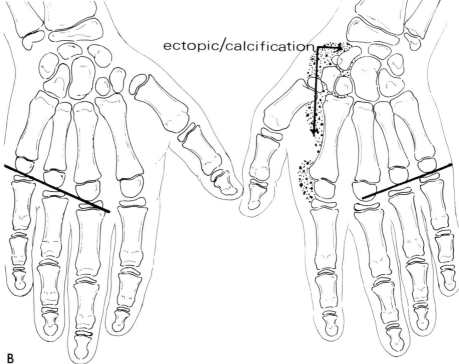

Figure 9–24 Pseudohypoparathyroidism. *A*, Dorsopalmar roentgenograph of both hands, showing ectopic calcification and short fourth and fifth metacarpals of the left hand. *B*, Sketch illustrating the same.

BIEMOND I

Cardinal features of this syndrome are cerebellar ataxia, nystagmus, and brachydactyly of the hands and feet. Biemond (1934) described this constellation in four generations of a family; only a few members possessed the full complex. Brachydactyly in this syndrome is due to dwarfing of the ulnar metacarpals. The trait is classed with the autosomal dominant phenotypes.

BRACHYCAMPTODACTYLY COMPLEX

Edwards and Gale (1970) described a kindred in which 28 persons presented the combined anomalies of brachymesophalangy and brachymetacarpia associated with flexion deformity of the digits. Many members had urinary incontinence. The offspring of affected cousins had severely dwarfed digits, syndactyly, polydactyly, deafness, and mental retardation, and one female possessed a vaginal septum.

CHROMOSOMAL ABERRATIONS

Infants born with aberrations of other than sex chromosomes are all dwarfs and have short digits; with the exception of 21 trisomics, these children usually die soon after birth. As a rule, infants with XO constitution (Turner's gonadal dysgenesis) survive and eventually evince the ensuing characteristics: short stature; pterygium colli with low hairline on the back of the neck; ovarian agenesis and infantile development of the vagina, uterus, and mammary glands; cubitus valgus; and short fourth and fifth metacarpals. The affected individual has 45 instead of 46 chromosomes, one X chromosome having been lost, thus producing an XO pattern in females. The latter are usually affected by this complex, although a number of cases of what is called Turner's syndrome in the male have been reported. Shortness of the two ulnar metacarpals is determined on a roentgenograph of the hand taken by dorsopalmar exposure. A tangential line touching the distal contours of the fifth and fourth metacarpal bones is drawn on the roentgenograph and is extended in the radial direction. Normally, this line does not pass through the head of the third metacarpal; in subjects with XO constitution, it does.

DE LANGE DWARFISM

In this form of primordial dwarfism, already mentioned, the thumb is said to be "proximally inserted" as a result of the abbreviated length of the first metacarpal. Not uncommonly, the hand lacks two or more digits, and one of the forearm bones may be missing. When there are five digits, the palm presents a simian crease (Fig. 9–25).

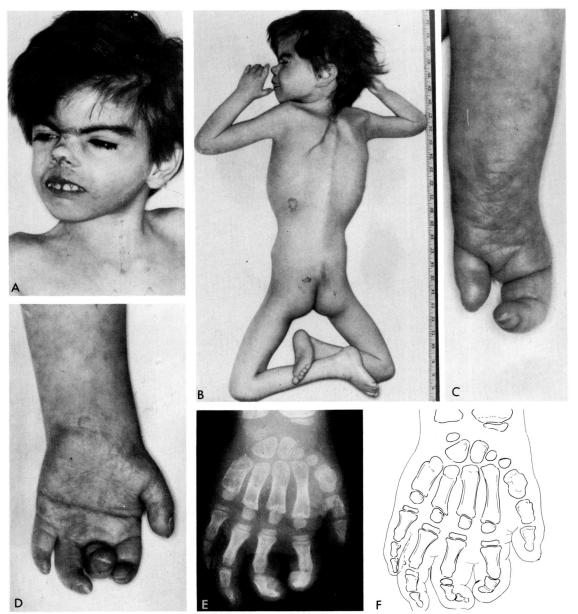

Figure 9–25 *A*, Frontal view of a six-year-old de Lange dwarf, showing leonine features. *B*, Dorsal view of the entire body. *C*, Palmar view of the bidactylic right hand. *D*, Palmar view of the left hand, showing simian crease of the palm, and a short thumb. *E*, Anteroposterior roentgenograph of the left hand, showing a short metacarpal and absence of epiphyses of the bones of the pollical ray. *F*, Sketch illustrating the same.

DIASTROPHIC DWARFISM

Diastrophic means tortuous. Lamy and Maroteaux (1960) used this adjective to distinguish a variety of dwarfism characterized by a twisted trunk and limbs; the affected infant has structural scoliosis, club foot, and dwarfed, distorted digits. In the hand, the first metacarpal suffers the greatest degree of dwarfing; it is oval or trapezoid in shape, causing the phalanges to incline in radial direction, assuming the stance of hitchhiker's thumb.

DU PAN SYNDROME (Fibula Aplasia and Complex Brachydactyly)

Martin Du Pan (1924) described a 14-year-old boy with bilateral absence of the fibula and brachydactyly of both hands: the middle phalanges of the third to fifth digits were dwarfed; the index fingers had no proximal phalanges, and the distal segments filled radially. The thumbs had short metacarpals and squat proximal phalanges. This case was sporadic. Grebe (1955) reported a brother and sister from a first-cousin marriage who had several short metacarpals, trapezoid middle phalanx of the index finger with radial deviation of the distal segment, bilateral absence of the fibula, and short toes. The inheritance in this instance was considered an autosomal recessive.

HAND-FOOT-UTERUS SYNDROME

In this complex, already discussed in Chapter Four, the first metacarpal suffers a great degree of dwarfing.

HYPOCHONDROPLASIA

This designation was introduced by Lamy and Maroteaux (1961) to denote a variant of achondroplasia in which the head is not affected. The fingers are short, but the hand is not of the trident type. McKusick (1968) stated that he knew of an affected father and daughter. Dorst et al (1969) presented a number of cases of hypochondroplasia. Patients with this condition each had short stature, a normal skull, shortening of the long bones, interpediculate narrowing of the lumbar and sacral spine, and short hands. Beals (1969) reported five kindreds with definite evidence of an autosomal dominant inheritance. Walker et al (1971) described 13 persons with this variety of "atypical" achondroplasia.

MULTIPLE EPIPHYSEAL DYSPLASIA

Fairbank (1945–1951) defined dysplasia epiphysealis multiplex as a rare congenital developmental error characterized by mottled, irregular density and deranged configuration of several developing epihyses. The affected individuals are moderate dwarfs and have short, stubby digits. The familial brachydactyly associated with degenerative hip disease described by Brailsford (1946) probably belongs to this group (Fig. 9–26).

MULTIPLE EXOSTOSES

In Chapter Four, it was pointed out that multiple exostoses may be accompanied by a variety of hand and forearm abnormalities—short metacarpals and isometric central three digits among others. The trait is transmitted as an autosomal dominant.

MYOSITIS OSSIFICANS PROGRESSIVA (MOP;
Fibrodysplasia Ossificans Progressiva; Munchmeyer's Syndrome)

It is now generally conceded that heterotopic ossification seen in early childhood has its inception in prenatal life. Helferich (1879) is credited with being the first to note the occurrence of dwarf digits in MOP. Digital dwarfing is considered a cardinal manifestation of MOP and a valuable early sign which appears long before calcification and ossification of muscles, tendons and fascia become detectable. Dwarfing affects primarily the thumbs and great toes. The affected thumb usually possesses one instead of two phalanges; it is presumed that the two segments have coalesced, producing a single bone which is shorter than the added length of the two unfused phalanges. When there are two unfused phalanges, these bones are again short, and the ungual phalanx is thin and spiked. Knorre (1955) and Lenz (1968) have described cases with short first metacarpals. MOP is classed with the autosomal dominant phenotypes.

OCULODIGITAL COMPLEXES

Weill (1922) reported a 42-year-old female with ectopia lentis, short stature, and small hands. This triad was described again by Marchesani (1939) and the complex has come to be known as Weill-Marchesani brachymorphia syndrome; it is regarded as an inverted form of Marfan's arachnodactyly. The dwarfing of the skeletal elements, including the tubular bones of the hand, is ascribed to hypochondroplasia. Meyer and Holstein (1941) reported four affected siblings in one family. The parents were first cousins. Inheritance of this trait is generally regarded as an autosomal recessive, although a few pedigrees with dominant transmission have been reported.

Sorsby syndrome consists of macular coloboma and apical dystrophy of the fingers. Sorsby (1935) reported four children with bilateral fissures on the inner surface of the retina at a point corresponding to the posterior pole of the eyeball

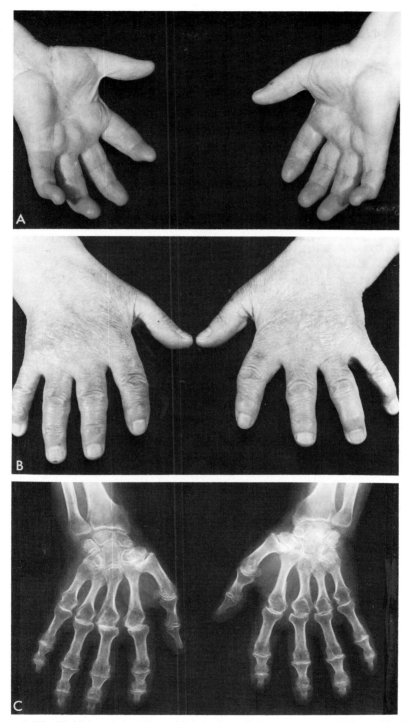

Figure 9–26 Multiple epiphysitis resulting in short digit premature arthritis and flexion contracture. *A*, Palmar view of the hands of an adult female who also has familial epiphysitis of hips, elbows, and knees. *B*, Dorsal view of the same. *C*, Dorsopalmar roentgenograph of the hands.

and, therefore, in the visual axis. All four children had apical dystrophy of the hands. The trait is listed with the autosomal dominant phenotypes.

Haney and Falls (1961) described a brother and sister with the following abnormalities: localized, cone-shaped curvature of the posterior corneal surface, pterygium colli, barrel chest, and brachydactyly. This complex is called keratoconus posticus circumscriptus cum brachydactyly, or Haney-Falls syndrome. It is probably transmitted as an autosomal recessive trait.

Both Tizzard (1933) and Hamilton (1938) noted the association between small cornea and dwarfed digit. The type of brachydactyly was not specified.

PERIPHERAL DYSOSTOSIS

In this disorder, the digits are short and stubby; they are spindle-shaped around interphalangeal joints and tapered at their tips. In growing children, the epiphyses of each phalanx is cone-shaped. The apex of this cone indents the basal rim of the metaphysis. The depression at the base of the phalangeal metaphysis has been likened to that seen at the bottom of old-fashioned wine bottles. The metaphyseal base flares out to accommodate the broad cone of the epiphysis. Since the epiphyseal piece has gained in girth around its base, the metaphyseal sheath enveloping it tends to splay like the fringes of a tent. In consequence, the finger appears thick at each epiphyseometaphyseal juncture. The affected bone matures precociously; the central axial process of the epiphyseal cone fuses with the shaft first, while the marginal portion continues to grow. As a result, the involved mature bone is short and its epiphyseal end is thick; when this broadened part enters into the composition of a joint with the comparatively smaller articular surface of the opposing bone, it causes untimely osteoarthritis. Comparable changes also affect the toes. Most authors emphasize the generalized nature of peripheral dysostosis and advise roentgenographic survey of other appendicular joints. Peripheral dysostosis is transmitted as an autosomal dominant trait.

Cone-shaped epiphyses, heretofore considered as being pathognomonic of peripheral dysostosis, are also seen in acrodysostosis, cleidocranial dysostosis, Ellis-van Creveld chondroectodermal dysplasia, tricho-rhino-phalangeal syndrome, and Weill-Marchesani brachymorphia, which are easily differentiated from peripheral dysostosis and from one another by concomitant findings (Fig. 9–27).

Graziansky (1934), who discussed Kaschin-Beck (also spelled Kashin-Bek) disease, featured a number of roentgenographs of the hands with cone-shaped phalangeal epiphyses. Kaschin-Beck disease is an acquired disorder; it is endemic in eastern Siberia and surrounding countries and is now known to be caused by a specific fungus — *Sporotrichella.*

Because of the fusiform swelling of the interphalangeal joint, H. Thiemann's (1909, 1910) disease is also considered in the differential diagnosis of peripheral dysostosis. Thiemann's disease is a form of osteochondritis of the phalangeal epiphyses. The disorder has its inception in childhood and early adolescence; it is akin to other avascular necroses of secondary growth centers. H. Thiemann should not be confused with H. H. Thiemann (1960), who observed the occurrence of cone-shaped epiphyses in Weill-Marchesani brachymorphia.

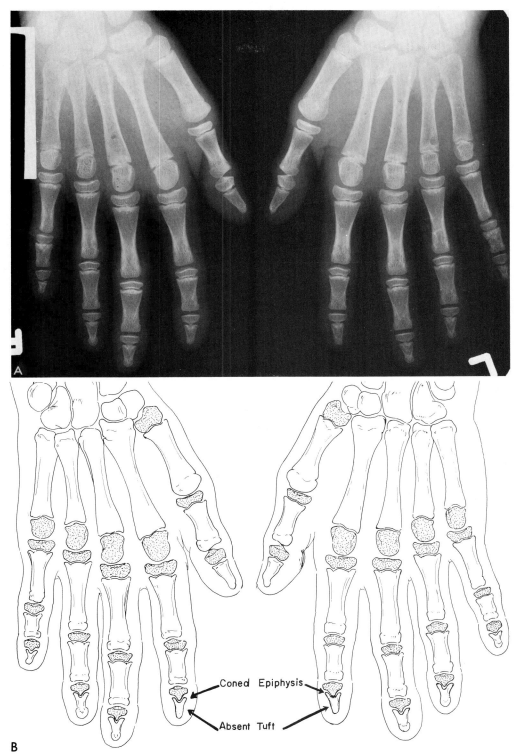

Figure 9–27 Peripheral dysostosis (coned epiphysis) in a growing child with cleidocranial dysostosis. *A*, Dorsopalmar roentgenograph of the hands. *B*, Sketch illustrating the same.

PYRUVATE KINASE DEFICIENCY AND SHORT METACARPALS AND METATARSALS

Valentine et al (1961) detected the deficiency of the enzyme called pyruvate kinase (PK). The deficiency of this enzyme is said to result in hemolytic anemia and hyperbilirubinemia. According to Bowman and Procopio (1963), severe hemolytic anemia will culminate in death during the first year of life if the affected infant is not treated with transfusions and splenectomy. Not all reported cases have been fatal, and it is possible that there are varying types or grades of congenital PK deficiency. Tanaka and Paglia (1971) considered the transmission of PK deficiency to be an autosomal recessive trait. As shown in Figure 1–2, a female teenager with PK deficiency had short ulnar metacarpals; she also had short fibular metatarsals (Fig. 9–28).

RENAL OSTEODYSTROPHY (Type E Brachydactyly Associated with Renal and Other Anomalies)

Temtamy (1966) discussed two sporadic cases with associated defects of the kidney and the hand. The first patient, a female, also had Klippel-Feil deformity of the cervical spine; the fourth metacarpal of her right, and the third and fourth metacarpals of her left hand were very short. The second patient, also female, had malformations of both ears, conductive deafness, short third and fourth metacarpals of the left hand and short first and fifth metacarpals of the right hand. Temtamy spoke of two other cases in which hypoplasia of the kidney was associated with digital dwarfing. In the first of these, there was bilateral stunting of the first metacarpal, Klippel-Feil deformity of the cervical spine, and bifid uvula; the second patient had short, webbed fingers and defective pectoralis major muscles.

TRICHO-RHINO-PHALANGEAL SYNDROME

Giedion (1966) described a constellation consisting of abnormally thin, slow-growing hair, a pear-shaped nose with a high filtrum, and changes involving both epiphyses and metaphyses. These skeletal aberrations resemble those seen in peripheral dysostosis with characteristic cone-shaped phalangeal epiphyses. The fingers are short and stubby. Giedion's patient was a female child. Her parents were unaffected. Murdock (1969) described a man who was short in stature and had precocious "male pattern baldness." Lateral x-ray view of the skull showed maxillary hypoplasia. Roentgenographs of the hands revealed irregularity of the proximal ends of the middle phalanges of the index and little fingers and shortness of the great toes. The proband's father also had precocious baldness. Murdock considered the possibility of an autosomal dominant transmission.

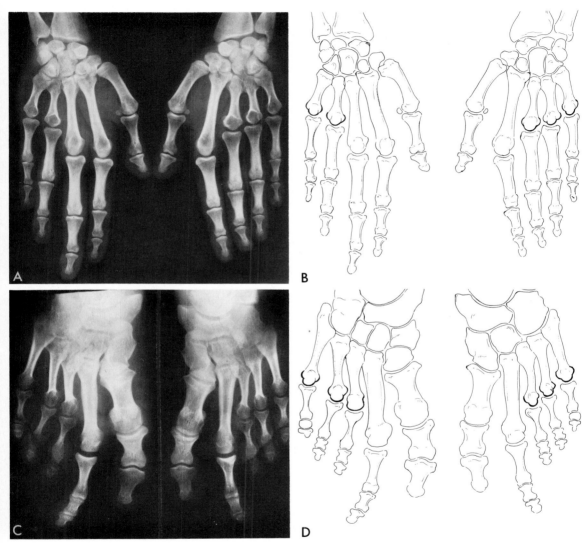

Figure 9–28 Short metacarpals and short metatarsals in a teenage female with congenital pyruvate kinase deficiency. *A*, Dorsopalmar roentgenograph of the hands. *B*, Illustrative sketch of *A*. *C*, Dorsoplantar roentgenograph of the forefeet. *D*, Illustrative sketch of the same. Note that shortness of the metatarsals is more symmetrical than the shortness of the metacarpals (the hands of this same patient were featured in Fig. 1–2).

TREATMENT

Surprisingly, very little has been written about the treatment of short digits. This means that most patients have not felt the need to have their fingers lengthened. Brachydactyly is often associated with axial deviations of one or more segments; only occasionally is osteotomy of the proximal bone performed to straighten the deviated distal segment. In order to correct the deviation of the terminal segment in a patient with delta-shaped middle phalanx of the index finger, Jones (1964) performed an osteotomy through the anomalous bone phalanx itself. This author prefers subcapital osteotomy of the proximal phalanx. In an occasional case of severe dwarfing of one of the metacarpals, an attempt is made to lengthen a single short digit by Z-osteotomy of the involved bone. Marcer (1949) surgically elongated a congenitally dwarfed fourth metacarpal by an intercalary bone graft. In a patient with bilateral Vidal type of brachydactyly of the index finger, the present author obtained satisfactory results after performing Z-type osteotomy and lengthening the second metacarpal; the osteotomized distal fragment is tilted toward the thumb until the forefinger comes to lie next to the long finger. Occasionally, one has to replace a functionally defunct short digital ray with a more powerful member (Figs. 9–29 to 9–35).

(*Text continued on page 279.*)

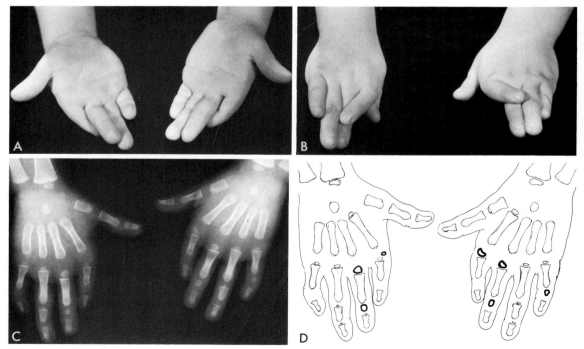

Figure 9–29   Bilateral brachyclinodactyly of the index finger. *A,* Palmar view of the hands of a 13-month-old male. *B,* Dorsal view of the same. *C,* Dorsopalmar roentgenograph, showing only one carpal bone (capitate) in each wrist, bilatarally dwarfed first metacarpals, and a small ossicle at the base of each index finger. *D,* Illustrates the same.

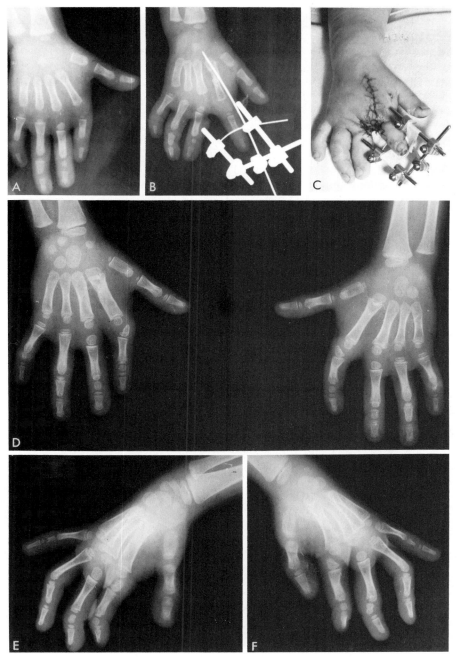

Figure 9–30 *A*, Preoperative dorsopalmar roentgenograph of the right hand of the child shown in Figure 9–29. *B*, The second metacarpal has been lengthened by Z-osteotomy; bone grafts have been inserted between the severed fragments, and improved position and length are maintained by an apparatus consisting of K-wires, side bars, and fixation nuts which can be adjusted and readjusted to assure the desired end result. *C*, Dorsal view of the hand with traction-fixation apparatus. The contracture on the ulnar aspect of the index finger was repaired by Z-plasty. Both hands were similarly operated on. *D*, Dorsopalmar roentgenograph of the hands four years after surgery. *E* and *F*, Oblique roentgenographs of the right and left hands, respectively.

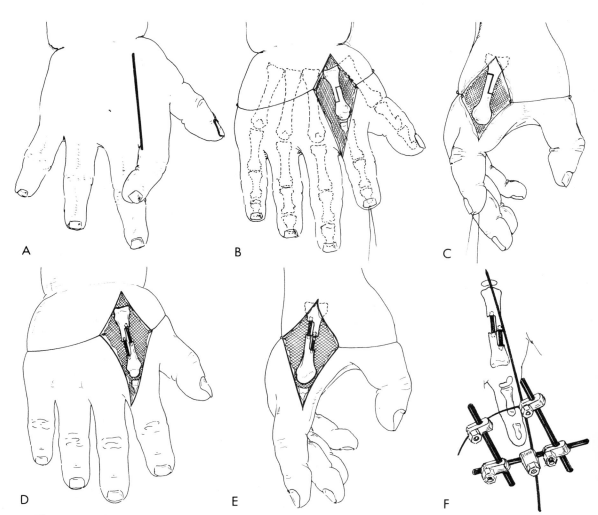

Figure 9–31 Sketches illustrating "bone carpentry" utilized in the preceding case (Figs.9–29 and 9–30) for correct-ing the ulnar angulation of the index finger and affording this digit a measure of augmented length. *A*, Incision. *B* and *C*, Z-osteotomy of the second metacarpal. *D* and *E*, Insertion of cortical bone grafts between the separated fragments of the first metacarpal. *F*, Apparatus to maintain length and corrected position.

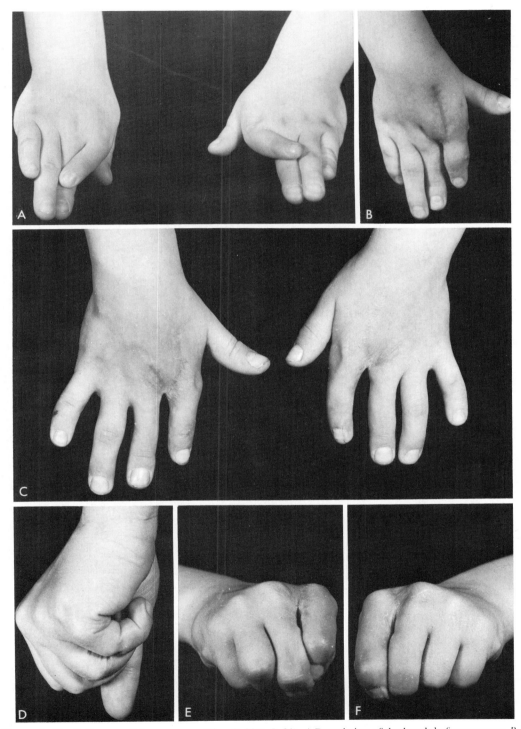

Figure 9–32 Follow-up of the same case (Figs. 9–29 to 9–31). *A*, Dorsal view of the hands before surgery. *B*, Dorsal view of the right hand soon after surgery. *C*, Dorsal view of the hands four years after surgery. *D*, Ulnar view of the clenched right hand. *E* and *F* show the action of making a fist with the right and left hands, respectively.

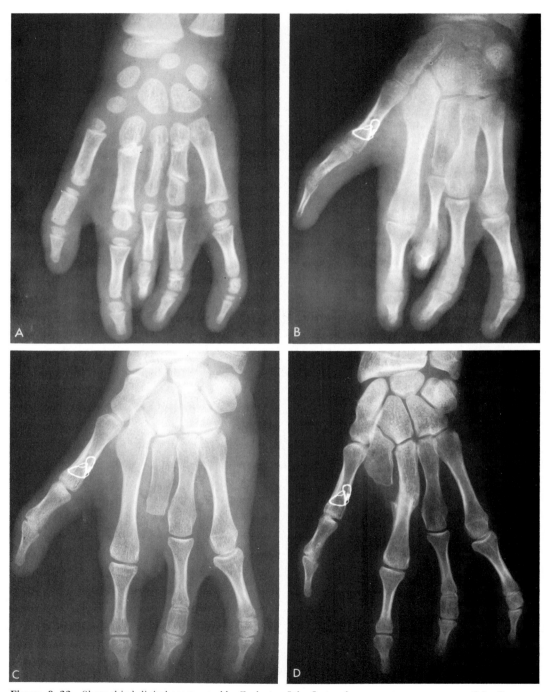

Figure 9–33 Short third digital ray treated by Z-plasty of the first webspace, rotary osteotomy of the first metacarpal, and shifting of the second ray onto the third in order to widen the first webspace and procure a longer finger. *A*, Dorsopalmar roentgenograph of the left hand of the same female child featured in Fig. 9–16 taken at six years of age. *B*, The first metacarpal has been subjected to rotation osteotomy. *C* and *D*, The vestigial third digit has been disarticulated, and the index finger with the distal two-thirds of its metacarpal has been grafted upon the third metacarpal.

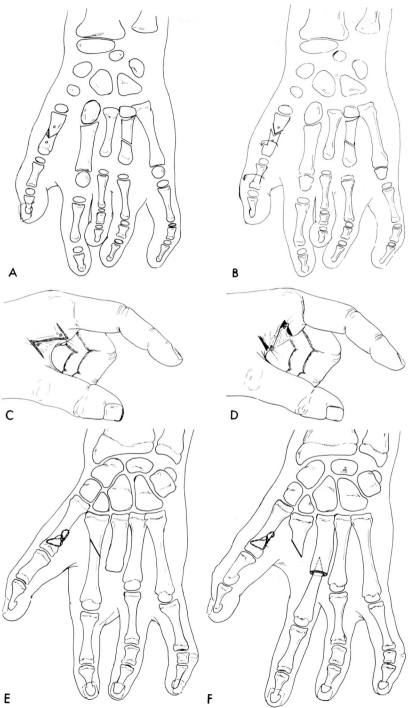

Figure 9–34 Sketches illustrating the procedures utilized for the case featured in Figure 9–33. *A* and *B* show the rotary osteotomy of the first metacarpal. *C* and *D* illustrate the Z-plasty for widening the first webspace. *E* and *F* show the shift of the second ray onto the third.

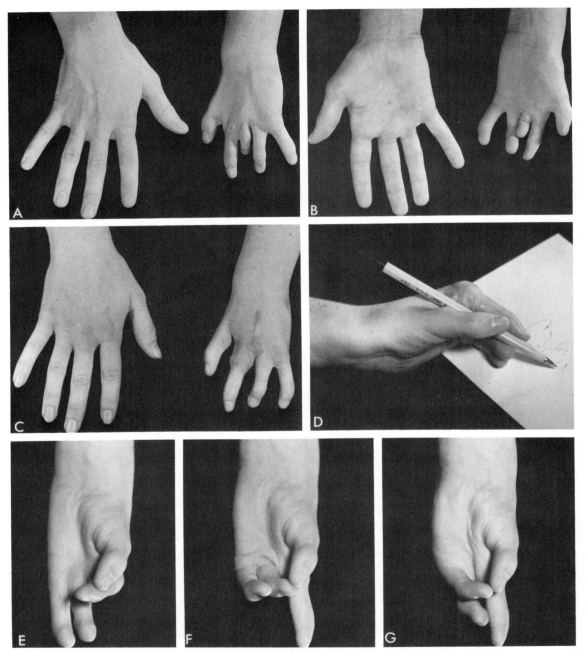

Figure 9–35 Results (Figs. 9–33 and 9–34). *A* and *B*, Dorsal and palmar views of the hands prior to surgery. *C*, Dorsal view of the hands soon after the completion of surgery. *D, E, F*, and *G* show that, postoperatively, the left thumb has gained relative and its ulnar neighbor absolute length; the rotated thumb can now effectively press its pulp against the pulps of the three fingers.

SUMMARY

Brachydactyly is an anomaly of transverse segmentation, either intercalary or terminal. To the latter category belongs the apical dystrophy of MacArthur and McCullough (1932), while the former includes brachymesophalangy, brachybasophalangy, brachymetacarpalia, and brachydactyly of hypersegmentation and symphalangism. The middle phalanges of the four ulnar digits are most commonly affected. The middle phalanges of the index and little fingers suffer the greater degree of dwarfing and distortion.

Brachydactyly is preeminently a genetic disorder and is usually transmitted as a dominant phenotype with slight variation. It may exist as an isolated anomaly or as part of a generalized disorder. All dwarfs have short digits.

Brachydactyly is an integral part of numerous syndromes. In some of these all the skeletal components of the digit are shortened; in others the dwarfing is selective. The thumb is short because of (a) premature ossification of the ungual phalanx; (b) shortness of the two phalanges with or without fusion; and (c) dwarfing of the first metacarpal. Premature ossification of the terminal phalanx results in stub thumb, which has been described in Chapter Eight. Apical dystrophy of the digits is a component of Sorsby's syndrome. Brachydactyly with cone-shaped epiphyses is encountered in cases of achondroplasia, acrodysostosis, cleidocranial dysostosis, Ellis-van Creveld chondroectodermal dysplasia, peripheral dysostosis, tricho-rhino-phalangeal syndrome, and Weill-Marchesani brachymorphia. In myositis ossificans progressiva, the thumb is short owing to dwarfing of its phalanges or the first metacarpal bone. Pre-axial brachymetacarpia is also seen in De Lange dwarfism, diastrophic dwarfism, Du Pan syndrome, hand-foot-uterus syndrome, myositis ossificans progressiva, and renal osteodystrophy. Postaxial brachymetacarpia is a feature of Albright's hereditary osteodystrophy, Banki syndrome, Biemond I, XO constitution, pyruvate kinase deficiency, and basal cell nevus syndrome.

Most cases of brachydactyly need no treatment. In Mohr-Wriedt type of brachymesophalangy of the index finger, the radial inclination of the distal segment is treated by subcapital osteotomy of the proximal phalanx. Z-osteotomy and lengthening of the second metacarpal is indicated in Vidal type of brachybasophalangy of the index finger.

References

Albright, F., Forbes, A. P., and Henneman, P. H.: Pseudo-pseudohypoparathyroidism. *Tr. Assn. Amer. Physicians, 65*:337–350, 1952.

Albright, F., Burnett, C. H., Smith, P. H., and Parson, W.: Pseudohypoparathyroidism—an example of 'Seabright-Bantam syndrome': report of three cases. *Endocrinology, 30*:922–932, 1942.

Algyogyi, H.: Ein seltener von Missbildung einer Oberextremitat. Brachydaktylie mit pero- und Ekrodaktylie. *Fortschr. Röntgenst., 16*:286–290, 1910–1911.

Archibald, K. M., Finby, N., and DeVito, F.: Endocrine significance of short metacarpals. *J. Clin. Endocrinol., 19*:1312–1322, 1959.

Arkless, R., and Graham, C. B.: An unusual case of brachydactyly. Peripheral dysostosis? Pseudo-pseudo-hyperparathyroidism? Cone epiphysis? *Am. J. Roentgenol., 99*:724–735, 1967.

Armstrong, H.: Digital deformities (hereditary deficiency of one, two, or all phalanges of one or more fingers). *Br. Med. J., 1*:1370, 1904.

Banki, Z.: Kombination erblicher Gelenk- und Knochenanomalien and der Hand. Zwei neue Röntgenzeichen. *Fortschr. Röntgenstr., 103*:598–604, 1965.

Barret: Brachymesophalangy and syndactyly in a Telegu. *Br. J. Radiol., 10*:817–821, 1937.

Bass, H. N.: Familial absence of middle phalanges with nail dysplasia: a new syndrome. *Pediatrics, 42*:318–323, 1968.

Bateson, W.: *Mendel's Principles of Heredity.* Cambridge, University Press, pp. 210–216, 1913.

Bauer, K. H., and Bode, W.: Brachydactylie. *In* Abel, W., et al, (eds.): *Erbiologie und Erhpathologie Korporlicher Zustande und Funktionen.* Berlin, J. Springer, pp. 171–176, 1940.

Beals, R. K.: Hypochondroplasia. A report of five kindreds. *J. Bone Joint Surg., 51A*:728–736, 1969.

Beck, E. B.: The problem of disforming endemic osteoarthritis in Baikal area. (Russian) *Ruskii Vrach, 5*:74–75, 1906.

Becker, P. E.: Unterschiedliche phanotypische Ausprägung der Anlage zur Brachymesophalangie in einer Sippe. *Z. menschl. Vererb. Konstitutionslehre, 23*:235–248, 1939.

Behr, F.: Über familiare Kurzfingrigkeit, Brachydaktylie, Klinodaktylie. *Fortschr. Röntgenstr., 44*:516–518, 1931.

Bell, J.: On hereditary digital anomalies: Part I - One brachydactyly and symphalangism. *In Treasury of Human Inheritance.* London, Cambridge University Press 5:1–31, 1951.

Biemond, S.: Brachydactylie. Nystagmus en cerebellaire Ataxie als familiair syndroom. *Nederl. T. Geneesk., 78*:1423–1431, 1934.

Birkenfield, W.: W. Über die Erblichkeit der Brachyphalangie. *Arch. Klin. Chir., 151*:611–631, 1928.

Block, J. B., and Glendenning, W. E.: Parathyroid hormone hyporesponsiveness in patients with basal-cell nevi and bone defects. *N. Engl. J. Med., 268*:1157–1162; Fig. 1, 1963.

Boorstein, S. W.: Symmetrical congenital brachydactylia: report of five cases. *Surg. Gynecol. Obstet., 43*:654–658, 1926.

Boston Medical and Surgical Journal: Rare anomalies of the phalanges shown by roentgen process. *Boston Med. Surg. J., 134*:198–199, 1896.

Bouet, O.: Symmetrische Brachydactylie und Hypophalangie in Hand und Fuss. *Acta Radiol., 15*:24–25, 1934.

Bowman, H. S., and Procopio, F.: Hereditary non-spherocytic hemolytic anemia of the pyruvate-Kinase deficient type. *Ann. Intern. Med., 58*:567–591, 1963.

Brailsford, J. F.: Familial brachydactyly. *Br. J. Radiol., 18*:167–172, 1945.

Brailsford, J. F.: Familial brachydactyly associated with bilateral coxitis. *Br. J. Radiol., 19*:127–130, 1946.

Brailsford, J. F.: *The Radiology of Bones and Joints.* Fifth edition. London, J. & A. Churchill Ltd. pp. 33; 71–73; 217; Figs. 22, 64, 1953.

Bucke, B.: Ein Beitrag zum fimiliären Auftren der Brachydaktylie. *Z. menschl. Vererb. Konstitionslehre, 37*:305–313, 1964.

Chesser, E. S.: Congenital deficiency of phalanges. *Br. Med. J., 2*:215, 1917.

Chevallier, P.: La brachymélie métapodiale congénitale. *N. Iconog. Salp., 23*:231–243; 429–443; 571–589; 685–694; Pl. 77, 78, 1910.

Chilton, N.: Hereditary deformity of the fingers. *Br. Med. J., 1*:15, 1927.

Clarke, D. S.: Congenital hereditary absence of some of the digital phalanges. *Br. Med. J., 2*:255, 1912.

Cloherty, J. P.: Brachydactyly Type C of Bell. *In* Bergsma, D., (ed.): *Birth Defects: Original Article Series.* New York, National Foundation—March of Dimes. Vol. 5, No. 3, pp. 78–80, 1969.

Cockayne, E. A.: An unusual form of brachydactyly and syndactyly with double proximal phalanx in the middle fingers. *J. Anat., 67*:165–167, 1933.

Cohn, B. N. E., and Raven, A.: An unusual case of brachydactyly. *J. Hered., 32*:45–48, 1941.

Colson, L.: Anomalie congénitale des mains, microdactylie. *Ann. Soc. Med. Gand., 61*:202–204, 1883.

Cotta, H., and Jaeger, M.: Ein besonderer Fall hereditärer Brachybasophalangie. *Z. Orthop., 100*:517–521, 1965.

Cragg, E., and Drinkwater, H.: Hereditary absence of phalanges in five generations. *J. Genet., 6*:61–89, 1916.

Crasselt, C., and Selzner, A.: Zur Differentialdiagnostik des brachymetakerpalen Mindwurschser. *Z. Orthop., 102*:295–305, 1966, 1968.

Cueva-Sosa, A., and Garcia-Segur, F.: Brachydactyly with absence of middle phalanges and hypostatic nails. *J. Bone Joint Surg.*, 53B:101–105, 1971.

De Lange, C.: Sur un type nouveau de dégénération (Typus Amstelodamensis) *Arch. Med. Enf.*, 36:713–719, 1933.

Dorst, J. P., Hall, J. G., and Murdock, J. L.: Hypochondrodysplasia. *In* Bergsma, D., (ed.): *Birth Defects: Original Article Series.* New York, National Foundation — March of Dimes. Vol. 5, No. 2, pp. 260–276, 1969.

Drinkwater, H.: An account of a brachydactylous family. *Proc. R. Soc. Edinb.*, 28:35–57, 1908.

Drinkwater, H.: Account of a family showing minor brachydactyly. *J. Genet.*, 2:21–40, 1913.

Drinkwater, H.: Minor brachydactyly. *J. Genet.*, 3:217–220, 1914.

Drinkwater, H.: A second brachydactylous family. *J. Genet.*, 4:323–340, 1915.

Drinkwater, H.: Hereditary abnormal segmentation of the index and middle fingers. *J. Anat. Physiol.*, 50:177–186, 1916.

Du Pan, M.: Absence congénitale du péroné sans déformation du tibia. Curieuses déformations congénitales des mains. *Rev. d'Orthop.*, 11:227–234, 1924.

Edwards, J. A., and Gale, R. P.: A kindred with unusual hand and foot anomaly. A new autosomal dominant trait with two probable homozygotes. *Am. J. Hum. Genet.*, 22:18, 1970.

Emanuele, L.: Sulla brachymetapodia. *Acta Ortop. Ital.*, 4:243–252, 1958.

Esau, P.: Die Brachyphalangie — eine erbliche Missbildung. *Arch. Klin. Chir.*, 130:786–792, 1924.

Fairbank, T.: Dysplasia epiphysialis multiplex. *Proc. R. Soc. Med.*, 39:315–317, 1945. Also in *Br. J. Surg.*, 34:225–232, 1946. Also in *An Atlas of General Affections of the Skeleton.* Edinburgh, E. & S. Livingstone, pp. 91–101, 1951.

Farabee, W. C.: Inheritance of digital malformation in man. *Papers of the Peabody Mus. Amer. Archaeol. Ethnol.* Harvard University, 3:69–70; Tables V–VI; Pl. 23–27, 1905.

Feil, A.: Brachydactylie par absence des phalanges de la main droite, avec atrophie de la main du bras et absence du grand pectorale droit. *Bull. Mém. Soc. Anat. Paris*, (6 s.), 93:578–583, 1923.

Féré, C.: Brachydactylie et polydactylie coincident sur le même membre. *Compt. Rend. Soc. Biol. Paris*, (10 s.), 2:420, 1885.

Ferrier, P. E., and Hindrichs, W. L.: Basal cell carcinoma syndrome. *Am. J. Dis. Child.*, 113:538–545, 1967.

Fischer, J., and Vendemark, E.: Bilateral symmetrical brachymetacarpalia and brachymetatarsalia: report of a case. *J. Bone Joint Surg.*, 27:145–148, 1945.

Fraccaro, M.: Contributo allo studio delle malattie del mesenchima osteopoetico. L'achondrogenesi. *Folia Hered. Path.*, 1:190–208, 1952.

Francois-Dainville, E., and Leonard, R.: Brachydactylie avec ectrodactylie et syndactylie de la main gauche et deux pieds. *Bull. et Mem. Soc. Anat. Paris*, (6 s.), 92:106–115, 1922.

Freund, L.: Ueber hypophalangie. *Z. Heilk.*, 24:333–341, 1905.

Freund, L.: Die Brachydaktylie durch Metakarpalverkurzung. *Z. Helk. Abth. Chir.*, 27:129, 1906.

Friedlaender, E.: Beitrage zur Kasuistik der Brachydaktylie. *Fortschr. Röntgenstr.*, 24:230–234, 1916–1917.

Friedrich, Schreiber, and Wilms: *Chirurgie der Oberen Extremitaeten.* Stuttgart, F. Enke, pp. 333–345, 1901.

Fuhrmann, W., Steffens, C., Schwarz, G., and Wagner, A.: Dominant erbliche Brachydactylie mit Gelenkplasien. *Humangenetik*, 50:337–353, 1965.

Garibaldi, G.: Una rara malformazione ereditaria del gruppo delle brachidattilie: la brachitelefalangia. Studio radiologico e tentativo de inquadramento genetico di uno caso. *Acta Genet. Med.*, 9:51–73, 1960.

Garn, S. M., Fells, S. L., and Israel, H.: Brachymesophalangia of digit five in ten populations. *Am. J. Phys. Anthrop.*, 27:205–210, 1967.

Gates, R.: A form of brachyphalangy in a cousin marriage. *Lancet*, 1:194, 1933.

Giedion, A.: Das Tricho-rhino-phalangeal Syndrom. *Helv. Paediat. Acta*, 21:475–582, 1966.

Glendenning, W. E., Herdt, J. R., and Block, J. B.: Ovarian fibromas and mesenteric cysts: Their association with hereditary basal cell cancer of the skin. *Am. J. Obstet. Gynecol.*, 87:1008–1012, 1963.

Gorlin, R. J., Yunis, J. J., and Tuna, N.: Multiple nevoid basal cell carcinoma, odontogenic keratocysts and skeletal anomalies; syndrome. *Acta Dermat. Venerol.*, 43:39–55, 1963.

Gorlin, R. J., Vickers, R. A., Kellin, E., and Williamson, J. J.: The multiple basal-cell nevi syndrome. An analysis of a syndrome consisting of multiple nevoid basal cell carcinoma, jaw cyst, skeletal anomalies, meduloblastoma, and hyporesponsibility to parathormone. *Cancer*, 18:98–104, 1965.

Grasselt, C., and Stelzner, A.: Zur Differentialdiagnostik des brachymetakarpalen. *Minderwurschesz. Orthop.*, 102:292–305, 1966.

Graziansky, W.: Die Kaschin-Becksche Krankheit im Rontgenbilde. *Fortschr. Röntgenstr.*, 40:367–376, 1934.

Grebe, H.: Die Achondrogenesis. Einfach rezessives Erbmerkmal. *Folia Hered. Path.*, 2:23–28, 1952.

Grebe, H.: *Chondrodysplasie.* Rome, Instit. Gregory Mendel, pp. 300–303, 1955.

Grebe, H.: Missbildungen der Gliedmassen: Brachyphalangie; Brachymetapodie; Symbrachydactylie. *In* Becker, P. E., (ed.): *Humangenetik.* Stuttgart, G. Thieme, Vol. 2:239–253, 1964.

Greene, S. N., and Saxton, A., Jr.: Hereditary brachydactylia and allied abnormalities in the rabbit. *J. Exp. Med.*, 69:301–314; Pl. 15–17, 1939.

Hamilton, J. B.: The significance of heredity in ophthalmology. Preliminary survey of hereditary eye disease in Tasmania. *Brit. J. Ophthal.*, 22:19–43; 83–108; 129–148, 1938.

Haney, W. P., and Falls, H. F.: The occurrence of congenital keratoconus posticus circumspectus in two siblings presenting a previously unrecognized syndrome. *Am. J. Ophthalmol.*, 52:53–57, 1961.

Hanflig, S. S.: A case of congenital asymmetrical shortening of metacarpals associated with marked lateral metatarsus atavicus. *J. Bone Joint Surg.*, 27:560–561, 1929.

Hann, R. C. d'A.: Familial abnormalities of the middle phalanges of each hand. *J. Anat. Physiol.*, 57:267–268, 1923.

Hasselwander, A.: Ueber 3 Falle von Brachy- und Hypophalangie und Hand u. Fuss. *Z. Morph. Anthrop.*, 6:511–526, 1903.

Haws, D. V.: Inherited brachydactyly and hypoplasia of the bones of the extremities. *Ann. Hum. Genet.*, 26:201–212, 1963.

Haws, D. V., and McKusick, V. A.: Farabee's brachydactylous kindred revisited. *Bull. Johns Hopkins Hosp.*, 113:20–30, 1963.

Helferich, H.: Ein Fall von sogenannter Myositis ossificans progressiva. *Arztliches Intel.-Blatt*, 26:485–492, 1879.

Herbert, P.: Atrophie congénitale du membre supérieur portant presque exclusivement sur les deuxièmes phalanges. *Rev. d'Orthop.*, (2 s.), 6:539–541; Pl. 25, 1905.

Hersh, A. H., DeMarinis, F., and Stecher, R. M.: On the inheritance and development of clinodactyly. *Am. J. Hum. Genet.*, 5:257–268, 1953.

Hertzog, K. P.: Shortened fifth medial phalanges. *Am. J. Phys. Anthrop.*, 27:113–118, 1967.

Hertzog, K. P.: Brachydactyly and pseudo-pseudohypoparathyroidism. *Acta Genet. Med.*, 17:428–437, 1968.

Hirrard, M. R.: Infantilisme asymétrique des doigts. Infantilisme apparent des doigts. Infantilisme real des métacarpiens. *Bull. Soc. Franc. Derm. et Syph.*, 43:1831–1835, 1935.

Jones, G. B.: Delta phalanx. *Bone Joint Surg.*, 46B:226–228, 1964.

Kellie: Short fingers. Extract from a letter from M. L. to Dr. Kellie. *Edinburg Med. Surg. J.*, 4:252–253, 1808.

Klaussner, F.: Ein Beitrage zur Casuistik der Brachydaktylie. *Beit. Klin. Chir.*, 70:236–252, 1910.

Klippel, M., and Rabaud, E.: Anomalie symétrique héréditaire de duex mains. (Bréveté d'un métacarpien). *Gaz. Hbd. Méd. Chir.*, 5:349–350, 1900.

Knorre, G.: Über die Myositis ossificans progressiva. *Z. menschl. Vererb. -u. Konstitutionslehre*, 33:85–95; Abb. 7, 1955.

Komai, T.: Three Japanese pedigrees of typical brachydactyly. *J. Hered.*, 44:78–85, 1953.

Lamy, M., and Maroteaux, P.: Le nanisme diastrophique. *Presse Méd.*, 68:1977–1980, 1960.

Lamy, M., and Maroteaux, P.: *Les Chondrodystrophies Génotypiques.* Paris, L'Expansion Scientifique Française, p. 26, 1961.

Leboucq, M.: De la brachydactylie et de l'hyperphalangie chez l'homme. *Bull. Acad. Roy. Méd. Belg.*, (4 s.), 10:344–361, 1896.

Lenz, W.: Zur Genese angeborenen Handfehlbildungen. *Chir. Plast. Reconst.*, 5:1–15; Abb. 5, 1968.

Lewis, T.: Brachydactylism. *In* Pearson, K., (ed.): *The Treasury of Human Inheritance.* London, Dulau & Co., Ltd., Vol. I, pp. 14–17, 1912.

Liebenam, L.: Beitrag zum familiären Auftreten der Brachydaktylie. *Z. menschl. Vererb. Konsitutionslehre*, 22:418–427, 1938.

Lobker, K.: Ein Fall von symmetrischer Brachydaktylie. *Mitt. a. d. Chir. Klin.*, Griefswald 1882–1883. Wien u. Leipzig, pp. 48–56, 1884.

Lossen, H.: Hyperphalangie der Mittelfinger bei beidseitiger partieller Brachydaktylie. (am I bis III Finger) *Fortschr. Röntgenstr.*, 58:428–438, 1937.

Lunghetti, B.: Sopra un caso di brachidattilia simetrica della mano. *Arch. di Ortop.*, 29:52–66, 1912.

MacArthur, J. W., and McCullough, E.: Apical dystrophy, an inherited defect of hands and feet. *Hum. Biol.*, 4:179–207, 1932.

Machol, A.: Beiträge zur Kenntnis Brachydaktylie. *Mitt. Grenzgh. Med. Chir.* [Suppl. III]: 717–766, 1907.

MacKinder, D.: Deficiency of fingers transmitted through six generations. *Br. Med. J.*, 2:845–846, 1857.

Mall, P.: On ossification centers in human embryos less than one hundred days old. *Am. J. Anat.*, 5:433–458, 1906.

Malloch, J. D.: Brachydactyly and symbrachydactyly. *Ann. Hum. Genet.*, 22:36–37; Pl. 1–5, 1956.

Mansour, A.: Metacarpal lengthening. A case report. *J. Bone Joint Surg.*, 51A:1638–1640, 1969.

Marcer, E.: Intervento per correggere la clinodattilia metacarpofalangia. *Clin. Ortop.*, 1:111–117, 1949.

Marchesani, O.: Brachydaktylie und angeborene Kugellinse als Systemerkrankung. *Klin. Mschr. Augenheilk.*, 103:392–406, 1939.

Margolis, E., Schwartz, A., and Falk, R.: Brachytelephalangy and brachymesophalangy in the same family. *J. Hered.*, 48:21–25, 1957.

Maroteaux, P., and Malamut, G.: L'acrodysostose. *Presse Méd.*, 76:2189–2192, 1968.

Marshall, R.: Note on a family with brachydactyly. *Arch. Dis. Child.*, 4:385–388, 1929.

Martino-Dubousquet, J., Burger-Wagner, A., and Burger, A. J.: Dysfaciobrachyclinodactylie. *Ann. Chir. Infantile, 4*:281–290, 1963.

Mathew, P. W.: A case of hereditary brachydactyly. *Br. Med. J., 2*:969, 1908.

McKusick, V. A.: *Mendelian Inheritance in Man*. Second edition. Baltimore, Johns Hopkins Press, p. 121, entry 1397, 1968. See also Third edition, p. 164, entry 14600, 1971.

McNutt, C. W.: Variability in expression of the gene for brachydactyly. *J. Hered., 37*:359–364, 1946.

Meyer, S., and Holstein, T.: Spherophakia with glaucoma and brachydactyly. *Am. J. Ophthalmol., 24*:247–251, 1941.

Mohan, J.: Brachydactyly in an Indian family. *J. Med. Genet., 6*:349–351, 1969.

Mohr, O. L., and Wriedt, C.: A new type of hereditary brachyphalangy in man. *Carnegie Institution of Washington, D. C. Publication*. No. 295, pp. 5–64, Pl. I–VII, 1919.

Mouchet, A.: Arrêt de développement des phalanges chez un foetus de cinq mois. *Bull. Soc. Anat. Paris, 71*:529–530, 1896.

Mouchet, A.: Atrophie congénitale de la main droite avec brachydactylie du pouce et du petit doigt. *Rev. d'Orthrop.* (2s.) *3*:53–55, 1902.

Müller, W.: *Die Angeborenen Fehlbildungen der Menschlichen*. Liepzig, G. Thieme, pp. 87–106, 1937.

Munchmeyer, F.: Über Myositis ossificans progressiva. *Z. Ration. Med.,* (3 s.), *34*:9–40, 1869.

Murdock, J. L.: Tricho-rhino-phalangeal dysplasia with possible autosomal dominant transmission. *In Birth Defects. Original Article Series*. New York, National Foundation—March of Dimes, pp. 218–219, 1969.

Nigst, P. F.: Brachydaktylie. *Schweiz. Med. Wschr., 8* (57 new number):88–91, 1927.

Nissen, K. I.: A study of inherited brachydactyly. *Ann. Eugen., 5*:281–310, 1933.

Nöller, F.: *Chirurgische-orthopädische Erkrankheiten im Gesets zur Verhutung erbkranken Nachwuches*. Jena, G. Fischer, pp. 34–35, 1942.

Pagenstecher, E.: Beitrag zu den Extremitatenmissbildungen. II. Brachydactyly—Pollex valgus—Luxation des radiuskopfchens und Missbildungen des Daumens U. S. W. *Dtsch. Z. Chir., 60*: 239–249, 1901.

Parenti, G. C.: La anosteogenesi. (Una varieta dell' osteogenesi imperfetta). *Pathologica, 28*:447–540, 1936.

Parrot, J.: Sur la malformation achondroplastique et le Dieu Ptah. *Bull. Soc. Anthrop.,* (3s.), *1*:296–308, 1878.

Pendergast, W.: Inheritance of short, stubby hands. *J. Hered., 27*:448, 1936.

Pfitzner, W.: Ueber Brachyphalangie und Verwandtes. *Verh. Dtsch. Anat. Ges., 12*:18–23, 1898.

Pippow, G.: Über das Zurammentreffen von Wirbelgelsnkoplasion und Brachydaktylie in einer Sippe. *Erbarzt, 10*:226–236, 1962.

Pol, R.: Die Formen der Brachydaktylie und ihre Bewertung. *Verh. Dtsch. Ges. Path.* (Jena), *17*:505–508, 1914.

Pol, R.: Die verschieden Formen der Brachyphalangie, Hypo- und Hyperphalangie und ihre Deutung. *Munch. Med. Wschr., 61*:1649–1650, 1914.

Pol, R.: "Brachydaktylie"—"Klinodaktylie"—Hyperphalangie und ihre Grandlagen. *Arch. Path. Anat. Phys., 229*:388–530, 1921.

Pol, R.: Brachydaktylie (Akrochondrodysplasie). *In* Schualbe, E., and Gruber, G. B., (eds.): *Die Morphologie der Missbildungen*. Jena, G. Fischer, 3 T., 17 Lief., 1Abt.; 7 kap., 1 Halfte, pp. 597–645, 1937.

Pryde, A. W., and Kiabatake, T.: Brachymesophalangism and brachymetapodia of the hand. *Atomic Bomb Casualty Commission, Technical Report*, pp. 18–59, 1959.

Quelce-Salgado, A.: A new type of dwarfism with various bone aplasias and hypoplasias of the extremities. *Acta Genet. Statist. Med.* (Basel), *14*:63–66, 1964.

Rieder, H.: Über gleichzeitiges Vorkommen von Brachy- und Hyperphalangie an der Hand. *Dtsch. Arch. Klin. Med., 56*:330–348, 1899.

Riedl, H.: Zur Kasuistik der Brachydaktylie: Ein Fall von doppelseitiger Verkruzung des III bis. V. Metakarpelknochens. *Fortschr. Röntgenstr., 11*:447–449; Tafel XXIII; Fig. 3, 1907.

Robinow, M., Pfeiffer, R. A., Gorlin, R. J., McKusick, V. A., Renuart, A. W., Johnson, G. F., and Summitt, R. L.: Acrodysostosis: A syndrome of peripheral dysostosis, nasal hypoplasia, and mental retardation. *Am. J. Dis. Child., 121*:195–203, 1971.

Robinson, G. C., Wood, B. J., Miller, J. R., and Baillie, J.: Hereditary brachydactyly and hip disease: Unusual radiological and dermatoglyphic findings in a kindred. *J. Pediatr., 72*:539–543, 1968.

Roche, A. F.: Clinodactyly and brachymesophalangia of the fifth finger. *Acta Paediatr.* (Upsala), *50*:387–391, 1961.

Roederer, C.: Brachydactylie isolée chez une scoliotique. *Rev. d'Orthop.,* (3s.), *5*:359–360, 1914.

Roughton, E. W.: A case of congenital shortness of metacarpal and metatarsal bones. *Lancet, 2*:19, 1897.

Sachs, D.: Familial brachyphalangy. *Radiology, 35*:622–626, 1940.

Schinz, H. R.: Erbtypen und Formen bei Brachydaktylie. *Arch. Klaus-stift. Vererb. Forsch., 18*:361, 1943.

Schmid, F., and Junker, F.: Die Brachymesophalangie des Kleinfingers. *A. Kinderheilk., 68*:399–407, 1950.

Selka, A.: Über Brachydaktylie kombiniert mit Syndaktylie. *Fortschr. Röntgenst., 12*:92–95, 1908.

Shafar, J.: Hereditary short digits (with report of two cases of chondro-osteo-dystrophy). *Br. J. Radiol., 14*:396–402, 1941.

Shoul, M. T., and Ritvo, M.: Roentgenographic and clinical aspects of hyperphalangism (polyphalangism) and brachydactylism: hereditary abnormal segmentation of the hand. *N. Engl. J. Med., 248*:274–278, 1953.

Smith, T. T.: A peculiarity in the shape of the hand in idiots of the mongol type. *Pediatrics, 2*:315–320, 1896.

Sorsby, A.: Congenital coloboma of the macula: Together with an account of the familial occurrence of bilateral macular coloboma in association with apical dystrophy of hands and feet. *Br. J. Ophthalmol., 19*:65–90, 1935.

Stecher, W. R.: Genealogical study of a case of symmetrical congenital brachydactylia. *Med. Rec., 144*:5–8, 1936.

Sternberg, J.: Zur Kenntnis der Brachydaktylie. *Wien Klin. Wschr., 15*:1060–1065, 1902.

Stiles, K. A.: The inheritance of brachymetapody. *J. Hered., 30*:87–91, 1939.

Tage-Hausen, E.: Arvelig Brachydactyli. *Hospitalstid, 81*:284–288, 1938.

Tanaka, K. R., and Paglia, D. E.: Pyruvate kinase deficiency. *Semin. Hematol., 8*:367–396, 1971.

Tanaka, K. R., Valentine, W. H., and Miwa, S.: Pyruvate kinase (PK) deficiency hereditary nonspherocytic hemolytic anemia. *Blood, 19*:269–295, 1962.

Temtamy, S. A.: *Genetic Factors in Hand Malformations.* Ph. D. Thesis. Baltimore, Johns Hopkins University, pp. 162–256, 1966.

Thiemann, H.: Juvenile epiphysen Störungen. *Fortschr. Röntgenstr., 14*:79–87, 1909–1910.

Thiemann, H. H.: Zapfenepiphysen in Kombination mit Teilsymptomen des Marchesani-Syndroms. *Förtschr. Röntgenstr., 93*:367–370, 1960.

Tillaye, P.: Ectrodactylie et brachydactylie. *Rev. d'Orthop.*, (2s.) *8*:295–297, 1907.

Tizzard, T.: Familial occurrence of macrocornea associated with brachydactyly. *Proc. R. Soc. Med., 27*:151, 1933.

Turner, H. H.: A syndrome of infantilism, congenital webbed neck and cubitus valgus. *Endocrinology, 23*:566–574, 1938.

Valentine, W. H., and Tanaka, K. R.: Pyruvate kinase deficiency hereditary hemolytic anemia. Second edition. *In* Stanbury, J. B., Wyngarden, J. B., and Frederickson D. S., (eds.): *Metabolic Bases of Inherited Diseases.* New York, McGraw-Hill Book Co., pp. 1051–1059, 1966.

Valentine, W. H., Tanaka, K. R., and Miwa, S.: Specific erythrocyte glycogenic enzyme defect (pyruvate kinase) in three subjects with congenital nonspherocytic hemolytic anemia. *Tr. Assn. Amer. Physicians, 74*:100–110, 1961.

Van der Werff ten Bosch, J. J.: The syndrome of brachymetacarpal dwarfism ("pseudopseudohypoparathyroidism") with and without gonadal dysgenesis. *Lancet, 1*:69–71, 1959.

Vidal, M. E.: Brachydactylie symétrique, et autres anomalies osseuses, héréditaires depuis plusieurs générations. *Bull. Acad. Med. Paris*, (3 s.), *63*:632–649, 1909.

Wagner, H.: Ein Beiträge zur Kenntnis Brachydaktylie. *Fortschr. Röntgenstr., 7*:94–98, 1903.

Walker, B. A., Murdock, J. L., McKusick, V. A., Langer, L. O., and Beals, R. K.: Hypochondroplasia. *Am. J. Dis. Child., 122*:95–104, 1971.

Walter, M. R.: Five generations of short digits. *J. Hered., 29*:143–144, 1938.

Webb, T. L.: A case of hereditary brachydactyly. *J. Anat. Physiol., 35*:487–488, 1901.

Weill, G.: Ectopie des cristallins malformations générales. *Ann. Oculist., 169*:21–44, 1922.

Wells, N. H., and Platt, M.: Hereditary phalangeal agenesis showing dominant Mendelian characteristics. *Arch Dis. Child., 22*:251–252, 1947.

Zurukzoglu, S.: Über eine erbliche Missbildung des kleinen Fingers (Klinodaktylie). *Arch. Klaus. Stift. Vererb. Fortschr., 4*:217–218, 1929.

Chapter Ten

HYPERPHALANGISM

In surveying the pedigrees of some hand anomalies, one is struck by the fact that different anatomical types are often interchangeable, one variety being transmitted from another. The progenitor of a pedigree may start with an increased number of digits, but some members of later generations will manifest other anomalies—for example, hyperphalangism. This variability of expression is especially prevalent in pre-axial polydactyly. Not uncommonly, in one and the same pedigree, bifid thumb is superseded by triphalangeal pollex. These two abnormalities may even coexist in the same individual, one anomaly affecting the right and the other the left thumb. Such close association has led some clinicians—Lapidus et al (1943), in particular—to postulate the theory that the surplus ossicle interposed between the proximal and distal phalanges of the triphalangeal thumb is derived from one of the two bones of the bifid distal segment. Watson and Boyes (1967) went so far as to consider the variety of hyperphalangism known as delta phalanx to be a manifestation of polydactyly. Ecke (1962) had reported a grandfather, son, and grandson who had twinning of the distal two phalanges of the thumb. McKusick (1971) discussed this pedigree in the entry entitled "Triphalangeal thumb with double phalanges."

It would perhaps be less confusing to call the anomaly described by Ecke and McKusick "polyphalangism" and reserve the designation hyperphalangism for digits which possess more than their normal quota of phalanges in proximodistal sequence. Polyphalangism is a variant of polydactyly—an anomaly of longitudinal dichotomy; in bifid or bifurcate forms of polydactyly, the surplus member lies to one side of its mate and often stands apart from it. Hyperphalangism is an anomaly of transverse segmentation; it is characterized by the interposition of an excess phalanx between two other phalanges; the supernumerary ossicle more or less lies in the same axial line as the phalanx behind and the one ahead. Hyperphalangism and polydactyly are sufficiently different to be put into separate classes.

When one speaks of hyperphalangism he generally has in mind excessive transverse segmentation of the thumb. Transverse hypersegmentation of the lesser digits has been reported by Leboucq (1896), Joachimsthal (1906), Drinkwater (1916), Hollander (1918), Pol (1921), Lossen (1937), and many more recent authors. The affected digit—usually the index or the middle finger—is short. A quadriphalangeal lesser digit with normal length is extremely rare. This fact alone accounts for the identification of hyperphalangism with triphalangeal thumb, and hypersegmentation of the lesser digits with brachydactyly. Triphalangeal thumb is considered to be a distinct anomaly, a well-defined deviation from the normal pollex with only two consecutive phalanges.

THE MISSING BONE IN BIPHALANGEAL POLLEX AND THE ADDED ELEMENT IN TRIPHALANGEAL THUMB

Jones (1944) gave the following as the normal phalangeal formula: $2 \cdot 3 \cdot 3 \cdot 3 \cdot 3$ — meaning the thumb has two while each one of the other digits has three phalanges. Jones conceded, as had most anatomists before him, that in the very remote past the thumb had lost an element. Presumably, the primordial mammalian pollex contained an additional skeletal element which disappeared during evolution. Like his professional predecessors, Jones wondered which bone had disappeared—the metacarpal or one of the phalanges?

This question has long been debated by both anatomists and anthropologists. In their turn, teratologists have wondered about the derivation of surplus bone in the triphalangeal thumb.

According to Galen (A.D. 165), Eudemius of Alexandria contended that the first bone of the pollical ray is metacarpal and that the thumb has two phalanges. Galen considered the thumb as consisting of three phalanges and lacking a metacarpal bone. This view is supported by the fact that while the epiphyses of the other metacarpals are located at their distal ends, the secondary growth center of the basal bone of the pollical ray is placed at its proximal end, as in phalanges. Struthers (1863) was perhaps the most influential propagator of this concept. "The position of the epiphysis is decisive in establishing the view that the bone which is wanting in the human thumb…is the metacarpal," Struthers wrote. In triphalangeal thumb, Struthers said, the additional bone was "placed in the position of the middle phalanx." In other words, the surplus bone did not replace the first metacarpal, which Struthers said had disappeared in phylogeny.

"When elements are lost in digits, and when digits themselves are lost in regular evolutionary series, it may be said that phylogenetic death of the member takes place from the free extremity backwards to the trunk. The metacarpal will persist long after the phalanges are lost," Jones (1944) argued. He spoke of the occasional appearance of the additional epiphysis at the distal end of the first metacarpal or at the proximal extremity of its ulnar neighbor. "These facts," he said, "teach us that we should not rely upon the dictum of Struthers that the position of epiphysis is decisive in establishing homologies."

Jones then turned his attention to the concept advanced by Uffelmann (1863) and Sappey (1888). These authors differed only in some of the minutiae. They considered the first metacarpal to be a composite structure derived from two bones, probably from the original metacarpal and the proximal phalanx of the primitive pollex. Their theory was popularized by Windle (1891). "The missing segment of the normal thumb is the proximal phalanx," Windle wrote. He thought it likely that the distal epiphysis of the original metacarpal took an independent development and gave rise to a supernumerary phalanx which would be the first—the one he suspected to have been lost in phylogeny.

"Windle's theory does not carry great conviction, even in connection with the work upon the anomalies of the thumb of which it was the outcome," Jones

(1944) wrote. "The başal member of the first digit is a true metacarpal . . . possessing no added element, but exhibiting an irregularity of ossification that may at times be shared by other metacarpals. . . ."

Humphry (1858) had written: "The first bone is neither truly a metacarpal bone nor a phalanx, but is intermediate between the two. Taking all things into consideration, it is perhaps most correct, as it is certainly most convenient for description, to continue to call it a metacarpal bone, and to consider that the second phalanx, with its flexor perforatus tendon, is the digital segment which is missing in the thumb." Perforatus is now called sublimis.

"Humphry," Jones (1944) wrote, "seems to have regarded this second phalanx as being altogether absent; but the more recent work of Pfitzner appears to make it very probable that it has been fused with the third or ungual phalanx to constitute the distal bony element of the first digit. I know of no fact derived from any study of normal and abnormal anatomy and paleontology which contradicts this finding...the first element of the first digit is the metacarpal...the second element is the first true phalanx, and the third, a compound, consisting of the ungual phalanx and the reduced phalanx, which has become incorporated with it."

Teratological evidence seems to support Pfitzner's (1890) view. "In all the cases of three-jointed thumb reported heretofore," Reynolds (1917) wrote, "the middle phalanx is the extra bone." McGregor (1926) drew attention to the fact that the terminal phalanx in the normal biphalangeal thumb is longer both relatively and absolutely than the terminal phalanges of the fingers. He ascribed this apparently disproportionate length of the ungual phalanx of the thumb to the fusion of the middle and distal phalanges of the primitive pollex. Gates (1946) related triphalangism of the thumb to failure of the last two bones of this digit to fuse (Fig. 10–1).

THE OCCURRENCE OF TRIPHALANGEAL THUMBS

Realdus Columbi (1559) spoke of a thumb with two interphalangeal joints. Dubois (1826) presented a hexadactylous infant whose thumb had three phalanges. Concerted interest in triphalangeal thumb appears to have been initiated by Struthers (1863) and was given added impetus by Windle (1891). Windle found 11 cases of triphalangeal thumb reported in the literature and added a case of his own. Of these 12 cases, four occurred in pentadactylous hands, and in the remaining eight, the thumb was replaced by two digits, one or both of which—more commonly the ulnar—had three phalanges. Windle said, "Heredity is met in several of the cases." His table showed only three cases with hereditary antecedents.

Dubreuil-Chambardel (1909) found 46 cases of triphalangeal thumb reported in the literature: 27 of these occurred in pentadactylous hands; 19 were associated with pre-axial polydactyly. Males and females were equally affected. Stieve (1916) collected 55 cases: in 39 of these, both thumbs were affected and in 16, only one thumb; 33 bilateral cases had hereditary antecedents; in none of the unilateral cases could a hereditary link be established.

In a later communication, Dubreuil-Chambardel (1925) cited 74 cases of triphalangeal pollex; 42 of these occurred in pentadactylous hands; in 32 the thumb was replaced by two digits. Swanson and Brown (1962) confined their list

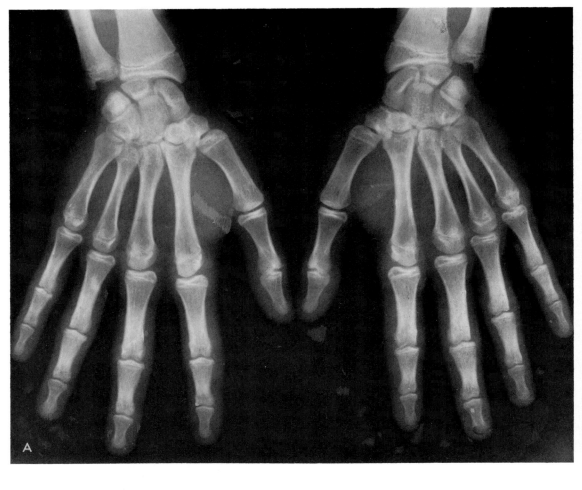

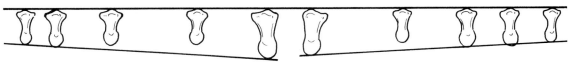

B

Figure 10–1 The length of ungual phalanges. *A*, Dorsopalmar roentgenograph of the hands of a 13-year-old female: note that the ungual phalanx of the thumb is longer than the corresponding bones of the lesser digits. *B*, Sketch illustrating the same.

to the cases that had been reported between 1930 and 1960; the total number of these cases was 58, and 51 of these were familial, hence hereditary; with the exception of one, all familial cases were bilateral.

Triphalangeal thumbs have been reported from many countries and no race appears to be immune from the taint. McGregor (1926) and Abramowitz (1959) noted its occurrence in the Bantu tribe in Africa; Fréré (1930), Lapidus and associates (1943), and Milch (1951) in American Negroes; Komai et al (1953) in Japanese; Sallam (1955) in Egyptians; and Girija (1958) in Hindus. Lapidus et al examined 75,000 draftees and found only three cases of triphalangeal thumb, which would give an incidence of one in 25,000. A number of pedigrees have been charted. The responsible gene manifests dominant behavior with variable expressions.

VARIETIES

Windle (1891) separated triphalangeal thumbs into two groups; in the first class he placed those that existed in pentadactylous hands; to the second category he relegated twin digits which had replaced the thumb and functioned as such. One of Windle's patients complained that he had "five fingers and no thumb" on one hand. But he could still turn the first or the most radial digit of this hand around and have it touch the volar surfaces of the ulnar digits. In other words, the triphalangeal first digit in this "five-fingered hand" was opposable. Numerous similar cases have since been reported in which the first digit failed to effect opposition. It became necessary to break Windle's first category into two classes: (1) single opposable triphalangeal pollex, and (2) single nonopposable first digit. Windle's second group—two opposable, finger-like radial digits which had replaced the thumb—has been classed with polydactyly by most recent authors.

OPPOSABLE TRIPHALANGEAL POLLEX

More than 100 years before the term *delta phalanx* became popular in orthopedic argot, Struthers (1863) jotted down the following notes about a patient: "In examining the thumbs I was surprised to find an additional joint, giving three phalanges beside the metacarpal bone.... The additional bone occupying the position of the middle phalanx is broader on the inner or radial side than on the side next to the index finger, having a triangular, or wedge-shaped figure which gives the distal phalanx an inclination towards the index.... The utility of the thumb is unimpaired."

Struthers taught in the Edinburgh School of Medicine. G. T. Beatson received his M.D. degree from the same school. They were not contemporaries; Beatson could not have attended Struthers' lectures. If Beatson ever read Struthers' article, he must have forgotten the reference to the triangular bone causing angulation of the distal segment of the thumb. When faced with a similar deformity, Beatson did not even suspect the existence of the anomalous bone wedged between the proximal and distal phalanges of the thumb. His patient was a female child. The terminal phalanx of her right thumb inclined in radial direction; the distal segment of her left thumb turned towards the index finger, as in Struthers' patient. "I confess the condition of the thumbs was new to me," Beatson (1897) wrote. Someone must have called Beatson's attention to an article by Morgan (1896) that had appeared during the preceding year, which featured one of the very first roentgenographs of an anomalous hand. Beatson decided to give the new diagnostic method a trial. A roentgenograph of the little girl's hands was taken. Beatson discovered what Struthers had described three decades earlier without the benefit of roentgenography. Beatson wrote: "Situated between the first and terminal phalanx of each thumb was, evidently, an extra bone of a wedge-shaped character, its broad base being on the inner side of the right thumb and the outer side of the left...."

A small triangular bone wedged between the first and the last phalanges does not increase the length of the thumb appreciably, but it does cause its distal segment to incline sideways. If the base of the wedge is on the radial side, the tip of the thumb will point towards the index finger. Conversely, a triangular piece with an ulnar base will cause the terminal segment to angle in the opposite direction. The former deformity is more common. The interposed bone is not always small or triangular; larger fragments are known to occur, and they are either rectangular or rhomboid in shape. Even the largest anomalous ossicle is not nearly as long as the middle phalanges of the next three ulnar digits. The surplus bone causes moderate augmentation of length. Triphalangeal thumb belonging to this category may reach the level of the proximal interphalangeal joint of the index but does not extend far beyond. Cases are known in which the interposed bone on one side is triangular in shape and on the other side has the configuration of a normal middle phalanx; the digit itself looks like a finger. In other words, opposable and nonopposable triphalangeal thumbs may concur in the same individual. These adjectives—opposable and nonopposable—need not be given rigid literal interpretation. Some subjects with a fingerlike first digit can effect a measure of opposition albeit limited. Conversely, thumbs with a triangular middle phalanx may attain only partial abduction and rotation and cannot adequately execute the act of opposition. Rarely, one finds three irregularly shaped ossicles between the metacarpal and the distal phalanx of the thumb and it is hard to say which one of these represents the proximal phalanx and which are the adventitious bones (Figs. 10–2 and 10–3).

NONOPPOSABLE TRIPHALANGEAL THUMB

A human manus with a nonopposable triphalangeal thumb is often called "five-fingered hand." This anomaly presents drastic structural deviation from the normal. These changes may be best appreciated if some of the pertinent features of the normal hand are reviewed.

In the human hand, the metacarpal bones of the lesser digits are long and slender. They bear their epiphyses at their distal ends. Proximally, their bases are snugged together and overlap each other. Interlacing capsular and stout interosseous ligaments bind these parts. The bases of the second and third metacarpals interlock with their respective carpal bones, and these two metacarpals are immovable. The fourth and fifth bones can be pushed in dorsal and palmar directions—the fifth to a greater extent than the fourth, because it is not flanked on its ulnar aspect by another bone. Distally, the heads of all four ulnar metacarpals are caught in the common bondage of volar transverse ligaments, both deep and superficial. The deep transverse ligament lies under the metacarpal heads and connects with the latter indirectly—through the intermediary of collateral ligaments and the capsules of the metacarpophalangeal joints. Each ulnar digit has three phalanges and each phalanx has an epiphysis at its base; the proximal phalanx is longer than the middle, and this in turn is longer than the distal bone.

The metacarpal of the thumb is shorter and thicker than any of its ulnar neighbors and, unlike them, it bears its epiphysis at its proximal extremity. This end of the first metacarpal connects with its own carpal bone, and the two together form a saddle-shaped joint with lax articular capsule. As all concavo-convex articulations, the first carpometacarpal joint permits motion in many directions—radial, ulnar, volar, and dorsal—as well as axial rotation. The base of

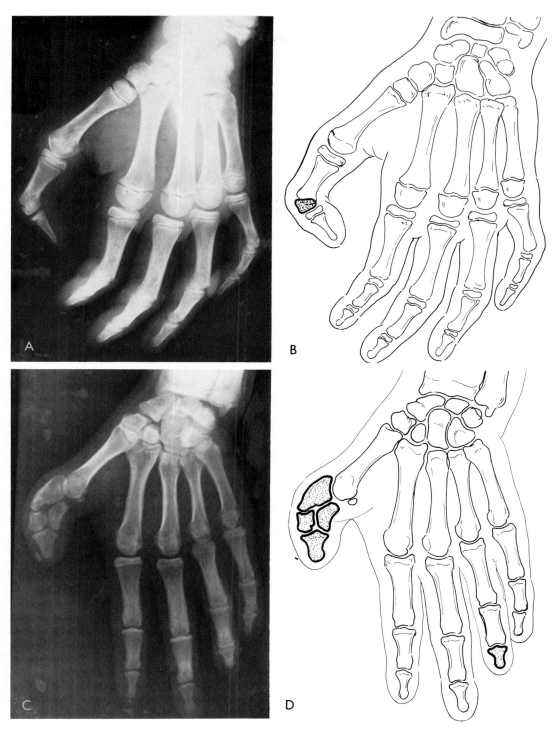

Figure 10–2 Usual and unusual forms of hyperphalangism of the thumb. *A*, Dorsopalmar roentgenograph of the left hand showing a single ossicle interposed between the proximal and distal phalanges of the thumb. *B*, Sketch illustrating the same. *C*, Dorsopalmar roentgenograph of another left hand with three irregularly shaped ossicles between the first metacarpal and the ungual segment of the thumb. *D*, Sketch illustrating the same.

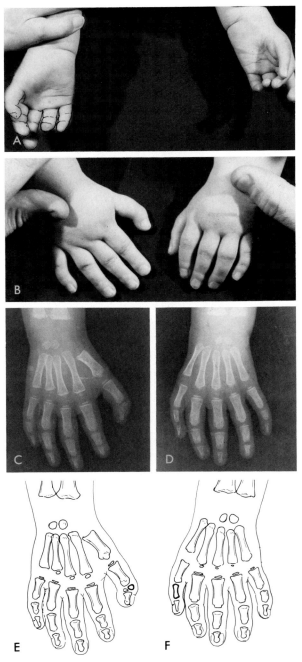

Figure 10–3 Inadequately opposable triphalangeal thumbs. *A,* Palmar view of the hands of a 10-month-old female: note that both thumbs only touch the middle phalanges of the index finger. *B,* Dorsal view showing that the ungual phalanx of the right thumb is tilted toward the index finger; it is flexed and its nail is only slightly sloped; the left thumb is longer and more slender; it resembles a finger but its nail is at a plane perpendicular to the plane of the fingernails. *C,* Roentgenograph of the right hand showing a triangular ossicle interposed between the proximal and distal phalanges of the thumb. *D,* Roentgenograph of the left hand: here the middle phalanx of the radialmost digit is rectangular in shape, causing no axial deviation of the ungual segment. *E* and *F* illustrate roentgenographs above each.

the thumb metacarpal is set at a distance from the base of the index metacarpal; it does not bear a side facet for this bone as do the four other metacarpals for one another, nor is it bound to the second metacarpal by an interosseous ligament. Proximally, then, the first metacarpal is free of the restraints imposed on the ulnar bones. Distally, its head lies outside the bondage of the deep transverse metacarpal ligament which tethers the heads of the other bones. The first phalanx of the thumb is shorter than the proximal phalanges of the next three fingers, but its terminal segment is longer than the ungual phalanges of the ulnar digits. Both phalanges of the thumb bear their epiphysis at their proximal ends. The thumb has no middle phalanx.

Owing to the abbreviated length of the first metacarpal and want of a phalanx, the normal thumb is short — when brought to the side of the index, it barely reaches the line of the first interphalangeal joint of this finger; as the thumb is radially rotated, its nail lies in a plane at a right angle to the plane of the other nails. From its position next to the index, the thumb may be made to sweep in ulnar direction, tracing an arc with its tip. This arc begins at a more distal point on the volar aspect of the first phalanx of the index, and ends at a proximal point in front of the fifth metacarpal head.

The webspace between the thumb and the index finger is wide, permitting the thumb to move in a radial direction. In preparation for the action pattern known as opposition, the right thumb rotates clockwise and the left, counterclockwise. At the same time, the thumb moves in ulnar direction until its volar surface comes opposite that of the finger with which it is to consummate the act of opposition. It requires two digits to effect a pinch. Obviously the shorter thumb cannot reach the distal segments of the three central fingers; these digits must bend towards the thumb. In pulp-to-pulp opposition, the thumb provides most of the power, but the opposing finger flexes to a greater degree. The thumb has its own intrinsic muscles, and its extrinsic motors are independent from those which move the fingers. This is especially true of the extensor pollicis longus which is unique in regard to both the separateness of its origin and the line of its pull (Figs. 10–4 to 10–7).

Abramowitz (1959) could find no account of "dissection of a triphalangeal thumb." He must not have made a serious search to find one. Voisin and Nathan (1902) dissected a five-fingered hand. They recorded the following findings: the first or the most radial digit had three phalanges and extended as far forward as the little finger; the thenar eminence was nonexistent, flat; the long abductor was absent; and the extensor pollicis longus arose from the common mass of digital extensors. The first digit had its own flexor. The flexor digitorum profundus supplied only the four ulnar digits; the sublimis sent separate tendons to all five digits, including the first. As in the fingers, the sublimis tendon of the radialmost digit split into halves, allowing the long flexor to pass under and reach the terminal phalanx. The lumbricals were present. The adductors were not mentioned. Nothing was said about the fixation of the first metacarpal base proximally, nor about the inclusion of its head in the common bondage of the transverse ligament complex.

Reynolds (1917) studied the hands of a boy with bilateral triphalangeal thumb. The left hand was affected more severely than the right. The thenar eminence was effaced. The first metacarpal of the right hand was relatively immobile; in the x-ray films, Reynolds noted "mortising" of the proximal end of the first metacarpal of the left hand. This metacarpal had two epiphyses — one at its

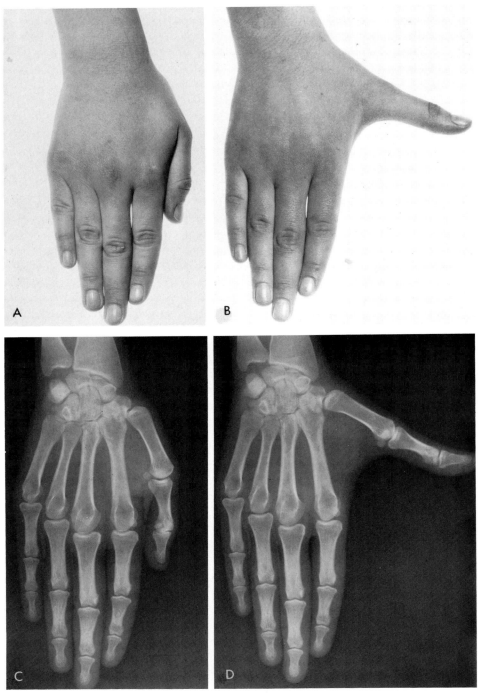

Figure 10–4   Range of adduction and abduction of a normal thumb. *A*, Dorsal photograph of the right hand with the thumb in adduction: the plane of the thumbnail is vertical to the plane of the fingernails. *B* shows the thumb in abduction: in this action the thumb supinates, bringing the plane of its nail closer to the plane of the fingernails. *C* and *D*, Dorsopalmar roentgenographs of the right hand with adducted and abducted thumb, respectively.

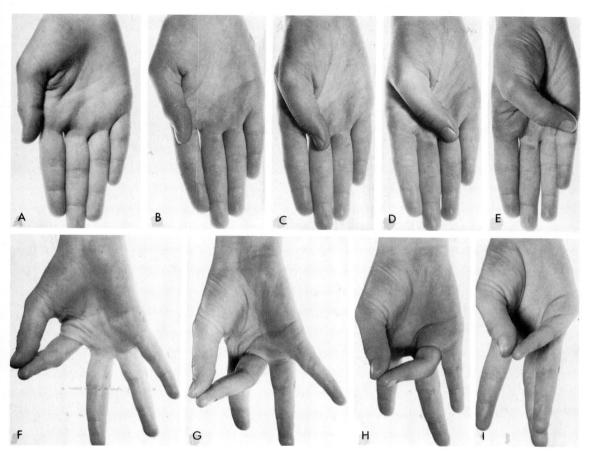

Figure 10–5   The sweep of the thumb across the palms and the act of pulp-to-pulp opposition with various fingers. *A, B, C, D,* and *E* show the arc traced by the tip of the thumb as it sweeps from the radial to the ulnar border of the hand. *F, G, H* and *I* demonstrate pulp-to-pulp opposition of the hand, using each ulnar digit: being longer, the fingers tend to flex to bring their pulps in contact with the pulp of the thumb.

proximal and another at its distal end. Reynolds thought two muscles were definitely absent in both hands: opponens and abductor pollicis brevis. In an analogous case, Ogilvie (1931) could find "no trace of an abductor pollicis or of separate extensor of the thumb." In this case, as in the one described by Voisin and Nathan (1902), the extensor of the most radial triphalangeal digit arose from the confluent mass of the extensor digitorum communis.

One needs to emphasize some other features. The first digit of the five-fingered hand is as long as the fifth. It is unrotated. Its nail lies in about the same horizontal plane as the nails of the other digits. The hand as a whole tends to tilt towards the radial side. Normally, the distal articular facet of the ulna lies proximal to the articular surface of the radius, and its styloid process does not project as far forward as the radial styloid. In the five-fingered hand, the ulna seems to have overtaken the radius and presents an overgrown styloid process. In comparison, the radial styloid is underdeveloped, which accounts for

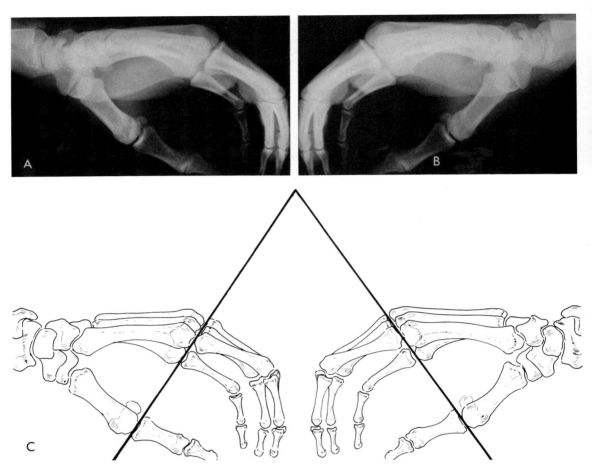

Figure 10–6 The first metacarpal is short but, when the thumb turns into oppositional position, the line passing through the first metacarpophalangeal joint passes through the corresponding articulations of the lesser digital rays. *A,* Lateral roentgenograph of the right hand in oppositional position. *B,* Analogous view of the left hand. *C,* Sketch illustrating the isosceles triangle formed by the lines passing through the metacarpophalangeal joints of the juxtaposed right hand and left hand with respective thumbs in oppositional position.

the radial deviation of the hand. The five-fingered hand may be regarded as a variant of radial ray defect.

The first metacarpal of the five-fingered hand is long and slender—it is often longer than the fifth metacarpal. As in other metacarpals, the first member bears an epiphysis at its distal end but will occasionally retain an additional growth center at its proximal extremity. In line with the first metacarpal, there are three well-formed phalanges, each with its own basal epiphysis. These phalanges can be flexed and extended; to a limited degree, the digit as a whole may be adducted and abducted. These last two movements take place at the metacarpophalangeal joint and not at the carpometacarpal articulation, as in the case of an opposable pollex. In the five-fingered hand, the webspace between the two radial digits is narrow. The first digit cannot move further away from the second, rotate around its own axis, and shift into a position for the fingers to bend towards it and effect pulp-to-pulp opposition (Fig. 10–8).

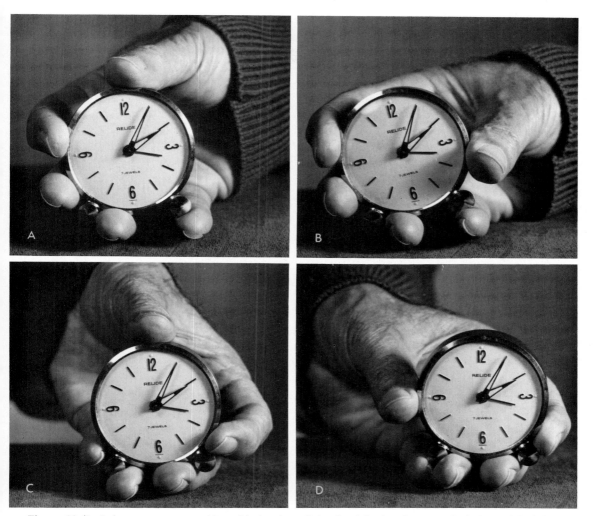

Figure 10–7 In its attempt at opposition with the ulnar digits, the right thumb rotates clockwise and the left coun- terclockwise. *A* and *B* show the right hand and *C* and *D*, the left.

ASSOCIATIONS

As noted, Windle (1891) considered twin digits which had replaced the thumb to be a variant of triphalangeal pollex. Hefner (1940) used the title "He- reditary polydactyly associated with extra phalanges in the thumbs," and McKu- sick (1971) employed the following headings: "Triphalangeal thumb with double phalanges" and "Triphalangeal thumb, opposable, with polydactyly." It would seem that polydactyly is the most common regional anomaly seen in connection with triphalangeal thumb. In the author's experience, triphalangeal first digit is more commonly associated with radial ray defects. Individuals with an absent or floating thumb in one hand will occasionally have triphalangeal pollex in the other. Triphalangeal thumbs have also been reported in connection with a number of more remote abnormalities (Figs. 10–9 to 10–11).

(Text continued on page 302.)

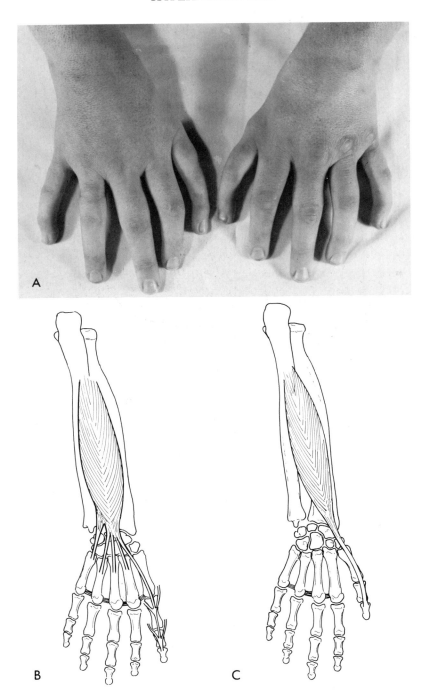

Figure 10–8 "Five-fingered hand." *A*, Dorsal view of the hands of a child with nonopposable first digits: the radialmost digits in both hands are long and slender and their nails barely slant; the first webspace is narrow. *B*, Sketch illustrating some of the anatomic features of five-fingered hand; namely, that the long extensors of the radialmost digit emanate from the common mass of extensors of the other digits and that the first metacarpal is caught in the common bondage of the deep transverse metacarpal ligament. *C*, Sketch illustrating analogous structures in a hand with opposable biphalangeal pollex.

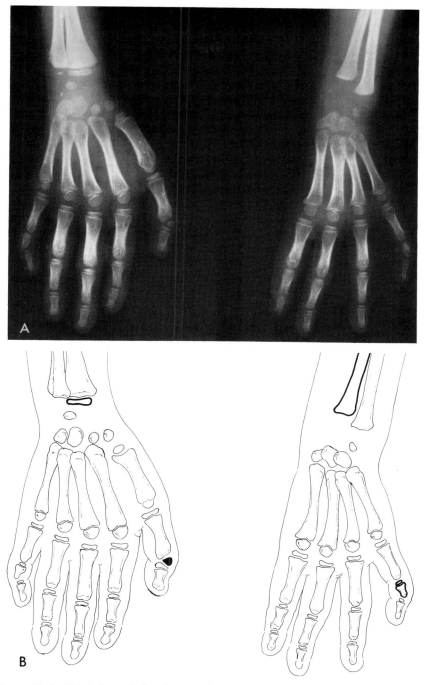

Figure 10–9 Triphalangeal thumb occurring in association with radial ray defect of the contralateral hand. *A*, Dorsopalmar roentgenograph of the distal forearms and the hands of a five-year-old boy, showing a triangular ossicle interposed between the proximal and distal phalanges of the right thumb. In the left hand, the radius is shorter than the ulna and the following bones are missing: the distal epiphysis of the radius, the lunate, the scaphoid, the trapezium, the first metacarpal, and the phalanges of the thumb. *B*, Sketch illustrating the same.

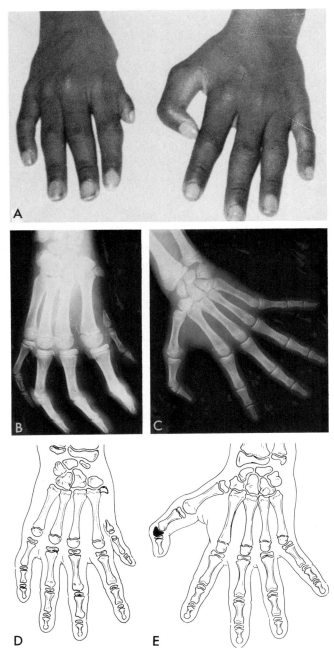

Figure 10–10 Triphalangeal thumb associated with intercalary defect of the first metacarpal of the opposite hand. *A*, Dorsal view of the hands of a 12-year-old male. *B*, Dorsopalmar roentgenograph of the right hand: note the absence of the proximal part of the first metacarpal. *C*, Dorsopalmar roentgenograph of the left hand, showing a triangular piece of bone wedged between the proximal and distal phalanges of the thumb. *D* and *E* illustrate roentgenographs above each.

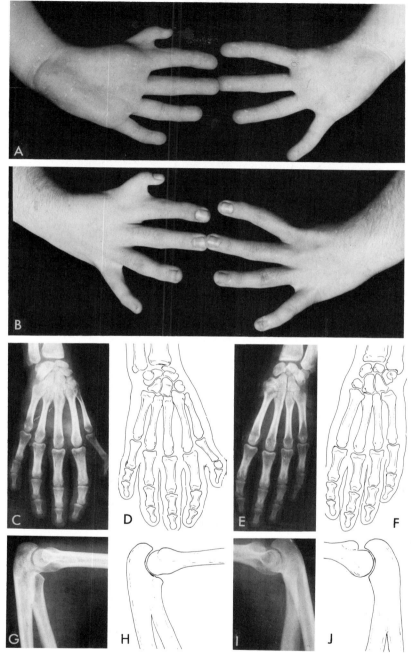

Figure 10–11 Triphalangeal webbed thumb associated with absence of the pollical ray of the opposite hand and bilateral proximal radioulnar synostosis. *A*, Palmar view of both hands of a 15-year-old female. *B*, Dorsal view, showing partial webbing of the right thumb and index finger. *C*, Dorsopalmar roentgenograph of the right hand: the first metacarpal is slender, and a small rectangular ossicle is interposed between the proximal and distal phalanges of the thumb. *D*, Sketch illustrating the same. *E*, Dorsopalmar roentgenograph of the left hand, showing absence of the pollical ray. *F*, Sketch illustrating the same. *G*, Lateral roentgenograph of the right elbow with radioulnar synostosis. *H*, Sketch illustrating the same. *I*, Lateral roentgenograph of the left elbow with radioulnar synostosis. *J*, Sketch illustrating the same.

ABSENT TIBIA AND TRIPHALANGEAL THUMB

The infant with nonopposable triphalangeal thumb examined by Voisin and Nathan (1902) had partial absence of the tibia. Pearson and Stocks (1913) reported a "thumbless but five-fingered woman" with absent tibia. Salzer's (1897) patient with defective tibia had triphalangeal thumb as did Reber's (1968). Eaton and McKusick (1969) presented a man with "five-fingered hands" and pre-axial polydactyly of the feet. His oldest daughter had five-fingered hands and pre-axial polydactyly of the feet; in addition, she showed syndactyly of the fourth and fifth manual digits, pedunculated postminimus on the left hand, and bilateral hypoplasia of the tibia. This woman had two affected daughters. One daughter had hypoplastic tibia and pre-axial polydactyly of the feet; she showed six digits on each hand, "none of which had the characteristics of a thumb." In the second daughter, the tibias were completely absent: there were eight toes on each foot; "each hand had six fingers plus a pedunculated postminimus." Pashayan et al (1971) reported a young woman with rudimentary tibias and pre-axial polydactyly of the feet. "Each hand had five fingers, each with three phalanges and a metacarpal bone." The proband's father was reported as having had absence of the tibia, polydactyly of the feet and, on each hand, "five fingers and no thumbs."

ANEMIA AND TRIPHALANGEAL THUMB

Erythrogenesis imperfecta, also called congenital hypoplastic anemia or pure red cell aplasia, is a deficiency affecting mainly the erythrocytic elements; leukocyte and platelet counts remain normal. It is said to result from a selective hypoplasia of the precursors of red blood cells in the bone marrow. Diamond et al (1961) reported a 25-year follow-up of 30 patients, one of whom had triphalangeal thumbs. Harvey (1966) described a six-week-old female with congenital hypoplastic anemia—"pure red cell aplasia"—and nonopposable triphalangeal thumbs. Aase and Smith (1969) reported the occurrence of congenital hypoplastic anemia and triphalangeal thumbs in two brothers, one of whom had congenital heart disease.

HOLT-ORAM CARDIOMELIC SYNDROME

Calo (1953) reported a patient who had triphalangeal thumb and showed evidences of drainage of two pulmonary veins into the right atrium. Holt and Oram (1960) described a mother and daughter, both of whom had atrial septal defect and thumbs with rudimentary proximal phalanges. The mother, in addition, had an "irregular growth of the ulna and the radius"—the latter being shorter than the former. McKusick et al (1961) reported a mother and daughter with atrial septal defect and triphalangeal or fingerlike thumb. The daughter gave birth to a male infant with upper extremity phocomelia and ventricular septal defect. Zetterquist (1963) listed the following triad as being characteristic of Holt-Oram syndrome: atrial septal defect, cardiac arrhythmia, and anomalous thumb. He presented a mother and son with combined anomalies. The mother had a triphalangeal thumb on one side and absent pollex on the other; the son had triphalangeal thumbs on both sides. Emerit et al (1965) reported six cases out of which only two presented the triad listed by Zetterquist; the other four had the same skeletal anomalies but different cardiac malformations. In the pedigrees reported by Gall et al (1966), Holt-Oram syndrome was transmitted as an autosomal dominant trait with essentially complete penetrance. These authors recorded the following anomalies of the hand: flattening and distal displacement of the thenar eminence, diminution of opposability of the pollex, and thumbs which "resembled triphalangeal digit."

In two families described by Holmes (1965), congenital heart disease was associated with three types of thumb abnormality characterized, respectively, as "finger-like," "vestigial," and "absent." Cascos (1967) described a mother and her four children with electrocardiographic changes; the mother had hypoplastic triphalangeal thumb on the right side and a malformed index finger; the youngest daughter had no thumb on the left side, and on the right hand there were two triphalangeal thumbs which were webbed together.

IMPERFORATE ANUS AND TRIPHALANGEAL THUMB

Stieve (1916) reported a sporadic case of bilateral triphalangeal thumb and atresia of the anus. In a family described by Townes and Brooks (1970), triphalangeal thumb was associated with skeletal abnormalities and imperforate anus. In this family, the trait seemed to be transmitted as an autosomal dominant.

THALIDOMIDE EMBRYOPATHY

Lenz et al (1964) stated that when the pregnant mother had taken thalidomide around the fiftieth day after her last menstruation the child was sometimes born with triphalangeal thumb.

TRIPHALANGISM OF THUMBS AND GREAT TOES AND MULTIPLE DEFECTS

Qazi and Smithwick (1970) reported a five-and-one-half-year-old boy who had triphalangism of the thumbs and great toes, with the ungual phalanges of the other digits being either absent or hypoplastic. The boy was a deaf mute and had hypoplastic nails and teeth; he was mentally retarded and subject to convulsive seizures.

TREATMENT

The problem of opposable triphalangeal thumb hinges on the angular deformity. The parents of the little girl who was brought to Beatson (1897) for consultation wanted to know what could be done to straighten her crooked thumbs. Beatson recommended extirpation of the triangular piece of bone which had become wedged between the proximal and distal phalanges of each pollex. He

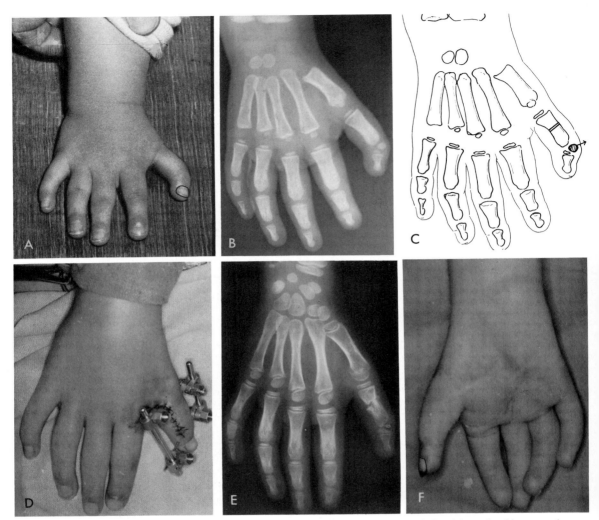

Figure 10–12   Triphalangeal thumb with contracted first webspace and a rounded ossicle wedged between the two phalanges of an inadequately rotated thumb, causing the ungual segment to tilt toward the index finger. This case was treated by widening the first webspace with a flap, removing the extraneous ossicle between the phalanges of the thumb, and performing abduction–radial rotation osteotomy of the first metacarpal. *A*, Preoperative dorsal view of the right hand. *B*, Dorsopalmar roentgenograph of the same. *C*, Sketch illustrating the site of osteotomy of the first metacarpal and the supernumerary ossicle to be removed. *D* shows the external fixation apparatus which was used to hold the thumb abducted and radially rotated. *E*, Roentgenograph taken six weeks after osteotomy of the first metacarpal and extirpation of the interphalangeal ossicle. *F*, Postoperative palmar view of the hand: compare the position of the thumbnail with that seen in *A*.

removed the anomalous ossicles from both thumbs and obtained "very satisfactory' results. This operation was repeated again by Milch (1951) and by Cotta and Jäger (1965). "If the diagnosis is established in infancy or childhood," Milch wrote, "the ossicle should be removed surgically. Only in this way can the deformity be overcome.... In the adult surgery is contra-indicated."

Excision of the ossicle is surely not the only way. Long ago, Herzog (1892) described an operation for the correction of this particular deformity — cuneiform osteotomy through the distal third of the first phalanx. Osteotomy is to be preferred when the interposed bone is too large or when it occurs in adults. Herzog also attempted excision of the articular ends of the bones entering into the joint at which angulation occurs. It was not stated whether the joint was fused after resection of the articular end of bones. Surgical fusion of the joint is another method. This operation is also applicable in adults. In an occasional case of triphalangeal pollex with triangular middle phalanx, the first webspace is narrow and needs to be widened by Z-plasty; rarely, the first metacarpal or the proximal phalanx is osteotomized to put the pollex in a better oppositional position (Fig. 10–12).

Nonopposable triphalangeal thumb or five-fingered hand presents two problems: inability of the first digit to move into an oppositional position and its inordinate length. The digit is shortened surgically by excision of a sizable segment from the midshaft of the metacarpal bone. The capital fragment is approximated to the basal bone; it is placed in such a position as would bring the digit away from the palm and opposite the index or the middle finger. The two fragments are transfixed with Kirschner wire. The webspace is widened with the aid of Z-plasty, local rotation, or distal flap. Zrubecky and Scharizer (1965) have supplemented this operation with an opponens transfer procedure (Fig. 10–13).

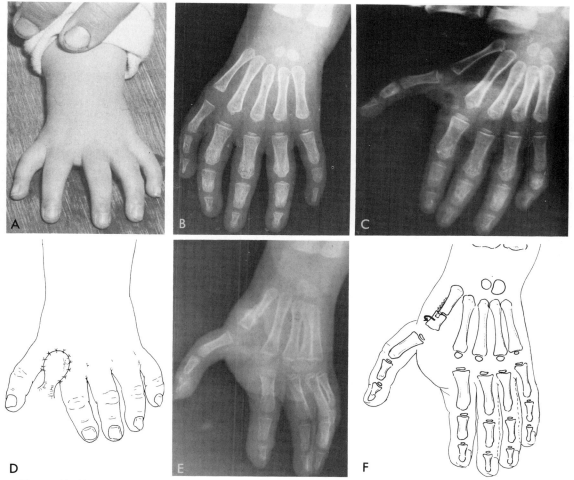

Figure 10–13 Procedure utilized for nonopposable triphalangeal thumb. *A*, Preoperative dorsal photograph of the left hand of the six-month-old child whose right hand is featured in Figure 10–12. *B*, Preoperative dorsopalmar roentgenograph of the same. *C*, Roentgenograph after the first webspace has been widened with the aid of an abdominal flap. *D*, Sketch illustrating the pedicled flap. *E*, Postoperative roentgenograph after shortening and rotation osteotomy of the first metacarpal. *F*, Sketch illustrating the same.

SUMMARY

Hyperphalangism as exemplified by triphalangeal thumb is an anomaly of transverse segmentation. It is thought that the human thumb attained its biphalangeal status by fusion of the middle and terminal phalanges of the primitive pollex, and triphalangism is due to failure of this coalescence. Two types of triphalangeal thumb are distinguished: opposable and nonopposable. Triphalangeal thumb may occur as an isolated anomaly or with other abnormalities of the ipsilateral or opposite upper limb; it is also seen in association with absent tibia, congenital anemia, congenital heart disease, thalidomide embryopathy, imperforate anus, and a complex consisting of triphalangeal hallux, dysplastic ungual phalanges of the lesser digits, deaf mutism, hypoplastic teeth and nails, mental retardation, and infantile epileptic seizures. Opposable triphalangeal thumb presents one main surgical problem—axial deviation of the distal phalanx. In the very young it is treated by excision of the triangular middle bone; in mature individuals the deformity is corrected by subcapital osteotomy of the proximal phalanx. Only occasionally does the first webspace need to be widened or the first metacarpal subjected to rotation osteotomy. Nonopposable first digit presents two problems: inordinate length and inability to shift radialward, turn around, and oppose the more ulnar digits. It is best treated by pollicization, a detailed technique of which will be taken up in Chapter Twenty-four.

References

Aase, J. M., and Smith, D. W.: Congenital anemia and triphalangeal thumbs, a new syndrome. *J. Pediatr.*, *74*:471–474, 1969.

Abramowitz, J.: Triphalangeal thumb in a Bantu family. *J. Bone Joint Surg.*, *41B*:766–771, 1959.

Abramowitz, J.: Triphalangeal thumb. A case report and evaluation of its importance in morphology and function of the thumb. *S. Afr. Med. J.*, *41*:104–106; Figs. 2 and 3, 1967.

Arquembourg, L.: Sur un cas de pouces à trois phalanges. *L'Echo Méd. du Nord* (Lille), *9*:613–615, 1905.

Beatson, G. T.: Congenital deformity of both thumbs. *Scott. Med. Surg. J.*, *1*:1083–1089, 1897.

Bellelli, F.: Un nuovo caso di pollice a tre falangi bilaterale. *Riforma Med.*, *55*:1001–1003, 1939.

Calo, A.: Cardiopatie congenite e malformazioni delgi arti. *Cuore Circ.*, *37*:303–313, 1953.

Campbell, D.: Dreigliedrige Daumen. *Fortschr. Röntgenstr.*, *39*:479–481, 1929.

Cascos, A. S.: Holt-Oram syndrome. *Acta Paediat. Scand.*, *56*:313–317, 1967.

Columbi, R.: *De Re Anatomica.* Libir XV, Venetiis ex Typog., N. Beuilacque, p. 485, 1559. Francofurdi Martinum Lechlerum sumptibus Petri Fischeri, 1593.

Cotta, H., and Jäger, M.: Die familiäre Triphalangie des Daumens und ihre operative Behandlung. *Arch. Orthop. Unfallchir.*, *58*:282–290, 1965.

Cotte, G.: Pouce bot varus congénital. *Rev. d'Orthop.*, (3 s.), *10*:411–413, 1923.

DeLaurenzi, V.: Pollice con tre falangi. *G. Med. Milit. 108*:149–152, 1958.

Diamond, L. K., Allen, D. M., and Magill, F. B.: Congenital (erythroid) hypoplastic anemia: 25-year study. *Am. J. Dis. Child.*, *102*:403–415, 1961.

Drinkwater, H.: Hereditary abnormal segmentation of the index and middle fingers. *J. Anat. Physiol.*, *50*:177–186, 1916.

Dubois, P.: Le pouce a de plus 3 phalanges. *Arch. Gén. Méd.*, *7*:148, 1826.

Dubreuil-Chambardel, L.: Un cas d'hyperphalangie du pouce. *Bull. Méd. Soc. d'Anthrop.* Paris, (5 s.), *19*:118–138, 1909. Also in *Gaz. du Centre, Tours*, *15*:25–29, 1910.

Dubreuil-Chambardel, L.: *Les Variations du Corps Humain.* Paris, Flammarion, pp. 128–135, 1925.

Eaton, G. O., and McKusick, V. A.: A seemingly unique polydactyly-syndactyly syndrome in four persons in three generations. *In* Bergma, D., et al., (eds.): *Birth Defects. Original Article Series.* New York, National Foundation – March of Dimes. Vol. V; No. 3:221–225, 1969.

Ecke, H.: Beitrag zu den Doppelmissbildungen in bereich der Finger. *Beitr. Klin. Chir.*, *205*:463–468, 1962.

Emerit, I., Grouchy, J. de, Laval-Jeantet, M., Corone, P., and Vernant, P.: Malformations complex des membres superieure associées a une cardiopathie congénitale. A propos de six observations. *Acta Genet. Méd. Gem.*, *14*:132–163, 1965.

Eudemius of Alexandria: quoted by Galen (A.D. 165).

Ferber, C.: Ein Beitrag zur Dreigliedrigkeit des Daumens. *Z. Orthop.*, *83*:55–64, 1952.

Fréré, J. M.: A case having thumbs with three phalanges simulating fingers. *South. Med. J.*, *23*:536–537, 1930.

Galen: *Oeuvres Anatomique. Physiologique et Médicales de Galden.* Par Ch. Daremberg. Paris, J. B. Balliere. Tome I, pp. 111–167, 1854. See also the section called "The wrist and the hand." In: *On the Usefulness of Parts of the Body.* Vol. I Translated by M. T. May. Ithaca, New York, Cornell University Press, 113–153, 1968. The original is said to have appeared around 165 A.D.

Gall, J. C., Jr., Stern, A. M., Cohen, M. M., Adams, M. S., and Davidson, R. T.: Holt-Oram syndrome: Clinical and genetic study of a large family. *Am. J. Hum. Genet.*, *18*:187–199, 1966.

Gates, R.: *Human Genetics.* Vol. I. New York, The Macmillan Co., pp. 385–469, 1946.

Gavani, J.: Deformita del pollice, eziologia e patogenesi. *Bull. Sci. Med.* (Bologna), *5*:66–73, 1905. See also *Rev. d'Orthop.* (2 s.), *6*:261–270, 1905.

Geelvink, P.: Über Hyperphalangie. *Arch. Psychiatr. Nervenkr.*, *52*:1015–1028, 1913.

Girija, A.: The occurrence of an additional phalanx in the thumb. *Indian J. Pediatr.*, *25*:374–376, 1958.

Grobelnik, S.: Dreigliedriger Daumenfinger. *Z. Orthop. Chir.*, *80*:294–298, 1950.

Grynkraut, B.: Pouce a trois phalanges (Essai de classification à propos d'un cas nouveau). *J. Radiol. Electrol.*, *11*:325–326, 1927.

Haas, S. L.: Three-phalangeal thumbs. *Am. J. Roentgenol.*, *42*:677–682, 1939.

Harvey, D. R.: On congenital hypoplastic anemia. *Proc. R. Soc. Med.*, London (Section of pediatrics), *59*:490–492, 1966.

Hefner, R. A.: Hereditary polydactyly associated with extra phalanges in the thumb. *J. Hered.*, *31*:25–27, 1940.

Hennig, C.: Von der Überzahl der Finger und Zehen und von dreigliedrigen Daumen. *Berl. d. Kinderheil.*, Leipzig, pp. 25–46, 1880.

Herzog, W.: Uber angeborene Deviationen der Fingerphalanges (Klinodaktylie). *Münch Med. Wochenschr.*, *39*:344–345, 1892.

Hilgenreiner, H.: Über Hyperphalangie des Daumens. *Beitr. Klin. Chir.*, *54*:585–629, 1907.

Hilgenreiner, H.: Neues zur Hyperphalangie des Daumens. *Beitr. Klin. Chir.*, *67*:196–221, 1910.

Hilgenreiner, H.: Zur Hyperphalangie resp Pseudohyperphalangie des dreigliedrigen Finger. *Z. Orthop. Chir.*, *35*:234–247, 1915.

Hollander, E.: Familiäre Finger Missbildungen (Brachydaktylie und Hyperphalangie). *Berl. Klin. Wochenschr.*, 57:472–474, 1918.

Holmes, L. B.: Congenital heart disease and upper-extremity deformities: A report of two families. *N. Engl. J. Med.*, 272:437–444, 1965.

Holt, M., and Oram, S.: Familial heart disease with skeletal malformations. *Br. Heart J.*, 22:236–242, 1960.

Humphry, G. M.: *A Treatise on the Human Skeleton (Including the Joints)*. Cambridge, Macmillan & Co., pp. 383–396, 1858.

Joachimsthal, G.: *Die Angeborenen Verbildungen der Oberen Extremitäten*. Hamburg, L. Grafe & Sillem, pp. 31–33, 1900.

Joachimsthal, G.: Verdoppelung des linken Zeigefingers und Dreigliederung des rechten Daumens. *Berl. Klin. Wochenschr.*, 37:835–838, 1900.

Joachimsthal, G.: Weitere Mittelungen über Hyperphalangie. *Z. Orthop. Chir.*, 17:462–472, 1906.

Jones, F. W.: *The Principles of Anatomy as Seen in the Hand*. Second edition. London, Balliere, Tindall & Cox, pp. 45–52, 1944.

Jurcié, F.: Ein Fall von Hyperphalangie beider Daumen. *Arch. Klin. Chir.*, 80:562–566, 1906.

Kessler, I.: Five-fingered hand: one-stage pollicization of the radial finger. *Isr. J. Med. Sci.*, 6:280–283, 1970.

Kirmission, E.: Pouces a trois phalanges symetriquement développées sur chacune des deux mains un jeune garçon de neuf ans. *Rev. d'Orthop.*, (2 s.), 10:249–253, Pl. II, 1909.

Komai, T., Ozaki, Y., and Inokuma, W.: A Japanese kindred of hyperphalangism of thumbs and duplication of thumbs and big toes. *Folia Hered. Pathol.* (Milano), 2:307–312, 1953.

Kristjansen, A.: Om "Hyperphalangia pollicis." *Hospstid.*, 69:109–119, 1926.

Krivanek, F.: Familial incidence of triphalangeal thumb. *Acta Chir. Orthop. Traumatol. Cech.*, 18:167–179, 1951.

Lapidus, P. W., and Guidotti, F. P.: Triphalangeal bifid thumb. *Arch. Surg.*, 49:228–234, 1944.

Lapidus, P. W., Guidotti, F. P., and Coletti, C. J.: Triphalangeal thumb: Report of six cases. *Surg. Gynecol. Obstet.*, 77:178–186, 1943.

Leboucq, H.: De la brachydactylie et de l'hyperphalangie chez l'homme. *Bull. Acad. R. Med. Belg.*, 5:344–361, 1896.

Lenz, W., Theopold, W., and Thomas, J.: Triphalangie des Daumens als Folge von Thalidomidschädigung. *Münch Med. Wochenschr.*, 106:2033–2041, 1964.

Lossen, H.: Hyperphalangie der Mittalfinger bei beidseitiger partieller Brachydaktylie. *Fortschr. Röntgenstr.*, 56:428–438, 1937.

Manzke, H.: Symmetrische Hyperphalangie der zweiten Fingers durch ein akzessorischen Metacarpale. *Fortschr. Röntgenstr.*, 105:425–427, 1966.

Maurizio, E.: Pollice varo, trifalangia del pollice e polidattilia radiale. *Arch. Putti Chir. Organi Mou.*, 19:449–456, 1964.

McGregor, A. L.: A contribution to the morphology of the thumb. *J. Anat.*, 60:259–263, 1926.

McKusick, V. A.: Medical genetics. *J. Chron. Dis.*, 14:1–198; Fig. 45, 1961.

McKusick, V. A.: *Mendelian Inheritance in Man*. Third edition. Baltimore, Johns Hopkins Press, Entry 19050, pp. 282–283, 1971, entry 19070, p. 283, 1971.

Milch, H.: Triphalangeal thumb. *J. Bone Joint Surg.*, 33A:692–697, 1951.

Morgan, G.: Skiagrams of a case of polydactylism. *Lancet*, 2:1599, 1896.

Mosengeil, K. V.: Subluxation des Os multangulum majus über das Niveau des Dorsum manus bei einer Hand, die stalt des Daumens einen dreiphalangigen Finger halte. *Arch. Klin. Chir.*, 12:723–724; Taf. X; Fig. 10, 1871.

Muller, W.: Beiträge zur Kenntnis des dreigliedrigen Daumens. *Arch. Klin. Chir.*, 185:377–386, 1936.

Ogilvie, W. H.: Congenital abnormalities of the hands. *Proc. R. Soc. Med.* (Section of Orthopaedics), 24:38–40, 1931.

Ottendorf: Zur Frage des dreigliedrigen Daumens. *Z. Orthop. Chir.*, 17:507–524, 1906.

Paltrinieri, M.: Nell variazioni numeriche delle falangi frequentemente la falange minute e la seconds. Ser. Med. in onore di Ugo Camer. *Ed. Min. Med.*, pp. 107–113, 1959.

Paltrinieri, M., and DeLucchi, G.: Rara deformita del pollice ereditariament transmissibile. *Bell. Sci. Med. Bologna*, 3:158–167, 1938.

Pashayan, H., Fraser, F. C., McIntyre, J. M., and Dunbar, J. S.: Bilateral aplasia of the tibia, polydactyly and absent thumb in father and daughter. *J. Bone Joint Surg.*, 53B:495–499, 1971.

Pearson, K., and Stocks, P.: An unusual case of digital anomaly. ("Thumbless but five-fingered woman." Absent tibia). *Biometrika*, 14:410–411, 1913.

Pfitzner, W.: Die Kleine Zehe. Eine anatomische Studie. *Arch. Anat. Entwickl.*, pp. 12–41, 1890.

Pol, R.: "Brachydaktylie" – "Klinodaktylie" – Hyperphalangie und ihre Grundlagen. *Arch. Path. Anat. Phys.*, 229:388–528, 1921.

Pol, R.: Hyperphalangie des Daumens, Klinodaktylie des Daumens (Pollex varus, pollex valgus). *In* Schwalbe, E., and Gruber, G. B., (eds): *Die Morphologie der Missbildungen des Menschen und der Tiere*. Jena, G. Fischer, 3 T., 17 Lief., 1 Abt., 7 Kap., 1 Halfte, pp. 646–654, 1937.

Poznanski, A. K., Garn, S. M., and Holt, J. F.: Thumb in the congenital malformation syndromes. *Radiology*, 100:115–129, 1971.

Qazi, Q. H., and Smithwick, E. M.: Triphalangy of thumbs and great toes. *Am. J. Dis. Child, 120*:255–257, 1970.

Ratichvili, G.: Pouce varus congenital à trois phalanges. *Rev. d'Orthop., 18*:228–231, 1931.

Reber, M.: Un syndrome osseux peu commun associant une heptadactylie et une aplasie de tibia (nonopposably triphalangeal thumb). *J. Genet. Hum., 16*:15–39, 1968.

Reynolds, L. R.: Hyperphalangism accompanied by supernumerary epiphyses and muscular deficiencies. *Anat. Rec., 13*:113–129, 1917.

Rieder, J.: Eine Familie mit dreigliedrigen Daumen. *Z. Morph. Anthrop., 2*:177–197, 1900.

Roberts, E.: Hereditary hyperphalangism of the thumb. *J. Hered., 34*:291–292, 1943.

Sallam, A. M.: Triphalangeal thumbs. *Arch. Surg., 71*:257–259, 1955.

Salzer, H.: Zwei Falle von dreighliedrigen Daumen. *Anat. Anz., 14*:124–131, 1897.

Sappey, Phd. .: *Traité d'Anatomie Descriptive*. Fourth edition. Paris, A. Delahaye et E. Lecroisier, Vol. I, pp. 423–426, 1888.

Schrader, E.: Dreigliedrige Daumen. *Fortschr. Röntgenstr., 40*:693–694, 1929.

Staderini, R.: Un pollice con tre falangi, una mano con sette dita nell'nono. *Monitore Zool. Ital.* (Firenze) 5:119–120, 1894.

Stieve, H.: Über Hyperphalangie des Daumens. *Anat. Anz., 48*:565–581, 1916.

Struthers, J.: On variations in the number of fingers and toes, and in the number of phalanges, in man. *Edinb. New Philos. J.* (n.s.), *18*:83–111, 1863.

Swanson, A. B., and Brown, K.: Hereditary triphalangeal thumb. *J. Hered., 53*:259–265, 1962.

Townes, P. C., and Brooks, E. R.: Imperforate anus and triphalangeal thumbs: a new autosomal dominant syndrome, abstracted. *Am. Pediatr. Soc. Inc. Soc. Pediatr. Research*, p. 129, 1970.

Uffelmann, J.: *Der Mittelhandknochen des Daumens*. Sein Entwicklungsgeschichte und Bedeutung. Gottingen, A. Rente, 1863.

Valenti, G.: Pollice ed alluci con tre falangi. *Mem. R. Acad. Sci. Inst.* (Bologna), *8*:491–503, 1900.

Voisin, R., and Nathan, M.: Malformations congénitales symétriques des membres. Pouce a trois phalanges. Absence partielle du tibia. Anomalies musculaires. *Bull. Soc. Anat.* (Paris), 77:843–845, 1902.

Watson, K., and Boyes, J. H.: Congenital angular deformity of the digits. Delta phalanx. *J. Bone Joint Surg., 49A*:333–338, 1967.

Weinisch, A.: *Ein Fall von dreigliedrigen Daumen*. Inaug. Diss. München, Druck der Kdg. Hofbruchdruckerei Kaster & Callwey, pp. 1–23, 1916.

Wertherman, A.: *Bewegungsapparat. Sechster Teil. Die Entwicklungstorungen der Extremitäten*. Berlin, Springer Verlag, pp. 163–167, 1952.

Weyers, H.: Die dreigliedrigkeit des Daumens, hyperphalangism of the thumb. *In* Diethelm. L., (ed): *Röntgendiagnostik der Skeleterkrankungen*. Berlin, J. Springer, Vol. V, Part 3:428–430, 1968.

Willert, H. G., and Henkel, H. L.: *Klinik und Pathologie der Dysmelie*. Berlin, Springer Verlag, pp. 14–16, 1969.

Willert, H. G., and Henkel, H. L.: Pathologisch-anatomische Prinzipien bei Extremitätenfehlbildungen dargertellt am Beispiel der Finger. *Z. Orthop., 107*:663–675; Abb. 6 (Teratologische Reihe der Triphalangie des Daumen), 1970.

Windle, C. A.: The occurrence of an additional phalanx in the human pollex. *J. Anat. Physiol., 26*:100–116, 1891.

Wittkower, B.: *Über Hyperphalangie am Daumen mit Valgusstellung der Endphalanx.* Berlin, O. Francke, pp. 1–32, 1903.

Zderkiewicz, W.: Familial occurrence of triphalangeal thumb. (Polish) *Warzad. Ruchu., 22*:551–553, 1957.

Zeller, R.: Über familiäres Auftreten von Hyperphalangie des Daumens und die Erblichkeit der Pseudoepiphysen. *Inaug. Diss*. Bonn, A. Brand, pp. 1–32, 1936.

Zetterquist, P.: The syndrome of familial atrial septal defect, heart arrhythmia and hand malformation (Holt-Oram) in mother and son. *Acta Pediatr., 52*:115–122, 1963.

Zrubecky, G., and Scharizer, E.: Die Triphalangie des Daumens. *Arch. Orthop. Unfallchir. 57*:45–50, 1965.

Chapter Eleven

SYMPHALANGISM

On June 18, 1873, Cunningham (1879) delivered a baby who had "no joints between the first and second phalanges of all the fingers of the left hand and also between the phalanges of all the fingers of the right hand except the index finger, which, with the thumbs of both hands, was natural." Cunningham described the deformity as congenital absence of phalangeal joints. Walker (1901) named it hereditary "anchylosis" of phalangeal joints. Cushing (1915) coined the term "symphalangism"; Drinkwater (1917), "phalangeal anarthrosis"; and Duncan (1917), "orthodactyly." German authors seem to prefer the designation aplasia of the interphalangeal joint. In England, the affected individuals are said to have Talbot fingers; in America, they are dubbed as being stiff- or straight-fingered; and in China, according to Hall (1928), they are called shovel-hands "because of their inability to pick up grain from a measure by grasping with pronated hand; instead, they tend to supinate the hand and scoop up the grain with a shoveling motion." Bloom (1937) proposed the designation hereditary multiple ankylosing arthropathy. Most authors seem content with Cushing's coinage, symphalangism.

THE NATURE OF THE DEFECT

In symphalangism, an intermediary element, a joint, is missing. The anomaly is to be regarded as an intercalary transverse defect. Two classes of symphalangism are distinguished—proximal and distal. In the former, the joint between the proximal and middle phalanx is eliminated; in the latter, the articulation between the middle and terminal phalanx is effaced. In the hand, proximal symphalangism prevails. When the comparatively uncommon distal variety occurs, it seems to favor the index and little fingers—more often the latter. As a rule, symphalangism does not affect both interphalangeal joints of the same digit. Proximal and distal varieties do not usually occur in the same hand of the same individual nor in various members of the same genealogical tree. There have been two exceptions. One of Walker's (1901) patients had ankylosis of both

interphalangeal joints of the little finger. In the pedigree of proximal symphalangism reported by Strasburger et al (1965), there was a young girl who had
distal interphalangeal fusion in the little finger on the right hand and proximal
interphalangeal fusion in the fifth digit of the left hand. Her ring finger on both
sides showed proximal interphalangeal fusion.

Symphalangism of the hand is predominantly bilateral and shows definite
predilection for the more ulnar digits. In the pedigree presented by Freud and
Slobody (1943), fusion of the proximal and middle phalanges became progressively less marked from the little to the index finger. Strasburger et al (1965)
wrote: "If any finger is affected, it is always the little finger." Most authors en-
dorse this edict. "The incidence of involvement decreases progressively from the
fifth to the second digit," Harle and Stevenson (1967) wrote.

In the pedigree reported by Savarinathan and Centerwall (1966), the
symphalangism affected only the interphalangeal joints of otherwise normal-ap-
pearing thumbs. In three cases, the roentgenographs revealed the presence of
joint space, suggesting fibrous rather than bony ankylosis. In this pedigree,
pollical symphalangism was associated with polydactyly and syndactyly. Pollical
symphalangism unassociated with other anomalies of the hand is extremely rare.
Harle and Stevenson (1967) ascribed the relative immunity of the thumb from
symphalangism to the lack of a middle phalanx in this digit (Fig. 11–1).

DEVELOPMENT

Much has been written about the propensity of the middle row of phalanges
to teratogenic disturbances. The vulnerability of these bones has been attributed
to their protracted period of differentiation. The middle row of phalanges are
the last bones of the hand to ossify; in this row, the more radially located elements differentiate earlier than those nearer the ulnar margin of the hand. The
last tubular bone of the hand to gain an ossific ring is the middle phalanx of the
little finger, and this digit is affected more often by symphalangism than its radial
neighbors.

At about the seventh week of embryonic life, the precartilaginous anlagen of
the consecutive phalanges of each digit are separated from one another by a
strip of condensed mesenchyme which marks the site of the future joint. Haines
(1947) named this strip "interzone." The interzone splits into three layers—two
dense strata destined to form hyaline joint surfaces and a loose intermediate
layer. The central portion of the intermediate layer breaks down and permits the
formation of minute spaces, which coalesce and form the joint cavity. Complete
cavitation is consummated between the ninth and tenth weeks of prenatal life. It
was previously thought that the formation of the articular cavity depended upon
motion. The onset of cavitation is now regarded as being independent of joint
motion; it is ascribed to an enzymic influence during early embryonic life.

Nowhere is it categorically stated, but after reading numerous articles on
this subject, one gets the impression that, like the tardily ossifying middle row of
phalanges, the proximal interphalangeal joints are also slow to undergo cavitation and that the postaxial articulations differentiate later than the pre-axial
joints. Inevitably, it is implied that the sluggishly differentiating joints show
greater tendency to symphalangism.

In the newborn, one does not, nor should he, expect to find solid bony

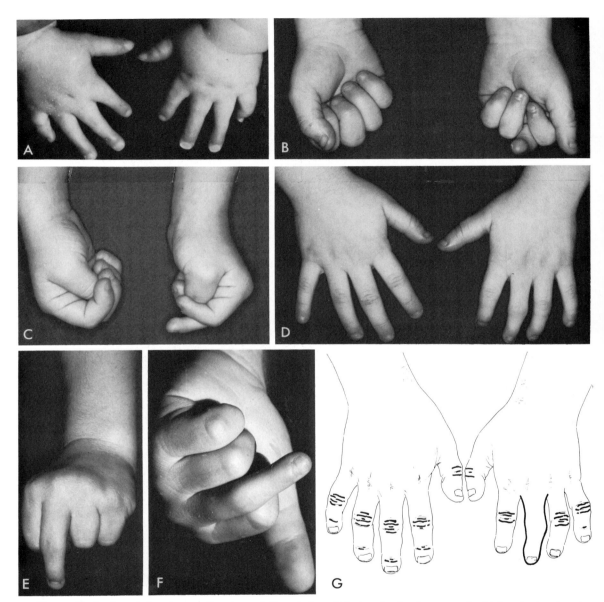

Figure 11–1 Symphalangism: earlier signs. *A*, Dorsal view of the hands of a three-month-old female showing absence of wrinkles on the back of the interphalangeal joints. *B*, Palmar view of the clenched hand three years later: the left middle finger fails to flex at both interphalangeal joints, and there is only minimal flexion at the distal articulations of the flanking digits. *C*, Radial view of the same. *D*, Dorsal view: here one notes the absence of transverse creases in the back of both interphalangeal joints of the left middle finger and the distal joints of the flanking digits. *E*, Dorsal view of the same hand at the age of five. *F*, Oblique view at six years of age: transverse lines over both interphalangeal joints of the left middle digit have not yet developed. *G*, Sketch illustrating *D*.

fusion between the two consecutive phalanges, since there is a cartilaginous epiphysis which must be ossified before bony continuity can be established. One merely finds absence of flexion creases on the volar aspect of the affected joint and absence of wrinkles on the extensor surface; there is also lack of motion at this juncture. Joint stiffness precedes osseous union — bony ankylosis develops insidiously over a period of years and is not completed until after the closure of the epiphysis. Phalangeal epiphyses are cartilaginous at birth and, hence, radiolucent. Prior to the period of skeletal maturation, roentgenography might show a narrowing of the joint space and the premature closure of the neighboring epiphysis. The latter fuses first to the shaft of the proximal phalanx and then to the distal bone. After the effacement of the growth cartilage line, the joint space narrows and eventually becomes obliterated. At the completion of this process, the two phalanges constitute a single bone with continuous marrow cavity and a homogeneous trabecular pattern (Figs. 11–2 to 11–4).

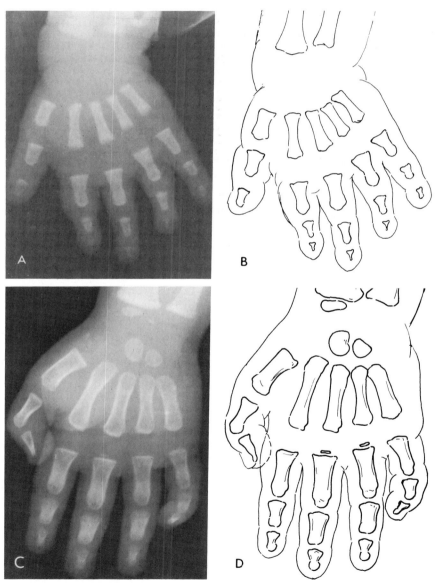

Figure 11–2 Development of symphalangism. *A,* Dorsopalmar roentgenograph of the left hand of the little girl shown in Figure 11–1—at the age of three months. *B,* Sketch illustrating the same. *C,* Roentgenograph of the hand at the age of 18 months, showing that the phalangeal epiphyses in the neighborhood of the symphalangism prone joints have not as yet ossified and a strip of radiolucent area intervenes between the shadows cast by two consecutive phalanges. *D,* Sketch illustrating the same.

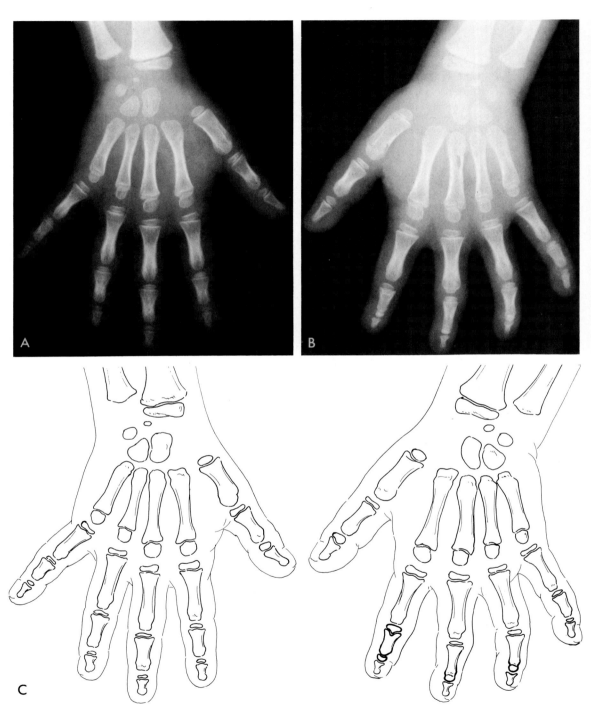

Figure 11–3 *A*, Dorsopalmar roentgenograph of the right hand of the same patient at the age of three years: note that a radiolucent area separates the epiphysis of each ungual phalanx from the diaphysis of the middle phalanx of each ulnar digit. *B*, Dorsopalmar roentgenograph of the left hand: here the epiphysis of the ungual phalanx of each central digit has begun to contact the diaphysis of the proximal bone. *C*, Illustrative sketch.

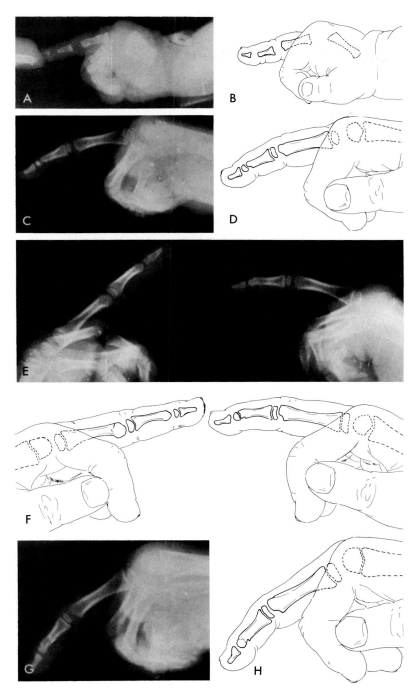

Figure 11–4 *A* and *B*, Lateral roentgenograph and sketch of the skeletal components of the middle finger of the same child at the age of three months: consecutive phalanges are separated by wide spaces. *C* and *D* illustrate the same at four years of age: the basal epiphysis of the ungual phalanx is beveled on its volar aspect. *E*, Lateral roentgenograph of the right and left middle fingers at the age of five, showing that the epiphysis of the ungual phalanx of the right middle finger has contacted the head of the middle phalanx. *F*, Sketch illustrating the same, *G* and *H*, Lateral roentgenograph and sketch of the right middle finger at the age of six, showing complete union of the ungual phalangeal epiphysis and the head of the middle phalanx.

The comparative immunity of the thumb to symphalangism is explained on the basis of the earlier development of this most pre-axial member. The formation of the interphalangeal joint of the thumb is said to precede the critical period of the action of the gene causing the symphalangism. This period is set at about the eighth week of embryonic development, at which time the gene responsible for the symphalangism is said to nullify the effect of the articular cavity–inducing enzyme. Two such genes, with separate loci, are incriminated—one for proximal and the other for distal symphalangism (Fig. 11–5).

PEDIGREES

There are now over 30 recorded pedigrees to prove that symphalangism is preeminently a genetic disorder. It is inherited as an autosomal dominant phenotype. Until recently, the pedigree described by Drinkwater (1917) was considered to be the most remarkable. Symphalangism was said to have been transmitted in the Talbot family through 14 generations, over a period of 500 years. Drinkwater claimed that the progenitor of the trait was John Talbot, first Earl of Shrewsbury, who figures in Shakespeare's *Henry VI* and was killed in battle near Bordeaux in 1453. Elkington and Huntsman (1967) recently cast doubt upon Drinkwater's claim. They reexamined the available documents and studied five living members of the Talbot family who had symphalangism. They suggested that the Talbot finger seen in living members of the family probably resulted from a more recent mutation.

Perhaps the most carefully documented pedigree of symphalangism is the one reported by Cushing (1915, 1916) and brought up to date by Strasburger et al (1965). The progenitor of this pedigree, William Brown, migrated from Scotland in 1740 and settled in southwest Virgina. Some of his descendants went to Ohio and others headed toward Texas. Strasburger et al wrote: "The family tree now spans ten generations including 684 individuals, of whom 350 are affected.... In the affected lines 50 percent have the trait." Families with symphalangism described by Duncan (1917), Hefner (1924), and Daniel (1936) are also of Scottish descent and are said to be related to Cushing's pedigree.

Almost all reported pedigrees of symphalangism have been in the white and yellow races. Freud and Slobody (1943) described a family in which nine out of ten members, in four generations, had proximal symphalangism. "Although this family at first glance was thought to be Negro, it should be emphasized that one of the progenitors was an American Indian," Freud and Slobody wrote.

The expression of the gene for symphalangism may be variable. In the pedigree of proximal symphalangism of the little fingers featured herewith, some members, especially females, showed no roentgenographic evidence of solid bony union of the two consecutive phalanges, but movement between them was practically nil. In all these cases in which roentgenographs revealed persisting joint space, the middle phalanx of the little—and in one case also of the ring—finger was short. Some affected and a few unaffected members of this kindred had stiff thumbs and limited pronation and supination of the forearm, but there was no radiological evidence of osseous union of the pollical bones or of radius and ulna. In one instance, the mother could not flex her little fingers at the first interphalangeal joints, in spite of radiological evidence of joint space between the proximal and middle phalanges. Her son had solid osseous union between the proximal ends of the radius and ulna. In this pedigree, the synostotic tendency seems to have been transmitted by both males and females, but the males were more severely affected (Figs. 11–6 to 11–13).

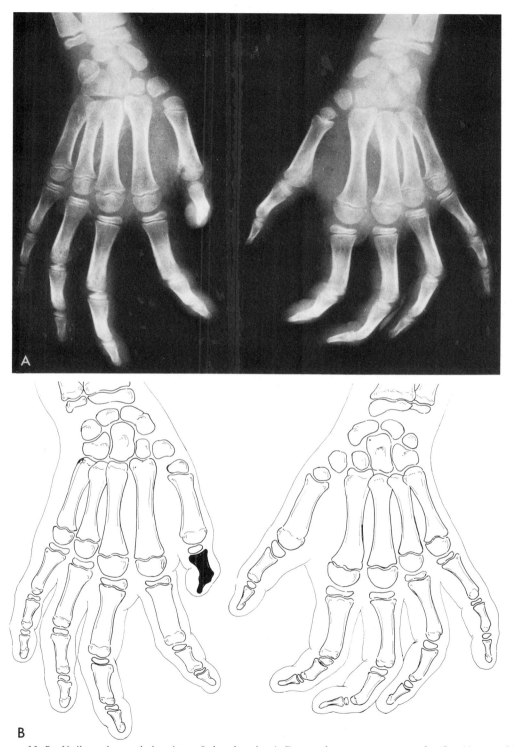

Figure 11–5   Unilateral symphalangism of the thumb. *A*, Dorsopalmar roentgenograph of a 12-year-old boy, showing symphalangism of the right thumb. *B*, Sketch illustrating the same.

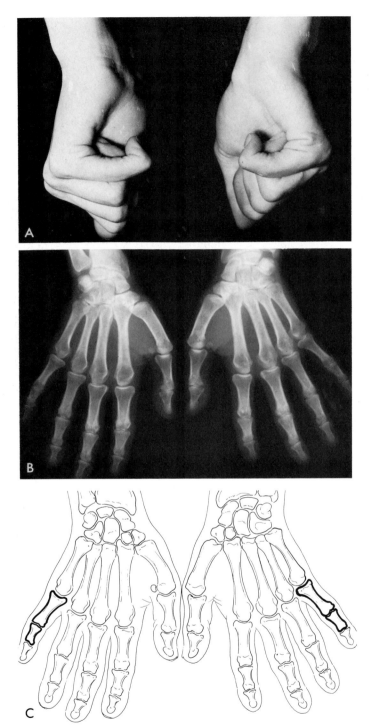

Figure 11–6   J. F., nee L., 34, female. *A*, Ulnar view of her fists: the little fingers fail to flex at the first interphalangeal joints. *B*, Dorsopalmar roentgenograph of the hands: the joint space between the proximal and middle phalanges of each little finger is narrow. *C*, Sketch illustrating the same. J. F. has three children—two sons and a daughter. One son has bilateral radioulnar synostosis. The other two children are unaffected. Her own parents were unaffected but her paternal grandfather had webbed toes.

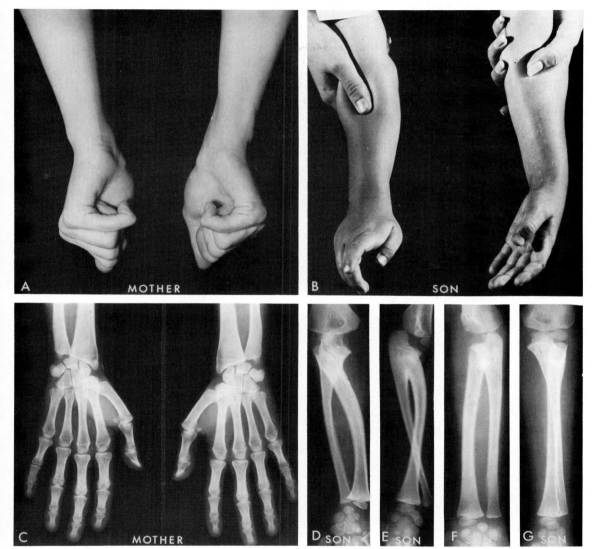

Figure 11–7 J. F. and her son with bilateral radioulnar synostosis. *A,* Ulnar view of J. F.'s fists with unbending little fingers. *B,* Radial view of the hands and forearms of her six-year-old son who could not pronate or supinate his forearms and hands but had no evidence of symphalangism. *C,* Dorsopalmar roentgenograph of mother's hands which have been sketched in Figure 11–6 *C. D, E, F,* and *G,* Anteroposterior and lateral roentgenographs of the son's forearms, showing complete bilateral radioulnar synostosis.

REGIONAL ASSOCIATIONS

In symphalangism, digital dwarfing is at times so drastic that many authors have been led to identify this form of end-to-end fusion of phalanges with brachydactyly. In classic brachymesophalanges, the rudimentary middle phalanx is at times fused with the terminal segment. In this type of brachydactyly there is diminution of stature. Generalized dwarfism is not a feature of proximal symphalangism.

Mercier (1838) associated symphalangism with absence of the metacarpal

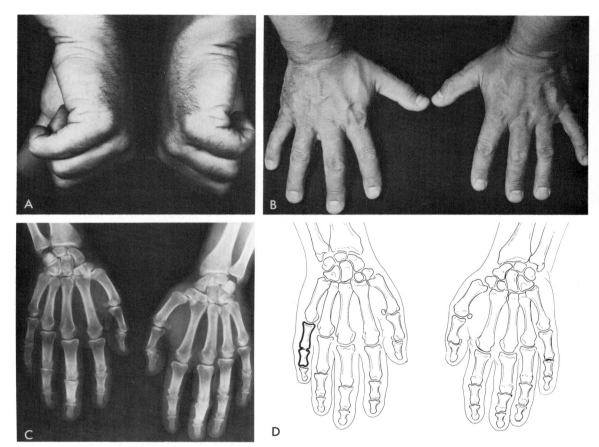

Figure 11–8 Senior C. L., 55, male—J. F.'s brother. *A*, Ulnar view of his fists: the right little finger barely bends at the first interphalangeal joint. *B*, Dorsal view of the hands showing absence of wrinkles in the back of the first interphalangeal joint of the right little finger. *C*, Dorsopalmar roentgenograph of both hands, showing narrowing of the first interphalangeal joint space of both little fingers, especially of the right. *D*, Sketch interpreting the same. Senior C. L. has seven children of whom only three are affected, as featured in Figures 11–9 to 11–11.

bone. In the case of split hand reported by Heath (1866) there was symphalangism of the thumb. Pervès (1932) presented a patient whose first metacarpal was dwarfed. Association of partial syndactyly and symphalangism was noted by Freud and Slobody (1943). In the pedigree reported by Savarinathan and Centerwall (1966), symphalangism of the thumb was associated with poly- and syndactyly. In Drey's (1912) cases, the terminal phalanges of the middle and ring fingers were missing. In the case reported by Révész (1916), symphalangism was accompanied by fusion between the trapezoid bones and the first metacarpals, which were inordinately short; in addition, the radial styloid was absent. The association of symphalangism with carpal or tarsal coalescence or both has been recorded by Miller (1922), Wilmoth (1930), Rochlin and Simonson (1932), Mastern (1934), Bloom (1937), Weber (1954), Geyer (1958), Strasburger et al (1965), Harle and Stevenson (1967), and Wildervanck et al (1967). Rochlin and Simonson (1932), Bloom (1937), Austin (1951), Weber (1954), and Geyer (1958) have noted the concurrence of symphalangism and anterior dislocation of the radial head. In the case reported by Mouchet and Saint Pièrre (1931), symphalangism

(*Text continued on page 325.*)

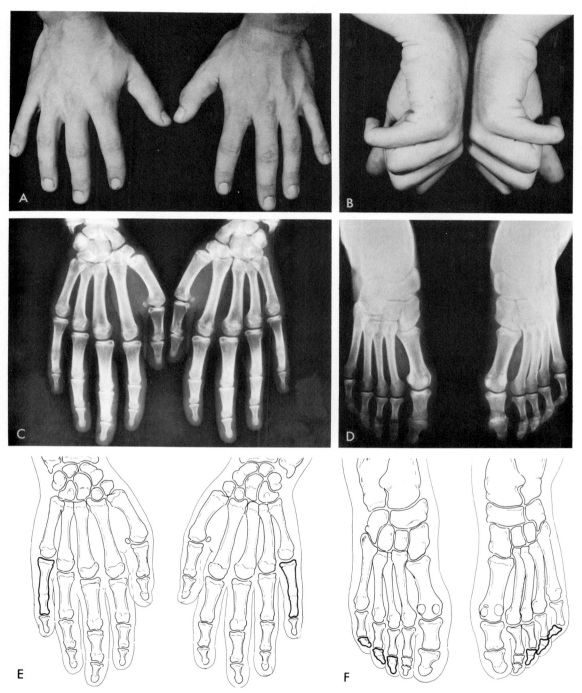

Figure 11–9 Junior C. L.—senior C. L.'s oldest son. *A*, Dorsal view of the hands, showing absence of creases in the back of the first interphalangeal joints of the little fingers. *B*, Ulnar view, showing absence of flexion at the proximal interphalangeal joints of the little fingers. *C*, Dorsopalmar roentgenograph of the hands, showing bony union of the proximal and middle phalanges of the little fingers. *D*, Dorsoplantar roentgenograph of the feet: here there is union between the middle and distal phalanges of three fibular digits of each foot. *E* and *F*, Sketches illustrating roentgenographs above each.

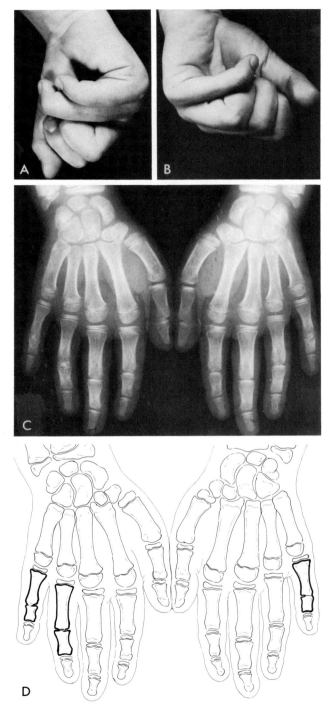

Figure 11–10   J. L. – senior C. L.'s younger son. *A*, Ulnar view of J. L.'s right fist: ring and little fingers barely flex at their first interphalangeal articulations. *B*, Ulnar view of the left fist: here only the little finger fails to flex. *C*, Dorsopalmar roentgenograph of both hands, showing narrowing of joint spaces between the proximal phalanges and the squat middle phalanges of the right ring and little fingers and left little finger. *D*, Sketch illustrating the same.

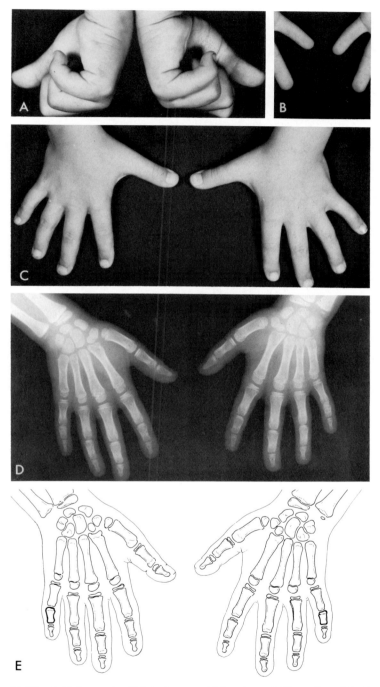

Figure 11–11 A. T. L. — senior C. L.'s six-year-old daughter. *A*, Ulnar view of the fists, showing only minimal flexion at the first interphalangeal joint of the right little finger and none at the corresponding articulation on the left side. *B*, Palmar view of the little fingers, showing absence of flexion crease in front of the first interphalangeal joints. *C*, Dorsal view of the hands, showing absence of wrinkles in the back of the first interphalangeal joints of both little fingers. *D*, Dorsopalmar roentgenograph of both hands, showing almost complete effacement of joint space at the first interphalangeal articulation of both little fingers, more on the left side, and also brachymesophalangy of each little finger. *E*, Sketch illustrating the same.

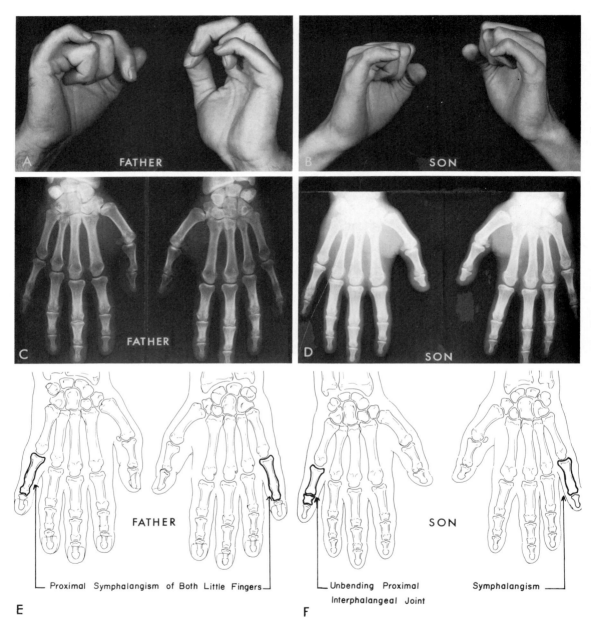

Figure 11–12 In this figure are featured the hands of E. L. and his son, A. L. The father is the paternal uncle of Mrs. J. F. and of senior C. L. *A,* Ulnar view of E. L.'s fists. *B,* Ulnar view of A. L.'s fists. *C,* Dorsopalmar roentgenograph of the father's hands. *D,* Dorsopalmar roentgenograph of the son's hands. Sketches *E* and *F* illustrate roentgenographs *C* and *D,* respectively. Note that the father has complete bilateral proximal symphalangism of both little fingers: there is a joint space between the proximal phalanx and dwarfed middle phalanx of the son's right little finger, but his left little finger shows solid bony union of these two phalanges. E. L. also had six other children. A deceased boy was a "mongolian" who had symphalangism of the little finger. One daughter was operated on for congenital anomaly of the spine (partial sacralization of the fifth lumbar vertebra).

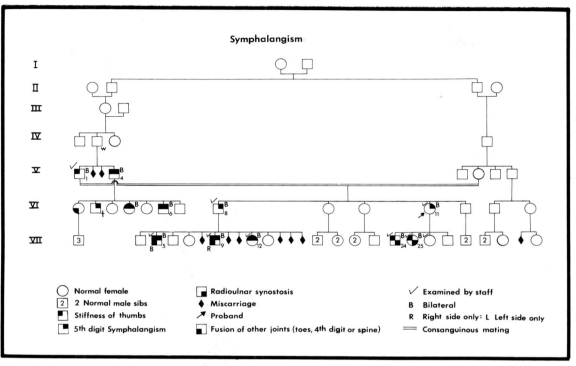

Figure 11-13 Pedigree of symphalangism.

was associated with fusion of the humerus and ulna. Wiles (1939) reported a case of multiple epiphyseal dysplasia with limited movement of the fingers.

A defective pectoral muscle is often reported as an accompaniment of symphalangism. Earlier authors—Walker (1901), Miller (1922), and Daniel (1936)—confused symphalangism with symbrachydactyly or short, webbed fingers; they included in their collective review of symphalangism cases complying with Poland's (1841) syndrome—syndactyly of the dwarfed digits associated with ipsilateral absence of the sternal head of the pectoralis major. In symbrachydactyly, the number of phalanges is reduced—usually the middle phalanges of webbed fingers are absent. In some cases of symbrachydactyly, the proximal phalanges are longer than normal, a condition which is presumed to have been produced by fusion of two phalanges. In about half of the reported cases, symbrachydactyly is associated with a defective pectoral muscle. Symbrachydactyly usually involves one hand and is reported only in sporadic cases. Symphalangism is usually bilateral and hereditary. Absence of the pectoral muscle is not a feature of hereditary symphalangism.

REMOTE ASSOCIATIONS

Symphalangism of the fingers is often accompanied by comparable changes in the four fibular toes; in the foot, the distal interphalangeal joints are more commonly involved. Kirmisson (1898) reported a case with symphalangism of the hand and bilateral varus deformity of the feet—*double pied bot varus*. In this case, varus deformity of the foot was due to tarsal coalescence, which is not an uncommon accompaniment of symphalangism. Pagenstecher (1901) described a patient with symphalangism and kyphosis of the spine. Bloom (1937) noted the association of symphalangism with flattening or wedging of the dorsal vertebrae. Dubois (1970) reported a female child with Nievergelt syndrome and symphalangism of the index, middle, and ring fingers. Although extremely rare by itself, symphalangism of the thumb is not an uncommon accompaniment of acrocephalosyndactyly, to be taken up in Chapter Twelve.

CONDUCTIVE DEAFNESS AND SYMPHALANGISM

Nessel (1960) reported the concurrence of symphalangism, strabismus, and hearing loss in a mother and daughter. Strasburger et al (1965) wrote: "Conductive deafness due to bony fusion of the stapes to the round window occurs sufficiently in patients with symphalangism and is otherwise sufficiently rare that one is forced to conclude that it is an effect of the same gene." In the literature, the constellation of congenital synostosis and conductive deafness is often referred to as Vessel-Forney syndrome. The patients—a mother and her two daughters—reported by Forney et al (1966)—had mitral insufficiency, short stature, fusion of the fifth and sixth cervical vertebrae, carpal coalescence, and conductive deafness.

DIASTROPHIC DWARFISM

McKusick and Milch (1964) and later McKusick (1966) alone reported a brother and sister with diastrophic dwarfism and symphalangism of the index, long, and ring fingers.

TREATMENT

At one period in the development of symphalangism, the epiphysis of the distal bone begins to contact the distal end of the proximal bone. The author has thought of preventing the union of the epiphysis of the distal bone with the shaft of the proximal bone by inserting a piece of silacsin between them. This operation is on trial.

SUMMARY

Symphalangism is preeminently a genetic disorder and is transmitted as an autosomal dominant phenotype. It is usually bilateral. Since an intermediary element—a joint—is missing, symphalangism is to be regarded as an intercalary defect. Two main varieties of symphalangism are distinguished: proximal and distal. The former is more common in the hand, and the incidence of involvement decreased progressively from the little to the index finger. The thumb appears to be relatively immune, and this immunity is attributed to the absence of a middle phalanx which, in the other digits, is regarded as most susceptible to teratogenic influence. Although rare as an isolated entity, symphalangism of the thumb often occurs in connection with acrocephalosyndactyly. Symphalangism is at times seen in connection with conductive deafness and diastrophic dwarfism. Classic symphalangism appears to be related to the other synostotic anomalies. It is possible that symphalangism, carpal and tarsal coalescence, radioulnar synostosis, humero-ulnar ankylosis, confluent vertebrae, and fusion of the stapes to the petrous bone are genetically related.

References

Aderholdt: Ein seltner Fall con angeborener Ankylose der Fingergelenke. *Münch. Med. Wochenschr.*, 53:125–126, 1906.

Ashner, B., and Engelmann, G.: *Konstitutionspathologie in der Orthopädie*. Wien, Berlin, J. Springer, pp. 64–84, 1928.

Austin, F. H.: Symphalangism and related fusions of the tarsal bones. *Radiology, 26*:883–885, 1951.

Bauer, B.: Eine bisher nicht beobactete kongenitale hereditäre Anomalie des Fingerskelettes. *Dtsch. Z. Chir., 86*:252–259, 1907.

Bauer, K. G., and Bode, W.: Aplasie von Interphalangealgelenken. *In* Abel, W., et al., (eds.): *Erbbiologne und Esbpathologie Kosposlicher Zustände und Funktionen*. Berlin, J. Springer, pp. 188–190. 1940.

Baumann: Verwachsung der Endphalangen mit den Mittelphalangen. Domonstration im arzlichen Verein Essen Ruhr. *Berl. Klin. Wochenschr., 1*:457, 1911.

Behr, K.: Ueber eine symmetrische Synostose der Hand- und Fusswurzelknochen. *Arch. Orthop. Unfallchir., 32*:12, 1932.

Bloom, A. R.: Hereditary multiple ankylosing arthropathy (congenital stiffness of the finger joints). *Radiology, 29*:166–171, 1937.

Bonney, T. C.: Congenital (hereditary) absence of middle joint of little finger. *Am. J. Roentgenol., 7*:336, 1920.

Brdiczka, V.: Vertebrare und angeborene multiple synostosen an zahlreichen Gelenken der oberen und unteren Extremität. *Fortschr. Röntgenstr., 58*:228–233, 1938.

Brucke: Ueber familiare Kongenitale Ankylosierung der Interphalangealgelenke Arztl Ver Hamburg. *Berl. Klin. Wochenschr., 1*:422, 1923.

Brugger, J.: Ueber angeborene Ankylosen der Fingergelenke. *Münch. Med. Wochenschr., 70*:874–875, 1923.

Cole, A. E.: Inheritance of a fused joint in the index finger. Ankylosis of the distal interphalangeal joint of the index finger. *J. Hered., 26*:225–228, 1935.

Comings, D. E.: Symphalangism and fourth digit hypophalangism. *Arch. Intern. Med., 115*:580–583, 1965.

Cunningham, A. V.: Congenital absence of phalangeal joints, with good use of fingers. *Va. Med. Mon., 6*:388, 1879.

Cushing, H.: Hereditary ankylosis of the proximal phalangeal joints (symphalangism). *Proc. Natl. Acad. Sci., 1*:621–622, 1915. Also in *J. Nerv. Ment. Dis., 43*:445, 1916; and in *Genetics, 1*:90–106, 1916.

Daniel, G. H.: A case of hereditary anarthrosis of the index finger, with associated abnormalities in the proportions of fingers. *Ann. Eugen., 7*:281–297, 1936.

Delamare, G., and Djemil, S.: Brachydactylie congenitale des index, atrophie et soudire phalanginophalangetiennes. *Bull. Mem. Soc. Anat.*, Paris, (6 s.), *20*:500–501, 1923.

Drey, J.: Hereditare Brachydaktylie, kombiniert mit Ankylose einzelner Fingergelenke. *Z. Kinderheilkd., 4*:553–556, 1912.

Drinkwater, H.: Phalangeal anarthrosis (synostosis, ankylosis) transmitted through fourteen generations. *Proc. R. Soc. Med.* (London), (Section on Pathology) *10*:60–68, 1917.

Dubois, H. J.: Nievergelt-Pearlman syndrome. Synostosis in feet and hands with dysplasia of elbows. *J. Bone Joint Surg., 52B*:325–329, 1970.

Duken, J.: Familiäre, kongenitale Aplasie der Interphalangealgelenke an Handen und Fussen mit histologischen Befunden. *Verh. Dtsch. Ges. Pathol. 18*:312–318, 1921.

Duken, J.: Ueber die Beziehungen Zwischen Assimilations-hypophalangie und Aplasie der Interphalangealgelenke. *Arch. Pathol. Anat. Phys., 233*:204–225, 1921.

Duncan, F. N.: Orthodactyly. *J. Hered., 8*:174–175, 1917.

Elkin, D. C.: Hereditary ankylosis in the proximal phalangeal joints. *J.A.M.A., 84*:509, 1925.

Elkington, S. G., and Huntsman, R. G.: The Talbot fingers: a study in symphalangism. *Br. Med. J., 1*:407–411, 1967.

Engel, H.: *Über kongenital Ankylosen an den Gelenken der Hände und Fusse*. Thesis. Berlin, Buckendruckerei v. G. Schade (Otto Francke), pp. 5–25, 1902.

Fiume, M.: Aplasia ed ipoplasia congenita ereditaria delle art culazioni interfalangee della mano. *Arch. Ortop., 66*:265–281, 1953.

Forney, W. R., Robinson, S. J., and Pascoe, D. J.: Congenital heart disease, deafness and skeletal malformations: a new syndrome. *J. Pediatr., 68*:14–26, 1966.

Freud, P., and Slobody, L. B.: Symphalangism. A familial malformation. *Am. J. Dis. Child., 65*:550–557, 1943.

Fuhrmann, W., Steffens, C., Schwartz, G., and Wagner, A.: Dominant erbliche Brachydaktylie mit Gelenkplasien. *Humangenetik, 1*:337–353, 1964–1965.

Geelhoed, G. W., Neel, J. V., and Davidson, R. T.: Symphalangism and tarsal coalition: a hereditary syndrome, report on two families. *J. Bone Joint Surg., 51B*:278–289, 1969.

Geyer, E.: Beitrag zu den Synostosenbildungen der Hand- und Fusswerzel. *Z. Orthop., 90*:395–408, 1958.

Goerlich, M.: Angeborene Ankylose der Fingergelenke mit Brachydaktylie. *Beitr. Klin. Chir.*, 59:441–446, 1908.

Goldflam, S.: Ein Fall von Kongenitaler, familiarer Ankylose der Fingergelenke. *Münch. Med. Wochenschr.*, 53:2299–2300, 1906.

Gorlin, R. J., Kietzer, G., and Wolfson, J.: Stapes fixation and proximal symphalangism. *Z. Kinderheilkd.*, 108:12–16, 1970.

Grebe, H.: Aplasie der Interphalangealgelenke. *In* Becker, P. E., (ed): *Humangenetik.* Stuttgart, G. Thieme, Vol. 2, pp. 285–294, 1964.

Haines, R. W.: The development of joints. *J. Anat.*, 81:33–35, Pl. 1–4, 1947.

Hall, G. A. M.: Hereditary brachydactylism and interphalangeal ankylosis. *Ann. Eugen.*, 3:365–368, 1928.

Harle, T. S., and Stevenson, J. R.: Hereditary symphalangism associated with carpal and tarsal fusions. *Radiology*, 89:91–94, 1967.

Heath, C.: Malformation of the hand. *Trans. Pathol. Soc. (London)*, 17:440–441, 1866.

Hefner, R. A.: Inherited abnormalities of the fingers. I. Symphalangism. *J. Hered.*, 15:323–329, 1924.

Hilgenreiner, H.: Zwei Fälle von angeborener Fingergelenksankylose, zugleich ein Beitrag zur Kenntnis der seltenen Spaltbildung der Hand. *Z. Orthop. Chir.*, 24:23–51, 1909.

Hilgenreiner, H.: Soltene Spatbildung der Hand und angeborene Fingergelenksankylose. *Prag. Med. Wochenschr.*, 11:162, 1909.

Hoffmeyer, H.: Beitrag zu den angeborenen Ankylosen Fingergelenke. *Münch. Med. Wochenschr.*, 53:1167, 1906.

Inman, O. L.: Four generations of symphalangism. *J. Hered.*, 15:329–334, 1924.

Kewesch, E. L.: Ueber hereditare Versch melzung der Hand- und Fusswurzelknochen. *Fortschr. Röntgenstr.*, 50:550–556, 1934.

Kirmisson, E.: Double pied bot varus par malformation osseuse primitive associe a des ankyloses congénitales des doigts et des orteils chez quatre membres d'une même famille. *Rev. d'Orthop.*, (1 s.), 9:392–398; Pl. 8–9, 1898.

Lamerias, H. I.: Ueber angeborene Ankylose der Fingergelenke. *Münch. Med. Wochenschr.*, 53: 2298–2299, 1906.

Lucke: Angeborene Fingergelenksankylose. *Münch. Med. Wochenschr.*, 53:2572, 1906.

Ludke, H.: Ueber Kongenital bilateral symmetriche Aplasie von Interphalangealgelenken. *Med. Klin.*, 31:208–209, 1935.

Mann, R. C. D'A: Familial abnormalities of the middle phalanges of each hand. *J. Anat.*, 57:267–268, 1923.

Mastern, J.: Erbliche Aplasie der Interphalangealgelenke (erbliche Phalanxsynostosen). *Z. Orthop. Chir.*, 61:421–422, 1934.

Mastern, J.: Erbliche Synostosen der Hand- und Fusswurzelknochen Erbliches os tibeale externum. *Röntgenpraxis.* 6:594–600, 1934.

McKusick, V. A.: *Heritable Disorders of Connective Tissue.* Third edition. St. Louis, C. V. Mosby Co., pp. 460–464; figs. 10–31, 1966. See also: *Mendelian Inheritance in Man.* Third edition. Baltimore, Johns Hopkins Press, Entry 22260; p. 366, 1971.

McKusick, V. A., and Milch, R. A.: The clinical behavior of genetic disease. *Clin. Orthop.*, 33:22–39, 1964.

Mercier, L. A.: Absence Héréditaire d'une phalange aux doigts et aux orteils. *Bull. Soc. Anat. (Paris)*, 13:35–36, 1838.

Miller, E. M.: Congenital ankylosis of joints of hands and feet. *J. Bone Joint Surg.*, 20:560–569, 1922.

Morgenstern, K.: Ueber kongenitale hereditäre Ankylosen der Interphalangealgelenke. *Beitr. Klin. Chir.*, 82:508–530, 1913.

Mouchet, A., and Saint Pièrre, L.: Ankylose congénitale héréditaire et symetrique de deux coudes. *Rev. d'Orthop.*, 18:210–220, 1931.

Moutard-Martin, and Pissavy, H.: Malformations congénitales multiples et héréditaires des doigts et des orteils. Fusion de la première et de la deuxième phalanges. *Bull. Soc. d'Anthrop. (Paris)*, 6:540–553, 1895.

Musser, J. H.: A note on symphalangism. *New Orleans Med. Surg. J.*, 83:325–326, 1930.

Nowak, H.: Die familiare Ankylose de Fingergelenke. *Dtsch. Med. Wochenschr.*, 63:937–938, 1937.

Oeynhausen, R. F.: Angeborene Synostosen (Kongenitale Ankylose, angeborene Gelenkaplasie). *In* Schwalbe, E., and Gruber, G. B., (eds.): *Die Morphologie der Missbildungen des Menschen und der Tiere.* Jena, G. Fischer, 3 T., 19 Lief, 1 Abt., 7 Kap., 2 Halfte, pp. 893–917, 1958.

O'Rahilly, R.: The development of joints. *Ir. J. Med. Sci.*, 382:456–461, 1957.

Pagenstecher, E.: Beitrage zu den Extremitätenmissbildungen. II. Brachydaktylie. *Dtsch. Chir.*, 60:239–249, 1901.

Paulicki: Congenitalen Ankylose beider Daumen. *Dtsch. Milit. -Artzl.*, 11:277–278, 1882.

Pervès, J.: Ankylose congénitale et fusion osseuse des phalanges. Maladie familiale (Etude de deux cas). *Rev. d'Orthop. Chir.*, l'App. Mot., 19:628–632, 1932.

Pol, R.: Aplasie der Finger- und Zehengelenke ("Angeborene steif Finger: "Geradfingergerigkeit"). *In* Schwalbe, E., and Gruber, G. B., (eds): *Die Morphologie der Missbildungen des Menschen und der Tiere.* Jena, G. Fischer, 3T., Abt. 1, Lief 17, Kap. 7, Halfte 1, pp. 655–682, 1937.

Poland, A.: Deficiency of the pectoral muscles. *Guy's Hosp. Rep.*, *6*:191–193, 1841.

Prieser: Ankylo e beider Daumen-Interphalangealgelenke. *Münch. Med. Wochenschr.*, *57*:1035, 1910.

Révész, V.: Beiträge zue Kenntnis der Entwicklungsanomalien der Hand. *Fortschr. Röntgenstr.*, *24*:143–144, 1916.

Rimbaud, L., and D'Allonnes, G. R.: Ankylose osseuse des articulations phalangino-phalanget. Tiennes de deux mains, trouble d'acroteophicité chez un adénomoidien. *N. Iconog. Salp.*,*28*:162–163, 1916.

Roasenda, F.: Sinostose interphalangea congenita: un case a carattere ereditario. *Atti S.I.O.T.*, *38*:363, 1953.

Rochlin, D. G.: Ueber die hereditäre symmetrische Gelenkhypoplasie. *Z. Konst. Lehre*, *13*:654–663, 1928.

Rochlin, D. G., and Simonson, S. G.: Ueber die angeborene Fingergelenkversteifung. *Fortschr. Röntgenstr.*, *46*:193–204, 1932.

Savarinathan, G., and Centerwall, W. R.: Symphalangism. A pedigree from South India. *J. Med. Genet.*, *3*:285–289, 1966.

Schniedewind: Anguilosis congenita de los dedos de la mano, bilaterale y familiare. *Semana Med.*, *31*:988–989, 1924.

Schreiber, A.: Symmetrische Fuss-Handwurzelsynostosen in u Generationen. *Z. Orthop.*, *104*:197–202, 1967.

Schwarz, P., and Rivellini, G.: Symphalangism. *Am. J. Roentgenol.*, *89*:1256–1259, 1963.

Schwarzweller, F.: Die erbliche Aplasie der Interphalangealgelenke und ihre Beziehungen zu den Gliedmassenplasien. *Arch. Orthop. Unfallchir.*, *40*:84–92, 1939.

Slater, P., and Rubinstein, H.: Aplasia of interphalangeal joints associated with synostosis of carpal and tarsal bones. *Quart. Bull. Sea View Hosp.*, *7*:429–443, 1942.

Stadaas, J.: Medfodt stivfinger (Congenital stiff fingers). *Tidsskr. Nor. Laegeforen.*, *85*:535–537, 1965.

Stecher, L.: Ueber Aplasie einzelner Interphalangealgelenke. *Arch. Klin. Chir.*, *134*:818–825, 1925.

Steinberg, A. G., and Reynolds, E. L.: Further data on symphalangism. *J. Hered.*, *39*:23–27, 1948.

Stiles, K. A., and Weber, R. A.: A pedigree of symphalangism. *J. Hered.*, *29*:199–202, 1938.

Strasburger, A. K., Hawkins, M. R., Eldridge, R., Hargrave, R. L., and McKusick, V. A.: Symphalangism: genetic and clinical aspects. *Bull. Johns Hopkins Hosp.*, *117*:108–127, 1965.

Sugiura, Y., and Inagaki, Y.: Symphalangism associated with carpal and tarsal fusions. *Jap. J. Hum. Genet.*, *5*:117–123, 1960.

Vessel, E. S.: Symphalangism, strabismus and hearing loss in mother and daughter. *N. Engl. J. Med.*, *263*:839–842, 1960.

Walker, G.: Remarkable cases of hereditary ankyloses, or absence of various phalangeal joints, with defects of the little and ring fingers. *Bull. Johns Hopkins Hosp.*, *12*:129–133, Pl. 27–28, 1901.

Weber, V.: Multiple symmetrische Synostosen an Hand und Fuss. *Arch. Orthop. Unfallchir.*, *46*:277–289, 1954.

Wildervanck, L. S., Goedhard, G., and Meijer, S.: Proximal symphalangism of fingers associated with fusion of os naviculare and talus and occurrence of two accessory bones in the feet. (Os paranaviculare and os tibiale externum) in an European-Indonesian-Chinese family. *Acta Genet. Statist.* (Basel), *17*:166–177, 1967.

Wiles, P.: Multiple epiphyseal dysplasia. *Proc. R. Soc. Med. (London)* (Section of orthopedica), *32*:279–281; fig. 3, 1939.

Wilgress, J. H. F.: A note on hereditary stiffness of the metacarpo-phalangeal joint of the thumb. *J. Anat. Physiol.* (London), *32*:753, 1898.

Wilmoth, C. L.: Hereditary joint abnormalities. *South Med. J.*, *23*:1001–1002, 1930.

Wolf: Zwei Fälle von angeboroun Missbildungen: Mangel beider Kniescheiben Fingerdeformität. *Münch. Med. Wochenschr.*, *47*:766–767, 1900.

Wray, J. B., and Herndon, C. N.: Hereditary transmission of congenital coalition of calcaneus and navicular (symphalangism associated with tarsal synostosis). *J. Bone Joint Surg.*, *45A*:370–372, 1963.

Chapter Twelve

SYNDACTYLY

The term syndactyly has gathered a great deal of moss since it first appeared in the literature about 150 years ago. Cruveilhier (1835) considered syndactyly as a form of congenital adhesion. The section on syndactyly in Velpeau's (1847) book bore the title "Adhesion of the fingers on their sides." In an extensive essay on this subject, Verneuil (1856) spoke of "the lateral adherence of fingers." Implicit in these allusions is the idea that digits which had been free from each other at an earlier period of prenatal life were somehow bruised and then became stuck together by scar tissue. This interpretation still persists in the continental literature, especially in connection with that type of syndactyly in which the digits are united at their tips but remain separated from each other proximally.

Adams (1836) advanced another concept. He ascribed the union of two digits to the persistence of the interdigital membrane, which presumably existed up to the second or third month of intrauterine life. Roblot (1906) stated that digits achieved their independence by a process of regression of the embryonic interdigital tissue from a distal point toward the palm. Browne (1933, 1939) defined syndactyly as a failure in the process by which the digits are carved out of the solid mass by atrophy of the intervening tissue. It is presumed that as the digits grow forward from the border of the embryonic handplate they drag with them a web of tissue which subsequently undergoes dissolution.

Around the sixth week of intrauterine life, the surface of the handplate is marked by five ridges which are destined to become digits. Four shallow notches appear along the free border of the handplate; these indentations represent the future interdigital commissures. According to Arey (1965), digital buds project forward rapidly away from the slowly growing palm, and their separation is accomplished by centrifugal extension and not by the centripetal atrophy of the intervening tissue.

Neither of the above concepts adequately explains why in syndactyly the intervening tissue tends to be selective in its localization. In both the foot and the hand the web joining two digits shows definite predilection for the first postaxial webspace. The axis of the foot traverses the second toe; that of the hand passes through the third digit. In most cases of syndactyly of the foot, the second and third toes are united; in the hand, the third and fourth digits are webbed. One

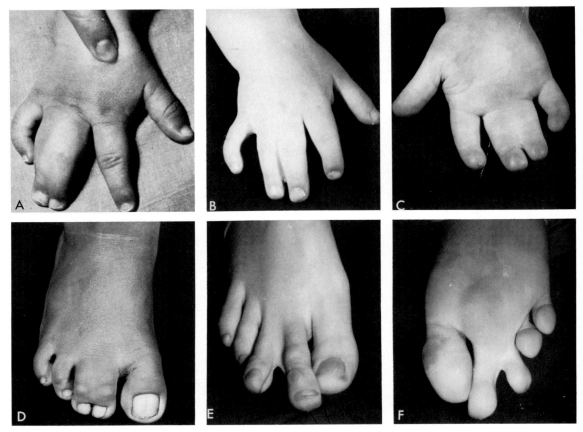

Figure 12–1   The axis of the hand traverses the third digit. The axis of the foot runs through the second toe. In both hand and foot, syndactyly favors the first postaxial space. *A*, Dorsal view of a hand with total syndactyly of the middle and ring fingers. *B*, Dorsal view of a hand with partial syndactyly of the middle and ring fingers. *C*, Palmar view of the same. *D*, Dorsal view of a foot with total syndactyly of the second and third toes. *E*, Dorsal view of a foot with partial syndactyly of the second and third toes. *F*, Plantar view of the same.

cannot explain this selectivity on the basis of lateral compression, bruising, and the subsequent union of the adjacent digits by scar tissue. This possibility is also precluded by the fact that syndactyly is often hereditary and that both hands and feet are affected in many instances (Fig. 12–1).

One must suppose that the gene in charge of syndactylism controls the growth or regression of the web between the middle and ring fingers in the hand and the second and third toes in the foot; this web either fails to undergo regression or grows forward with the advancing digits. To explain the sundry varieties of syndactyly, one must also presume that the provoking gene is capable of diversified phenotypical expressions. It is also conceivable that different genes control various forms of webbed digits.

INHERITANCE

Adams (1836) thought syndactyly was very frequently hereditary. Fort (1869) did not think heredity played as great a role in syndactyly as it did in polydactyly. Mirabel (1873) reviewed about a dozen cases of familial polydactyly and could only cite two instances of hereditary syndactylism. Familial syndactyly of the hand has since been reported by a number of authors. Davis and German (1930) estimated that about 80 per cent of the cases of syndactyly reported in the literature were without hereditary antecedent. Inherited polydactyly appears to be more common.

Straus (1925) is often quoted concerning the mode of transmission of hereditary syndactylism. This trait is said to manifest one of the following genetic behaviors: sex-linked dominant, simple dominant, mutant, and recessive. At the time Straus wrote his article, a characteristic which appeared more often in one sex than in the other was considered sex-linked; reduced penetrance was confused with recessiveness. In the pedigree recorded by Davis and German (1930), syndactyly appeared at least once in each successive generation and no mention was made of consanguineous marriage on the part of the parents. Davis and German thought that syndactyly in this pedigree manifested "a recessive character." It would now be interpreted as a dominant trait with reduced penetrance. In most of the pedigrees recorded, syndactyly is transmitted as an autosomal dominant phenotype with variable expression (Fig. 12–2).

OCCURRENCE

Polaillon (1884) quoted Moreau to the effect that he had not seen a single case of syndactyly among 3000 newborn babies. MacCollum (1940) gave the ratio of occurrence of syndactyly as one in 2000 to one in 2500 births. Cutler (1942) considered fusion of the adjacent fingers as the "most frequent of all congenital deformities of the hand." In the first edition of his book, Bunnell (1944) pronounced syndactyly as "the most common deformity" of the hand. According to Barsky (1958), syndactyly is "the most common congenital deformity" of the hand. Patterson (1964) also regarded webbing of digits as "probably the commonest single abnormality." In the more recent editions of Bunnell's book revised by Boyes (1964, 1970), polydactyly was considered to be "probably the most common of all hand anomalies" and syndactyly "the next most common." Flynn (1966) regarded polydactyly as "the commonest of hand anomalies and webbing of the digits...probably the second most common."

One notes the recurrence of the word "probably" in the above quotations and wonders if it would not have been better to avoid comparisons and simply say that polydactyly and syndactyly are two of the more common hand anomalies which are brought to the surgeon's attention. If a comparison need be made, it would be that polydactyly often occurs along the radial and ulnar margins of the hand, while syndactyly affects mainly the central digits, favoring especially the middle and ring fingers.

Davis and German (1930) attested that 68 per cent of their patients with syndactylism were males. MacCollum (1940) gave the preponderance of males as 66 per cent; Nylen (1957), 84 per cent; Barsky (1958), 56 per cent; Kettelkamp and Flatt (1961), 60 per cent; Emmett (1963), 66 per cent. It would seem that syndactyly is more common in males than in females. Out of 50 cases reported by Davis and German (1930), 46 were in white patients and four in black: syndactylism appears to be 10 times more common in white than in black people. The converse is true of polydactylism.

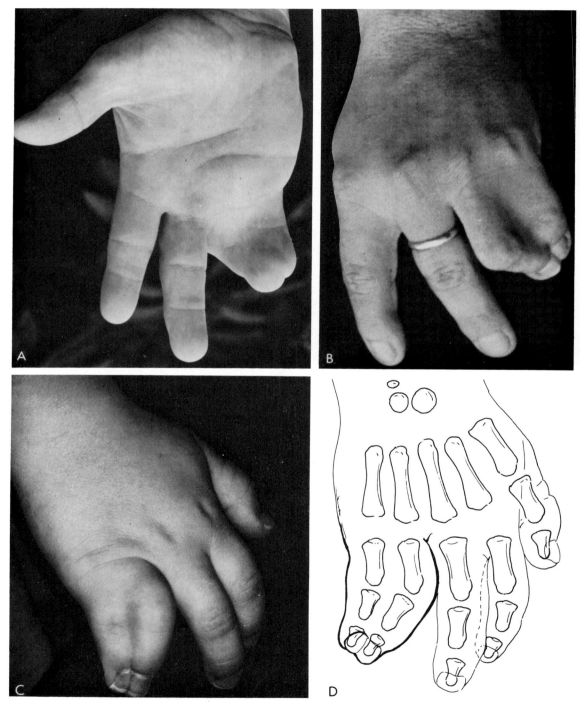

Figure 12–2   Father-to-son transmission of syndactyly of the ring and little fingers. *A*, Palmar view of the father's right hand. *B*, Dorsal view of the father's left hand. *C*, Dorsal view of the son's right hand. *D*, Sketch illustrating the skeletal components of the son's right hand.

ALLOCATION

Fort (1869) collected 27 cases of syndactyly of the hand. There were almost twice as many bilateral involvements as unilateral, and the middle and ring fingers were affected most frequently. In MacCollum's (1940) series, 48 per cent of the patients had syndactyly of both hands; in 35 per cent, the toes were also webbed. "In our own series of cases," Barsky and associates (1964) wrote, "unilateral involvement occurred almost twice as often as bilateral. The middle and ring fingers were most frequently involved."

Almost every author since Fort has considered the space between the middle and ring fingers to be the most common site of webbing. Kettelkamp and Flatt (1961) surveyed 69 patients with syndactylism of the hand; in 50 per cent of this series the middle and ring fingers were involved; in 28 per cent, the ring and the little fingers; in 15 per cent, the middle and index fingers; and in 7 per cent, the index finger and the thumb. The earlier separation of the thumb from the embryonic handplate may account for its infrequent involvement in syndactyly.

VARIETIES

Cases of syndactyly have been classified according to the external appearance of the webbed digits or deeper changes. They are categorized as being genetic and nongenetic in origin; they have also been graded and assorted into numbered types. Somehow these numbered grades and types fail to elicit clear pictures. Classifications are useless unless they evoke distinctive images in the surgeon's mind. The surgeon needs to visualize definite patterns and plan accordingly. The following types of syndactyly pose their own peculiar problems and necessitate diversified surgical attack: (1) soft tissue syndactyly of two digits which are almost equal in length; (2) syndactyly of two digits of unequal length; (3) syndactyly of three or more digits; (4) syndactyly of dwarfed digits; (5) acrosyndactyly; (6) syndactyly associated with diminished number of digits (oligo- or ectrosyndactyly); (7) syndactyly associated with increased number of digits; and (8) syndactyly complicated by bony union, of which two subgroups are known: (a) simple variety in which the conjoined bones, usually the terminal phalanges, have retained their regular contour and alignment, and (b) osseous syndactyly with irregularly shaped and misaligned bones. Osseous syndactyly may occur in the pentadactylous hand as well as in hands with too many or too few digits (Figs. 12–3 to 12–5).

REGIONAL ASSOCIATIONS

Syndactyly occurs in association with the following local or regional abnormalities: polydactyly; mirror hand or ulnar dimelia; brachydactyly; side-to-side fusion of phalanges, metacarpals, and carpal bones; anomalies of digital posture; annular grooves and terminal transverse defects; simian crease of the palm; split

(*Text continued on page 339.*)

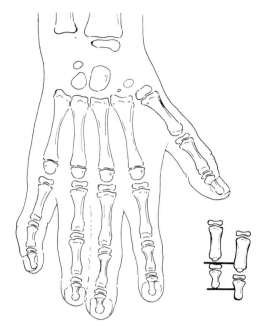

Syndactyly Of Equal Digits: Third With Fourth

A

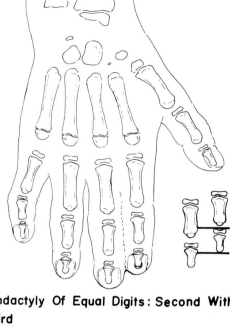

Syndactyly Of Equal Digits: Second With Third

B

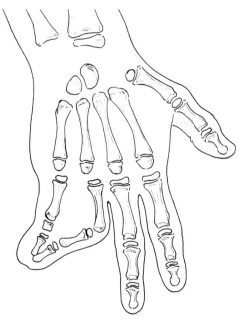

Postaxial Syndactyly Of Unequal Digits

C

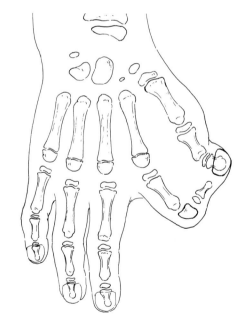

Preaxial Syndactyly Of Unequal Digits

D

Figure 12-3

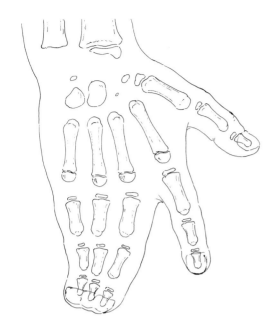

Syndactyly Of More Than Two Digits

A

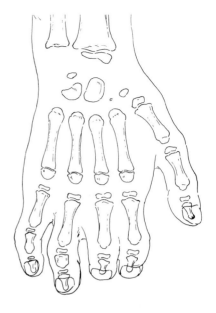
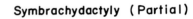

Symbrachydactyly (Partial)

B

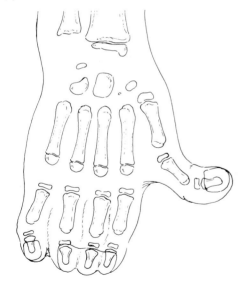

Symbrachydactyly Of Four Digits

C

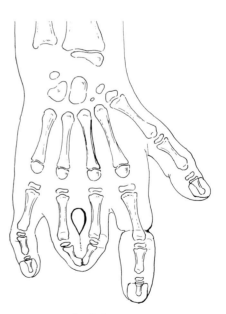

Acrosyndactyly

D

Figure 12–4

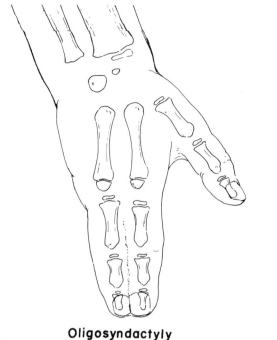

Oligosyndactyly

A

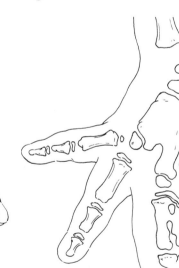
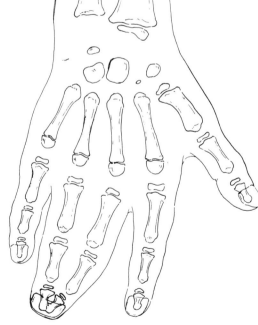

Syndactyly With Bony Fusion : Simple

C

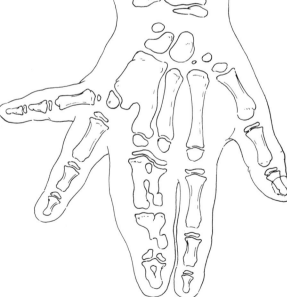

Syndactyly + Polydactyly

B

**Osseous Syndactyly With Irregularly
Shaped Misaligned Bones**

D

Figure 12–5

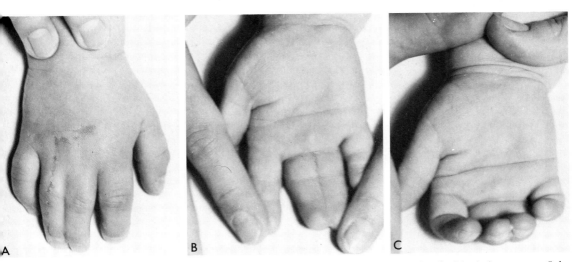

Figure 12–6 Syndactyly of the right middle and ring fingers of an infant, associated with simian crease of the palm. *A*, Dorsal view of the hand. *B*, Palmar view, with fingers forced into extension. *C*, Same, with fingers in semiflexed position.

hand; macrodactyly; radial and ulnar ray defects; phocomelia; dislocation of the radial head; and radioulnar synostosis. Besides the fact that in a number of cases there is also webbing of the toes, syndactyly of the hand can claim many remote and syndromic associations (Figs. 12–6 to 12–12).

ACRO-PECTORO-VERTEBRAL DYSPLASIA

Gross et al (1969) described a family in which eight members in three generations were affected in varying degrees by the following abnormalities: broad, short, malformed thumbs with incipient distal phalangeal duplication; syndactyly of the thumb and index finger with radial deviation of the latter; an extra bone or bony bridge between the webbed mass; carpal coalescence, usually capitate with hamate; comparable changes in the toes; prominent sternum with a pectus excavatum component; and spina bifida occulta of the fifth lumbar or first sacral vertebra. The trait was inherited in an autosomal dominant manner.

CHROMOSOMAL ABERRATIONS

Böök and Santesson (1960) described a male infant who was born of a 30-year-old mother. The father was 29 years old. The parents were unrelated; they had another son without any detectable defect. Along with other abnormalities—hypoplastic jaw, multiple lipomas, and thin legs—the affected child had cutaneous as well as bony syndactyly of the hands and feet. The total number of chromosomes was 69. In another communication, Böök (1961) featured photographs of a two-year-old boy with syndactyly of the middle and ring fingers.

(Text continued on page 345.)

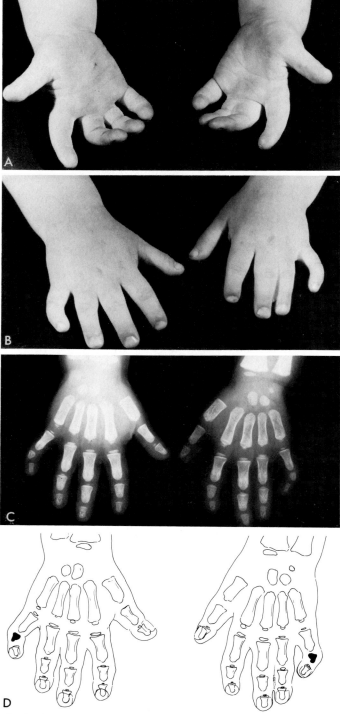

Figure 12–7 Syndactyly associated with brachymesophalangy and clinodactyly of the little finger. *A* and *B*, Palmar and dorsal views of the hands of a two-year-old male with partial syndactyly of the right middle and ring fingers and almost total syndactyly of the same digits of the left hand. *C*, Dorsopalmar roentgenograph of the hands: note that the middle phalanx of each little finger is dwarfed and has a longer ulnar border, causing the ungual segment to tilt in the radial direction *D*, Sketch illustrating the same.

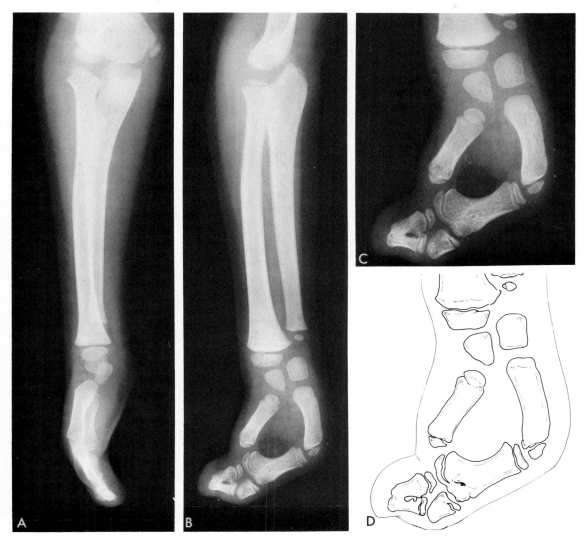

Figure 12–8 Oligosyndactyly associated with short ulna, subluxation of the radial head at the elbow, and anomalous fusion of the hand bones. *A*, Lateral roentgenograph of the left elbow, forearm, and hand. *B*, Dorsovolar roentgenograph of the same. *C*, Roentgenograph of the hand alone. *D*, Sketch illustrating the same.

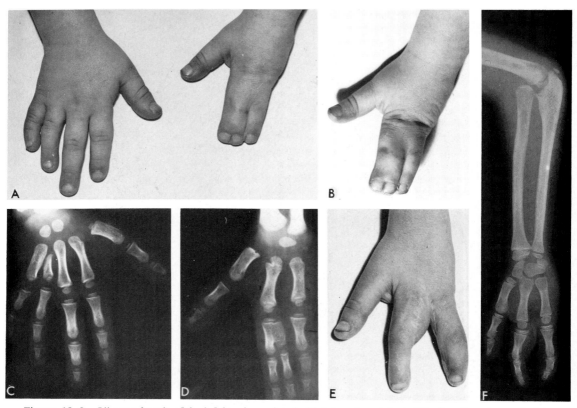

Figure 12–9 Oligosyndactyly of the left hand associated with intercalary defect of the fourth metacarpal of the opposite hand and dislocation of the radial head of the ipsilateral limb. *A,* Dorsal photograph of both hands. *B,* Preoperative photograph of the left hand alone. *C,* Dorsopalmar roentgenograph of the right hand, showing that the fourth metacarpal is defective proximally. *D,* Dorsopalmar roentgenograph of the left hand: here a digital ray, probably the fifth, is missing; what is taken to be the middle finger has three phalanges without a metacarpal to support them, and the basal phalanx of this digit is fused with the corresponding bone on its radial aspect. These were removed and the index and ring fingers were separated from one another as shown in *E* and *F*. Note that in *F* the radial head is dislocated.

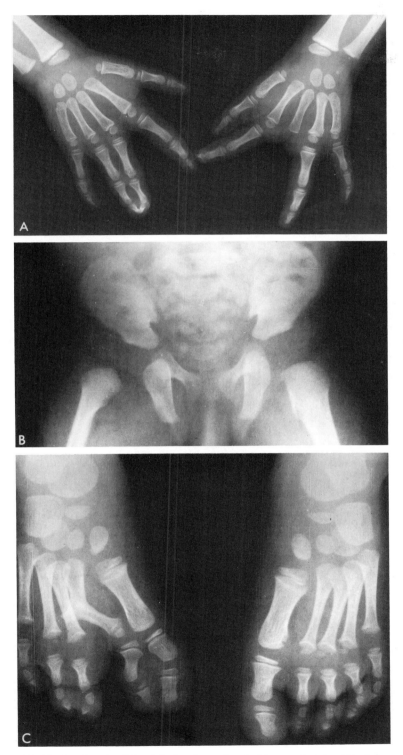

Figure 12–10 Syndactyly of the right hand associated with ectrodactyly of the left manus, acetabular dysplasia of the right hip, and cloven right foot. *A*, Dorsopalmar roentgenograph of the hands. *B*, Anteroposterior roentgenograph of the pelvis. *C*, Dorsoplantar roentgenograph of the feet of the same patient taken at a date later than the preceding roentgenographs.

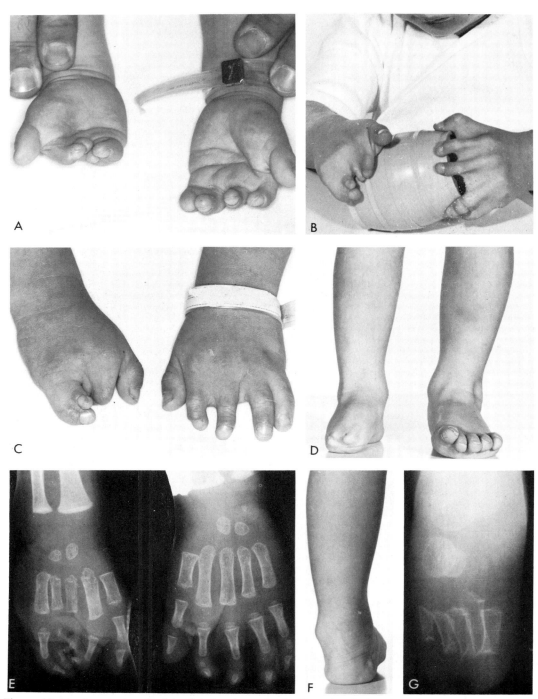

Figure 12–11   Acrosyndactyly of the right hand associated with symbrachydactyly of the left hand, varus deformity of the left heel, and terminal transverse defect of the left toes. *A*, Palmar view of the hands. *B* shows the hands in action, bringing into better view the interdigital webs, especially of the left hand. *C*, Dorsal view of the hands. *D*, Frontal view of the legs and feet. *E*, Dorsopalmar roentgenograph of the hands: the index and little fingers have diminutive middle phalanges and ring fingers have no middle phalanges. *F*, Dorsal view showing varus deformity of the right heel. *G*, Roentgenograph of the right foot, showing absence of phalanges.

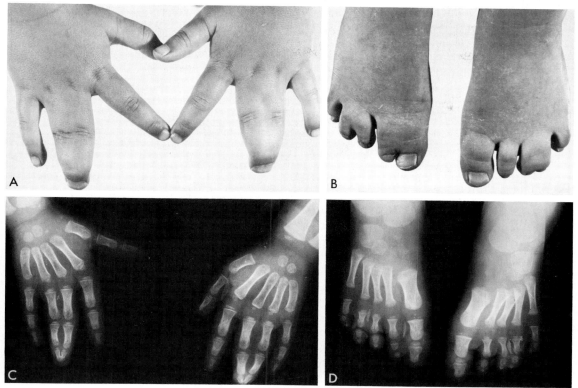

Figure 12–12 Syndactyly of the hands and feet. *A,* Dorsal view of the hands of a three-year-old boy. *B,* Dorsal view of the feet. *C,* Dorsopalmar roentgenograph of the hands. *D,* Dorsoplantar roentgenograph of the feet.

According to Breg (1969), syndactyly is common in *cri-du-chat* syndrome. This syndrome owes its name to the fact that the affected infant emits a catlike wail. It is attributed to the deletion of a portion of the short arm of a B-group chromosome. The subject usually has small hands with dwarfed metacarpal bones and crooked little fingers.

CONGENITAL HEART DISEASE AND SYNDACTYLY

Oppenheimer et al (1949) noted the association of interatrial septal defect and syndactyly. Calo (1953) described a number of patients who suffered from cyanosis due to ventricular septal defect, and who had syndactyly of the hands.

CRANIOSYNOSTOSIS

A number of designations are used in describing deformities of the skull. Acrocephaly signifies elevation of the calvarium to a summit; this term is often used interchangeably with dolichocephaly, turricephaly, oxycephaly, and hypsicephaly, which respectively mean long, tower-shaped, sharp, and peaked head. Sphenocephaly means wedge-shaped, and trigencephaly denotes a triangular head. When the head is compressed from side to side and bears a resemblance to a boat, the term scaphocephaly is used. Brachycephaly, meaning short skull, is often employed in this connection to describe the diminished anteroposterior diameter of the head. Brachybasocephaly relates to the contracted base of the skull. When the head is lopsided with two unequal lateral halves, the designation plagiocephaly is used.

The primary disturbance causing these various configurations is thought to be defective development of the basal portion of the skull while it is being formed by endochondral ossification; premature closure of sutures of the basal portion of the skull results in stenosis of the floor of the cranial cavity. The membranous vault is pushed up by the pressure of the fast-growing brain. The contraction of the base of the skull and disproportionate expansion of the membranous calvarium are progressive and dynamic. The following are consequential: increased intracranial pressure, atrophy of the optic nerve, protruding eyes, nystagmus, diminished hearing, and dulled sense of smell.

Two classes of craniosynostosis are recognized: isolated and syndromic. Syndactyly is the most common hand anomaly which occurs in association with syndromic craniosynostosis. According to Degenhardt (1950), the arrest in development of both the skull and the digit occurs between the twenty-ninth and thirty-fifth day of embryonic life. The extent of syndactyly is taken to be an index of the early or late origin of the symptom complex. When the syndactyly is complete, the teratogenic phase occurs around the sixth week; when there is only partial webbing of the fingers, the syndrome is said to start during the eighth or the beginning of the ninth week.

Troquart (1886) described a newborn infant with a voluminous head, prominent frontal bosses, and syndactyly of the digits. Combination of acrocephaly and syndactyly was described again by Beno (1886), Magnan and Galippe (1892), and Camus (1903). Apert (1906) gave a more detailed description and introduced the designation acrocephalosyndactyly.

In Apert's acrocephalosyndactyly, the vertex rises to a peak; the occiput is flat; the fingers and toes are short and webbed, and they are often united by bone. The thumb is usually free, but shows varying degrees of distortion. The proximal phalanx of the thumb is triangular or trapezoidal in shape with a broad ulnar base, which causes the distal segment to tilt in the radial direction; eventually these two phalanges become fused together. The central digits are affected extensively; there may be one or two phalanges, or even a finger, missing. The conjoined digits may have individual nails or share a common nail. The webbed fingers are often stiff and flexed; the palm is cupped, resembling a spoon. Comparable changes also occur in the feet. Patients with Apert's disease eventually suffer from hydrocephalus, optic atrophy, and visual disturbances; they die early. They are repulsive in appearance and are not likely to find marital mates and procreate. Nonetheless, hereditary cases have been reported. Weech (1927) described a Negro mother and her child with Apert's syndrome. The trait is considered to be dominant. Most cases of Apert's acrocephalosyndactyly are sporadic and are ascribed to new mutation. As in achondroplasia, advanced paternal age is considered to be a factor.

Apert's is the most common form of acrocephalosyndactyly and is deservedly given the epithet classic. There are a number of other forms. In Carpenter's (1901, 1909) acrocephalopolysyndactyly, besides distortion of the calvarum and

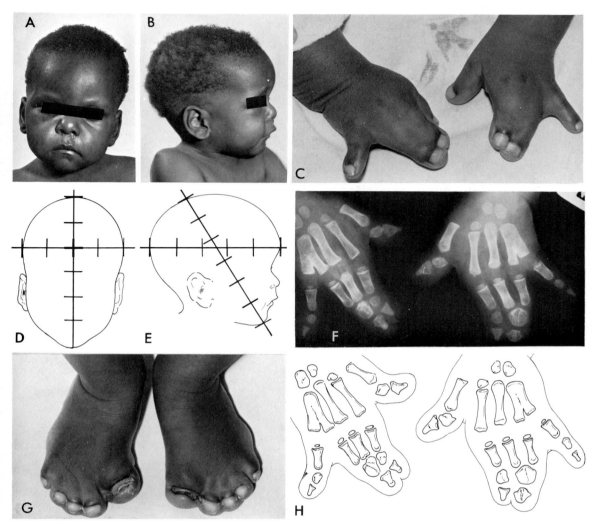

Figure 12–13 Acrocephalosyndactyly. *A* and *B,* Frontal and right profile views of the head. *C,* Dorsal view of the hands. *D* and *E* illustrate dimensions of the calvarium. *F,* Dorsopalmar roentgenograph of the hands. *G,* Dorsal view of the feet. *H,* Sketch illustrating the roentgenograph above it.

syndactyly in the hands and feet, there is duplication of the great toes, and the inheritance is considered to be an autosomal recessive trait. Noack's (1959) acrocephalopolysyndactyly is said to differ from Carpenter's in that it is transmitted as an autosomal dominant phenotype.

Greig (1926) used the designation oxycephaly to denote a peculiar configuration of the skull in the form of an expanded cranial vault leading to a high forehead and bregma. He reported a mother and her daughter, both of whom had syndactyly of both hands. The daughter had bifid thumbs and great toes; her intelligence was normal, even above average. Temtamy and McKusick (1969) described a family in which ten members in four generations and six sibships were similarly affected; these authors considered the trait to be fully penetrant and autosomal dominant.

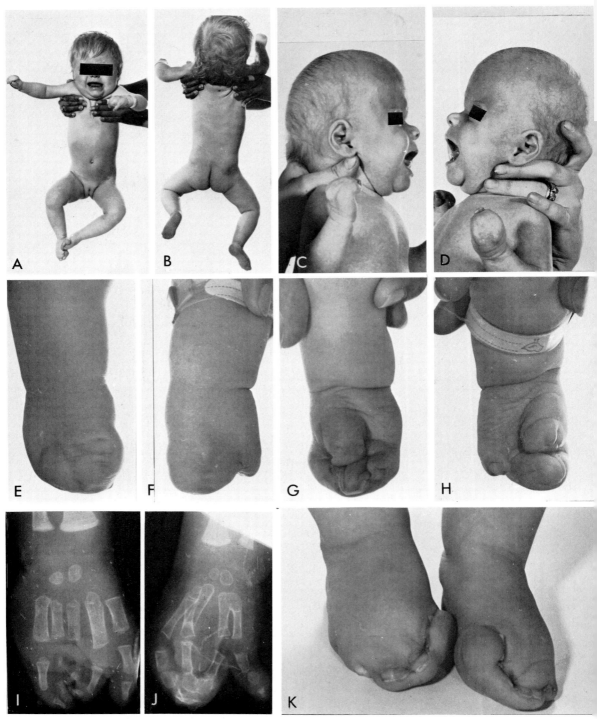

Figure 12–14 Acrocephalosyndactyly. *A* and *B*, Frontal and dorsal views of the child. *C* and *D*, The right and left profiles. *E* and *F* are dorsal and *G* and *H* palmar views of the right and left hands, respectively. *I*, Dorsopalmar roentgenograph of the right hand. *J*, Dorsopalmar roentgenograph of the left hand. *K*, Dorsal view of the feet.

Acrocephalosyndactylies bearing Chotzen's and Vogt's names have one characteristic in common: the facial features of the affected individual are suggestive of Crouzon's craniofacial dysostosis, displaying hypertelorism, exophthalmos, parrot-beaked nose, hypoplastic maxilla, and relative prognathism. In a family described by Chotzen (1932), the father and two sons were affected; they had elongated heads with constricted circumferences—brachycephaly—and were mentally unbalanced; their fingers were webbed. Vogt (1933) described two cases with a less severe degree of webbing of the fingers and toes than that seen in Apert's syndrome; the syndactyly affected only the three central digits, leaving the marginal members free.

In Saethre's acrocephalosyndactyly, the syndactyly is of the soft tissue variety, there being no coalescence of bones, and unlike cases with Apert's syndrome, the affected individual does not have a flat, precipitous occiput. Saethre (1931) described a mother and two daughters, one of whom was illegitimate and affected more severely than her half-sister. The mother's brother and her great-grandmother had similar deformities. In the Waardenburg type of acrocephalosyndactyly, syndactyly is likewise of the soft tissue variety; the affected digits are only partly webbed; in addition to acrocephaly, there are malformations of the orbits. Waardenburg (1934) traced the pedigree of a family in which eight members—and probably five others—were affected, and four out of seven affected individuals had asymmetrical heads or plagiocephaly. In the acrocephalosyndactyly named after Mohr, only two ulnar digits are webbed and the toes are not affected. Mohr (1939) described an affected father, five of whose nine children inherited the trait.

Michail et al (1957) had reported a boy with an elongated cranium, "Cyrano type of nose and insipid smile." The boy also had funnel chest and cryptorchidism, and was mentally retarded. Roentgenographs of his hands showed that each thumb had a wedge-shaped proximal phalanx, with the base of the triangular bone lying on the ulnar side, causing the terminal phalanx to incline radially.

Pfeiffer (1964) described a similar syndrome which now bears his name. He reported a family in which eight members in three generations were affected. The proximal phalanx of the thumb in affected individuals was either triangular or trapezoidal, and in some cases it was fused with the distal segment. The thumb pointed away from the other digits. The big toes were broad and short. Even though none of the digits were webbed, Pfeiffer considered this anomaly to be a variant of acrocephalosyndactyly, and many other authors have categorized it as such. In a later communication, Pfeiffer (1969) stated that the chief deformity of Apert's syndrome was limited to a dysplasia of the proximal phalanx of the thumb which acquired a triangular or trapezoidal shape before being fused with the terminal phalanx.

Six years after the publication of Apert's (1906) article on acrocephalosyndactyly, Crouzon (1912) came out with the description of a syndrome which he called hereditary craniofacial dysostosis. Many authors in the past—more recently Cruveiller (1954)—have identified this complex with Apert syndrome and have even hyphenated Crouzon with Apert. It is perhaps safe to say that in Crouzon's craniofacial dysostosis heredity features prominently, and such insigniae as hypertelorism, exophthalmos, divergent strabismus, parrot-beak nose, and out-jutting chin are accentuated, while appendicular abnormalities, especially of the lower extremities, are comparatively uncommon.

Two out of five patients with craniofacial dysostosis reported by Dodge et al

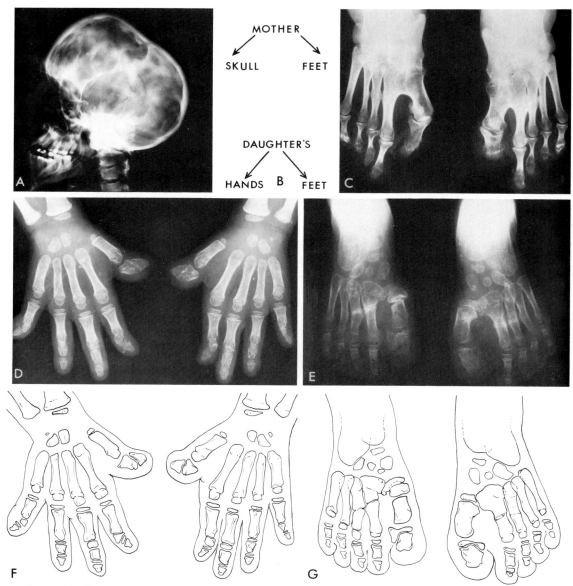

Figure 12–15 Acrocephalosyndactyly Type V or Pfeiffer syndrome: mother-to-daughter transmission. *A*, Lateral roentgenograph of the mother's skull. *B*, Explanatory notes. *C*, Dorsoplantar roentgenograph of the feet, showing inter-metacarpal fusions and coalescence of the phalanges of the big toes. *D*, Dorsopalmar roentgenograph of the daughter's hands: note the triangular proximal phalanges of the thumbs and hitch-hiker position of these digits and anomalous middle phalanges of the fingers. *E*, Dorsoplantar roentgenograph of the daughter's feet: note the anomalous transverse lines across three tibial metatarsals and the short stubby big toes. *F* and *G* illustrate sketches above each.

(1959) had syndactyly of the fingers and toes. Shiller (1959) described a family of which 23 members were affected in four generations. Syndactyly was a feature of the family reported by Alfieri et al (1967) in which Crouzon's craniofacial dysostosis was transmitted as an autosomal dominant phenotype.

Herrmann et al (1969) described a boy who had an elongated, bitemporally flattened head, pronounced hypertelorism, and partial cutaneous syndactyly of

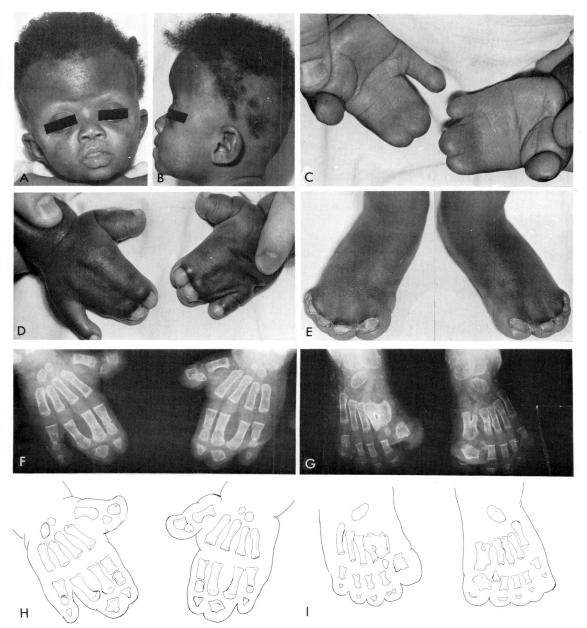

Figure 12–16 Craniosynostosis, possibly Crouzon's type. *A* and *B*, Frontal and left profile views of the head. *C*, Palmar view of the hands. *D*, Dorsal view of the hands. *E*, Dorsal view of the feet. *F*, Dorsopalmar roentgenograph of the hands. *G*, Dorsoplantar roentgenograph of the feet. *H* and *I* illustrate roentgenographs above each.

the short ulnar digits, the shortness being due to hypoplastic or aplastic middle phalanges. He had only one toe—the hallux—on each foot. His mother was 34 and his father 37 years of age at the time of conception. Because of the advanced paternal age, it was thought that the trait probably represented a dominant new mutation (Figs. 12–13 to 12–16).

ECTODERMAL DYSPLASIA

Clouston (1939) distinguished two major forms of hereditary ectodermal dysplasia and named them respectively hidrotic and anhidrotic. The hidrotic variety is characterized by profuse sweating and a non-sex-linked dominant mode of inheritance. The anhidrotic variety is characterized by the following features: diminished sweating, defective teeth, dysplasia of the nails, hypotrichosis, and a recessive mode of inheritance. Rosselli and Gulienetti (1961) reported that four patients with ectodermal dysplasia "displayed serrate syndactyly with fusion of bony elements of the third and fourth fingers, strangulation of the second at the level of the ungual phalanx of the left hand; syndactyly of the same type between the first, second and fourth fingers of the right hand." Another patient had "palmate syndactyly, bilateral and symmetrical between the third, fourth and fifth fingers of the hands." Robinson et al (1962) described a pedigree in which several members suffered from sensorineural deafness and hidrotic ectodermal dysplasia with associated dystrophy of the teeth and nails. In some, the primary and secondary dentitions were delayed, many teeth were missing, and those present were misshapen. The finger and toe nails were small and irregularly shaped. The propositus had syndactyly.

FOCAL DERMAL HYPOPLASIA
(Goltz-Gorlin Syndrome; FDH)

Goltz et al (1962) described a complex consisting of atrophy and linear pigmentation of the integument, herniation of fat through thinned-out areas of the skin, multiple papillomas of the mucous membrane, and cracked lips, hypoplastic teeth, and skeletal abnormalities. Among the latter are included syndactyly of the fingers, polydactyly, axial deviations of the digits, and ectrodactyly.

Gorlin and associates (1963) presented two female patients. The left hand of the first patient exhibited bifid distal phalanx of the thumb and syndactyly of the latter with the index finger; these two digits were distorted and diverged away from the middle finger, which in turn was webbed with the fourth digit. The nails were thin, brittle, and deformed; the right hand manifested divergence of the third and fourth digits. The hands of the second patient were also asymmetrically deformed: there were polydactyly and syndactyly of the right hand; on the left side, the two last ulnar digits and their metacarpals were completely absent; and the index was webbed with the middle finger. Gorlin et al (1963) cited 13 cases from the literature. Syndactyly appears to be the most common anomaly of the hand associated with focal dermal hypoplasia; polydactyly comes next; transverse terminal defects of the digits and clinodactyly seem to occur only occasionally; dystrophy of the nails is seen in almost half of the reported cases. Focal dermal hypoplasia is listed with X-linked phenotypes.

MÖBIUS SYNDROME

This complex described by Möbius (1888) consists of paralysis of ocular and facial muscles in the newborn, presumably due to nuclear aplasia. Henderson

(1939) reviewed 61 cases of Möbius syndrome; some of these had associated abnormalities of the upper extremity, and short webbed fingers were evident among others. In three cases, the homolateral pectoral muscles were defective, suggestive of Poland's syndrome. Hellström's (1949) patient—a child with congenital facial diplegia—had a cousin on the mother's side with syndactyly and a maternal aunt with polydactyly. Richards (1953) described an infant with Möbius syndrome and bilateral symbrachydactyly. Evans (1955) reported a similar case. One of the three patients with congenital facial diplegia reported by Harrison and Parker (1960) had "syndactyly of both hands." Möbius syndrome is transmitted as an autosomal dominant trait. In hereditary cases, the digital abnormality is sometimes suppressed.

OCULODIGITAL COMPLEXES

Syndactyly has been reported in connection with the following abnormalities: congenital cataract—by Ginestous (1922): anophthalmia or microphthalmia—by Ciotola (1938), Berliner (1941), Meyran (1949), and Betetto (1958); aniridia—by Hamilton (1938); retinal degeneration—by Albrectsen and Svendsen (1956); and Holmes-Adie syndrome—by Littlewood and Lewis (1963).

Oculodentodigital dysplasia (ODD), also called oculodento-osseous syndrome, is a definite clinical entity; the affected individual has a thin nose with hypoplastic alae, microphthalmos, hypoplasia of the enamel, and digital abnormalities—mainly syndactyly and camptodactyly of the ring and little fingers. Gillespie (1964) reported two siblings—a boy and a girl—with a history of consanguinity of the maternal grandparents. There was another girl in the family who was normal. The affected children had bilateral microphthalmia and defective teeth, and were born with syndactyly of the fourth and fifth digits of each hand. Gillespie suggested an autosomal recessive transmission of the trait. The case reported by Gorlin (1969) had (a) "typical facies characterized by pinched nose, microcornea," and (b) "typical 4-5 syndactyly with ulnar deviation of the involved fingers. . . ." Taybi et al (1971) described a 23-month-old boy with bilateral syndactyly of the fourth and fifth digits of the hands.

ORODIGITAL COMPLEXES

Sinclaire and McKay (1945) reported a four-week-old female with absent anterior half of the tongue and split posterior portion; all her fingers were short and webbed. Fulford et al (1956) described a five-week-old male infant with aglossia congenita; the vestibular mucosa was directly continuous with the floor of the mouth; the anterior alveolar margin of the mandible was depressed; his left hand presented syndactyly of the index with the middle finger and of the ring with the little finger. All these digits were diminutive. Bünnige (1960) reported a case with ankyloglossia and symbrachydactyly of both hands.

Birch-Jensen (1959) reported two unrelated subjects with cleft lip-palate and symbrachydactyly. The first patient, a boy, had harelip and cleft palate; his right index and middle fingers were rudimentary, and the ring and little fingers were confluent. In the left hand, the central three digits were short and webbed.

The second patient, also a boy, had left harelip and cleft palate. The middle and ring fingers of his left hand were dwarfed and webbed, and his right middle finger presented a hypoplastic ungual phalanx. Fogh-Anderson (1942) described a male infant with median harelip and short, webbed fingers. Fuhrman and Vogel (1960) presented a female infant with median cleft of the upper lip, partial syndactyly of the index with the middle finger and of the ring with the little finger. The mother had syndactyly of the fingers and a split, ankylosed tongue. Several members of her family had syndactyly of the fingers. Klein (1963) described a mother and daughter with cleft palates and fistulas of their lower lips. The mother, also had syndactyly of the middle and ring fingers, unilateral popliteal webbing, talipes equinovarus, and a dysplastic nail on one of her big toes. The son had syndactyly of both middle and ring fingers. Transmission of this trait appears to be autosomal dominant.

On its internal aspect, each lip is connected to the corresponding gum by a median fold of mucous membrane called frenulum. In orofaciodigital (OFD) syndrome, the hypertrophied frenulum extends backward and causes an incomplete cleavage of the jaw; the tongue is lobulated, and the upper lip is split in the middle. The fingers manifest various malformations—trident arrangement, brachydactyly, polydactyly, and axial deviation, but, most commonly, syndactyly. Two types of OFD syndromes are now recognized. In the more common type described by Papillon-Léage and Psaume (1954, 1964), called OFD I, only females are affected and the trait is transmitted as an X-linked phenotype. In the variety described by Mohr (1941), OFD II, the trait is inherited as an autosomal recessive.

Pierre Robin syndrome consists of a triad of defects: micrognathia, cleft palate, and glossoptosis. Smith and Stowe (1961) reviewed 39 cases and listed syndactylism as an associated anomaly.

POLAND'S SYNDROME

After examining a convict who complained that "he could never draw his left arm across his chest," Poland (1841) recorded the following findings: "The whole of the sternal and costal portions of the pectoralis major muscle were deficient but its clavicular origin was quite normal. . . . The pectoralis minor muscle was wholly absent; not a vestige of it is to be seen. The serratus magnus was also, for the most part deficient . . . . In the left hand, the middle phalanges were absent in all the fingers except the middle finger, where a ring of bone, a quarter of an inch in length, supplied its place. The web between the fingers extended to the first phalangeal articulation so that only one phalanx remained free on the distal extremity of each finger. The left thumb was quite normal. The left hand was shorter than the right, by the length of the middle phalanges."

The syndrome, consisting of unilateral deficiency of the pectoral muscles and ipsilateral symbrachydactyly, described by Poland, and named after him, has since been reported by the following authors: Berger (1878), Stinzing (1889), Sklodowski (1890), Benario (1890), Young (1894), Hoffmann (1896), Martirené (1903), Jean and Solcard (1923), Stöhr (1927), Brown and McDowell (1940), Resnick (1942), Sorderberg (1949), De Gennaro (1960), De Benedetti and Chia-

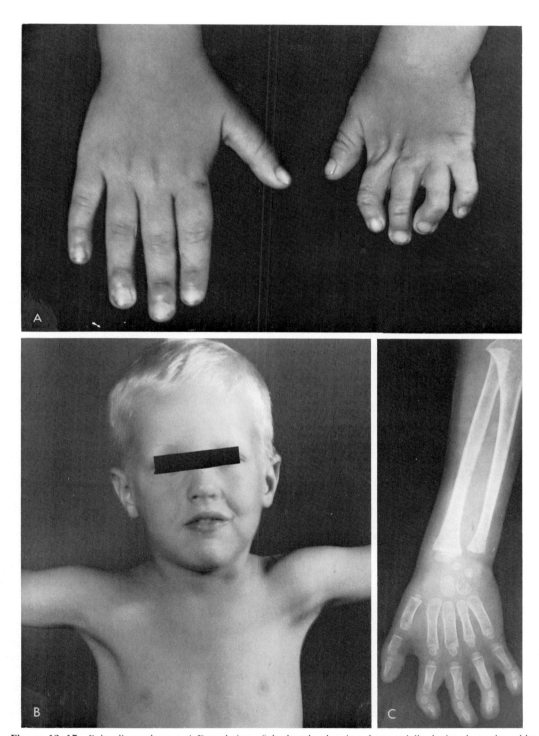

Figure 12–17   Poland's syndrome. *A*, Dorsal view of the hands, showing short, axially deviated, partly webbed left digits. *B* shows absence of the anterior fold of the left axilla, denoting absence of the costo-abdominal portion of the pectoralis major muscle. *C*, Dorsopalmar roentgenograph of the left forearm and hand: note the dwarfed middle phalanges of the fingers.

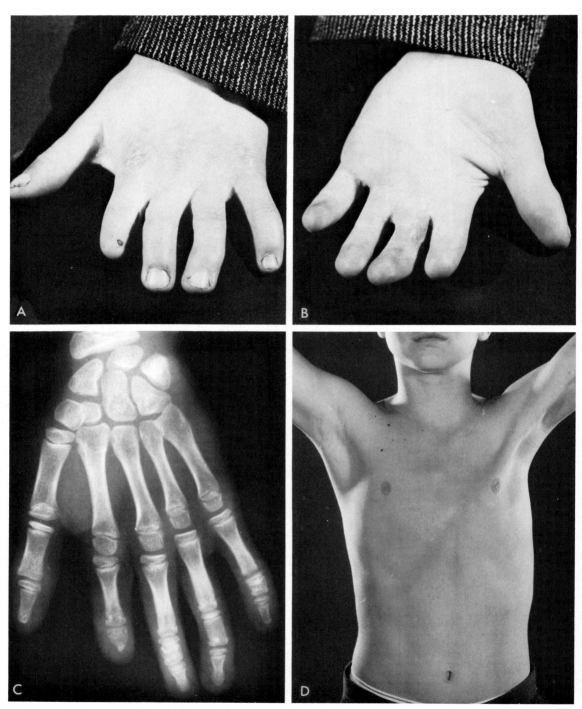

Figure 12–18   Poland's syndrome. *A* and *B*, Dorsal and palmar views of the left hand, showing partial syndactyly of the index and middle fingers. *C,* Dorsopalmar roentgenograph of the left hand: the first metacarpal has two epiphyses; the index finger lacks a middle phalanx, and its ungual bone is spiked; the middle phalanges of the ulnar three digits, especially of the little finger, are dwarfed. *D* shows that the costo-abdominal portion of the pectoralis major muscle has been reduced to a cord.

puzzo (1960), Clarkson (1962), Gellis and Feingold (1965), Baudinne et al (1967), Anger and Strube (1969), Chamberlain (1969), Walker et al (1969), Brooksaler (1971), Pearl et al (1971), and perhaps by some others. When the pectoralis major is defective, the nipple on the same side is atrophic. It should be noted that deficiencies of pectoral muscles are also seen in some other anomalies of the hand in addition to symbrachydactyly (Figs. 12–17 to 12–19).

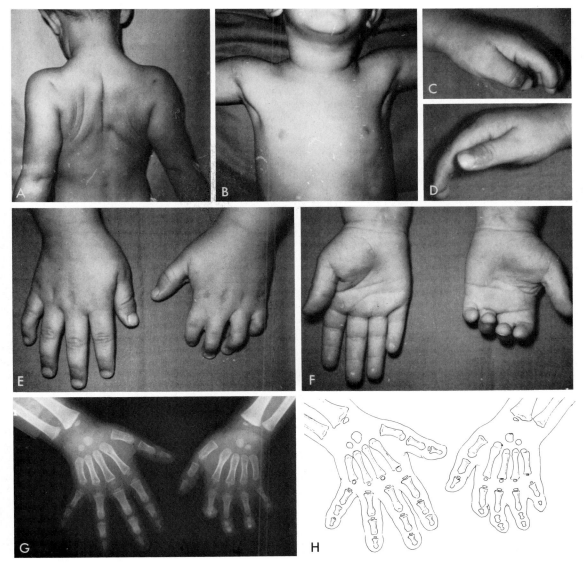

Figure 12–19   Poland's syndrome. *A,* Dorsal view showing a well-defined dimple in the back of each shoulder. *B,* The anterior fold of the left axilla is reduced considerably. *C,* Radial view of the left hand. *D,* Radial view of the right hand. *E,* Dorsal view of the hands. *F,* Palmar view of the same. *G,* Dorsopalmar roentgenograph of the hands. *H,* Sketch illustrating the same.

SCLEROSTENOSIS

Falconer (1937) described a patient with cortical sclerosis of the tubular bones, partial syndactyly of the ulnar digits, and deformed terminal phalanges of both index fingers. Higinbotham and Alexander (1941) reported four siblings with generalized osteopetrosis; all of them had partial syndactyly of the fingers. Truswell (1958) described the two cases. The metacarpals of the first patient "appeared oblong, lacking the normal tublation of the shafts. A similar thickening was present in the phalanges, but the distal phalanges of the index fingers were hypoplastic." Truswell's second patient presented "cutaneous syndactylism between the left ring, middle and index fingers and between the right index and middle fingers. . . . Both index fingers appeared to have only two phalanges, with the distal ones angled outwards. Most of the nails were short."

GENERAL PRINCIPLES OF TREATMENT

There are over three dozen surgical procedures on record for the repair of syndactyly of the fingers. The most durable procedures are based on the combined contributions of a few pioneers: Zeller (1810), who devised the triangular dorsal flap to establish a commissure between the two conjoined digits; Kummer (1891), who employed a distant flap for the repair of a complicated case; Lennander (1891), who utilized free skin graft to cover the raw surfaces resulting from the separation of webbed fingers; and Pieri (1920), who condemned straight incisions and recommended Z-cuts. In the more modern operations for the repair of syndactyly, the free border of the commissural flap is rounded, the tips of the small triangles incident to the zigzag incision are blunted, and streamlined methods of calibrating free skin grafts are used. No new basic principle has been added.

The aim of the surgical treatment of syndactyly is to separate the conjoined digits from each other to see thay they remain separated without deformity. Establishment of an adequate commissure between the bases of the separated digits is paramount. Prevention of binding scars is equally important. "The main object to be aimed at in an operation for such a deformity is avoidance of cicatrical contraction and the least possible interference with the palmar surface of the fingers," Bidwell (1895) wrote. Palmar cuts cause contractures, especially if they are longitudinally disposed and cross the flexion creases.

SOFT TISSUE SYNDACTYLY OF DIGITS OF EQUAL LENGTH

Syndactyly affects adjacent members, and no two neighboring digits are equal in length. The most frequently webbed pair—the middle and ring fingers—are unequal in length, but the difference between them is negligible. The tip of the ring finger reaches a point past the level of the last interphalangeal joint of the middle finger. In syndactyly of this pair, the last interphalangeal joint of the middle finger is adequately splinted by the ungual phalanx of the ring finger, and angular deformity of the distal segment of the longer member is prevented. For practical purposes, side-to-side union of these two digits—or the less common coalescence of the index and middle fingers—may be considered as syndactyly of two digits of equal length. Since there is no imminent danger of deformity, one can wait a year or more before attempting surgical separation of the confluent digits.

The surgical repair of soft tissue syndactyly consists of the following steps: (1) development of the commissural flap; (2) separation of the digits; (3) surfacing of the denuded areas; and (4) postoperative management. The operation is carried out under general anesthesia and with the aid of a tourniquet. During surgery, the tourniquet is released at intervals and hemostasis is secured. At the end of the operation, before the pressure dressing is applied, the tourniquet is released and the return of circulation in the fingers is observed: if a digit remains pale or is bluish, stitches at the base of the ischemic or congested digit are removed.

The commissural flap is raised with the aid of a horeshoe incision on the back of the hand. The incision overlies the distal segments of the metacarpal bones of the conjoined fingers. Its location is somewhat proximal to that described in most books and articles. The reason for this is that as children grow the web between the fingers advances forward. In anticipation of this hazard, it is deemed advisable to start with a deeper commissure. As the flap is elevated from its distal border backward toward its base, it is made thicker. This precaution is taken in order to provide the flap with adequate circulation and also, in reconstructing a new commissure, to simulate the dorsopalmar slope of the normal interdigital web.

The separation of the syndactylized fingers is initiated by two interdigital, longitudinally disposed, undulating incisions—one dorsal and the other volar. On the dorsal aspect there is usually an interdigital groove which is not often present on the palmar side. After the dorsal curvilinear incision has been made, several straight needles are inserted until they emerge on the palmar aspect. The points of the needles on the palmar side serve as guideposts. The palmar incision starts where the dorsal cut ends, between the tips of the conjoined fingers; it is traced toward the palm in a curvilinear fashion. The palmar cut must avoid crossing the flexion creases between the phalanges. In the distal palm, the incision turns toward the ulnar border of the hand for a distance of about half a centimeter. In placing this cut, the surgeon must again bear in mind the dorsopalmar slope of the normal interdigital web. In the palm, the web between the middle and ring fingers—or between the ring and little fingers—inclines from a distal radial point to a proximal ulnar point.

The palmar interdigital incision is deepened. The neurovascular bundle of each finger is identified. The fingers are spread apart. The deep transverse metacarpal ligament lies behind the bifurcation of the common digital artery. This vessel and the accompanying digital nerves are retracted volarward; the transverse metacarpal ligament is severed. This ligament connects with the overlying metacarpal head through the capsular structures of the metacarpophalangeal joints. As the metacarpal bones grow forward, the transverse ligament advances and pushes the overlying integument ahead. This is obviated by cutting the transverse metacarpal ligament between the bases of the conjoined fingers.

The commissural flap is now turned toward the palm and sutured to the palmar incision, using a single No. 34 stainless steel suture. The threads of this stitch are not tied but are twisted together until they bring the skin edges into close contact. The wire suture is supplemented by 5-0 absorbable surgical (polyglycolic acid or Dexon) suture. The denuded sides of the separated digits are surfaced with full-thickness free skin graft. For the small amount of skin needed, it is not necessary to use a dermatone. The needed piece of skin may be expeditiously dissected out with a scalpel. A hairless area is chosen from the medial aspect of the upper arm or the volar surface of the forearm, slightly distal to the cubital crease. (In females, the inner aspect of the thigh is preferred.) An elliptical piece of skin is cut along the longitudinal axis of the arm; the defect thus created is closed by undermining the margins or by performing Z-plasty. The skin removed is turned with its raw surface up; it is spread on a tongue depressor and tied to it under tension. Every bit of fat and areolar tissue is scraped from its seam; it is serrated in several places like a pie crust. Two such grafts are prepared—one for each finger. Each graft is brought to its respective recipient area, raw surface turned down, and sutured to the margins of the wound.

The postoperative care consists of mild pressure dressing and immobilization of the operated fingers in a widely spread-out position. A fine Kirschner wire is inserted intracutaneously on the unoperated side of each finger and pushed proximally though the soft tissues into the palm. The protruding ends of the Kirschner wires are held apart by a connecting spreader bar. The space between the two fingers is packed with fine mesh gauze. The other interdigital spaces are also packed. The hand is enclosed in an elastic bandage, allowing the tips of the fingers to be seen. This dressing is not to be disturbed for three weeks. The wire suture transfixing the commissural flap is then untwisted and removed. The extraction of the percutaneous Kirschner wire causes no pain. MacCollum (1940) advised splinting the hand for six months and carrying out prolonged physical therapy. These are not necessary (Figs. 12–20 to 12–23).

SYNDACTYLY OF TWO DIGITS WITH GREAT DISPARITY IN LENGTH

In syndactyly of the thumb and the index finger, both interphalangeal joints of the longer digit remain unsplinted; the last two segments of the index finger are pulled by the short but stronger thumb and angulate toward the radial border of the hand. In long-standing cases, the middle phalanx of the index finger assumes a triangular shape and may even slip to the ulnar side of the main axis of the digit; therefore such patients should be operated on early in infancy. Three procedures are dovetailed: (1) separation of the coalesced digits; (2) widening of the first webspace with the aid of a pedicled flap or Z-plasty; and (3) correction of the angular deformity of the ulnar digit by subcapital osteotomy of the proximal phalanx.

The little finger barely reaches the level of the last interphalangeal joint of the ring finger. In syndactyly of the fourth and fifth digits, the last interphalangeal joint of the longer finger remains unsplinted and the segment beyond it tends to incline toward the shorter digit. If left alone, permanent disability is inevitable. These patients should also be operated upon early in infancy. When the angulation of the terminal phalanx of the ring finger has already become established and roentgenographic studies reveal slanting of the interdigital articular surfaces, a two-stage operation is required. During the first session, the fingers are separated as outlined for simple syndactyly of the middle and ring fingers. At a later date, the deformity of the ring finger is corrected by subcapital osteotomy of the middle phalanx (Fig. 12–24).

(Text continued on page 366.)

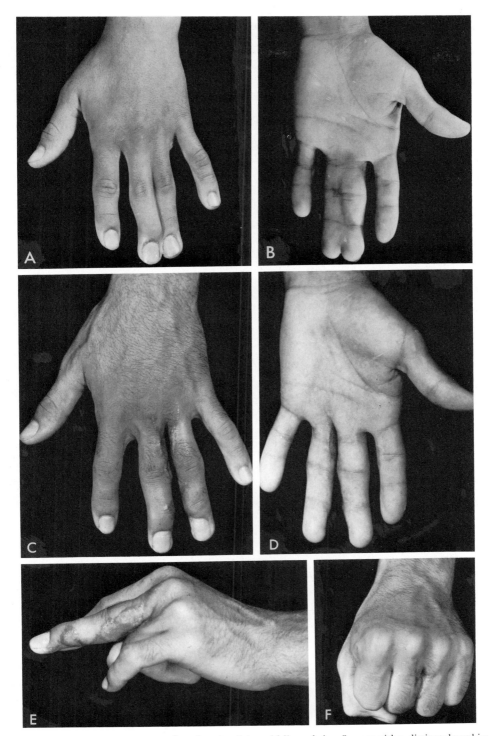

Figure 12–20   Treatment of syndactyly of the middle and ring fingers with a distinct dorsal interdigital groove. *A,* Preoperative dorsal view of the left hand of an 18-year-old male. *B,* Palmar view of the same. *C* and *D,* Dorsal and palmar views of the same hand six months after surgery. *E,* Ulnar aspect of the extended middle finger. *F,* Flexion of the digits after operation.

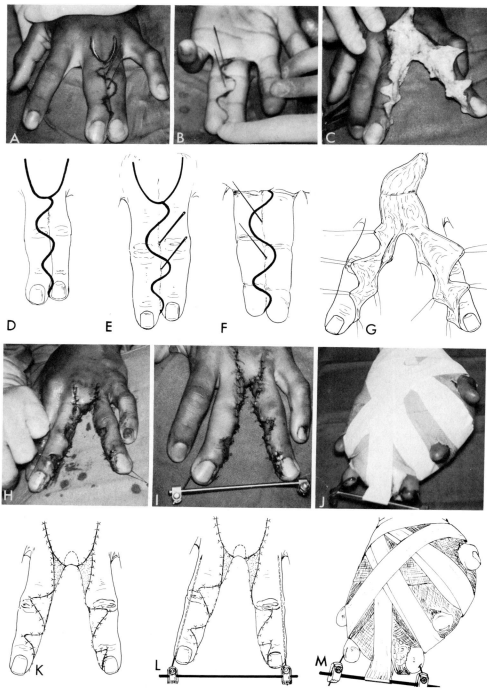

Figure 12–21 Procedures utilized for the preceding case (Fig. 12–20). *A*, Undulating dorsal incision with two straight needles marking the two convex flaps. *B*, Undulating volar incision which stays shy of the flexion creases. *C*, Elevated flaps. *D, E, F,* and *G* illustrate photographs above each. *H,* Closure of the flaps which had been supplemented by small patches of full-thickness free grafts. *I,* Spreader splint anchored to two percutaneously inserted Kirschner wires (K-wires) and holding the separated digits apart. *J,* Postoperative pressure dressing. *K, L,* and *M* illustrate photographs above each.

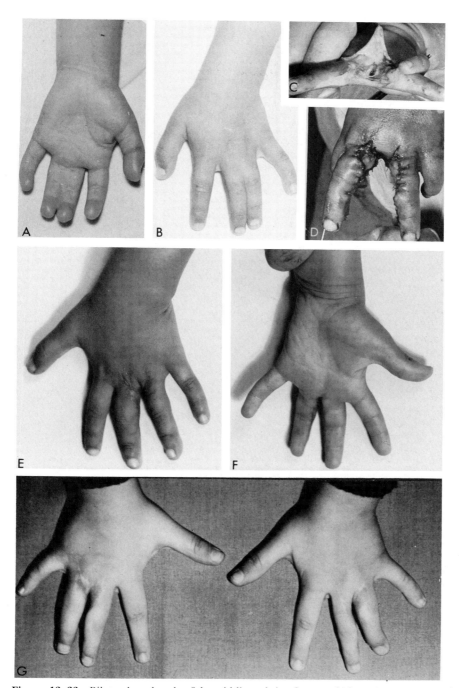

Figure 12–22 Bilateral syndactyly of the middle and ring fingers of a boy who was operated on when he was only 13 months old. *A* and *B*, Preoperative palmar and dorsal views of the left hand. *C* shows the dorsal triangular flap, separation of webbed digits, and exposure of the deep transverse metacarpal ligament, which must be cut to prevent recurrence. *D*, Establishing a wide and deep commissure and surfacing the raw areas on the sides of the separated digits with free full-thickness graft: note also the percutaneous K-wires which had been inserted on the nonoperated sides of the separated digits. The projecting ends of the K-wires were connected to a spreader bar. *E* and *F*, Dorsal and palmar views of the left hand three months after surgery. The right hand was similarly operated on at the same sitting. *G*, Dorsal view of both hands five years after surgery.

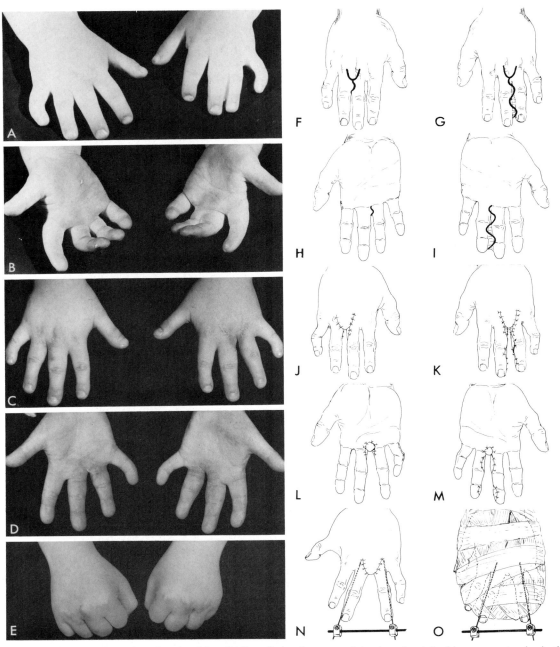

Figure 12–23   Bilateral syndactyly of the middle and ring fingers – minimal on the right side, more extensive in the left hand. *A* and *B*, The hands before surgery. *C, D,* and *E,* Postoperative cosmetic and functional results. *F, H, J,* and *L* illustrate procedure utilized for the right hand. *G, I, K,* and *M* show the method used for the left hand. *N,* Percutaneous K-wires and spreader bar. *O,* Pressure dressing.

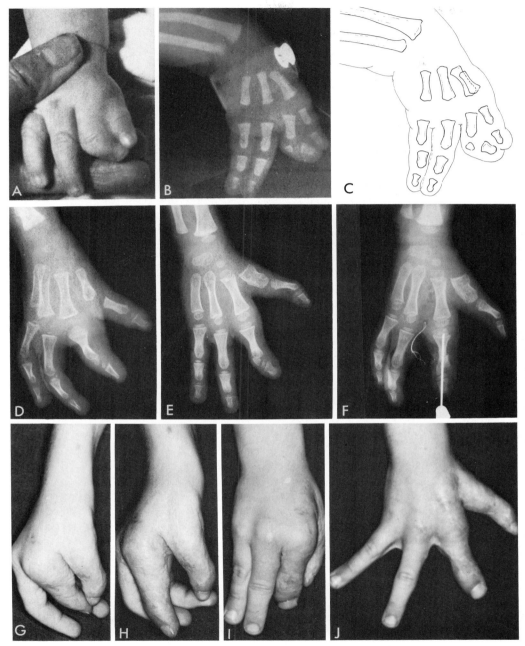

Figure 12–24   Syndactyly of the index and pollex in a three-month-old child with four digits only. *A*, Dorsal view of the right hand. *B*, Dorsopalmar roentgenograph of the hand: note the triangular middle phalanx of the index finger. *C*, Sketch illustrating the same. *D*, Roentgenograph after separation of the webbed digits and deepening of the first webspace with the aid of an abdominal flap. After this operation the thumb did not abduct adequately; the first metacarpal was subjected to abduction osteotomy. *E*, Roentgenograph two years after osteotomy of the first metacarpal. *F* shows that the proximal phalanx of the index finger has been osteotomized to correct the radial inclination of the ungual segment; the fractured fragments are held in corrected position with the aid of an axially inserted K-wire. The index finger appeared short: to procure physiological length for this digit, the second webspace was deepened using a dorsal flap which was sutured to the palmar skin with the aid of a wire suture seen between the index and middle fingers. *G*, *H*, *I*, and *J* show the functional results seven years after the initial surgery.

SYNDACTYLY OF THREE OR MORE DIGITS

Syndactyly may involve three or more digits. When coalescence affects four or five digits, the hand assumes the configuration of a shallow cup or a deep spoon, as in acrocephalosyndactyly. Tridigital syndactyly usually involves the last three ulnar digits, in which case the middle and ring fingers tend to incline in the ulnar direction.

Dessaix (1761) seems to have been the first to operate on an infant with massive or pentadigital syndactyly of the hands. The baby's hands resembled two fleshy masses; each hand bore a single transversely disposed nail. Dessaix carved out four digits from each mass. As attested by Velpeau (1847), when he grew, this patient could write and manage most types of manual feats. Brabazon (1854) described another case of massive coalescence of the digits. The patient was a 12-month-old female child whose left hand resembled "the paddle of a seal, rather than the hand of a human being." Brabazon separated the two marginal digits—the thumb and little finger—and obtained "favorable" functional results.

The author now attempts to separate all webbed digits and carry on the surgical procedure on each pair at different sessions, with an interval of two to three months between each session. Priority is given to the syndactyly of marginal pairs—two webbed digits with great disparity of length. The thumb is separated from the index very early in infancy, and the little finger is isolated from its immediate ulnar neighbor soon after. The separation of the index from the middle and the latter from the ring finger may be postponed. At no time are the three central digits separated from one another during a single session; one pair is subjected to surgery at a time. In some cases of massive syndactyly of the hand, one of the separated digits may seem to have precarious blood supply and appear deprived of muscular control. The skeletal elements of the vestigial digit are enucleated, and viable skin yielded by this procedure is utilized to cover the raw surface of the commissure of the adjacent finger. There have been a number of patients with massive syndactyly of the hand in whom the limb as a whole appears atrophic; the hand is flexed at the wrist and, even when together, the digits barely move. These patients are left alone (Figs. 12–25 and 12–26).

SYMBRACHYDACTYLY

This anomaly is defined as webbing of digits which possess less than their normal quota of phalanges and are consequently short. Pol (1921) collected 33 cases from the literature. Symbrachydactyly occurs sporadically, without any hereditary antecedent, and is usually unilateral, although in an occasional case there may be a transverse terminal defect in the opposite hand or in one or both feet. In most cases, the thumb is free and opposable. When the thumb is unrotated and held in adducted position, one needs to widen the first webspace by Z-plasty; the first metacarpal is subjected to osteotomy in order to bring the thumb into more effective opposition. Movement of the ulnar digits is enhanced by deepening the commissures between them (Figs. 12–27 to 12–33).

(Text continued on page 376.)

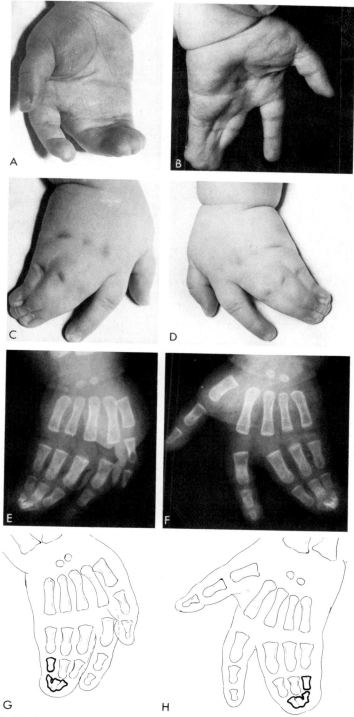

Figure 12–25 Syndactyly of three ulnar digits. *A*, Palmar view of the right hand of an 11-month-old female. *B*, Palmar view of the left hand. *C*, Dorsal view of the right hand. *D*, Dorsal view of the left hand. *E*, Dorsopalmar roentgenograph of the right hand. *F*, Dorsopalmar roentgenograph of the left hand. *G* and *H* illustrate roentgenographs above each.

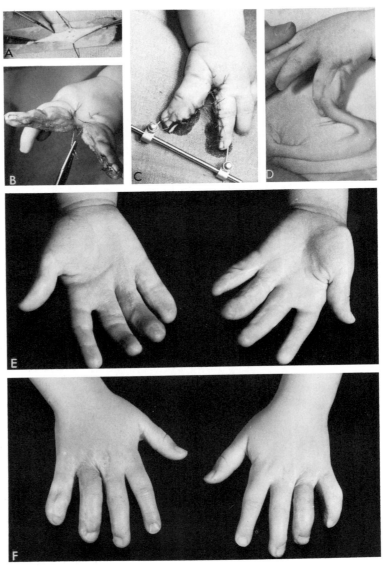

Figure 12–26 Procedures utilized for the preceding case (Fig. 12–25) and results obtained after two-stage operation for each hand. *A,* Free full-thickness skin graft with raw surface up, to be utilized to surface the denuded sides of the separated middle and ring fingers. *B,* Left hand after separation of the middle and ring fingers and closure of the commissure with a dorsal flap. *C,* Right hand after separation of the middle and ring fingers and surfacing of the raw areas. *D,* Marsupialized end of an abdominal tube has been inserted between the ring and little fingers of the right hand; later, the interdigital flap was utilized to establish a commissure and to surface raw areas left after separation of these digits which seemed attenuated. *E,* Palmar view of both hands three years after the last surgery. *F,* Dorsal view.

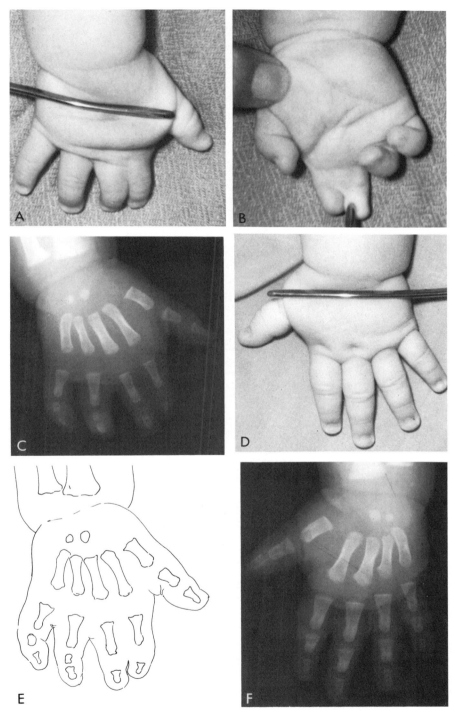

Figure 12–27 Symbrachydactyly of the right hand of an eight-month-old male infant. *A*, Dorsal view of the hand. *B*, Palmar view. *C*, Dorsopalmar roentgenograph showing absence of a middle phalanx in the index and middle fingers. *D*, Dorsal view of the left hand. *E*, Sketch illustrating the roentgenograph above it. *F*, Dorsopalmar roentgenograph of the left hand.

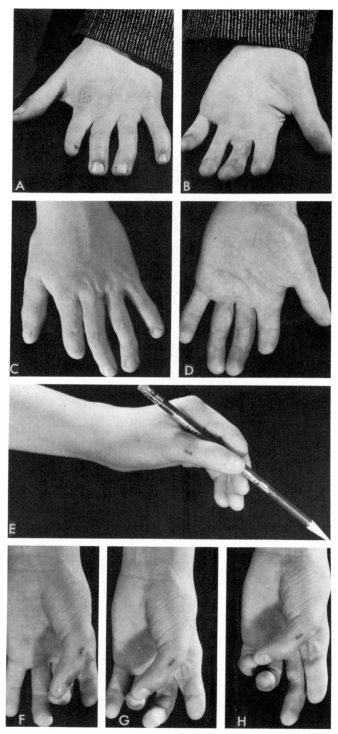

Figure 12–28 Symbrachydactyly treated by deepening the second and third commissures. *A,* Preoperative dorsal view of the hand. *B,* Preoperative palmar view. *C,* Postoperative dorsal view. *D,* Postoperative palmar view. *E, F, G,* and *H* show the functional results.

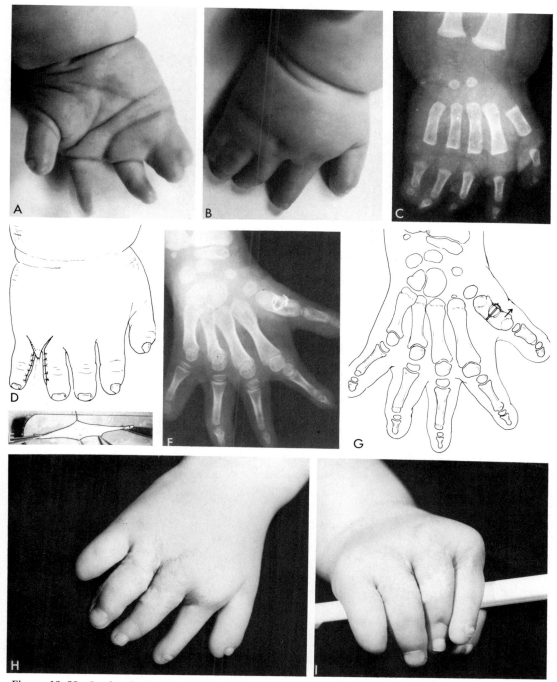

Figure 12–29 Symbrachydactyly with insufficiently rotated thumb. *A,* Palmar view of the right hand of a six-month-old female. *B,* Dorsal view. *C,* Dorsopalmar roentgenograph showing an absence of the middle phalanx in each finger. *D,* Sketch illustrating the separation of the webbed ring and little fingers and deepening of the interdigital commissure between the third and fourth digits. *E,* Full-thickness skin graft which was bisected and the halves utilized to surface the raw areas on the contiguous sides of the separated digits. *F,* Dorsopalmar roentgenograph after rotary osteotomy of the first metacarpal which was performed at the age of seven. *G,* Sketch illustrating the same. *H* and *I* show postoperative results: note the deepened interdigital commissures and the position of the thumbnail.

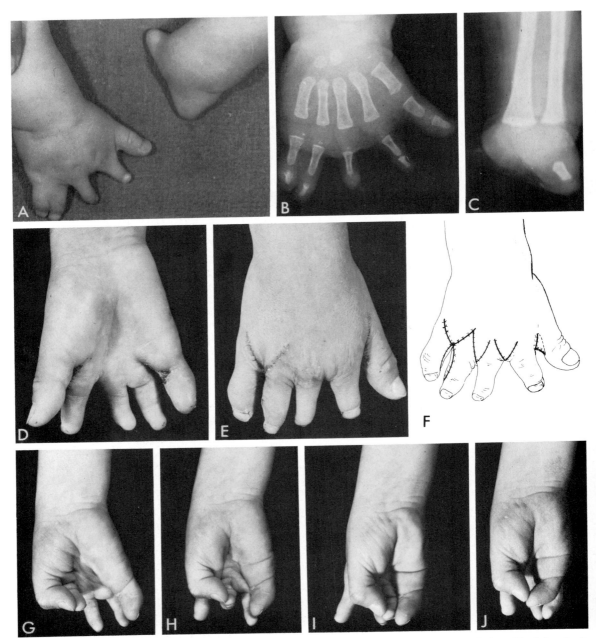

Figure 12–30 Symbrachydactyly associated with absence of the contralateral hand. *A,* Dorsal view of both hands. *B,* Dorsopalmar roentgenograph of the right hand. *C,* Dorsopalmar roentgenograph of the left distal forearm and wrist. *D,* Palmar view of the hand after separation of the webbed digits and deepening of all five interdigital clefts. *E,* Dorsal view. *F,* Sketch showing the incision lines for separating the webbed fourth and fifth digits and for deepening the interdigital clefts. *G, H, I,* and *J* demonstrate the postoperative functional results.

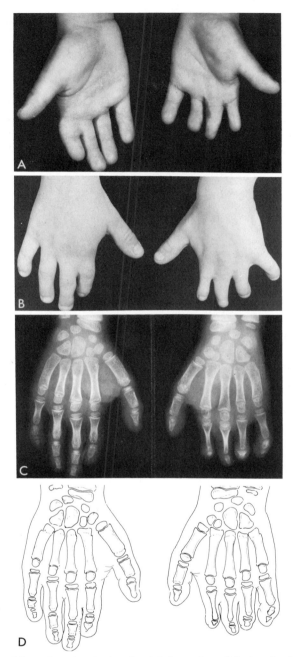

Figure 12–31 Bilateral symbrachydactyly. *A*, Palmar view of the hands of a nine-year-old boy. *B*, Dorsal view. *C*, Dorsopalmar roentgenograph of the hands: note the diminutive ungual and middle phalanges of the right index and little fingers. In the left hand, the ungual phalanges of the ulnar four digits are short and thin, the central three digits lack middle phalanges, and the ungual phalanges of the index and little fingers lack epiphyses. *D*, Sketch illustrating the same. The webbing of the right and left index and middle fingers was treated by simple syndactyly repair. The right hand needed no further care. In order to procure physiological length for the ulnar digits of the left hand, the commissures between each pair of fingers were deepened. The fifth webspace healed with binding scars: it needed to be redeepened. The left thumb would not abduct or rotate sufficiently (see Fig. 12–32).

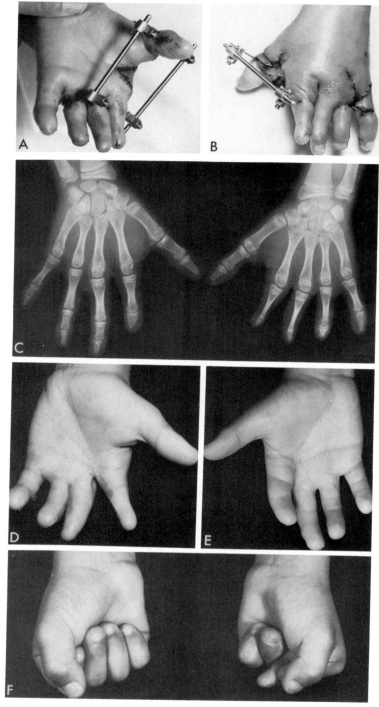

Figure 12–32   Z-plasty to widen the first webspace of the left hand shown in Figure 12–31, and final results. *A*, Palmar view of the hand after Z-plasty and incorporation of the external fixation apparatus to maintain position. *B*, Dorsal view of the same. *C*, Dorsopalmar roentgenograph of the hands two years after the initial surgery. *D*, *E*, and *F*, Final functional and cosmetic results.

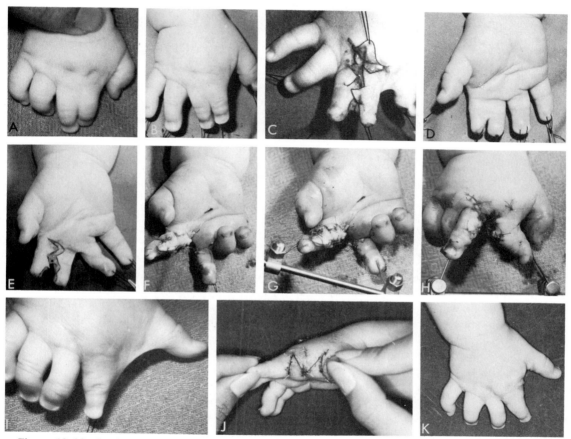

Figure 12–33 Symbrachydactyly of the right hand of a six-month-old boy with partial webbing of the thumb and the index and middle fingers and flexion contractures of the three radial digits. *A*, Preoperative dorsal view of the hand. *B*, Same, when the child was under anesthesia and the digits were straightened by traction sutures through the terminal pulps. *C*, Dorsal commissural flap and zig-zag incision between the index and middle fingers. *D*, Palmar view of the hand prior to separation of the index and middle fingers. *E*, Palmar zig-zag incision. *F*, The radial side of the middle finger has been closed by Z-plasty and the ulnar side of the index finger surfaced with free full-thickness graft. *G* and *H*, Palmar and dorsal views of the spreader bar hooked to K-wires inserted percutaneously into the unoperated aspects of the separated digits. *I*, Dorsal view of the hand three months after separation of the index from the middle finger, showing the web between the thumb and the index finger; this web extended as far forward as the base of the ungual phalanx of the thumb. It was recessed by performing Z-plasty as shown in *J*. *K*, Final postoperative result.

ACROSYNDACTYLY

Longuet (1876) appears to have been the first to describe what is variously called lattice form, amniotic, cicatrical, fenestrated, exogenous, or terminal syndactyly or acrosyndactyly. Longuet was followed by Kirmisson (1889), Dervaux (1909), and Assali (1921). There have been numerous reports since. In most recorded cases, webbing of the digits is associated with transverse terminal defects and annular grooves. The thumb may be stunted, but it is rarely caught in the massive confluence. Usually, the central digits are affected, and the ends of two neighboring members are united by soft tissue. The ungual phalanges are often absent. The severance of a soft-tissue bridge between the ends of conjoined digits offers no difficulty. The raw areas left after separation are surfaced by full-thickness free skin grafts. The interdigital webspace between dwarfed digits may have to be deepened (Figs. 12–34 to 12–36).

SYNDACTYLY ASSOCIATED WITH DIMINISHED NUMBER OF DIGITS

This anomaly is variously called ectrosyndactyly or oligosyndactyly. It is often associated with radial and ulnar ray defects, dislocations of the radial head, radioulnar synostosis, and split hand. In radial ray defect, the thumb may be missing, and the index finger is occasionally confluent with the middle finger. In the latter instance, the index finger should be separated from its immediate ulnar neighbor and pollicized by rotation osteotomy of its metacarpal. In defects of the ulnar ray, the fourth and fifth digits are usually absent, and the index and middle fingers are webbed; occasionally, the thumb is held in fixed adduction or is unrotated. Repair of the syndactyly in this instance is dovetailed with widening of the first webspace or abduction-rotation osteotomy of the thumb metacarpal. In the ectrosyndactyly of split hand, correction of syndactyly may need to be coupled with closure of the palmar cleft (Figs. 12–37 to 12–44).

(Text continued on page 387.)

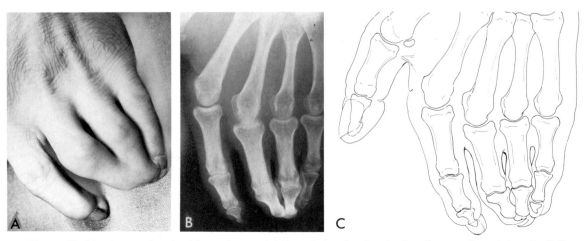

Figure 12–34 Acrosyndactyly with two fenestra. *A*, Dorsal view showing the four fingers of an adult male. *B*, Dorsopalmar roentgenograph of the same digits. *C*, Sketch illustrating the skeletal components of the hand.

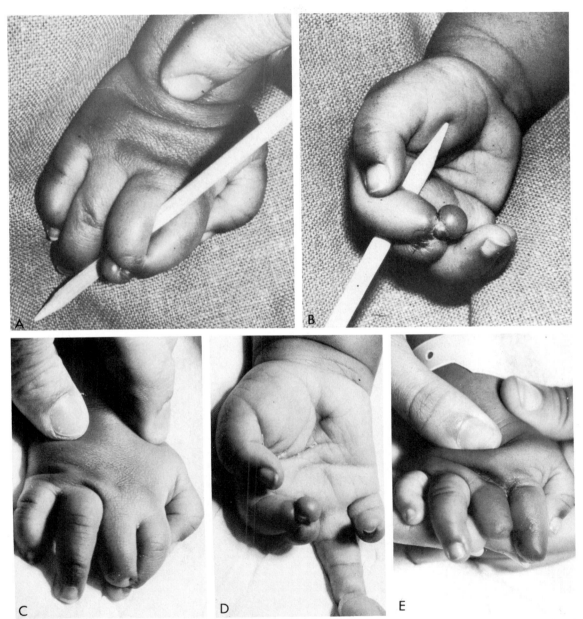

Figure 12–35 Acrosyndactyly with a single fenestrum. *A, B, C,* and *D,* The right hand of a four-month-old male with acral syndactyly of the index and middle fingers and large enough proximal fenestrum to admit a pencil. *E* shows the postoperative appearance of the separated digits: note that both digits lack terminal segments and also nails.

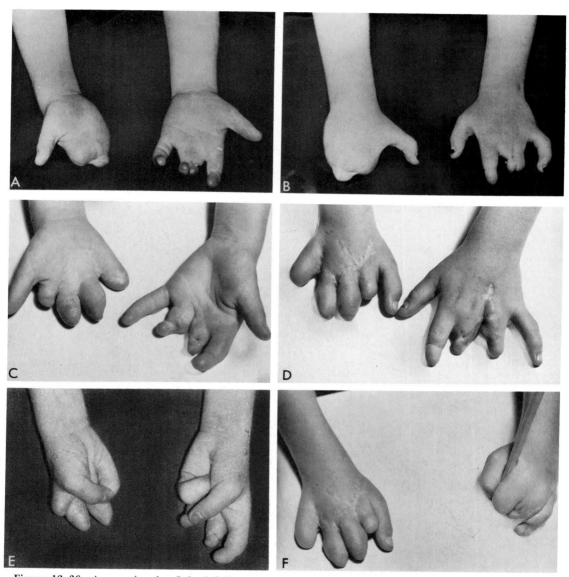

Figure 12–36 Acrosyndactyly of the left hand associated with terminal transverse defect of the right manus treated by deepening the interdigital clefts. The deepened commissures and the raw surfaces of the separated digits were covered with distant flaps. *A* and *B*, Palmar and dorsal views of both hands. *C* and *D*, Corresponding postoperative views. *E* and *F*, Functional results.

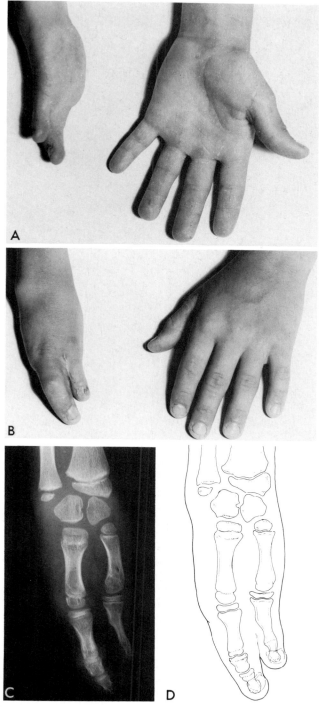

Figure 12–37 A hand with only two digits which are webbed and contain anomalous bones. *A* and *B*, Photographs of both hands; the affected limb was short and the right hand failed to completely supinate. Dislocation of the radial head is a common accompaniment of oligosyndactyly; it was present in this case. *C*, Dorsopalmar roentgenograph of the right hand, showing that the ulnar styloid has extended as far forward as the radial. The ulnar digit possesses three phalanges, one of which, the middle, is short; the radial digit possesses a single long phalanx which probably was produced by the fusion of three small phalanges. *D*, Sketch illustrating the same.

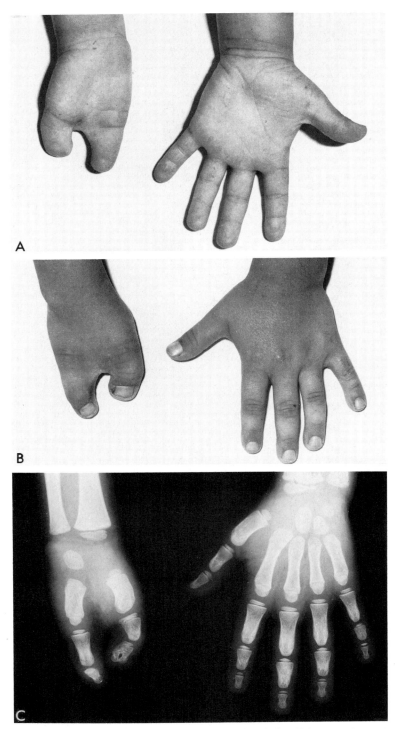

Figure 12–38   Syndactyly of a hand with only two thumblike digits. *A*, Palmar view of both hands. *B*, Dorsal view: note that the two digits of the right hand are thick and their nails are on the same horizontal level. *C*, Dorsopalmar roentgenograph of both hands: each digit of the right hand possesses a metacarpal and two phalanges; the epiphysis of the ulnar metacarpal is located at its proximal extremity, and the ungual phalanx of this digit is bifid.

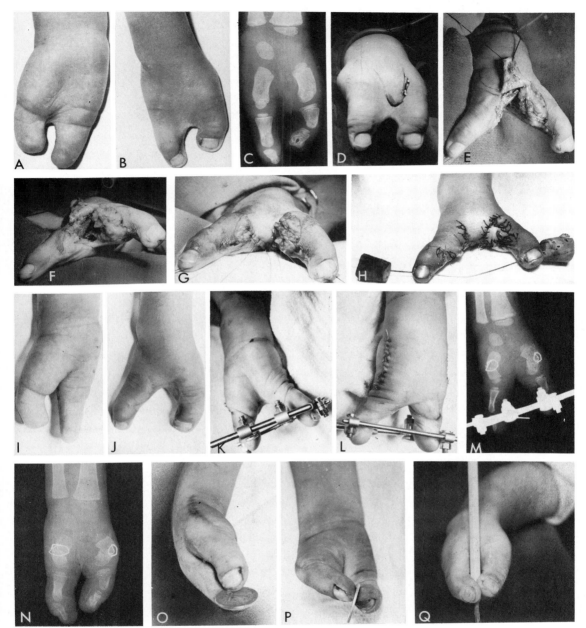

Figure 12–39 Two-stage procedure for the treatment of the right hand shown in Figure 12–38. The first stage consisted of separation of the webbed digits, and during the second session the digits were made to turn and face one another. *A* and *B*, Preoperative photographs of the hand. *C*, Preoperative roentgenograph. *D*, Delineation of the dorsal flap. *E*, Elevation of the dorsal flap and separation of the webbed digits. *F*, Deepening of the interdigital commissure. *G*, Dorsal flap has been sutured to establish a broad webspace. *H*, Remaining raw areas have been surfaced by Z-plasty on the ulnar digit and free full-thickness graft on the radial digit; K-wire is passed through the ungual phalanges to keep the separated digits apart. *I* and *J*, The results of the first stage, showing that a deep interdigital cleft has been created, but the separated digits remain unrotated and cannot effect pulp-to-pulp opposition. As shown in *K*, *L* and *M*, the metacarpals of each digit were subjected to rotary osteotomy and the digits held in opposition. *N* shows healing of osteotomized bones. *O*, *P*, and *Q* demonstrate functional results.

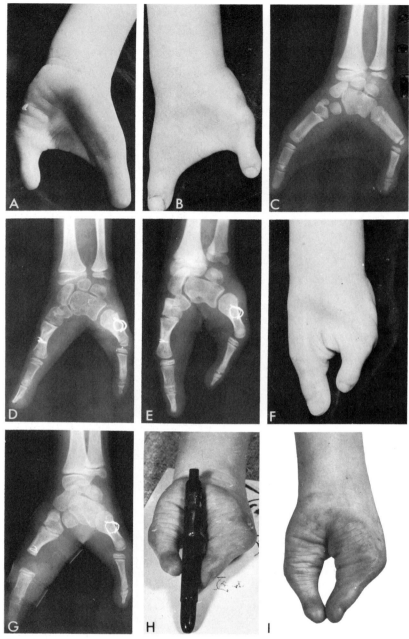

Figure 12–40   Oligosyndactyly of the left hand of an 11-year-old female with two thumblike digits and a wide interdigital web. *A,* Palmar view of the hand. *B,* Dorsal view: the nails of the two surviving digits are on the same horizontal plane, indicating failure of rotation of the radial digit. *C,* Dorsopalmar roentgenograph of the hand, showing coalescence of capitate and hamate bones and a biphalangeal little finger. *D,* Roentgenograph after the interdigital commissure had been deepened and the two marginal metacarpals subjected to rotary osteotomy using stainless steel wire for coaptation of the fragment. *E* and *F* show that six months after surgery the digits fail to oppose because of an unbending pollex. *G,* Roentgenograph after resection of thumb metacarpal head. *H* and *I,* Final functional results — procurement of pinch.

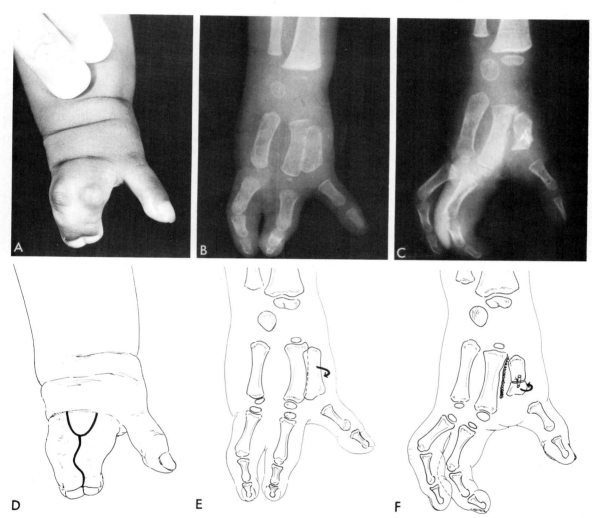

Figure 12–41 Oligosyndactyly associated with side-to-side fusion of metacarpals. *A*, Dorsal view of the hand. *B*, Dorsopalmar roentgenograph after repair of syndactyly. *C*, Separation of the two fused metacarpals from one another and osteotomy of the metacarpal of the thumb. The interspace between the two separated metacarpals was packed with Oxycel gauze. *D*, *E*, and *F* illustrate various procedures utilized for separation of the webbed digits and fused bones, and for rotary osteotomy of the first metacarpal.

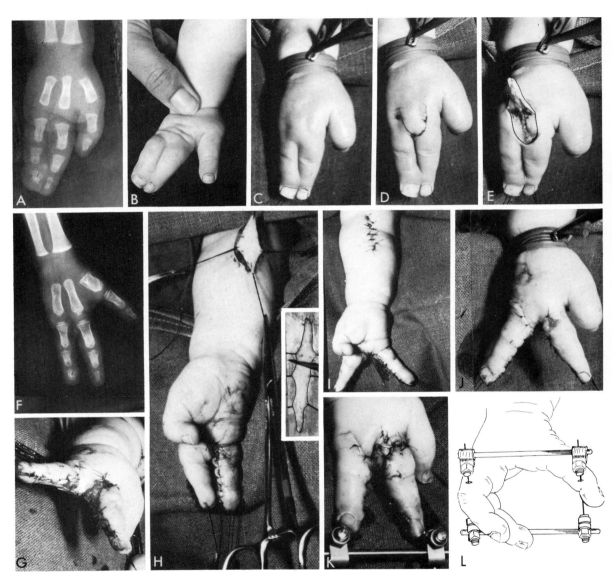

Figure 12–42 The infant boy whose hands are featured in this and the next two illustrations had bilateral oligodactyly and insufficient rotation of both thumbs. He had only two ulnar digits in each hand. The ulnar digits of the right
hand, presumably the index and middle fingers, were webbed. In this figure, the procedures utilized for repair of the
right hand are shown. *A*, Dorsopalmar roentgenograph of the hand. *B*, Dorsal view showing webbing of two fingers: note
that the thumbnail is almost on the same plane as the plane of the fingernails. *C*, Rubber catheter used as a tourniquet. *D*,
Incision for the dorsal commissural flap. *E*, Elevation of the flap. *F*, Dorsopalmar roentgenograph after separation of the
webbed digits. *G*, Surfacing the deepened interdigital commissure with the dorsal flap. *H*, Lifting an elliptical piece of
skin from the forearm which is turned raw side up (see inset) and scraped free of fat and areolar tissue. *I*, Closure of the
donor site of the forearm by Z-plasty. *J*, Surfacing the raw areas on the sides of the separated digits. *K*, Spreader bar attached to the percutaneous wires to keep the fingers apart. *L*, Sketch illustrating the apparatus used after rotation osteotomy of the first metacarpal.

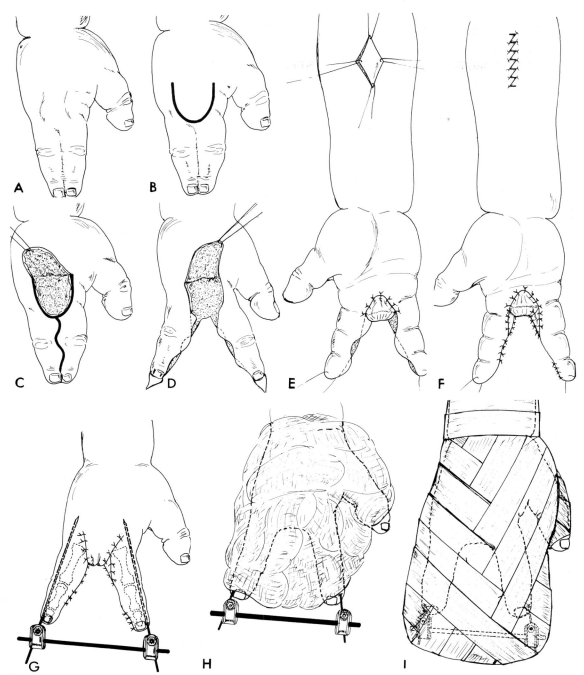

Figure 12–43 Sketches illustrating some of the procedures utilized for separation of the webbed digits of the right hand shown in Figure 12–42. *A*, Sketch of the hand. *B*, Dorsal horseshoe-shaped incision. *C*, Elevation of the dorsal flap. *D*, Separation of the digits by undulating incision. *E*, Suturing the dorsal flap to the skin of the palm and lifting a free graft from the volar aspect of the forearm. *F*, Closure of the donor site with Z-plasty and surfacing the raw areas on the sides of the separated digits. *G*, Digits held apart with the aid of percutaneous K-wire and spreader bar. *H*, Packing the interdigital spaces and surrounding the hand with fluffy fine-meshed gauze. *I*, Pressure dressing.

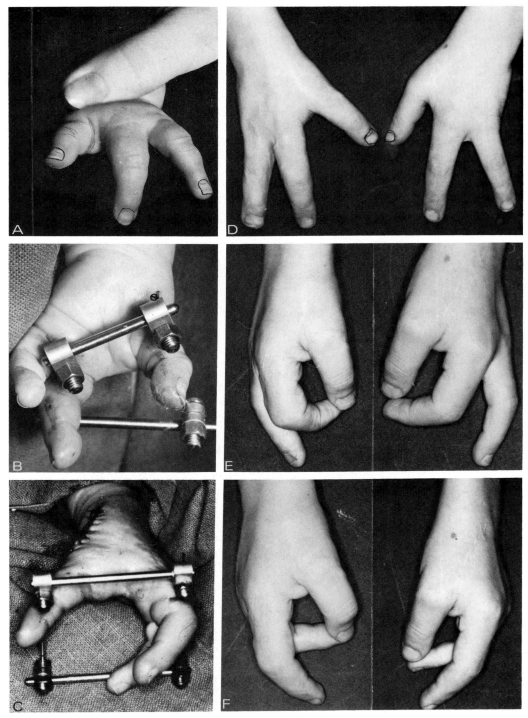

Figure 12–44   The same case—continued. *A*, Dorsal view of the left hand: the thumbnail lies on the same horizontal plane as the plane of the fingernails. *B*, Ulnar view of the right hand after rotation osteotomy of the thumb metacarpal and institution of external fixation apparatus. *C*, Radial view of the left hand after similar procedure. *D*, *E*, and *F*, Cosmetic and functional results four years after the initial surgery.

SYNDACTYLY ASSOCIATED WITH INCREASED NUMBER OF DIGITS

Two confusing terms crop up in the literature — polysyndactyly and sympolydactyly. Some authors use the term polysyndactyly to describe webbing of three or more digits of pentadactylic hands, reserving the designation sympolydactyly for webbing of fingers in hands with supernumerary digits. Another group employs these terms interchangeably; and a third, consisting mainly of geneticists, insists that the term polysyndactyly should be used for cases in which the supernumerary digit is pre-axial and the word sympolydactyly for those in which the extra member is on the postaxial side. Albeit redundant, the designation used at the head of the present section is less confusing.

Association of polydactyly and syndactyly is a feature of mirror hand or ulnar dimelia. Syndactyly and polydactyly are often seen together without any malformations of the forearm. The anomaly is usually bilateral and is referred to as the Haas type of syndactyly. The malformation was described by Harker (1865), Rahon (1892), Audebert (1896), Rasch (1897), Boissard (1898), Jacobsohn (1909), Bonnet (1928), and by many others before the article by Haas (1940) was published. Heredity features prominently. In most reported cases, the trait is transmitted as an autosomal dominant.

The surgical management of a hand with six or more webbed digits does not differ much from that utilized for the treatment of massive syndactyly of a pentadactylic hand. Again an attempt is made to insulate the thumb and the little finger as early as possible. Digits with attenuated skeleton and absent muscular control are filleted out and the available skin is utilized to cover in part the raw surface of their more robust neighbor's. It will be noted in Chapter Thirteen that in some instances the supernumerary digit shares the same sets of tendons and neurovascular bundles as its neighbor, and caution must be exercised not to sacrifice these structures (Figs. 12–45 and 12–46).

SYNDACTYLY COMPLICATED BY BONY UNION

Webbing of two fingers with bony fusion of the terminal phalanges requires early surgical intervention. The fused bones are split evenly with a sharp osteotome, and are then surfaced with full-thickness skin grafts. Free grafts adhere to bone and may contract and cause angular deformity. At a later date it may be necessary to replace the adherent free grafts with cross-finger or distant skin flaps. In most instances, the conjoined fingers share one nail. The latter is split in the middle, and the cut edges are trimmed (Figs. 12–47 and 12–48).

Syndactyly complicated by irregularly shaped, misaligned, fused bones is difficult to treat. Kummer (1891) introduced three principles which have since been used for this type of complicated syndactyly: (1) realignment of the remaining bones; (2) resection of articular ends to promote motion; and (3) the use of distal flaps for coverage. In some instances, it might be necessary to sacrifice a digit whose bones are difficult to bring into proper alignment (Figs. 12–49 and 12–50).

(*Text continued on page 393.*)

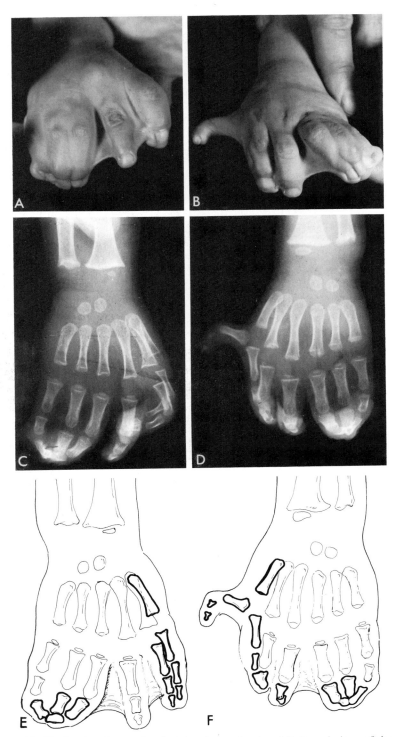

Figure 12–45 Syndactyly associated with polydactyly. *A* and *B*, Dorsal views of the right and left hands of a two-year-old female. *C* and *D*, Dorsopalmar roentgenographs of the right and left hands. *E* and *F* illustrate roentgenographs above each. The left hand is still under surgical care.

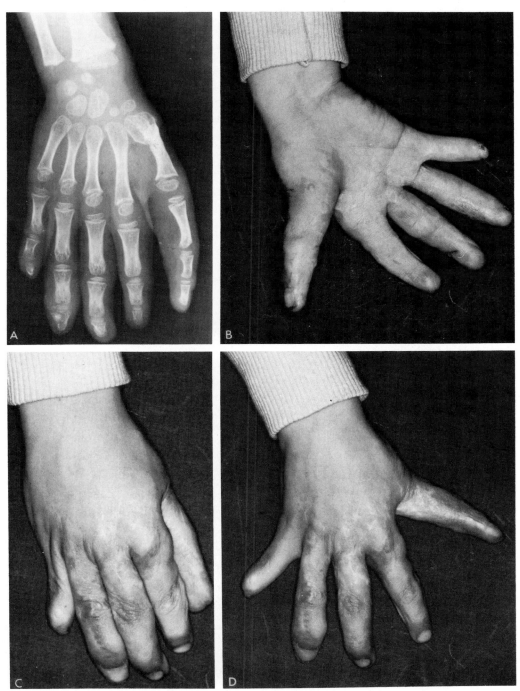

Figure 12–46   The outcome of surgery on the right hand of the little girl featured in Figure 12–45. The radialmost ray was removed, leaving only its proximal end, and the next ray was shifted radially and anchored to this piece. Each pair of digits was disengaged at different sessions. *A*, Dorsopalmar roentgenograph of the right hand four years after initial surgery. *B*, Palmar view of the hand with outstretched digits. *C*, Dorsal view with digits close together. *D*, Same, with outstretched digits.

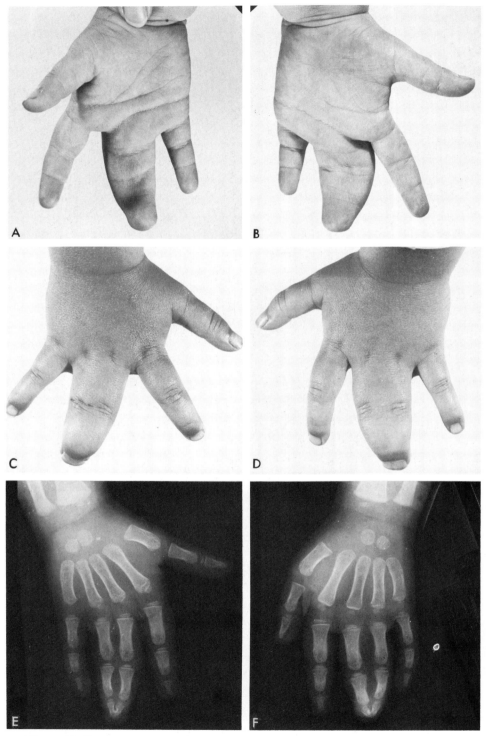

Figure 12–47 Bilateral syndactyly of the middle and ring fingers of a two-year-old male without dorsal and volar grooves and with osseous union of ungual phalangeal tips. *A* and *B*, Palmar view of the hands. *C* and *D*, Dorsal view of the same. *E*, Dorsopalmar roentgenograph of the right hand. *F*, Dorsopalmar roentgenograph of the left hand.

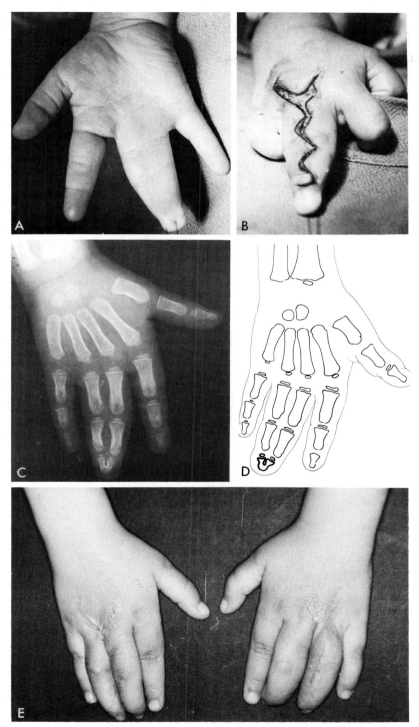

Figure 12–48 The hands of the boy shown in Figure 12–47. *A*, Palmar view of the right hand. *B*, Dorsal view of the hand, showing an already deepened incision. *C*, Dorsopalmar roentgenograph of the right hand. *D*, Sketch illustrating the same. *E*, Postoperative appearance of the right and left hands.

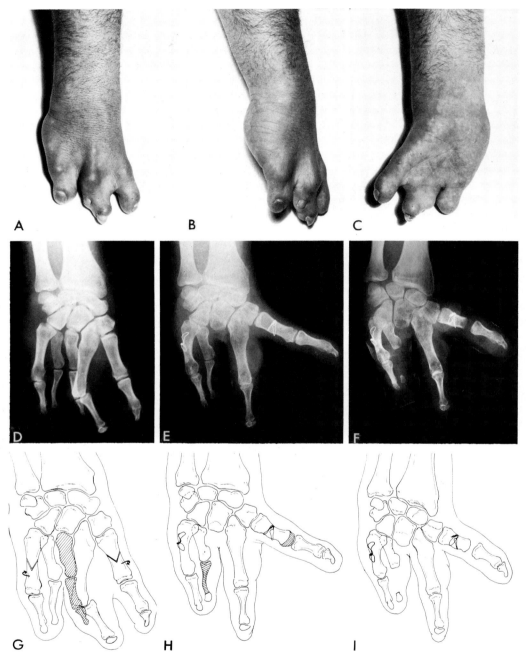

Figure 12–49 Massive syndactyly associated with short third and fourth metacarpals, absent proximal and middle phalanges of the fingers, symphalangism of an unrotated thumb, and stiff unbending joints treated by excision of the third and fourth digital rays, rotary osteotomy of the marginal metacarpals, and arthroplasty of the metacarpophalangeal joint of the thumb. *A, B,* and *C,* Various views of the right hand. *D,* Preoperative dorsopalmar roentgenograph. *E,* Roentgenograph of the right hand after removal of the third digital ray and rotary osteotomy of the marginal metacarpals. This operation failed to procure opposition. *F,* Roentgenograph after arthroplasty of the pollical metacarpophalangeal joint. *G, H,* and *I* illustrate rotary osteotomy of the marginal bones and excision of some of the central digital rays and resection of the distal articular and of the first metacarpal.

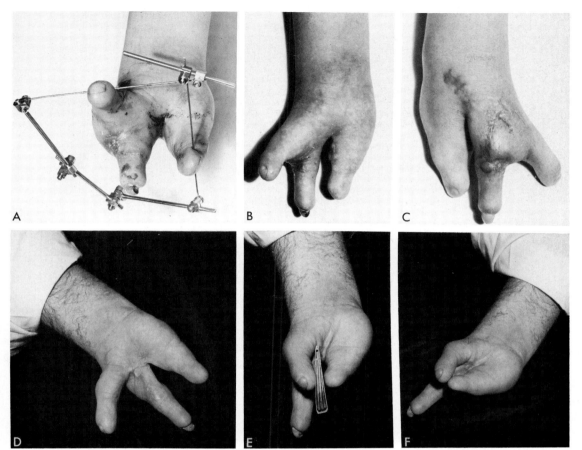

Figure 12–50 The same case as shown in Figure 12–49. *A*, External fixation apparatus applied after removal of some of the central digital rays and rotary osteotomy of the marginal metacarpals. *B* and *C*, Palmar and dorsal views of the hand following first attempt at correction. *D*, *E*, and *F*, Functional results after the second attempt.

SYNDACTYLIES WHICH ARE BEST LEFT ALONE

Roentgenography was discovered in 1895—four years after Kummer performed his operation. The first x-ray film of a hand with osseous syndactyly appeared in connection with an article by Lund (1897), who reported a complicated case. Lund characterized the disposition of the bones in the affected hand as being "irregularly irregular." He advised against surgery, reasoning that the conjoined fingers moved in unison; after separation they might fail to move individually. It might be advantageous to heed this advice in some cases. Surgery should also be avoided when the webbed digits have no muscular control and when there is massive syndactyly of vestigial digits with fixed flexion deformity at the wrist (Figs. 12–51 to 12–54).

In craniosynostosis with syndactyly, it may be worthwhile to separate the webbed fingers. Decompression of the skull is advised for patients with very early closure of coronal sutures or when loss of vision becomes imminent.

(*Text continued on page 398.*)

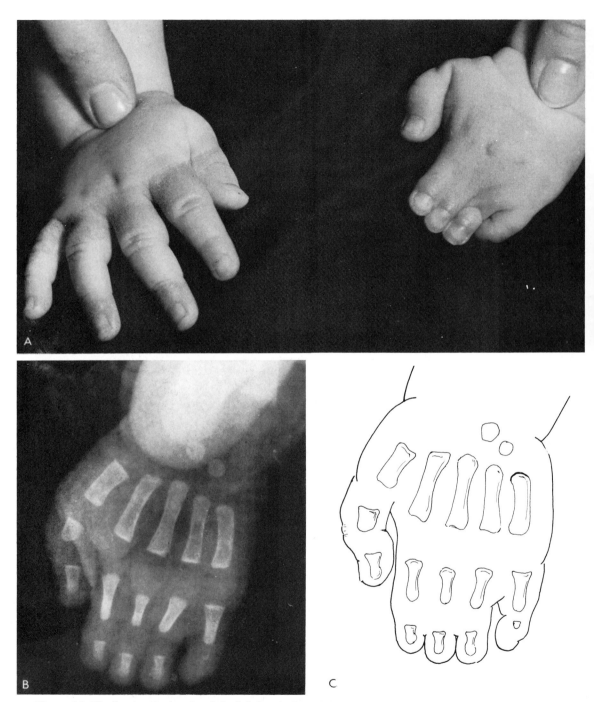

Figure 12–51 Symbrachydactyly of the left hand of a child with diminutive webbed central digits which fail to move, even together, indicating absence of muscular control. *A*, Dorsal view of both hands. *B*, Dorsopalmar roentgenograph showing absence of middle phalanges of all fingers and vestigial ungual phalanx of the little finger. *C*, Sketch illustrating the same.

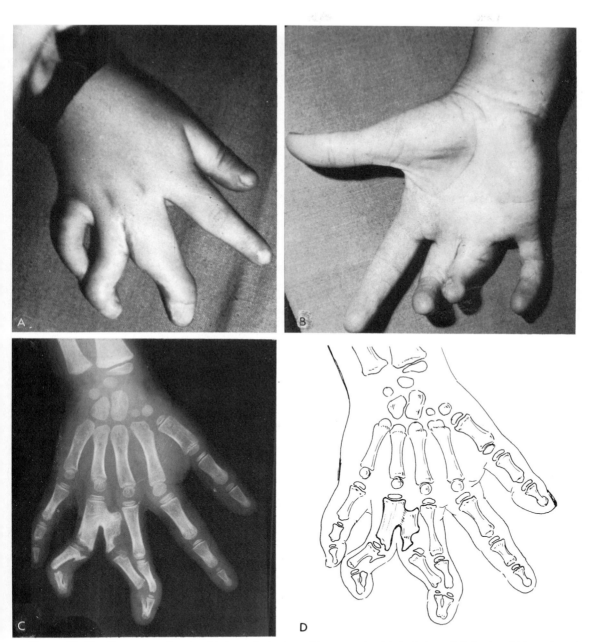

Figure 12–52 Osseous syndactyly with irregularly shaped bones and axial deviation of digits, in which coalesced members move well enough together and might not when separated. *A* and *B*, Dorsal and palmar views of the left hand of a five-year-old boy. *C*, Dorsopalmar roentgenograph of the hand. *D*, Sketch illustrating the same.

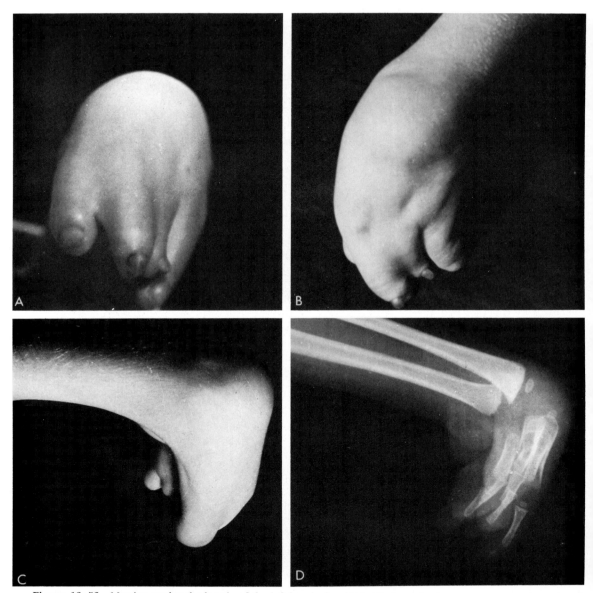

Figure 12–53 Massive symbrachydactyly of the left hand of a child with fixed flexion contracture at the wrist. *A,* Dorsal view of the confluent digits. *B,* Dorsal view of the wrist and hand. *C,* Ulnar view of the same. *D,* Lateral roentgenograph showing that most of the (probably middle) phalanges are missing and the remaining digital bones are sliver-thin.

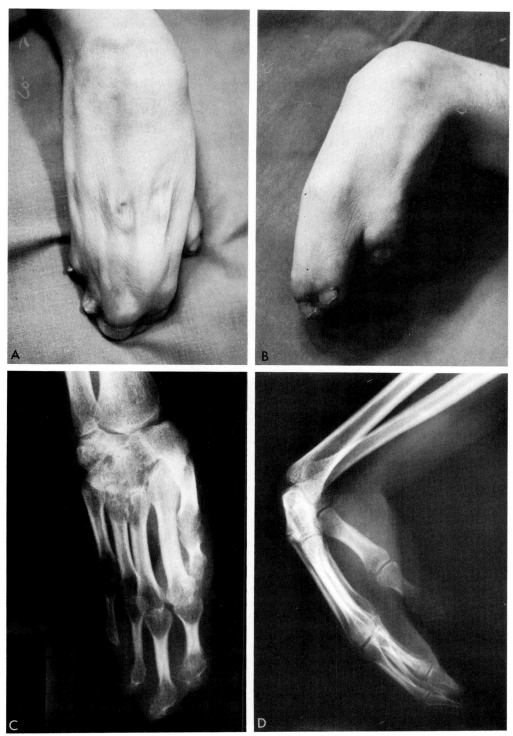

Figure 12–54 Massive symbrachydactyly of the right hand of an adult with fixed flexion contracture at the wrist. *A*, Dorsal view of the hand. *B*, Radial view. *C*, Dorsopalmar roentgenograph: note the massive fusion of the carpus and the carpometacarpal fusion on the ulnar aspect. *D*, Lateral roentgenograph.

SUMMARY

Syndactyly is a common anomaly. It tends to affect mainly the central digits, showing a distinct predilection for the middle and ring fingers; the first postaxial — or the third — webspace is obliterated. Syndactyly is more common in males than in females, and more prevalent in white than in black people. Only occasionally is syndactyly hereditary, being transmitted as a dominant phenotype. Acrosyndactyly and symbrachydactyly are sporadic. Acrosyndactyly is usually associated with annular grooves and transverse terminal defects. Symbrachydactyly is occasionally seen in connection with aglossia, ankyloglossia, cleft lip-palate, Poland's syndrome, and the facial diplegia named after Möbius. In craniosynostosis with syndactyly, two or more ulnar digits are webbed together, and the terminal bones of two neighboring fingers may be confluent. In syndactyly with an excessive number of digits, the supernumerary members are at times without tendons, and caution is required when determining which digits should be sacrificed. Syndactyly of digits of unequal length, such as the thumb and index or the ring and little fingers, requires early surgical repair. In ordinary cases, the best results are obtained by using the combined methods of dorsal flap to establish a commissure and free skin graft to cover the parietes of the separated digits.

References

Adams, R.: Congenital malformations of the hand. *In* Todd, R. B., (ed.): *The Cyclopaedia of Anatomy and Physiology.* London, Longman, Brown, Green, Longmans & Roberts, Vol. II, p. 519, 1836.

Aiken, W. A. E.: Syndactylism. *Can. Med. Rev.* (Toronto), 7:106–110, 1898.

Albert, H.: The inheritance of syndactylism. *Science, 41*:951, 1915.

Albrectsen, B., and Svendsen, T. B.: Hypertrichosis syndactyly and retinal degeneration in two siblings. *Acta Derm. Venereol., 36*:96–101, 1956.

Alfieri, A., Abu, C., and Ceccarini, M.: Dysostose cranio-faciale hereditaire et syndactylie. *J. Genet. Hum., 16*:1–14, 1967.

Alvary, G.: Bilateral symmetrical syndactylism. *U.S. Armed Forces Med. J., 3*:569–573, 1952.

Alvord, R. M.: Zygodactyly and associated variations in a Utah family. *J. Hered., 38*:49–53, 1947.

Anger, C., and Strube, G.: Das Poland-syndrom. *Schweiz. Med. Wochenschr., 99*(1):483–485, 1969.

Annandale, T.: *The Malformations, Diseases and Injuries of the Fingers and Toes.* Philadelphia, J. B. Lippincott & Co., pp. 41–61, 1866.

Apert, E.: De l'acrocéphalosyndactylie. *Bull. Soc. Méd. Hôp. Paris, 23*:1310–1330, 1906.

Avery, L. B.: *Developmental Anatomy: A Textbook and Laboratory Manual of Embryology.* Seventh edition. Philadelphia, W. B. Saunders, pp. 210–212, 1965.

Assali, J.: Amputation digitales, syndactylie, ectrodactylie et sillons congénitaux, déterminés par brides amniotiques, malformations portant sur les deux mains et le pied gauche. *J. Méd. Bordeaux, 51*:107–109, 1921.

Audebert: Syndactylie et polydactylie héreditaires. *Soc. Anat. Physiol. Norm. Pathol. Bordeaux, 17*:129–131, 1896.

Bailey, S. d'A.: A pedigree of syndactylism. *J. Hered., 29*:467–468, 1938.

Barsky, A. J.: *Congenital Anomalies of the Hand and Their Surgical Treatment.* Springfield, Illinois, Charles C Thomas, pp. 26–47, 1958.

Barsky, A. M., Kahn, S., and Simon, B. E.: *Principles and Practices of Plastic Surgery.* Second edition. New York, Blakiston Div., McGraw-Hill Book Co., pp. 702–708, 1964.

Basler, A.: Über die Häufigkeit der Zygodaktylie bei Tübinger Bevölkerung. *Z. Morphol. Anthropol., 26*:59–67, 1927.

Baudinne, P., Bovy, G. L., and Wasterlain, A.: Un cas de syndrome de Poland. *Acta Paediatr. Belg., 21*:407–410, 1967.

Bauer, T. B., Tondra, J. M., and Trusler, H. M.: Technical modification in repair of syndactylism. *Plast. Reconstr. Surg., 17*:385–391, 1956.

Bell, J.: On syndactyly and its association with polydactyly. *Treasury of Human Inheritance, 5*:33–50, 1953.

Benario, J.: Ueber einen Fall von angeborenem Mangel des Musculus pectoralis major und minor mit Flughautbildung und Schwimmhautbildung. *Berl. Klin. Wochenschr., 27*:225–227, 1890.

Benassi, V., and Trabucchi, L.: Terapia chirurgica della deformita congenite della mano. *Chir. Organi Mov., 51*:177–195, 1962.

Benedict, A. L.: Syndactylus. *Med. News,* Philadelphia, *63*:126–127, 1893.

Beno, J.: *Essai sur la Syndactylie Congénitale.* Thèse. Nancy, Imp. Lorraine, pp. 43–49, 1886.

Berger, O. v.: Angeborener Defect der Brustmuskeln. *Arch. Pathol. Anat. Physiol., 72*:438–444, 1878.

Bérigny: Sur des cas de palmidactylism se reproduisant dans une même famille pendant plusier générations. *C. R. Acad. Sci., 57*:743–744, 1863.

Berliner, M. L.: Unilateral microphthalmia with congenital anterior synechiae and syndactyly. *Arch. Ophthalmol. 26*:653–660, 1941.

Bidwell, L. A.: An operation for webbed fingers. *Lancet, 1*:1640–1641, 1895.

Bigot, C.: *L'Acrocéphalo-Syndactylie (Dysostose Cranienne Congénitale avec Syndactylie).* Thèse. Paris, A. Legrand, pp. 9–105, Figs. 1–4, 1922.

Bilhaut, M.: Doigts palmés, procédés anciens: Procédé nouveau. *Ann. Chir. d'Orthop., 17*:257–263, 1904.

Birch-Jensen, A.: *Congenital Deformities of the Upper Extremities.* Translated from the Danish by E. Aagesen. Commission, Andlesbogtrykkerrei i Odense Det Danske Forlag., pp. 127–233, 242, 243, 1959.

Bittner, W.: Zwei Fälle von totaler Syndaktylie der Hand. *Prager Med. Wochenschr., 41*:465, 1895.

Blackfield, H. M., and Hause, D. P.: Syndactylism. *Plast. Reconstr. Surg., 16*:37–46, 1955.

Blank, C. E.: Apert's syndrome (A type of acrocephalosyndactyly)—observations on a British series of thirty-nine cases. *Ann. Hum. Genet., 24*:151–164, 1960.

Böcs, G. and Dévényi, I.: Combined occurrence of syndactyly and polydactyly. Data on the inheritance of this condition. (Hungarian) *Orv. Hetil., 105*:747–748, 1964.

Boissard: Polydactylie et syndactylie hereditaire. *Bull. Soc. Obst. Paris, 2*:232–235, 1899.

Bonnet, L.: Syndactylie et polydactylie à caractére familial. *Bull. Mém. Soc. Chir.* (Paris), *20*:677–681, 1928.

Bonnet, P.: Dysostose cranio-faciale et syndactylie. Signes oculaires chez une fillet de 13 ans. *Bull. Soc. Ophtalmol.* (Paris), pp. 665–667, 1947.

Böök, J. A.: Clinical cytogenetics. *In* Gedda, L., (ed.): *De Genetica Medica*. Rome, Apud Mendelianum Inst. Pars tertia, pp. 21–57; fig. 11, 1961.

Böök, J. A., and Santesson, B.: Malformation syndrome in man associated with triplody (60 chromosomes). *Lancet, 1*:858–859, 1960.

Boppe, M.: Syndactylie plastic par greffe cutanée libre. *Mem. Acad. Chir., 63*(1):503–504, 1937. Also in *Paris Mèd., 111*:522–527, 1939.

Boucaud (de): Syndactylie par accolement des doigts sous le peau. *Bull. Soc. Anat. Physiol. Norm. Pathol. Bordeaux, 17*:1539, 1896.

Boudet, and Reverdy: Syndactylie congénitale generalisée, avec clinodactylie et anomalies diverses du squelette. *Bull. Soc. Sci. Méd. Biol.* (Moutpollier). 7:279–283, 1925–1926.

Boyes, J. H., (ed.): *Bunnell's Surgery of the Hand*. Fourth edition. Philadelphia, J. B. Lippincott Co., pp. 80–90, 1964. See also the fifth edition, pp. 85–91, 1970.

Brabazon, A. B.: Case of congenital malformation of the hand, with remarks. *Dublin Hosp. Gaz., 1*:375–376, 1854.

Breg, W. R.: Cri-du-chat syndrome. *In* Gardner, L. I., (ed.): *Endocrine and Genetic Disease of Childhood*. Philadelphia, W. B. Saunders Co., pp. 632–638, 1969.

Brites, G.: Syndactylie totale et hypophalangie de la main. *Folia Anat. Univ. Conimb., 5*(No. 7):1–5; Pl. I, II, 1930.

Brizio, L.: Il trattamento chirurgico della sindattila congenita della mano. *Boll. Mem. Soc. Tosco-umbra Chir., 12*:605–608, 1952.

Brohl: Beseitigung der narbigen Syndaktylie mittels Thiersch'scher Transplantationen. *Dtsch. Med. Wochenschr., 19*:866, 1893.

Brooksaler, F. S.: Poland's syndrome. *Am. J. Dis. Child., 121*:263–264, 1971.

Brown, J. B., and McDowell, F.: Syndactylism with absence of pectoralis major. *Surgery, 7*:599–601, 1940.

Brown, J. B., and McDowell, F.: *Skin Grafting*. Third edition. Philadelphia, J. B. Lippincott Co., pp. 149–150, 1958.

Browne, D.: Congenital malformations. *Practitioner, 131*:20–32, 1933.

Browne, D.: Congenital abnormalities of the extremities. *Practitioner, 142*:270–277, 1939.

Bruno: Demonstration eines Falls von doppelseitiger Klumphand, Radius and Daumendefekt und Syndactylie. *Münch. Med. Wochenschr. 52*:724, 1905.

Bunnell, S.: *Surgery of the Hand*. Philadelphia, J. B. Lippincott Co., pp. 609–647, 1944.

Bünnige, M.: Angeborene Zungen-Munddach-Verwachsung (Ankyloglossum superius congenitum). *Ann. Paediatr., 195*:173–180, 1960.

Busachi, T.: Sindattilia completa della mano destra es viluppodi un dito del quale manca il metacarpo. *Arch. Ortop., 9*:102–104, 1892.

Calo, A.: Cardiopatie congenite e malformazioni degli art. *Cuore Circ. 37*:303–313, 1953.

Camus, M.: Accumulation de stigmates physiques chez un dégénéré. *C. R. Soc. Biol., 55*:1555–1557, 1903.

Carpenter, G.: Two sisters showing malformations of skull and other congenital abnormalities. *Rep. Soc. Study Dis. Child., 1*:111–118, 1901.

Carpenter, G.: Case of acrocephaly, with other congenital malformations. *Proc. R. Soc. Med.* (Sect. Study Dis. Child.), Vol. II, Part 1:45–53, 199–201, 1909.

Cenani, A., and Lenz, W.: Totale Syndaktylie und totale radioulnare Synostose bei zwei Bründern. *Z. Kinderheilkd., 101*:181–190, 1967.

Chamberlain, J. L.: Poland's syndrome. *Clin. Proc. Child. Hosp. D.C., 25*:10–11, 1969.

Chauvenet, Daraignez, and Ducassou, J. L.: Syndactylie compléte des mains et des pieds chez un enfant de deux ans. *Rev. d'Orthop. Chir. L'App. Mot., 33*:157, 1947.

Chotzen, F.: Eine eigenartige familiäre Entwicklungsstörung, (Akrocephalosyndaktylie, Dysostosis craniofacialis und Hypertelorismus). *Monatsschr. Kinderheilkd., 55*:97–122, 1932.

Ciotola, G.: Microftalmo e malformazion della dita (Sindattilia, polidattilia). *Boll. Ocul., 17*:855–867, 1938.

Clark, W. E., and Le, G.: A case of hereditary syndactyly. *Lancet, 2*:434, 1916.

Clarkson, P.: Poland's syndactyly. *Guy's Hosp. Rep., 111*:335–346, 1962.

Clouston, H. R.: The major forms of hereditary ectodermal dysplasia. *Can. Med. Assoc. J., 40*:1–7, 1939.

Cogswell, H. D., and Trusler, H. M.: A modified Agnew's operation for syndactylism. *Surg. Gynecol. Obstet., 64*:793, 1937.

Cohn, B. N. E.: True oxycephaly with syndactylism: case report. *Am. J. Surg., 68*:93–99, 1945.

Coleman, H. A.: Coexistence of congenital amputations and syndactylism. *J.A.M.A., 83*:1164–1165, 1924.

Collette, A. T.: A case of syndactylism of the ring and little finger. *Am. J. Hum. Genet., 6*:241–243, 1954.

Conway, H., and Bowe, J.: Congenital deformities of the hand. *Plast. Reconstr. Surg., 18*:460–468, 1956.

Cozzolino, A.: Sulle sindattilie congenite. *Arch. Ortop., 67*:319–338, 1954.

Cramer, H.: Un cas de brachydactylie avec syndactylie osseuse et membrane. *Rev. Med. Suisse Romande, 51*:365–371, 1931.

Cronin, T. B.: Syndactylism. *Tristate Med. J.*, *15*:2869–2871, 2884, 1943.

Cronin, T.: Syndactylism: Results of zigzag incision to prevent postoperative contracture. *Plast. Reconstr. Surg.*, *18*:460–468, 1956.

Cross, H. E., Lerberg, D. B., and McKusick, V. A.: Type II syndactyly. *Am. J. Hum. Genet.*, *20*:368–380, 1968.

Crouzon, O.: Dysostose cranio-faciale héréditaire. *Bull. Mém. Soc. Méd. Hôp.* (Paris), 3 s., *33*:545–555, 1912.

Cruveilhier, J.: *In Anatomie Pathologique du Corps Humain.* Tome II, 38 e livreson, pp. 1–4, 1835.

Cruveiller, J.: *Maladie d'Apert-Crouzon.* Thèse. Paris, R. Vezin, pp. 1–138, 1954.

Cutler, C. W.: *The Hand. The Disabilities and Diseases.* Philadelphia, W. B. Saunders Co., pp. 413–423, 1942.

Davis, G. G.: The operative correction of webbed fingers. *Tr. Am. Orthop. Assoc.*, *11*:184, 1898.

Davis, J. S., and German, W. J.: Syndactylism. *Arch. Surg.*, *21*:32–75, 1930.

De Benedetti, M., and Chiapuzzo, A.: Malformazione unilaterale dei muscoli pettoral. *Arch. Ortop.*, *73*:408–417, 1960.

Degenhardt, K. H.: Zum entwicklungsmechanischen Problem der Akrocephalosyndaktylie. *Z. menschl. Vererb. Konstitutionslehre*, *29*:791–819, 1950.

De Gennaro, P. F.: L'assenza congenita del muscoli pettorali. *Arch. Putti*, *13*:371–390, 1960.

Dervaux, M.: Syndactylie terminale des deux mains et syndactylie d'un pied. Intervention. *Bull. Soc. Obstet.* (Paris), *12*:316–317, 1909.

Dessaix: Extrait d'un observation intéressant sur un vice conformation. *Gaz. Salutaire ou Feuille Hebd.*, No. 22:2–3, 1761.

Diaday, H. A.: V. Das Wissenswertheste aus den neuesten Zeitschriften und Werken. Ueber ein neuces Operatives Verfahren gegen die angeborene Verwachsung der Finger oder die digiti palmati. *J. Kinderheilkd.*, *14*:470–475, 1850.

Dickson, J.: Treatment of webbed fingers. *In Frank E. Bunts Institute Lectures.* pp. 72–74, 1937. Also in: *Cleveland Clin. Quart.*, *6*:72–74, 1939.

Didot, A.: Note sur la séparation des doigts palmés et sur un nouveau procédé anaplastique destiné a prevenir la reproduction de la difformité. *Bull. Acad. R. Med. Belg.*, *9*:351–356, 1849–1850.

Dodge, H. W., Jr., Wood, M. W., and Kennedy, R. L. J.: Craniofacial dysostosis: Crouzon's Disease. *Pediatrics*, *23*:98–106, 1959.

Dorrance, G. M., and Bransfield, J. W.: The treatment of webbed fingers, congenital or acquired. *Ann. Surg.*, *78*:532–533, 1923.

Dowd, C. N.: Webbed fingers. *Ann. Surg.*, *31*:393–404, 1900.

Ebskov, B., and Zachariae, L.: Surgical methods in syndactylism. Evaluation of 208 operations. *Acta Chir. Scand.*, *131*:258–268, 1966.

Eckinger, W.: Dag bild der gog. Symbrachydaktylie. *Arch. Orthop. Unfall. Chir.*, *38*:662–669, 1938.

Edwards, J. G.: Syndactylism. *Med. J. Aust.*, *2*:319, 1916.

Ehringhaus: Zur Pathologie und Therapie der Syndaktylie. *Berl. Klin. Wochenschr.*, *49*:421–422, 1912.

Emmett, A. J. J.: Syndactylism of the hand: a review of 60 cases. *Br. J. Plast. Surg.*, *16*:357–375, 1963.

Engdahl, F.: A new surgical procedure for cutaneous syndactylie (In Swedish). *Hygiea.*, *1*:681–683, 1888.

Esser, J. F. S.: Il trapiento epiteliale libro nel trattamento della sindattilie. *Ortop. Tram. App. Mot.*, *6*:158–162, 1934.

Esser, J. F. S., and Raoul: Operation des syndactylies par "Epithelial Inlay." *Rev. Chir. Plast.*, *3–5*:21–32, 1933–1935.

Evans, P. R.: Nuclear agenesis. Möbius syndrome. The congenital facial diplegia syndrome. *Arch. Dis. Child.*, *30*:237–243, 1955.

Falconer, A. W., and Ryrie, B. J.: Report on a familial type of generalized osteosclerosis. *Med. Press Circular*, *195*:12–20, 1937.

Faniel, H.: Syndactylie: modification du procédé de Didot. *Le Scalpel*, *64*:254–258, 1911.

Félizet, G.: Opération de la syndactylie congénitale (procédé autoplastique). *Rev. d'Orthop.*, (1 s.), *3*:49–61, 1892.

Fergesson: Webbed fingers. *Lancet*, *1*:425, 1857.

Fieschi, D.: Contributo alla cura della sindattilie. *Arch. Ital. Chir.*, *37*:204–208, 1934.

Flatt, A.: Treatment of syndactylism. *Plast. Reconstr. Surg.*, *29*:336–341, 1962.

Flynn, J. E.: Congenital anomalies. *In* Flynn, J. E., (ed.): *Hand Surgery.* Baltimore, Williams & Wilkins Co., pp. 29–41, 1966.

Fogh-Anderson, P.: *Inheritance of Harelip and Cleft Palaté.* Copenhagen. Nyt Nordisk Forlag, Arnold Buschk, pp. 11–266; in particular, fig. 68, 1942.

Forni, I.: Il trapiato "a sigaretta" nel trattamento della sindattilia. *Minerva Ortop.*, *9*:197–199, 1958.

Forques, L. D.: Syndactylie membraneuse congénitale du medius et de l'annulaire de deux main; operation. *Arch. Méd. Pharm. Mil.* (Paris), *27*:128–133, 1896.

Fort, J. A.: *Des Difformites Congénitales et Acquises des Doigts.* Paris, A. Delahaye, pp. 61–70, 1869.

Fourrier, P.: Intérét des graffes dermo-épidérmiques dans le traitement des syndactylies. *Rev. Chir. Orthop.*, *39*:370–377, 1953.

Fraccaro, M.: Zigodattilia recessive con manifestaziono differente in due fratelli. *Folia Hered. Pathol.*, *3*:113–114, 1907.

Fuhrmann, W., and Vogel, F.: Zur Genetik der Kombination von Lippen-Kiefer-Gaumen-Spalten und Syndaktylie. *Mschr. Kinderheilkd., 108*:20–23, 1960.

Fulford, G. E., Ardran, G. M., and Kemp, F. H.: Aglossia congenita: Cineradiographic findings. *Arch. Dis. Child., 21*:400–407, 1956.

Fusari, A.: Plastica per sindattilia membranosa. *Minerva Ortop., 5*:260–261, 1954.

Gaudier, and Debeyre: Syndactylie; hypophalangie (Brachydactylie) et index bifide. *Rev. d'Orthop.,* (2 s.), *87*:335–346, 1906.

Gellis, S., and Feingold, M.: Poland's syndactyly. *Am. J. Dis. Child., 110*:85–86, 1965.

Gentés, and Aubaret: Main droite attente de syndactylie congénitale. *J. Méd. Bordeaux, 30*:134, 1900.

Gentés, and Aubaret: Dissection d'une main atteinte de syndactylie. *J. Méd. Bordeaux, 30*:152–153, 1900.

Gentés, and Aubaret: Sur la syndactylie. *Gaz. Hebd. Sci. Méd. Bordeaux, 21*:124–128, 136–138, 1900.

Georg, H.: Technik und Zeitpunkt der operativen Behandlung angeborener Fingermissbildungen. *Ann. Chir. Plast., 9*:170–175, 1964.

Ghisellini, F., and Silva, E.: Die Teknik der "Zigaretten-Plastik" zur Kommissurbildung der Trennung von Syndaktylien. *Z. Orthop., 103*:115–117, 1967.

Gillespie, F. D.: A hereditary syndrome: dysplasia occulo-dento-digitalis. *Arch. Ophthalmol. 71*:187–192, 1964.

Ginestous, E.: *Ophthalmologie Infantile.* Paris, Librairie Octave Doin. pp. 348–349; 455–460, 1922.

Goltz, R. W., Peterson, W. C., Jr., Gorlin, R. J., and Ravitz, H. G.: Focal dermal hypoplasia. *Arch. Dermatol., 86*:708–717, 1962.

Goodman, R. M.: A family with polysyndactyly and other anomalies. *J. Hered., 56*:37–38, 1965.

Gorlin, R. J.: Some facial syndromes. *In* Bergsma, D., (ed.): *Birth Defects: Original Article Series.* New York, National Foundation – March of Dimes, Vol. V. No. 2:65–76; fig. 5, 1969.

Gorlin, R. J., Meskin, L. H., and Geme, J. W.: Oculodentodigital dysplasia. *J. Pediatr., 63*:69–75, 1963.

Gorlin, R. J., Meskin, L. H., Peterson, W. C., Jr., and Goltz, R. W.: Focal dermal hypoplasia syndrome. *Acta Derm. Venereol., 43*:421–440, 1963.

Grebe, H.: Untersuchungen über Papillarlinienveränderungen bei Syndaktylie und Polydaktylie. *Z. Morphol. Anthropol., 39*:62–78, 1940.

Grebe, H.: Syndaktylie, Missbildungen der Gliedmassen. *In* Becker, P. E., (ed): *Humangenetik.* Stuttgart, G. Thieve, pp. 297–304, 1964.

Greig, D. M.: Oxycephaly. *Edinb. Med. J., 33*:189, 280, 357, 1926.

Greig, D. M.: Acrodysplasia. Type: syndactylic oxycephaly. *Edinb. Med. J.,* (n.s.), *42*:537–560, 1935.

Grilli, F. P.: Il trattamento chirurgico della sindattilia congenita della mano. *Arch. Putti, 11*:328–353, 1959.

Grilli, F. P.: La sindattilia congenita della mano. *Arch. Putti, 111*:55–71, 1959.

Gross, F. R., Hermann, J., and Opitz, J. M.: The F-form of acropectoro-vertebral dysplasia: the F-syndrome. *In* Bergsma, D., (ed.): *Birth Defects: Original Article Series.* New York, National Foundation – March of Dimes, Vol. V., No. 3:48–63, 1969.

Groves, E. W. H.: An unusual case of syndactylism. *Br. J. Surg., 1*:143–144, 1913.

Gyergyai, A.: Fall von Syndaktylie, operirt und Geheilt unter dem Lister'schen Verbande. *Cent. Chir.,* No. *1*:1–3, 1879.

Haas, S. L.: Bilateral complete syndactylism of all fingers. *Am. J. Surg., 50*:363–366, 1940.

Hamilton, J. B.: The significance of heredity in ophthalmology, preliminary survey of hereditary eye diseases in Tasmania. *Br. J. Ophthalmol., 22*:19–43; 83–108, 129–148, 1938.

Harker, J.: Malformation of the hands. *Lancet, 2*:389, 1865.

Harrison, M., and Parker, N.: Congenital facial diplegia. *Med. J. Aust., 1*:650–653, 1960.

Heim, W.: Neuere Ansichten über die Enstehung und Behandlung der Syndactylie. *Med. Welt., 14*:481–483, 1940.

Hellström, B.: Congenital facial diplegia. *Acta Paediatr., 37*:464–473, 1949.

Henderson, J. L.: The congenital facial diplegia syndrome: clinical features, pathology and aetiology. A review of 61 cases. *Brain, 62*:381–403, 1939.

Henriet: Syndactylie. *Progrés Méd.* (Paris), *8*:172, 1880.

Hensge, J., Schubert, M., and Stelle, W.: Behandlungsergebnisse einfacher Syndaktylien. *Verh. Dtsch. Orthop. Ges., 55*:421–425, 1948.

Herrmann, J., and Opitz, J. M.: An unusual form of acrocephalosyndactyly. *In* Bergsma, D., (ed.): *Birth Defects: Original Article Series.* New York, National Foundation – March of Dimes, Vol. V. No. 3:39–42, 1969. See also the article entitled "Craniosynostosis and craniosynostosis syndromes" by Herrmann, J., Pallister, P. D., and Opitz, J. M.: *Rocky Mountain Med. J., 66*:45–56, 1969.

Heupel, P.: Syndactylie. *Mntschr. Geburtsh. Gynäk., 63*:11–118, 1923.

Higinbotham, N. L., and Alexander, S. F.: Osteopetrosis. Four cases in one family. *Am. J. Surg., 53*:444–454, 1941.

Hilton: Webbed fingers in a young man. *Lancet, 2*:627, 1857.

Hoffmann, v.: Ein Fall von angeborenem Brustmuskeldefect mit Atrophie des Armes und Schwimmhautbildung. *Arch. Path. Anat. Physiol., 146*:163–172, 1896.

Hsu, C. K.: Hereditary syndactylie in a Chinese family. *Chin. Med. J., 84*:482–485, 1965.

Hurlin, R. G.: A case of inherited syndactyly in man. *J. Hered., 11*:334–335, 1920.

Iselin, F.: Traitement chirurgical des syndactylies congénitales. Résultats d'après 42 observations. *Rev. Prat., 10*:2611–2620, 1960.

Jacobsohn, E.: Ueber Kombinierte Syn- und Polydaktilie. *Beitr. Klin. Chir., 61*:332–350, 1909.

Jayle, and Jarvis: Ectrodactylie des deux pieds, ectrodactylie et syndactylie de la main droite. *Bull. Soc. Anat.* Paris, (5 s.), *12*:139–143, 1898.

Jean, G., and Solcard: Absence partielle du grand pectoral s'accompagnant de brachydactylie et de syndactylie. *Bull. Soc. Anat.* (Paris), *93*:496–497, 1923.

Jeanbrau, L.: Note sur le traitement de la syndactylie, par la procédé de Didot perfectionné. *Rev. d'Orthop.*, (2 s.), 2:39–44; 232–233, 1901.

Joachimsthal, G.: Eine ungewöhnliche Form von Syndaktilie. *Arch. Klin. Chir., 56*:332–338, 1898.

Johnston, O., and Davis, R. W.: On the inheritance of hand and foot anomalies in six families. *Am. J. Hum. Genet., 5*:356–372, 1953.

Johnston, O., and Kirby, V. V.: Syndactyly of the ring and little finger. *Am. J. Hum. Genet., 7*:80–92, 1955.

Jorns, G.: Die Syndaktilie—Operation nach R. Klapp. *Chirurg, 28*:369–373, 1957.

Kettelkamp, D. B., and Flatt, A.: An evaluation of syndactylia repair. *Surg. Gynecol. Obstet., 133*:471–478, 1961.

Kirchmair, H.: Eim Syndaktilie-Stammbaum. *Munch. Med. Wochenschr., 83*:605–606, 1936.

Kirmisson, E.: La syndactylie envisagée au point de vue pathogénique. Deux grand variétes: 10 la syndactylie par arrêt de developpement; 20 la syndactylie d'origine pathologique. *Rev. d'Orthop.*, (1 s.), *10*:271–278; Pl. XV, 1899.

Kirmisson, E.: Un cas de syndactylie membraneuse associée à la brachydactylie. *Rev. d'Orthop.*, (3 s.), 6:409–411, 1919.

Kite, J. H.: Congenital syndactylism of fingers. *S. Afr. Med. J., 51*:160–164, 1958.

Klapp, R.: Demonstrationen aus der praktischen Chirurgie. Die Operation der Syndaktilie. *Arch. Klin. Chir., 177*:688–695, 1933.

Klein, D.: Un cureiux syndrome héréditaire: cheilopalatoschizis avec fistules de la lévre inferieure associé à une syndactylie, une onychodysplasie particuliére, un pterygion poplité unilateral et des pieds varus equins. *J. Genet. Hum., 11*:65–71, 1962–1963.

Klippel, M., and Rabaud, E.: Étu e d'un cas de polysyndactylie. *N. Iconog. Salp., 27*:246–250, 1915.

Könner, D.: Ein Beitrag zur Syndaktilie und ihrer Vererbung. *Mitt. Anthropol. Ges. Wein., 63*:84–90, 1924.

Kremer, K.: Plastische Syndaktiliebehandlung mit einem intrakutan geschnittenen, modifizierten Thiersch'schen Lappen. *Zbl. Chir., 75*:1534–1548, 1950.

Kummer, E.: Syndactylie congénitale; anaplasite d'après la méthode Italienne. *Rev. d'Orthop.*, (1 s.), 2:129–133, 1891.

Lajos, N.: Syndaktilia and perodactylia (Hungarian). *Gyogyaszat., 39*:138, 1899.

Lauber, H. J.: Beitrag zur Behandlung der Syndactylie. *Chirurg.* 7:598–599, 1935.

Legendre, L. Q.: Syndactylie des cinquiemes doigts et absence du cinquieme orteil. *C. R. Soc. Biol.*, (2 s.), *4*:93–94, 1858.

Lehmann, U.: Uber eine Familie mit multiplen Missbildungen an Handen und Fussen: Hochgradige Syndaktilie fehlen einen Binnenstrahles verdopp. u. Brachydaktilie. *Acta. Gen. Med. Gem.* (Roma), 2:87–103, 1953.

Lennander, K. G.: Fall af kongenital syndaktyli, opereradt, med hjelp af Thiersch's hudtransplantationsmetod. *Upsale Lak., Forhandlingar, 26*:151–152, 1891.

Lerno, R.: Note sur un cas de syndactylie congenitales de quatre extremites. *Flandre Med.* (Gand.), 2:225–232, 1 pl., 1895.

Liceaga, F. J.: Un cas de syndactylie complete des mains et des pieds et autres deformations. *Arch. Med. Enf., 4*:448–452, 1937.

Littlewood, J. M., and Lewis, G. M.: The Holmes-Adie syndrome in a boy with acute juvenile rheumatism and bilateral syndactyly. *Arch. Dis. Child., 38*:86–88, 1963.

Lloyd, F. E., and Washburn, F. L.: An instance of webbed fingers in men. *Pop. Sci. Month., 47*:856, 1895.

Longhi, L.: Malformizioni congenite dell mani. *Arch. Ortop., 55*:183–212, 1939.

Longuet, M.: Peids-bots, syndactylie, sillons cutanes, amputation spontanee, survenus pendant la vie intrauterine; lesion d'origine nerveuse. *C. R. Soc. Biol., 28*:100–166, 1876.

Luaces, E. G.: Sindactilia congenita seguida en varias generaciones. *La Ped. Espan., 6*:88–90, 1917.

Lueken, K. G.: Uber eine Familie mit Syndaktilie. *Z. menschl. Vererb. Konstitutionslehre, 22*:152–159, 1938.

Lund, F. B.: A case of web-fingers, associated with curious anomalies of the phalanges, metacarpal bones and fingernails. *Boston Med. Surg. J., 136*:157–158, 1897.

MacCollum, D. W.: Webbed fingers. *Surg. Gynecol. Obstet., 71*:782–789, 1940.

Maeder, G.: Héméralopie et syndactylie familiales. *Ophthalmologica, 111*:278–284, 1946.

Magnan, and Galippe: Accumulation de stigmates physiques chez un debile. Brachycéphalie, plagiocéphalie, acrocéphalie, asymetrie faciale, astrésie buccale, syndactylie des quatre extrémites. *C. R. Hebd. Seances Mém. Soc. Biol., 44*:277–287, 1892.

Maisels, D. O.: Acrosyndactyly. *Br. J. Plast. Surg., 15*:166–171, 1962.

Malhotra, K. C., and Rife, D. C.: Syndactyly and clinodactyly within an Indian kindred. *J. Hered.*, 55:219–220, 1963.

Mallock, J. D.: Brachydactyly and symbrachydactyly. *Ann. Hum. Genet.*, 22:36–37; Pl. 1–5, 1956.

Mancini, G.: Trattamento della sindattilia con trapianto libero. *Minerva Orthop.*, 3:21–22, 1952.

Mansfield, O. T.: Syndactyly. *Br. J. Plast. Surg.*, 13:249–252, 1960–1961.

Manson, J. S.: Hereditary syndactylism and polydactylism. *J. Genet.*, 5:51–63, 1916.

Manson, J. S.: Hereditary syndactylism and polydactylism description of recent additions to pedigree. *Br. Med. J.*, 2:1044 1934.

Manzoni, S., and Lanzi, F.: Note tecniche sul trattamento chirurgico della sindattilia congenita della mano. *Arch. Orthop.*, 76:243–254, 1963.

Martirené, M.: Absence congénitale des muscles pectoraux. *Rev. d'Orthop.*, (2 s.), 4:215–217, 1903.

Messerschmidt, G.: *Über Syndactylie.* Inaug. Diss. Greifswald, Druck von C. Sell, pp. 1–31, 1885.

Meyer-Burgdorff, H.: Eine einfache Plastik bei Syndaktylie. *Zentralbl. Chir.*, 58(1):998–1000, 1931.

Meyran, J.: Report of a case of microphthalmos associated with syndactyly. *Ann. Soc. Mex. Oftal.*, 23:48–52, 1949.

Michail, J., Matsoukas, J., and Theodorou, S.: Pouce bot arcué forte abduction extension et autre symtoms concomitans. *Rev. d'Orthop.*, 43:142–146, 1957.

Miller, P. R.: Syndactyly. *N. Engl. J. Med.*, 269:112–113, 1963.

Minor, L. S.: Several cases of hereditary web-fingers in one family (Russian). *Vrach. St. Petersb.*, 9:121–124, 1888.

Minor, L. S.: Dix-sept cas de syndactylie héréditaire dans une même famille. *Rev. Gen. Clin. Therap.*, 2:113–115, 1888.

Mirabel, A.: *Des malformations des Doigts et des Orteild dans leur Rapports avec l'Hérédité.* Paris, Imp. Nouvelle, pp. 1–60, 1873.

Miyata, P.: Über einen seltenen Fall von Syndaktylie. *Z. Orthop. Chir.*, 29:257–262, 1911.

Möbius, P. M.: Über angeborene doppelseitige Abducens-facialis Lähmung. *Münch. Med. Wochenschr.*, 35:91–94; 108–111, 1888.

Mohr, O. L.: Dominant acrocephalosyndactyly. *Hereditas.*, 25:193–203, 1939.

Mohr, O. L.: A hereditary lethal syndrome in man. *Avh. Norske Videnkad.* (Oslo), 14:1–18, 1941.

Monet, M.: Amputation congénitale et syndactylie. *Bull. Mèm. Soc. Chir.* (Paris), 20:272, 1894.

Montagu, M. F. A.: A pedigree of syndactylism of the middle and ring fingers. *Am. J. Hum. Genet.*, 5:70–72, 1953.

Montgomery-Smith, W. S.: A family history of digital deformities (absence of thumbs and syndactyly of ulnar digits). *Guy's Hosp. Rep.* (35), 30:115–116. 1888.

Morel-Lavallèe, M.: Cas de syndactylie chez l'homme. *C. R. Sea Mém. Soc. Biol.*, pp. 166–167, 1850.

Morestin, H.: Syndactylie. *Bull. Mém. Soc. Chir.* (Paris), 36:762–769, 1910.

Mosongeil, K. V.: Ein Fall von Syndaktylie an den vier Extremitäten. *Arch. Klin. Chir.* 16:522–583, 1874.

Mouchet, A.: Un puzzle osseux dans une syndactylie mèdius et de l'annualire de la main droite. *Press. Méd.*, 48:917, 1940.

Murphy, D. P.: Five successive generations of webbed-finger deformity. *J.A.M.A.*, 84:576–577, 1925.

Nèlaton, A.: *Éléments de Pathologie Chirurgicale.* Tome Sixième. Paris, G. Bailliére et Cie, pp. 1019–1023, 1884.

Nicita: Sindattilia congenita. *Minerva Med.*, 1:346–352, 1936.

Noack, M.: Ein Beitrag zum Krankheitsbild der Akrozephalosyndactylie (Apert). *Arch. Kinderheilkd.*, 160:168–171, 1959.

Norton, A. T.: A new and reliable operation for the cure of webbed fingers. *Br. Med. J.*, 2:931–932, 1881.

Norvig, J.: To Tilfaelde af Akrocephalosyndaktylie hos Soskende. *Hospitalstid.*, 72:165–178, 1929.

Nové-Josserand, C.: Sur une variété anormal de syndactylie. *Rev. d'Orthop.*, 6:405–407, 1918.

Nylen, B.: Repair of congenital finger syndactyly. *Acta. Chir. Scand.*, 113:310–319, 1957.

Oldfield, M. C.: The "horse-shoe" web flap in the treatment of syndactyly. *Br. J. Plast. Surg.*, 1:69–72, 1949.

Ombrédanne, L.: *Technique Chirurgicale Infantile.* Paris, Masson et Cie, pp. 271–274, 1912.

Ombrédanne, L., and Févre, M.: *Précis Clinique et Opératoire de Chirurgie Infantile.* Cinquième edition. Paris, Masson et Cie, pp. 708–713, 1949.

Oppenheimer, B. S., Blackman, N. S., and Grishman, A.: The association of the interatrial septal defect and anomalies of osseous system. *Trans. Assoc. Am. Physicians*, 62:284–293, 1949.

Otto, A. W.: *Monstrorum Sexcontorum Descriptio Anatomicum.* Vratislavia, pp. 313–314; Tab. XXI; figs. 1–12, 1841.

Overman, P.: *Syndaktylie, ihre wesen und ihre Behandlung.* Inaug. Dis.. Bonn, Kolnes, pp. 1–35, 1891.

Owen, W.: Webbed fingers; Norton's operation. *Med. Press Circ.*, (n.s.), 46:59, 1888.

Palma, R.: Modificazione al metodo di Zeller per la cura della sindattilia. *Ann. Ital. Chir.*, 13:1068–1074, 1934.

Papillon-Léage, E., and Psaume, J.: Une malformation héréditaire de la muqueuse buccale brides in freins anormaux. *Rev. Stomatol.*, 55:209–277, 1954.

Papillon-Léage, E., and Psaume, J.: Une nouvelle malformation héréditaire. Dysmorphie des freins buccaux. Huit observations. *Actualites Odento-Stomatol.*, 27:7–27, 1954.

Papillon-Léage, E., and Psaume, J.: Dysplasie bucco-digito-faciale. *Ann. Chir. Infant,* 5:145–150, 1964.

Parham, F. W.: Webbed fingers associated with other congenital deformities. *New Orleans Med. Surg. J.,* (n.s.), *14*:755–757, 1886–1887.

Park, E. A., and Powers, G. F.: Acrocephaly and scaphocephaly with symmetrically distributed malformations of the extremities: a study of the so-called "acrocephalosyndactylism." *Am. J. Dis. Child.,* 20:235–314, 1920.

Park, R.: Syndactylus. *Med. News,* (New York), *68*:41, 1896.

Patterson, T. J. S.: Classification of the congenitally deformed hand. *Br. J. Plast. Surg.,* *17*:142–144, 1964.

Patterson, T. J. S.: Syndactyly and ring constrictions. *Proc. R. Soc. Med.* (Sect. Plast. Surg.), *62*:51–53, 1969.

Pearl, M., Chow, T. F., and Friedman, E.: Poland's syndrome. *Radiology, 101*:619–623, 1971.

Penrose, L. S.: Inheritance of zygodactyly. *J. Hered., 37*:285–287, 1946.

Perkoff, D.: Syndactylism in four generations. *Br. Med. J.,* 2:341–342, 1938.

Peterson, D.: Zur pathogenese der syndaktylie. *Verh. Dtsch. Orthop. Ges., 54*:448–451, 1968.

Pfeiffer, R. A.: Dominant erbliche Akrocephalosyndaktylie. *Z. Kinderheilkd., 90*:301–320, 1964.

Pfeiffer, R. A.: Associated deformities of the head and hands. *In* Bergsma, D., (ed.): *Birth Defects: Original Article Series.* New York, National Foundation–March of Dimes. Vol. V, No. *3*:18–34, 1969.

Picqué, R.: Considerations anatomo-pathologiques, pathogéniques, et opératoires sur la syndactylie. *Rev. d'Orthop.,* (2 s.), *4*:25–47, 1903.

Pieri, G.: Plastica cutanea per retrazioni cicatriziali delle ditta. *Chir. Organi. Mov., 4*:303–306, 1920.

Pieri, G.: Processo operatorio per la cura sindattilia grave. *Chir. Ital., 3–4*:258–265, 1949.

Pipkin, S. B., and Pipkin, A. C.: Two new pedigrees of zygodactyly. Variation of expression of polydactyly. *J. Hered., 37*:93–96, 1946.

Pol, R.: Reduktion der mittelphalangen in kombination mit syndaktylie (einseitige symbrachydaktylie). *Arch. Pathol. Anat. Physiol., 229*:447–472, 1921.

Polaillon: Doigt. *In* Dechambre, A., (ed.): *Dictionaire Encyclopédique de Sciences Médicales.* Paris, G. Masson & P. Asselin et Cie, 30:115–353, 1884.

Poland, A.: Deficiency of the pectoral muscles. *Guy's Hosp. Rep., 6*:191–193, 1841.

Pooley, J. H.: Congenital union of the fingers, with two other cases of the hand. *Illust. Med. Surg.* (New York), 2:119–122, 1883.

Princeteau, M. L.: Nouveau procédé opératoire pour la cure de la syndactylie congénitale. *Rev. Chir., 32*:675–676, 1905.

Radulesco, A. D.: Un nouveau procédé opératoire digito-commissural comme traitement de la syndactylie congénitale. *Rev. d'Orthop.,* (3 s.), *10*:499–502, 1923.

Rahon, J.: Sex-digitaire attent de syndactylie partielle. *Bull. Soc. d'Anthrop.,* (4 s.), *3*:334–336, 1892.

Rasch, H.: Ein fall von Kongenitaler kompleter Syndaktylie un Polydaktylie. *Beitr. Klin. Chir., 18*:537–544, 1897.

Regis, E.: Syndactylie ectrodactylie, clinodactylie chez un demente precose degénéré. *Iconog. Salp., 21*:401–411, 1908.

Resnick, E.: Congenital unilateral absence of pectoral muscles often associated with syndactylism. *J. Bone Joint Surg., 24*:925–928, 1942.

Richards, R. N.: The Möbius syndrome. *J. Bone Joint Surg., 35A*:437–444, 1953.

Robin, P.: Cas de syndactylie. *Bull. Soc. d'Anthrop.,* (3 s.), *12*:124, 1889.

Robinson, G. C., Miller, J. R., and Bensimon, J. R.: Familial ectodermal dysplasia with sensori-neural deafness and other anomalies. *Pediatrics, 30*:797–802, 1962.

Roblot, G.: *La Syndactylie Congénitale.* Paris, Maulde, Doumenc et Cie, pp. 1–45, 1906.

Rocher, Forton, and Guérin: Quatre cas de malformation congénitales de la main. *J. Méd. Bordeaux, 55*:257–260, 1928.

Romer, H.: Einseitige symbrachydaktylie. *Dtsch. Z. Chir., 174*:1–9, 1922.

Roskoschny, E.: Summetrische syndaktylie beider hand und fuss. *Dtsch. Med. Wochenschr., 44*:350–351, 1918.

Rosselli, A., and Gulienetti, R.: Ectodermal dysplasia. *Br. J. Plast. Surg., 14*:190–204; figs. 2 and 25, 1961.

Rosselli, G. S.: La sindattilia chirurgica temporanea nella cura delle retrazioni cicatriziali delle dita. *Minerva Chir., 95*:1280–1285, 1961.

Routier, A.: Syndactylie–Opération par la methode à lambeau dorsal. Guérison. *France Méd., 26*:465–466, 1870.

Rudtorffer, F. S.: *Abhandlung über die Einfachste und Sicherste Operations-Methode eingesperrter leistenund Sghenkelbrüche.* Wien, in der Degenschen Buchhandlung. II Band. pp. 472–487, 1908.

Russo-Travali, G.: Sopra un caso di sindattilia. *Sicilia Med.* (Palermo), *1*:237–240, 1889.

Saethre, H.: Ein beitrag zum turmschadelproblem (Pathogenese, erblichkeit und Symptomatologie). *Dtsch. Z. Nervenheilkd., 119*:533–555, 1931.

Saint-Germain, de: Syndactylie: opération par lá methode a lambeau dorsal; Guérison (Rap. par A. Routier). *France Méd.,* 26:465, 1879.

Savariand: Sur la syndactylie. *Bull. Mém. Soc. Chir.,* (n.s.), *37*:330–331, 1911.

Savariand: Syndactylie par fusion osseuse des dernier phalanges; operation par un procédé special. *Bull. Mém. Soc. Chir.,* (n.s.), *40*:314, 1914.

Schatzki, P.: Über verdeckte syndaktylie, Polydaktylie und über "Triangelbildung" in der menschlichen Mittelhand. *Arch. Orthop. Unfallchir.*, *34*:637–652, 1934.

Schauerte, E. W., and St. Aubin, P. M.: Progressive synosteosis in Apert's syndrome (acrocephalosyndactyly) with a description of the roentgenographic changes in the feet. *Am. J. Roentgenol.* 97:67–73, 1966.

Scherer, F.: Über einen fall von symmetrischen poly- und syndaktylie. *Arch. Kinderheilkd.*, *17*:244–250, 1893–1894.

Schlatter, C.: Die Mendel'Schen Vererbungsgesetze beim Menschen un Hand zweier Syndaktylie—Sämmbäume. *Schweiz. Arzt.*, *44*:255–261, 1914.

Schmitt, E., and Lyrakos, A.: Bericht über einen Fall von tetrameller poly-Syndaktylie kombiniert mit ausgeprager Brachydaktylie. *Z. Orthop.*, *108*:669–678, 1971.

Schultz, A. H.: Zygodactyly and its inheritance. *J. Hered.*, *13*:113–117, 1922.

Scott, W.: Syndactylism with variations. *J. Hered.*, *24*:240–244, 1933.

Senn, N.: Syndactylism. *Chicago Clin. Rev.*, *6*:172, 1896–1897.

Shiller, J. G.: Craniofacial dysostosis of Crouzon. A case report and pedigree with emphasis on heredity. *Pediatrics, 23*:107–112, 1959.

Sibut, P. S.: *De la Syndactylie Congénitale au Point de Vue Opératoire.* Thèse. Strasbourg, E. Huder, pp. 1–33, 1868.

Sigal, E.: Case of syndactyly, ectrodactylie, gigantonychia (Czech). *Casop. Lek. Cesk.*, *71*:329–333, 1932.

Sinclaire, J. G., and McKay, J.: Median harelip, cleft palate and glossal agenesis. *Anat. Rec.*, *91*:155–160, 1945.

Sjovall, H.: Beitrag zur Technik der Syndactylie-Operation. *Chirurg, 17–18*:35, 1946.

Sklodowski, J.: Ueber einen Fall von angeborenem rechtsseitigem Mangel der Musculi pectorales major et minor mit gleichzeitigen Missbildungen der rechten Hand. *Arch. Pathol. Anat. Physiol.*, *121*:600–604; Taf. X; fig. 2, 1890.

Skoog, T.: Syndactyly. A clinical report on repair. *Acta Chir. Scand.*, *130*:537–549, 1965.

Slingenberg, B.: Missbildungen extremitäten. *Arch. Pathol. Anat. Physiol. 193*:1–92, Taf. I and II (Fenestrated syndactyly), 1908.

Smith, J. L., and Stowe. F. R.: The Pierre Robin syndrome (glossoptosis, micrognathia, cleft palate). *Pediatrics, 27*:128–133, 1961.

Sorderberg, B. N.: Congenital absence of the pectoral muscle and syndactylism: a deformity association sometimes overlooked. *Plast. Reconstr. Surg.*, *4*:434–438, 1949.

Stapff, R.: Über eine familie mit erblicher Syn- und Polydaktylie (Hyperphalangie pollicis). *Fortschr. Röntgenstr.*, *34*:531–538, 1926.

Stenstrom, J. D.: Congenital malformations of the extremities. *Can. Med. Assoc. J.*, *51*:325–334, 1944.

Stephan, H.: Beitrag zur operativen behandlung der syndaktylie. *Zentralbl. Chir.*, *68*:794–796, 1939.

Stiles, K. A., and Hawkins, B. A.: The inheritance of zygodactyly. *J. Hered.*, *37*:16–18, 1946.

Stinzing, R.: Der angeborene und erworbene Defect der Brustmuskeln, zugleich ein klinischer Beitrag zur progressiven Muskelatrophie. *Dtsch. Arch. Klin. Med.*, *45*:205–232, 1889.

Stöhr, F. J.: Ein Fall von einseitiger Symbrachydaktylie und Brustwanddefekt mit Amastie als seltener Missbildung. *Z. Morphol. Anthropol.*, *26*:384–390, 1927.

Straus, W. L., Jr.: The nature and inheritance of webbed toes in man. *J. Morphol.*, *41*:427–439, 1925.

Streeter, G. L.: Focal deficiency in fetal tissues and their relation to intrauterine amputation. *Carnegie Inst.*, Washington, Publ. No. 414. 22:1–144, 1930.

Stucke, K.: Über die erscheinungsformen der Symbrachydaktylie und ihre operativen behandlung. *Arch. Klin. Chir.*, *261*:215–232, 1948.

Stucke, K., and Glansmüller, O.: Zur Klassifizierung, Klinik und Behandlung der Syndaktylie. *Arch. Klin. Chir.*, *260*:77–108, 1947.

Stucke, K., and Helbig, H.: Syndaktylie. *In* Schwalbe, E., and Gruber, G. B., (eds.): *Die Morphologie der Missbildungen des Menschen und der Tiere.* Jena, G. Fischer, T 3, Lief. 19, Abt. 1, Kap. 7, Hälfte. 2:809–843, 1958.

Taybi, K., Say, B., Firat, T., and Gürsu, G.: Oculodentodigital dysplasia syndrome. *Acta Paediatr. Scand.*, *60*:235–238, 1971.

Temtamy, S. A.: Carpenter's syndrome; acrocephalopolysyndactyly. An autosomal recessive syndrome. *J. Pediatr.*, *61*:111–120, 1966.

Temtamy, S. A., and Hall, J. G.: Carpenter syndrome (acrocephalopolysyndactyly). *In* Bergsma, D., (ed.): *Birth Defects: Original Article Series.* New York, National Foundation—March of Dimes, Vol. V., No. 3:204–206, 1969.

Temtamy, S. A., and McKusick, V. A.: Synopsis of hand malformations with particular emphasis on genetic factors. *In* Bergsma, D., (ed.): *Birth Defects: Original Article Series.* New York, National Foundation—March of Dimes, pp. 125–184, 1969.

Thomson, J. B.: Hereditary transmission of webbed fingers. *Edinburgh Med. J.*, pp. 501–502, 1858–1859.

Tréves, A.: Syndactylie et polydactylie a charactére familial. *Bull. Mém. Soc. Chir.*, *20*:677–681, 1928.

Troquart, M.: Syndactylie et malformations diverses. *Soc. Med. Chir. Bordeaux Mèm. Bull.*, *61*:61, 1886.

Truswell, A. S.: Osteopetrosis with syndactyly. A morphological variant of Albers-Schonberg's disease. *J. Bone Joint Surg.*, *40B*:208–218, 1958.

Tschudy, E.: Ein Fall von angeborener vollständiger Verwachsung aller 5 Finger. *Dtsch. Z. Chir.*, *35*:567, 1893.

Tubby, A. H.: An operation for webbed fingers. *Br. Med. J.*, *2*:1464–1466, 1912.

Turner, A. H.: Webbed hand with abnormalities of bones. *Br. Med. J.*, *2*:479, 1925.

Valentin, B.: Klinischse Beitrag zum Wesen der Missbildungen. *Arch. Orthop. Unfallchir.*, *28*:385–397; Abb. 1 ("Endogene syndaktylie") Abb. 2 ("amniogene syndaktylie"), 1930.

Velpeau, A. A. L. M.: *New Elements of Operative Surgery*. Translated by P. S. Townsend. New York, Samuels & Wood, Vol. I, pp. 385–387, 1847.

Verdelet, L., and Chavannaz, J.: Un cas de polysyndactylie congénitale. *Arch. Franco-Belge. Chir.*, *25*:934–937, 1922.

Verneuil: Chirurgie de la main — adherence latérale des doigts. *J. Connaissances Medico-Chir.*, *4*:33–38; 113–120; 171–176; 197–202; 421–424; 477–480, 1856.

Viannay: Un cas de syndactylie membraneuse bilateral. *Loire Med.* (St. Etienne), *37*:79–81, 1933.

Villechaise, H. M., and Jean, G.: Quelques points de technique concernant la chirurgie de la syndactylie. *Rev. d'Orthop.*, (3 s.), *14*:241–243, 1927.

Vogel, K.: Über familiäres Auftreten von Polydaktylie und Syndaktylie. *Fortschr. Röntgenstr.*, *20*:443–447, Taf. XXI, 1913.

Vogel, M.: Elastic ligature for cure of webbed fingers. *Am. J. Med. Sci.*, *7*:261–262, 1875.

Vogt, A.: Dyskephalie (Dysostosis craniofacialis, Maladie de Crouzon 1912) und eine neuaritige kombination dieser krankheit mit syndaktylie der 4 extremitäten (dyskephalodaktylie). *Klin. Monatsbl. Augenheilkd.*, *90*:441–454, 1933.

Waardenburg, P. J.: Eine merkwürdige Kombination von angeborene Missbildungen: Doppelseitiger Hydrophthalmus verbunden mit Akrokephalosyndaktylie, Herzfehler, Pseudohermaphroditismus und anderen Abweichungen. *Klin. Monatsbl. Augenheilkd.*, *92*:30–45, 1934.

Walker, J. D., Jr., Meijer, R., and Aranda, D.: Syndactylism with deformity of the pectoralis muscle: Poland's Syndrome. *J. Pediatr. Surg.*, *4*:569–572, 1969.

Walsh, R. J.: Acrosyndactyly. A study of twenty-seven patients. *Clin. Orthop.*, *71*:99–111, 1970.

Weech, A. A.: Combined acrocephaly and syndactylism occurring in mother and daughter. *Bull. Johns Hopkins Hosp.*, *40*:73–76, 1927.

Weidenreich, E.: Die zygodaktylie und ihre Vererbung. *Z. Abstammungsl.*, *32*:304–311, 1923.

Wightman, J.: A pedigree of syndactylie. *J. Hered.*, *28*:421–423, 1937.

Wolff, F.: Ein Fall dominanter Vererbung von Syndaktylie. *Arch. Rass. Gessel. Biol.*, *13*:74–75, 1921.

Wolfflin, E.: Ueber einen Stammbaum von Syndaktylie. *Arch. Rass. Gessel. Biol.*, *17*:412–413, 1925.

Young, E. H.: Absence of sternal origin of the pectoralis major. *Lancet*, *1*:19, 1894.

Zachariae, L.: Syndactyly. *J. Bone Joint Surg.*, *37B*:356, 1955.

Zarnoff, N.: Note sur l'opération de la syndactylie. *Rev. Gén. Clin. Therup.*, *2*:115, 1888.

Zeller, S.: *Abhandlung über die ersten Erscheinungen venerischer Lokalkrankheits-Formen und deren Behandlung, Sammt einer Kurzen Anzeigo zweier neuen Operations-Methoden, nämlich: die angeborenen verwachsenen Finger und die Kastrazion*. Wein, J. G. Binz. pp. 107–111, 1810.

Chapter Thirteen

POLYDACTYLY

On the human hand, digits in excess of five are considered anomalous. The resulting abnormality is called hyper- or polydactyly; it is also referred to as supernumerary digits. The surplus member may have its own separate metacarpal or may stem from the same common basal bone as its neighbor. In many instances, the terminal two phalanges alone are duplicated.

THE THEORY OF ATAVISM AND THE CONCEPT OF DICHOTOMY

In polydactyly there are usually six digits per hand, but a greater number has often been reported. Kerckringii's (1670) polydactylous dwarf had seven digits on the right hand and eight on the left; there were eight toes on the right foot, while the left displayed the heretofore unheard of fecundity of nine—"dexter enim octo, sinister novem inaudita hactenus ostendi foecunditate." We read in the London Medical Gazette (1834) that Thomas Copsey had 14 fingers and that one of his sisters had two surplus digits removed from each hand. Such overabundance of digits has led more than one author to think of polydactylism as an expression of atavism—reversion to the multirayed manus of an earlier animal.

"As the transient forms of the foetus are for the most part comparable to the persistent forms of the lower animals," Vrolik (1849) wrote, "the malformations occasioned by impeded development often acquire a brute appearance." This concept has since been incorporated in the theory of recapitulation, according to which phylogenetic forms are reproduced temporarily during ontogenetic development. Vrolik's statement implies more: it says in effect that phylogenetic forms persist as malformations.

In his discussion of polydactylism, Darwin (1868) expressed indebtedness to Vrolik. Darwin considered supernumerary digits to be "the result of reversion to a remote ancestor." The theory of atavism, sponsored by Darwin, is often evoked in connection with congenital anomalies, but especially in discussion of polydactylism. Advocates of atavism—Verrier (1885), Boinet (1898), Smith and Boulgakoff (1924), Seiferle (1927), among many — regarded polydactylism in man as the racial harking back to a multidigitate manus which presumably existed in a lower species on the evolutionary scale. It is assumed that the five finger formula in man is the result of reduction from a greater number of digits.

Gegenbaur (1880) argued vehemently against Darwin's contention that excess digits were due to reversion to an earlier form; he ascribed surplus fingers and toes to "reduplication" of already existing parts. Jones (1944) had this to say more recently: "Babies are sometimes born with two heads, but this fact affords no safe ground for believing that our single head had been derived from a former condition of polycephaly. In his five fingers and toes, man . . . displays a condition that . . . is the absolute bedrock of mammalian primitiveness." Jones contended that polydactylism in man is caused by addition to the primitive pentadactylic hand rather than by reduction from a multirayed manus. The increase in the number of digits is brought about either by "serial addition" or by "fission of individual members," Jones concluded. Polydactylism is now generally ascribed to an excess of longitudinal segmentation during embryonic life — a process described variously as twinning, duplication, or dichotomy.

THE CONCEPT OF REGENERATION OF DISARTICULATED SUPERNUMERARY DIGIT

It is well known that, in some lower forms, when a segment of the body is severed, the remainder will reproduce the missing part by regeneration. Darwin (1868) thought that amputated supernumerary digits would likewise regenerate. He cited a patient whose surplus digit had twice been "removed by its socket-joint" but again "grew and reproduced a nail." As with the theory of atavism, in fact with almost all his contentions, this view of Darwin allured numerous, unquestioning sophomoric supporters. Once again, Gegenbaur (1880) demurred; he referred to a large number of cases, communicated by German surgeons, "in which there was no regeneration of supernumerary fingers after they had been once amputated." Obviously when a surplus phalanx is removed, leaving its cartilaginous epiphysis behind, the latter will produce bone, but surely no nail as claimed by Darwin.

INCIDENCE

According to Tapie (1885), during the year 1884 in the Maternity Hospital of Paris, 2200 babies were born and five of these were polydactylous. Shapiro et al (1958) surveyed 30,398 consecutive births between January 1, 1952, and December 31, 1955, and found 2 white and 78 black polydactylous babies. Simpkiss and Lowe (1961) estimated that 1.4 per cent of babies born in Mulaga Hospital, Kampala, Uganda, were polydactylous.

Polydactylism has been reported from almost every country and continent. No race is immune. Johnston (1910) found polydactylism to be more common among black than white or yellow peoples; it was especially prevalent among Bahama Negroes. Danforth (1918) described a pedigree of pedunculated postminimus and regarded this type of extra digit as common among Negroes. Handforth (1950) found 14 cases of polydactyly among 5842 Chinese prisoners in Hong Kong. Frazier (1960) surveyed the records of live births in Baltimore between the years 1954 and 1958: there were 200 polydactylous babies, 179 of which were black and 21 white; the incidence of polydactylism among Negroes was 3.4 per 100. Mellin (1963) estimated that the incidence of polydactylism per 10,000 was 106.8 among the Negro population, but only 15.6 among the white population. "The occurrence of polydactylia is obviously more common in the Negro race," Mellin wrote. He placed the incidence among Orientals between the rates for blacks and whites. Polydactylism is said to occur twice as often in males as in females.

ENDEMIC POLYDACTYLISM

Devay (1862) credited a scientist by the name of A. Potton with the story that toward the end of the eighteenth century, in Izeaux, in the mountains of Isere, the entire population consisted of hexadactylous members. Devay ascribed this preponderance of polydactylism to consanguineous marriages. Boinet (1898) mentioned a family named Foldi from one of the isolated Arab tribes of Hyamites. All members of this family were hexadactylous; when, on occasion, a child was born with five fingers, it was considered an *adulterin*, a bastard. Dubreuil-Chambardel (1925) traced this story to a report given by Dr. Avia in 1886. The patriarchal family of Foldi, we are told, lived on the southern tip of the Arabian peninsula.

Sysak (1928) spoke of the hearth of polydactyly in the Poltava government. He particularized a village called Jitnik. This village was populated mainly by a large family bearing the surname Jetniki. There was another family by the name of Siomak. "The family Siomak (*siomy* means seven in Ukranian) had received this surname because each member . . . had seven fingers on each hand," Sysak wrote. "When the Jetnikis married Siomaks and the Siomaks married Jetnikis the children born from such marriages had six fingers." Siomaks then went to live in the village of Krivak, and there produced a generation of men and women with six to seven digits on each hand.

DeLinares (1930) visited the town of Cervera de Buitrago, near Madrid. This small community consisted of only 150 members, and more than 100 of them were hexadactylous. The supernumerary finger sprang from the side of the thumb. It was "sometimes united with it at the second phalanx and sometimes separated from it." Daisy Bates (1938) spoke of "six-fingered and six-toed" aborigines who had lived between Eucla and Eyre, in Australia. They were seen around this area as late as the 1860s. "They later came down from the Peterman Ranges and inter-married with five-fingered groups. These men were believed to have transmitted their peculiarity to their offspring," Bates wrote.

It may well be that the gene responsible for endemic polydactylism eventually becomes disseminated. Bénard (1916 to 1918) recorded the pedigree of a polydactylous family. The progenitor of this family originally came from the village of Colombes in Isere, not far from Izeaux, the center of polydactylism mentioned by Devay (1862). Almost 100 years after Devay's report, Lyonnet (1961) reported another polydactylous family whose ancestors came from

Izeaux. Shevkenek and Thomson (1933) charted the pedigree of a hexadacty-lous family in Saskatchewan. Previous generations of this family had lived in Bukowina, which is not far from the hearth of polydactylism in Poltava mentioned by Sysak (1928). Isolated cases of polydactyly are ascribed to mutant genes. Recessive polydactyly is usually syndromic.

POLYDACTYLISM IN THE EMBRYO AND IN TWINS

Lineback (1921) studied a 22-mm. embryo which showed an extra thumb. Bossy and Sabby (1966) reported a 48-mm. embryo with a bifid pollex. "A healthy woman of 25 gave birth to twin sons at her first labor," Veitch (1928) wrote. "Not content with this munificence, she had given to each twin six toes on each foot and one well-formed supernumerary finger, whilst one had also the rudiments of a second supernumerary finger. . . . There has been no case of polydactylism in the mother's family but the father had one brother who was born with supernumerary thumb." Ruhl (1938) described another pair of twins, each one of whom had bilateral postminimus.

PEDIGREES

In 1930 in the city of Batum, Manoiloff (1931) saw a man who bore the same name as the Roman general Scipio Africanus (185–129 B.C.). Manoiloff's patient had six fingers on each hand and six toes on each foot. The patient admitted that the peculiarity was transmitted hereditarily in his family. His ancestors had originally come from Italy to Poland and then to Russia. "The origin of this family at large," Manoiloff wrote, "is said to have been traced to Scipian the African, who lived over 200 years before our era and according to the historical data, had likewise six fingers and six toes." If this story could be verified, Gates (1946) commented, it would follow that hexadactyly had been transmitted in this line for over 2000 years and that the name Scipio had survived through some 80 generations.

Manoiloff's might be the longest pedigree, but the one recorded by Morand (1773) is more instructive. It concerns a Maltese family named Kalleia. Gratio Kalleia was born with six fingers on each hand and six toes on each foot. He had three sons and one daughter named, respectively, Salvadore, George, André, and Marie. Salvadore had twelve fingers and twelve toes like his father. George's surplus digit was fused with his thumb; he also had bifid great toes. André was unaffected. Marie had bifid thumbs and big toes like George. Salvadore had three sons and one daughter: the two sons and the daughter each had twelve fingers and twelve toes like their father and grandfather. Salvadore's third son was unaffected like his uncle André. George had three daughters and one son. Two daughters were affected like their grandfather; the third daughter had six toes on one foot only; the son was unaffected. André had numerous children; they were all unaffected like himself. Marie had two daughters and two sons, and only one son was partly affected—like his cousin George's daughter, he had six toes on one foot only. The responsible gene in this pedigree appears to be dominant, with variable expressivity and reduced penetrance in Marie's progeny.

There are now over 100 recorded pedigrees of polydactyly. In the great majority of these, the trait is transmitted as an autosomal dominant. Snyder (1929) reported a Negro family with postaxial polydactyly. He spoke of "a set of critical matings" involving a woman who had several normal children by a normal man whose family had never shown polydactylism; she had one illegitimate polydactylous child by a man who himself showed the abnormality. Snyder thought the evidence in this pedigree met the criteria of recessiveness. Shevkenek and Thomson (1933) reported a white family, several members of which had partially duplicated little fingers. The trait in this family was said to be "inherited as a simple autosomal recessive." These authors confused reduced penetrance with recessiveness. Postaxial polydactyly is a feature of several recessive syndromes: Ellis-van Crevald chondroectodermal dysplasia and Laurence-Moon-Bardet-Biedl syndrome, among others.

MORPHOLOGICAL TYPES

In the hand, the surplus digit lies either on the side of the thumb or on the side of the little finger. In the former location, it is said to be pre-axial; in the latter situation, it is described as being postaxial. Duplication of one of the central digits was given the epithet *intercalary* by Béchet (1851) and is qualified by the adjective *central* by more recent authors. This variety is rare in the hand and when it occurs, it seems to favor the index or the ring finger. Most bifid or bifurcated terminal phalanges are marginal, either pre- or postaxial. Occasionally, pre- and postaxial polydactyly will occur in the same hand. Rarely one hand presents pre-axial and the other postaxial polydactyly (Figs. 13–1 to 13–10).

Horne (1838) described a woman who had "six fingers on each hand. That which occupies the natural situation of the thumb resembles the index finger; or, in other words, that which ought to be a thumb is a finger of three phalanges, on the radial side of which is a sixth or supernumerary digit, precisely similar in size and shape to the little finger so that instead of fourteen phalanges and five metacarpal bones, there are eighteen phalanges and six metacarpal bones." Patients with two pre-axial digits, each equipped with its own metacarpal and three phalanges and acting as thumbs, have also been reported by Vidal (1865), Damourette (1890), Desnoyers and Ill (1924), and Penhallow (1928). James and Lamb (1963) described a father and two sons with hexadactylic hands and no thumbs (Fig. 13–11).

In the literature, one runs across the recurrent controversy as to whether pre- or postaxial polydactyly is more prevalent. Müller (1937), who studied mainly German patients, considered pre-axial polydactyly more frequent than the postaxial variety. Handforth (1950) found duplication of the thumb most common in the southern Chinese. In Barsky's (1958) series, probably consisting mostly of Caucasians, pre-axial polydactyly prevailed. As noted, polydactyly is 10 times more common in blacks than in whites, and blacks seem to have been excluded from these statistics, as has syndromic polydactyly, which is preeminently postaxial.

In either pre- or postaxial polydactyly, the surplus digit may contain well-

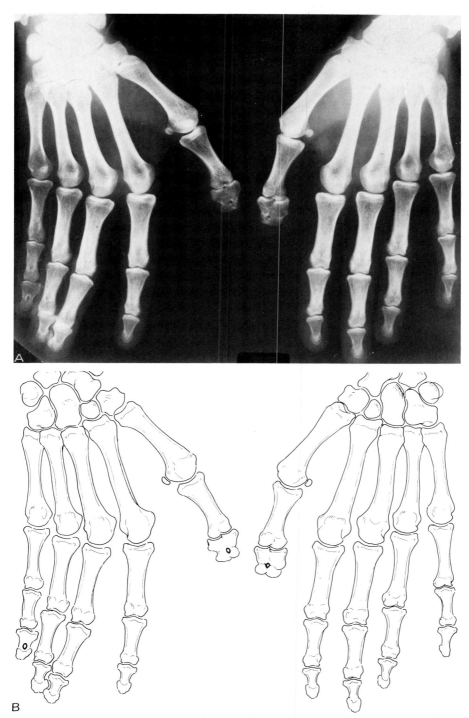

Figure 13–1 Pre-axial polydactyly: incipient form. *A*, Dorsopalmar roentgenograph of the hands, showing broad perforated distal phalanges of the thumbs. The ungual phalanx of the right little finger is also perforated. The right middle and ring fingers were webbed in this case; both thumbs have partly duplicated (or partly coalesced) short ungual phalanges, giving the effect of stubbing. *B*, Interpretative sketch.

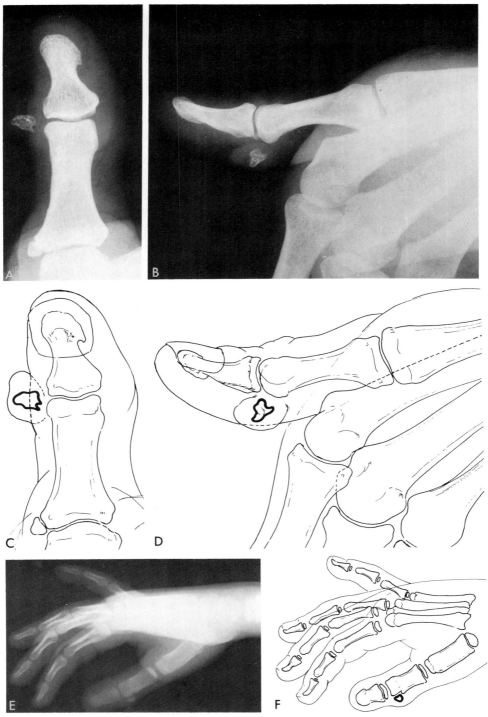

Figure 13–2 Pre-axial polydactyly: abortive and concealed forms. *A*, Dorsal roentgenograph of the right thumb of an adult. *B*, Side view of the same. *C* and *D* are sketches illustrating *A* and *B*, respectively. *E*, Lateral roentgenograph of the hand of a six-year-old male who has had a "bump" on the side of his right thumb since birth: note the ossicle on the radial aspect of the distal end of the proximal phalanx of the thumb. *F*, Sketch illustrating the same.

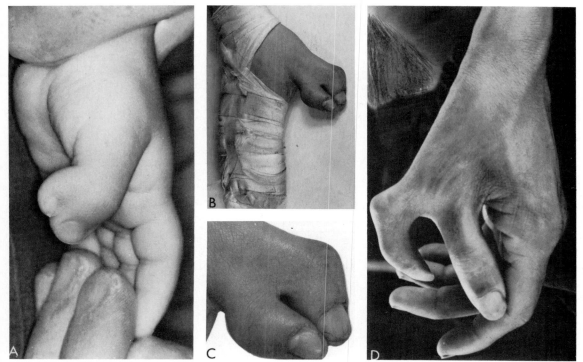

Figure 13–3 Pre-axial polydactyly: bifid and bifurcate thumbs. *A,* Bifid left thumb. *B,* Bifurcate right thumb (the bandage covers lacerated ulnar digit). *C,* Enlarged view of the terminus of the same. *D,* Bifurcate left thumb with deeper commissure and diverging sets of phalanges.

formed phalangeal bones or thin slivers. Pedunculated postminimus is usually devoid of an osseous core and may hang by a threadlike pedicle. Bifid digits may share the same nail or support separate nails. Two sets of phalanges may be enveloped in a single sleeve of skin or each may have its own individual encasement and diverge from its mate, the two together forming a V. In some instances, a pair of digits will assume the configuration of parentheses. More commonly, one digit lies along the axis of the metacarpal, while the other slants sideways. Popham (1867) reported a trifid little finger, and Desnoyers and Ill (1924) described a trifid thumb. Trifid digits are very rare.

Béchet (1851) stated that bifurcated digits shared common extensor and flexor tendons. Lorain (1852) dissected a hand with a supplementary thumb. He found that both digits were supplied by collateral nerves and arteries; the flexor pollicis longus ran directly to the central thumb; the long extensor did the same, but sent a small fibrous band to the marginal pollex; the long abductor and the short extensor were attached to the surplus thumb; and the thenar muscles were atrophic. Chuquet (1876) described a bifurcated thumb in which the common flexor tendon split in two to supply the diverging digits; the terminal segments of the thumb could flex only in unison, never independently. The radial artery was very thin and terminated at the level of the anatomical snuffbox; the ulnar artery was sizable and supplied the whole hand.

(Text continued on page 422.)

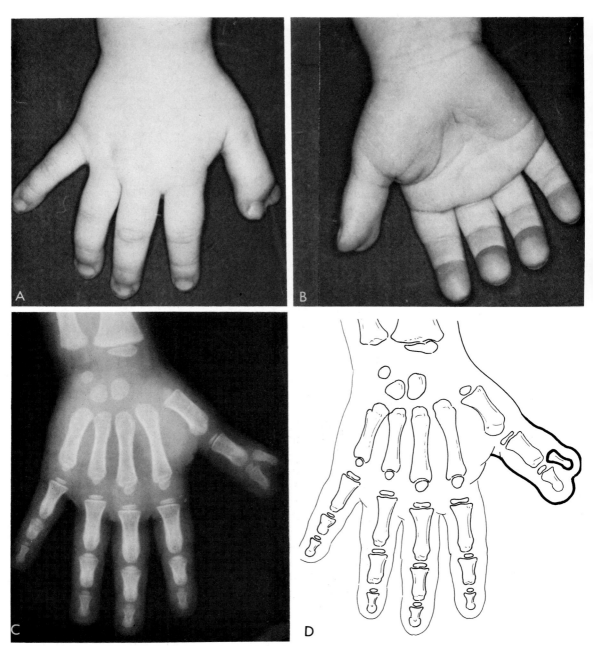

Figure 13-4 Bifid thumb. *A*, Palmar view of the right hand of a three-year-old child. *B*, Dorsal view of the same. *C*, Dorsopalmar roentgenograph: note that the ulnar component of the bifid ungual digit has an epiphysis while its radial neighbor lacks one. *D*, Sketch illustrating the same.

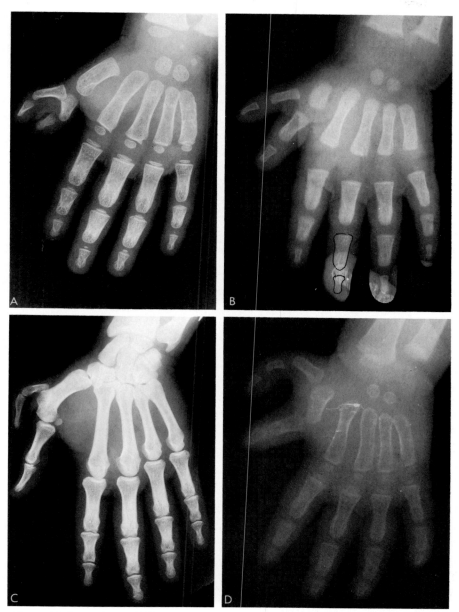

Figure 13–5 Varieties of bifurcate thumb as seen in roentgenographs. In *A*, the base of the radial component of the bifurcate thumb barely reaches the line of the metacarpophalangeal joint; in *B*, it approaches, and in *C*, it bypasses the head of the first metacarpal. In *D*, the radial component of the bifurcate pollex has its own metacarpal which extends as far proximally as the carpometacarpal junction.

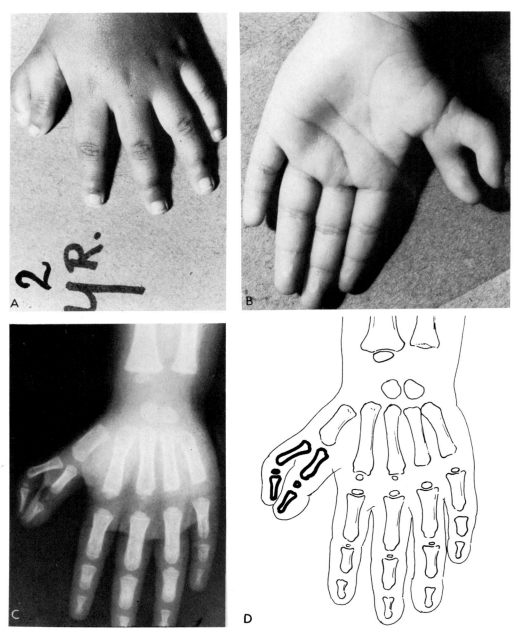

Figure 13–6 Bifurcate thumb. *A*, Dorsal photograph of the left hand of a three-year-old male. *B*, Palmar view. *C*, Dorsopalmar roentgenograph. *D*, Illustrative sketch.

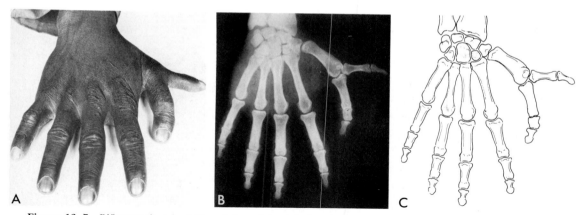

Figure 13–7   Bifurcate thumb. *A*, Dorsal view of the right hand of an adult. *B*, Dorsopalmar roentgenograph of the same: note that the ulnar component of the bifurcate digit has three phalanges. *C*, Sketch illustrating the same.

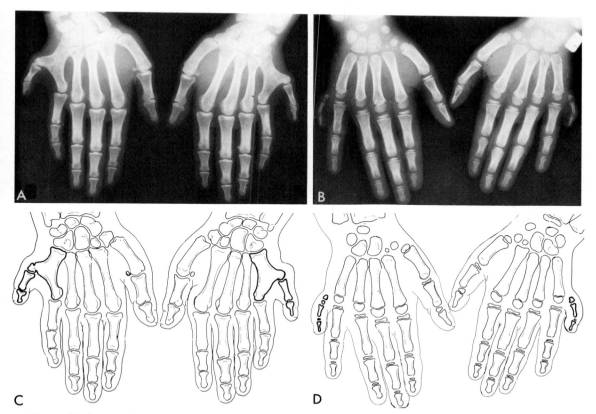

Figure 13–8   Postaxial polydactyly. *A*, Dorsopalmar roentgenograph of the hands, showing bilateral, bifurcated little fingers stemming from a massive forked metacarpal. *B*, Bilateral, dangling, surplus postaxial digits containing vestigial bones. *C* and *D*, Sketches illustrating the roentgenograph above each.

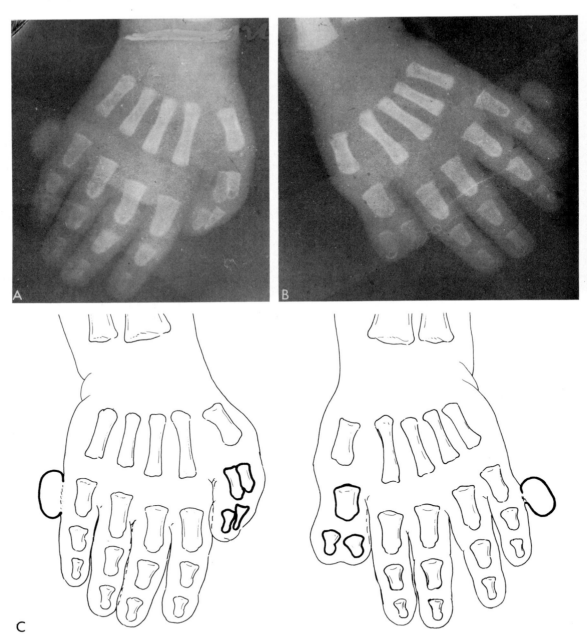

Figure 13–9   Pre-axial polydactyly associated with pedunculated postminimus of each hand. *A* and *B*, Dorsopalmar roentgenographs of the hands of a newborn infant. *C*, Sketches illustrating the same.

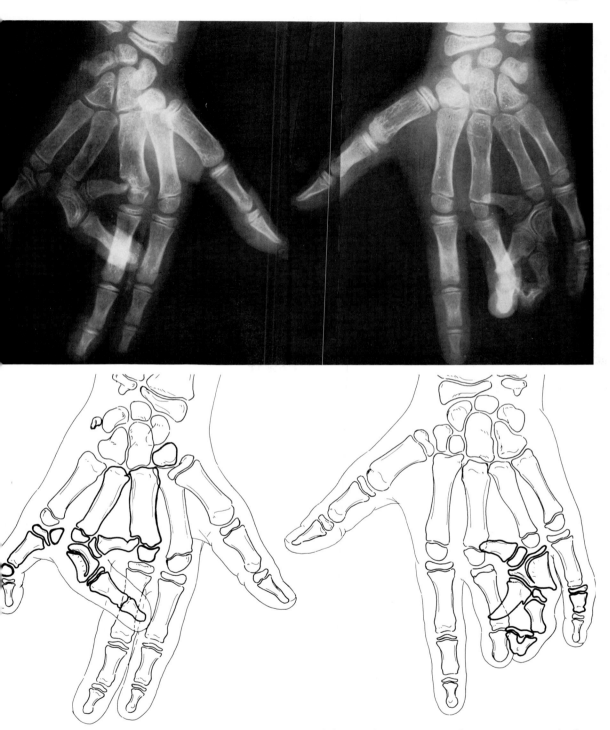

Figure 13–10 Central polydactyly: bilateral polyphalangy of the ring finger. *A*, Dorsopalmar roentgenograph of the hands: note that only a single supernumerary phalanx sprouts from a semicircular bone which is taken to be the proximal phalanx of the right ring finger; from the corresponding basal bone of the left ring finger emanate two extra phalanges, and the ungual segment of this digit is bulky — it probably represents two phalanges which have effected side-to-side osseous union. *B*, Sketch of *A*.

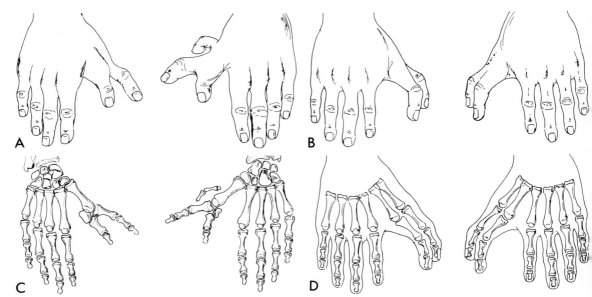

Figure 13–11   Pre-axial opposable extra digits. *A*, Drawing of the hands described by Desnoyers and Ill (1924). *B*, Drawing of the hands of Penhallow's (1928) case. *C* and *D* are sketches of the roentgenographs of the hands above each.

ASSOCIATIONS

Polydactyly is often bilateral and frequently exhibits serial homology affecting both hands and feet. In some instances, only one limb is affected; in others, two, three, or even four extremities are polydactylous. The giant of Goth mentioned in the Bible (II Samuel 1:20) "had on every hand six fingers and on every foot six toes." As pointed out by Hutchinson (1893), Kerckringii's (1670) "monstrum polydactylum" was a short-limbed dwarf (Figs. 13–12 to 13–16).

Polydactyly is seen in association with several regional anomalies of the hand. Perhaps the most common local accompaniment of polydactylism is syndactyly. In some cases, the thumb is missing, being replaced by two opposable triphalangeal digits. Triphalangeal thumb is not an uncommon contralateral accompaniment of polydactyly. Cases of mirror and multiple hands—to be taken up in Chapter Fourteen—are *ipso facto* polydactylous. Polydactyly is also seen in a number of syndromes (Figs. 13–17 to 13–20).

CHROMOSOMAL ABERRATIONS

Bartholini (1657) spoke of a child with absent eyes, a maldeveloped mouth, and six digits on each hand and foot. Anophthalmia (microphthalmia) and hexadactyly, with or without cleft lip-palate, has since been reported in cases of trisomy 13–15. Patau et al (1960) presented a female child whose chromosome count was 47; the extra unit seemed to belong to the group of medium-sized

(Text continued on page 431.)

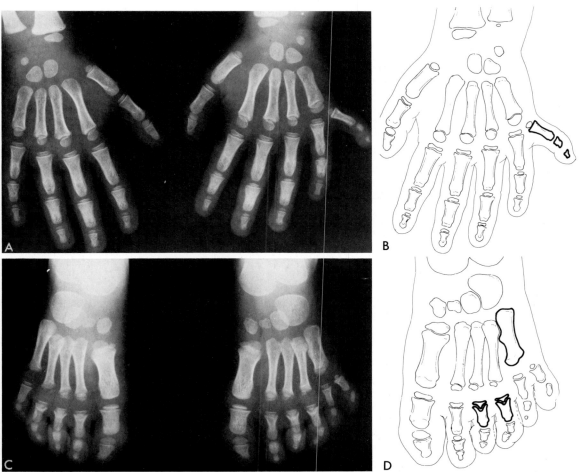

Figure 13–12   Unilateral postaxial polydactyly of the hand associated with an extra digit on the postaxial aspect of the ipsilateral foot. *A*, Dorsopalmar roentgenograph of the hands. *B*, Sketch illustrating the skeletal components of the left hand. *C*, Dorsoplantar roentgenograph of the feet. *D*, Sketch illustrating the skeletal components of the left foot; note the irregularly shaped fifth metatarsal and the cone-shaped epiphyses of the basal phalanges of the third and fourth toes.

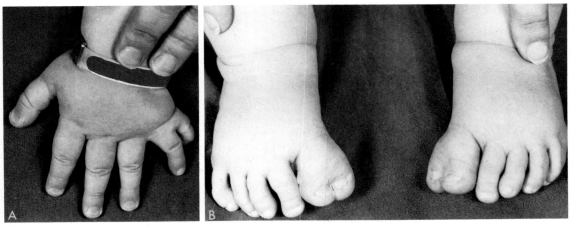

Figure 13–13   Unilateral postaxial polydactyly of the hand associated with bilateral pre-axial polydactyly of the feet. *A*, Dorsal view of the hand of a 13-month-old infant. *B*, Dorsal view of the feet.

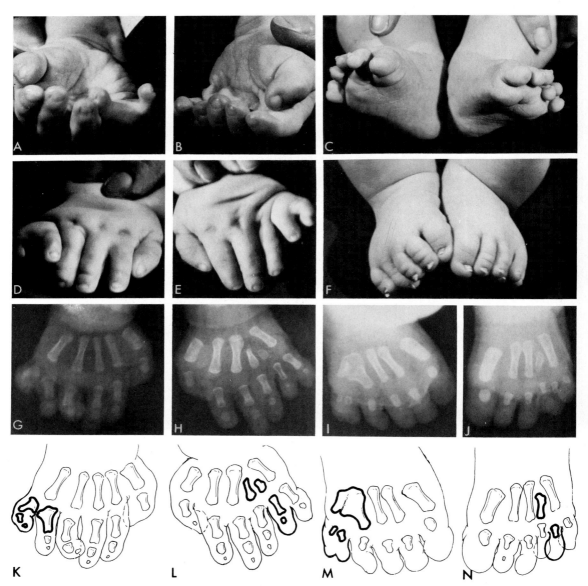

Figure 13–14   Postaxial polydactyly of the hands, simulating serial homology. *A* and *B*, Frontal views of the right and left hands of a two-month-old female infant. *C*, Frontal view of the feet. *D*, Dorsal view of the right hand. *E*, The same of the left hand. *F*, Oblique view of the feet. *G*, Dorsopalmar roentgenograph of the right hand, showing postaxial polydactyly. *H*, Dorsopalmar roentgenograph of the left hand: the fourth and fifth metacarpals have no proximal halves. *I*, Dorsoplantar roentgenograph of the right foot, showing confluence of the fourth and fifth metatarsals and bifid little toe. *J*, Roentgenograph of the left foot, showing a vestigial fourth digital ray and bifid little toe. *K, L, M,* and *N* illustrate roentgenographs above each.

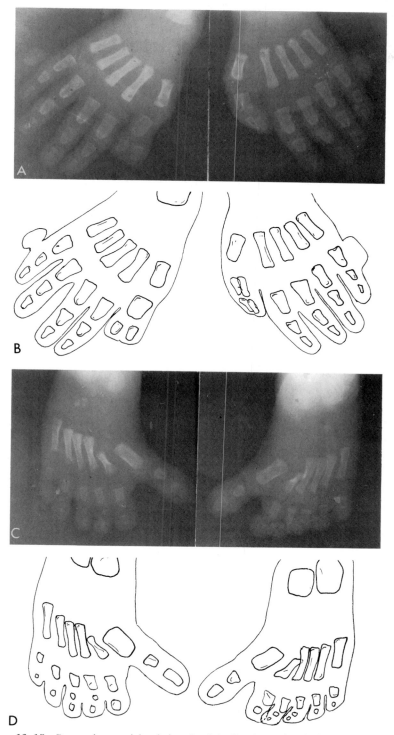

Figure 13–15   Pre- and postaxial polydactyly of the hand associated with bilateral hallux varus and central polydactyly of the feet. *A*, Dorsopalmar roentgenograph of the hands of a newborn infant. *B*, Sketch illustrating the same. *C*, Dorsoplantar roentgenograph of the feet. *D*, Sketch illustrating the same.

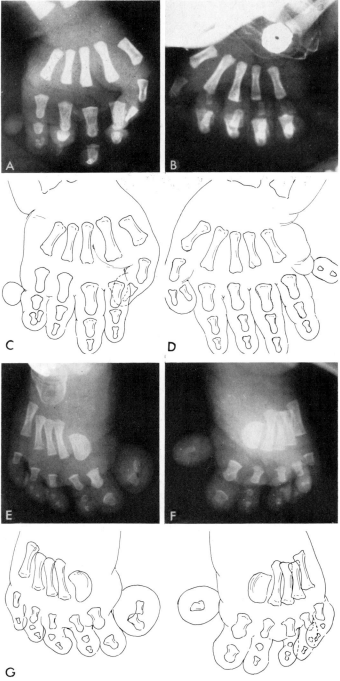

Figure 13–16   Pre- and postaxial polydactyly of the hands associated with pedunculated pre-axial polydactyly of the feet. *A*, Dorsopalmar roentgenograph of the right hand, showing pedunculated boneless postminimus; the distal segment of the little finger contains two phalanges. *B*, Dorsopalmar roentgenograph of the left hand with bifid thumb and a postminimus which contains two small ossicles. *C* and *D* illustrate roentgenographs above each. *E*, Dorsoplantar roentgenograph of the right foot, showing an extra bulbous toe which contains two bones and has a proximal ring constriction. *F*, Here the extra pre-axial toe is also pedunculated and tumefied but contains only one bone. *G* illustrates *E* and *F*.

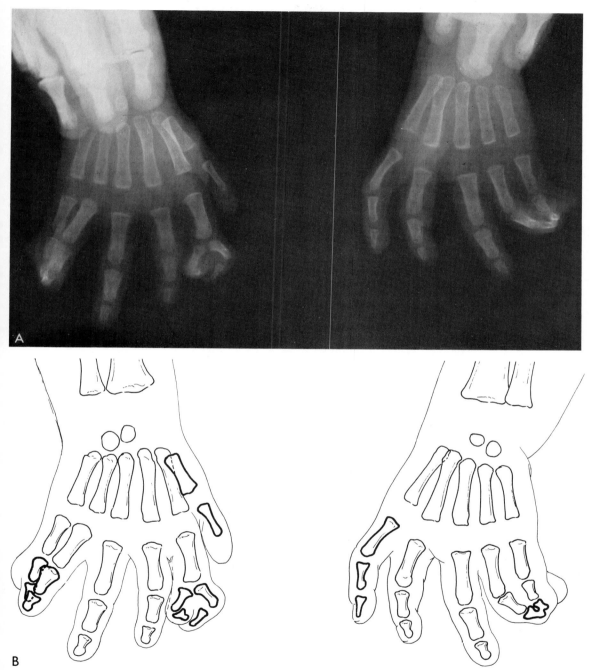

Figure 13–17 Child with six digital rays in the right hand: the radialmost digit of this hand has a short metacarpal and only a proximal phalanx; the second digit is bifurcate, and the last two ulnar digits are webbed. The left hand has five digital rays, the most radial of which has three phalanges, and the ungual phalanges of the fourth and fifth are fused. There is a fleshy tumescence on the ulnar tip of the fifth ray. *A*, Dorsopalmar roentgenograph of the hands. *B*, Sketch illustrating the same.

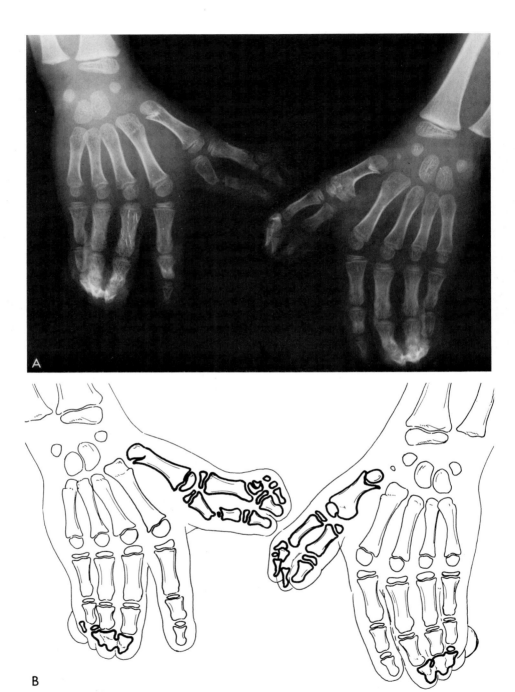

Figure 13–18 Pre-axial polydactyly associated with terminal osseous syndactyly of the last three ulnar digits of each hand. *A*, Dorsopalmar roentgenograph of the hands. *B*, Sketch illustrating the same.

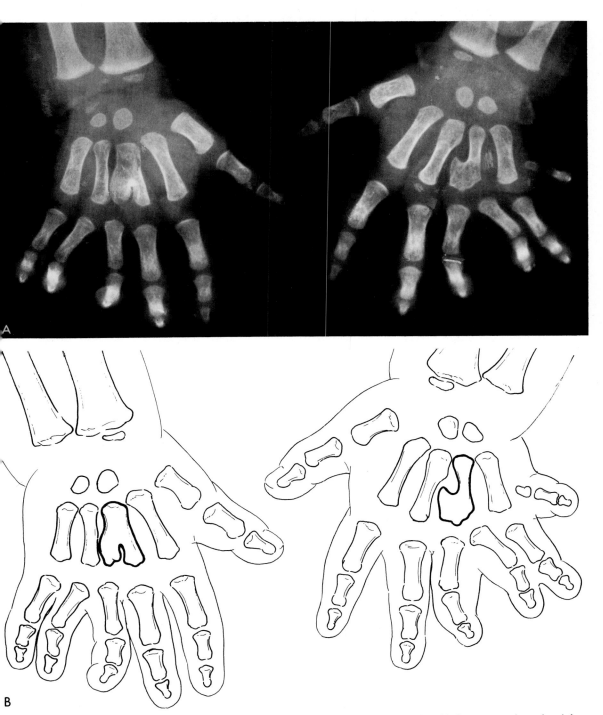

Figure 13–19 Postaxial polydactyly associated with attempts at duplication of the third metacarpal on the right hand and the fourth metacarpal on the left hand. *A,* Dorsopalmar roentgenograph of the hands of a two-year-old child. *B,* Sketch illustrating the same.

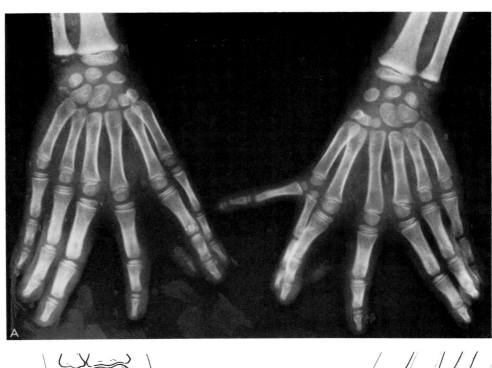

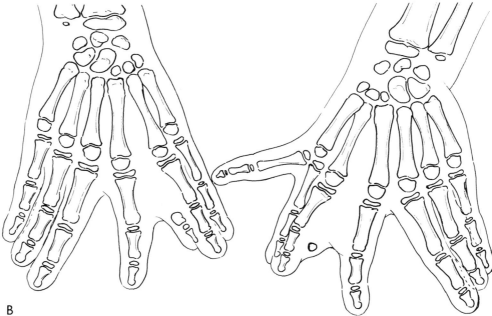

Figure 13–20   Polydactyly associated with syndactyly. *A*, Dorsopalmar roentgenograph of the hands of a seven-year-old child with pre-axial polydactyly and a supernumerary carpal bone. *B*, Sketch illustrating the same.

acrocentric autosomes — the D or 13–15 group. The child reported by Lubs et al (1961) had polydactyly of both hands and the left foot. Erkman et al (1965) described another child with extra rudimentary digits on both hands. Fogh-Anderson (1967) reported two cases of trisomy 13–15 with facial cleft and postaxial polydactyly. This complex is variously referred to in the literature as Bartholini-Patau syndrome, Patau syndrome, trisomy 13–15, or D_1 trisomy.

Popham (1867) described a polydactylous infant who had a fissure in the occipital bone through which protruded the membrane of the brain. Morton (1947) reported a neonate with arhinencephalia (absence of the olfactory lobe) who had "six digits on each limb and absence of testes." The auricles were of the cauliflower type; the pupils showed bilateral medial coloboma; the occiput was edematous and discolored; and radiological examination revealed defects in the posterior and superior parts of the parietal bones. A newborn boy described by Biles et al (1970) had similar malformations: his cytogenic and autoradiographical studies showed a D_1 ring chromosome in 88 per cent of the metaphases; both hands were "clinodactylous with extra digits."

DEFECTIVE TIBIA AND POLYDACTYLY

Pedal polydactyly is not an uncommon accompaniment of an absent or hypoplastic tibia. In the hand, nonopposable triphalangeal thumb is more common. Reber (1968) described a patient whose extra little fingers had been amputated. In the family reported by Eaton and McKusick (1969), a one-day-old female had "polydactyly of all four limbs and very hypoplastic tibia."

ELLIS-VAN CREVELD CHONDROECTODERMAL DYSPLASIA

Baisch (1931) described a child with congenital anonychia, irregular eruption of the teeth, and postaxial polydactyly of both hands. McIntosh (1933) reported a white girl with "hereditary ectodermal dysplasia, associated with polydactylism and chondrodystrophy." The proband had short arms and legs, defective teeth, and rudimentary nails. Ellis and van Creveld (1940) presented three patients with ectodermal dysplasia affecting the hair, teeth, and nails; postaxial polydactyly; chondrodysplasia; and congenital morbus cordis. Two patients were female and one was male; the parents of two cases were first cousins. No similar condition had been seen in the relatives. The trait is an autosomal recessive. Numerous cases of Ellis-van Creveld syndrome have since been reported from many countries, involving almost all races. The Amish of Lancaster County, Pennsylvania, contain the largest concentration of this trait. The pedigree of this clan was detailed by McKusick et al (1964) (Figs. 13–21 and 13–22).

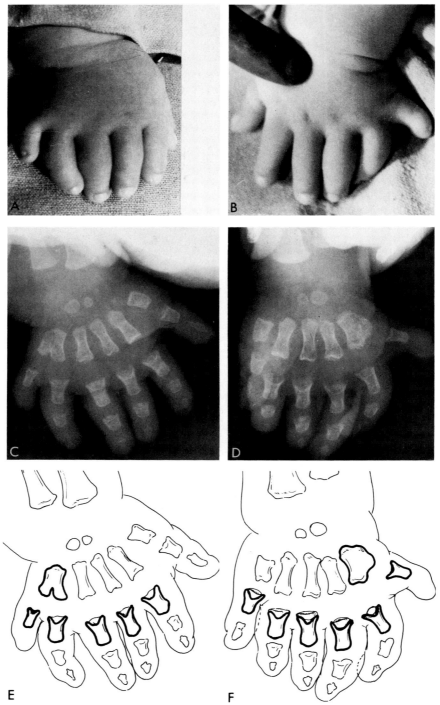

Figure 13–21 Ellis-van Creveld chondroectodermal dysplasia. *A* and *B*, Dorsal views of the right and left hands of an eight-month-old female with postaxial polydactyly. *C*, Roentgenograph of the right hand, showing incomplete fusion of the fifth and sixth metacarpals; the supernumerary digit possesses only one phalanx. *D*, Roentgenograph of the left hand: here there is complete fusion of the fifth and sixth metacarpals. In both *C* and *D*, metaphyses of the proximal and middle phalanges are cup-shaped. *E* and *F* illustrate roentgenographs above each.

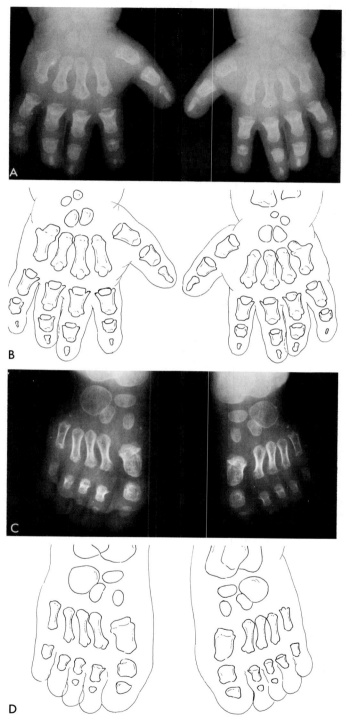

Figure 13–22 Ellis-van Creveld syndrome. *A*, Dorsopalmar roentgenograph of the hands of a five-year-old child with incipient postaxial polydactyly represented by the following: a spur emanating from the base of each fifth metacarpal, a thick metacarpal of each thumb and its proximal phalanx, thick proximal and middle phalanges of the lesser digits, cone-shaped epiphyses, and attenuated ungual phalanges. *B*, Sketch illustrating the same. *C*, Dorsoplantar roentgenograph of the feet, showing chondrodystrophic changes of some tubular bones but no polydactyly. *D*, Sketch illustrating the same.

INFANTILE THORACIC DYSTROPHY
(Familial Asphyxiating Thoracic Dystrophy; Jeune's Syndrome)

This complex is probably a variant of Ellis-van Creveld chondroectodermal dysplasia. In both, the inheritance is autosomal recessive and polydactyly is postaxial; congenital heart disease and defective teeth and nails are other common features. In infantile thoracic dystrophy, chondrodystrophic changes seem to affect the ribs most severely, resulting in a diminutive thoracic cage which is responsible for extraordinary respiratory distress and consequent pulmonary infections. The affected child usually dies soon after birth. Survival was reported by Maroteaux and Savart (1964) and by Hanissian et al (1967).

INTERATRIAL SEPTAL DEFECT AND POLYDACTYLY

Oppenheimer et al (1949) described a man who had achondroplasia, polydactyly of the hands, and interatrial septal defect. His grandson presented the following anomalies: achondroplasia, polydactyly, syndactyly, interatrial septal defect, and mitral stenosis. This complex may be another variant of Ellis-van Creveld chondroectodermal dysplasia.

OCULODIGITAL COMPLEXES

Polydactyly of the hand has been reported in association with anophthalmia/microphthalmia by Collins (1886), Heinberg (1926), Yudkin (1928), Hippel (1934), Harris and Thomas (1937), Ciotola (1938), and Appelbaum and Marmelstein (1943); with aniridia by Bornstein (1952); and with congenital cataract by Appenzeller (1884), Manson and Nettleship (1917), and Rieger (1941). Feichtinger (1943), Ullrich (1951), and some other German authors have described a syndrome called dyscranio-pygo-phalangy. This complex is said to consist of microphthalmia with deep-set eyes and narrow fissures between the lids, broad nose with depressed root, distorted auricle and deafness, micrognathia, masklike face, malformation of the genitals (in males, cryptorchidism and hypospadias; in females, vaginal septa), spina bifida, and hexadactyly of the hand. Smith (1969) thought that some of the cases reported in the past as dyscranio-pygo-phalangy were probably those of trisomy 13–15.

Another controversial syndrome is the one called Biemond II. Biemond (1934) described a syndrome consisting of coloboma of the iris, mental retardation, obesity, hypogenitalism, and postaxial polydactyly. This constellation is considered developmentally akin to the Laurence-Moon-Bardet-Biedl (LMBB) syndrome, but it is genetically distinct. LMBB syndrome is transmitted as a recessive trait. The inheritance of the Biemond II syndrome is said to be irregularly dominant.

LMBB syndrome is the best known of all oculodigital complexes that are accompanied by polydactyly. Laurence and Moon (1866) saw a little, "fat, flat-featured and heavy-looking" girl who could not see well, especially at night; ophthalmoscopic examination revealed retinitis pigmentosa. Her parents had normal vision. She had three brothers with normal eyesight, and three others and one sister with defective vision. One affected brother, aged 18, was examined by Mr. Little — probably of Little's disease fame — who reported that the boy was short, "the height being only four feet six inches"; his genital organs were "those of a boy five years old." In the original report, the following features of LMBB syndrome were indicated: retinitis pigmentosa, obesity, moderate dwarfism, genital dystrophy, and familial occurrence. Bardet (1920) added polydactyly to this complex, and Biedl (1922) expanded the syndrome to include mental retardation.

The LMBB syndrome consists of the following pentad: obesity, mental deficiency, polydactyly, retinitis pigmentosa, and genital dystrophy. Blumel and Kniker (1959), who reviewed the literature, gave the following figures: obesity in 83 per cent of reported cases; mental deficiency in 80 per cent; polydactyly in 75 per cent; retinitis pigmentosa in 68 per cent; and genital dystrophy in 60 per cent. About half of the reported cases have been familial. Kalbian (1956) described a boy who had six fingers on each hand and six toes on each foot. The hands were flat and spadelike. The testes were small and the penis was infantile. He was the product of a consanguineous marriage.

ORODIGITAL COMPLEXES

Roux (1847) reported a father and his son. The father had a unilateral harelip and six digits on each limb; the son had the same anomaly of the hands and feet and a double harelip. Thurston (1909) described a 20-year-old Hindu male who had a central notch on his upper lip, six fingers on each hand, and six toes on each foot. The polydactyly of the hands was postaxial. This man had a five-year-old brother who possessed seven fingers on each hand, six toes on the left foot, and the normal number of digits on the right foot; he also had a median harelip. The parents were normal. Consanguinity was not mentioned. Lyons (1939) described a female infant with cleft palate, harelip, and "six sets of phalanges and five metacarpals" on the right hand.

Dysostosis acrofaciales (DAF) is the name given by Weyers (1952, 1953) to the symptom complex consisting of hexadactyly, cleft mandible, and a diminished number of teeth. The word "acra" denotes terminal point; in this instance it refers to the digits of the hand. "While on the jaw malformations lead to malfusion and oligodentia, extremities show excess formation like polydactyly with prevalence on the left side," Weyers wrote.

As noted in Chapter Twelve, syndactyly is the most common accompaniment of OFD (oral-facial-digital) syndrome, characterized by hypertrophied frenula, incomplete cleavage of the jaw, lobulated tongue, split upper lip, and digital anomalies. Two classes of OFD syndrome are recognized: OFD-I and OFD-II. According to Rimoin and Edgerton (1967), unilateral polydactyly distinguishes OFD-I syndrome from OFD-II syndrome. This concept was corroborated by Thuline (1969). A case of OFD reported by Segmi et al (1970) had postaxial polydactyly and contracted, axially deviated digits.

POIKILODERMA AND PARAPSORIASIS
WITH POLYDACTYLY

Heggs (1936) reported a man with atrophic areas of the skin and pre-axial polydactyly. A first cousin who was the offspring of a marriage between the proband's sister and his mother's brother was said to have "a similar anatomical deformity of the hand." Jacobsohn, who discussed this report, considered the skin lesion as being akin to parapsoriasis.

POLYDACTYLY/IMPERFORATE
ANUS/VERTEBRAL ANOMALIES SYNDROME

Say and Gerald (1968), Fuhrmann (1968), and Say et al (1971) described a complex consisting of imperforate anus, various types of vertebral anomalies (including an excess number of vertebrae, hemivertebrae, and sacral agenesis), and polydactyly.

RENAL-ACRAL COMPLEX

Simpoulous et al (1967) described three newborn male siblings with polycystic kidneys, internal hydrocephalus, and polydactyly. The parents were not cousins. The trait was possibly transmitted as an X-linked phenotype.

SMITH-LEMLI-OPITZ SYNDROME

Smith et al (1964) described three unrelated children with microcephaly, mental defect, hypertonicity, growth retardation, incomplete development of the external genitals, syndactyly of some of the toes, and rudimentary polydactyly of the hand. These children presented with peculiar facies; they had high-arched palates, receding chins, epicanthal folds, low-set ears, and turned-up nostrils. The infant reported by Gellis and Feingold (1968) had postaxial polydactyly of the left hand.

TUBEROUS SCLEROSIS AND ACCESSORY
THUMB

Classic tuberous sclerosis consists of the following triad: epilepsy, mental retardation, and adenoma sebaceum. Fibromas under or at the margin of the nails have been reported by many authors. The metacarpals and phalanges of the hand may show cortical erosions caused by the pressure of an extraosseous fibroma; there may be intraosseous cysts and localized periosteal reaction. The patient described by MacCarthy and Russell (1958) had an accessory thumb.

TREATMENT

In the treatment of polydactylism, amputation is optional. In most instances, the aim of surgery is cosmetic improvement. One need not hesitate to dispose of a functionally defunct, flail postaxial appendage which has been added to a pentadactylous hand. However, one should exercise caution in contemplating amputation of a supernumerary digit which enhances the functional propensity of the hand.

The question often arises as to which one of the two adjoining fingers should be sacrificed. Prior to the advent of roentgenography, it was customary to remove the marginal digit and retain the central. Roentgenographic studies have since revealed many skeletal aberrations, some of which were suspected in the past but could not be confirmed. In many instances, the marginal digit is equipped with a more substantial skeletal framework than its central mate; occasionally, bifurcated digits share a common epiphysis, a common proximal phalanx, or a common metacarpal. In all these variants there may be an unequal distribution of tendons, which should be regrouped to reinforce the power of the thumb to be saved.

The function of the finger depends as much upon its soft tissue content as upon the skeletal equipment, if not more. Roentgenographs fail to demonstrate the presence or absence of the former. Roentgenographic findings should be correlated with the functional potential of the digit. The polydactylous infant must be examined periodically and carefully studied both when awake and active and when asleep. Children tend to clench their fists in sleep; the more powerful digit will take part in this action, while the weaker member dangles away from the palm. Not uncommonly, a seemingly malformed digit will perform with greater efficacy than its more normal looking neighbor; the former should be preserved, notwithstanding its appearance. When one of the two adjoining digits has greater flexion power and the other excels in extension, the latter is amputated and its extensor tendon is transferred to the former. Syndactyly often complicates polydactylism, and the conjoined digits may share a common tendon and nerve. These two structures must be saved when the skeletal elements of the superfluous finger are shelled out.

For obvious reasons, the surgeon exercises greater caution in contemplating amputation of a pre-axial supernumerary digit. The duplication of the thumb may be partial or complete. To the former category belong bifid and bifurcate thumbs. Bifurcate thumb splits away at either the interphalangeal or metacarpophalangeal joint; it may even stem from the shaft of the first metacarpal. In all these variants, there may be an unequal distribution of tendons which should be regrouped to reinforce the power of the thumb to be saved (Figs. 13–23 and 13–24).

For the treatment of duplication beyond the distal interphalangeal joint of the thumb, Bilhaut (1890) devised an operation which is still being practiced by many surgeons. A V-shaped segment, including skin, nail, and bone, is removed from between the two adjoining phalanges; the remaining parietal portions are brought to the midline and sewed together to form a tapered terminal thumb segment (Fig. 13–25).

There have been numerous modifications of the Bilhaut procedure. When performing any of them in growing children, one runs of the risk of damaging the epiphyseal plates, which will result in growth disturbance and deformity. In order to obviate these hazards, Stelling (1967) recommended surgical syndactyly

(*Text continued on page 442.*)

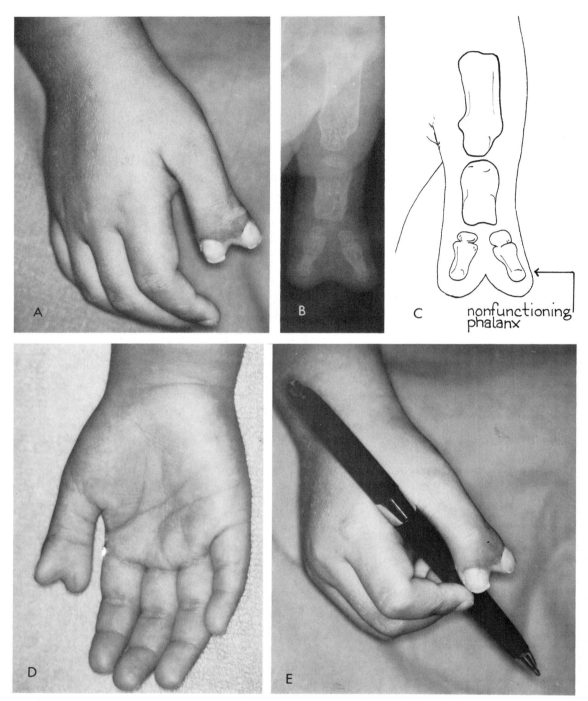

nonfunctioning
phalanx

Figure 13–23   Duplicated webbed ungual phalanges of the thumb in which the ulnar phalanx appears to function well and should be preserved. *A*, Dorsal view of the right hand. *B*, Dorsopalmar roentgenograph of the thumb. *C*, Sketch illustrating the same. *D*, Palmar view of the hand. *E*, The act of wielding a pen: the radial component of the bifid thumb does not seem to take part in this most important action and may well be sacrificed.

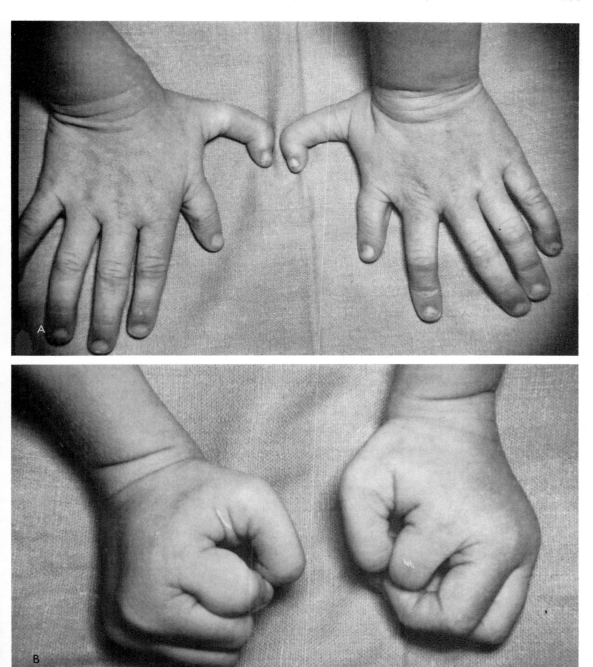

Figure 13–24 Pre-axial polydactyly in which the radialmost digit does not look like a thumb: it is thin and contracted but borders a broad webspace and is rotated. The digit on its ulnar aspect is unrotated and is separated from its ulnar neighbor by a narrow webspace. *A*, Dorsal view of the hands. *B*, Radial view showing that the radialmost digit partakes in the action of opposition and is preserved, notwithstanding its anomalous posture: it functions better than its ulnar neighbor, which is sacrificed.

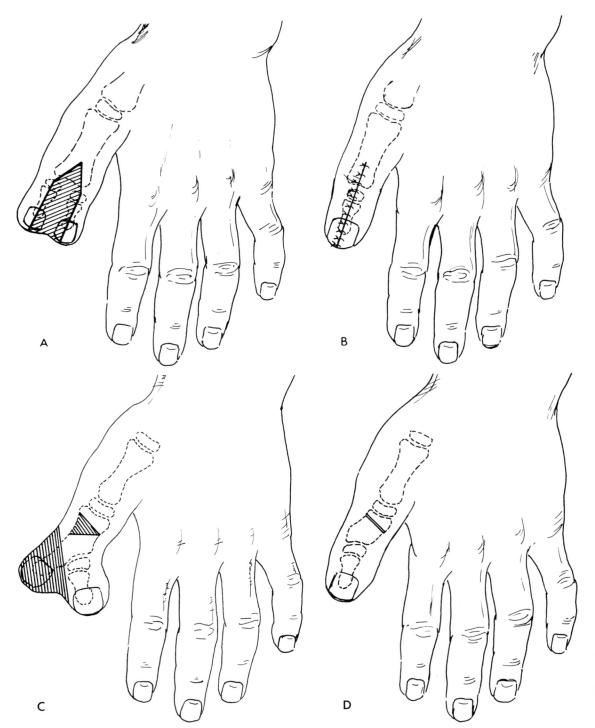

Figure 13–25 Sketches illustrating the Bilhaut procedure and its modification. *A* and *B*, The classic operation. *C*, and *D*, Modification—the removal of the surplus ungual bone is supplemented by cuneiform osteotomy of the proximal phalanx of the thumb.

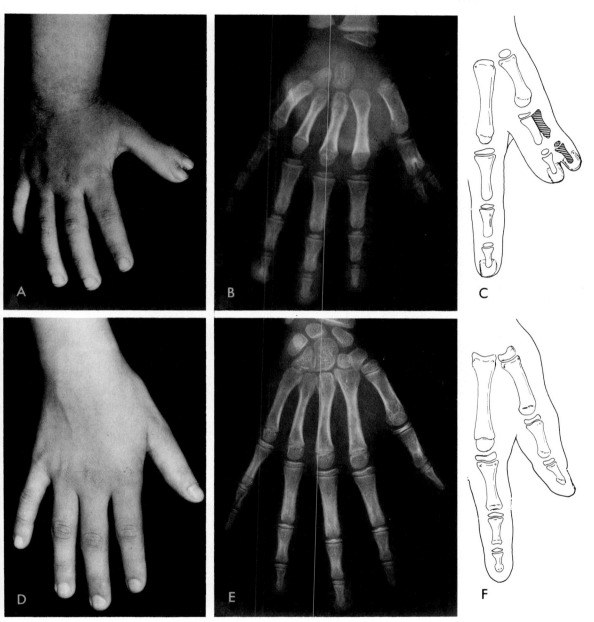

Figure 13–26   Bifid thumb treated by Bilhaut operation in infancy and subsequent subcapital osteotomy of the proximal phalanx at the age of four. *A,* Dorsal view of the right hand of a two-year-old girl. *B,* Dorsopalmar roentgenograph of the same. *C,* Sketch illustrating the preoperative osseous content of the bifid pollex. *D,* Dorsal view of the hand at the age of eight. *E,* Postoperative roentgenograph at the same age. *F,* Sketch illustrating the osseous content of the thumb six years after surgery.

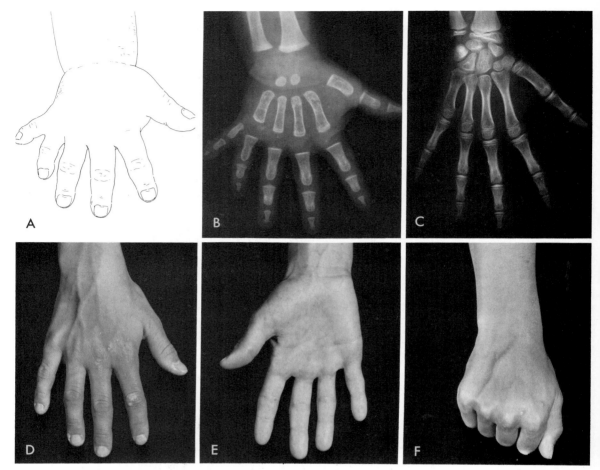

Figure 13–27 Disarticulation of postaxial surplus digit. *A*, Sketch of the right hand of an 11-month-old girl. *B*, Preoperative dorsopalmar roentgenograph. *C*, Roentgenograph six years after surgery. *D*, Dorsal photograph six years after surgery, showing the digits in extension. *E*, Palmar view of the same. *F*, Clenched fist.

of the diverging digits, delaying more definitive surgery until the age of maturity. Stelling did not mention the psychological injury a child of school age would suffer on account of his broad, stubby thumb, which is not likely to escape the ridicule of other children.

Egawa (1966) thought that the Bilhaut operation could be carried out as early as one month after birth. He considered postoperative ulnar or radial deviation of the terminal phalanx rare, and said that this deformity could be corrected in the future either by subcapital osteotomy of the proximal phalanx or by fusion of the joint. When dichotomy occurs at the proximal interphalangeal joint, the weaker digit is removed, and its tendons are transferred to the remaining member. At a later date—usually six months after the first operation—the curvature of the phalanx is corrected by osteotomy (Fig. 13–26).

Karchinov (1962) presented two cases of almost total duplication of the thumb. For the first case he utilized the principle of preservation of the neurovascular bundle and transposed the pulp and the nailplate, together with a broad volar band, from the functionally defunct central thumb to the marginal,

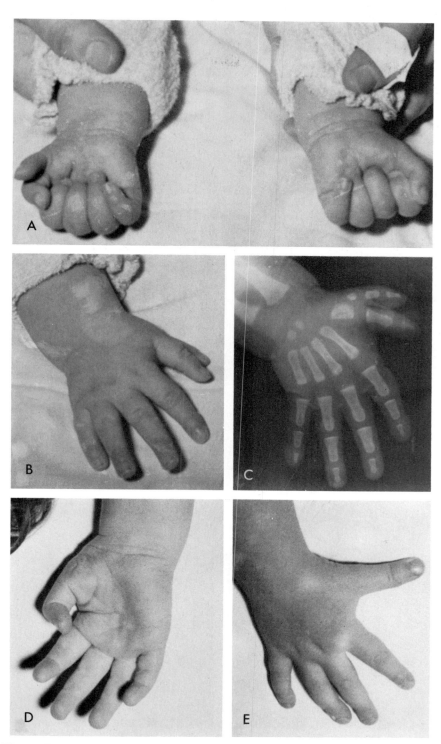

Figure 13–28 Disarticulation of pre-axial surplus digit. *A.* Palmar view of the clenched hands of a seven-month-old female infant: the second digit of the polydactylous right hand participates in the clenched fist. *B,* Dorsal view of the same. *C,* Preoperative dorsopalmar roentgenograph. *D,* Post-operative palmar view, showing flexion and adduction of the preserved thumb. *E,* Postoperative dorsal view, showing extension and abduction of the thumb.

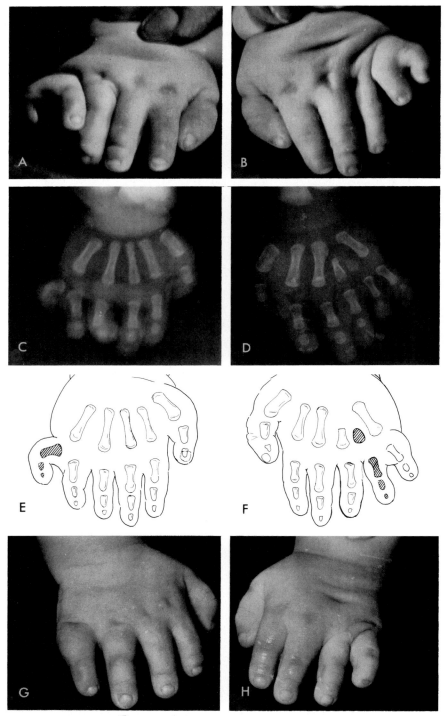

Figure 13–29   Postaxial polydactyly of the right hand and central polydactyly of the left hand of a newborn female infant. *A*, Dorsal view of the right hand. *B*, Dorsal view of the left hand. *C*, Dorsopalmar roentgenograph of the right hand. *D*, Dorsopalmar roentgenograph of the left hand: note the intercalary defect of the fourth and fifth metacarpals. *E* and *F*, Sketches showing the elements (shaded) removed. *G*, Postoperative dorsal view of the right hand. *H*, Postoperative dorsal view of the left hand.

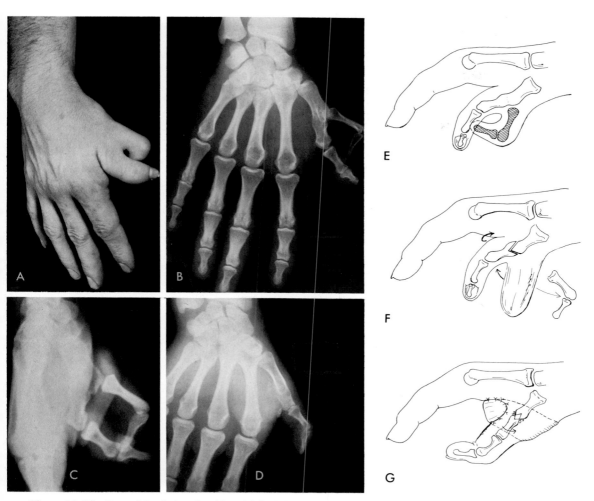

Figure 13–30 Pre-axial polydactyly with axial deviation of the two radial digits. *A*, Dorsal view of the right hand. *B*, Dorsopalmar roentgenograph of the same. *C*, Lateral roentgenograph of the thumb. *D*, Dorsopalmar roentgenograph of the hand after surgery which consisted of filleting the two nonfunctioning radial phalanges and utilizing the skin thus made available for widening the first commissure, transmetacarpal rotation, and shortening osteotomy of the preserved pollex. *E*, Sketch showing the two phalanges to be removed. *F* and *G* show removal of the bony contents utilization of the available skin for widening the first commissure, and osteotomy of the first metacarpal.

seemingly accessory, pollex which had muscular power but no nail. Karchinov's second patient had two individually inadequate thumbs. He combined these two thumbs by side-to-side bony fusion of the phalanges and surgical syndactyly, hoping to augment the power of the reconstructed single thumb.

The treatment of hands possessing a pair of triphalangeal digits which have replaced the thumb and are opposable is optional. These digits may look like fingers, but functionally they are thumbs. In a laboring man, they should be left alone or syndactylized. In females, the surgery on these digits is motivated entirely by cosmetic considerations. In this operation, the weaker digit is amputated and its tendons are transferred to the digit which is preserved. In the event that the latter is too long, it may be shortened by resection of a segment from the metacarpal shaft. If necessary, the distal fragment is rotated for better opposition (Figs. 13–27 to 13–30).

SUMMARY

Polydactyly ranks with syndactyly as one of the more common anomalies of the hand. In contrast to syndactyly, polydactyly is seen more often in the Negro: it is the most common congenital hand anomaly in black people. Polydactyly commonly affects the radial and ulnar borders of the hand rather than the central portion. Sporadic and endemic cases have been reported. Hereditary polydactyly is usually transmitted as an autosomal dominant trait with variable expression. The polydactyly which occurs in association with Ellis-van Creveld chondroectodermal dysplasia and Laurence-Moon-Bardet-Biedl complex pursues a recessive pattern of inheritance. Syndromic polydactyly is usually postaxial. Amputation of the surplus digit is standard treatment. Not the best looking, but functionally the most effective, digit is preserved, and its nonfunctioning or weaker neighbor is sacrificed. Some cases of pre-axial polydactyly present special problems. One tries to procure a member which is equipped with adequate motor power and has sufficient mobility to carry out the actions of pinch and grasp.

References

Acker, R. B.: Generalized polydactylism with concurrent syndactylism. *J. Bone Joint Surg.*, (n.s.), *13*:580–582, 1931.

Albers: Ein Fall von Polydactylie. *Berl. Klin. Wochenschr.*, *30*:230–232, 1893.

Ammon, F. A. V.: *Die angeborenen Chirurgischen Krankheiten des Menschen.* Berlin, F. A. Herbig, pp. 99–101, 1842.

Amrein, G.: *Ein Fall von Hereditärer Hexadaktylie nebst sechs weiteren Fallen von Polydaktylie.* Inaug. Diss. Basel, Schweizer, Venlags-Drukerri, pp. 5–53; Taf. I, II, 1903.

Appelbaum, A., and Marmelstein, M.: Congenital bilateral anophthalmos vera with unilateral polydactyly and cleft palate. Report of a case. *Arch. Ophthalmol.*, *29*:258–265, 1943.

Appenzeller, G. F. A.: *Ein Beitrag zur Lehre von der Erblickeit der Grauen Staars.* Inaug. Diss. Tubingen, H. Laupp, pp. 4–27, 1884.

Archambault, L.: *De La Polydactylie, au Point de Vue Héréditaire Coincidence des Malformations avec les Tares Nevropathiques.* Thèse. Paris, A. Maloine, pp. 1–69, 1896.

Arps, G. F.: Polydactylism and the phenomenon of regeneration. *J.A.M.A.*, *74*:873–874, 1920.

Artusi, G.: La polidattilia peduncolata dei bambini. *Policlinico (Prat.)*, *31*:1267–1268, 1924.

Atkinson, E. M.: A case of hereditary polydactylism occurring in four generations and many members of the same family. *Br. J. Surg.*, *9*:298–301, 1921.

Atkinson, J. B.: Some cases of polydactylism and syndactylism occurring in one family. *St. Barth.'s Hosp. J.*, *8*:189, 1901.

Attlee, W. H. W.: A case of supernumerary digits. *Lancet*, *2*:163, 1907.

Atwood, E. S., and Pond, C. P.: A polydactylous family. *J. Hered.*, *8*:96–97, 1917.

Audebert, and Lasaigues: Note sur un case de polydactylie héréditaire. *Toulouse Méd.*, (2 s.), *6*:128, 1904.

Audoin, P.: Polydactylie des mains et des pieds. *Bull. Mèm. Soc. Anat.*, (6 s.), *1*:1072–1073, 1899.

Baisch, A.: Anonychia congenita, Kombinert mit Polydaktylie und verzögertem abnormen Zahndurchbruch. *Dtsch. Z. Chir.*, *232*:450–457, 1931.

Balico, G.: Pollice bifido. *Chir. Plast.*, *5*:128–130, 1939.

Ballowitz, E.: Über die Hyperdaktylie des Menschen. *Klin. Jb.*, *13*:143–153, 1904. Also published as a separate pamphlet, Jena, G. Fischer, pp. 1–108, 1904.

Ballowitz, E.: Über hyperdactyle Familien und die Vererbung der Vielfingerigkeit des Menschen. *Arch. Rassen. Gesellsch. Biol.* (Berlin), *1*:347–365, 1904.

Ballowitz, E.: Welchen Aufschluss geben Bau and Anordung der Weichteile hyperdaktyler Gliedmassen über die aetiologie und Morphologische Bedeutung der Hyperdaktylie des Menschen. *Arch. Pathol. Anat. Physiol.*, *178*:1–25, 1904.

Ballowitz, E.: Das Verhalten der Ossa sesamoiden an den Spaltgliedern bei Hyperdaktylie des Mensch. *Arch. Pathol. Anat. Physiol.*, *178*:164–169, 1904.

Barbacci, G.: Un raro reporto di pollice bifido. *Red. Med.*, *9*:938–942, 1928.

Bardeleben, K. V.: *Hand und Fuss.* Wien, *Verh. Anat. Ges.*, *8*:337–357, 1892.

Bardet, G.: *Sur un Syndrome d'Obésité Congénitale avec Polydactylie et Hetinite Pigmentaire.* Thèse. Paris. A. Legrand, pp. 1–107, 1920.

Barge: Über einen Fall von extremer Hyperdaktylie. *Z. Anat.*, *93*:253–296, 1930.

Barrer, L. A.: Unilateral hexadactyly in man. *J. Hered.*, *38*:345–346, 1947.

Barsky, A. J.: *Congenital Anomalies of the Hand.* Springfield, Illinois, Charles C Thomas, pp. 48–64, 1958.

Bartholini, T.: *Historian Anatomicum Rarorum.* Amsterdam, Centura III, Observato 47, p. 95, 1657.

Bates, D.: *The Passing of the Aborigines.* London, J. Murray, pp. 121–122, 1938.

Beauvais, de: Observation de polydactylie. *Bull. Soc. Méd. Paris*, *10*:34–40, 1876.

Béchet, M.: Doigt surnuméraire. *Bull. Soc. Anat.*, (1 s.), *26*:247–249, 1851.

Beckmann, E., and Widdlund, L.: On inheritance of poly- and syndactyly in man. *Acta Genet. Med. Gem.*, *11*:43, 1962.

Bell, J.: Some new pedigrees of hereditary disease. A polydactylism and syndactylism. B. Blue sclerotics and fragility of bone. *Ann. Eugen.*, *4*:41–49, 1930.

Bell, J.: Three further cases of hereditary digital anomaly seen in the out-patient department of Great Ormond Street Hospital for Sick Children. *Ann. Eugen.*, *4*:233–237, 1931.

Bénard, R.: Neuf cas de polydactylie héréditaire au cours de cinq générations. *N. Iconog. Salp.* *28*:147–161, 1916–1918.

Beranger: Doits supplémentaires sur le bord cubitale de chaque main. *Bull. Soc. d'Anthrop.*, (3 s.), *10*:600–603, 1887.

Bergmann: Missbildungen an einem Kinde, mit besonderer Berucksichtigung der Polydaktylie. *Z. Orthop. Chir.*, *17*:131–149, 1906.

Bernhardi: Extra fingers and toes. *Med. Times Gaz.*, *2*:628–629, 1856.

Biedl, A.: Geschwisterpaar mit adiposo-genitaler Dystrophie. *Dtsch. Med. Wochenschr.*, *48*:1630, 1922.

Biemond, A.: Het syndroom von Laurence-Biedl en een aanverwand, nieuw Syndroom. *Ned. Tijdschr. Geneesk.*, *78*:1801–1814, 1934.

Bienvenue, F.: Un cas de pouce supplémentaire à trois phalanges. *Rev. d'Orthop.*, (3 s.), *3*:91–96, 1912.

Biles, A. R., Jr. Luers, T., and Sperling, K.: D_1 ring chromosome in a newborn with peculiar face, polydactyly imperforatanus, and arrhinencephaly and other malformations. *J. Med. Genet.*, *7*:399–401, 1970.

Bilhaut, M.: Guérison d'un pouce bifide par un nouveau procédé opératoire. *Congr. Fr. Chir.*, *4*:576–580, 1890.

Bjerkners, W.: Et tilfaelde av Kombineret Poly- og Brachydaktylie. *Norsk. Mag. Loe Gev.*, *83*:517–523, 1922.

Blankenburg, H.: Die Polydaktylie. *Beitr. Orthop. Traumatol.*, *14*:160–165, 1967.

Blasi, B.: Su di un caso di polidattilia. *Policlinico*, *38*:954–957, 1931.

Bloome, G.: *Considérations sur la Polydactylie*. Thèse. Paris, L. Boyer. pp. 1–46, 1901.

Blumel, J., and Kniker, W. T.: Laurence-Moon-Bardet-Biedl syndrome. Review of the literature and a report of five cases including a family group with three affected males. *Texas Rep. Biol. Med.*, *17*:391–410, 1959.

Boinet, E.: Polydactylie et atavism. *Rev. Méd.*, *18*:316–328, 1898.

Boissard: Polydactylie et syndactylie héréditaire. *Bull. Soc. d'Obstet.*, *2*:232–235, 1899.

Bolk, L.: Over een belamgwekkenden voen van minimus bifidus, en over het onstaan van polydactylie in het algemeen. *Ned. Tijdschr. Geneesk.*, *9*(1):391–396, 1904.

Bonnevie, K.: Polydactyli i norske bygdeslegter. *Norsk. Mag. Lagev.*, *17*:601–632, 1919.

Bornstein, N. B.: Aniridie bilatérale avec polydactylie. Rélations des anomalies oculaires du type colobomateux associées à des malformations squelettiques avec les formes atypiques du syndrome de Bardet-Biedl. *J. Genet. Hum.*, *1*:211–226, 1952.

Bossy, J., and Sabby, J. P.: Les points d'ossification de la main chez un embryon de 48 mm (V.C.) porteus d'un pouce bifide. *Arch. Anat. Pathol.*, *14*:92, 1966.

Boulian: Polydactylie opération. *Rec. Mèm. Méd. Milit.*, (3 s.), *13*:67–71, 1865.

Bourgin: Polydactylie familiale héréditaire. *Bull. Soc. Sci. Méd. Biol. Montpellier*, *3*:264, 1921–1922.

Bouteiller, M.: Pouce surnuméraire. *Bull. Soc. Anat.*, (1 s.), *26*:231–233, 1851.

Boyd, C.: A six-fingered family. *Br. Med. J.*, *1*:154, 1887.

Brandeis, J. W.: Polydactylism as a hereditary character. *J.A.M.A.*, *64*:1640–1642, 1915.

Brault, J.: Note sur quelques cas de polydactylie, de luxations congénitales des doigts et d'ecrodactylie. *Arch. Prov. Chir.* (Paris), *7*:363–366, 1898.

Braus, H.: Entwicklungsqueschichtliche Analyse der Hyperdaktylie. *Münch. Med. Wochenschr.*, *55*:386–390, 1908.

Br. Med. J.: A six-fingered family. *1*:30, 1887.

Broca, H. M.: Sur la polydactylie, une travail par M. Lenglen. *Bull. Acad. Méd.* (Paris), pp. 1312–1314, 1877.

Brody, L. J.: Polydactylism in five generations. *Am. J. Dis. Child.*, *47*:701–702, 1934.

Brown, H. M.: Report of a case of polydactylism recurring through four generations. *Weekly Med. Rev.* (Chicago), *9*:35, 1884.

Bruncher: Polydactylie chez un indigène Algérien. *Prov. Méd.* (Paris), *22*:494–495, 1911.

Bunge, R. G., and Bradbury, J. T.: Two unilaterally cryptorchid boys with spermatogenic precocity in the descended testis, hypertelorism and polydactyly. *J. Clin. Endocrinol.*, *19*:1103–1109, 1959.

Cabot, A. T.: Supernumerary fingers. Surgical cases of Dr. Warren. *Mass. Gen. Hosp. Med. Surg. J.*, *95*:271–273, 1876.

Callan, R.: Polydactyly in a Negro family. *J. Hered.*, *33*:229–232, 1942.

Carlisle, A.: An account of a family having hands and feet with supernumerary fingers and toes. *Phil. Trans. R. Soc.*, *104*:94–101, 1814.

Cazeaux: Existence d'un doigt surnuméraire. *Gaz. Méd.* (Paris), p. 271, 1850.

Chamayon: Note sur un cas de polydactylie. *Gaz. Hop.* (Toulouse), *12*:57, 1898.

Christiaens, L., Laude, M., and Fontaine, G.: Les polydactylies: à propos d'un case familial. *Pédiatrie*, *18*:709–714, 1963.

Chuquet: Cas de polydactylie: deux pouces sur un seul métacarpien. Anomalie des artères de l'avantbras. *Bull. Soc. Anat.*, (4 s.), *1*:725–726, 1876.

Ciotola, G.: Microftalmo e malformazioni della dita (sindattilia, polidattilia). *Boll. Ocul.*, *17*:855–867, 1938.

Collins, E. T.: On anophthalmos. *Ophthalmic Hosp. Rep.* (London), *11*:429–455, 1886.

Constantini, G.: Considérations sur la valeur morphologique de la polydactylie. *N. Iconog. Salp.*, *24*:81–89, 1911.

Contze, W. A.: *Polydactylie.* 8°. Dissertation. Bonn, Druck von Ernst Heydorn, pp. 1–29, 1893.

Cooke, W.: Cases of supernumerary thumbs. *Lancet*, *1*:406, 1885.

Corneli, F.: Osservazioni sopra un caso di polidattilia. *Ortop. Traum. App. Mot.*, *22*:495–502, 1954.

Corrigan, S. H.: An unusual type of supernumerary digit. *Can. Med. Assoc. J.*, *19*:342, 1928.

Crawford, R.: On supernumerary fingers and toes. *Monthly J. Med. Sci.* (London & Edinburgh), *13*:356–357, 1851.

Cummins, H.: Spontaneous amputation of human supernumerary digits: pedunculated postminimi. *Am. J. Anat.*, *51*:381–416, 1932.

Damourette: Vice de la conformation de la main droite (deux index supplémentaires au lieu de pouce). *Arch. Gén. Méd.*, (7 s.), *20*:666–675, 1890.

Danforth, C. H.: A comparison of the hands of a pair of polydactylic Negro twins. *Amer. J. Phys. Anthropol.* 2:147–165, 1918.

Darbois: La polydactylie. *Bull. Soc. Radio. Méd.* (Paris), *3*:188, 1911.

Darwin, C.: *The Variation of Animals and Plants under Domestication*. Second edition. New York, D. Appleton & Co., Vol. I, pp. 457–460, 1896. The first edition was published in 1868.

Da Silva Leal, M., and De Espregueira Mendes: Quelques cas de polydactylie. *Folia Anat. Univ. Conimb.* 7(No. 17):1–3; pl. I-III, 1932.

Dawson, W. J. F.: Hereditary polydactylism in three generations. *Tr. Med. Soc. Calif.*, 28:74–75, 1898.

DeBauvais: Observation de polydactylie. *Gaz. des Hôp.*, 48:379–381, 1875.

Dehus, D., and Snyder, L. H.: Dominance in man, with especial reference to polydactylism. *Ohio. J. Sci.*, 32:232–260, 1932.

DeLinares, L. G.: Collective polydactylism in a small town. *J.A.M.A.*, 94:2080–2081, 1930.

DeMarinis, F., and Sobbota, A.: On inheritance and development of preaxial and postaxial types of polydactyly. *Acta Genet.*, 7:215–216, 1957.

DeMarinis, F., and Wildervanck, L. S.: Pre-axial polydactylie (verdubbelde duim) en trifalangie. *Ned. Tijdschr. Geneesk.*, 104:2169–2171, 1960.

Demme: Zwei Fälle von symmetrischer Polydactylie und Syndactylie. *Verh. Berl. Med. Ges.*, 25:210; pl. I, 1895.

DeMussy, G.: Doigt surnuméraire à la partie interne du pouce gauche. *Bull. Soc. Anat.*, (1 s.), *13*:40, 1838.

Desnoyers, and Ill.: Pouces surnuméraire et pouces bifides. *Rev. d'Orthop.*, 2:343–348, 1924.

Devay, F.: *Du Danger des Mariages Consanguins sous le Rapport Sanitaire*. Second edition. Paris, V. Masson et Fils, pp. 105–107, 1862.

Dixon: Superfluous fingers occurring in five generations. *Med. Times Gaz.*, 1:59, 1859.

Douarre: Pouce bifide. *Bull. Soc. Acad.*, (6 s.) *18*:293–294, 1921.

Drake-Brochman, H. E.: Remarkable cases of polydactylism. *Br. Med. J.*, 2:1167–1168, 1892.

Drewry, W. F.: Supernumerary digits. *Med. News* (Philadelphia), *54*:418, 1889.

Dubreuil-Chambardel: *Les Variations du Corps Humain*. Paris, E. Flammarion, pp. 100–112, 1925.

Dunker, D.: Drei Fälle von unvollstadinger Polydaktylie der Aussenseite von Hand und Fuss. *Z. Orthop. Chir.*, 47:547–552, 1926.

Duschl, J.: Eine seltene form von Polydaktylie. *Münch. Med. Wochenschr.*, 44:827–828, 1917.

Eaton, G. O., and McKusick, V. A.: A seemingly unique polydactyly-syndactyly syndrome in four persons in three generations. *In* Bergsma, D., (ed.): *Birth Defects. Original Article Series*. New York, National Foundation—March of Dimes, Vol. V, No. 3:221–225, 1969.

Ebstein, E.: Über den Pollex bifidus (sog. "doppelter Daumen." "Daumenschere"). *In* Angeborene familiäre Eskrankungen an dem Nageln. *Derm. Wochenschr.*, 68:113–124, 1919.

Ecke, H.: Beitrag zu den Doppelmissbildungen im Bereich der Finger. *Beitr. Klin. Chir.*, 205:463–468, 1962.

Egawa, T.: Polydactyly. (Japanese). *Jap. J. Plast. Reconstr. Surg.*, 9:97–105, 1966.

Ellis, R. W. B., and van Creveld, S.: A syndrome characterized by ectodermal dysplasia, polydactyly, chondrodysplasia and congenital morbus cordis. Report of three cases. *Arch. Dis. Child.*, 15:65–84, 1940.

Erkman, R., Bassur, V. R., and Conen, P. E.: D/D translocation and "D" syndrome. *J. Pediatr.*, 67:270–282, 1965.

Fabris, U.: La etiopatogenesi della polidattilia in rapporto con la patologia comparata. *Gaz. Internat. Med. Chir. Napoli*, 29:3–13; 45–47, 1926.

Feichtinger, H.: *Ein neurer typischer, vorwiegend die Akran betreffender Fehlbildungskomplex*. Inaug. Diss. Med. Rostock, typescript pp. 1–35, 1943.

Ferreira de Magalhaes, A.: Pollegar bifurcado. *Brasil Med.*, 32:290, 1918.

Flatt, A. E.: Problems in polydactyly. *In* Cramer, L. M., and Chase, R. A., (eds.): *Symposium on the Hand*. Saint Louis, C. V. Mosby Co., 3:150–167, 1971.

Fogh-Anderson, P.: Genetic and non-genetic factors in the etiology of facial clefts. *Scand. J. Plast. Surg.*, 1:22–29; figs. 3a, 3b, 4a, 4b, 1967.

Fort, J. A.: *Des Difformités Congénitales et Acquisés des Doigts*. Thèse. Paris, A. Delahaye, pp. 12–43, 1869.

Frazier, T. M.: A note on race-specific congenital malformation rates. *Am. J. Obstet. Gynecol.*, 80:184–185, 1960.

Frentzel, O.: Untersuchung einer Kinder mit 6 Fingern an beiden Handen und Fussen. *Arch. Pathol. Anat. Physiol.*, 119:566–569, 1890.

Freund, L.: Die Hyperdaktylie. *Z. Thiermed.*, 10:110–117, 1905.

Fuhrmann, W. A.: A new polydactyly/imperforate-anus/vertebral anomalies syndrome. *Lancet*, 2:918–919, 1968.

Fumarola, G.: Contribution a l'étude des difformités congénitales associées des mains (ectro-poly-macro-syndactylie et micro-thoraco-mélie unilateral). *N. Iconog. Salp.*, 24:329–334, 1911.

Gaillard, L.: Note sur les doigts surnuméraires. *Gaz. Méd. Paris*, No. 43:665–666, 1892.

Gates, R. R.: *Human Genetics.* New York, The Macmillan Co., Vol. II, pp. 385–469, 1946.

Gazeaux, M.: Existence d'un doigts surnuméraire. *Gaz. Méd. Paris,* No. 43:271–272, 1862.

Gegenbaur, C.: Kritische Bemerkungen über Polydactylie als Atavismus. *Morph. Jahrb.,* 6:584–596, 1880. See also the translation in *J. Anat. Physiol. Norm Pathol.,* 16:615–622, 1882.

Gegenbaur, C.: Über polydactylie. *Morph. Jahrb.,* 14:394–406, 1888. See also a review of this article in: *Rev. Sci. Méd. en France et á L'Etranger,* 34:46–47, 1889.

Gellis, S. S., and Feingold, M.: Picture of the month: denouement and discussion of Smith-Lemli-Opitz syndrome. *Am. J. Dis. Child.,* 115:603–604, 1968.

Girard, A.: Polydactylie provoquée chez Pleurodeles Waltlii Michahelles. *C. R. Soc. Biol.,* (10 s.), 2:789–792, 1895.

Goodman, R. M.: A family with polydactyly and other anomalies. *J. Hered.,* 56:37–38, 1965.

Gougenheim, M.: Deux phalangettes supplémentaire. *Bull. Soc. Anat.,* (2 s.), 9:61, 1864.

Graeffenburg, E.: Die entwicklungsgeschlichtliche Bedeutung der Hyperdactylie menschlicher Gliedmassen. *Studein Z. Pathol. Entwicklung.,* 5:565–619, 1920.

Grandclément: Polydactylie et syndactylie chez un ouvrier vigneron de quarante-quatre ans. *Gaz. Hôp. Civ. Mil.,* No. 124:555, 1861.

Grandieu, E. H.: Prenatal deformity of arm and hand. *Am. J. Obstet.,* 20:425–426, 1887.

Graper, L.: Zur Genese der Polidactylie. *Arch. Entwklngschn. Organ.,* 107:154–161, 1926.

Grebe, H.: Polydaktylia. *In* Becker, P. E., (ed.): *Humangenetik.* Stuttgart, G. Thieme, Band 2:182–202, 1964.

Green, S. H. Supernumerary digits and a history of heredity. *Lancet,* 2:859–860, 1907.

Gressot: Polydactylie. *Lyon Méd.,* 5:182–184, 1870.

Gross: Quatre cas de polydactylie. *Rev. Med. d'Est.,* 11:276–277, 1879.

Grote, L. R.: Über vererbliche Polydaktylie. *Z. Menschl. Vererb. Konstitutionslehre,* 9:47–59, 1923.

Gruber, G. B.: Hyperdaktylie (Polydaktylie), Diplocherie und Diplopodie, Hypermelie, Oligodaktylie und Defekte von Rohrenknochen. II. Menschlicher Betrachtungskreis. *In* Schwalbe, E., and Gruber, G. B., (eds.): *Die Morphologie derMissbildungen des Menschen und der Tier.* Jena, G. Fischer. 3 T 3, 19 Lief, Abt. 1, Kap. 7:720–808; fig. 70–84, 1958.

Gruber, W.: Zur Duplicität des Daumens. *Prakt. Heilk.,* 11:836–840, 1865.

Gruber, W.: Zusammenstellung veröffentlichter fälle von polydactylie, mit 7–10 fingern an der hand. Melanges Biol. *Acad. Imp. Sci. St. Petersburg,* 7:523–552, 1870.

Guermonprez, F.: Sur divers faits de polydactylie. *Bull. Mèm. Soc. Chir.,* 11:581–587, 1885. See also *Rev. Mens. Mal. l'Enf.,* 4:118–124, 1886.

Guerreiro. L.: Sobre a polidactylia. *Arq. Anat. Antropologia,* 10:431–492. 1926.

Guyon: Polydactylie irréguliere. *Gaz. des Hôp. Civil.,* p. 539, 1865. See also *Bull. Soc. Imp. Chir.,* (2 s.), 6:485–488, 1866.

Hallopeau, H.: Sur une deuxiéme cas de polydactylies suppuratives récidivantes. *Bull. Soc. Franc. Dermat. Syph.* (Paris), 3:200–204, 1892.

Haman, C. R.: Multiple anomalies. *Radiog. Clin. Photog.,* 12:19; figs. 2–5, 1892.

Handforth, J. R.: Polydactylism of the hand in Southern Chinese. *Anat. Rec.,* 106:119–125, 1950.

Hanissian, A. S., Riggs, W. W., Jr., and Thomas, D. A.: Infantile thoracic dystrophy—a variant of Ellis-van Creveld syndrome. *J. Pediatr.,* 71:855–864, 1967.

Hare, P. J.: Rudimentary polydactyly. *Br. J. Derm.,* 66:407–408, 1954.

Harris, H. A., and Thomas, G. C.: Persistent truncus arteriosus communis with microphthalmos, orbital cyst and polydactyly. *Arch. Dis. Child.,* 12:59–66, 1937.

Heggs, G. M.: Poikiloderma with polydactyly. *Proc. R. Soc. Med.* London (Sect. Dermat.), 29:717–720, 1936.

Heinberg, C. J.: Congenital bilateral anophthalmos and polydactylism with report of a case. *J. Florida Med. Assoc.,* 12:253–256, 1926.

Hersent, D.: Vice de conformation des phalanges du doigt annulaire de la main droite. *Bull. Soc. Anat.,* (1 s.), 18:42, 1843.

Hey, H. D.: Supernumerary digits. *Br. Med. J.,* 1:1254, 1904.

Hippel, E. v.: Ueber die Beziehungen von Mikrophthalmus mit Unterlidcyste zu allgemeinen Missbildungen, besonder zum Lindauschen Symptomenkomplex. *Graefes Arch. Ophthalmol.,* 132:256–264, 1934.

Hjelmman, J. V.: A case of polydactyly (Finnish). *Finska Lak.-Sallsk Handl.* (Helsingfors), 35:705–711, 1893.

Horne, A.: Hereditary malformations—supernumerary digits. *Lancet,* 1:115, 1838.

Horne, A.: Excessive development of fingers and toes. *Dublin J. Med. Sci.,* 73:239–240, 1882.

Horwitz, S.: Seltener Fall von Polydaktylie. *Dtsch. Med. Wochenschr.,* 54:829, 1928.

Houzel: Polydactylie: amputation des doigts surnuméraires (Rap. de P. Berger). *Bull. Mèm. Soc. Chir. Paris,* (n.s.), 10:885–891, 1884.

Hurlin, R. G.: A case of inherited polydactyly. *J. Hered.,* 11:334, 1921.

Hutchinson, J.: A short-limbed polydactylous dwarf. *Arch. Surg.,* 4:302–303; Pl. XCII, 1893.

Hutchinson, J.: Superfluous thumb on one hand—history of the same deformity in the same hand, in a single individual, in three generations. *Arch. Surg.,* 4:307–312, 1893.

Ivanhoff, E.: Inherited malformation (extra fingers). (Russian) *Voyenno-med J. St. Petersb.,* 188:541–545, 1897.

Jackson, V. W.: Four generations of polydactyly. *J. Hered.*, *28*:267–268, 1937.

James, J. I., and Lamb, D. W.: Congenital abnormalities of the limbs. *Practitioner*, *191*:159–172, 1963.

Jeney, A.: Ueber einen cigenartigen Fall von Kombination einer Polydaktylie mit Syndaktylie nebst daraus resultierenden Bemarkungen zur Lehr der Polydaktylie. *Wien Med. Wochenschr.*, *1*:2365–2368, 1903.

Jeune, M., Beraud, C., and Carron, R.: Dystrophie thoracique asphyxiante de caractère familial. *Arch. Franc. Pediatr.*, *12*:886–891, 1955.

Jeune, M., Carron, R., Beraud, C., and Loaec, Y.: Polychondrodystrophie avec blocage thoracique d'evolution fatale. *Pediatrie*, *9*:390–392, 1954.

Jin, S.: Congenital bilateral polydactylism: case. *Taiwan Lgakki Zassi.*, *38*:112, 1939.

Joachimsthal, G.: Ein weiterer Beiträg von der Polydaktylie. *Fortschr. Röntgenstr.*, *4*:112–113, 1900–1901.

Johnson, A. A.: Case of polydactylism, in which nine toes existed on one foot. *Tr. Pathol. Soc. London*, *9*:427–430, 1858.

Johnson, J. G.: Supernumerary fingers, hereditary for five generations. *Am. Med. Times*, *1*:275, 1860.

Johnston, H. H.: *The Negro in the New World.* London, Methuen & Co., pp. 9 and 300, 1910.

Johnston, O., and Davis, R. W.: On the inheritance of hand and foot anomalies in six families. (2. Polydactyly). *Am. J. Hum. Genet.*, *5*:356–372, 1953.

Joly, N.: Nouveau cas de polydactylie chez un mulet, observé à Toulouse. *C. R. Acad. Sci.* (Paris), *50*:1137–1139, 1860.

Jones, F. W.: *The Principles of Anatomy as Seen in the Hand.* Second edition. London, Balliére, Tindall & Co., pp. 30–44, 1944.

Kalbian, V. V.: Laurence-Moon-Biedl syndrome in an Arab boy: familial incidence. *J. Clin. Endocrinol.*, *16*:1622–1625, 1956.

Karchinov, K.: The treatment of polydactyly of the hand. *Br. J. Plast. Surg.*, *15*:362–376, 1962.

Kelly, J. E.: On a case of polydactylism. *Proc. R. Irish Acad. Dublin*, (2 s.), *2*:539–546, 1875–1877.

Kemp, T., and Ravn, J.: Über erbliche Hand- und Fuss deformitäten in einem 140-köpfigen Geschlecht, nebst einigen Bemerkungen über Poly- und Syndaktylie beim Menschen. *Acta Psych. Neurol.*, *7*:275–296, 1932.

Kerchringii, T.: *Spicilegivm Anatomicvm.* Amstelodami, A. Frisii, pp. 51–53, 1670.

Kollmann, J.: Handskelett und hyperdaktylie. *Anat. Anz.*, *3*:515–530, 1888.

Lafforgue, E.: La polydactylie et les influences héréditaire. *Rev. Méd. Pharm. Afrique Nord.* (Alger), *2*:79–95, 1899.

Langran, B.: Supernumerary fingers and malformations of foetal hand. *Lancet*, *1*:619–620, 1896.

Laurence, J. Z., and Moon, R. C.: Four cases of "retinitis pigmentosia" occurring in the same family and accompanied by general imperfections of development. *Ophthalmol. Rev.*, *2*:32–41; fig. 210, 1866.

LeConte, J.: A case of inherited polydactylism. *Science*, *8*:166, 1886.

Ledoux-Lebard, R., and Hérbert, G.: Un cas de polydactylie. *J. Radiol. Electrol.* (Paris), *3*:129, 1918.

Lehmann, W., and Witteler, E. A.: Zwillingsbeobachtung zur Erbpathologie der Polydactylie. *Zentralbl. Chir.*, *62*:2844–2852, 1935.

LeMarec, B., and Coutel, Y.: La polydactylie: maladie ou symptome? *Pediatrie*, *25*:735–746, 1970.

Lenglen: Sur la polydactylie héréditaire. *Bull. Acad. Méd.*, *5*:1312–1314, 1877.

Lenz, F.: Polydactyly or polydactylism. *In* Baur, E., Fischer, E., and Lenz, F., (eds.): *Human Heredity.* Third edition. Translated by E. Paul and C. Paul. New York, The Macmillan Co., pp. 285–297, 1931.

Lepoutre, C.: Malformations congénitales des extrémités (polydactylie, ectrodactylie, syndactylie, pouce à trois phalanges, etc.) chez un enfant et chez sa mère. *Rev. d'Orthop.*, (3 s.), *10*:237–244, 1923.

Lewis, T.: Polydactylism. *Treasury of Human Inheritance*, *1*:10–14, 1912.

Lineback, P. E.: A case of unilateral polydactyly in a 22 mm. embryo. *Anat. Rec.*, *20*:313–319, 1921.

Liston, R.: *Lectures on the Operations of Surgery.* Philadelphia, Lea & Blanchard, pp. 389–391, 1846.

Lobligeois: Sur un cas de polydactylie. *Bull. Mém. Soc. Radiol. Méd.* (Paris), *3*:187–188, 1911.

Lombard, P.: Bifurcation héréditaire et familiale de la main par fusion de deux métacarpeins en un os unique bifide—doigts surnuméraires. *Rev. d'Orthop.*, (3 s.), *5*:135–146, 1914.

Londe, A., and Meige, H.: Radiographies des extrémités d'un sexdigitaire. *N. Iconog. Salp.*, *10*:39–44, 1897.

London Med. Gaz.: A many toed and fingered family. *14*:65, 1834.

Longuet, M.: Un cas de pouce bifide: de la bifidité du pouce. *Rev. d'Orthop.*, (1 s.), *3*:290–303, 1892.

Lorain, P.: Note sur un cas de doigt surnuméraire chez un nouveau-né. *Gaz. Méd. Paris*, pp. 317–318, 1852. See also: *C. R. Soc. Biol.*, (1 s.), *4*:38–39, 1852.

Lovelady, R.: Bilateral duplicity (polydactylia) of the fifth digit. *Med. Radiog. Photog.*, *24*:85, 1948.

Löwy, M.: Ein Fall von vererbter Polydaktylie. *Prag. Med. Wochenschr.*, *23*:123, 1898.

Lubs, H. A., Jr., Koenig, E. U., and Brandt, I. K.: Trisomy 13–15, a clinical syndrome. *Lancet*, *2*:1001–1002, 1961.

Lucas, R. C.: On a remarkable instance of hereditary tendency to the production of supernumerary digits. *Guy's Hosp. Rep.*, (3 s.), *25*:417–419, 1881.

Lücker, F. C.: Uber Vererbung von Missbildungen, insbesonderer Hasenscharte und Polydaktylie, und ihre Beziehungen Geburtshilfe. *Monatsschr. Geburtsh. Gynäk.*, 66:327–336, 1924.

Lyonnet, R.: Cinq polydactyles dans la même fraterie grandpére maternel lui-même polydactyle et originaire de Izeaux. *Bull. Féder. Soc. Gynecol. Obstet. Langue Franc.*, 13:298–299, 1961.

Lyons, D. C.: Skeletal anomalies associated with cleft palate and harelip. *Am. J. Orthodent.*, 25:895–897, 1939.

MacCarthy, W. C., Jr., and Russell, D. G.: Tuberous sclerosis: report of a case with ependymoma. *Radiology*, 71:833–839, 1958.

MacPhail, D.: Child with double thumbs in each hand. *Glascow Med. J.*, 41:143–146, 1894.

Manoiloff, E. O.: A rare case of hereditary hexadactylism. *Am. J. Phys. Anthropol.*, 15:503–508, 1931.

Manson, J. S., and Nettleship, E.: Hereditary lamellar cataract and digital deformity in the same pedigree. *Trans. Ophthalmol. Soc. U.K.*, 32:45–53, 1917.

Marjolin, M.: Doigts surnuméraires. *Bull. Soc. Imp. Chir.*, (2 s.), 6:490–492, 1865.

Maroteaux, P., and Savart, P.: La dystrophie thoracique asphyxiante. Ètude radiologique et rapports avec le syndrome d'Ellis et van Creveld. *Ann. Radiol.*, 7:332–338, 1964.

Marsh, F.: A case of double polydactylism, double harelip, complete cleft palate, and double talipes varus. *Lancet*, 2:739, 1889.

Martin, E.: Deux soeurs atteintes de polydactylie. *Rev. Med. Suisse Romande*, 19:645–648, 1899.

Marzolo, F.: Interno ad una famiglia de sedigiti. *Mem. r. First Veneto di Sci., Lett. ed Arti.*, 20:457–484, 1876–1879.

Mauny: Pouce surnuméraire: disarticulation. *Bull. Soc. Anat.* (Paris), 65:252, 1890.

Mazzuca, R. C.: Considerazioni su di un caso di pollice soprannuerario. *Arch. Putti*, 23:462–466, 1964.

McClintic, B. S.: Five generations of polydactylism. *J. Hered.*, 26:141–144, 1935.

McCurdy, S. Le R.: Three generations of six-fingered anomalies. *Am. Med. Surg. Bull.* (New York), 10:240, 1896.

McIntosh, R.: Hereditary ectodermal dysplasia associated with polydactylism and chondrodystrophy. *In Holt's Diseases of Infancy and Childhood.* Tenth edition. Revised by L. E. Holt, Jr., and R. McIntosh. New York, D. Appleton-Century Co., p. 362; fig. 47, 1933.

McKellar, P. H. M.: Hereditary malformation of extremities. *Glascow Med. J.*, 2:390–391, 1870.

McKusick, V. A., Egeland, J. A., Eldridge, R., and Krusen, D. E.: Dwarfism in the Amish. I. The Ellis-van Creveld syndrome. *Bull. Johns Hopkins Hosp.*, 115:306–336, 1964.

Meige, H.: Un cas de polydactylie symétrique des mains et des pieds. *J. Conn. Méd. Prat.*, 65:114–116, 1897.

Mellin, G. W.: The frequency of birth defects. *In* Fishbein, M., (ed.): *Birth Defects.* Philadelphia, J. B. Lippincott Co., pp. 1–17, 1963.

Ménaché: Polydactylie héréditaire. *Bull. Soc. Obstet. Gynecol.* (Paris), 20:393–394, 1931.

Menning, K.: *Beitrag zur Kenntnis des anatomischen Verhaltens bei Hyperdaktylie.* Inaug. Diss. Wurzburg, P. Scheiner's Buchdruckerei, pp. 1–25, 1892.

Michalski, A.: Polydactylie. Doigts surnuméraires du bord cubital des deux mains. *Gaz. Hop. Div. Milit.*, No. 82:1–2, 1871.

Miles, A. E.: A case of hereditary polydactylism occurring in four generations and many members of the same family. *Br. J. Surg.*, 9:293–301, 1921.

Milford, F.: Case of congenital double thumb of the right hand. *New South Wales Med. J. Gaz.*, 3:381–383, 1872.

Mill, G. S.: A case of polydactylous hand. *Br. Med. J.*, 2:630, 1892. See also *Lancet*, 2:772, 1892.

Milles, B. L.: The inheritance of human skeletal anomalies (Polydactylism Type I and II.) *J. Hered.*, 19:28–46, 1928.

Millesi, H.: Fingerverformung nach Operationen wegen Polydaktylie. *Klin. Med. Wien.*, 22:266–272, 1967.

Mitchell, A.: Case of hereditary polydactylism. *Med. Times Gaz.*, 2:91, 1863.

Miura, M.: Die Poly- und Syndaktylie. *Mitthl. Med. Fac. Jap. Union.* (Tokyo), 4:13–15, 1898.

Mohan, J.: Postaxial polydactyly in three Indian families. *J. Med. Genet.*, 6:196–200, 1969.

Moncorvo: Nota sombre am caso de polydactylia. *Uniano Med. Rio di Jan.*, 3:531–535, 1883.

Morand, M.: Recherches sur quelques conformations monstrueses des doigts dans l'homme. *Hist. Acad. R. Sci. Année* (1770), pp. 137–150, Paris, 1773.

Morestin, H.: Pouce bifide. *Bull. Mèm. Soc. Anat.*, (6 s.), 5:519–520, 1903.

Morestin, H.: Double pouce. *Bull. Mèm. Soc. Anat.*, (6 s,), 12:150–152, 1910.

Morgan, G.: Skigrams of a case of polydactylism. *Lancet*, 2:1599, 1896.

Morrish, W. J.: Polydactylism. *Lancet*, 2:369, 1907.

Morton, W. R. M.: Arrhinencephaly and multiple developmental anomalies occurring in a full-term foetus. *Anat. Rec.*, 98:45–58, 1947.

Mouchet, A., and Lumiere, F.: Pouces surnuméraires et pouces bifides. *Rev. d'Orthop.*, (3 s.), 7:177–180, 1920.

Mouchet, A., and Noureddine, B.: Sur une variété de polydactylie: doigts supplémentaire aberrant pédicule. *Bull. Soc. Anat.*, 94:213–218, 1924.

Muir, J. S.: Note of a curious instance of abnormal development of adventitious fingers and toes, as illustrating the influence of heredity in five consecutive generations. *Glascow Med. J.*, 21:420–423, 1884.

Müller, W.: *Die Angeborenen Fehlbildungen der Menschlichen Hand.* Leipzig, G. Thieme, pp. 45–60, 1937.

Mussy, G. de: Doigt surnuméraire. *Bull. Soc. Anat.,* (1 s.), *13*:40, 1838.

Nigst, P. F.: Die polydaktylie. *Schweiz. Med. Wochenschr.,* 8:98–106, 1927.

Noël, H.: *Contribution à l'Étude des Doubles Pouces.* Thèse. Paris, Vig. Frères, pp. 90–95, 1913.

Noël, P.: Polydactylie et hérédité. *Presse Méd., 32*:1049–1050, 1942.

Noller, F.: *Chirurgisch-Ostopadische Erbkrankheiten im Gesetz vorbutung arbkranten Nachwuches.* Jena, G. Fischer, pp. 30–32, 1942.

Nourse, W. E. C.: Six-fingered persons. *Br. Med. J., 1*:251, 1887.

Nylander, E. S.: Präaxiale Polydaktylie in fünf Generationen einer schwedischen Sippe. *Upsala Läk. Forn., 36*:275–292, 1931.

Odiorne, J. M.: Polydactylism in related New England families. *J. Hered., 34*:45–55, 1943.

Ogle, J. A.: On hereditary transmission of structural peculiarities. *Brit. Foreign Med. Chir. Rev., 59*:500–521, 1872.

Ohkura, K.: Clinical genetics of polydactylism. *Jap. J. Hum. Genet., 1*:11, 1956.

Oliver, C. P.: Recessive polydactylism, associated with mental deficiency. *J. Hered., 31*:365–367, 1940.

Oppenheimer, B. S., Blackmann, N. S., and Grishman, A.: The association of the interatrial septal defect and anomalies of the osseous system. *Trans. Assoc. Am. Physicians, 62*:284–293, 1949.

Parhon, C., and Urechia, C.: Contribution casuistique a l'étude de la polydactylie chez les aliénés. *N. Iconog. Salp., 24*:391–397, 1911.

Parker, R. W., and Robinson, H. B.: Inherited congenital deformity of hands and feet. *Lancet, 1*:729–730, 1887.

Patua, K., Therman, E., Smith, D. W., Inhorn, S. L., and Wagner, H. P.: Multiple congenital anomalies by an extra autosome. *Lancet, 1*:790–793, 1960.

Pattarin, P.: Sopra un caso di polidattilia. *Monitor Zool. Ital., 39*:251–254, 1928.

Pelacz Vellegas, P. L.: La polidactilia es una deformidad o un fenomeno de atavisme? *Ciencia Med. Madrid, 4*:454–456, 1897.

Penhallow, D. P.: An unusual case of polydactylism. *J.A.M.A., 91*:564–565, 1928.

Péraire, M.: Un cas de polydactylie avec épreuve radiographique. *Bull. Soc. Anat.,* (5 s.), *12*:151, 1898.

Pfitzner, W.: Beiträg zur Kenntniss der Missbildungen des menschlichen Extremitätenskelets. *Morphol. Arbeit., 8*:304–340, 1898.

Phocas, M.: Difformités congénitales des doigts et pouce bifide. *Le Nord. Méd., 4*:26–29, 1898. Also in *Ann. Chir. Orthop., 9*:46–52, 1898.

Pigné, P.: Étiologie des doigts surnuméraires et autres organes externes. *J. Chir. Melgaigne.* Paris, P. Dupot et Cie, *4*:216–217, 1846.

Pigné, P.: Doigt surnuméraire. *Bull. Soc. Anat.,* (1 s.), *21*:205–210, 1846.

Pipkin, S. B., and Pipkin, A. C.: Variation of expression of polydactyly. *J. Hered., 37*:93–96, 1946.

Pires de Lima, J.: Polydactylie transitoire. *C. R. Soc. Biol., 83*:1190–1192, 1920.

Pires de Lima, J.: Un nouveau cas d'heptadactylie. *Ann. Anat. Pathol., 10*:1215–1216, 1933.

Pokorny, L.: Zur Klinik und Aetiologie der Polydaktylie. *Med. Klin., 29*:1486–1488, 1933.

Pol, R.: Hyperdaktylie (Polydaktylie), Diplocheirie und Diplopodie, Hypermelie, Oligodaktylie und Defekte von Rohrenknochen. *In* Schwalbe, E., and Gruber, G. B., (eds.): *Die Morphologie der Missbildungen des Menschen und der Tiere.* Jena, G. Fischer, T. 3, Apt. 1, Kapital 7:683-719, 1958.

Polonskaja, R.: Anatomische Eigenschaften der Menschen mit Polydaktylie. *Folia Morphol., 7*:114–120, 1936.

Popham, J.: Hemicephalic infant—protrusion of the membranes of the brain through a fissure of the occipital bone—supernumerary fingers and toes. *Dublin Quart. J. Med. Sci., 44*:481–483, 1867.

Porter, F. T.: Congenital malformation of the hand. *Dublin J. Med. Sci., 62*:68, 1876.

Pouillet, A.: Doigts surnuméraires du bord cubital de la main. *Courrier Méd., 23*:245–246, 1873.

Prakash, C., and Singh, S.: Coarctation of the aorta with hypertelorism, pilonidal sinus and polydactyly. *J. Indian Med. Assoc., 35*:267, 1960.

Prentiss, C. W.: Extra digits and digital reductions. *Pop. Sci. Monthly, 68*:336–348, 1906.

Rahon, J.: Sex-digitaire atteinte de syndactylie partielle. *Bull. Soc. d'Anthrop.,* (4 s.), *3*:334–336, 1892.

Reber, M.: Un syndrome osseux peu commun associant une heptadactylie et un aplasie des tibia. *J. Genet. Hum., 16*:15–39; fig. 9, 1968.

Reeves, R. S.: Supernumerary distal phalanx of the right thumb. *U.S. Naval Med. Bull., 14*:265–266, 1920. Also in *Penn. Med. J., 23*:720–721, 1920.

Refior, H. J.: Beiträge zur postaxialen familiaren Polydaktylie. *Arch. Orthop. Unfallchir., 63*:293–301, 1968.

Regnault, J.: Pouce supplémentaire remplacant le sésamoide externe. *Bull. Mèm. Soc. Anat.,* (6 s.), *13*:286–287, 1911.

Renard, F.: Note sur deux cas de polydactylie. *Ann. Orthop. Chir. Prat.* (Paris), *5*:213–227, 1892.

Ricaldoni, A., and Isola, A.: Maladie congénitale et familiale caracterisée par une dystrophio-adiposo-génitale associée e une rétinite pigmentaire et une polydactylie. *Arch. Méd. Enfants, 32*:27–35, 1929.

Ricciardi, L.: La polidattilia transitoria. *Clin. Ortop., 6*:441–447, 1954.

Richet, M.: Pouce surnuméraire de la main gauche. Amputation dans l'articulation métacarpophalangienne. Guérison. Conservation des movements dans le pouce restant. *Bull. Soc. Chir.*, (2 s.), *2*:227–232, 1862.

Rieder, H.: Über verdoppelung der Endphalanx des Daumens usw. *Internat. Photogr. Monatsschr. Med.*, *3*:49–55, 1900.

Rieger, H.: Erfgragen in der Augenheilkunde. *Arch. Ophthalmol.*, *143*:277–299, 1941.

Rimoin, D. L., and Edgerton, M. T.: Genetical and clinical heterogeneity in the oral-facial-digital syndromes. *J. Pediatr.*, *71*:94–102, 1967.

Rochlin, G. D.: Zum Problem der Hyperdaktylie. *Z. Anat. Entwicklungsgesch.*, *78*:148–160, 1926.

Rörberg: Ueberzahlige Finger und Zehen. *J. Kinderkrank.*, *35*:426, 1860.

Rosbach, H.: *De Numero Digitorum Adaucto*. Inaug. Diss. Bonnae, Typis Caroli Georgil, pp. 1–35, 1838.

Rosenverg, T., Palombini, B. C., and Peterson, N.: Simultaneous occurrence of spherocytosis and polydactyly in a Brazilian family. *Acta Gen. Med. Gelmellal*, *11*:55–72, 1962.

Rouby: Observations d'un index supplémentaire. *Gaz. Méd. Lyon*, *15*:364–365, 1863.

Roux: Bec-de-lièvre unilateral. *Gaz. Hop.*, p. 247, 1847.

Rudert, I.: Über die Vererblichkeit der präazialen Polydaktylie. *Z. menschl. Vererb. Konstitutionslehre*, *21*:545–557, 1937.

Rüdinger: Ueber Polydaktylie. *Sitz. Ges. Morphol. Physiol.*, *2*:119–120, 1886.

Ruhl, H.: Über Polydaktylie bei Zwillingen. *Zentralbl. Gynäk.*, *62*:2706–2709, 1938.

Say, B., and Gerald, P. S.: A new polydactyly/imperforate anus/vertebral anomalies syndrome. *Lancet*, *2*:688, 1968.

Say, B., Balci, S., Tugrul, P., and Tuncbilek, E.: A new syndrome of dysmorphogenesis: imperforate-anus associated with poly-oligodactyly and skeletal (mainly vertebral) anomalies. *Acta Paediatr. Scand.*, *60*:197–202, 1971.

Scherer, F.: Ueber einen Fall von symmetrischer Poly- und Syndaktylie. *Arch. Kinderheilkd.*, *17*:244–250, 1893–1894.

Schönenberg, H.: Polydaktylie. *In Über Missbildungen der Extremitäten*. Bibliotheca Paediatrica, Fasc. 80. Basel (Schweiz); New York, pp. 9–11, 1962.

Schoo, H. J. M.: Ueber ungleiche Bifurkation des kleinen Finger. *Arch. Pathol. Anat. Physiol.*, *205*:113–121, 1911.

Schoolfield, B.: Bilateral polydactylism with multiple syndactylism: case report. *South Med. J.*, *49*:716–717, 1956.

Schurmeier, H. L.: Congenital deformities of drafted men. *Am. J. Phys. Anthropol.*, *5*:51–60, 1922.

Sédillot, C.: Note sur l'amputation des doigts surnuméraires. *C. R. Mem. Biol.*, *5*:145–146, 1854.

Segmi, G., Serra, A., Mastrangelo, R., Polidori, G., and Massasso, J.: Sindrome OFD in un Maschio. Rilivi sulla genetica della sindrome OFD dell analisi 33 famiglie. *Acta Genet. Med. Gem.*, *19*:546–566, 1970.

Seiferle, E.: Atavismus u Polydaktylie der hyperdaktylen Hinterpfoten des Haushundes. *Morph. Jahrb.*, *57*:313–380, 1927.

Shapiro, R. N., Eddy, W., Fitzgibbon, J., and O'Brien, G.: The incidence of congenital anomalies discovered in the neonatal period. *Am. J. Surg.*, *96*:396–400, 1958.

Sharma, N. L., Singh, R. N., and Anand, J. S.: Polydactylo-syndactylism with unusual skeletal anomalies in mother and her six children. *Indian J. Pediatr.*, *32*:233–237, 1965.

Shevkenek, W., and Thomson, W. P.: A case of recessive polydactylism. *Trans. R. Soc. Canada*, Sec. V. *27*:169–171, 1933.

Shull, A. F.: *Heredity.* Fourth edition. New York, McGraw-Hill Book Co., pp. 110–112, 1948.

Simpkiss, M., and Lowe, A.: Congenital abnormalities in the African newborn. *Arch. Dis. Child.*, *36*:404–406, 1961.

Simpoulos, A. P., Brennan, G. G., Alwan, A., and Fidis, N.: Polycystic kidneys, internal hydrocephalus and polydactylism in newborn siblings. *Pediatrics*, *39*:931–934, 1967.

Sinha, S.: Polydactylism and tooth color. *J. Hered.*, *9*:96, 1918.

Sjostedt, G.: Beschereibung einer Familie mit Polydaktylie. *Acta Chir. Scand.*, *83*:269–286, 1940.

Smith, D. W.: The 18 trisomy and D_1 trisomy syndromes. *In* Gardner, L. T. (ed.): *Endocrine and Genetic Diseases of Childhood*. Philadelphia, W. B. Saunders Co., pp. 638–652, 1969.

Smith, D. W., Lemli, L., and Opitz, J. M.: A newly recognized syndrome of multiple congenital anomalies. *J. Pediatr.*, *64*:210–217, 1964.

Smith, S., and Boulgakoff, B.: A case of polydactylia showing certain atavistic characters. *J. Anat.*, *58*:350–367, 1924.

Smith, W. A. De W.: Case of supernumerary digits. *Med. News* (Philadelphia), *54*:307–308, 1889.

Snedecor, S. T., and Harryman, W.: Surgical problems in hereditary polydactylism and syndactylism. *J. Med. Soc.* (New Jersey), *37*:443–449, 1940.

Snyder, A.: A recessive factor for polydactylism in man. Studies in human inheritance III. *J. Hered.*, *20*:73–77, 1929.

Sobbota, A., and De Marinis, F.: On the inheritance and development of preaxial and postaxial types of polydactylism. *Acta Genet. Med. Gem.*, *6*:85–93, 1957.

Sommer: Bemerkungen zu einem Fall von vererber Sechsfingergkeit. *Klin. Psych. Krank.*, *5*:197–308, 1910.

Sorrel, E., and Oberthur, H.: Deux cas de polydactylie. *Bull. Soc. Anat.*, (6 s.), *19*:241–243, 1922.

Stapff, R.: Über eine Familie mit erblicher Syn- und Polydaktylie (Hyperphalangie pollicis). *Fortschr. Röntgenstr.*, *34*:531–538, 1926.

Stein, J.: Ein Fall von Polydaktylie. *Prag. Med. Wochenschr.*, *10*:224, 1885.

Stelling, F.: *In* Ferguson, A. B., (ed.): *Operative Surgery in Infancy and Childhood.* Second edition. Baltimore, Williams & Wilkins, Co., pp. 282–339; Third edition, pp. 292–334, 1967.

Stevenson, A. C., Johnston, H. A., Stewart, M. J. P., and Golding, D. R.: Malformations of limbs and extremities: polydactyly. *Bull. World Health Org.* (Geneve), *34*:58–59, 1966.

Stocquast: Note sur un cas de polydactylie bilatérale. *Bull. Soc. Anthrop.* Bruxelles, *14*:335, 1895–1896.

Struthers, J.: On variation in the number of toes, and in the number of phalanges, in man. *New Philos J.* Edinburgh, (n.s.), *18*:83–111, 1863.

Sutton, J. B.: Rudimentary supernumerary pollex. *Proc. Anat. Soc.* Great Britain & Ireland, p. XIII, 1892–1893.

Sverdrup, A.: Postaxial polydactylism in six generations of Norwegian family. *J. Genet.*, *12*:217–240, 1922.

Sysak, N.: About hearths of polydactyly in the Poltava government. *Z. menschl. Vererb. Konstitutionslehre*, *12*:463–468, 1928.

Tapie, J.: *De la Polydactylie.* Thèse. Paris, A Parent, pp. 5–54, 1885.

Tarnier, M.: Une phalange supplémentaire enlèvée à la racine du pouce. *Bull. Soc. Anat.*, (2 s.), *2*:209, 1857.

Tattoni, A.: *Scritti Medici in onore di Aristide Busi.* Bologna, L. Cappelli, Parte I, pp. 748–760, 1931.

Tatum, T.: Supernumerary little finger in an adult; removal. *Lancet*, *1*:93–94, 1863.

Tessari, L.: Sulla polidattilia. *Arch. Ortop.*, *74*:1186–1196, 1961.

Thienot, J.: Les familles sexdigitaires. *L'Indépend. Med.* Paris, *6*:18, 1900.

Thomsen, O.: Einige Eigentümlichkeiten der erbliche Poly- und Syndaktylie bei Menschen. *Acta Med. Scand.*, *65*:609–644, 1927.

Thorpe, G.: Two cases of congenital deformity. *Lancet*, *2*:817, 1890.

Thouret, T.: Pouce surnuméraire tenant à l'éminence thénar par un pédicule non-osseux. *Bull. Soc. Anat.*, (1 s.), *2*:17, 1844.

Thuline, H. C.: Current status of a family previously reported with the oral-facial-digital syndrome. *In* Bergsma, D., (ed.): *Birth Defects: Original Article Series.* New York, National Foundation—March of Dimes, Vol. V, No. 2:102, 1969.

Thurston, E. O.: A case of median harelip associated with other malformations. *Lancet*, *2*:996–997, 1909.

Tissot, J.: Une famille de sexdigitaires. *Méd. Mod.* (Paris), *9*:497–498, 1898.

Tomlinson, H. A.: The existence of supernumerary fingers running through three generations. *Med. Times* (Philadelphia), *10*:212–213, 1879–1880.

Tornier, G.: Über Hyperdaktylie, Regeneration und Vererbung mit Experimentaten. *Arch. Entwickg. v. Roux.* *3*:469–476, *4*:180–210, 1896.

Treiger, J.: Ein Fall von Polydaktylie. *Fortschr. Röntgenstr.*, *27*:419–422; Taf. XXVI; fig. 1–4, 1921.

Ullrich, O.: Der Status Bonnevie-Ullrich im Rahmen anderer Dyscranio-Dysphalangien. *Ergebn. Inn. Med. N. F.*, *2*:412–466, 1951.

Van Neck, M.: Pouce bifide opéré par la procédé de Cloquet. *Arch. Franco-Belge. Chir.*, *28*:607–608, 1925.

Veitch, H. C. V.: Polydactylism in twins. *Lancet*, *1*:650, 1928.

Verrier, M. E.: Des anomalies symétriques des doigts et du rôle que l'on pourrait attribuer à l'atavisme dans ces anomalies. *C. R. Acad. Sci.*, *100*:865–869, 1885.

Vidal, J. P. I.: Note explicative sur un pouce double d'Annamite. *Rec. Mèm. Méd., Chir. Pharm. Milit.*, (3 s.), *13*:71–74. 1865.

Vogel, K.: Über Familiares Auftreten von Polydaktylie und Syndaktylie. *Fortschr. Röntgenstr.*, *20*:443–447, 1913.

Vrolik, W.: Teratology. *In* Todd, R. B., (ed.): *The Cyclopedia of Anatomy and Physiology.* London, Longman, Brown, etc., Vol. IV, pp. 942–976, 1849.

Wachowski, T. J.: Familial polyphalangia and duplicity (polydactylie). *Med. Radiog. Photog.*, *24*:85–87, 1948.

Wakley, T.: Cases of supernumerary thumb, imperforate vagina, and imperfect development of the ear, in children. *Lancet*, *2*:421, 1861.

Walker, J. T.: A pedigree of extra-digit-V polydactyly in a Batutsi family. *Ann. Hum. Genet.*, *25*:65–68, 1961.

Wassel, H. D.: The results of surgery for polydactyly of the thumb. A review. *Clin. Orthop.*, *64*:175–193, 1969.

Watson, W. S.: Specimen of a supernumerary finger removed from the little finger. *Trans. Pathol. Soc.* (London), *18*:281, 1867.

Weingrow, S. M.: Supernumerary distal phalanx of the thumb. Case report. *Am. J. Roentgenol.*, *23*:206–207, 1930.

Wertheim-Salomonson, J. K. A.: Ein seltener Fall von Polydactylie. *Fortschr. Röntgenstr.*, *4*:42–43, 1900–1901.

Weyers, H.: Über eine korrelierte Missbildung der Kieferund Extremitätenakren (Dysostosis acrofacialis). *Fortschr. Röntgenstr.*, 77:562–567, 1952.

Weyers, H.: Hexadactylie, Unterkieferspalt und Oligodontie ein neuer Sympton Komplex. Dysostosis acrofacialis. *Ann. Paediatrici.*, 181:45–60, 1953.

Wilson, G.: Hereditary polydactylism. *J. Anat. Physiol.*, 30:437–449, 1896.

Windle, C. A.: The occurrence of an additional phalanx in the human pollex. *J. Anat. Physiol.*, 26:100–116, 1891.

Withrow, O. C.: A case of supernumerary digits. *Lancet*, 2:558, 1907.

Wood, V. E.: Duplication of the index finger. *J. Bone Joint Surg.*, 52A:569–573, 1970.

Wood, V. E.: Treatment of central polydactyly. *Clin. Orthop.*, 74:196–205, 1971.

Woolf, C. M., and Woolf, R. M.: A genetic study of polydactyly in Utah. *Am. J. Hum. Genet.*, 22:75–88, 1970.

Yano, M., and Soma, H.: A kindred of polydactyly. *Jap. J. Hum. Genet.*, 6:124–126, 1961.

Young, R. F.: Hereditary polydactylism. *Br. Med. J.*, 1:91, 1922.

Yudkin, A. M.: Congenital bilateral microphthalmus accompanied by other malformations of the body. *Am. J. Ophthalmol.*, 11:128–131, 1928.

Zabolotikov, P. V.: On the problem of polydactylia (Russian). *Arkh. Anat.*, 50:91–93, 1966.

Zampa, G.: Pollice bifidi e pollice suprannumerari. *Chir. Organi Mov.*, 13:195–212, 1928.

Zeller, R.: *Über familiäres Auftreten von Hyperphalangie und Polydaktylie des Daumens und die Erblichkeit der Pseudoepiphysen.* Inaug. Diss. Bonn, A. Brand, pp. 1–32, 1936.

Zweig, W.: Polidattilia famigliare. *Radiol. Med.* (Milano), 25:735–739, 1938.

Chapter Fourteen

MULTIPLE AND MIRROR HANDS

In most communications, multiple and mirror hands are discussed in connection with polydactyly and are, in fact, considered as extreme forms of the latter. In both anomalies there is an excessive number of digits, but here the resemblance ends. A sizable body of literature has now grown around mirror hand; however, the bibliography of this anomaly remains buried in the more extensive lists of references pertaining to polydactyly. Salvaging this material provides additional justification for allotting a chapter to mirror hand. Not enough has been written about multiple hands to justify the assignment of a separate chapter. This abnormality bears closer affinity to mirror hand than to any other anomaly; hence, its inclusion here.

MULTIPLE HANDS

Only six authenticated cases of multiple hands have thus far been reported. Grandin (1887) described the deformity of a 13-month-old female infant as follows: "The upper arm of the right side consisted of two humeri, each articulating with a radius and an ulna. Between these two radii and ulnas were a third radius and ulna. . . . There were three hands. . . . Each hand moved separately. . . . The father's aunt of this infant had two thumbs on each hand; another relative, again on the father's side, had some peculiarity in the joints of one hand; the child's brother had a rudimentary tail."

Faltin (1904) featured the photograph of a boy whose left arm had an additional hand with two fingers, two metacarpals, and a long bone which ran parallel to the humerus; the surplus hand sprouted from the ulnar side of the upper arm. Pol (1914) described a young girl with a surplus vestigial arm and hand jutting out from the left shoulder. Alonso (1939) reported a child with two separate forearms and two hands. One forearm had a radius and an ulna; in the other, these two bones appeared to have been fused. Alonso amputated the less functional of the two hands.

The patient presented by Stein and Bettmann (1940) was a 52-year-old woman with a massive arm and forearm which terminated in three hands. X-ray showed double scapuli, two humeri, two radii, and three ulnas. The fingers on one hand appeared normal; on the other two, they were in fixed flexion; one thumb served two conjoined hands. The third hand was free and had its own thumb. There were altogether 16 digits. Kruckenmeyer's (1958) case had an extra arm and hand emanating from the right side of the neck.

MIRROR HANDS OR ULNAR DIMELIA

In contrast to the relatively rare appearance of multiple hands, tens times as many—about 60—cases of mirror hands have been reported; several individually incomplete but collectively fairly comprehensive reviews have been published by Morand (1773), Taruffi (1886), Dwight (1892, 1893), Bateson (1894), Santero (1936), O'Rahilly (1951), Bonola (1955), Perini (1955), and Burman (1968). Rueff (1587) is credited as having described the first case of mirror hand or ulnar dimelia. His book contains a plate showing a boy who has twinned hands and twinned feet; each twinned manus is shown to consist of two components and each one of these contains five digits, four fingers and the thumb. The hands are joined together by their ulnar margin, which is contrary to the present day concept of ulnar dimelia.

With but slight modification this same drawing reappeared in Aldrovandi's (1642) book. Du Cauroi (1696) reported an infant with eight fingers on the right hand, of which two indices were joined together. There were seven fingers on the left hand. Carré (1838) described an adult who had five fingers and two thumbs on his right hand, and his forearm contained an "additional radius." Erichsen (1873, 1885) included a drawing in his book which showed a massive bifid index finger flanked on either side by three normal looking ulnar digits. There was no comment in the text beyond the statement that "in some rare cases, as in that from which the annexed drawing was taken, two hands appear to be fused into one." Clutton (1896) featured a similar drawing which was said to have been copied from a specimen in the St. Thomas Hospital Museum.

Many authors have since cast doubt on the authenticity of some of the above cases and have dismissed the rest for lack of adequate description. Carré's (1838) contention that the hand he described contained an additional thumb and that there was an excess radius in the forearm has been questioned. Carré probably mistook the surplus ulna in the forearm for a radius, and the two thumbs he mentioned represented, respectively, the little and ring fingers of the fused hands. In every case of mirror hand which has been subjected to careful dissection or roentgenographic study, the radius and the thumb are found to be absent, and the ulna and the distal components of the ulnar ray have been duplicated. Occasionally in an older individual, as in the 63-year-old woman reported by Appelrath (1922), the carpal articular end of the pre-axial ulna will undergo adaptive changes and broaden, simulating the distal end of the radius; the two surplus digits on the sides will function as thumbs, and in doing so they will thicken. In all such cases, what appears as a radius near the wrist has been shown to have an olecranon process at the elbow; the digits functioning as thumbs often have three phalanges and a sublimis tendon but no thenar muscles.

The first definitely authenticated, and perhaps most thoroughly documented, case of ulnar dimelia with mirror imaging of the fingers was reported by Jackson (1853) and later described in greater detail by Dwight (1892, 1893).

"There is one central index finger, and upon each side of it a middle, ring and little finger, seven altogether, and perfectly formed, the index being no longer than natural. The subject of this case was a German machinist, aged thirty-seven years; and the hand was not merely useful in the way of his business, but gave him some advantage . . . in playing the piano. . . . The three upper fingers . . . were used efficiently as a thumb to oppose the three others," Jackson wrote. When the man died, his limb was dissected. In the forearm, there were two ulnas and no radius or radial artery. In the wrist, no trace of the scaphoid and the trapezium could be found. The other carpal bones were duplicated, making a total of 10 ossicles. In the hand, the metacarpal and phalanges of the thumb were absent; there were seven metacarpals and an equal number of fingers arranged in two groups facing one another. The radial group consisted of three partially webbed fingers; the ulnar set had four fingers. All digits were flexed at the interphalangeal joints, and the hand was bent volarward at the wrist and radially deviated. "The malformation seems to consist of the fusion by the radial edge, of two very imperfectly developed extremities. . . . In the forearm . . . there are two ulnas, but no radius," Jackson concluded. Dwight had this to say: "The hand is flexed and somewhat pronated. . . . A very curious feature of this extremity is the evident attempt of the extra ulna to imitate a radius. . . . Still more curious is the origin from the musculo-spiral nerve of a branch in place of the radial which becomes an ulnar. . . . "

Jardine Murray's (1863) patient was "a well-developed, healthy, active and intelligent woman." She was 38 years old, married, and had a seven-year-old child who was "normal in every respect." On the left hand she had eight fingers radiating from a common palm; Murray considered the anomaly to be a "double hand." The middle and ring fingers on the "supernumerary hand" were webbed, the flexion at the elbow was limited, and the forearm and the wrist were thick. "I feel sure," Murray wrote, "that the duplicity of the bony structure begins at the carpus."

Giraldes (1866, 1869) described a child with no thumb and eight fingers on the right hand. Neither Murray nor Giraldes made any mention of an absent radius or a duplicated ulna. The patient presented by Bruce (1868) was a middle-aged man whose left hand had no thumb, its place being occupied by three ulnar digits "belonging to the right hand, whilst the index-finger is bifid, and evidently consists of two fingers incompletely united together. . . . The forearm has very limited powers of pronation or supination which seems the result of a second ulna," Bruce wrote.

No mention was made of duplication of the ulna in the cases reported by Fumagalli (1871), Kuhnt (1872), Gherini (1874), Langalli (1875), and Giärth (1903). Jolly's (1891) patient was a 24-year-old male whose left upper limb was affected. It was shorter than his right; the movements at the elbow were limited. Pronation and supination of the forearm were nil; the hand had six, or two groups of three, fingers, each consisting of the middle, ring, and the little fingers. Jolly was inclined to think that the ulnar parts of two forearms and hands were fused together, while the radial constituents had been suppressed.

Ballantyne (1893) presented a male infant with flexion contracture of the elbow and the wrist and pronated position of the forearm. "There are," Ballantyne wrote, "seven digits, and these are divided into two groups, a radial and an ulnar, by an interdigital sulcus, which is somewhat deeper than any of the others. The ulnar group consists of four digits, each made up of three phalanges; the innermost of these is no doubt the little finger; then followed the ring, middle and index as one passes towards the radial side of the hand. The thumb is wanting.

This group of digits no doubt constitutes the right hand proper of the infant, whilst the fingers on the radial side are supernumerary, and make up the deformity. This radial group consists of three digits, of which that on the radial side is the little finger while the other two are the ring and the middle fingers. Each has three phalanges, but the ring and middle fingers are webbed in the region of their proximal phalanges. . . . In addition to the deformity of the hand there is an abnormal condition of the elbow on the same side. . . . It seems as if the ulna is dislocated inwards."

Dwight (1892, 1893) regarded the absence of the radius and thumb and the duplication of the ulna and the distal components of the ulnar ray as the salient features of "polydactylism resulting from fusion of the ulnar portions of the hands. . . . In all these cases, which are adequately described," Dwight wrote, " . . . the hands are fused by corresponding sides. There is no instance of the ulnar side of one hand being joined to the radial side of the other." According to Bateson (1894), in what had been described as a "double hand," the two groups stood as a complementary pair, the one being the optical image of the other, and an ulna-like bone took the place of the radius.

Since the introduction of radiography, in cases of mirror imaging of the hand, it has been possible to demonstrate duplication of the components of the ulnar ray and suppression of the radial elements. With some slight variation, these changes have been present in the cases reported by the following authors: Fischer (1912), Restemeier (1920), Mau (1922), Appelrath (1922), Vincent (1922), Weil (1924), Nitsche (1931), Hueber and Pollitzer (1931), Kanavel (1932), Santero (1936), Fusari (1936), Buettner (1938), Cornacchia (1950), Priessnitz (1954), Bonola (1955), Perini (1955), Mukerji (1957), Davis and Farmer (1958), Hopf (1959), Entin (1959), Harrison et al (1960), Salzer (1961), Kelley (1962), Manaresi (1962), Guerzoni and Lenzi (1963), Pintilie et al (1964), Buck-Gramcko (1964), Laurin et al (1964), Tünte and Kersting (1967), Keiser (1968), Störig (1968), and Rinaldi (1968). In the cases reported by Priessnitz and Rinaldi, the humeral head at the shoulder was dislocated.

O'Rahilly (1951) considered the duplication of the ulna and of the distal components of the ulnar ray as the most constant feature of mirror hands; conversely, the components of the radial ray, including the radius, the scaphoid, the trapezium, the first metacarpal, and the phalanges of the thumb, are absent. "The hemimelic pattern," O'Rahilly wrote, "is dependent on the successive longitudinal development of the embryonic limb, as follows from the experimental observations of Saunders. In particular, the radius, scaphoid, trapezium, first metacarpal and thumb form a radial ray in a sense that they display close ontogenic interdependence. . . . The association of radial hemimelia with ulnar dimelia is probably an example of mutational inhibition of differentiation in the region of overlap of competing limb fields."

It may be remembered that on the basis of his experimental investigation, Saunders (1948) evolved the theory of apical ectodermal control of limb development. His findings have since been confirmed by Zwilling (1955, 1956), Amprino and Comosso (1955), Zwilling and Hansborough (1956), and some others. Saunders et al (1957) wrote: "The apical ectodermal ridge exercises an inductive action on the subjacent mesoderm bringing about the formation of the terminal limb parts. . . . This influence affects the regional character of morphological differentiation and inductive specificity of the mesoderm with respect to proximo-distal axis of the limb. . . ." Tschumi (1957) said: "The apical ridge of proliferation lays down the prospective limb segments in a proximo-distal direction."

Several clinicians have evoked this theory in their attempt to explain the polydactyly of ulnar dimelia. In the embryo, the border of the limb bud which is to form the elements of the radial ray is closer to the head. This pre-axial border is said to influence the development of ulnar components which are relegated to a caudal position. If the pre-axial sector of the apical ridge is destroyed or has undergone focal necrosis, the elements of the radial ray fail to develop; the post-axial area, which has been quiescent during the supremacy of the pre-axial portion, induces the differentiation of two groups of ulnar digital rays, making a total of six, seven, or eight fingers.

Polydactyly of ulnar dimelia differs from the ordinary variety of supernumerary digits in more than one respect. The thumb is absent in ulnar dimelia, its place being taken by two or more digits which collectively conduct the function of opposition, but are individually weaker than the normal pollex. The carpal and metacarpal bones are arranged in an arc with a deep palmar concavity, and the fingers radiating from them turn their volar surface toward one another. Most fingers maintain a flexed position; some of them are webbed. The hand is flexed at the wrist and it is often deviated to one side, usually in the radial direction. The wrist and the elbow are thick, and the arm as a whole is short. In older individuals, the carpal epiphyses of the two ulnas are broad; in the young, they are small and usually lack styloid processes. At the elbow, the articular end of each ulna has turned around on its axis so as to make its olecranon fossa face the corresponding notch of its mate; the distal articular end of the humerus lacks a capitulum and is composed of two ill-defined trochleas (Figs. 14–1 and 14–2).

In varying degrees, cases of ulnar dimelia present the following surgical

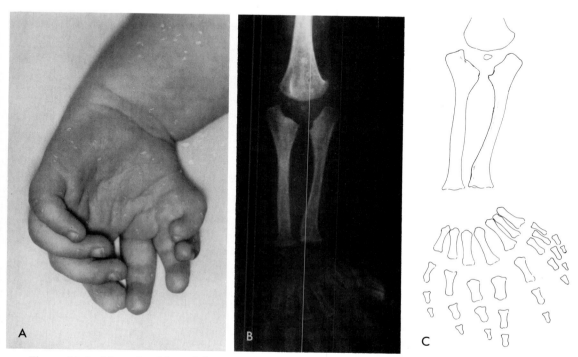

Figure 14–1 Mirror hand in an infant. *A*, Palmar view of the right hand. *B*, Anteroposterior roentgenograph of the right forearm, showing two ulnae. *C*, Sketch illustrating the skeletal components of the forearm and hand.

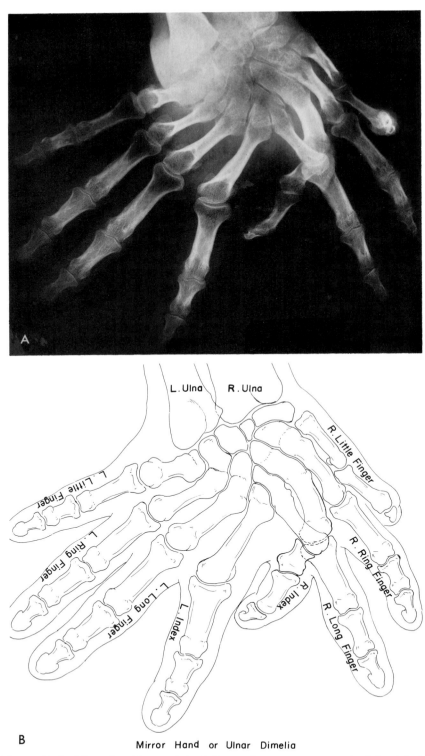

Figure 14–2   Mirror hand in an adult. *A*, Dorsopalmar roentgenograph of the right hand. *B*, Sketch illustrating the same.

problems: digits in excess of the normal formula of five, weak apposition of fingers, syndactyly of some fingers, limited extension at the wrist, limited movements at the elbow, and curtailed pronation and supination of the forearm and hand.

In the infant he reported, Giraldes (1866, 1869) reduced the number of digits from eight to five by amputation of three radial fingers. After reading Murray's (1863) article about an adult with good functional propensity, Giraldes regretted his surgical venture. Erichsen (1873, 1885) did not think any operation could advantageously be practiced upon the deformity, which he called "fusion of hands." Despite these reports, operations (usually amputation of surplus digits) continued to be practiced during the latter half of the nineteenth and earlier decades of the twentieth centuries. In a child with eight digits on one hand, Giärth (1903) "removed three fingers and one metacarpus, leaving a well-developed hand with five fingers without thumb or stump."

Mau (1922) seems to have been the first to attempt pollicization of one of the remaining five fingers. Santero (1936) introduced the concept of excising the proximal articular end of one of the ulnas to enhance flexion and extension of the elbow and to promote freer pronation and supination of the forearm and the hand. Fusari (1936), and after him Bonola (1955), transferred the most potent extensor tendon of one of the amputated digits to the pollicized finger. Priessnitz (1954) combined the principle of resection of one of the olecranon processes with pollicization of the most radial of the five remaining fingers. Cornacchia (1950) retained two radial digits and enclosed them in a common sleeve of skin; he corrected the flexion deformity of the wrist by cuneiform osteotomy of the distal ulna.

The principle of syndactylizing two weak radial digits to procure a strong thumb was utilized again by Davis and Farmer (1958). Entin (1959) removed the first and third radial digital rays and used the flap of skin thus made available to establish a broad web between the second and fourth digits; he then performed rotation osteotomy at the base of the second metacarpal and held the pollicized digit in position with a strut bone graft between its metacarpal and the metacarpal of the next ulnar finger. After amputation of the surplus digits, pollicization of the most radial of the remaining five fingers was practiced again by Kelley (1962), Manaresi (1962), Boyes (1964, 1970), Buck-Gramcko (1964), and Pintilie et al (1964).

SUMMARY

Polymelia—or multiple arms and hands—appears to be extremely rare. Ulnar dimelia or mirror hand is comparatively more common. This latter anomaly may be defined as a defect of the radial ray, with duplication of the ulna and the distal digital components of the ulnar ray, giving the impression that two hands with total longitudinal defect of the radial ray have become fused along their pre-axial margins. The abnormality is unilateral and does not seem to be hereditary. It poses two surgical problems: limited pronation and supination of the forearm and absence of a thumb. When the hand is in marked pronation, it may be brought into neutral position by rotary osteotomy of one or both ulnas. Excision of the olecranon process of one of the ulnas, usually the pre-axial bone, will also enhance the rotary movements of the forearm and the hand. A thumb or oppositional member is reconstructed from the most powerful finger of the pre-axial hand; the surplus digits are disposed of and their tendons are utilized to reinforce the pollicized finger.

References

Aasar, Y. H.: A heptadactylous human hand. *J. R. Egyptian Med. Assoc., 26*:337–339, 1943.

Aldrovandi, U.: Vititia Manuum, et digitorum vonformatio. *In Monstrorum Historia.* Bonn, Marcus Antonius Bernia, pp. 495–497, 1642.

Alonso, S.: Malformacion asimetrica doble. Aplasia de la clavicula. *Rev. Med. Rosaria, 29*:786–793, 1939.

Amprino, R., and Comosso, M.: Recherche sperimental sulla morfugens; deligiarti nel pollo. *J. Exp. Zool., 129*:453–493, 1955.

Andersen, K. S., and Rovsing, H.: Diplòpedia. *Acta Orthop. Scand., 42*:291–295, 1971.

Appelrath: Zur Kenntnis des Doppelbildungen einzelner Gliedmassen. *Fortschr. Röntgenstr., 29*:57–59, 1922.

Aschner, B.: Zur Erbbiologie der Skeletsystems. *Z. menschl. Vererb. Konstitutionslehre, 14*:129–211, 1929.

Ballantyne, J. W.: An infant with a bifid hand. *Edinburgh Med. J., 38*:623–626, 1893.

Bateson, W.: *Materials for the Study of Variation.* London, Macmillan and Co., pp. 324–356, 1894.

Bonola, A.: Sulla correzione chirurgica del raddoppiamenti speculari della mano. *J. Ortop. Traum. App. Mot., 23*:713–721, 1955.

Born, W.: Monsters in art. *Ciba Symposia, 9*:684–696, 1947.

Boyes, J. H.: *Bunnell's Surgery of the Hand.* Fourth edition. Revised by J. H. Boyes. Philadelphia, J. B. Lippincott Co., pp. 77–79; 99–102; figs. 99–102, 1964. Also in Fifth edition, pp. 83–85, 1970.

Brandt, W.: *Lehrbuch der Embryologie.* Basel, S. Karger, pp. 603–607, 1949.

Bruce, A.: Remarkable malformation of the left hand. *Trans. Pathol. Soc.* (London), *19*:452, 1868.

Buck-Gramcko, D.: Operative Behandlung einer Spiegelbild-Deformitat der Hand (Mirror Hand – doppelte Ulna mit Polydaktylie). Traitement operatoire d'une difformite en miroir de l'avantbras (Dedoublement du cubitus et des doigts cubitaux). *Ann. Chir. Plast., 9*:180–183, 1964.

Buettner, G.: Ulnar Polydaktylie bei Ulnaverdoppelung und Radius defekt. *Z. menschl. Vererb. Konstitutionslehre, 22*:428–440, 1938.

Bunnell, S.: *Surgery of the Hand.* Second edition. Philadelphia, J. B. Lippincott Co., pp. 815–820, 1948. Also in: Third edition, pp. 935–939, fig. 913, 1956.

Burman, M.: An historical perspective of double hands and double feet. The survey of cases reported in the 16th and 17th centuries. *Bull. Hosp. Joint Dis., 29*:241–254, 1968.

Carré: Communication. Séance publique de la *Soc. R. Méd. Chir. Pharm. Toulouse,* pp. 28–30, 1838.

Clutton, H. H.: Supernumerary digits. *In* Treves, F., (ed.): *A System of Surgery.* London, Cassel and Co. Ltd. Vol. II, pp. 85–87; fig. 523, 1896.

Cornacchia, M.: Rara malformazione congenita dell-arto superiore e sui trattamento chirurgico. *Bull. Sci. Med. Bologna, 3*:265–276, 1950.

Damman, J.: Ein Weiterer Fall von angeborener Ulnaverdoppelung (Spiegelelle). *Beitr. Orthop. Traum., 9*:181–188, 1962.

Davis, R. G., and Farmer, A. W.: Mirror hand anomaly: a case presentation. *Plast. Reconstr. Surg., 21*:80–83, 1958.

Du Cauroi: Extrait d'une lettre de Monsieur de Cauroi. Medicine de la Ville de Beauvais. *J. des Scavans* (pater superseded by J. des Savants), pp. 82–85, 1696.

Dwight, T.: Fusion of hands. *Mem. Boston Soc. Nat. Hist., 4*:473–486; pl. 43, 44, 1892. Also in *Anat. Anz., 8*:60–69, 1893.

Entin, M.A.: Reconstruction of congenital abnormalities of the upper extremity. *J. Bone Joint Surg., 41A*:681–700; fig. 8 A-H, 1959.

Ercolani, G. B.: Della polydactylia della polymelia nell homo e nei vertebrati. *Mem. Acad. Sci. Inst. Bologna, 3*:265–276, 1950.

Erichsen, J. E.: *The Science and Art of Surgery.* Seventh edition. Henry C. Lea, Vol. II, p. 330; fig. 420, 1873, Also in Eighth edition, p. 506; fig. 626, 1885.

Faggiana, F.: Sulla genesi dei raddoppiamonti speculari delgi arti superiori. *Ortop. Traum. App. Mot., 17*:349–365, 1949.

Faltin, R.: Ein Fall von Missbildungen der oberen Extremität dürch Ueberzahl. *Pflugers Arch. Anat. Physiol.,* pp. 350–371, 1904.

Fischer, H.: *Zahlreiche Missbildungen an einem Foetus und ein Fall einer doppelten Ulna-Bildung.* Inaug. Diss. Bonn, H. Ludwig, pp. 42–45; figs. 14–15, 1912.

Fumagalli, C.: Sulle deformita congenite della dita. *Ann. Univ. Med. Milano, 216*:305–321, 1871.

Fusari, A.: Dichiria e doppia ulna con assenza del radio. *Bull. Mem. Soc. Piemontese Chir., 6*:541–555, 1936.

Gandolfi, M., and Guerzoni, P. L.: La diplopedia. *Minerva Ortop., 16*:404–409, 1965.

Gherini, A.: Di una deformita congenita per eccesso alle mani e ai piedi. *Gaz. Med. Italiana-Lonbardia,* No. 51:401–402, figs. I-IV, 1874.

Giärth, D. J.: Child with eight fingers on one hand. *Amer. Med., 6*:463, 1903.

Giraldes, J.: Fusion de deux mains. *Bull. Soc. Chir. Paris,* (2 s.), *2*:505–507, 1866. See also *Lecons Cliniques sur les Maladies Chirurgicales des Enfants.* Paris, A. Delahaye, pp. 42–44; fig. 3, 1869.

Grandin, E. H.: Prenatal deformity of arm and hand. *Am. J. Obstet., 20*:425–426, 1887.

Guerzoni, P. L., and Lenzi, L.: Raddoppiamento speculare dell'arto inferiore. *Chir. Organi. Mov., 52*:202–208, 1963.

Hamburger, V.: Monsters in nature. *Ciba Symposia, 9*:666–683, 1947.

Harrison, R. G., Pearson, M. A., and Roaf, R.: Ulnar dimelia. *J. Bone Joint Surg., 42B*:549–555, 1960.

Hartz, B.: Ananiotische Entwicklungsstörung mit Hypermelie und Gliedmassenverpflazung. *Beitr. Pathol. Anat., 94*:606–610, Abb. 1, 1935.

Hopf, A.: Die Polydaktylie hoheren Grades: Handverdoppelungen *In* Hohmann, G., Hackenbroc, M., and Lindemann, K., (eds.): *Spezielle Orthopädie obere Extremität of Handbuch der Orthopädie.* Stuttgart, G. Thieme, Band 3:444–445; Abb. 16, 1959.

Hueber, E., and Pollitzer, G.: Missbildung der linken oberen Extremität (Polymelie oder Schizomelie). *Münch. Med. Wochenschr., 38*:134–135, 1931.

Jackson, J. B.: Malformation in an adult subject, otherwise well formed, consisting of apparent fusion of two upper extremities. *Am. J. Med. Sci.,* (n.s.), 25:91–93, 1853. See also *Descriptive Catalogue of the Warren Anatomical Museum,* Harvard University. Boston, A. Williams & Co., Entry 917, pp. 137–138, 1870.

Jolly, F.: Ueber Polydaktylie mit Missbildung des Armes. *Internat. Beitr. Will. Med., 1*:617–630; fig. 1–3, 1891.

Kanavel, A. B.: Congenital malformations of the hand. *Arch. Surg., 25*:1–53; 282–320; fig. 45, 1932.

Keiser, D. V.: Doppelbildungen. *In* Diethelm, L., (ed.): *Skeletanatomie (Röntgendiagnostik).* Berlin, Springer, Bd. IV; Teil 2:211–213; figs. 17 and 18, 1968.

Kelley, J. W.: Mirror hand. *Plast. Reconstr. Surg., 30*:374–377, 1962.

Kruckenmeyer, K.: Seltene Anomalie der Overarmentwicklung (Notomelie?) *Zbl. Alg. Pathol., 95*:60–64, 1958.

Kuhnt: Eigenthumliche Doppelbildung an Handen und Fussen. *Arch. Pathol. Anat. Physiol., 56*:268–269; Taf. VI, 1872.

Langalli: An account of wax model of a girl's right hand found in a museum: four fingers of three phalanges represent the normal hand; the other four represent the absent thumb. *La Scienze e la Practica.* Pavia, 1875; cited by Dwight (1892) and Bateson (1894).

Lange, B.: Polydaktylie mit Radiusdefekt und Unnaverdoppelung. Inaug.-Diss. Breslau, Schles. Volkszeitung, pp. 1–34, 1923.

Laurin, C. A., Fevreau, J. C., and Labelle, P.: Bilateral absence of the radius and tibia with bilateral duplication of the ulna and fibula. *J. Bone Joint Surg., 46*:137–142, 1964.

Manaresi, C.: La dimelia ulnare e il sui trattamento. *Chir. Organi. Mov., 51*:76–83, 1962.

Matzen, P. F., and Fleissher, H. K.: *Orthopedic Roentgen Atlas.* New York, Grune & Stratton, Inc., pp. 387–474; figs. 599a and 599b, 1970.

Mau, C.: Ein weiterer Fall von Doppelbildung der Ulna bei fehlendem Radius. *Z. Orthop. Chir., 42*:355–366, 1922.

Minssen, A.: Ein weiterer Fall von angeborener Doppelbildung der Ulna. *Z. Orthop. Chir., 78*:570–574, 1949.

Morand, M.: Recherches sur quelques conformations monstreuses des doigts dans l'homme. *Hist. Acad. R. Sci.* Année 1770, (Paris), pp. 137–150, 1773.

Mukerji, M.: Congenital anomaly of hand: "mirror hand." *Br. J. Plast. Surg., 9*:222–227, 1957.

Müller, W.: *Die Angeborenen Fehlgildunger der Menschlichen Hand.* Leipzig, G. Thieme, pp. 56–60, 1937.

Murray, J. J.: Case of a woman with three hands, illustrated by analogous malformations of the lower animals. *Medico-Chir. Trans. London, 46*:29–32; pl. II; fig. 1–3, 1863.

Newman, H. H.: *The Physiology of Twinning.* Chicago, University of Chicago Press, pp. 200–205, 1923.

Nitsche, F.: Über lokalisierte Doppelmissbildungen und ihre Genesse. *Z. Orthop. Chir., 55*:601–617, 1931.

O'Rahilly, R.: Morphological patterns in limb deficiencies and duplications. *Am. J. Anat., 89*:135–187, 1951.

Perini, G.: Dimelia ulnare e suo trattamento chirurgico. *Arch. Putti, 6*:363–372, 1955.

Péterffy, P., and Jona, S.: Zwei Fälle von seltener Anomalie der Oberarmentwicklung. *Z. Chir., 69*:878–896; fig. 9–16, 1942.

Pintilie, D., Hatmanu, D., Olaru, I., and Panoza, G.: Double ulna with symmetrical polydactyly. *J. Bone Joint Surg., 46B*:89–93, 1964.

Pol, R.: Die Hypermelie beim Menschen. *Münch. Med. Wochenschr. 60*:2924–2925, 1913.

Pol. R.: Die Vertebratenhypermelie, mit 44 Abbildungen. *In* Meyer, R., and Schwalbe, E., (eds.): *Studies zur Pathologie der Entwicklung.* Jena, G. Fischer, 1 Bd., 1 H., pp. 71–84, 1914.

Pol, R.: Die Diplocheirie und Diplopodie und ihre Bezlehungen zur Hyperphalangie und einfachen Hyperdaktylie des ersten Strahles. Naturforsch. u. Med. Ges. zu Rostock. *Münch. Med. Wochenschr.,* No. 43:71, 1330, 1923.

Pol, R.: Missbildungen der Extremitäten. Hyperdaktylie (Polydaktylie), Diplocheirie und Diplopodie, Hypermelie, Oligodaktylie und Defekte von Röhreknochen. *In* Schwalbe, E., and Gruber, G. B., (eds.): *Die Morphologie der Missbildungen des Menschen und der Tiere.* Jena, G. Fischer, 3 T., 19 Lief., 1 Abb., 7 kap., 2 Halfte:683–719, 1958.

Priessnitz, O.: Ein neuer Fall von Ulnarer Polydaktylie (Spiegelhand) bei Ulnaverdopplung, Radiusdefekt und angeborener Schulterluxation. *Arch. Orthop. Unfall-chir., 46*:569–577, 1954.

Przibram, H.: Die Bruch Dreifachbildung im Tierreiche. *Arch. Entwicklungsmechanik., 48*:205–446; Taf. III, bis XXI, 1921.

Rausch, E.: Zur Frage der Hyperdaktylie und Diplocheirie (Diplopodie). *Med. Diss.,* Gottingen, 1946.

Restemeier: Eine Missbildung der Hand und des Unterarmus infolge Doppelbildung der Ulna bei Fehlendem Radius. *Dtsch. Z. Chir., 155*:121–135, 1920.

Rinaldi, E.: Su di un caso di lussazione congenita della spalla e dimelia ulnare omolaterale. *Arch. Putti, 23*:457–461, 1968.

Rueff, J.: Hand with twelve fingers. Two hands joined by ulnar side, each with five fingers. (Latin) *In De Conceptu.* Frankfort, as moenum, p. 43, fig. 8, 1587.

Salzer, M.: Die angeborene Ulnaverdoppelung beim Radiusdefekt. *Z. Orthop., 94*:429–435, 1961.

Sandrow, R. E., Sullivan, P. D., and Steel, H. H.: Hereditary ulnar and fibular dimelia with peculiar facies. *J. Bone Joint Surg., 52A*:367–370, 1970.

Santero, N.: Dichiria con duplicita dell ulna e assenza del radio. *Arch. Ital. Chir., 43*:173–193, 1936.

Saunders, J. W., Jr.: The proximo-distal sequence of origin of the parts of the chick wing and the role of ectoderm. *J. Exp. Zool., 108*:363–404, 1948.

Saunders, J. W., Jr., Cairns, J. M., and Gesseling, M. T.: The role of the apical ridge of ectoderm in the differentiation of the morphological structure of inductive specificity of limb parts in the chick. *J. Morphol., 101*:57–87, 1957.

Saviard, B.: *Nouveau Recueil d'Observation Chirurgicales.* Paris, J. Collombat, pp. 516–517, Table des Observation CXVII. D'un enfant qui avait tout les doigts doubles. 1702.

Scalabrino, F., and Coletta, C.: Polidattilia e raddioppiamenti speculari delgi arti superiori. *Acta. Ortop. Italica, 6*:123–140, 1960.

Schenk, R., and Jacquemain, B.: Hochgradige numerische Plusvariante an Hand und Fuss. *Z. Orthop., 105*:515–527, 1968.

Simonds, M.: Untersuchungen von Missbildungen mit Holfe des Rötgenverfahrene (Chondrodystrophie, Aneucephalie, Dicephalus, Sympus, extrauterine entwickelter Foetus). *Fortschr. Röntgenstr., 4*:197–211, 1901.

Stein, H. C., and Bettmann, E. H.: Rare malformation of the arm; double humerus with three hands and sixteen fingers. *Am. J. Surg.,* (n.s.), *50*:336–342, 1940.

Stöer, F. H.: Die Extremitätenmissbildungen und ihre Beziehungen zum Bauplan der Extremität. *Z. Anat. Entwickl. Ges., 108*:136–160, Abb. 16, 1938.

Storig, E.: Mohrfachildungen der Extremitäten Grades. *In* Diethelm, L., (ed.): *Röntgendiagnostik der Skeleter-Krankunger,* Berlin, Springer, Teil 3:698–703, 1968.

Taruffi, C.: *Storia della Teratologica.* Bologna, Regia Tipografia, Parte prima, Tome III, pp. 408–457, 1886.

Tilley, A. R.: Segmental duplication of ulnar elements of the hand and forearm. *Med. Radiog. Photog., 30*:58, 1954.

Tschumi, P. A.: The growth of the hindlimb bud of Xenopus leavis and its dependence upon the epidermis. *J. Anat. London, 91*:149–173, 1957.

Tünte, W., and Kersting, D.: Spiegelbildliche Verdoppelung von Ulna und ulnarem Handenteil bei fehlendem Radius ("mirror hand"). *Z. Orthop., 103*:490–498, 1967.

Vincent, E.: Main double à sept doigts cubitaux sans pouces accompangée de malformations congénitales curieuses de tout le membre supérieur. Étude pathogénique. Problèmes orthopédiques. *Rev. d'Orthop.,* (3S.), *9*:47–59, 1922.

Weil, S.: Diplocheirie und Diplopodie. *Z. Orthop. Chir., 43*:595–607, 1924.

Weiman: Double ulna syndrome. (Polish). *Chir. Narzad. Ruchu. Ortop. Pol., 29*:547–549, 1964.

Werthemann, A.: *Die Entwicklungsstörungen der Extremitaten.* Berlin, Springer-Verlag, pp. 37–56, 1952.

Wirtensohn, J.: A human monster with four hands and four feet in the Berlin Museum. *Dissertation.* Berlin, 1855. Cited by Dwight (1886–1893).

Zwilling, E.: Ectoderm-mesoderm relationship in the development of chick embryo limb bud. *J. Exp. Zool., 128*:423–438, 1955.

Zwilling, E.: Interaction between limb bud ectoderm and mesoderm in chick embryo II. Experimental limb duplication. *J. Exp. Zool., 132*:173–187, 1956.

Zwilling, E.: Interaction between limb bud ectoderm in the chick embryo IV. Experiments with wingless mutant. *J. Exp. Zool., 132*:241–253, 1956.

Zwilling, E.: Inductive mechanism. *In First International Conference on Congenital Malformations.* Philadelphia, J. B. Lippincott Co., pp. 133–139, 1961.

Zwilling, E., and Hansborough, L. A.: Interaction between limb bud, ectoderm and mesoderm in chick embryo. *J. Exp. Zool., 132*:219–240, 1956.

Chapter Fifteen

SPLIT HAND COMPLEX

Reduction of digits from the normal number of five is known under the generic name ectrodactyly. By way of analogy with cloven palate, a variety of ectrodactyly—characterized by suppression of one or more central digital rays and cone-shaped fissure of the palm—is called cleft hand. In the literature, one also runs across the ensuing designations: crayfish-claw, crab-claw, lobster-claw, pincer, monodactyly, oligodactyly, metacarpophalangeal hypodactyly, didactyly or bidactyly, peromanus, and forked or bifurcated hand. Kanavel (1932) called this anomaly "median" hypoplasia of the hand. Since the axis of the hand passes through the third digital ray, which is often absent, O'Rahilly (1951) suggested the term axial adactylia. The author has chosen the designation split hand, since in many cases there is a deficiency of the radial digital rays only, and there is no central cone-shaped palmar cleft tapering proximally. The hand appears spliced obliquely and what remains is one or two ulnar digital rays or none at all. In most cases, especially cases with hereditary antecedent, there is also comparable deformity involving both feet; hence, the qualifying word *complex* is added.

IDENTIFICATION OF SUNDRY FEATURES

Ambroise Paré (1575) reported a nine-year-old "monster" with a deformed right forearm, two fingers in the corresponding hand, and two toes on the left foot. Hartsinck (1770) described a Negro tribe called Touvinga. The members of this clan had two large fingers on each hand and two large toes on each foot, resembling the claws of a crab—*Kraften Schaar*. Otto's (1816) patient had only a fifth digit. Ménière (1828)—of Ménière's disease fame—dissected a pair of feet with marginal toes only. Béchet (1829) described the first well-documented pedigree of split hand complex. Walther (1829) reported a sporadic case.

Cruveilhier (1835) featured a number of excellent drawings of two-fingered hands and two-toed feet; in the text he used the expression *pince de homard*, which means lobster-claw. Excellent drawings of split hand and split foot are to be found also in Otto's (1841) book which, in addition, contains drawings of dissected specimens, showing deficiencies of the deeper structures of the affected hands. Scoutetten (1857–1858) reported familial cases and noted the occurrence of syndactyly in subjects with split hand. Heath's (1866) patient, a young woman, had only a thumb and a little finger on her hand and "the joint between the first and second phalanges of the thumb was anchylosed." Nicaise (1875) demonstrated the presence of a crossbone in one hand of a cadaver; the other hand had two separate metacarpal bones supporting a single digit. The first roentgenographs of split hand were published by Dowd (1896) and showed coalescence of two metacarpal bones.

Variability is perhaps the most constant feature of split hand complex. Variations are more common in the hand than in the foot. Exceptionally in split hand, which is classed with ectrodactyly, all five digits are present and there is widening of the second interdigital space. As a rule, one or more digits are absent. When phalanges are missing, the corresponding metacarpals are absent or rudimentary. The converse—absence of proximal bone and persistence of the distal element—does not occur in split hand. The palmar cleft, when present, gapes distally; proximally, it converges to a point. The span between the diverging distal ends of the metacarpal bones is at times bridged by a crossbone, which is regarded as the displaced remnant of the metacarpal or proximal phalanx of the missing digit. In the literature, one encounters the statement that crossbone does not occur in the foot. This is not true.

In cloven hand, the digits on either side of the cleft are usually thick and long; their distal segments tend to incline toward the central fissure. When more than two digits are present, the neighboring members are frequently webbed together. In some instances, the proximal interphalangeal joints of the remaining digits are stiff and unbending. The thumb is often absent. Less commonly, the pre-axial digits present the appearance of having been spliced along an oblique line beginning at a distal point on the ulnar border of the hand and ending proximally at about the base of the thumb. There may not even be a single digital ray, and the hand appears as if it had been amputated across the metacarpal bones. Tetramelic deformities are not uncommon. Split hand complex manifests a marked tendency to become hereditary (Figs. 15–1 to 15–7). (*Text continued on page 474.*)

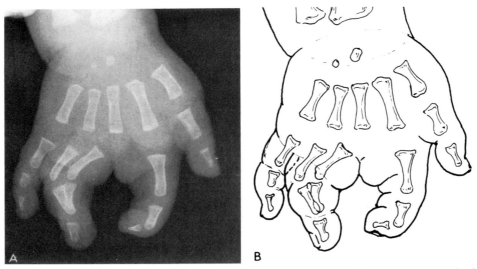

Figure 15–1 Monomelic split hand with no ectrodactyly. *A,* Dorsopalmar roentgenograph of a five-month-old infant with deep second interdigital commissure, syndactyly of the third and fourth digits, absence of an ungual phalanx in the confluent mass, and axial deviation of the remaining distal phalanx, as well as axial deviation of the ungual phalanx of the index finger. *B,* Sketch of same.

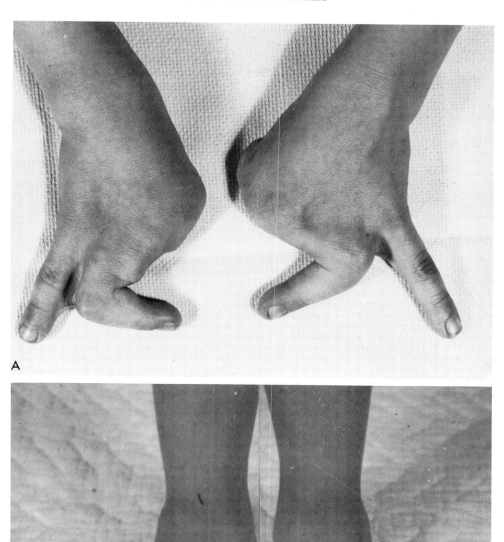

Figure 15–2 Tetramelic split hand complex showing that the lobster-claw deformity is more characteristic of the feet than of the hands. *A*, Dorsal view of the hands, showing oblique splicing of the radial digits. *B*, Dorsal view of the feet with lobster-claw deformity.

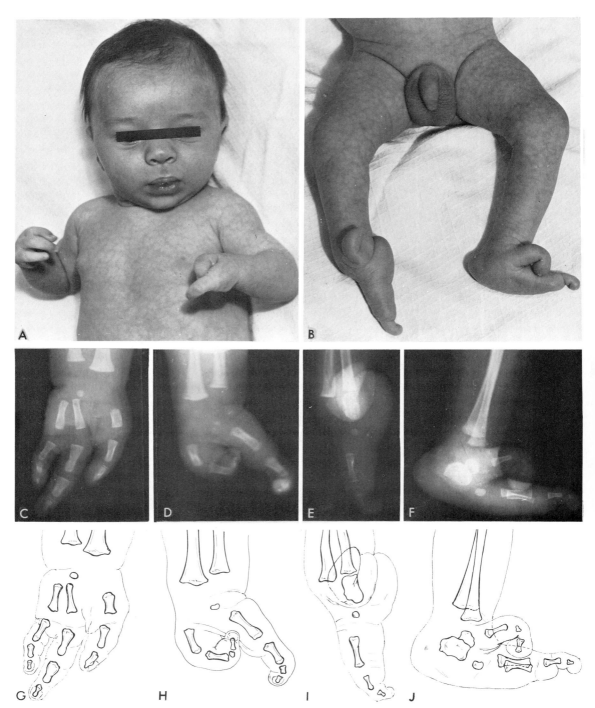

Figure 15–3 Tetramelic split hand complex of a three-month-old male infant with three digits on the right hand and two on the left hand. *A*, Photograph of the upper half of the body. *B*, Photograph of the lower half. *C*, Dorsopalmar roentgenograph of the right hand. *D*, Dorsopalmar roentgenograph of the left hand. *E*, Roentgenograph of the right foot. *F*, Roentgenograph of the left foot. *G*, *H*, *I*, and *J* are sketches illustrating roentgenographs above each.

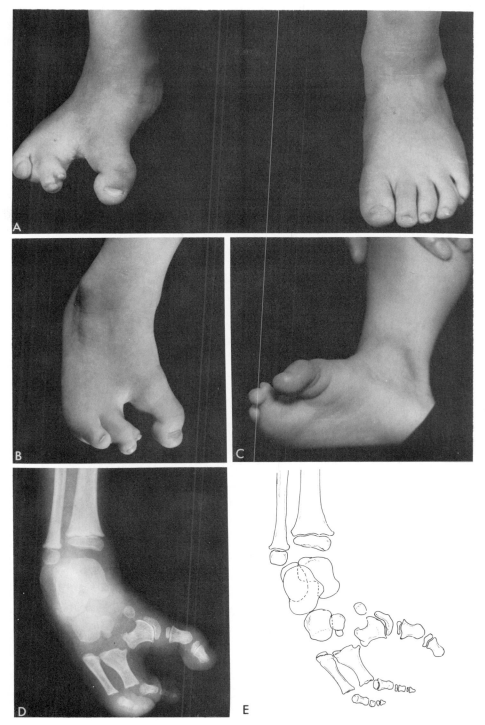

Figure 15–4 Unilateral split foot with crossbone. *A*, Dorsal view of the feet of a six-year-old female. *B*, View of the right foot. *C*, Oblique plantar view of the same. *D*, Dorsoplantar roentgenograph of the right foot. *E*, Interpretative sketch.

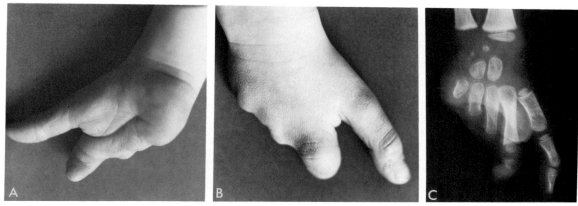

Figure 15–5 Obliquely spliced ulnar digits with a deep palmar groove. *A*, Palmar view of the right hand of a four-year-old boy. *B*, Dorsal view of the same. *C*, Dorsopalmar roentgenograph of the hand.

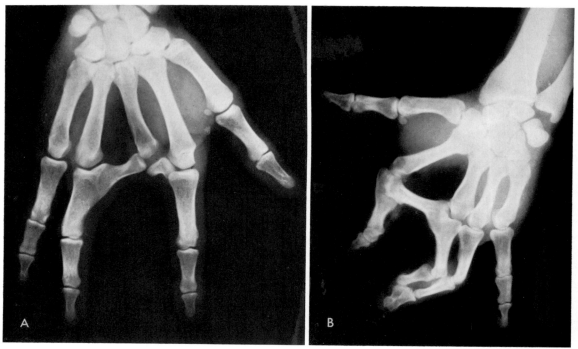

Figure 15–6 Hands with crossbones. *A*, Dorsopalmar roentgenograph of the right hand of a woman with monomelic deformity. *B*, Dorsopalmar roentgenograph of the left hand of a man, also with monomelic malformation.

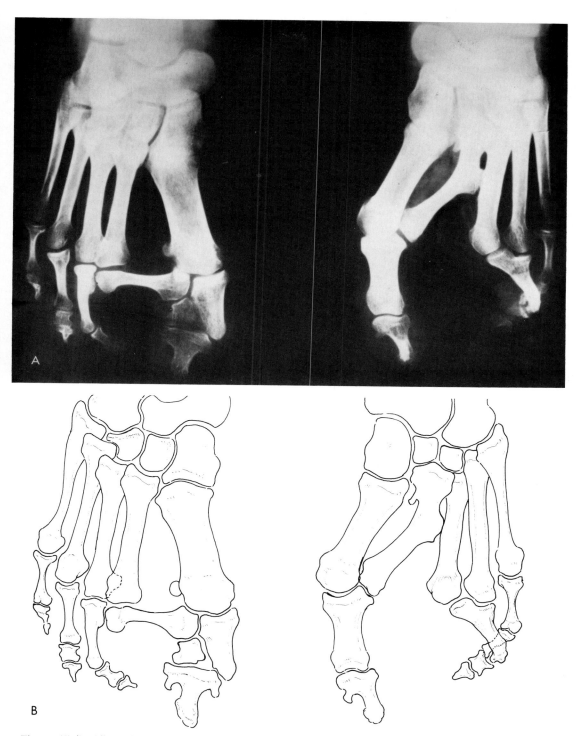

Figure 15–7 Bilateral split foot with crossbone on one side and irregularly shaped and aligned bones on the other. *A*, Dorsoplantar roentgenograph of the feet. *B*, Sketch illustrating the same.

CLASSIFICATION

Lange (1936, 1937) distinguished typical from atypical split hand, and this distinction was maintained by Birch-Jensen (1949), Barsky (1964), and many others. In typical variety, so it is said, there is absence of one or more central digital rays; there is cone-shaped palmar cleft which tapers as it approaches the wrist; some remaining digits may be webbed; comparable deformities also occur in the feet; and, in familial cases, the inheritance is dominant. Atypical split hand is said to occur sporadically, involving only one hand. Vogel (1958) also recognized the existence of two varieties of split hand deformity: (1) the type with constant involvement of feet and regular autosomal dominant inheritance; (2) the type with inconsistent involvement of the feet and irregular inheritance. As with all attempts in separating bizarre, overlapping anomalies into discrete categories, the classification of split hand complex leaves much to be desired.

INCIDENCE

Kümmel (1895) published the first collective review of split hand complex. He cited 17 cases. Perthes (1902) raised this number to 59, and Haim (1904) listed 67. Lewis and Embleton (1908) collected 180 cases from the literature; out of these, all but 13 cases were familial. Birch-Jensen (1949) estimated that "typical" split hand occurred once in about 90,000 births and once in about 112,000 in the population. He gave the figures for "atypical" split hand as once in about 150,000 births and once in about 200,000 in the population.

HEREDITY

The section of Béchet's (1829) essay dealing with split hand complex was reviewed by *Lancet* (1830), which reads: "Victoire Barre . . . was admitted . . . into the obstetrical institution of M. Maygrier. . . . Her extremities were peculiarly malformed; . . . she had on each hand one finger only, the other fingers, and their metacarpal bones, with the exception of imperfect rudiments of the two of the latter, were entirely wanting." Her feet resembled "the claws of a lobster." In 1827, Victoire gave birth to a female child. This infant presented the following malformations: "On each hand, four fingers and three metacarpal bones were wanting; the fifth, which was apparently the little finger, was supported by one metacarpal bone. . . . On each foot there was one toe, with three phalanges." In 1829, Victoire gave birth to a second girl with exactly the same deformities as her sister. In 1825, prior to the birth of these two defective girls, Victoire had given birth to a boy, but "the father of this boy was not . . . the father of the girls also." Victoire's own mother was free of any malformation. Victoire's father and his sister "had on each foot the fifth toe only and on the left hand one finger. . . ."

Numerous pedigrees of split hand complex have since been recorded. The responsible gene is considered to be autosomal dominant with variable expression: the differences in manifestation are ascribed to the influence of modifying genes. In hereditary cases, the lobster-claw deformity breeds true more constantly in the foot. The deformity of the hand is extremely variable (Figs. 15–8 to 15–10).

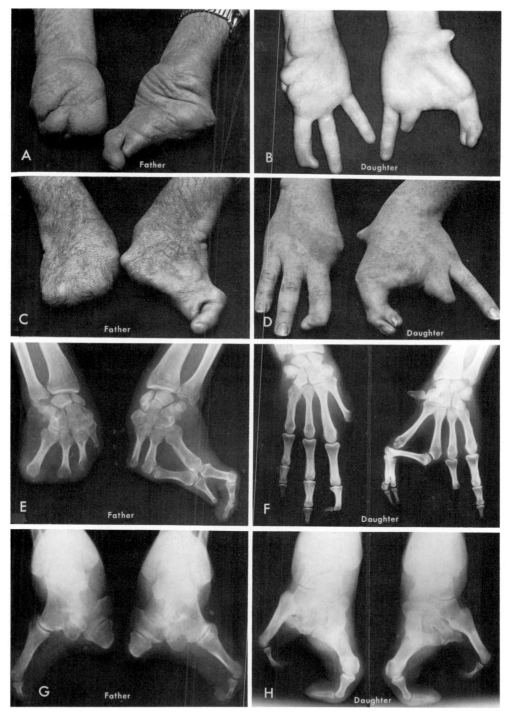

Figure 15–8 Split hand complex. Father-to-daughter transmission. *A*, Palmar view of the father's hands. *B*, Palmar view of the daughter's hands. *C*, Dorsal view of the father's hands. *D*, Dorsal view of the daughter's hands. *E*, Dorsopalmar roentgenograph of the father's hands. *F*, Dorsopalmar roentgenograph of the daughter's hands. *G*, Dorsoplantar roentgenograph of the father's feet. *H*, Dorsoplantar roentgenograph of the daughter's feet. One notes the variability of expression of the trait.

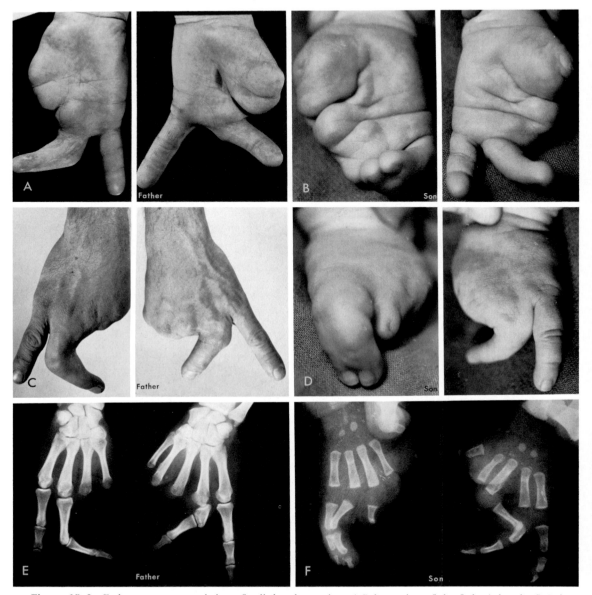

Figure 15–9   Father-to-son transmission of split hand complex. *A,* Palmar view of the father's hands. *B,* Palmar view of the son's hands. *C,* Dorsal view of the father's hands. *D,* Dorsal view of the son's hands—note the syndactyly of the two ulnar digits of the right hand. *E,* Dorsopalmar roentgenograph of the father's hands. *F,* Dorsopalmar roentgenograph of the son's hands.

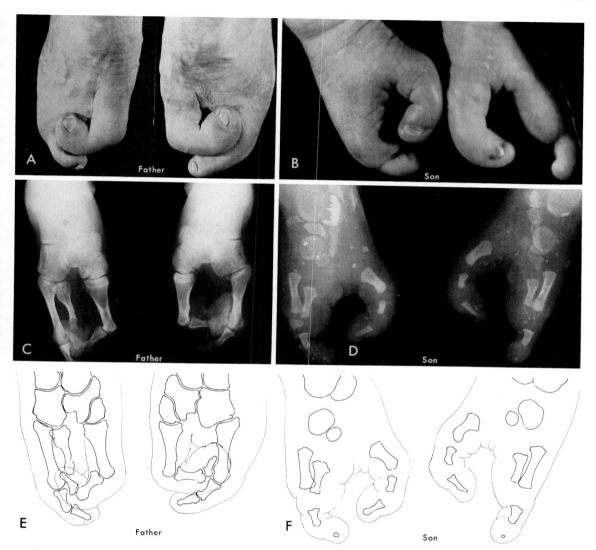

Figure 15–10 The feet of the father and son shown in Figure 15–9. *A,* Dorsal view of the father's feet. *B,* Dorsal view of the son's feet. *C,* Dorsoplantar roentgenograph of the father's feet. *D,* Dorsoplantar roentgenograph of the son's feet. *E* and *F* illustrate the roentgenographs of the father's and son's feet, respectively.

CONFUSION WITH MIRROR HANDS

The title "bifurcated hand" is used indiscriminately for both split and mirror deformities. Under the heading "Bifuraction of the hand," Lombard (1914) described a pedigree of bilateral deformity characterized by four metacarpal bones and five digits in each hand. The middle and ring fingers were supported by a single, massive, bifurcated metacarpal; these digits diverged from each other in the form of a V. Lombard drew an analogy between the probands he described and the cases of mirror hands reported in the literature. He also noted some similarity between the hands of his patients and the forked hand described by Kümmel (1895) and the cleft hand reported by Dowd (1896). Not long after

Lombard, Bircher (1918) described a similar case with a bifurcated fourth metacarpal supporting two diverging digits. Bircher used the title *Gabelhand*, which means forked hand. More than one compiler has included Lombard's cases in his tabulation of mirror hands or ulnar dimelia.

Split hand and mirror hands have several features in common. In both, the hand assumes the appearance of having been divided into two parts; the central digits diverge from one another and the marginal pairs are usually webbed together. Here the resemblance ends. In almost all reported cases of mirror hand, the ulna is duplicated. Polydactylism is the rule, and the involvement is unilateral. The feet are not implicated, and hereditary is not a factor.

CONFUSION WITH MACRODACTYLY

Ribeiro (1954) reported a case of bilateral macrodactyly. His communication was entitled "Lobster-claw hands." As noted, in split hand, fingers bordering the palmar cleft will occasionally appear oversized. But these digits never attain the gigantic size seen in macrodactyly. Macrodactyly is not known to affect the hands and feet of the same individual, and it is without hereditary antecedent.

CONFUSION WITH SYNDACTYLY

In *Eugenical News* (1930), there is an article which bears the title "Syndactylism in F-family." The cases described are those of split hand. The author of this article seems to have seen the tree and overlooked the forest. Syndactyly is a feature of split hand and not the other way around.

DIFFERENTIATION OF SPLIT HAND FROM OTHER FORMS OF ECTRODACTYLY

Almost every author writing about split hand complex avoids an important question: in what respect does split hand differ from other forms of ectrodactyly? Lewis and Embleton (1908) considered it an invariable rule that in split hand deformity a proximal bone is never absent when the corresponding distal one is present. When a finger is missing in split hand, the corresponding metacarpal is absent, underdeveloped, or fused with its neighbor. In many cases of split hand, the carpal bones are coalesced but the bones of the forearm are present. Suppression of one or two marginal digits does not belong to the category of split hand when the remaining central members have intact metacarpals, when the feet do not show comparable deformities, and when there is no hereditary antecedent. Dominantly inherited tetramelic deformities, such as those described by Hegdekatti (1939), do belong to the category of split hand even though the malformations in some members of this pedigree simulate terminal transverse defects.

Ectrodactyly is a feature of radial as well as of ulnar defect. When the thumb is missing, usually trapezium and scaphoid bones of the wrist are either absent or diminutive, and there may be aplasia or hypoplasia of the radius. In ulnar ray defect, one or two ulnar digits may be missing, and there is usually dislocation of the radius at the elbow.

REGIONAL ASSOCIATIONS

Most authors consider syndactyly as an integral part of split hand complex. The same may be said about axial deviation of the digits flanking the palmar cleft. Stiff interphalangeal joints and even symphalangism are known to occur with split hand. One or more nails may be absent or atrophic. Other common local accompaniments include: crossbone; two metacarpals supporting one digit, or one bifurcated basal bone supporting two digits; side-to-side fusion of the neighboring metacarpals; carpal coalescence; and radioulnar synostosis (Figs. 15–11 and 15–12).

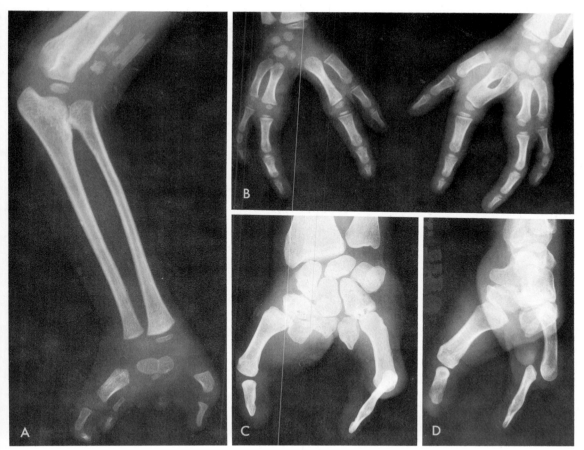

Figure 15–11   Cases of split hand with synostosis. *A*, Dorsopalmar roentgenograph of the right hand of a two-year-old boy with monomelic deformity: note the incipient proximal radioulnar synostosis and coalescence of carpal bones. *B*, Dorsopalmar roentgenograph of the hands of a four-year-old girl, showing partial coalescence of the left second and third metacarpal bones. *C*, Dorsopalmar roentgenograph of an adult male, showing symphalangism of the little finger of the left hand. *D*, Oblique view of the same: the confluent phalangeal rod is dislocated at the metacarpophalangeal joint.

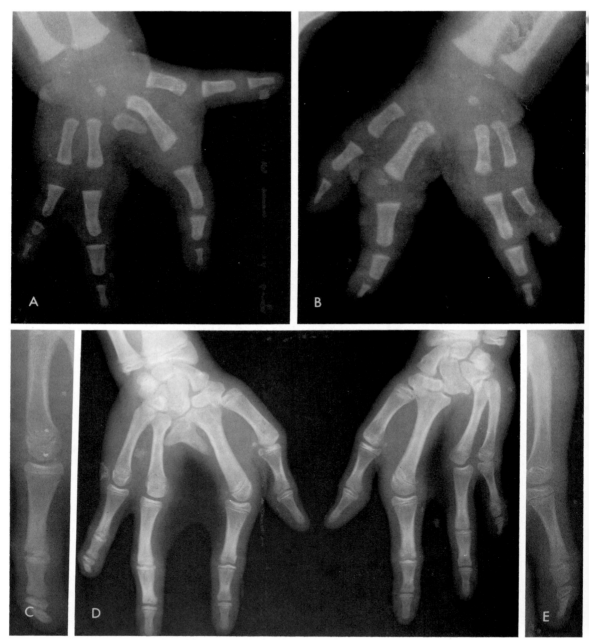

Figure 15–12   Bilateral split hand of a three-month-old male infant who insidiously developed bilateral Kirner's deformity of the little fingers. *A*, Dorsopalmar roentgenograph of the right hand, showing a dwarfed middle phalanx of the little finger. *B*, Dorsopalmar roentgenograph of the left hand: the little finger is short and its middle and ungual phalanges are very small. *C*, Enlarged dorsopalmar roentgenograph of the right little finger taken at age 10, showing brachymesophalangy and dystelephalangy. *D*, Dorsopalmar roentgenograph of both hands. *E*, Enlarged dorsopalmar roentgenograph of the left little finger with dwarfed middle phalanx and dystelephalangy or Kirner's deformity.

REMOTE ASSOCIATIONS

In most cases of split hand, the opposite manus is affected and there is usually split foot. Raymond and Janet (1897) reported a case of split hand in an epileptic with asymmetrical development of the two halves of the body. Orth (1910) presented a patient with split hand complex and absence of the pectoral muscles. Goll and Kahlich-Koenner (1940) noted the association of split hand and acrocephaly. Jäger (1967) described a case of bilateral split hand with "localized giantism" of one foot. Fèvre and Hannouche (1968) reported a patient who had a number of missing ribs on the right side and only two digits on the right hand. In the literature, one finds a number of more constant remote associations of split hand complex (Figs. 15–13 and 15–14).

DEFECT OF THE TIBIA AND SPLIT HAND COMPLEX

Largot (1924) described a boy with partial absence of the right tibia and bilateral split hand—*main en fourché*. The patient described by Schwarzweller (1939) had an absent left tibia, short left lower leg, and cloven hands. Andersen (1942) reported a mother and daughter with split hands. The daughter had total absence of the tibia and talipes equinovarus. Roberts (1967) reported a family in which several members in four generations had unilateral split hand with missing middle digits and flexed ring fingers. Some other members had, in addition, absent tibias. One child had only leg deformity; another, absent forearms together with malformed legs. The absent tibia with split hand complex in this family was considered to be an autosomal dominant trait with variable expression.

DE LANGE DEGENERATION

Monodactyly, bidactyly, and cloven palms are often seen in de Lange dwarfs (Figs. 15–15 and 15–16).

OCULODIGITAL COMPLEXES

Savin and Sorsby (1935) described two brothers, members of a family with split hand. The younger brother had aniridia and congenital subluxation of the lenses; he was blind but had no skeletal defects. The older brother had normal vision and split hand. Karsch (1936) reported two cases of congenital cataract associated with split hand complex. One patient had an absent middle finger and cloven palm on the right hand; the other had only one digit on each hand.

(Text continued on page 485.)

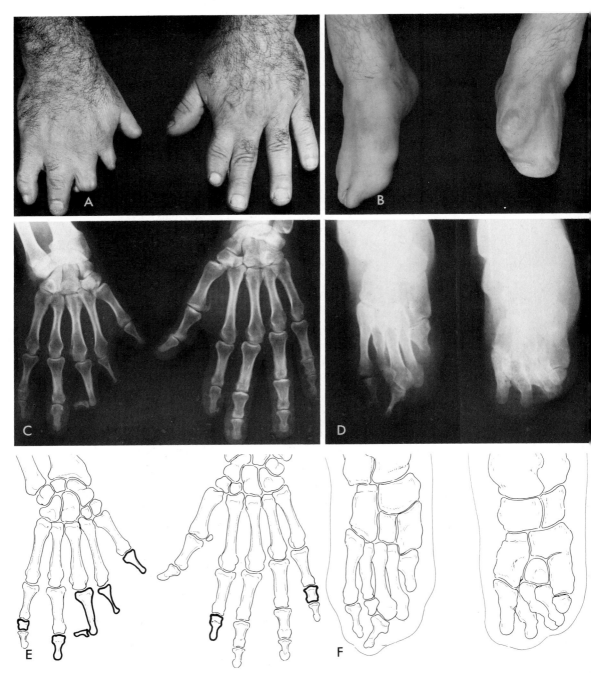

Figure 15–13   Tetramelic malformation which simulates some of the features of split hand (oblique splicing of the three radial digits of the right hand) and is associated with syndactyly and brachymesophalangy of the opposite hand and transverse terminal defect of the feet. *A*, Dorsal view of the hands. *B*, Dorsal view of the feet. *C*, Dorsopalmar roentgenograph of the hands. *D*, Dorsopalmar roentgenograph of the feet. *E* and *F* illustrate roentgenographs above each.

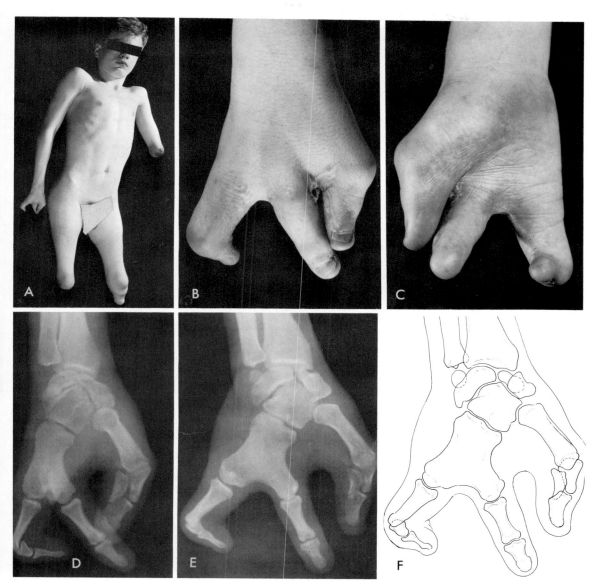

Figure 15–14 Tetramelic malformation with split right hand and transverse terminal deficiency of the other limbs. *A*, Frontal view of a 14-year-old boy. *B*, Dorsal view of the right hand. *C*, Palmar view of the same. *D* and *E*, Oblique and dorsopalmar roentgenographs of the right hand, showing coalescence of carpal bones. There are fusion of two ulnar metacarpals and duplication of the middle phalanx of the thumb. *F*, Sketch illustrating *E*.

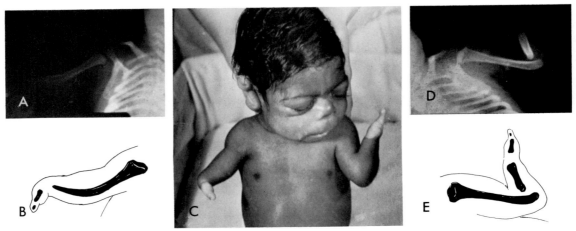

Figure 15–15 Monodactylous de Lange dwarf. *A*, Roentgenograph of the right upper limb. *B*, Interpretative sketch. *C*, Frontal view of the upper part of the body: note the bushy eyebrows and hirsutism. *D*, Roentgenograph of the left upper limb. *E*, Sketch illustrating same.

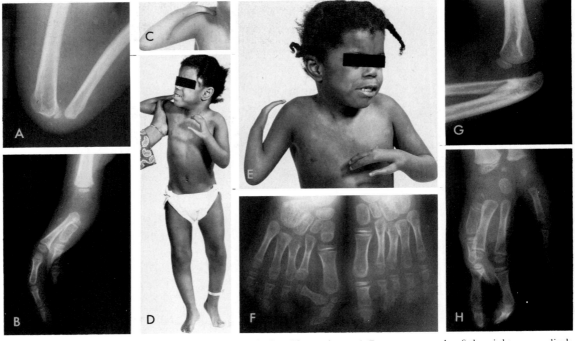

Figure 15–16 De Lange dwarf with asymmetrical malformations. *A*, Roentgenograph of the right upper limb, showing a single bone in the forearm. *B*, Lateral roentgenograph of the right wrist and hand, showing no carpal bones and two digital rays. *C*, Photograph of the right hand, showing two digits. *D*, Frontal view of the entire body. *E*, Frontal view showing the upper part of the body. *F*, Roentgenograph of both feet: note the crossbone on the right side. *G*, Roentgenograph of the left elbow, showing radioulnar synostosis. *H*, Dorsopalmar roentgenograph of the left wrist and hand, showing a more mature radial epiphysis, four carpal bones, and four digital rays.

ORODIGITAL COMPLEXES

Split hand complex has been reported in association with anodontia or hypodontia by Brendt (1948) and Temtamy (1966). Split hand is more commonly associated with cleft lip-palate. This association has been recorded by Eckoldt and Martens (1804), Fronhofer (1896), Cockayne (1936), Birch-Jensen (1949), Schonenberg (1955), Fraser (1961), Walker and Clodius (1963), Jaworska and Papiolek (1968), Berndorfer (1970), and Rüdiger et al (1970). In the familial cases, such as those reported by Cockayne, Walker and Clodius, and Berndorfer, the constellation was transmitted as an autosomal dominant trait. In the case reported by Rüdiger et al, cleft lip-palate and split hand complex were associated with ectodermal dysplasia.

OTODIGITAL COMPLEX
(Deafness and Split Hand; Wildervanck Syndrome)

Birch-Jensen (1949) reported an isolated case of deaf-mutism associated with split hand. Wildervanck (1963) described two brothers with perceptive deafness associated with split hand and split foot. An older brother was unaffected, as were the parents, who were not related. There was no history of deafness or of split hand in the family. Wildervanck ascribed the constellation to a rare recessive gene.

TREATMENT

Dowd (1896) operated on a patient with a complicated case of split hand. The case presented four surgical problems, each of which needed individualized attention: (1) ulnar deviation of the ring and small fingers, (2) the cleft between middle and ring fingers, (3) partial syndactyly between each pair of digits flanking the palmar fissure, and (4) flexion contracture of the three central digits. To correct all these deformities, Dowd utilized a number of procedures and completed the whole reconstructive work at several sessions. He performed subcapital cuneiform osteotomy of the fourth and fifth metacarpals to correct the ulnar deviation of the ring and little fingers. The gap between the diverging rays was effaced by promoting side-to-side osteosynthesis between the distal ends of the corresponding metacarpal bones. Syndactyly of each pair of digits was repaired with the aid of dorsal triangular flaps. To correct the flexion contracture of the central digits, Dowd excised the tight cutaneous bands, resected the palmar fascia, and surfaced the raw areas with free skin grafts.

Kanavel (1932) also completed the reconstructive work on split hand in several sessions. He considered the correction of the anomalous alignment of the digits to be far more important than the repair of the syndactyly. Kanavel advised tackling the former problem first. He distinguished two varieties of split hand: (1) cases in which the cleft extended into the palm, and (2) cases without palmar fissure. In the former, he removed transversely disposed and rudimentary bones from the cleft and approximated the diverging metacarpals by chromic catgut suturing of the periosteum and the capsules of the neighboring

(*Text continued on page 489.*)

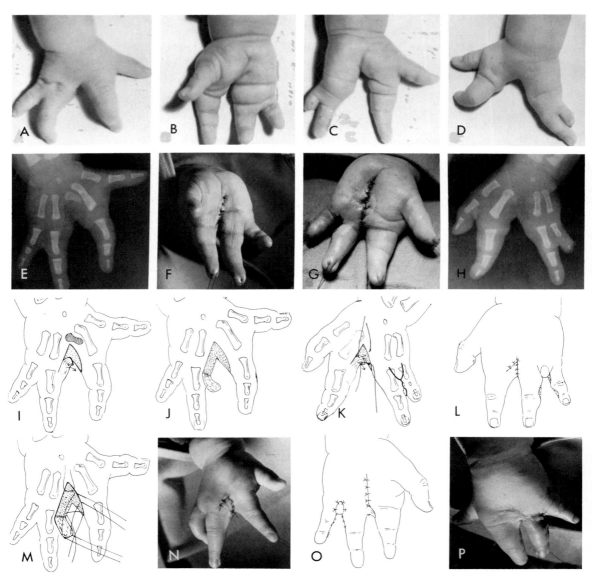

Figure 15–17   *A*, Dorsal view of the right hand of a three-month-old boy. *B*, Palmar view of the same. *C*, Palmar view of the left hand: note the webbing of the ring and little fingers. *D*, Dorsal view of the same. *E*, Dorsopalmar roentgenograph of the right hand. *F*, Palmar view of the right hand after the repair of the cleft. *G*, Postoperative palmar view of the left hand. *H*, Dorsopalmar roentgenograph of the left hand, showing comparatively diminutive middle and ungual phalanges of the little finger. *I*, Elevation of a rectangular skin flap from across the apex of the palmar cleft of the right hand. *J*, A rectangular flap has been developed to its base on the radial aspect of the ring finger. *K*, A similar flap has been raised on the left hand and is being resutured: this sketch also shows the incision for the repair of the syndactyly between the ring and little fingers. *L* shows closure of the left palmar cleft and separation of the webbed fingers. *M*, Sketch showing closure of the right palmar cleft. *N*, Postoperative dorsal view of the right hand. *O*, Palmar view sketch showing closure of the left palmar cleft and repair of syndactyly. *P*, Postoperative dorsal view of the left hand.

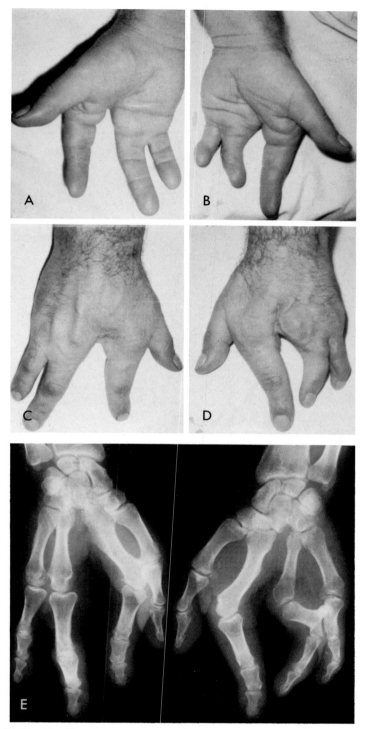

Figure 15–18 Bimelic split hand with partial syndactyly and angular deformity of some of the digits. *A* and *B*, Palmar view of the hands of an adult male. *C* and *D*, Dorsal view of the same. *E*, Dorsopalmar roentgenograph of the hands.

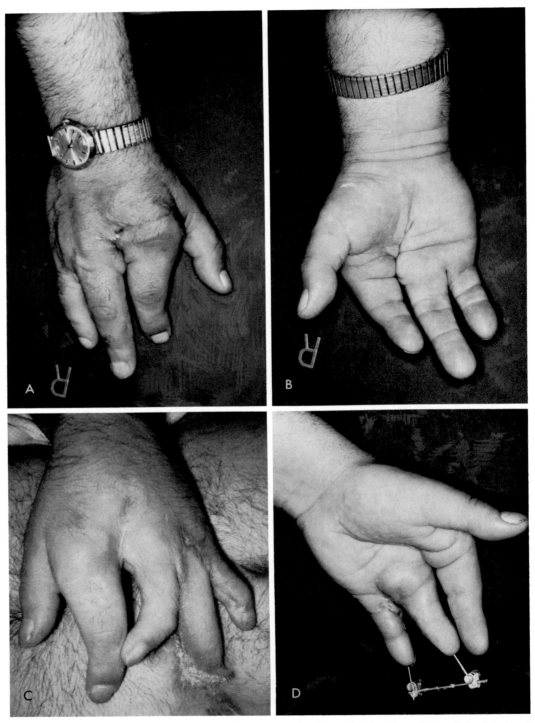

Figure 15–19   The outcome of surgery in the patient shown in Figure 15–18. *A*, Dorsal view of the right hand after closure of the palmar cleft. *B*, Palmar view of the same. *C*, Dorsal view of the left hand after the ring and little fingers were separated and an abdominal flap was interposed between them—preliminary to corrective osteotomy of the metacarpal and proximal phalanx of the ring finger and the middle phalanx of the little finger. *D* shows K-wire holding the angulated digits of the left hand in corrected position.

metacarpophalangeal joints. In the cases without palmar fissure, he again removed the intervening bone, dissected the index finger free, and transferred this digit over to a prepared bed beside the ring finger. Kanavel repaired the syndactyly at a later date by using free full-thickness skin graft.

Kelikian and Doumanian (1957) introduced a minor modification for the purpose of establishing a web between the bases of the diverging digits. They fashioned a rectangular flap from one side of the palmar cleft; the pedicle of this flap was on a level with the analogous commissure between two fingers of the opposite hand. This flap was turned distally so that it bridged the gap near the bases of the divergent digits, thus forming a web. The remaining skin of the cleft was trimmed away, and the palmar and dorsal edges approximated. In the young patients, the diverging metacarpals will come together after the intervening rudimentary bone is removed. When there are only two digits and their nails lie on the same horizontal level, one or both metacarpals may be osteotomized and the digits placed in opposition. When the proximal interphalangeal joints are interlocked or stiff, it is sometimes necessary to excise the head of the basal phalanx to create sufficient space for motion (Figs. 15–17 to 15–19).

In patients with only a single digit—usually the small finger—the surgeon has two alternatives: (1) transfer a toe to the hand, or (2) create a composite pedicled tube to provide an oppositional strut. The first method was practiced by Reid (1960); the second was advised by Barsky (1964). Both these procedures come under the general heading of reconstruction of the thumb, which will be discussed in Chapter Twenty-Four.

SUMMARY

Typical split hand complex is a genetic disorder and is transmitted as an autosomal dominant phenotype; as a rule, both hands are affected and the feet show comparable deformities. The atypical variety is sporadic; it is unilateral and the feet are unaffected. Distinction is made between split hand and other forms of ectrodactyly. In split hand, when a digit is missing, its metacarpal is absent or stunted; the converse—intercalary defect of the proximal element and intact distal segments—does not occur. Split hand is found in connection with nail defects, defects of the teeth, deafness, congenital cataract, facial clefts, and defective tibia. The treatment of the malformed hand is directed toward separating the webbed fingers, correcting the axial deviation of the digits, and eliminating the cleft in the palm. Since the thumb is missing in many instances, one or both marginal digits may need to be shifted around or rotated in order to restore the function of fingertip-to-fingertip pinch.

References

Ammon, F. A. v.: *Die angeborenen chirurgischen Krankheiten des Menschen.* Berlin, F. A. Herbig, Vol. 4, Part I, pp. 96–98,1842.

Anders, E.: Zwei Fälle von anomaler Extremitätenbildung. *Jb. Kinderheilkd.,* 16:435–436, 1881.

Andersen, J.: Über einen Fall von Spalthand in Kombination mit schwerer Missbildung der unteren Extremitäten in der Descendenz. *Z. menschl. Vererb. Konstitutionslehre,* 25:545–552, 1942.

Anderson, W.: Congenital malformation of the hands and feet transmitted through four generations. *Br. Med. J.,* 1:1107–1108, 1886.

Apfelthaller, M.: Drei Fälle von angeborenen Missbildungen der Hand. *Arch. Pathol. Anat. Physiol.,* 262:565–571, 1926.

Arquellada, A. M.: Un caso de deformidad congenita de manos y pied. *Pediat. Espan.,* 7:377–382, 1918.

Auerbach, C.: A possible case of delayed mutation in man. *Ann. Hum. Genet.,* 20:266–269, 1956.

Ayer, A. A., and Rao, V. S.: Split hand and split foot. *J. Indian Med. Assoc.,* 24:108–112, 1954.

Barsky, A. J.: Cleft hand: classification, incidence, and treatment; review of the literature and report of nineteen cases. *J. Bone Joint Surg.,* 46A:1707–1720, 1964.

Béchet, J.: *Essai sur les Monstruosités Humaines ou Vices Congénitaux de Conformation.* Thèse. Paris, Didot le Jeune, pp. 32–35, 1829.

Bédart: Ectrodactylie quadruple des pieds et des mains se transmettant pendant trois génerations. *C. R. Soc. Biol.,* 4:367–371, 1892.

Bell, J.: Cloven feet and hands. *Lancet,* 1:24, 1911.

Berger, P.: Quelques faits d'ectrodactylie sur une observation de M. le Dr. Guermonprez de Lille, intitulée; ectrodactylie avec conservation partielle de pouce et de l'auriculaire. *Bull Mém. Soc. Chir. Paris,* 10:721–733, 1884.

Berndorfer, A.: Gesichtsspalten gemeinsam mit Hand- und Fussspalten. *Z. Orthop.,* 107:344–354, 1970.

Bibergeil, E.: Über Spalthand. *Charité-Ann,* 34:762–768, 1910.

Bindseil, W.: Bericht über einen Fall von erblicher Spaltbildung an Händen und Füssen. *Z. menschl. Vererb. Konstitutionslehre,* 26:357–364, 1942–1943.

Bindseil, W., and Grimm, H.: Über Papillarmuster bei einem Fall von erblicher Spaltbildung an Händen und Füssen. *Z. menschl. Vererb. Konstitutionslehre,* 26:365–375, 1942–1943.

Bircher, E.: Die Gablehand, zugleich ein Beitrag zur Theorie der Missbildungen. *Beitr. Klin. Chir.,* 111:187–205, 1918.

Birch-Jensen, A.: *Congenital Deformities of the Upper Extremities.* Translated from the Danish by Aagesen. Commission: Andelsbogtrykkereit i Odense and det Dandke Forlag, Copenhagen, Ejnar Munksgaard, pp. 16–18; 46–74; 141–143; 171–192, 1949.

Blankenburg, H.: Spalthand- und Spaltfussbildungen in typischen und atypischen. *Beitr. Orthop. Traum.,* 14:209–215, 1967.

Boinet, E.: Ectrodactylie symétrique. *Gaz. Hebd. Sci. Med.* (Montpellier), 11:337–353, 1889.

Bosshardt, M.: Über einen Fall von hereditärem Defekt von Fingern und Zehen. *Mschr. Geburtsh. Gypäk.,* 44:154–163, 1916.

Bousquet, H.: Un cas de malformation de la main; pince de homard et syndactylie. *Progrès Méd.* (Paris), 7:108–109, 1903.

Bradley, W. N.: Report of a case of congenital deformity of both hands and both feet. *Arch. Pediatr.,* 32:276–277, 1915.

Brancadoro, P., Galluzzo, A., and Siciliano, A.: Studio clinico-radiologico e genetico di un ceppo familiare de "ectrodattila." *Nuntius Radiol.,* 32:1137–1546, 1966.

Branciforti, S.: Un caso raro di deformita congenite della mani e dei piedi. *Chir. Organi Mov.,* 37:66–70, 1950.

Brandenberg, F.: Missbildung und Heredität. *Z. Orthop. Chir.,* 21:54–69, 1908.

Brendt, H.: Case report of partial anodontia connected with missing and stunted phalanges of hands and feet. *Oral Surg. Oral Med. Oral Pathol.,* 1:283–290, 1948.

Cardi, G.: Condiderazioni sopra un caso di malformazione congenita della mano. *Arch. Ortop.,* 52:426–433, 1936.

Chaleix: Cas de malformation congénitale des mains—Main gauche en patte d'ecrevisse—Main droite rameuse—Ectrodactylie—Brachydactylie—Syndactylie—Clinodactylie. *J. Méd. Bordeaux,* 19:291–293; pl. I, 1890.

Clark, R. K.: Case of congenital malformation (split hand). *Boston Med. Surg. J.,* 82:413, 1870.

Cockayne, E. A.: Cleft palate, harelip, dacrocystitis and cleft hand and feet. *Biometrika,* 28:60–63, 1936.

Cook, R.: Too few fingers—and too many. Some notes on genes and pigs-feet-in-the-diet agents to produce digital abnormalities. *J. Hered.,* 26:457–462; fig. 13, 14, 1935.

Cruveilhier, J.: Maladie des extrémités. *Anatomie Pathologique du Corps Humain.* 58e livraison, 2:1–4, pl. I, 1835.

David, M., and Lipliarsky, S.: Zur Aetiologie der Spalthand. *Dtsch. Med. Wochenschr.,* 29:431–433, 1903.

Delthil: Ectrodacytlie symétrique de deux medius. *Bull. Mèm. Soc. Méd. Chir. Prat. Paris,* pp. 50–53, 1894.

Dowd, E. N.: Cleft hand: a report of a case successfully treated by the use of periosteal flaps. *Ann. Surg.*, *24*:211–216, 1896.

Druillet, J.: *De l'Ectrodactylie.* Thèse, Paris, Ollier-Henry, pp. 7–44, 1886.

Eckoldt, J. G., and Martens, F. H.: *Über eine sehr kompicierte Hasenscharte.* Leipzig, Steinacker, 1804, cited by Walker and Clodius (1963).

Epstein, J.: Perodactylism, syndactylism, and cleft extremities in a child. *New York Med. J.*, *109*:153–156, 1919.

Eugenical News: Syndactylism in F-family. *Eugen. News*, *15*:72–74, 1930.

Ewh, H.: *Ueber angeborene Defekte der Extremitäten.* Inaug. Diss. Witten, C. L. Krüger, pp. 1–17; figs. 1–3, 1890.

Faber: Verg. Karsch: Spalthand, Spaltfuss und erbliche Augenmissbildungen. *Verh. Dtsch. Orthop. Ges.*, *66*:105–107, 1937.

Fetscher, R.: Ein Stammbaum mit Spalthand. *Arch. Rass. Ges. Biol.*, *14*:176–177, 1922.

Fèvre, M., and Hannouche, D.: Les breches thoraciques par aplasie ou par anomalies costales. *Ann. Chir. Infantile*, *9*:153–166; fig. 14, 1968.

Fischer-Wasels, J.: Eine seltene Form von Spalthandmissbildung. *Arch. Orthop. Unfallchir.*, *46*:259–262, 1954.

Flamain: Ectrodactylie de la main droite. *Bull. Soc. Anat. Paris*, (2 s.), *14*:166–167, 1879.

Fortunatoff, A. M.: On hereditary ectrodactylism in man (Russian). *Protok. Zasaid, Russk. Anthrop. Obsh. p. Imp. St. Petersb. Univ.*, *3*:61–64, 1892.

Fotherby, H. A.: The history of a family in which similar hereditary deformity appeared in five generations. *Br. Med. J.*, *1*:975–976, 1886.

Fraser, F. C.: Congenital clefts of the face. *In* Gedda, L., (ed.): *De Genetica Medica.* pars tertia. Rome, Apud Mendelianum Inst., pp. 289–295, fig. 2, 1961.

Fronhofer, E.: Die Entstehung der Lippen-Kiefer-Gaumen Spalte in Folge Ammitscher Adhäsionen. *Arch. Klin. Chir.*, *52*:883–901, Taf. XII, 1896.

Gaillard: Difformité congénitale des quatre extremités; luxations, atrophies; réunions parties divisées par la méthode de M. Jules Cloquet. *Gaz. Méd. Paris*, *14*:787–788, 1859.

Gallez: Un cas d'ectrodactylie . . . chez un enfant de 8 mois. *Bull. Acad. Méd. Belgique*, *11*:992–996, 1868.

Goldmann, E. E.: Beitrag zur Lehre von den Missbildungen der Extremitäten. *Beitr. Klin. Chir.*, Taf. VI-VII, *7*:239–256, 1890.

Goll, H., and Kahlich-Koenner, D. M.: Akrocephalosyndaktylie mit Spalthand bei einem Partner eines eineiigen Zwillinspaares. *Z. menschl. Vererb. Konstitutionslehre*, *24*:516–535, 1940.

Goriainowa, R. W.: Zur Fräge der Heredität der Ectrodactylie. *Fortschr. Röntgenstr.*, *50*:289–294, 1934.

Graham, J. B., and Badgley, C. E.: Split hand with unusual complications. *Am. J. Hum. Genet.*, *7*:44–50, 1955.

Grand, M. J. H., and Dolan, D. J.: Heredofamilial cleft foot. *Am. J. Dis. Child.*, *51*:338–348, 1936.

Grebe, H.: Zur Ätiologie ein und doppelseitiger Gliedmassenmissbildungen. *Z. menschl. Vererb. Konstitutionslehre*, *32*:126–142, 1954.

Grebe, H.: Spalthand-Spaltfuss, Ektrodaktylie. *In* Schwalbe, E., and Gruber, G. B., (eds.): *Die Morphanangie der Missbildungen des Menschen und der Tiere.* Jena, G. Fischer, 3 T., 19 Lief., 1 Abt., 7 Kap., 2 Halfte: 844–892, 1958.

Grebe, H.: Spalthände und Füsse. *In* Becker, P. E., (ed.): *Humangenetik.* Stuttgart, G. Thieme, pp. 304–316, 1964.

Grynkraut, B.: L'os transversal de la main. *Presse Méd.*, *32* (2, annex):1433, 1924.

Haim, E.: Über Spalthand und Spaltfuss. *Arch. Orthop. Mech. Unfallchir.*, *1*:375–380, T. X-XII, 1904.

Hallipré: Main en pince de homard: radiographic. *Rev. Méd. Normandie*, *4*:47, 1903.

Hanhart, E.: Stark unregelmässige Dominanz einer Anlage zu Spalthand auf Grund eines schwachen entwicklungslabilen Gens. *Arch. Klaus-Stift. Vererb. Forsch.*, *20*:96–118, 1945.

Hartsinck, J. J.: *Beschryving van Guiana, of de wilde Kust in Zuid-America.* Amsterdam, G. Tielenburg, *2*:811–812, 1770.

Heath, C.: Malformation of the hand. *Pathol. Coc. London*, *17*:440, 1866.

Hegdekatti, R. M.: Congenital malformations of hands and feet in man. *J. Hered.*, *30*:191–196, 1939.

Herwig, P.: Ein Fall von beiderseitiger Spalthand verbunden mit Syndaktylie. *München Med. Wochenschr.*, *56*:1383–1384, 1909.

Hilgenreiner, H.: Zwei Fälle von angeborener Fingergelenkankylose zugleich ein Beitrag zur Kenntnis der seltenen Spaltbildungen der Hand. *Z. Orthop. Chir.*, *24*:23–51, 1909.

Hofmann, M.: *Vererbung von Spalthand und Spaltfuss Beobachtungen an 2 Familien.* Inaug. Diss. München, Bilger-Druckerei, pp. 1–31, 1936.

Howard, W. T.: Congenital symmetrical deformity of both hands and feet. *Memphis Med. J.*, *24*:57–58, 1904.

Huet, E., and Infroit, C.: Ectrodactylie de deux pieds, ectrodactylie et syndactylie de la main droit. *Bull. Soc. Anat. Paris*, (5 s.), *12*:139–143. Also in *Presse Méd.*, *1*:105, 1898.

Jäger, M.: Gleichzeitiger Vorkommen eines angeborenen Defekts der Hand und angeborener Hyperplasie des Fusses. *Arch. Orthop. Unfallchir.*, *61*:206–210, Abb 2, 3:1967.

Jaworska, M., and Popiolek, J.: Genetic counseling in lobster-claw anomaly: discussion of variability of genetic influence in different families. *Clin. Pediatr.* *7*:396–399, 1968.

Joachimsthal, G.: *Die Angeborenen Verbild. der oberen Extremität.* Hamburg, L. Grafe & Sillem, pp. 33–36, 1900.

Johnston, O., and Davis, R. W.: On inheritance of hand and foot anomalies in six families. *Am. J. Hum. Genet.,* 5:356–372, pl. 1–4, 1953.

Kanavel, A. B.: Congenital malformations of the hand. *Arch. Surg.,* 25:1–53; 282–320, 1932.

Karsch, J.: Erbliche Augenmissbildung in Verbindung mit Spalthand und Fuss. *Z. Augenhlk.,* 89:274–279, 1936.

Karsch, J.: Zur Klinik und Erbbiologie des angeborenen Stars, insbesondere des Schichtstars. *Z. Augenhlk.,* 92:322–335, 1937.

Kelikian, H., and Doumanian, A.: Congenital anomalies of the hand. Part I. *J. Bone Joint Surg.,* 39A:1002–1019, fig. 6–8, 1957.

Kellner, A. W.: Über Spalthand und Fuss mit Oligodaktylie. *Klin. Wochenschr.,* 13:1507–1709, 1934.

Khorsovani, H.: Malformations des mains et des pieds (ectrodactylie) à travers cinq générations successives dans un grande famille Vaudoise. *J. Génét. Human.,* 8:1–60, 1959.

Klages, F. L., and Jacob, R.: Anatomische und erbbiologische Untersuchungen an einer mit Spaltfüssen und Missbildungen der Hände behafteten Sippe. *Z. Orthop.,* 70:265–281, 1940.

Klaussner, F.: *Uber Missbildungen der Menschlichen Gliedmassen.* Wiesbaden, J. F. Bergmann, pp. 41–53, 1900.

Klein, T. J.: Hereditary ectrodactylism in siblings. *Am. J. Dis. Child.,* 43:136–142, 1932.

Köster, H.: *Zur Frage der Zahn- und Haaranomalien bei syndaktyler Spalthand und Spaltfussbildung.* Inaug.-Diss. Göttingen; Druck der Dietrichschen Universitäts-Buchdruckerei, W. Fr. Kaestner, pp. 1–15, 1936.

Krabbe, H.: Nedarvet Mangel af Fingre of Täer. *Nord. Med. Ark.,* 12:1–2, 1880.

Kümmel, W.: *Die Missbildungen der Extremitäten durch Defekt. Verwachsung und Überzahl.* Bibliotheca Medica, Section E, Vol. III. Cassel, Verlag Th. G. Fischer & Co., pp. 21, 47–48, 1895.

Lallement, G. A.: Ein Beitrage zur Kenntnis des Spalthand. *Fortschr. Röntgenstr.,* 19:387–388, Taf. XXVI, fig. a, 1912–1913.

Lancet: Remarkable case of hereditary monstrosity. *Lancet,* 1:791–792, 1830. See also *Lancet,* 1:743–744, 1908.

Lange, M.: *Erbbiologie der Angeborenen Körperfehler.* Stuttgart, F. Enke, pp. 84–85, Abb. 28, (Spalthände und Spaltfüsse bei einem 2 jährigen Kind), 1935. See also *Z. Orthop. Chir.,* 63:84–85, 1935.

Lange, M.: Grundsätzliches über die Beurteilung der Entstehung und Bewertung atypischer Hand- und Fussmissbildung. *Verh. Dtsch. Orthop. Ges.,* 31:80–87, 1936. Also in *Z. Orthop.,* 66:8–87, 1937.

Largot, F.: Absence congénitale partielle du tibia. Main en foruche. *Rev. d'Orthop.,* (3 s.), 11:437–442, 1924.

Leboucq, H.: Description anatomique d'une monstruosité de la main. *Ann. Soc. Méd. Gand.,* 57:49–61, 1879.

Lehmann, W.: Über eine Familie mit multiplen Missbildungen an Händen und Füssen. *Acta. Genet. Med. Gem. Roma,* 2:87–102, 1953.

Lemaire, J.: Malformations congénitales, familiales, héréditaires des mains et des pieds. *Rev. d'Orthop.,* (2 s.), 10:267–273, pl. III-IV, 1909.

Lepoutre, C.: Malformations congénitales des extrémités (polydactylie, ectrodactylie, syndactylie, pouce trois phalanges, etc.) chez un enfant et chez sa mere. *Rev. d'Orthop.,* 10:237–244, 1923.

Lereboullet, P., and Allard, F.: Un cas de malformation digitale dite en "pince de homard." *N. Iconog. Salp.,* 13:250–252, 1909.

Lewis, T.: Hereditary malformations of the hands and feet. *In* Pearson, K., (ed.): *Treasury of Human Inheritance.* London, Dulau & Co., Vol. I, pp. 6–10, 1912.

Lewis, T., and Embleton, D.: Split hand and split foot deformities, their types, origin and transmission. *Biometrika,* 6:26–58, 1908.

Liebenam, L.: Beitrag zum familiären Vorkommen von Spalthänden und Spaltfüssen. *Z. menschl. Vererb Konstitutionslehre,* 22:136–151, 1939.

Lombard, P.: Bifurcation héréditaire et familiale de la main par fusion de deux metacarpiens en un os unique bifide. — Doigts surnuméraires. *Rev. d'Orthop.,* (3 s.), 5:135–146, 1914.

Lorenz, H.: Ektrodaktylie aller vier Extremitätenzeigen. *Wien. Klin. Wochenschr.,* 16:1344, 1903.

MacKenzie, H. J., and Penrose, L. S.: Two pedigrees of ectrodactyly. *Ann. Eugen.,* 16:88–96; figs. 5–6, 1951.

Magnanini, N.: Déformations congénitales des quatre membres: lesions symétriques des mains et des pieds. *Rev. Chir.,* 27:349–360, 1903.

Maisels, D. O.: Lobster-claw deformity of the hand. *The Hand,* 2:79–82, 1970.

Martens, F. H.: Über eine sehr komplicirt Hasenscharte oder einen sogenannten Wolfsrachen, mit einer an demselben Subjekte befindlichen merkwürdigen Missaltung der Hände und Füsse. Operiert von Dr. Johann Gottlob Eckoldt, abgebildet und beschrieben von Dr. Franz Heinrich Martens. Leipzig, E. F. Steinacher, 1804.

Mauclaire, P., and Bois: Ectrodactylie et syndactylie; main et pied fourchus. *Bull. Soc. d'Anthropol.,* (4 s.), 5:123–158, 1894.

Mayer, C.: Zur Casuistik der Spalthand und des Spaltfusses. *Beitr. Pathol. Anat.,* 23:20–41, 1898.

McKnight, H. A.: Congenital lobster-claw deformity. *Med. Surg., 1*:30–33, 1917.

McMullan, G., and Pearson, K.: On inheritance of the deformity known as split foot or lobster-claw. (Second papers). *Biometrika, 9*:381–390, 1913.

McWilliams, C. A.: Some congenital anomalies of the hands and feet. *Am. J. Med. Sci., 133*:602–607, 1907.

Meller, J.: Ein Fall von angeborener Spaltbildung der Hände und Füsse. *Berl. Klin. Wochenschr., 30*:232–233, 1893.

Menegaux, G.: Un nouveau cas d'ectrodactylie. *Rev. d'Orthop.*, (3 s.), *13*:239–242, 1926.

Ménière, P.: Observations sur quelques difformités congénitales des pieds et des mains. *Arch. Gén. Méd., 16*:364–380, 1828.

Meyerding, H. W., and Upshaw, J. E.: Heredofamilial cleft foot deformity (lobster-claw foot or split foot). An operation devised for correction of the deformity. *Am. J. Surg., 74*:889–892, 1947.

Morel-Lavallée: Bidactylie ou les deux mains et le pied droit en pinces d'écrevisse; absence du second orteil au pied gauche. *Bull. Soc. Chir. Paris, 2*:409–412, 1861.

Müller, W.: *Die angeborenene Fehlbildungen der menschlichen Hand.* Leipzig, G. Thieme, pp. 119–127, 1937.

Nardelli, R.: Ectrodattilia: reversione atavica? *Atti de XI Cong. Med. Internaz. 1894*, Roma, 4:125–188, 1895.

Neugebauer, H.: Spalthand und -fuss mit familärer Besonderheit. *Z. Orthop. Chir., 95*:500–506, 1962.

Nicaise: Note sur l'ectrodactylie. *Gaz. Méd. Paris*, (4 s.), pp. 499–502, 1875.

O'Rahilly, R.: Morphological patterns in limb deficiencies and duplications. *Am. J. Anat., 89*:135–193, 1951.

Orth, O.: Beiderseitiger Spaltfuss and Spalthand, kombiniert mit partiellem rechtsseitigen Pectoralisdefekt. *Arch. Klin. Chir., 91*:282–294, 1910.

Otte, P.: Malformation congénitales. *J. Radiol. Electr., 12*:507, 1928.

Otto, A. W.: *Seltene Beobachtungen zur Anatomie, Physiologie und Pathologie.* Breslau, A. Holeufer, pp. 58–59, 1816.

Otto, A. W.: *Monstrorum Sexentorum Descriptio Anatomica.* Bratislava, F. Hirt, pp. 147–149, No. 256: Tab. XVIII-XX, 1841.

Packard, F. A.: Congenital anomaly of both hands. *Trans. Am. Pathol. Soc., 13*:9–11, 1887.

Paré, A.: Des monstres et des prodiges: Exemple du défaut de la quantité de la semence. *In* Malagaigne, J. F., (ed.): *Oeuvres Complètes.* Paris, J. B. Bailliere, Vol. II, p. 21, 1841. See also *Oeuvre de M. Ambrose Paré.* Paris, Gabriel Buon, p. 825, 1575.

Parker, R. W., and Robinson, H. B.: A case of inherited congenital malformation of the hands and feet: plastic operation of the feet; with a family tree. *Trans. Clin. Soc. London, 20*:181–189, 1887.

Paster, C.: Angeborene Missbildung and Händen und Füssen bei einem Chinesen. *Arch. Pathol. Anat., 104*:54–58, Taf. I, 7:1886.

Paul, E.: Eine vierfingerige Hand mit Verbildung der Handwurzel. *Dtschr. Z. Chir., 151*:174–190, fig. 1, 2, 1919.

Paulicky, A.: Über kongenitale Missbildungen. *Dtsch. Milit. Z., 11*:199–234: Beobachtung III, 1882.

Pearson, K.: On inheritance of the deformity known as split foot or lobster-claw. *Biometrika, 6*:69–79, 1908–1909.

Pearson, K.: On the existence of the digital deformity—so-called "lobster-claw"—in the apes. *Ann. Eugen., 4*:339–340; pl. I-X, 1931.

Pélissier, G.: Un cas d'ectrodactylie de la main gauche. Bifurcation de la main gauche. *Bull. Soc. Anat. Paris., 16–17*:167–170, 1920.

Perthes, G.: Über Spalthand. *Dtsch. Z. Chir., 63*:132–148, 1902.

Pokorny, L.: Zur Klinik un Aetiologie der Spalthand. *Fortschr. Räntgenstr., 32*:274–280, 1924.

Popenoe, P.: Splithand. *J. Hered., 28*:174–176, 1937.

Pott, R.: Beitrag zu den symmetrischen Missbildungen der Finger und Zehen. *Jb. Kinderhelk., 21*:392–407, 1884.

Potter, E., and Nadelhoffer, L.: A familial lobster-claw: deformity of the feet and hands in a mother and two children. *J. Hered., 38*:331–335, 1947.

Pye: Symmetrical malformation of both hands and both feet. *Lancet, 2*:1119–1120, 1889.

Ray, A. K.: Another case of split foot mutation in two sibs. *J. Hered., 61*:169–170, 1970.

Raymond, F., and Janet, P.: Malformations des mains en "pinces de homard" et asymétrie du corps chez une épileptique. *N. Iconog. Salp., 10*:370–373, 1897.

R. C.: Other pedigrees of syndactyly and "lobster-claw." *J. Hered., 24*:243–244, 1933.

Régis, E.: Syndactylie, ectrodactylie, clinodactylie chez un dément précoce dégénéré. *N. Iconog. Salp., 21*:401–411, 1908.

Reid, D. A. C.: Reconstruction of the thumb. *J. Bone Joint Surg., 42B*:444–465, 1960.

Renaut: Sur deux cas d'ectrodactylie et un cas d'hémimelie. *Bull. Soc. Anat. Paris, 15*:224–225, 1870.

Ribeiro, A. L.: Lobster-claw hands. *Br. Med. J., 1*:1209, 1954.

Riedinger, J.: Ein Fall von Spalthand. *Monatsschr. Med. Naturwiss, 3*:327–332, 1896.

Roberts, A. S.: A case of deformity of the forearm and hands, with an unusual history of hereditary congenital deficiency. *Trans. Pathol. Soc. Philadelphia, 13*:4–9, 1887.

Roberts, J. A. F.: *An Introduction to Medical Genetics.* Fourth edition. London, Oxford University Press, pp. 264–266, 1967.

Rohlederer: Topographische Resonderheiten des Spaltfusses. *Z. Orthop., 66*:107–115, 1937.

Roloff: Über den Spaltfuss, *Fortschr. Röntgenstr., 3*:179–182, 1899.

Roth, W. E.: Animism and folklore of Guiana Indians. *In Bureau of American Ethnology.* Report No. 153, p. 364, 1911–1912.

Roucayrol, E.: Contribution a l'étude de la syndactylie et de l'ectrodactylie. *Rev. d'Orthop.,* (2 s.), *6*:85–91, 1905.

Rüdiger, R. A., Haase, W., and Passarge, E.: Association of ectrodactyly, ectodermal dysplasia and cleft lip-palate: the EEC syndrome. *Am. J. Dis. Child., 120*:160–163, 1970.

Rutherford, W. J., and Crawford, B. G. R.: Hereditary malformation of the extremities. *Lancet, 1*:979–980, 1919.

Savin, L. H., and Sorsby, A.: Two brothers, members of a family with "lobster-claw" (split-hand, split-foot deformity) one showing skeletal deformity, the other anirida. *Proc. R. Soc. Med., 28*:525, (Sect. Ophthal.), 1935.

Schade, H.: Zur endogenen Entstehung von Gliedmassendefekten. *Z. Morphol. Anthropol., 36*:375, 1937.

Schade, H.: Untersuchungen zur Frage der Erblichkeit von Mangelund Fehlbildungen der Gliedmassen. *Der Erbarzt., 8*:239–256, 1940.

Schäfer, W.: Über kongenitale Defekte an Händen und Füssen. *Beitr. Klin. Chir., 8*:436–462; Tab. X, 1892.

Scheffen, P.: Drei Fälle von Extremitätenmissbildungen. *Dtsch. Z. Chir., 112*:206–220, 1911.

Scholtz, A.: Über mannigfaltige Fehlbildungen an Händen und Füssen. *Z. Orthop., 72*:231–237, 1941.

Schonenberg, H.: Über die Kombination von Lippen-Kiefer-Gaumenspalten. *Z. Kinderheilk., 76*:79–90, 1955.

Schonenberg, H.: *Über Missbildungen der Extremitäten Bibliotheca Paediatrica.* Fasc. 80. Basel (Schweiz) New York, pp. 79–82, 1962.

Schroeder, E.: Entstehung und Vererbung von Missbildungen an der Hand eines Hypodaktylie Stammbaumes. *Mschr. Gebutsh. Gynäk., 48*:210–222, 1918.

Schultze, E.: Familiäre symmetrische Monodaktylie. *Dtsch. Med. Wochenschr., 30*:1689, 1904.

Schwalbe, E.: Über Extremitätenmissbildungen (Spalthand, Spaltfuss, Syndaktylie, Adaktylie, Polydaktylie). *Münch. Med. Wochenschr., 53*(1):493–496, 1906.

Schwarzweller, F.: Ein Beitrag zur Genese und Systematik der Gliedmassen-Missbildungen. *Arch. Orthop. Unfallchir., 39*:400–419, 1939.

Scoutetten, H.: Observations de difformités congénitales des pieds et des mains. *Bull. Acad. Imper. Méd., 23*:97–101, 1857–1858.

Secheyron, L.: Ectrodactylie quadruple. *Gaz. Med. Chir. Toulouse, 23*:105, 1891.

Selby, E. R.: Hereditary transmission of physical defects in the EMB family. *Can. Med. Assoc. J., 66*:439–441, 1952.

Smith, G. H.: Hereditary malformations of the hands and feet. *Lancet, 1*:358–359, 1941.

Smith, W. R., and Norwell, J. S.: Hereditary malformations of the hands and feet; with operation on one subject. *Br. Med. J., 2*:8–11, 1894.

Steininger, F.: Erbliche Missbildungen der Hände und Füsse, *Umschau., 38*:512, 1934.

Stevenson, A. C., and Jennings, L. M.: Ectrodactyly—evidence in favour of a disturbed segregation in the offspring of affected males. *Ann. Human. Genet., 24*:89–96, 1960.

Stieve, H.: Über Ektrodaktylie. *Z. Morphol. Anthropol., 20*:73–110, 1917.

Stiles, K. A., and Pickard, I. S.: Hereditary malformations of the hands and feet. *J. Hered., 34*:341–344, 1943.

Ströer, W. F. H.: Familiäres Auftreten von Hand- und Fussabweichungen in fünf Generationen. *Genetica, 17*:299–312, 1935.

Temtamy, S. A.: Absence deformities: ectrodactyly. *In Genetic Factors in Hand Malformations.* Ph. D. Thesis. Baltimore, Johns Hopkins University, pp. 15–32; 50–75; 160–162, 1966.

Thévenot, and Mouriquand, E.: Ectrodactylie des mains et des pieds. *Rev. d'Orthop.,* (2 s.), *8*:287–294, 1907.

Thibierge, G.: Une "femme homard": mains et pieds a deux doigts. *N. Iconog. Salp., 21*:472–474, 1908.

Thomson, J. D.: Congenital malformations of hands and feet. *Br. Med. J., 1*:1188–1190, 1892.

Tilanus, C. B.: Over een zeldzamm gevel van ectrodactylie. *Nederl. T. Geneesk., 2. R. 31*:934–938, 1895. See also *Z. Orthop. Chir., 4*:186–190, 1896.

Tomesku, T.: Syndaktylie, Synektrodaktylie (unvollständige Spalthand). *Fortschr. Röntgenstr., 36*:629–631, 1927.

Tubby, A. H.: A case of "lobster-claw" deformity of the feet and partial suppression of the fingers, with remarkable hereditary history. *Lancet, 1*:396–398, 1894.

Unterrichter, L.: Beiträge zur Kenntnis der angeborenen Anomalien der Extremitäten. *Z. menschl. Vererb. Konstitutionslehre, 18*:317–338, 1934.

Verschuer, O. F.: Woran erkennt man die Erblichkiet körperlicher Missbildungen? *Arch. Klin. Chir., 193*:185–213, Abb. 2, 1938.

Vogel, F.: Verzögerte Mutation beim Menschen? Einige kritische Bemerkungen zu Ch. Auerbachs Arbeit (1956). *Ann. Human. Genet.*, *22*:132–137, 1958.

Vogel, K.: Spalthand und Spaltfuss. *Fortschr. Röntgenstr.*, *6*:13–17, 1903.

Walker, J. C., and Clodius, L.: The syndrome of cleft lip, cleft palate with lobster-claw deformities of hands and feet. *Plast. Reconstr. Surg.*, *32*:627–636, 1963.

Walther, P.: Über die Exarticulation der Finger mit ihren Mittelhandbeinen aus den Handwurzelgelenken. *J. Chir. Augenheilk.*, *13*:351–374, 1829.

Wildervanck, L. S.: Perceptive deafness associated with split hand and foot, a new syndrome? *Acta Genet. Statist. Med.* (Basel), *13*:161–169, 1963.

Willard, De F., and Singer, B. L.: Multiple hand and foot deformities in the third, fourth, seventh, and ninth children of the same family; the others being normal and parents normal. *Am. J. Orthop. Surg.*, *7*:319–325, 1909.

Williams, E. P.: A case of hereditary deformity. *Illustr. Med. Surg.*, *2*:183–184, 1883.

Yap, S. E., and Pineda, E. V.: Two intersting cases of ectrosyndactyly. *Phillipine J. Sci.*, *20*:1–11, 1922.

Chapter Sixteen

ANNULAR GROOVES AND ALLIED ACRAL ABSENCES

In connection with webbed fingers, it was noted that terminal syndactyly and annular grooves often occur in the same hand. It was also pointed out that, in acrosyndactyly, conjoined digits are defective at their ends—in the language of teratologists, they have suffered intrauterine amputation. Annular grooves and acral absences are associated with each other often enough to suggest an intimate relation—a common cause. What that cause is remains controversial. More than one etiological agent has been incriminated.

CONSTRICTION BY UMBILICAL CORD

Simpson (1836) cited 10 cases of what he called circular depression. In one patient, two transverse grooves were placed at different levels on the same arm. Simpson contended that such multilevel defects could only be caused by the umbilical cord. This contention was not questioned for three-quarters of a century. Many authors have since pointed out that a small, slippery digit would not stay in one position long enough to be snared by a cord many times larger in caliber, and that annular grooves are too narrow to have been produced by the thick umbilical cord.

AMNIONIC COMPRESSION

Montgomery (1833) described a deep depression surrounding the limb. It had the appearance of a groove, such as would be made by tying a string with great force around the plump limb of a child. Although Montgomery did not see any constricting band, he surmised that there must have been a ligamentous thread formed out of "organized lymph" which, in turn, was said to have been derived from "prolongations of the egg membrane"—meaning the amnion.

496

The amniogenic theory of annular grooves and acral absences has now survived for more than a century. Ombrédanne (1913) and his followers — Brindeau et al. (1952) and many others — consider the following to be diverse manifestations of amniotic disease: intrauterine amputations, annular grooves, skin defects, dimples, and scars. Dennis Browne (1957) visualized perforations in the attenuated amnion, with fetal parts poking through these holes and being strangulated in the process. Köhler (1962) described a child who presented multiple lesions, ranging from relatively shallow, circular grooves around digits to complete separation of a leg with a raw and ragged bony stump. The mother of this child had reported trickling of liquid during her pregnancy. Köhler thought that this loss of amniotic fluid was consistent with the hypothesis which incriminates the hole in the amniotic membrane as the culprit of constriction. Torpin (1968) offered a considerable body of observations to support this view.

FAULTY GENESIS

Simpson (1836) reported a patient with the following defects: annular grooves involving the fingers, discrepancy between the length of the right and left arm, and unequal development of the two sides of the chest. Simpson argued that such multiple abnormalities could result only from a primary lack of growth potency on the part of embryonic tissue. Roberts (1894) presented a three-month-old female whose left forearm exhibited a constriction near the wrist; the three central digits of the left hand were stunted and coalesced, forming a single triangular mass. Roberts wondered about the possibility of faulty development in this instance. Abbe (1916) reported a Negro male who had whittled terminal phalanges and short fingers with circular grooves around them; he attributed these deformities to "nondevelopment." Pers (1963) considered it significant that aplasia of the skin, ring constriction, and spontaneous amputation are often observed together with amniotic bands. He ascribed all these anomalies to the failure of the cells surrounding the embryo to differentiate during the first three months of gestation. The implication is that both the conceptus and its covering have been simultaneously damaged by the same genetic determinant.

Streeter (1930) put the entire blame upon the embryo. He contended that what had previously been described as amniotic bands were the residue of a focal necrosis of the tissue derived from the embryo itself and not from the surrounding membrane. Streeter said, in effect, that (1) annular grooves and acral absences owed their origins to the imperfect histogenesis of embryonic tissue leading to focal necrosis, (2) they were predetermined in the germ cell, and (3) focal necrosis might appear to show preference for mesenchymal elements, but it also involved ectodermal derivatives, the skin in particular. He also held that the extent of damage depended upon the location of the focal necrosis. In acral absences, the terminal part sloughed off; in annular grooves, intermediary soft tissues were mainly affected and parts distal became isolated. If the groove was deep enough to interrupt the circulation of the distal part completely, the latter dropped off; a shallow groove did not seriously affect distal parts.

Streeter's view was supported by many. Blackfield and Hause (1951) considered the theory that amniotic strands were the cause of annular grooves to have been completely explained into oblivion by Streeter's concept of embryogenic focal necrosis. McKusick (1968) wrote: "Since the work of Streeter . . . the causative role of the amniotic bands has been discounted and the malformations, both the bands and the associated absence deformities, are thought to result from tissue necrosis probably on a vascular basis." McKusick (1971) appears to have changed his mind after the publication of Torpin's (1968) book. He conceded the plausibility of "a modified form of the amniotic band theory." The question as to whether annular grooves are caused by disturbances of the fetal membrane or result from defects inherent in the embryo itself remains unsettled.

ANNULAR GROOVES (Ring Constrictions; Congenital Ainhum; Spontaneous Dactylolysis)

In the upper limb, annular grooves are seen most often on the fingers; they also occur in the palm and forearm. The groove may be deep or shallow. In some cases, it spans the entire circumference of the part; in others, it traces a segment of a circle. As a rule, annular grooves are transversely disposed. Oblique grooves have been recorded by Abbe (1916), Stenstrom (1944), and Patterson (1961). Oblique annular grooves seem to favor the metacarpal region. Most annular grooves are unilateral. In the less frequent bilateral cases, the two sides are affected differently. Most rudimentary digits consist of bubblelike fleshy masses, some of which contain slivers of bone and may even have vestigial nails. These rudimentary digits usually have constricted bases and rightly belong to the category of intercalary defects (Figs. 16–1 to 16–9).

Annular grooves are known to recur. Hiller (1927) reported a 37-year-old woman who had been born with annular grooves on her right forearm, hand, and fingers, and also on her lower leg. The grooves had gradually become deeper and occasioned periodic attacks of numbness, pain, cyanosis, and coldness in parts distal to the grooves. Amputation of the right foot had been performed 17 years earlier; sometime later, because of recurrent pain, the leg was amputated at a point 7 cm. above the right knee joint. Shortly after this operation, another groove appeared just proximal to the end of the stump, with the result that the distal tissues became periodically cyanosed, cold, painful, and tender. The groove above the right wrist also deepened and was accompanied by cyanosis and coldness of parts distal. Inglis (1952) reviewed this case and considered the formation of the annular grooves to be a dynamic process.

Annular grooves of the hand and forearm are at times accompanied by elephantoid enlargement of parts distal. Coupland and Balding (1881) exhibited the plaster model of an infant's hand with an annular groove at the base of a short finger. This digit measured "a quarter of an inch in diameter at the seat of the constriction and two thirds of an inch in diameter beyond the constriction." Farmer (1948) noted "astonishing degrees of lymphedema" in connection with "a tight constricting band higher in the limb." Blackfield and Hause (1951) spoke of stasis and enlargement occurring in parts distal to the annular grooves. In Patterson's (1961) series of 52 cases, three showed lymphedema of parts distal to the annular groove (Fig. 16–10).

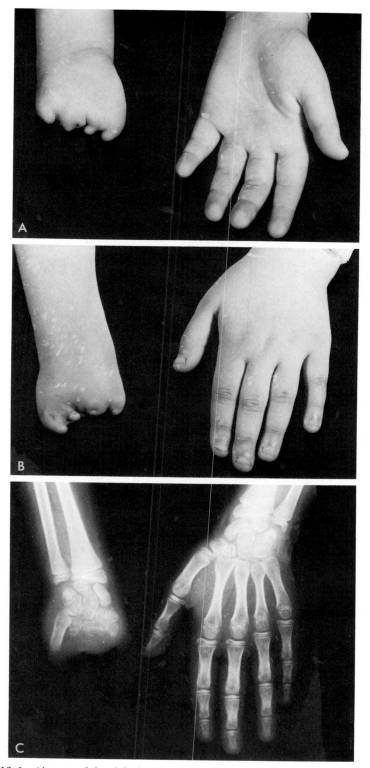

Figure 16–1 Absence of the right hand with small terminal buds bearing miniature nails. *A*, Palmar view of the hands of a 12-year-old girl. *B*, Dorsal view. *C*, Dorsopalmar roentgenograph of the hands.

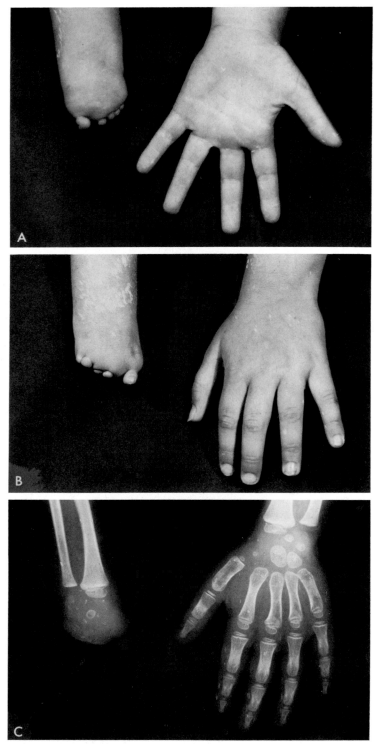

Figure 16–2   Absence of the right hand with rudimentary digits bearing vestigial nails. *A*, Palmar view of the hands of a four-year-old female. *B*, Dorsal view. *C*, Dorsopalmar roentgenograph showing one carpal ossicle in the affected limb as compared to five bones in the opposite wrist.

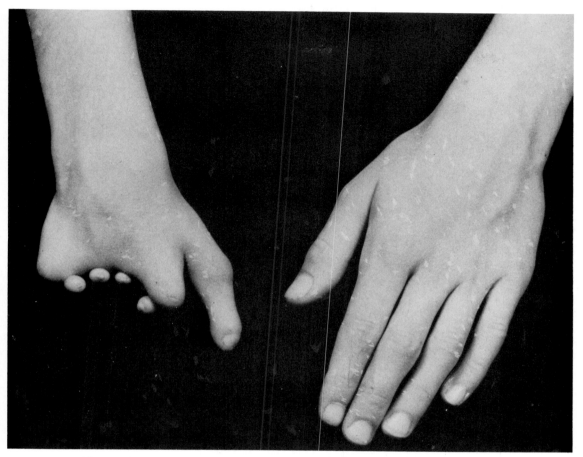

Figure 16–3 Rudimentary digits ("bubbles") of the right hand of a 14-year-old boy.

Compression of nerves with consequent motor paralysis or loss of sensation has been reported in connection with annular grooves. Meyer and Cummins (1941) described a newborn baby with a deep annular groove around the middle of the upper arm. The infant had a definite wrist drop due to the compression of the radial nerve. The child with annular groove of the forearm and skin defect reported by Pers (1963) also had radial nerve paralysis. Barenberg and Greenberg (1942) and Blackfield and Hause (1951) presented patients with anesthesia of parts distal to the annular groove. Neurotropic ulcers of the terminal parts often occur in association with annular grooves of the lower extremity. They are rare in the upper limb.

Analogies have often been drawn between congenital annular grooves, pedunculated postminimus, *pouce flottant* or floating thumb, and ainhum and ainhum-like inanitions seen in sundry disorders. Cummins (1932) gave pedunculated postminimus as a salient example of congenital annular groove. Gupta (1963) reported a pedunculated postminimus which had become gangrenous beyond the constricted pedicle. The analogous deformity on the radial side of the hand is represented by *pouce flottant*, which is regarded as an intercalary defect of the radial ray. The base of the floating thumb is encircled by a deep

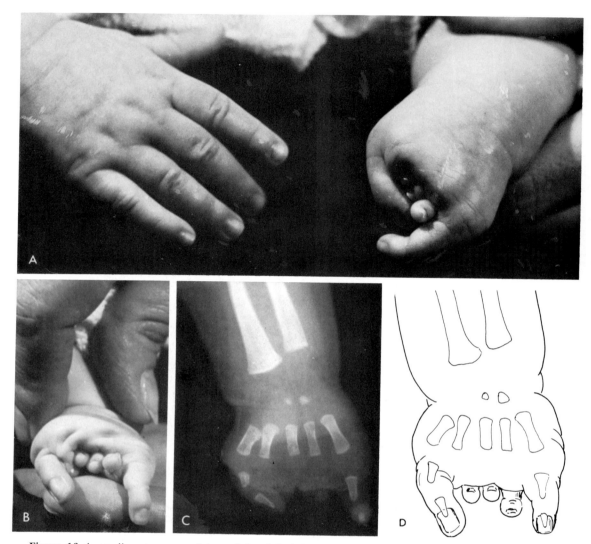

Figure 16–4   Rudimentary central three digits of the left hand, each with a small nail. *A,* Dorsal view of the hands of a five-month-old child. *B,* Frontal view of the left hand. *C,* Dorsopalmar roentgenograph of the left hand. *D,* Sketch illustrating the same.

groove; proximally, a bone—the first metacarpal in part or as a whole—is missing. In annular groove proper, parts proximal are present.

Da Silva Lima (1867) described a condition characterized by an insidiously deepening groove around the little toe and the eventual withering of its terminal portion. This disease occurs predominantly in African Negroes, mainly in males. To this condition, Da Silva Lima attached the name *ainhum,* which in the language of the natives means "to saw," or "sawed off." Menzel (1874) reported several cases of congenital annular groove of the fingers and called this anomaly dactylolysis spontanea. Beauregard (1875) added the adjective *essential* to distinguish dactylolysis of ainhum from other forms of digital inanition. This distinction was overlooked by later authors who identified spontaneous dactylolysis with ainhum. Abbe (1916) considered congenital ring constriction analogous to ainhum. Streeter (1930) was also impressed by the similarity of congenital dac-

(Text continued on page 506.)

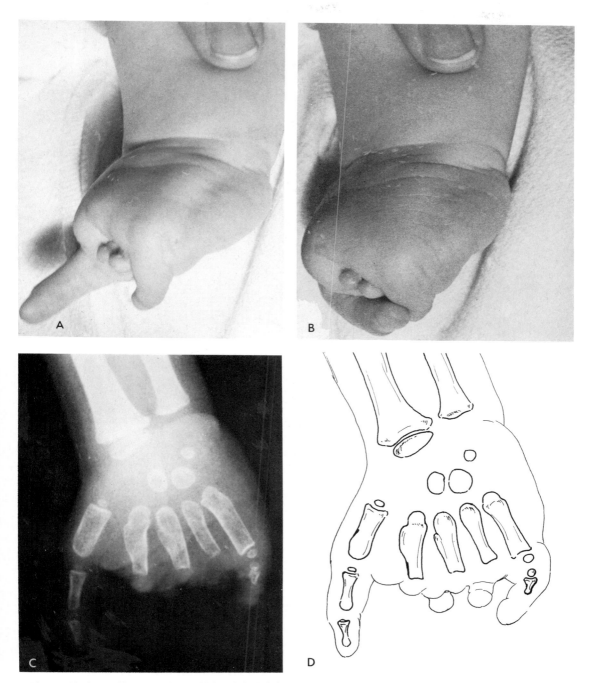

Figure 16–5 Rudimentary lesser digits of the left hand. *A* and *B*, Frontal views of the left hand of a 13-month-old female. *C*, Dorsopalmar roentgenograph. *D*, Sketch illustrating the same.

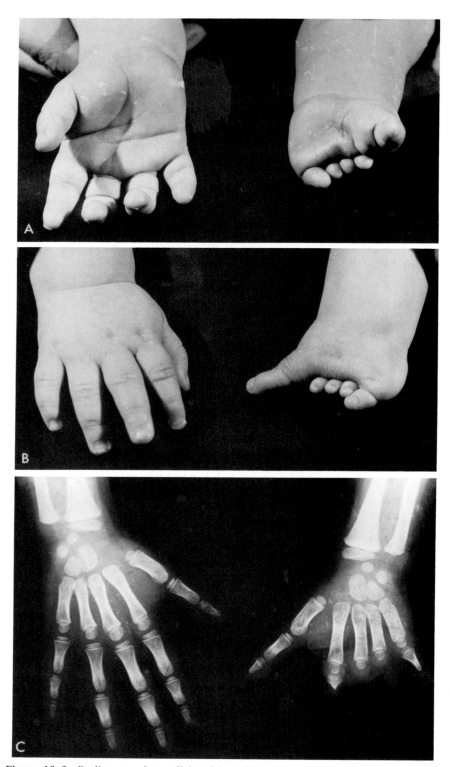

Figure 16–6 Rudimentary lesser digits of the left hand bearing small nails. *A*, Palmar view of the hands of a four-year-old boy. *B*, Dorsal view. *C*, Dorsopalmar roentgenograph.

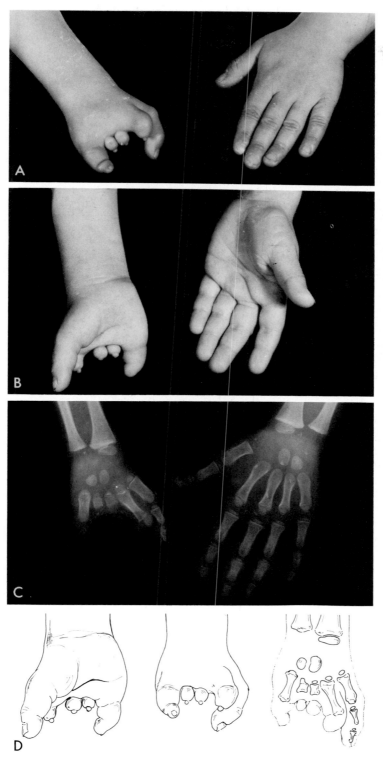

Figure 16–7 Rudimentary ulnar digits of the right hand bearing small nails. *A*, Dorsal view of the hands of a two-year-old male. *B*, Palmar view. *C*, Dorsopalmar roentgenograph. *D*, Illustrative sketches.

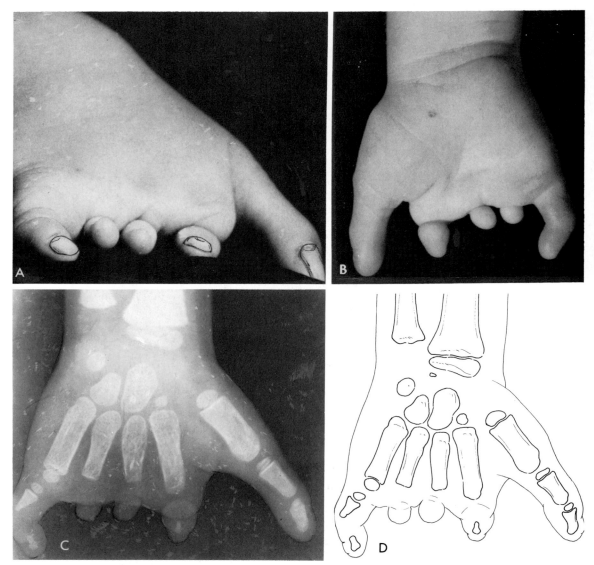

Figure 16–8 Rudimentary lesser digits of the right hand. *A*, Dorsal view of the right hand of a four-year-old boy: vestigial index and little fingers bear nails and, as shown by the roentgenograph (*C*), these same digits contain remnants of ungual phalanges. *B*, Palmar view. *C*, Dorsopalmar roentgenograph of the hand: the vestigial index finger has only a diminutive phalanx, probably ungual; the longer little finger has two phalanges—proximal and distal. *D*, Sketch illustrating the same.

tylolysis and ainhum. Bluefarb (1948) reported an annular groove around the little finger of a nine-year-old white girl. The constricting band involved the skin just proximal to the first interphalangeal joint. This abnormality had been present since birth.

Annular grooves may also be simulated by the following conditions: leprosy, scleroderma, syphilis, metabolic diseases, cicatrices, umbra pilaris, syringomyelia, and *mal de Meleda*. The last disorder consists of symmetrical cornification of the palms and soles. It is said to be common among the inhabitants of the island of Meleda, Dalmatia. Mal de Meleda is transmitted as an autosomal recessive trait.

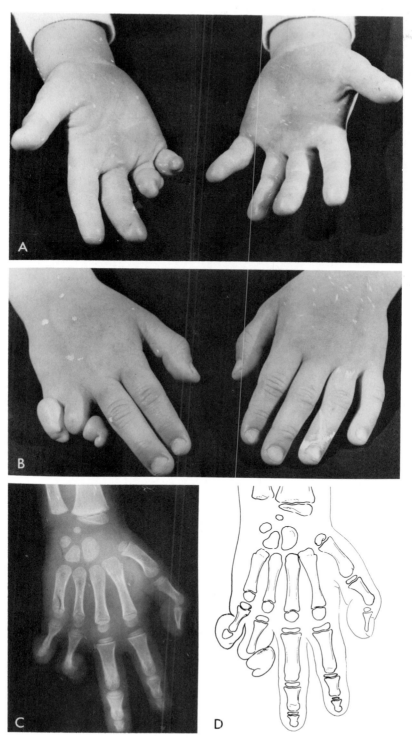

Figure 16–9 Annular grooves of the right ring and little fingers associated with absence of middle and ungual phalanges. *A*, Palmar view of the hands of a four-year-old boy. *B*, Dorsal view. *C*, Dorsopalmar roentgenograph of the right hand. *D*, Sketch illustrating the same.

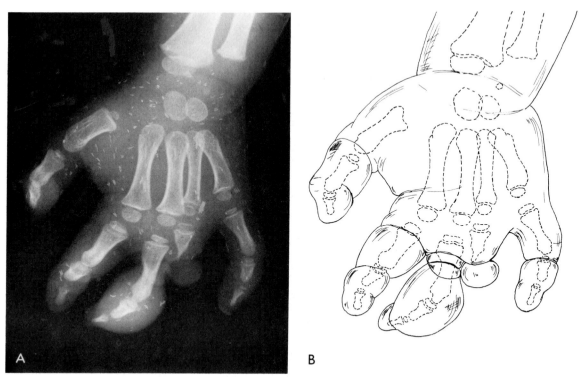

Figure 16–10   Annular groove causing bulbous tumefaction of parts distal. *A*, Dorsopalmar roentgenograph of the left hand of a two-year-old female with elephantine enlargement beyond annular grooves; the two phalanges of the ring finger are missing. *B*, Sketch illustrating the same.

ACRAL ABSENCES (Intrauterine Amputations; Peripheral Absences)

The term *terminal transverse defect* is used for absences in which the limb or the digit seems to have been severed from one border to another and parts distal do not exist. Absence of the entire limb is called *amelia;* when half or nearly half of the limb is missing the designation *transverse hemimelia* is used; absences of the hand, digital rays, and phalanges are called *acheiria, adactylia,* and *aphalangia,* respectively (Figs. 16–11 to 16–14).

Earlier authors classed acral absences with congenital amputations. Two types of congenital amputation were distinguished and labeled, respectively, developmental and spontaneous. The former is now classified with endogenous and the latter with exogenous defects. Endogenous amputation is said to present the ensuing distinctive features: rudimentary digits, with or without nails, at the end of the defective limb; well-padded stump; roentgenographically demonstrable bone defects; involvement of multiple parts, the defects being at times bilateral but not symmetrical; and the presence of such associated anomalies as annular grooves, cutaneous dimples, and clubbing of the feet. The following findings are said to be indicative of exogenous amputation: lopped-off, stunted digits which, unlike the bubblelike rudiments seen in the endogenous variety, contain sizable bones and are equipped with tendons; associated acrosyndactyly;

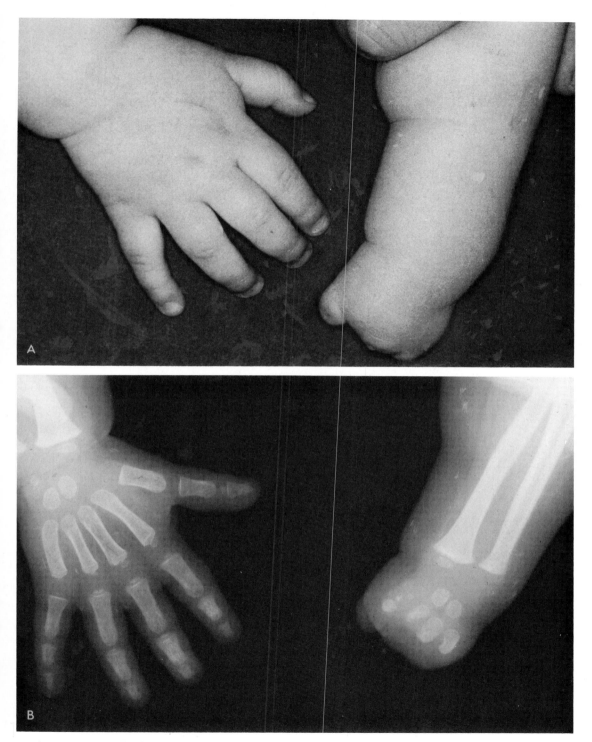

Figure 16–11   Acheiria. *A*, Dorsal view showing absence of the left hand of an 18-month-old male. *B*, Dorsopalmar roentgenograph of the same.

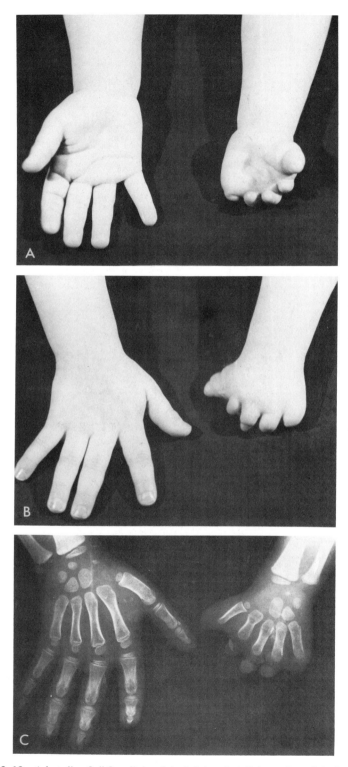

Figure 16–12   Adactylia of all five digits of the left hand. *A*, Palmar view of the hands of a four-year-old female. *B*, Dorsal view. *C*, Dorsopalmar roentgenograph of the hands.

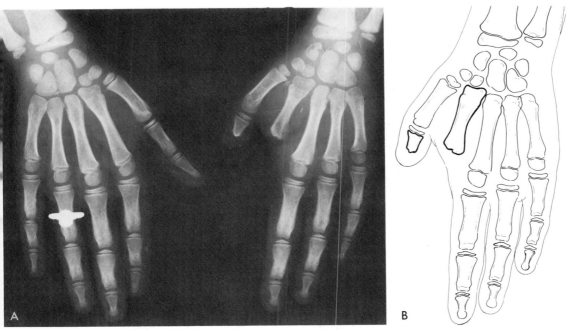

Figure 16–13 Adactylia of the left index finger associated with absence of the distal end of the proximal phalanx and absence of the ungual phalanx of the left thumb. *A*, Dorsopalmar roentgenograph of the hands of an 11-year-old female. *B*, Sketch illustrating the left hand.

scar formation; and firm, tapered stumps which at times permit the bone to protrude. The distinction between endogenous and exogenous acral absences is, at best, conjectural.

By far the majority of reported cases of acral absences have been sporadic and unilateral. Koehler (1936) described a Brazilian family in which four members had no hands and feet. The parents were unaffected; they were consanguineous. Inheritance in this instance is considered to be autosomal recessive. Köhler (1962) presented twin sisters, one of whom had no skeletal abnormalities; the other sister's left hand was missing. The parents were unaffected, but a paternal uncle had a missing hand; he was the father of eight surviving children, and they were all unaffected. Köhler considered two genetic interpretations: recessive transmission of the trait and dominant inheritance with reduced penetrance. Toledo and Saldaha (1969) reported two sibships with acheiropody. In both families, the affected members were closely consanguineous. The pattern of inheritance in these families seemed to be recessive.

ASSOCIATIONS

Annular grooves and acral absences are seen in a number of regional anomalies of the hand. Acrosyndactyly is often accompanied by annular grooves

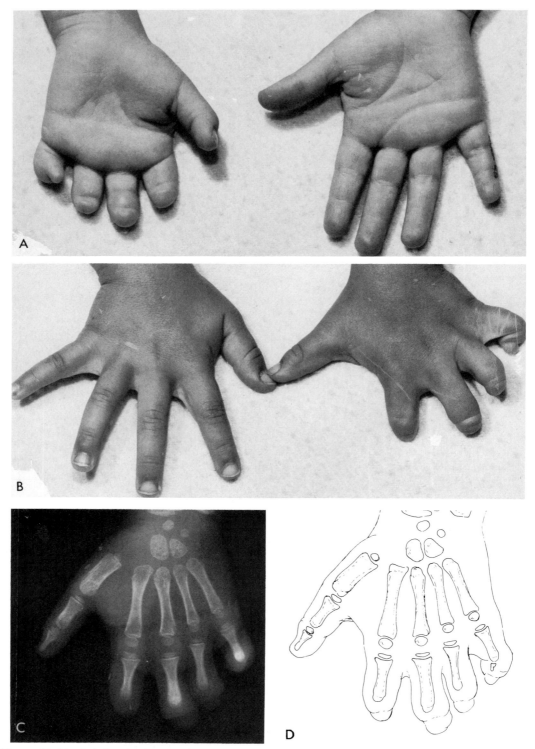

Figure 16–14 Aphalangia: absence of distal two rows of phalanges of the lesser digits of the left hand. *A*, Palmar view of the hands of a four-year-old female. *B*, Dorsal view. *C*, Dorsopalmar roentgenograph of the left hand. *D*, Sketch illustrating the same.

as well as by terminal transverse defects. Terminal transverse defect of the four ulnar digits is a feature of Type B brachydactyly—also known as apical dystrophy. In more severe forms of split hand complex, all digits or even digital rays may be missing. In acheiria, carpal bones eventually become fused with one another or with the remaining bases of the metacarpals. In some cases of acral absences of the hand, the costosternal portion of the ipsilateral pectoralis major is defective. Occasionally, the opposite hand is also affected. Trimelic and tetramelic malformations are comparatively uncommon. No two limbs are affected to the same extent. Annular grooves and acral absences are known to occur in a few syndromes (Figs. 16–15 to 16–28).

BIRD-HEADED DWARFISM

Seckel (1960) listed the following main features of this complex as follows: low birth weight, extremely short stature, small head and small brain, mental retardation short of true idiocy, beaklike protrusion of the central face and a receding chin, and frequent association with multiple congenital malformations. Among the latter is included deep circular cutaneous creases of the forearm. Bird-headed dwarfism is transmitted as an autosomal recessive trait.

(*Text continued on page 527.*)

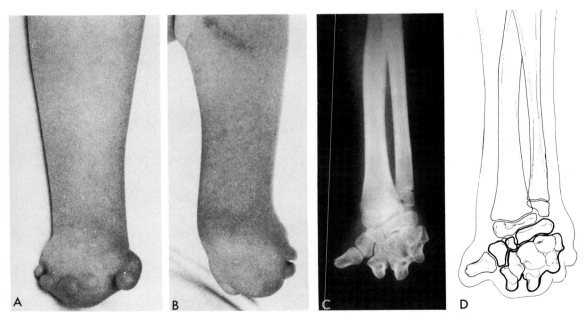

Figure 16–15 Fusion anomalies incident to acral absences. *A*, Palmar view of the left forearm and wrist of a 13-year-old male. *B*, Dorsal view. *C*, Dorsovolar roentgenograph: in the proximal row, lunate and triquetral bones are fused; in the distal row, carpal bones are fused with the bases of four ulnar metacarpals. *D*, Sketch illustrating the same.

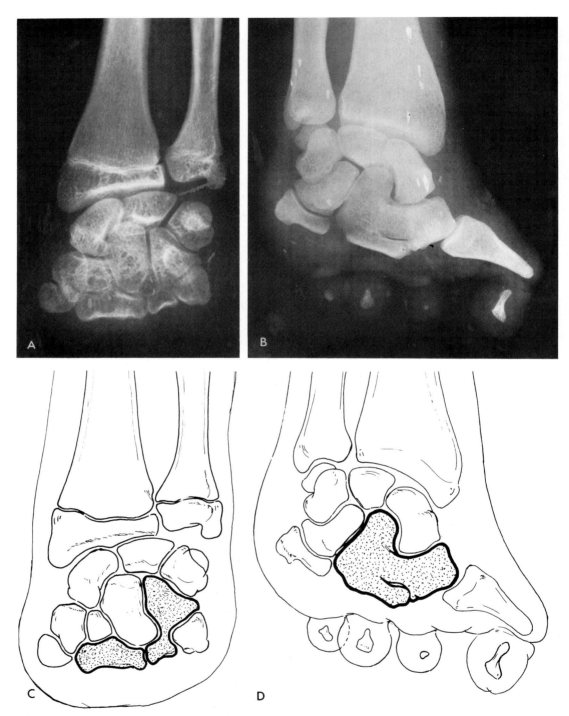

Figure 16–16   Fusion anomalies occurring in acral absences. *A*, Roentgenograph of the right wrist of a boy with transverse terminal defect, showing fusion of the bases of the third and fourth metacarpals. *B*, Roentgenograph of the right wrist of an adult with transverse intercalary absence: here the trapezium, trapezoid, capitate, and the bases of the second and third metacarpals have formed a solid mass, and the bases of the fourth and fifth metacarpals have coalesced. *C* and *D* illustrate the roentgenograph above each.

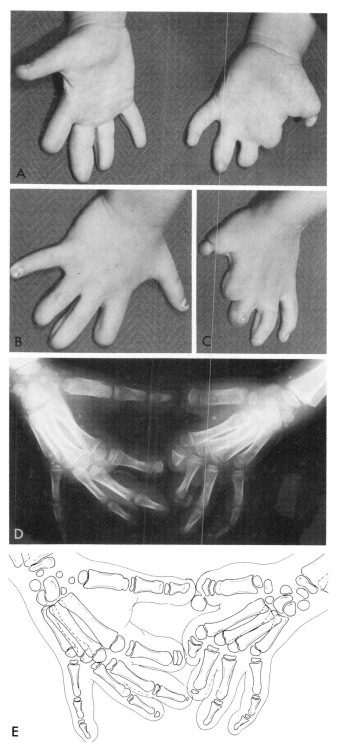

Figure 16–17 Bilateral asymmetrical absence of phalanges. *A*, Palmar view of the hands of a six-year-old female. *B*, Dorsal view of the right hand. *C*, Dorsal view of the left hand. *D*, Oblique roentgenograph of the hands. *E*, Sketch illustrating the same.

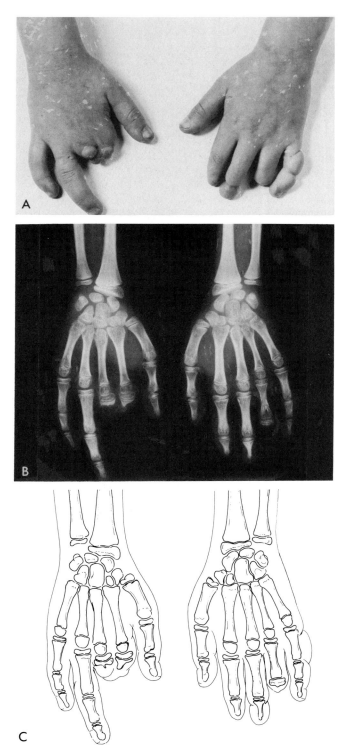

Figure 16–18   Bilateral annular grooves and acral absences. *A*, Dorsal view of the hands of an eight-year-old female. *B*, Dorsopalmar roentgenograph. *C*, Sketch illustrating the same.

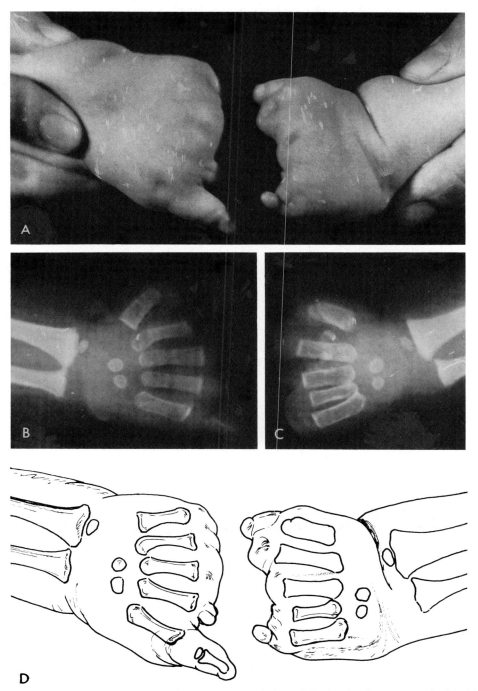

Figure 16–19 Bilateral acral absences. *A*, Dorsal view of the hands of an 11-month-old girl with bilateral asymmetrical absence of digits. *B*, Dorsopalmar roentgenograph of the right hand. *C*, Dorsopalmar roentgenograph of the left hand. *D*, Sketch illustrating the roentgenographs of the right and left hands.

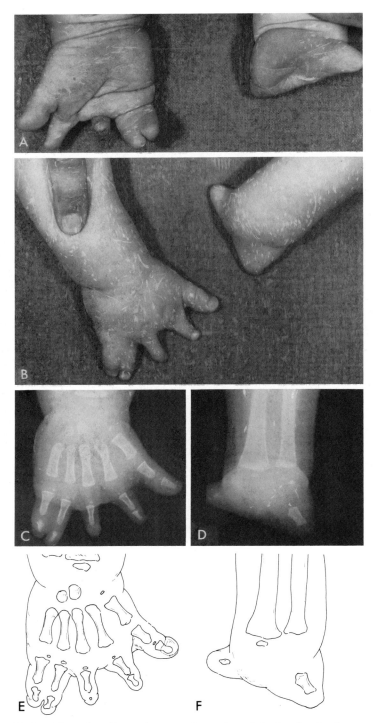

Figure 16–20   Bilateral malformation. *A*, Palmar view of the hands of a three-year-old male with symbrachydactyly of the right hand and absence of the left hand. *B*, Dorsal view. *C* and *D*, Dorsopalmar roentgenographs of the right and left hands. *E* and *F* illustrate the roentgenograph above each.

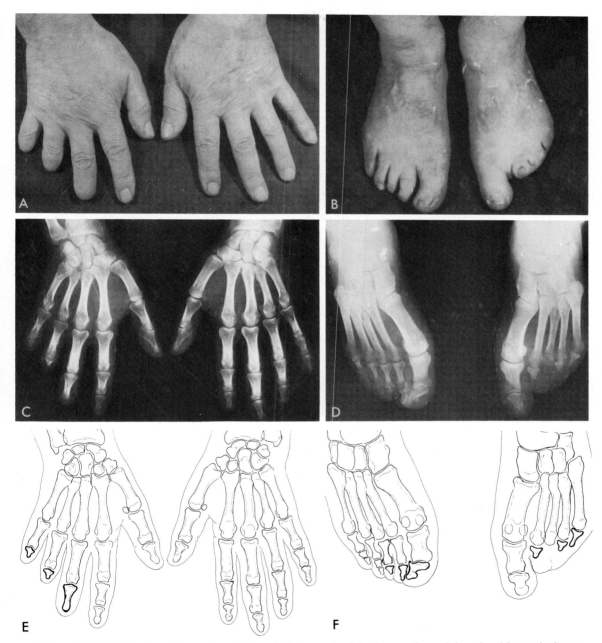

Figure 16–21 Trimelic malformation. *A*, Dorsal photograph of the hands of an adult male with terminal transverse defects of the right ring and little fingers. *B*, Dorsal view of both forefeet, showing acral absence of the right second and third toes and of the four fibular digits of the left foot. *C*, Dorsopalmar roentgenograph of both hands: the right ring and little fingers lack ungual phalanges, and the middle phalanx of each is represented by a small conical ossicle. *D*, Dorsoplantar roentgenograph of the forefeet: here the right second and third toes lack ungual phalanges; the left third toe has no phalanges, and the second, fourth, and fifth toes have diminutive phalanges. *E* and *F* illustrate the roentgenograph above each.

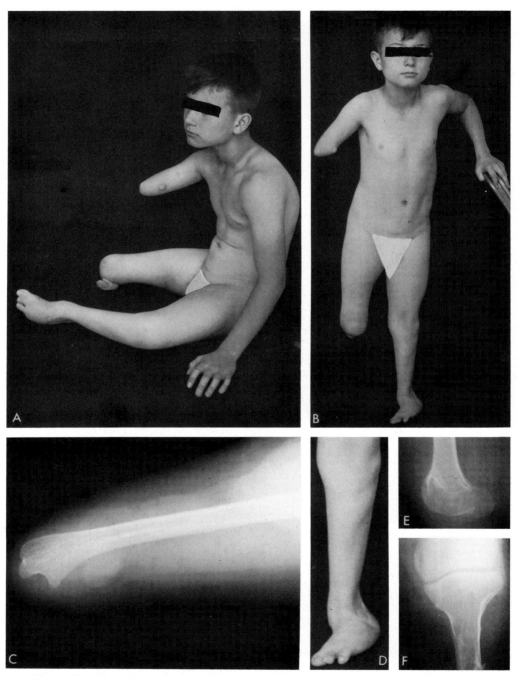

Figure 16–22   Trimelic malformation. *A*, Side view of a teenage male with absence of the right forearm and hand, absence of the right leg and foot, absence of the left fibula, syndactyly of the first and second toes, and absence of the fourth and fifth toes of the left foot. *B*, Frontal view. *C*, Roentgenograph of the right humerus taken when the patient was in his thirties. *D*, Enlarged photograph of the left leg which had later been amputated. *E*, Lateral roentgenograph of the right distal femur. *F*, Anteroposterior roentgenograph of the stump of the amputated left leg, showing absence of the fibula.

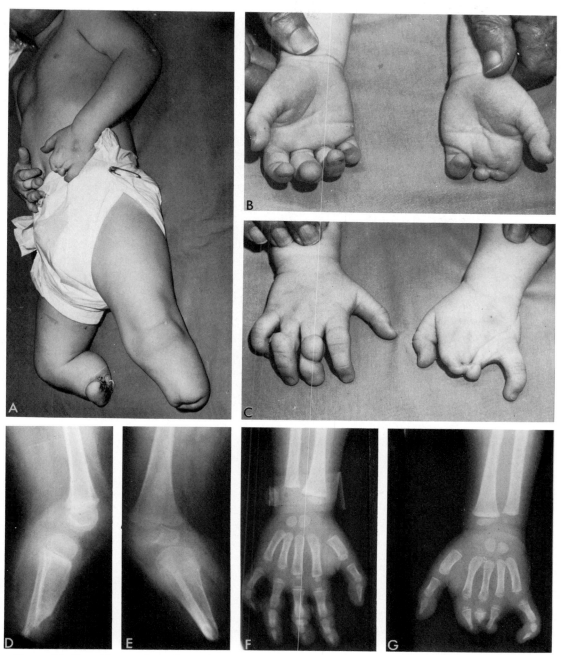

Figure 16–23   Tetramelic malformation. *A*, Side view of a young man with annular grooves of the middle and ring fingers of the right hand, acrosyndactyly of the central three digits of the left hand, and bilateral absence of the lower legs and both feet. *B*, Palmar view of the hands. *C*, Dorsal view. *D* and *E*, Lateral roentgenographs of the right and left legs after revision of the stumps. *F* and *G*, Dorsopalmar roentgenographs of the right and left hands, taken at the age of two.

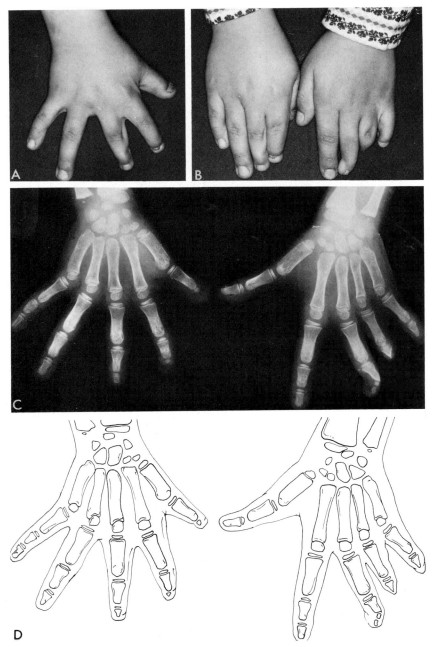

Figure 16–24   Tetramelic malformation. *A*, Dorsal photograph of the right hand of an eight-year-old boy with defective nails of the three radial digits and partial syndactyly of the index and middle fingers. *B*, Dorsal view of both hands, showing defective three ulnar digits on the left hand. *C*, Dorsopalmar roentgenograph of both hands: in the right hand, the ungual phalanges of the three radial digits are rudimentary, but each phalanx gains some bulk as one approaches the middle finger. In the left hand, the three ulnar digits are affected and the defect becomes more severe as one approaches the ulnar border of the hand. *D*, Sketch illustrating the same.

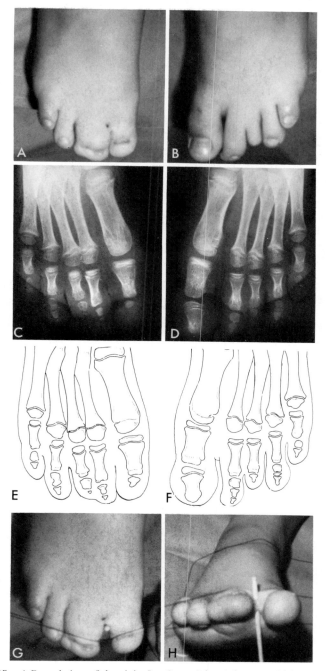

Figure 16–25 *A*, Dorsal view of the right forefoot of the eight-year-old featured in Figure 16–24: there is complete syndactyly of the right second and third toes and fenestrated syndactyly of the right first and second toes. *B*, Dorsal view of the left forefoot: the second and third toes are partially webbed; the second toe has a dystrophic and the third, no nail. *C*, Dorsoplantar roentgenograph of the right foot, showing vestigial ungual phalanges of the three tibial digits. *D*, Roentgenograph of the left forefoot: note that the second toe has a diminutive and the third toe, no ungual phalanx. *E* and *F* illustrate the roentgenograph above each. *G* and *H* show the fenestrum between the webbed first and second toes of the right foot.

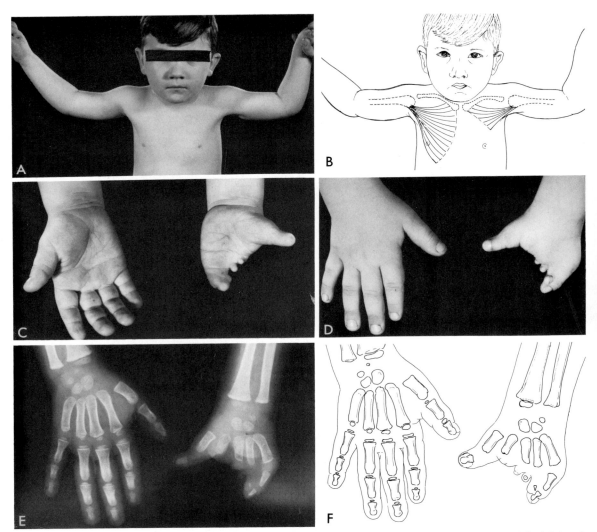

Figure 16–26   Absence of central digits, absence of a phalanx in both the thumb and the little finger of the left hand, and disharmonious development of the carpal bones associated with absence of the sterno-abdominal head of the ipsilateral pectoralis major muscle. *A*, Frontal view of the upper body of a four-year-old boy. *B*, Sketch illustrating the defective portion of the left pectoralis major muscle. *C*, Palmar view of the hands. *D*, Dorsal view. *E*, Dorsopalmar roentgenograph of the hands, showing defective development of the bones in the left wrist and hand. *F*, Sketch illustrating the same.

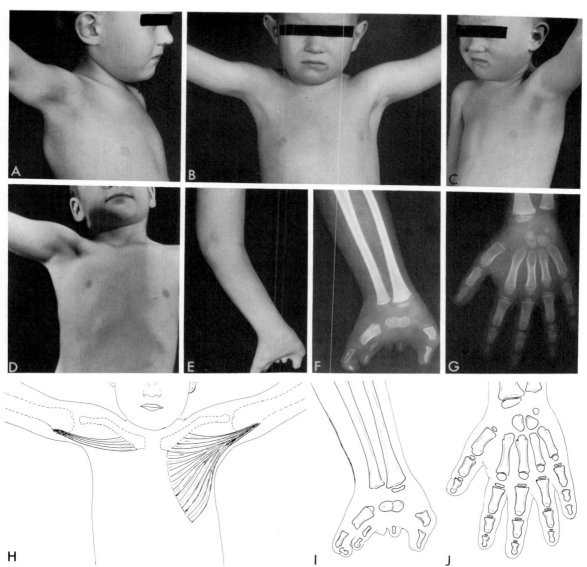

Figure 16–27　Central adactylia of the hand, simulating split hand, in a four-year-old boy with absent costosternal head of the ipsilateral pectoralis major muscle. *A*, Right axilla. *B*, Frontal view showing that the right anterior axillary fold is absent. *C*, Left axilla. *D*, The fold formed by the clavicular head of the pectoralis major muscle. *E*, Dorsal view of the right forearm and hand. *F*, Dorsopalmar roentgenograph of the left hand. *G*, Dorsopalmar roentgenograph of the right hand. *H*, Sketch illustrating the absence of the costosternal head of the right pectoralis major muscle. *I* and *J* illustrate the roentgenograph above each.

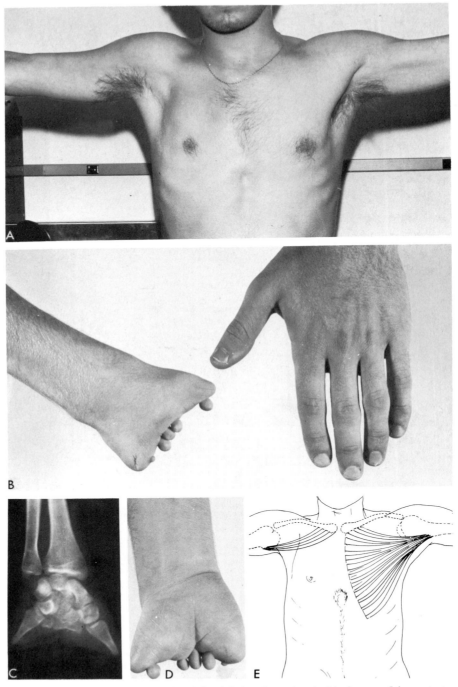

Figure 16–28   Rudimentary digits of the right hand associated with absence of the costosternal head of the ipsilateral pectoralis major muscle. *A*, Frontal view of the chest and axillae of a 14-year-old male. *B*, Dorsal view of the hands: the right hand has five bubbles and there is a dimple near its ulnar border. *C*, Dorsopalmar roentgenograph of the right hand. *D*, Palmar view of the right hand. *E*, Sketch illustrating the absence of all but the clavicular head of the pectoralis major muscle.

CRANIOSYNOSTOSIS AND TERMINAL TRANSVERSE DEFECT

As noted in Chapter Twelve, in most cases of acrocephalosyndactyly, the webbed digits are defective at their ends and in an occasional case the hand resembles an amputated stump. Garcin et al (1933) described a 23-month-old girl with characteristic features of Crouzon's craniofacial dysostosis: strabismus, hypertelorism, exophthalmos, short upper lip, arcuate parrot-beaked nose, hypoplastic maxilla, and relative mandibular prognathism. She had no digits on the right hand. Roentgenography revealed terminal transmetacarpal defect.

DEFECT OF THE SCALP, SKULL, AND DIGITS

Pincherle (1938) presented a patient with congenital defect of the scalp and absent terminal phalanges of the second to fifth digits of the left hand. Adams and Oliver (1945) reported a family in which eight members had congenital defects of the scalp, skull, and extremities. The proband had transverse terminal defects of both legs below the midcalf and absence of all the digits, and some of the metacarpals, of the right hand. The father was born with absence of the four fibular toes on the left foot and with short terminal phalanges of the fingers. Adams and Oliver considered the trait to be an autosomal dominant with variable expression. A newborn infant reported by Kahn and Olmedo (1950) had a defect of the scalp, vestigial toes with absent terminal phalanges, and an absent terminal phalanx of an index finger.

HANHART'S ABSENCE DEFORMITY OF THE LIMBS WITH MICROGNATHISM (Peromelia-Micrognathia Complex)

Hanhart (1950) described a six-year-old girl with hypoplastic mandible and absence of both hands. Her relatives were said to have many degenerative signs; both her parents came from an inbred community. Hanhart's second case with micrognathia was a 39-year-old female. She had a birdlike profile: her chin receded, sloping down into her neck. She presented terminal transverse defect of the right thigh and left forearm and ectrodactyly of the right hand. The trait is an autosomal recessive.

OROMELIC COMPLEXES

Anonychia-ectrodactyly syndrome was described in Chapter Seven. Anodontia-adactylia syndrome was taken up in Chapter Fifteen.

Absence or underdevelopment of the tongue is at times accompanied by defective digits—symbrachydactyly, but more often terminal transverse defect.

The complex is called aglossia-adactylia. Kettner (1907) described a four-year-old male who had, instead of a tongue, a small mass of tissue in the floor of his mouth. He also had bilateral absence of the index and long fingers; with the exception of the right little finger, the other digits of both hands were deformed.

Rosenthal's (1932) patient was a three-year-and-three-month-old girl who was born with almost complete absence of the tongue. Her right hand had only one digit, which was interpreted as being a thumb containing two bones, a metacarpal and a vestigial proximal phalanx; there was also a rudimentary fifth metacarpal. On her left hand, the three last ulnar digits were normal. The thumb possessed a broad but short proximal phalanx and an underdeveloped distal phalanx; the index finger had a rudimentary middle and no terminal phalanx. The patient reported by Shear (1956) had underdeveloped maxillae, microglossia, diminished number of teeth, absent terminal phalanx of the right thumb, and almost complete absence of four ulnar digits; the phalanges and metatarsals of both feet were nonexistent. Patterson (1961) described a baby boy with aglossia congenita and bony ankylosis of the jaws. There was no nail on his left thumb. The right thumb was poorly developed; the second digits of both hands had only two phalanges. Gorlin and Pindberg (1964) featured the photographs of a child with no tongue and terminal transverse defect of both forearms.

In ankyloglossum superior or glossopalatine ankylosis, there is congenital fusion of the tongue to the hard palate or upper alveolar ridge. This anomaly is occasionally accompanied by symbrachydactyly but more often by terminal transverse defect of the digits. Phelip (1920) reported a female child with this anomaly; she had only a thumb and little finger on her left hand. Cosack's (1953) patient had unilateral facial palsy and terminal transverse defect of both feet and of the left index finger. The patient reported by Wilson et al (1963) had terminal transverse defect of the right index and long fingers.

Rocher and Pesme (1945) described an infant with bilateral cleft lip, coloboma of the left iris, and complete absence of the left upper limb. Tower (1953) reported a 15-year-old girl with the following associated anomalies of the right side of the face and right upper extremity: coloboma of the nasal third of the lower lid, absence of the lower lacrimal junction and caruncle, unilateral harelip, partial coloboma of the choroid, and terminal transverse defect of the ring and little fingers.

OTODIGITAL COMPLEXES

Drummond (1939) described a 19-year-old deaf mute female with annular grooves around the three fingers of both hands. Nockemann (1961) reported a family in which four members in four generations presented the following constellation: congenital deafness; keratosis palmaris and plantaris, which became manifest around the age of two; thickening of the skin over the elbows and knees; and insidiously developing annular grooves around the central fingers and toes. Gibbs and Frank (1966) presented a 19-year-old girl who suffered from mild, bilateral, high-frequency hearing loss which was neural in character. Since the age of three months she showed marked thickening of the skin on the hands and feet, right elbow, and both knees; subsequently, an "ainhum-like constriction" had developed around all toes near the posterior nailfold. Her deceased father was reported to have had hearing loss and a similar cutaneous condition on the palms and soles. The trait consisting of congenital deafness, keratopachyderma, and annular grooves of the fingers and toes is an autosomal dominant.

TYLOSIS (Keratosis Palmo-Plantaris)

Wigley (1929) reported a case of "ainhum-like constriction" which occurred in connection with keratosis palmo-plantaris. The patient was a 10-year-old white girl. The thickening of her palms and soles had been noticed at the age of three months, but the constricting bands around her fingers first appeared when she was seven years old.

TREATMENT

The surgical effacement of an annular groove around the forearm or the finger resolves itself to the proper application of Z-plasty. In cases of precarious circulation of the peripheral parts, it may be judicious to close the gap in two sessions, repairing one-half of the circular groove at one time and the other at a later date. In many cases, the first web is narrow and the fingers are short and stubby and bent forward. Effacement of the annular grooves may have to be supplemented by widening the first web space, deepening the commissures between the rudimentary fingers, and correcting flexion contractures (Figs. 16–29 to 16–36).

The treatment of acral absences varies in accordance with the level of the defect. When the line of severance runs across the proximal ends of the metacarpals, the central carpal bones—the capitate, lunate, and trapezoid bones—are removed and a cleft is created between the remaining marginal sets. The insertions of extensor carpi radialis longus and extensor ulnaris are crossed over with the hope of procuring a side-to-side pinch.

In an occasional case, when only short stubs of proximal phalanges remain, the interdigital commissure is deepened. In this operation, the transverse metacarpal ligament is severed in each intermetacarpal space, and the interdigital commissure is recessed. In cases in which the tips of the remaining proximal phalanges are unpadded, the dorsal skin of each vestigial digit is turned toward the volar aspect and the denuded areas are surfaced with the aid of a pedicled graft; sufficient skin is piled up on the hand to be used for deepening the interdigital commissures and for covering the sides of the separated rudiments. Skin supplied by a pedicled graft is not used to cover the tips or the palmar surfaces of newly fashioned digits because this type of transposed integument is devoid of sensation.

When the middle and ungual phalanges are missing and only the proximal

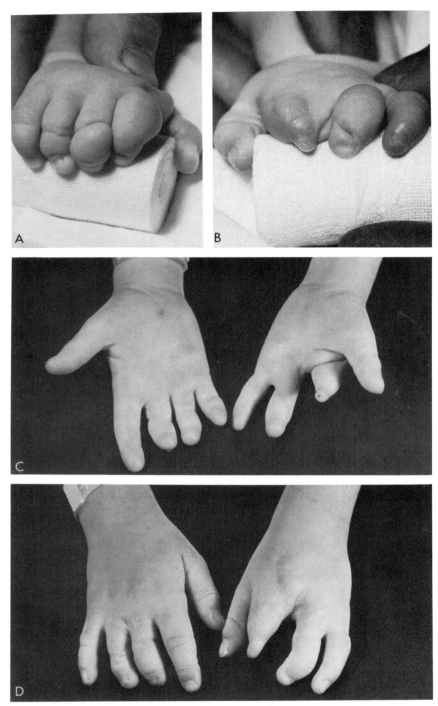

Figure 16–29   Annular grooves of the lesser digits of both hands associated with a missing digit in the left hand — treated by Z-plasty. *A* and *B*, Preoperative dorsal views of the right and left hands of a newborn male infant, showing tumefaction distal to the grooves which, in the left hand, was located at the bases of the three ulnar digits. *C*, Postoperative palmar view. *D*, Postoperative dorsal view.

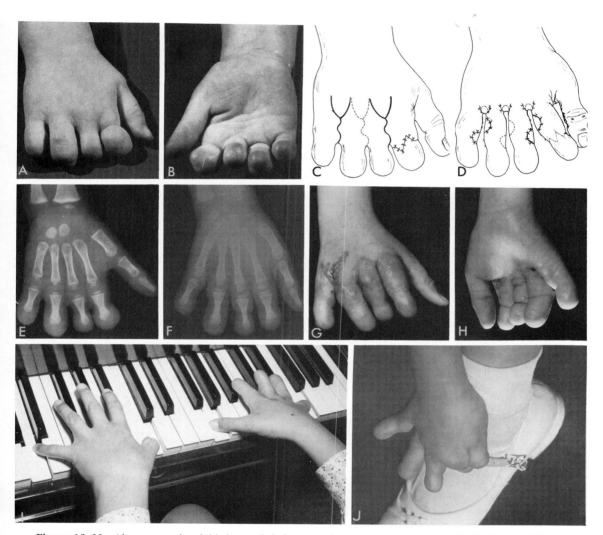

Figure 16–30 Absent second and third row of phalanges and annular grooves—treated by Z-plasty and deepening of the interdigital commissures. *A* and *B*, Preoperative dorsal and palmar views of the right hand of a 13-month-old female. *C* and *D*, Sketches illustrating the operative technique. *E*, Preoperative dorsopalmar roentgenograph. *F*, Postoperative roentgenograph. *G* and *H*, Postoperative dorsal and palmar views. *I*, Playing piano at the age of six years. *J*, Hooking a shoe strap.

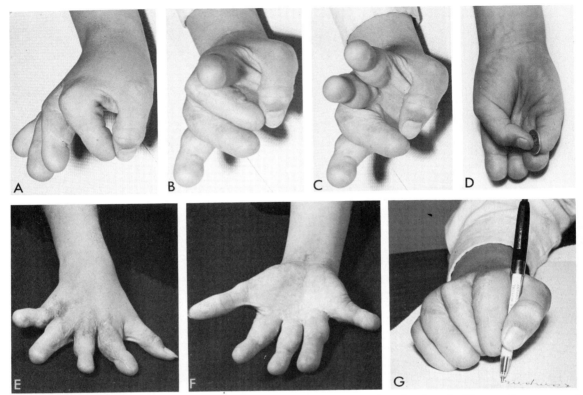

Figure 16-31   The right hand of the same girl shown in Figure 16–30: functional results 10 years after surgery. *A, B, C,* and *D,* Opposition with index, middle, ring, and little fingers. *E,* Abduction of the fingers. *F,* Adduction. *G,* Wielding a pen.

phalanx of the finger remains, an inch of the dorsal skin is turned volarward, and the denuded surface is covered with a distant pedicled flap. The latter is weaned six weeks later, and cylindrical pouches are fashioned at the end of each vestigial digit. Individual bone pegs are inserted into each pouch. Three bone pegs are obtained from the tibia; they undergo atrophy if they are not anchored firmly to the recipient bone and if the elongated digit is not activated soon after bony union.

In children, the author has often utilized the proximal phalanges of the lesser toes as free grafts. The donor toe is stabilized by surgical syndactyly with its neighbor. In his earlier attempts, the author reversed the direction of the transported toe phalanx and connected its distal nonepiphyseal end with the phalanx of the recipient digit. The transferred phalanx did not grow appreciably, and its epiphysis closed within a year. The author now inserts the phalangeal graft into the previously prepared pouch at the end of each short digit and transfixes it with a Kirschner wire. The author has not as yet attempted extensions of tendons to the grafted phalanx (Figs. 16–37 to 16–43).

A Krukenberg type of bifurcation operation has been tried for more proximal transverse defects. One questions the advisability of this operation in children. Prosthesis offers another alternative.

In the majority of cases, terminal transverse defect of the forearm and hand is unilateral, and it occurs more often on the left side. Aitken and Frantz (1955)

(*Text continued on page 537.*)

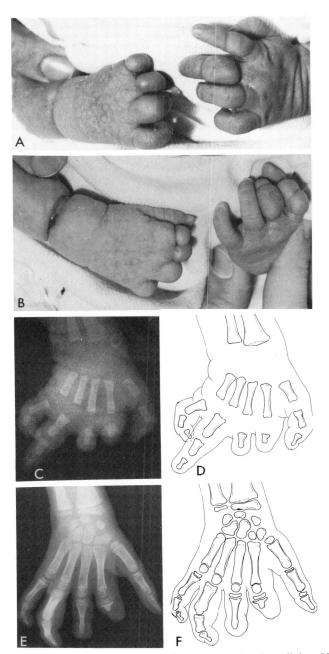

Figure 16–32 Annular grooves of the right forearm and the ulnar digits of both hands with agenesis of the intermediate and ungual phalanges of the right index and middle fingers. *A*, Dorsal view of the right forearm and both hands of a newborn female infant. *B*, The same, with the wrist flexed, showing a deep annular groove of the forearm. *C*, Dorsopalmar roentgenograph of the right hand. *D*, Sketch illustrating the same. *E*, Dorsopalmar roentgenograph of the right hand taken at the age of seven years, showing precocious closure of the phalangeal physis of the ring finger. *F*, Sketch illustrating the same.

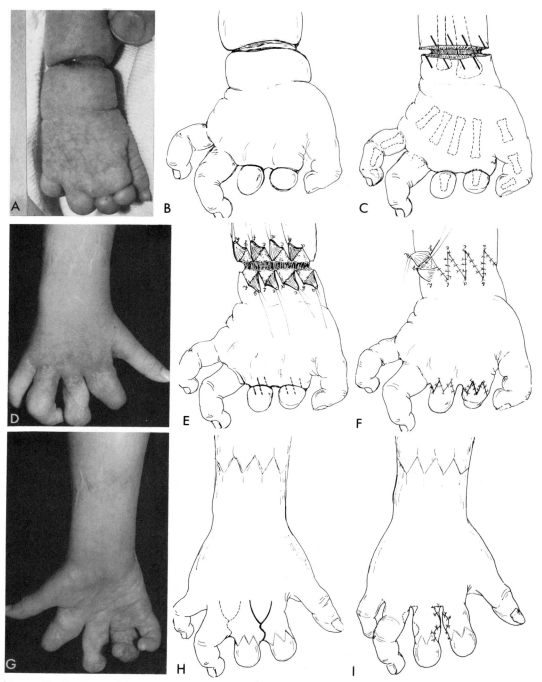

Figure 16–33   Some of the procedures utilized for the treatment of the right forearm and hand of the female child featured in Figure 16–32. *A*, Dorsal view of the distal forearm and the hand. *B*, Sketch illustrating the same. *C*, Sketch showing the initiation of Z-plasty for effacement of the annular groove of the forearm. *D*, Dorsal view after effacement of annular grooves of the forearm and of the vestigial index and middle fingers and deepening of the cleft between these two digits. *E* and *F* illustrate subsequent steps of Z-plasty. *G*, Postoperative palmar view of the hand. *H* and *I* illustrate the procedures utilized for deepening the interdigital clefts of the vestigial index and middle fingers.

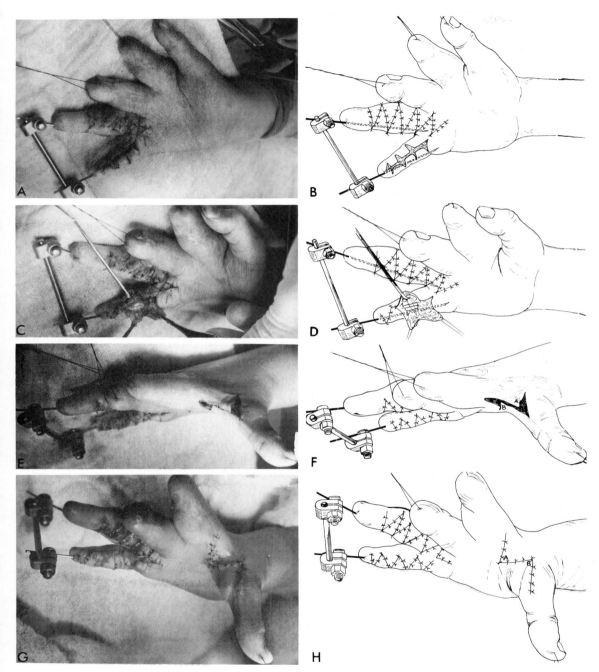

Figure 16–34 Additional surgery for the correction of the flexion contracture of the ring and middle fingers and adduction contracture of the thumb of the right hand of the female child shown in Figures 16–32 and 16–33. *A* and *B* show various stages of Z-plasty on the flexed ring and little fingers. *C* and *D* show the exposure for anterior capsulotomy of the first interphalangeal joint of the little finger. *E*, *F*, *G*, and *H* show the Z-plasty for widening the first webspace.

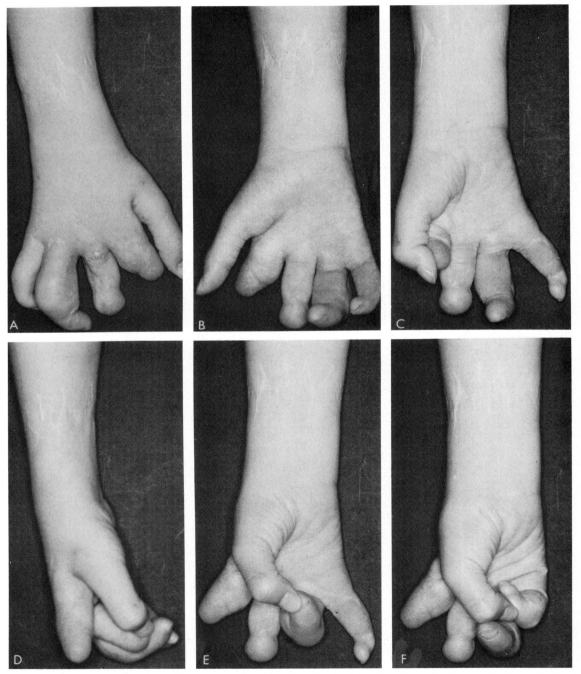

Figure 16–35   Results obtained after surgery on the right hand of the child shown in Figures 16–32 to 16–34. *A* and *B*, Postoperative dorsal and palmar views of the hand. *C*, *D*, *E*, and *F* show the functional results.

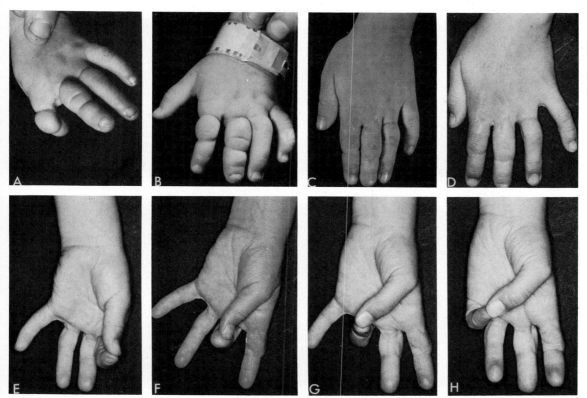

Figure 16–36 The left hand of the child featured in Figures 16–32 to 16–35 had no skeletal defects but only flexion contracture of the index finger and annular grooves around all four lesser digits which were remedied by Z-plasty. *A*, Preoperative dorsal view of the hand. *B*, Same, after correction of the flexion contracture of the index finger. *C*, After elimination of annular grooves around the index and middle fingers. *D*, After effacement of the groove at the base of the ring finger. *E*, *F*, *G*, and *H* show functional results six years after the initial surgery.

found this anomaly to be slightly more prevalent in females. There are two types of artificial hands: cosmetic and functional. The former is preferred by females. Since most individuals are right-handed, there would seem to be little need for functional prosthesis. In bilateral cases, functional prosthesis is indispensable. According to Aitkin and Frantz, most children prefer the split-hook type of terminal device on the prosthesis. They recommended that these juvenile amputees be fitted with a prosthesis at four years of age, at which time "the self-help patterns requiring two-handed skills are developing. A child fitted and trained at four years will have one year of wearing before he begins formal schooling of kindergarten," Aitken and Frantz wrote.

A number of myoelectric upper-extremity prostheses have been devised in recent years. These provide adequate cosmetic disguise and procure the function of fingertip prehension. Their effectiveness depends upon the number and the contractility of controlling muscles. "Using muscle action potentials for control of signals provides an excellent means of establishing communication between man and machine," Gingras (1966) wrote. He expressed the hope that future designs would provide the means of controlling motor-function prostheses either with electric power or in combination with other forms of external energy.

(*Text continued on page 546.*)

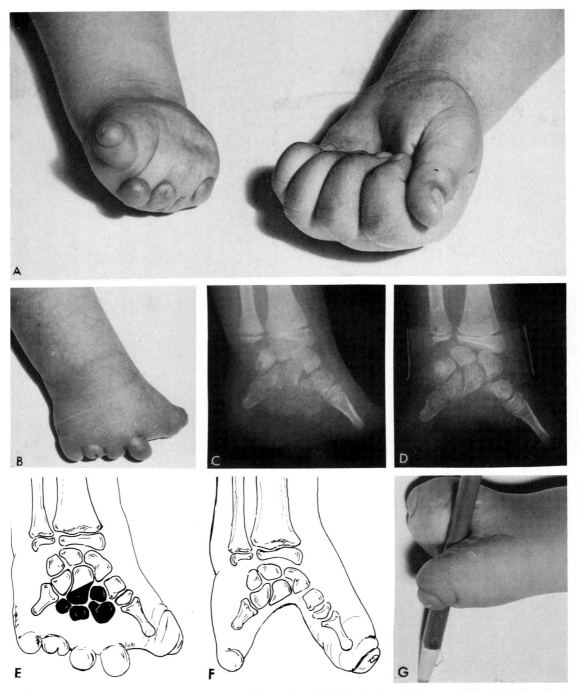

Figure 16–37　Acheiria treated by clefting. *A*, Palmar view of the hands of an eight-year-old female. *B*, Dorsal view of the right hand. *C*, Preoperative roentgenograph of the same. *D*, Postoperative roentgenograph. *E* and *F* illustrate *C* and *D*, respectively. *G*, Functional result.

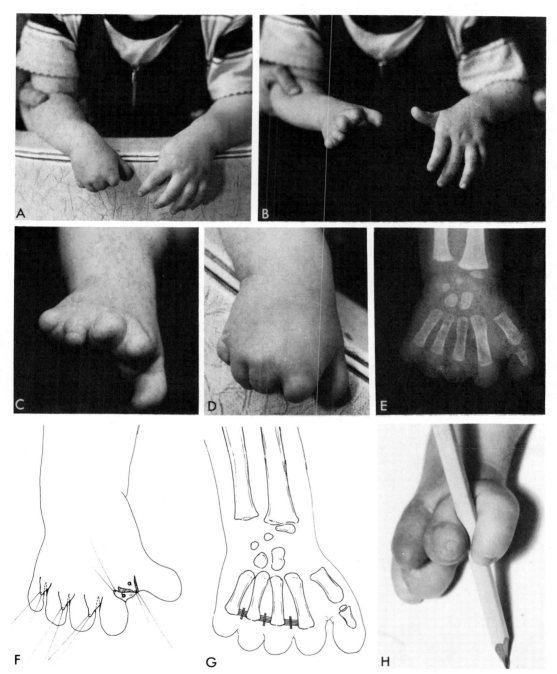

Figure 16–38 Rudimentary digits—treated by Z-plasty of the first webspace and deepening of the other three commissures by severing the intermetacarpal segments of the deep transverse ligament and covering the raw surfaces with dorsal flaps. *A* and *B*, Sundry views of both hands. *C*, Frontal view of the right hand. *D*, Dorsal view. *E*, Dorsopalmar roentgenograph. *F*, Sketch showing the Z-plasty of the first web and elevation of the dorsal triangular flaps between the heads of the second to fifth metacarpals. *G*, Sketch showing the severance of the deep transverse metacarpal ligament between the distal ends of the deep transverse ligament. *H*, Final result.

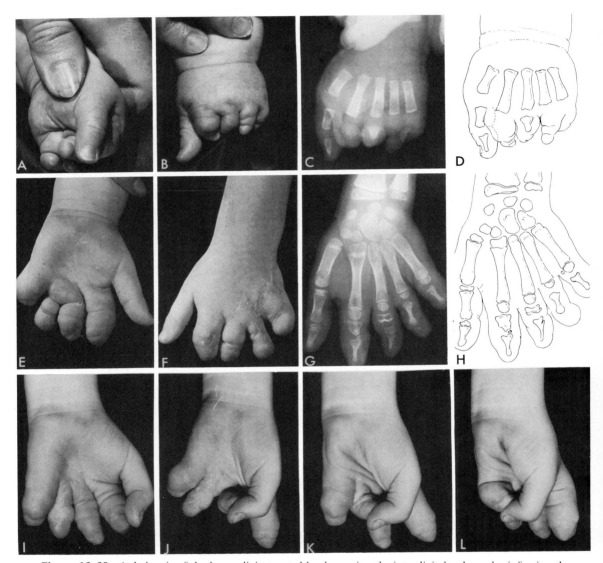

Figure 16–39 Aphalangia of the lesser digits treated by deepening the interdigital webs and reinforcing the vestigial fleshy masses with autogenous bone grafts consisting of middle phalanges of the toes. *A* and *B*, Palmar and dorsal views of the left hand of a newborn male infant. *C*, Dorsopalmar roentgenograph of the hand. *D*, Sketch illustrating the same. *E* and *F*, Palmar and dorsal views of the hand three years after recessing the interdigital webs. *G*, Roentgenograph after transplantation of pedal phalanges; these bones were transposed with their epiphyses but the growth line of each became effaced within nine months after the transposition operation, which was performed between the ages of five and eight. *H*, Sketch illustrating postoperative roentgenograph. *I*, *J*, *K*, and *L*, Postoperative results.

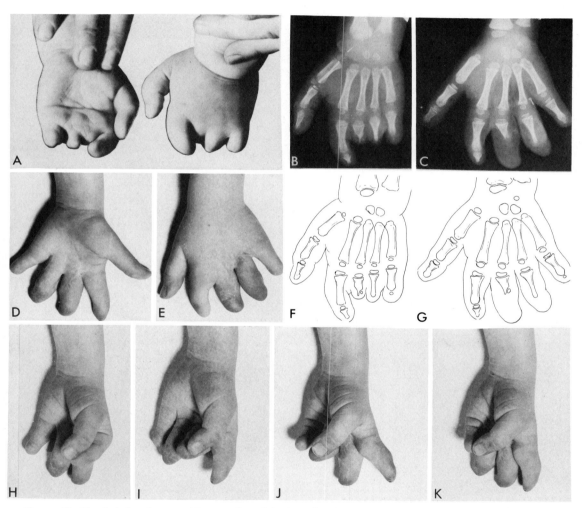

Figure 16–40 Aphalangia treated by recession of the interdigital webs. *A,* Preoperative palmar and dorsal views of the left hand of a 12-month-old female. *B,* Dorsopalmar roentgenograph of the same. *C,* Dorsopalmar roentgenograph a year after deepening the interdigital clefts. *D* and *E,* Postoperative palmar and dorsal views of the hand. *F* and *G* illustrate the roentgenograph above each. *H, I, J,* and *K,* Functional results at four years of age.

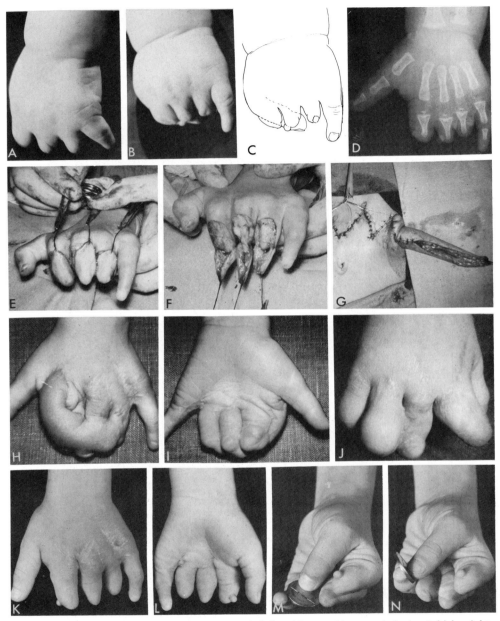

Figure 16–41 Stubby uniphalangeal central digits with taut skin over their tips (which might impede the forward growth of the remaining phalanges)—treated by turning three dorsal flaps forward and covering the denuded surfaces with a distant flap; the interdigital clefts were also deepened. *A*, Dorsal view of the left hand of a seven-month-old male infant. *B*, The thumb fails to reach the tip of the fourth digital bud. *C*, Sketch illustrating the same. *D*, Dorsopalmar roentgenograph. *E*, Incisions for elevation of dorsal digital flaps. *F*, Flaps have been turned down and forward and the tips of the proximal phalanges have been freed. *G*, Petal flap which was sutured to the deepened first web and made to cover the raw areas shown in the preceding photograph. *H*, The flap was weaned from the donor site six weeks after it was sutured to the hand. *I*, Palmar view of the hand at this stage. *J*, The index finger was separated from the third finger, and the little finger was isolated from the fourth digit. *K*, The middle finger was later separated from the fourth digit. *L*, Palmar view of the same. *M* and *N*, Functional results.

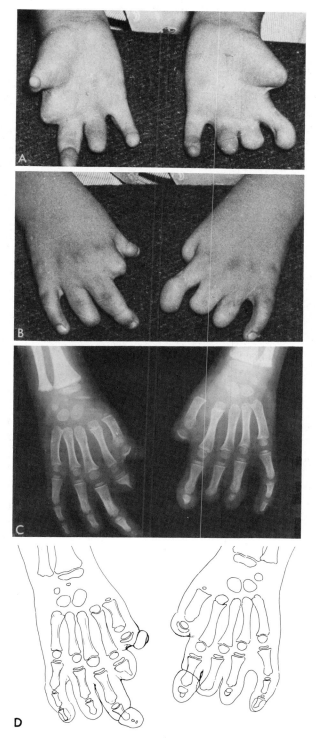

Figure 16–42 Bilateral acral defect involving most severely the thumb and the index finger. *A*, Palmar view of the hands. *B*, Dorsal view. *C*, Dorsopalmar roentgenograph of the hands. *D*, Sketch illustrating the same.

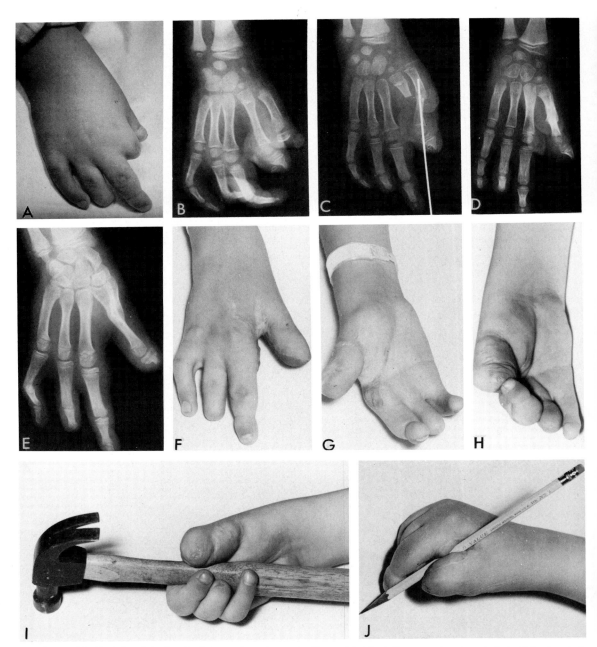

Figure 16–43   The right hand of the patient shown in Figure 16–42. *A,* Preoperative dorsal view of the hand. *B,* Preoperative dorsopalmar roentgenograph. *C,* Roentgenograph showing that the second metacarpal has been grafted onto the first and transfixed with a K-wire. *D,* Roentgenograph after solid osteosynthesis. *E,* Roentgenograph after removal of the remnants of the second metacarpal, widening of the webspace between the thumb and the middle finger, and abduction rotation osteotomy of the first metacarpal. *F, G, H, I,* and *J,* show the functional and cosmetic results.

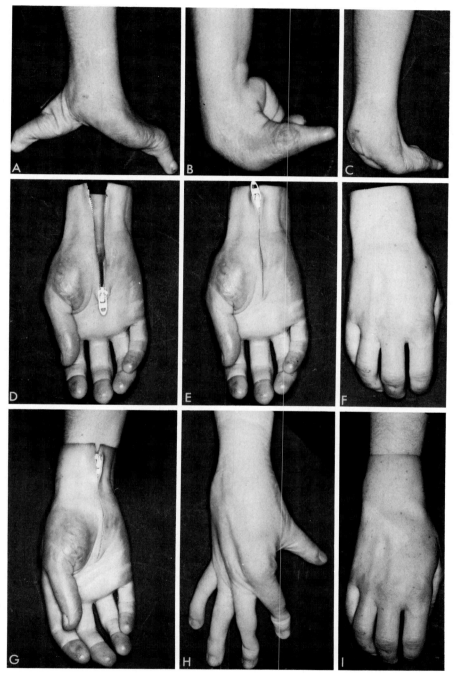

Figure 16–44 Cosmetic glove. *A*, Dorsal view of the right hand of a 16-year-old female who was born with absent central digits and vestigial marginal members. At four years of age the central metacarpals and corresponding carpal bones were removed, and the extensor carpi tendons were crossed and anchored to the bases of the marginal metacarpals. *B*, Radial view showing the range of flexion and fairly effective pinch. *C*, Ulnar view showing the range of extension. *D* and *E*, Palmar views of the unzipped and zipped glove. *F*, Dorsal view of the same. *G*, *H*, and *I*, Sundry views of the gloved hand.

SUMMARY

Annular grooves and acral absences of the limb may be regarded as intercalary and terminal variants, respectively, of transverse defect. In the former, soft tissues are involved; in the latter, both soft tissue and skeletal elements are affected. It is now generally conceded that enodgenous influences (focal necrosis) and exogenous factors (amniotic adhesions or apertures) may be responsible for either defect. In hereditary cases, which are comparatively uncommon, one must suspect a genetic influence. Genetic factors are also responsible for syndromic deficiencies. By far, the majority of isolated cases of annular groove and acral absences have been sporadic or without hereditary antecedent. In the very few familial cases reported, the transmission seems to follow a recessive pattern. Annular grooves are effected by Z-plasty. The treatment of acral absences varies according to the level of the defect. Females with acheiria prefer a cosmetic prosthesis. Males seem satisfied with a prosthesis that has a split-hook type of end device. Myoelectric upper-extremity prostheses provide adequate cosmetic disguise and enable the patient to effect a measure of finger-tip prehension. They do not procure sufficient motor power for grasp or grip. It is hoped that a future design will augment the power of the myoelectric prosthesis by supplying it with some form of external energy.

References

Abbe, T.: So-called congenital amputation. *Am. J. Obstet., 73*:118–119, 1916. See also Report of a case of congenital amputation of fingers. *Am. J. Obstet. Dis. Women Children, 73*:1089–1092, 1916.

Adams, F. H., and Oliver, C. P.: Hereditary deformities in man due to arrested development. *J. Hered., 36*:3–7, 1945.

Aitken, G. T., and Frantz, C. H.: Congenital amputation of the forearm. *Ann. Surg., 141*:519–522, 1955.

Ajinka, Y. N.: Intra-uterine amputations and annular constrictions in a living infant, now a child of 4, due to amniotic adhesions resulting from oligohydramnios. *J. Obstet. Gynecol. Br. Emp., 45*:692–695, 1938.

Anderson, J. J.: Notes of a case of intra-uterine amputation. *Br. Med. J., 2*:78, 1881.

Aubertin, Tessier, and Boulat: Gangrène symétrique des doigts (M.S.) chez un nouveau-né de vingt-six jours. *J. Med. Bordeaux, 25*:496–497, 1945.

Audebert: Sillons congéniteaux et amputations congénitales. *Echo Med. Toulouse*, (2 s.), *14*:235–237, 1900.

Ayer, J.: Intra-uterine amputation. *Boston Med. Surg. J., 101*:905–906, 1879.

Bailey, H.: Report of a case of hemimelus or so-called congenital amputation. *Am. J. Obstet. Gynecol., 3*:72–76, 98–99, 1922.

Baker, C. J., and Rudolph, A. J.: Congenital ring constrictions and intra-uterine amputations. *Am. J. Dis. Child., 121*:393–400, 1971.

Bar, P.: Enfant né d'une mère syphilitique et presentant a l'avantbras un malformation qui semble être une amputation congénitale. *Ann. Dermat. et Syph.*, (3 s.), *9*:357–358, 1898.

Barenberg, L., and Greenberg, B.: Intra-uterine amputations and constriction bands. Report of a case with anaesthesis below constriction. *Am. J. Dis. Child., 64*:87–92, 1942.

Barwell, R.: Two cases of truncated arms bearing at the ends of foetal hands voluntarily mobile. *Trans. Pathol. Soc. London, 32*:280–281, 1881.

Bassetta, A.: Amputation congénitale, sillon congéniteaux et pieds bots. *Rev. d'Orthop.*, (2 s.), *9*:45–68, 1908.

Battle, I. P.: Amputation of the human forearm in utero (letter to the editor). *Med. Rec., 73*:360, 1908.

Baylac, J.: Amputation congénital de la main. *Toulouse Méd., 2*:303, 1900.

Beatty: Foetus with left arm partly amputated by the funis coiled around it. *Dublin Quart. J. Med. Sci., 2*:533, 1846.

Beauregard, G.: *Des Difformities des Doigts (Dactylolyses)*. Paris, J. B. Bailiere et Fils., pp. 1–111; pl. I–IV, 1875.

Bennett, E. H.: A comparison of the pathological changes in intra-uterine amputations with those produced by ordinary amputation. *Trans. Roy. Acad. Med.* (Ireland), *1*:363, 1888.

Bertwistle, A. P.: Intra-uterine amputation. *Lancet, 2*:1120–1121, 1939.

Bilhaut, M.: Malformations multiples chez un nouveau-né; double pied bot varus equin: amputation congénitale de petit doigt (main gauche); sillons à la première phalanx de l'index, du medius et de l'annulaire de la même main. *Ann. d'Orthop. Chir. Pract.* (Paris), *8*:289–296, 1895.

Blackfield, H. M., and Hause, D. E.: Congenital constricting bands of the extremities. *Plast. Reconstr. Surg., 8*:101–109, 1951.

Blancard, C.: *Sur le Role de l'Amnios Dans les Malformations Congénitales.* Thèse. Paris, Impremerie F. Deveron, pp. 7–62, 1902.

Bluefarb, S. M.: Constriction of finger simulating ainhum: Report of a congenital case. *Arch. Dermatol. Syph., 57*:741–743, 1948.

Bohomoletz, M.: Further light on the handless and footless family in Brazil. *Eugenical News, 10*:1943–1945, 1930.

Bom, G. S.: Operative treatment of congenital amniotic anomalies. (Russian). *Ortop. Travmat.*, (Kharkoff), *8*:41–42, 1934.

Boncour, P.: Arrêts de développement: amputations congénitales. *Bull. Soc. Anat. Paris, 2*:613–615, 1877.

Borchman, H.: Der angeborene Handdefekt. *Fortschr. Röntgenstr.*, 5:149–160; Taf. X, 1917.

Bottomley, A. H.: Myoelectric control of powered prostheses. *J. Bone Joint Surg., 47B*:411–415, 1965.

Braun, G.: Ueber spontane Amputationen des Foetus und ihre Beziehungen zu den amniotischen Bändern. *Z. Ges. Aerzte Wien, 10*(2):192, 1854.

Braun, G.: Neuer Beitrag zur Lehre von den amniotischen Bandern und deren Einfluss auf die fotale Entwickelung. *Med. Jb., 4*:3–15, 1862.

Braun, G.: Die strangförmige Aufwickelung des Amnion um den Nabelstrang des reifen Kindes—eine seltene Ursache des intrauterinen Foetaltodes. *Oest. Z. Prakt. Heilk., 11*:181–183, 1865.

Bremmenkamp, H.: *Ueber einen Fall von amniotischen Schlingen an den Extremitaten beim Foetus.* Thesis. Marburg, Univ. Buchdruckerei, pp. 1–20, 1889.

Brindeau, A., Lantuejoul, P., and Chappaz, G.: Des malformations d'origine amniotique: (Arrêts de developpement ou maladies de la membrane amniotique). *Sem. Hop. Paris, 28*:2769–2775, 1952.

Broca, A.: Bride amniotique et amputations congénitales. *Bull. Soc. Anat.* (Paris), *65*:476–484, 1890.

Brown, B. Jr.: Case of a child with amputated upper and lower extremities. *Trans. Obstet. Soc.* (London), *8*:102, 1886.

Browne, D.: The pathology of congenital ring constrictions. *Arch. Dis. Child., 32*:517–519, 1957.

Buchanan, A. H.: A case illustrative of etiology of spontaneous amputation of the limbs of the foetus in utero. *Trans. Tennessee Med. Soc., 10*:41, 1839.

Buhrer, C. E.: *Ueber einen Fall von amniotischer Amputation.* Thesis. Berlin, H. Blanke Buchdruckerei, pp. 1–29, 1914.

Caesar, R. T.: Case of amelus or limbless monster. *Br. Med. J., 1*:525, 1889.

Calderini, G.: Adattilia congenita unilaterale dell' arto superiore. *Ann. Ostet.* (Milano), *45*:341–372, 1923.

Caratozzolo, A.: Un caso raro di emimelia. *Arch. Ortop., 52*:435–439, 1936.

Chaves, D. A.: Molesta amniotica. *Rev. Med. Cir. Brasil, 47*:183–199, 1939.

Chiari, H.: The relation of amnion to the origin of human malformations. *Bull. Johns Hopkins Hosp., 32*:35–39, pl. iii, IV, 1911.

Chiariello, A.: Contribution a l'ètude de l'hémimélie. Absence de la main. *Rev. d'Orthop., 15*:242–251, 1928.

Clap, L.: Ectrodactylie totale de la main droite. *Bull. Mém. Soc. Anat., 16–17;* 50–54, 1920.

Cleisz, L., and Bret, J.: Les gangrènes seches du nouveau-né; a propos d'un cas d'amputation spontanée des deux membres inferieurs dans les suites immédiates de naissance et de deux cas de plaises du cuir chevelu en cours de cicatrisation observées a la naissance. *Gynecol. Obstet., 47*:204, 1948.

Cholmogoroff, S.: Ein Fall von Amelus. *Zentralbl. Gynäkol., 12*:819–824, 1888.

C. O. H.: Two examples of intra-uterine amputations. *Polyclinic* (London), *6*:154–158, 1902. See also: An example of intra-uterine amputation. *Polyclinic* (London), *6*:516, 1902.

Coles, W.: An obstetrical case: intra-uterine amputations. *St. Louis Med. Surg. J., 39*:316–322, 1880.

Coll de Carrera, and Battle: Amputations congénitales et sillons par brides amniotique. *Bull. Soc. Obstet. Gynec., 23*:308–309, 1934.

Collins, R. J., and Nichols, D. H.: Congenital fetal anomalies: intra-uterine amputation and annular constriction bands. *N. Y. State J. Med., 50*:1403–1405, 1950.

Coote: Congenital absence of the greater part of the left arm in a girl, the middle humerus forming a conical stump. *Lancet, 2*:509, 1863.

Cormack, J. R.: Remarks on what is usually called the spontaneous amputation of limbs of the foetus in utero. *London Med. Gaz., 1*:410–411, 1838.

Cosack, G.: Die angeborene Zungen-Munddach-Verwachsung als Leitmotiv eines Komplexes von multiplen Abartungen. (Zur Genese des Ankyloglossum superius). *Z. Kinderheilkd. 72*:240–257, 1953.

Coupland, S., and Balding, M.: Congenital malformations of hands and feet. *Trans. Pathol. Soc. London, 32*:190–192, 1881.

Courtois, J., Lelièvre, and Brière: Une variété rare de malformation congenitale chez un foetus à terme. *Gynec. Obstet., 45*:122, 1946.

Cummins, H.: Spontaneous amputation of human supernumerary digits: pedunculated postminimi. *Am. J. Anat., 51*:381–416, 1932.

Dareste, M. C.: Sur le rôle de l'amnios dans la production des anomalies. *C. R. Acad. Sci., 94*:173–175, 1882.

Da Silva Lima, J. F.: Estudo Sobre o—"Ainhum"—molestia ainda nao descripta, peculiar a raca Ethiopica, e affectando dedos minimos dos pes. *Gaz. Med. Bahia, 1*:146–151, 1867.

Delmanto, A.: Un caso de enctromelia con auscencia completa de todos os membros. *Pub. Med., 25*:63–65, 1955.

Dock, G.: Intra-uterine amputations. *Trans. Assoc. Am. Physicians, 29*:528–534, 1914.

Dresher, C. S., and MacDonnell, J. A.: Total amelia. *J. Bone Joint Surg., 47A*:511–516, 1965.

Drummond, M.: A case of unusual skin disease. *Ir. J. Med. Sci.,* (6 s.), No *157*:85, 1939.

Engen, T. J.: Restoration of function in upper extremities by external power. *Phys. Med. Rehab., 47*:182–189, 1966.

Engen, T. J., and Ottinat, L. F.: Upper extremity orthotics: a project reported. *Orthotics and Prosthetics, 21*:112–127, 1967.

Eustache, G.: Des amputations congénitales. *J. Sci. Med. Lille, 1*:481–492, 1895.

Farmer, A. W.: Congenital elephantiasis associated with constriction by anomalous bands. *J. Bone Joint Surg., 30B*:606–612, 1948.

Frantz, C. H., and Aitken, G. T.: Management of the juvenile amputee. *Clin. Orthop., 14*:30–49, 1959.

Frasson, U.: Un caso di amelia in feto vivo e vitale. *Ginecologia, 13*:88–95, 1947.

Freire-Maia, N., and Freire-Maia, A.: Congenital malformations of the extremities. *Lancet, 2*:1363–1364, 1961.

Freire-Maia, N., Quelce-Salgado, A., and Kohler, R. A.: Hereditary bone aplasias and hypoplasias of the upper extremities. *Acta Genet. Statis. Mod., 9*:33–40, 1959.

Frenkel, H.: Amputation congénitale de la main. *Echo Med. Toulouse,* (2 s.), *15*:61–63, 1901.

Froelich, R.: Hypertrophie ou éléphantiasis congénitale due a des brides amniotiques. Syndactylie et ectrodactylie de même origine. *Rev. d'Orthop.,* (2 s.), *1*:77–85, 1900.

Fussell, M. H.: Intra-uterine amputation. *J.A.M.A., 29*:25–26, 1897.

Garcia Otero, R. G.: Un caso de "amelio." *Rev. Clin. Esp., 12*:117–124, 1944.

Garcin, R., Thurel, R., and Rudaux, P.: Sur un cas isolé de dysostose cranio-faciale (Maladie de Crouzone), avec ectrodactylie. *Arch. Méd. Enfants, 36*:359–365, 1933.

Gasne, G.: Un cas d'hémimélie chez un fils de syphilitique. *N. Iconog. Salp., 10*:31–35, 1897.

Gatty, W. H.: Some remarks on the causes of amputations of foetal limbs occurring within the uterus. *London Med. Gaz.,* (n.s.), *12*:627–633, 1851.

Gibbs, R. C., and Frank, S. B.: Keratoma hereditaria mutilans (Vohwinkel). *Arch. Dermatol., 94*:619–625, 1966.

Gingras, G.: Canadian experience with the Soviet myoelectric upper-extremity prosthesis. *J. Orthop. Prosthetic Appliances, 20*:294–304, 1966.

Giraudeau, C.: Malformation congénitale d'un membre superieur. Absence du metacarpe et des phalanges. *Bull. Soc. Anat., 6*:271, 1881.

Glessner, J. R., Jr.: Spontaneous intra-uterine amputation. *J. Bone Joint Surg., 45A*:351–355, 1963.

Goetzen, C.v.: Amniogene Gliedmassenmissbildung: Amputation der rechten oberen Hemmung an der übrigen Extremität. *Zentralbl. Gynäkol., 44*:225–230, 1920.

Goldstein, D., and Kiptenko, N. D.: Ueber amniogene Missbildungen der Extremitäten. *Arch. Orthop. Unfallchir., 32*:225–244, 1932.

Gorlin, R. J., and Pindberg, J. J.: *Syndromes of the Head and Neck.* New York, Blakiston Division, McGraw-Hill Book Co., pp. 37–40, 1964.

Gourdon, J.: Trois cas d'absence congénital de la main. *Gaz. Hebd. Sci. Med. Bordeaux, 45*:790, 1924.

Gourdon, J.: Ectromélie thoracic bilateral héréditaire. *J. Méd. Bordeaux, 109*:20–22, 1932.

Grassi, R.: Di un caso amelia completa. *Ann. Ostet. Ginecol., 31*:553–560, 1909.

Gravely, H.: Case of amelus or limbless monster. *Br. Med. J., 1*:1280, 1889.

Grisel, P.: Amputations congénitales et sillons congéniteaux. *Rev. d'Orthop.,* (2 s.), *4*:72–91; 139–163, 1903.

Gruber, G. B.: Angeborene Amputation, amniotische Amschnürung, hypoplastische Gliedmassen-Stummel, Peromelie. *Münch. Med. Wochenschr., 83*:259, 1936.

Gruber, G. B.: Hypoplasie, Mikromelie, Phokomelie, Amelie, Peromelie (einschl. der sog. "Spontanamputationen"). *In* Schwalbe, E., and Gruber, G. B., (eds.): *Die Morphologie der Missbildungen des Menschen und der Tiere.* Jena, G. Fischer, 3 T, 17 Lief. 1 Abt., 7 Kap, 1 Halfte: 300–328, 1937.

Gruber, G. B.: Ueber Wesen und Abgrenzung amniogener Missbildungen. *Arch. Dtsch. Pathol. Ges., 1938. 31*:228, 1939.

Gruber, W.: Ueber Missbildungen der Finger an beiden Händen eines Lebenden. *Arch. Pathol. Anat. Physiol., 47*:303–307; T. VIII (fig. 1), 1869.

Günther: Beschreibung einer Missgeburt. Amputatio Spontanea. *Dtsch. Klin., 6*:412–414, 1854.

Günther, R.: Zur Frage der angeborenen Amputationen. *Z. menschl. Vererb. Konstitutionslehre, 23*:736–758, 1939.

Gupta, M. L.: Congenital annular defects of the extremities and the trunk. *J. Bone Joint Surg., 45A*:571–575, 1963.

Haase, F.: Beitrage zur Kenntnis der Entstehungsursachen amniotischer Stränge. *Monatsschr. Geburtsh. Gynaekol., 32*:21–23, 1910.

Haberland, H. F. O.: Angeborene Amputation. *Münch. Med. Wochenschr., 83*(1):55, 1936.

Hanhart, E.: Uber die Kombination von Peromelie mit Mikrognathie, ein neues Syndrom beim Menschen, entsprechend der Akroteriasis congenita von Wriedt und Mohr beim Rinde. *Arch. Klaus-Stift, 25*:531–540, 1950.

Hardy, S. L.: Spontaneous amputation of the forearm in utero. *Dublin Hosp. Gaz., 7*:131–133, 1860.

Harris, H. E.: Intra-uterine amputation of three extremities; webbed fingers on the hand of the only limb. *Br. J. Child. Dis., 1*:502, 1904.

Hastings, C.: Description of a monster, in which the upper and inferior extremities were entirely wanting. *Med. Chir. Soc. Edinburgh, 2*:39–41, 1826.

Hedenstedt, S.: Zwei Fälle von totaler Amelie. *Acta Obstet. Gynecol. Scand., 24*:271–277, 1944.

Heidler, H.: Ein Fall von Missbildung mit amniotischen Strängen. *Zentralbl. Gynakol., 9*:363–364, 1922.

Hellner, H.: Untersuchungen über die amniogene Entstehung der Gliedmassenmissbildungen. *Arch. Klin. Chir., 172*:133–225, 1933.

Herrinalon, C.: A case of adactylism. *St. Bartholomew Hosp., 30*:192, 1922–1923.

Hiller, B.: Congenital constriction of limbs. *Med. J. Australia, 1*:283, 1927.

Hovorka, O.v.: Ueber Spontanamputationen. *Z. Orthop. Chir., 15*:40–59, 1906.

Hutchinson: A child born without extremities, and on whom intra-uterine amputation of all the limbs had probably been performed. *Trans. Path. Soc. London, 5*:343, 1853–1854.

Hutchinson, J.: Portrait of a case of congenital absence of both upper extremities. *Trans. Path. Soc. London, 17*:435–436, 1866.

Hutchinson, J.: Intra-uterine amputation of the digits on one hand. *Arch. Surg., 8*:359–360, 1897.

Hutchinson, J.: Intra-uterine amputation of the digits of the left hand in three members of the same family. *Arch. Surg., 8*:360–361, 1897.

Ilberg, G.: Fötus ohne Arme und Beine (Amelos). Zusammenstellung von Beobachtungen über Amelie. *Z. Geburtsh. Gynakol. 114*:174–184, 1937.

Illemann-Larsen, G.: Et Tilfaelde af Komplet Ameli. *Ugeskr. Laeger, 116*:928, 1954.

Inglis, K.: The nature of agenesis and deficiency of parts. *Am. J. Pathol.*, 28:449–475, 1952.

Isidor: Note sur un cas d'amputation congénitale de l'avant-bras droit avec ectrodactylie de la main gauche. *Rev. d'Orthop.*, (1 s.), 4:205–208, 1893.

Jansen, M.: The amnion considered as an etiologic factor in congenital deformities. *Proc. Staff Meet. Mayo Clin.*, 9:345–348, 1934.

Jeannel, J.: Contribution à l'étude des sillons congénitaux et des amputations spontanées. *Gaz. Hebd. Méd. Chir.*, 23:569–571; 587–590, 1886.

Johnson, H. M.: Congenital cicatrizing bands: report of a case with etiologic observations. *Am. J. Surg.*, (n.s.), 52:498–501, 1941.

Jumon, H.: Un cas d'ectrodactylie. *Rev. d'Orthop.*, (3 s.), 2:279–282, 1911.

Kahn, E. A., and Olmedo, L.: Congenital defect of the scalp, with a note on the closure of large scalp defects in general. *Plast. Reconstr. Surg.*, 6:435–440, 1950.

Kanski-Bacos: Ein Fall von Amelie. *Münch. Med. Wochenschr.*, 50(2):1641, 1903.

Kettner: Kongenitaler Zungendefekt. *Dtsch. Med. Wochenschr.*, 33:532, 1907.

Kiewe, L.: Zur Frage der Ätiologie der Sogenannten "Spontanamputationen." *Z. Orthop. Chir.*, 58:20–42, 1933.

Killingsworth, P. W., and Engledow, R.: Congenital absence of the four extremities. Am. J. Dis. Child., 63:914–918, 1942.

King, C.: A case of congenital deficiency of the fingers. *Internat. Med. Mag.*, 5:91–92, 1897.

Kirmisson, E.: Amputation congénitale de la jambe gauche; sillon profound de la jambe droite, syndactylie de la main gauche malformations des orteils. *Rev. d'Orthop.*, (2 s.), 1:67–70; pl V, 1900.

Klippel, M., and Bouchet, P.: Hémimélie avec atrophie numeriques des tissues. *N. Iconog. Salp.*, 20:290–333; 396–417, 1907.

Klippel, M., and Feil, A.: Étude clinique et pathogénique de l'hémimélia: a propos d'un nouveau cas. *Paris Medicale*, 49:207–213, 1923.

Klippel, M., and Rabaud, E.: Étude sur les malformations congénitales des membres. *N. Iconog. Salp.*, 27:333–359, 1914–1915.

Knowles, J. B., Stevens, B. L., and Howe, L.: Myo-electric control of hand prostheses. *J. Bone Joint Surg.*, 47B:416–417, 1965.

Knox, D. N.: Intra-uterine amputation of fingers and toes. *Glasgow Med. J.*, (n.s.), 10:572, 1878. See also *11*:20–24, 1879.

Koehler, G.: Die hand- und fusslosen brasilianischen Geschwister. Ein Beitrag zur Frage der Erbbedingtheir angeborener Missbildungen. *Z. menschl. Vererb. Konstitutionslehre*, 19:670–690, 1936.

Köhler, H. G.: Congenital transverse defects of limbs and digits ("intra-uterine amputation") *Arch. Dis. Child.*, 37:263–276, 1962.

Köhler, H. G.: Die intra-uterine Amputation. Eine medizin-historische und biographische Betrachtung. Part I, *Med. Mschr.*, 17:696, 1963; Part II, *Med. Mschr.*, 18:18–21, 1964.

Krückmeyer, K.: Ueber Anomalien des Extremitätenskelettes (ein Beitrag zur Kenntnis der Amelie). *Zentralbl. Alg. Pathol.*, 93:262–266, 1955.

Lamb, D. S., MacNaughten, A. K. M., and Fragiakis, E. G.: Congenital absence of the upper limb and hand. A review of benefits and bimanual function by early prosthetic replacement. *The Hand*, 3:193–199, 1971.

Lange, M.: Abschnürungsdefekte an den Gliedmassen (Spontanamputationen) Erbbiologie der angeborenen Körperfehler. Stuttgart, F. Enke. *Z. Orthop. Chir.*, 63:89–99, 1935.

Lannelongue: Anomalie de trois membres par défaut: amputation congénitale des anteurs. *Arch. Méd. Gen.*, (7 s.), 9:157–168, 1882.

Lanzi, F.: Considerazione patogenetiche sulle malformazione congenite a tipo cicatriziale. *Arch. Ortop.*, 78:431–446, 1965.

Latta, J. S.: Spontaneous intra-uterine amputations. *Am. J. Obstet. Gynecol.*, 10:640–648, 1925.

Laurence, H. M.: Intra-uterine amputations. *Clin. Sketches* (London), 1:19–20, 1895.

Laurence, R. F., and Sherman, D.: A case of intra-uterine amputation due to external trauma. *Br. Med. J.*, 2:425, 1948.

Lebec, M.: Arrêt de developpement des doigts de deux mains. Pieds bots varus. Sillons cutanés. *Bull. Soc. Anat. Paris*, (3 s.), 2:21–22, 1877.

Leboucq, H.: Description anatomique d'un monstrosité de la main. *Ann. Soc. Méd. Gand.*, 57:49–61, 1879.

Legendre, E. Q.: Cas d'amputation spontanée des doigt et section incomplète d'un bras; mechanism de cet lésion observé sur un foetus de 7 mois. *C. R. Soc. Biol.* (Paris), 19:70–71, 1858.

Leigh, T.: Congenital deformity in a girl four years of age. *Illust. Med. News*, 5:40–41, 1889.

Lennon, G. G.: Some aspects of foetal pathology (with special reference to the role of amniotic bands). *J. Obstet. Gynaecol. Br. Emp.*, 54:830–837, 1947.

Leopold: Angeborene spontane Amputation des rechten Vorderarmes. *Arch. Gynaekol.*, 9:323–325, 1879.

Levasseur, C.: *Des Amputations Congenitales et des Sillons Congénitaux*. Thèse. Paris, H. Jouve, pp. 1–80, 1903.

Levy, F.: Fötale Amputation der linken Hand. *Dtsch. Med. Wochenschr.* 34:169, 1908.

Levy, J. L.: Girl born without legs and without arms: Report of a case. *South. Med. J.*, 34:1085. 1941.

Levy-Valensi, and Feil, A.: Ectrodactylie des quatre derniers doigts. *Sem. Hop. Paris*, 6:61–62, 1930.

Lhomme, R.: *Recherches sur les Amputations Congénitales.* Thèse. Paris, H. Jouve, pp. 1–87, 1893.

Lindemann, K.: Peromelie und erbliche Missbildung. *Münch. Med. Wochenschr., 86*:513–514, 1939.

Lindemann, K.: Zur Prognose und Therapie schwerer Gliedmassenfehlbildungen. *Acta Orthop. Scan., 32*:298–306, 1962.

Lodes, R.: Ueber Erfahrungen an Armamputierten mit Sauerbruch-Prothesen. *Verb. Dtsch. Orthop. Ges., 53*:329–338, 1965.

Louyot, C.: Lesion mutilant congénitale de la main. *Rev. Med. Nancy, 66*:822–826, 1938.

Lukjanow, G. N.: Ein Fall von Amelia totalis. *Z. Ges. Anat.* (Avt. 1), *93*:645–659, 1930.

Lyman: Spontaneous amputation in utero. *Boston Med. Surg. J., 104*:396, 1881.

Macan, A. V.: Case of intra-uterine amputation. *Dublin J. Med. Sci., 59*:55–63, 1875.

Maher, J.: Intra-uterine amputations; probably caused by fibrin abnormally present in the liquor amnii. *J.A.M.A., 37*:547–548, 1901.

Mansfield, O. T., and Knight, J. S.: The treatment of congenital amputations through the forearm. *Br. J. Plast. Surg., 16*:23–31, 1963.

Marquardt, E.: The Heidelberg pneumatic arm prostheses. *J. Bone Joint Surg., 47B*:425–434, 1965.

Martin, E. A.: Ueber Selvstamputation beim Fötus. *Jeanische. Ann. Physiol. Med., 1*:333–358, 1850.

Martius, G., and Walter, S.: Periomelie und Mikrognathie als Missbildungskombination (Hanhartsches Syndrome). *Geburtsch. Frauenheilkd., 14*:558–563, 1954.

Mason, R. O.: Amniotic bands as a cause of amputation in utero. *Am. J. Obstet., 4*:747, 1872.

Mattei: Sur l'amputation spontanée d'un membre par le cordon ombilical pendant le cours de la vie intra-utérine. *Bull. Soc. d'Anthrop. Paris,* (3 s.), *1*:146–147, 1878.

McKenzie, D. S.: The clinical application of externally powered artificial arms. *J. Bone Joint Surg., 47B*:399–410, 1965.

McKenzie, D. S.: The Russian myo-electric arm. *J. Bone Joint Surg., 47B*:418–420, 1965.

McKusick, V. A.: *Mendelian Inheritance in Man.* Second edition. Baltimore, Johns Hopkins Press, Entry 2127, p. 248, 1968. See also Third edition, Entry 21710, p. 349, 1971.

McLaurin, C. A.: External power in upper-extremity prosthetics and orthotics. *J. Orthop. Prosthetic Appliances, 20*:145–151, 1966.

Menzel, A.: Spontane Dactylolyse, eine eigenthümliche Erkrankung der Finger. *Arch. Klin. Chir., 16*:667–680, Taf. XIX, 1874.

Meunier, H.: Amélie, description du type et considerations pathogéniques au suject d'un cas nouveau. *N. Iconog. Salp., 10*:15–30; Pl. III, 1897.

Meyer, H., and Cummins, H.: Severe maternal trauma in early pregnancy. Congenital amputations in the infant at term. *Am. J. Obstet. Gynecol., 42*:150–153, 1941.

Monod: Amputation congénital et syndactylie. *Bull. Mém. Soc. Chir. Paris, 20*:272–275, 1894.

Montgomery, W. F.: Observations on the spontaneous amputation of the limbs of the foetus in utero, with attempt to explain the occasional cause of its production. *Dublin Med. Chem. Sci. J., 1*:140–148, 1832.

Montgomery, W. F.: Further observation on spontaneous amputations of the limbs of the foetus in utero. *Dublin Med. Chem. Sci. J., 2*:49–51, 1833.

Montgomery, W. F.: Foetus. *In* Todd, R. B., (ed.): *The Cyclopaedia of Anatomy and Physiology.* London, Longman, Brown, Green, Longman & Roberts, Vol. III, pp. 316–338, 1836–1839.

Moreau, L.: Absence congénitale de la main et du poignet gauches. *Bull. Mém. Soc. Anat. Paris, 16–17*:308–310, 1920.

Mouchette, J.: Hemimélie et amputation congénitale. *Bull. Mém. Soc. Anat. Paris, 4*:742–763, 1902.

Movers, F.: Zur Frage der amniogenen fetalen Missbildungen. *Arch. Gynaekol., 168*:22–25, 1939.

Muir, T. R.: Intra-uterine amputations. *Polyclinic* (London), *7*:170–171, 1903.

Müller, W.: Die verschiedenen Fehlbildungstendenzen am Vorderarm. *Arch. Orthop. Unfallchir., 39*:541–557, 1939.

Munde, P.: Report of a case of partial spontaneous amputation of metacarpus in utero, with explanatory remarks. *Boston Med. & Surg. J., 80*:409–414, 1869.

Newmann, A.: Pseudoainhum: report of congenital case involving several fingers and the left wrist. *A.M.A. Arch. Dermatol. Syph., 68*:421–427, 1953.

Nockemann, P. F.: Erbliche Hornhautverdickung mit Schnürfurchen an Fingern und Zehen und Innenohrschwerhörigkeit. *Med. Welt, 2*:1894–1900, 1961.

Ombrédanne, L.: Malformations congénitales par brides amniotiques. *Rev. d'Orthop.,* (3 s.), *4*:277–280, 1913.

Ombrédanne, L., and Lacassie: La maladie ulcéreuse intra-utérine. *Arch. Méd. Enfants, 33*:199–211, 1930.

Ombrédanne, L., and Langeron, J.: Un nouveau cas de maladie ulcéreuse amniotique en évolution. *Arch. Méd. Enfants, 39*:228–232, 1936.

Osmond, M.: *Contribution a l'Étude des Amputations Congénitales.* Thèse. Paris, H. Jouve, pp. 1–98, 1892.

Osmont, M.: Amputation congénitales multiples. *Bull. Soc. Obstet., 3*:267–271, 1900.

Otero, R. G.: Un caso di "amelio." *Rev. Clin. Esp., 12*:117–124, 1944.

Packard, F. A.: Eight cases of malformation of the hands and feet. *Arch. Pediatr., 15*:357–365, 1898.

Patterson, T. J. S.: Congenital ring constrictions. *Br. J. Plast. Surg., 14*:1–31, 1961.

Patterson, T. J. S.: Ring constrictions. *The Hand, 1*:57–59, 1969.

Pers, M.: Congenital absence of skin: Pathogenesis and relation to ring constriction. *Acta Chir. Scand.*, *126*:388–396, 1963.

Peterka, H. M., and Karon, I. M.: Congenital pseudoainhum of fingers. *Arch. Dermatol.*, *90*:12–14, 1964.

Petersen, D.: Pathogenese der Peromelie. *Ergeb. Chir. Orthop.*, *53*:145–175, 1970.

Petit, P., and Bedouelle, J.: Maladie amniotique. *Malformations Congénitales des Membres. In Encyc. Med. Chir.*, Vol. 3, No. 152000, B10, pp. 1–4, 1955–1957.

Petterson, C.: Aglossia congenita with bony fusion of the jaws. Report of one case. *Acta Chir. Scand.*, *122*:93–95, 1961.

Pfotenhauer, G.: Familiarsuchung bei zwei Fällen von angeborener Amputation. *Der Erbarzt, 1*:11–12, 1936.

Phelip, J. A.: Ankyloglosse supérieure congénital. *Arch. Med. Enfants, 23*:243–244, 1920.

Pillay, V. K.: Congenital constriction bands in Singapore. *Singapore Med. J.*, *5*:198–202, 1964.

Pillay, V. K., and Hesketh, K. T.: Intra-uterine amputations and annular limb defects in Singapore. *J. Bone Joint Surg., 47B*:514–549, 1965.

Pincherle, B.: Nouveau-né avec ulcération congénitale du cuir chevelu, mutilations multiples de pha-langes et syndactylie partielle (Contribution à la maladie ulcéreuse amniotique d'Ombrédanne). *Arch. Méd. Enfants, 41*:96–99, 1938.

Pires de Lima, J. A.: Alguns atrophias congenitas dos membros. *Arg. Anat. Anthropol., 10*:403–429; Fig. 4, 7, 8, 9, 1926.

Pires de Lima, J. A.: Amputation par bride amniotiques. *Folia. Annat. Univ. Conimbr., 5*(No. 1):1–5; pp. I-VI, 1930.

Pires de Lima, J. A.: A propos d'un cas d'ectromélie. *Soc. Anat. Paris*, Séance de Juin, pp. 830–832, 1933.

Plotkin, D.: Congenital cicatrizing fibrous hands. *Arch. Pediatr., 68*:120–125, 1951.

Poidevin, L. O. S.: Amelia. Review of the literature and report of a case. *J. Obstet. Gynaecol. Br. Emp., 60*:922–925, 1953.

Poirer da Clisson: Amputation congénitale des doigts. *Bull. Soc. Obstet. Paris, 6*:9, 1903.

Pomerance, H. H., and Soifer, H.: Amelia: Review of literature and report of a case. *J. Pediatr., 34*:465–469, 1949.

Popov, B.: The bioelectrically controlled prostheses. *J. Bone Joint Surg., 47B*:421–424, 1965.

Portniaghine, C.: *Bride Amniotiques Circulaires et Sillons Congénitaux.* Thèse. Paris, Ollier-Henry, pp. 1–19, 1924.

Powell, H. H.: Report of a case of amniotic band causing amputation of a finger. *Cleveland Med. J., 1*:39, 1902.

Price, J.: Two cases of intra-uterine amputation of the forearm. *Trans. Am. Assoc. Obstet. Gynecol., 2*:41–44, 1889.

Price, M. D.: Baby without arms or legs (brief history with pathograph). *J. Indiana State Med. Assoc., 21*:250, 1928.

Radtke, E.: *Zwei Fälle von intra-uteriner Spontan-Amputation.* Inaug.-Diss. Königsberg, E. Eratis, pp. 1–48, 1894.

Reclus, P.: Amputations congénitales. *Sem. Méd., 3*:293–294, 1883.

Redard, P.: Sillon congénital du membre inferieur gauche: anomalies multiplex des doigts de deux mains (syndactylie, ectrodactylie): excision de bride; Guerson. *Gaz. Méd. Paris*, (7 s.), *4*:61, 1887; *5*:329, 1889.

Reed, J. M.: A case of intra-uterine amputation. *J.A.M.A., 87*:1213, 1926.

Renard, M.: Contribution à l'étude des amputations congénitales du membre superieur. *Rev. d'Orthop., 4*:50–58, 1893.

Riggles, J. L.: Case of intra-uterine amputation during foetal growth. *V. Med. Mon.*, (n.s.), *19*:325, 1914.

Roberts, C. H.: Curious congenital deformity. *Trans. Obstet. Soc. London, 36*:341–343, 1894.

Robinson, H. B.: Congenital cicatrices, a problem in antenatal pathology. Reports of the *Society for the Study of Diseases in Children.* *1*:63, 1900–1901.

Rocher, H. L.: Deux cas d'ectrokeyrie par abortement de la main. *J. Méd. de Bordeaux, 116*(2):115–117, 1939.

Rocher, H. L., and Ayguesparsse: Sillon congénital sus-malleclaire et amputations congénitales mul-tiplex (Doigts et orteils). *J. Méd. Bordeaux* 91 Année (n.s.) 91–97, 1920.

Rocher, H. L., and Pesme: Bec-de-lievre compliqué bilatéral, compliqué de coloboma bilatéral pal-pebral et de coloboma irien gauche. Ectromélie totale du membre superieur droit. *J. Méd. Bor-deaux, 25*:493–495, 1945.

Rocher, H. L., Lasserre, and Lataste: Mutilations congénitales multiples par brides amniotiques por-tant sur les quatre membres. *Bull. Mém. Soc. Méd. Chir. Bordeaux*, pp. 173–174, 1923.

Rockwell, A. H.: Intra-uterine amputation. *Trans. Michigan St. Med. Soc., 14*:399–400, 1890.

Rodriquez, J. M.: Caso de amputacion intrauterina (Prof. D. L. Munoz' case). *Gaceta Med. Mexico, 7*:34–38, 1872.

Roederer, M.: Hemimélie partielle transversal de deux membres inferieures. Amputation congénital d'un avant-bras. *Bull. Soc. Ped. Paris, 24*:144–146, 1926.

Roger, L.: Maldevelopment of the wrist and hand. *Edinburgh Med. J.*, (n.s.), *32*:407–409, 1925.

Rosenthal, R.: Aglossia congenita. Report of a case of the condition combined with other congenital malformations. *Am. J. Dis. Child.*, *44*:383–389, 1932.

Roth, J.: Zur Frage der "angeborenen Amputationen." *Der Erbarzt*, 58–59, 1936.

Rousseau, A.: *Contribution à l'Étude des Brides Congénitales des Membres*. Thése. Paris, Impm. de la Faculté de Medicine, 1. Boyer, pp. 1–76, 1901.

Schade, H.: Untersuchungen zur Frage der Erblichkeit von Mangelund Fehlbildungen der Gliedmassen. *Der Erbarzt*, *8*:239–256, 1940.

Schönenberg, H.: Ueber die quere Extremitätendysplasie. *Z. Kinderheilkd.*, *104*:331–348, 1968.

Seckel, H. P. G.: *Bird-headed Dwarfs. Studies in Developmental Anthropology Including Human Proportions.* Springfield, Illinois: Charles C Thomas, p. 41; fig. 12, 1960.

Seligman, S. A.: Ectromelia: a case report. *Arch. Dis. Child.*, *36*:658–660, 1961.

Shear, M.: Congenital underdevelopment of the maxilla associated with partial adactylia, partial anodontia and microglossia. Report of a case. *J. Dent. Assoc. S. Africa.* *11*:78–83, 1956.

Shore, L. R.: Two cases of congenital deformity of upper limb. *J. Anat.*, *62*:118–120, 1927.

Sim, F. L.: Intra-uterine amputations. *Memphis Med. Mon.*, *8*:457–461, 1888.

Simonhart: Note sur les amputations spontanées. *J. Connaissance Méd.*, pp. 327–330, Juin 1846. See also: *Arch. Med. Belg.*, pp. 112–119, 1846.

Simpson, D. C.: Artificial hands. *The Hand*, *3*:211–212, 1971.

Simpson, D. C., and Lamb, D. W.: A system of powered prostheses for severe bilateral upper arm deficiency. *J. Bone Joint Surg.*, *47B*:442–447, 1965.

Simpson, J. Y.: Cases illustrative of the spontaneous amputation of the limbs of the foetus in utero, with remarks. *Dublin J. Med. Sci.*, *10*:220–241, 1836.

Simpson, J. Y.: On rudimentary reproduction of extremities after their spontaneous amputation. In: *Diseases of Women*. Edinburgh, A. C. Black, *1*:129, 1871.

Sjostedt, J. E.: Amelia totalis. A case report. *Riv. Ostet. Ginecol.*, *12*:173–179, 1957.

Slingenberg, B.: Missbildungen von Extremitäten. *Arch. Pathol. Anat. Physiol.*, *193*:1–92; Taf. I-XII, 1908.

Souques, A., and Marinesco, G.: Lésions de la moelle épinière dans un cas d'amputation congénitale des doigts de la main. *Presse Med.*, *45*:250–253, 1897.

Souto, V.: Sobre un caso de feto amputacaon congenital e syndactylia. *Brazil Med.*, *32*:172–173, 1918.

Stenstrom, J. D.: Congenital abnormalities of the extremities. *Can. Med. Assoc. J.*, *51*:325–334, 1944.

Stevenson, T. W.: Release of circular constricting scar by Z-flaps. *Plast. Reconstr. Surg.*, *1*:39–43, 1946.

Stowell, W. L.: Intrauterine amputations and amniotic bands. *Arch. Pediatr.*, *22*:342–345, 1905.

Street, D. M., and Cunningham, F.: Congenital anomalies caused by intra-uterine bands. *Clin. Orthop.*, *37*:82–97, 1964.

Streeter, G. L.: Focal deficiencies in fetal tissues and their relation to intra-uterine amputation. Carnegie Inst. of Washington, Pub. 414, *Contrib. Embryol.*, *22*:1–44, 1930.

Strouzer, W.: Aplasies congénitales multiples. Hémimélies transverses, symétriques des extrémités édentations. *J. Radiol. Electrol.*, *23*:169–170, 1939–1940.

Swanson, A. B.: Restoration of hand function by the use of partial or total prosthetic replacement. *J. Bone Joint Surg.*, *45A*:276–288, 1963.

Swanson, A. B.: The Krükenberg procedure in the juvenile amputee. *J. Bone Joint Surg.*, *46A*:1540–1549, 1964.

Swanson, A. B.: Treatment of congenital limb malformations. *Kobe J. Med. Sci.*, *11*(Suppl.):41–53, 1965.

Templeton, G.: Intra-uterine amputation of fingers. *Clin. J. London*, *11*:175–176, 1897–1898.

Terruhn, E.: Ueber die Entstehung amniogener Hautdefekte während der Schwangerschaft mit besonderer Berücksichtigung des Schädels beim Neugeborenen. *Arch. Gynäkol.*, *140*:428–460, 1930.

Tilanus, C. B.: Amputatio antebrachii congenita. *Ned. T. Geneesk.*, *2*:1893–1894, 1915.

Toledo, S. P. A., and Saldaha, P. H.: Radiological and genetic investigation of acheiropody in a kindred including six cases. *J. Genet. Hum.*, *17*:81–94, 1969.

Torpin, R.: *Fetal Malformations Caused by Amnion Rupture during Gestation*. Springfield, Illinois: Charles C Thomas, pp. 1–165, 1968.

Tournier, C.: Note sur deux cas d'amputation congénitale de l'avantbras sans autre malformation. *Rev. d'Orthop.*, (1 s.), *2*:272–276, 1891.

Tower, P.: Coloboma of lower lid and choroid, with facial defects and deformity of the hand and forearm. *Arch. Ophthalmol.*, *50*:33–343, 1953.

Trasler, D. C., Walker, B. E., and Fraser, F.: Congenital malformations produced by amniotic puncture. *Science*, *124*:439, 1956.

Troisier: Hémimélie thoracique du côté droite. Examen de la moelle épinière. *Bull. Soc. Anat. Paris*, (2 s.), *15*:140–150, 1874.

Tronchet: Amputation congénitale de doigts. Bull. Soc. Anat. Bordeaux, 6:31, 1885.

Turner, E. J.: Intra-uterine constriction band. *J. Pediatr.*, *57*:590–591, 1960.

Unterrichter, L.: Ueber angeborene Gliedmassenstummel. *Der Erbarzt*, *7*:104–115, 1939.

Unterrichter, L.: Die Peromelie. *Fortschr. Erbpath.*, *6*:32–54, 1942.

Vecchione, F.: Sulle cosidette "amputazioni congenite dell' avanbraccio." *Arch. Ortop.*, *59*:24–47, 1940.

Vaidya, D. R.: Amelia. *Indian Med. Gaz.*, *26*:286–287, 1939.

Variot, G., and Chicotot, G.: Un cas d'amputations congénitales multiples des doigts et des orteils ètudié par le méthode radiographique. *Bull. Soc. Méd. Hôp.*, (3 s.), *15*:838–841, 1898.

Variot, G., and Leconte, M.: Amputation congénitale des doigts et des orteils avec syndactylie; sillon congénitale des jambes. *Bull. Soc. Ped.* (Paris), *9*:106–109, 1907.

Ware, C. E.: Spontaneous amputation in utero. *Boston Med. Surg. J.*, *66*:27, 1862.

Waterman, J. A.: Amputation of fingers in utero. *Caribbean Med.*, *15*:31, 1953.

Wells, T. L., and Robinson, R. C. V.: Annular constrictions of the digits. Presentation of an interesting example. *A.M.A. Arch. Dermatol. Syph.*, *66*:569–572, 1952.

Wigley, J. E. M.: Case of hyperkeratosis palmaris and plantaris associated with Ainhum-like constriction of the fingers. *Br. J. Dermatol. Syph.*, *41*:188–191, 1929.

Williams, C. L.: A case of multiple intra-uterine amputations. *Med. Rep.* (Calcutta), *2*:239–240, 1893.

Wilson, R. A., Kliman, M. R., and Hardyment, A. F.: Ankyloglossia superior (palato-glossal adhesion in newborn infant). *Pediatrics*, *31*:1051–1054, 1963.

Witt, A. N., and Jäger, M.: Die operative Behandlung der peripheren Hypoplasie der Hand. *Arch. Orthop. Unfallchir.*, *64*:52–63, 1968.

Wittwer, E.: Ueber eine bisher selten beobachtete Entstehung sursache amputierender und umschnürender amniotischer Faden und Stränge. *Strassburger Med.*, *14*:127–129, 1917.

Wix, M.: *In Les Sillons Congénitaux Dits par Brides Amniotiques.* Thèse. Paris, Vigot Frères, pp. 11–102, Pl. 1–11, 1936.

Wolff, J.: Intra-uterine Spontanamputationen an den oberen Extremitäten bei eimen 5 Monate alten Fötus mit vollständiger Erhaltung des die Amputation bedingenden Amniosfädens. *Arch. Gynäkol.*, *1*:281–290, 1900.

Wong, W. W.: Congenital cicatrix. *Plast. Reconstr. Surg.*, *6*:79–83, 1950.

Wood, W. A.: Congenital amputations and constrictions. *Med. J. Australia*, *9*:516, 1904.

Wossidle: Fall von Selbstamputation durch die Natur. *Arch. Klin. Chir.*, *6*:792–793, 1865.

Young, J. K.: The etiology of congenital absence of parts. *Lancet-Clinic*, *115*:248–250, 1916.

Young, O. H.: A case of spontaneous amputation in utero. *Med. Rec.*, *1*:27, 1866.

Chapter Seventeen

ANOMALIES OF DIGITAL POSTURE

Discrepancies in digital alignment often accompany other anomalies of the hand. Some of these have already been discussed; others will be taken up in succeeding chapters. In this chapter, an attempt will be made to clarify a few moot points concerning the postural abnormalities of the thumb and the fingers. Traditionally, fixed deviation of the digit or its phalanges toward the radial or ulnar border of the hand is called *clinodactyly*, and the term *camptodactyly* is used for flexion contractures for which, with no valid justification, such abstruse designations as campylodactyly, streblodactyly, and gampsodactyly are often flaunted.

FLEXION AND ULNAR DEVIATION OF THE THUMB DUE TO DEFICIENT EXTENSORS AND LONG ABDUCTOR MUSCLES (Thumb-Clutched Hand; Congenital Clasped Thumb)

Tamplin (1846) said he had seen a case of congenital flexion adduction deformity of the thumb. In the illustration featured, the thumb is shown pulled into the palm with the lesser digits closed upon it. During dissection of a limb, Shattock (1881) noted the absence of an extensor tendon of the thumb. Kirmisson (1898) presented a case in which the thumb deviated from the carpometacarpal joint and lay flat in the palm, its tip pointing toward the ulnar border of the hand. Zadek (1934) operated on a young child with flexion deformity of both thumbs at the interphalangeal joint. Surgical exploration disclosed an attenuated extensor pollicis longus tendon. One of the patients operated on by Miller (1943) lacked extensor pollicis brevis as well as abductor pollicis longus tendons. Similar cases have since been reported by White and Jensen (1952), Giordani (1954), Allaria (1956), Loomis (1957), Broadbent and Woolf (1964), Namba and associates (1965), Crawford et al (1966), Weckesser et al (1968), and Gold and Perlman (1968). In most of these, the extensor pollicis brevis has been found most often to be wanting or weak.

The short extensor of the thumb is inserted into the dorsal base of the proximal phalanx; it stabilizes the metacarpophalangeal joint, extends the basal phalanx, and abducts the thumb as a whole without rotating it. When this muscle is missing or is functionally defunct, the thumb is flexed at the metacarpophalangeal joint; both phalanges are pulled into the palm, and the tip of the thumb comes to lie on the volar aspect of the third metacarpal. The abductor pollicis longus is inserted into the radial base of the first metacarpal and pulls this bone in the radial direction. When it is functionally ineffective, all three segments of the pollical ray are pulled into the palm and the tip of the thumb extends further toward the ulnar border of the hand than it does in the deformity resulting from a nonfunctioning short extensor alone. The long extensor of the thumb, whose main function is to extend the ungual phalanx, is inserted into the dorsal base of the distal phalanx. Because of the oblique disposition of its tendon, the long extensor rotates the thumb—counterclockwise on the right and clockwise on the left side—to bring its nail closer to a horizontal plane. When the long extensor is not functioning, the distal phalanx remains flexed and the thumb is supinated (Fig. 17–1).

The deformity caused by the absence of any of the above three muscles, either alone or in combination, is usually bilateral and symmetrical. It is often hereditary, and the trait is transmitted as an autosomal dominant phenotype. The deformity caused by an absent or attenuated extensor pollicis longus is often mimicked by the one due to the nodular thickening of the long flexor, or trigger thumb. The differential diagnosis between these two conditions should not be difficult. Aplasia or hypoplasia of thumb extensors and long abductor often occurs in arthrogryposis. This disorder presents sundry generalized manifestations: stiff joints, multiple dislocations, attenuated bones, retarded growth, and crippling. Flexion adduction contractures of the thumb also follow upper motor neuron lesions, in which case the affected individual shows other signs of spasticity.

It is often difficult to establish a definite diagnosis of nonarthrogrypotic, congenital flexion-adduction deformity of the thumb in newborn infants. Even when awake, the infant holds its thumb clasped in the palm. It is not until three months after birth—sometimes even later—that the child attempts to clear its thumb out of the palm and grasp an object. After the establishment of the grasping reflex when the child is awake and active, the thumb does not stay in one position unless it is voluntarily held immobile, or it is paralyzed or malformed. The thumb can only be said to have assumed an anomalous posture when, as a whole or in segments, it remains stationary or changes position to a limited degree.

In infants, because of the hereditary antecedent when one suspects congenital insufficiency of the extensors or long abductor of the thumb, immobilization of the pollex in the functional position should be carried out until the advent of the grasping reflex. Bearing the possibility of hypoplastic muscles in mind, one may continue periodic splinting of the thumb for several months. In older children, immobilization of the thumb is carried out intermittently, and functional exercises are encouraged when the hand is freed from splintage. None of these measures avail if the muscles are aplastic. Often, the exact condition of the involved muscles and tendons cannot be ascertained unless the hand is surgically explored and examined.

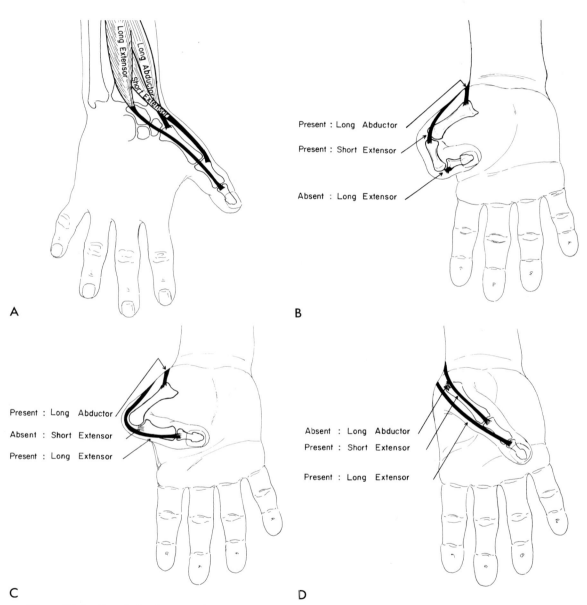

Figure 17–1 Correlation between absence of extensor pollicis longus and brevis and abductor pollicis longus and the position of the thumb. *A*, Sketch of the dorsal aspect of the thumb, showing the insertion of the three muscles. *B*, The thumb is flexed at the interphalangeal joint when the action of the long extensor is nullified. *C*, The thumb is flexed at the metacarpophalangeal joint and drops into the palm when the extensor pollicis brevis is ineffective. *D*, When the abductor pollicis longus fails to function, the thumb is pulled nearer to the ulnar border of the hand.

Numerous operative procedures have been recommended for the treatment of congenital flexion-adduction contracture of the thumb: tendon transfers, intermetacarpal bone graft, and arthrodesis of the joint proximal to the flexed or adducted segment. A tendon transfer operation provides the thumb with the needed motor power; arthrodesing procedures will procure a stable position. In old, untreated cases in which contractures have already become established, one may have to perform Z-plasty to widen the first webspace. It may even be necessary to release the adductors and perform capsulotomy of the contracted joint. At times, one may have to carry out abduction and derotation osteotomy of the first metacarpal bone, or even to fuse the first metacarpophalangeal joint.

Not every case will benefit from the same treatment. A female child with bilateral absence of the extensor pollicis longus came under the author's care. Her mother had the same defect of the hands, marked scoliosis, and absent sternocleidomastoid muscle on one side. The daughter's sternocleidomastoid muscle was missing on both sides, and she began to develop scoliosis at about the age of 10 years. Three other children in the family were unaffected. The daughter with the absent extensor pollicis was subjected to surgery when she was six years of age. The area in the back of the second metacarpal of one hand was explored: the extensor indicis proprius was missing. The extensor carpi ulnaris was utilized as a motor, and the gap between it and the terminal phalanx of the thumb was spanned with a free graft obtained from the long extensor of the fourth toe. Both sides were operated on (Figs. 17–2 to 17–4).

FLEXION DEFORMITY OF THE THUMB DUE TO BLOCKED FLEXOR POLLICIS LONGUS TENDON (Notta's Node; Congenital Trigger Thumb)

Notta (1850) was probably the first to describe this condition. He suspected the presence of a nodule which had formed on the long flexor tendon of the thumb, interfering with its gliding mechanism and arresting its excursion. Since newborn infants hold their thumbs flexed, the condition is not suspected until one of the parents attempts to extend the thumb passively—at which time definite resistance is experienced, although it seldom snaps. The acquired form of this condition favors the lesser digits; the congenital variety shows a distinct predilection for the thumb. Only rarely, an infant is seen with flexion contracture of one of the lesser digits due to blocked flexor tendons (Fig. 17–5).

White and Jensen (1953) presented nine cases of trigger thumb in infants, two of whom had "a definite family history." Most reported cases have been sporadic. The thumb is bent at both the metacarpophalangeal and interphalangeal joints. The treatment is surgical. The tendon sheath of the flexor pollicis longus is slit longitudinally at about the level of the metacarpophalangeal joint of the thumb, and the nodule on the tendon is shaved. Care is taken not to injure the volar digital branches of the median nerve whose filaments flank the tendon sheath and lie in a more palmar plant (Figs. 17–6 to 17–8).

(Text continued on page 564.)

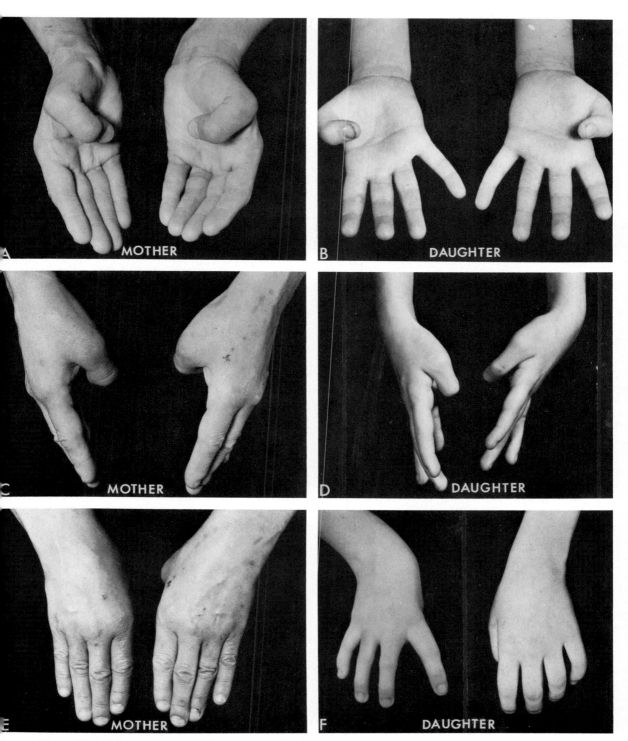

Figure 17–2 Bilateral absence of the extensor pollicis longus: mother-to-daughter transmission. *A*, Palmar view of the mother's hands. *B*, Palmar view of the daughter's hands. *C*, Radial view of the mother's hands. *D*, Radial view of the daughter's hands. *E*, Dorsal view of the mother's hands. *F*, Dorsal view of the daughter's hands.

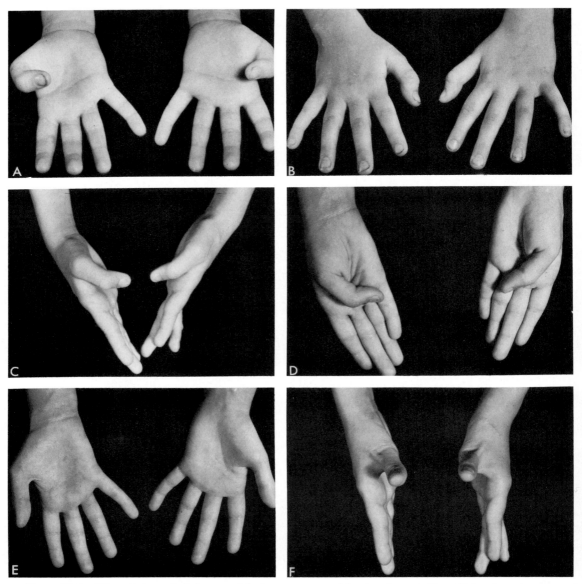

Figure 17–3 Bilateral congenital absence of the long extensor of the thumb treated by utilizing the extensor carpi ulnaris as a motor and spanning the gap between the detached tip of its tendon and the base of the ungual phalanx of the thumb with a graft obtained from the fourth extensor tendon of the foot. *A*, Preoperative palmar view of the hands of the daughter featured in Figure 17–2. *B*, Preoperative dorsal view. *C*, Preoperative radial view. *D*, The left thumb, which was operated on first, is contrasted with the as yet unoperated right thumb. *E*, Palmar view of the hands one year after surgery on the left hand and six months after surgery on the right hand. *F*, Postoperative radial view of both hands.

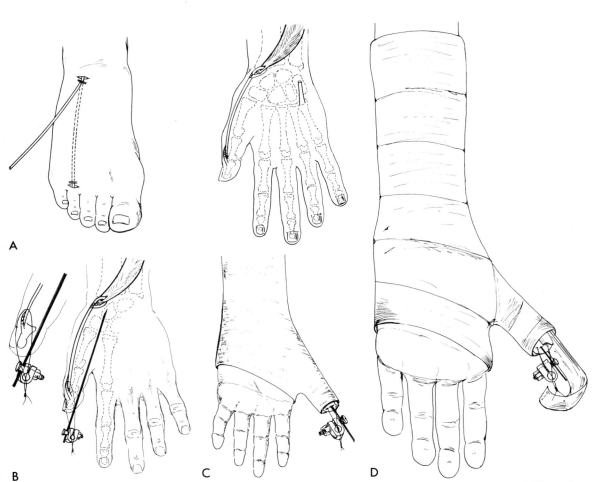

Figure 17–4   Procedures utilized in the treatment of the preceding case (Figs. 17–2 and 17–3). *A*, Sketch illustrating utilization of the extensor carpi ulnaris as a motor and bridging the gap between it and the ungual phalanx of the thumb with a free tendon graft taken from the extensor of the fourth toe. *B*, Suturing the distal end of the graft to the periosteocapsular flap lifted from the dorsal aspect of the interphalangeal joint; inset shows utilization of a pull-out wire which is anchored to a nut which, in turn, is hooked to a percutaneous K-wire used for immobilization. *C*, Additional immobilization is obtained by a circular cast. *D*, Hood incorporated in the cast for protective purposes.

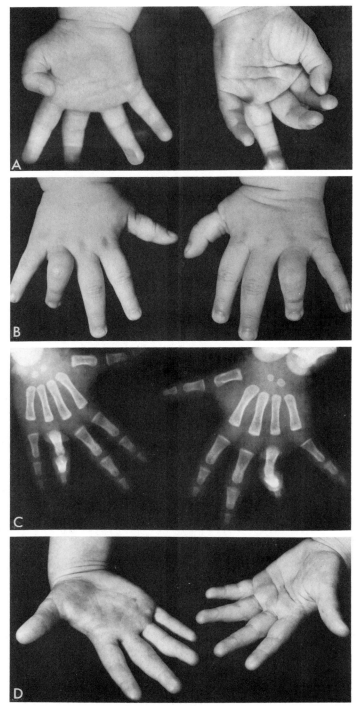

Figure 17–5   Bilateral flexion contracture of the ring finger treated by splitting the sheath of the flexor tendons. *A*, Preoperative palmar view of the hands of a six-month-old female infant with the ring fingers forced passively into extension. *B*, Preoperative dorsal view. *C*, Dorsopalmar roentgenograph of the hands. *D*, Postoperative palmar view, showing active extension of the ring fingers.

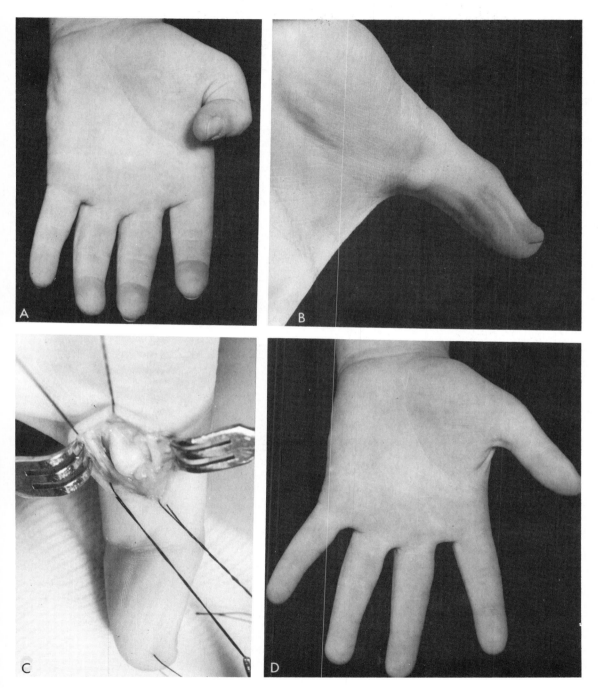

Figure 17–6 Blocked long flexor of the thumb. *A*, Palmar view of the left hand of a two-year-old female with flexion deformity of the thumb which had been present since birth. *B*, The child was put under anesthesia and the thumb was forced into extension by a traction suture through the distal pulp. *C*, Exposure of the tumor (Notta's node). *D*. Postoperative result.

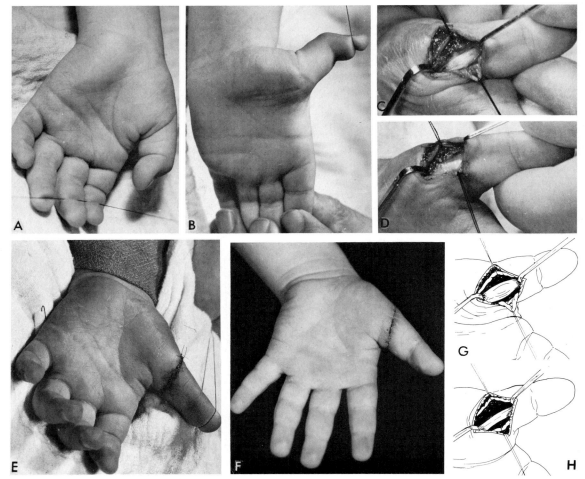

Figure 17–7   Blocked flexor hallucis longus tendon. *A*, Preoperative palmar view of the left hand of an 11-month-old male. *B*, Same, when the child was under anesthesia and an attempt was made to passively extend the ungual phalanx of the thumb. *C*, Exposure of the nodule on the tendon. *D*, The same, after shaving the nodule. *E*, Immediate postoperative result. *F*, Result after removal of the stitches. *G* and *H* illustrate *C* and *D*, respectively.

ADDUCTION CONTRACTURE OF THE THUMB DUE TO THE ANCHORAGE OF THE FIRST METACARPAL BY THE DEEP METACARPAL LIGAMENT

Occasionally, as in nonopposable triphalangeal and, less frequently, in biphalangeal pollex, the deep transverse ligament extends radially and tethers the first metacarpal or the proximal phalanx of the thumb. This condition is often accompanied by narrowing of the first webspace, which needs to be widened by stripping the more distal fibers of the first interosseous muscle, and performing Z-plasty of the first web skin. At the same time, the metacarpal and the proximal phalanx of the thumb are freed from the deep transverse ligament. Z-plasty of the first web skin and dehiscence of the underlying tissues are occasionally supplemented with abduction osteotomy of the first metacarpal (Fig. 17–9).

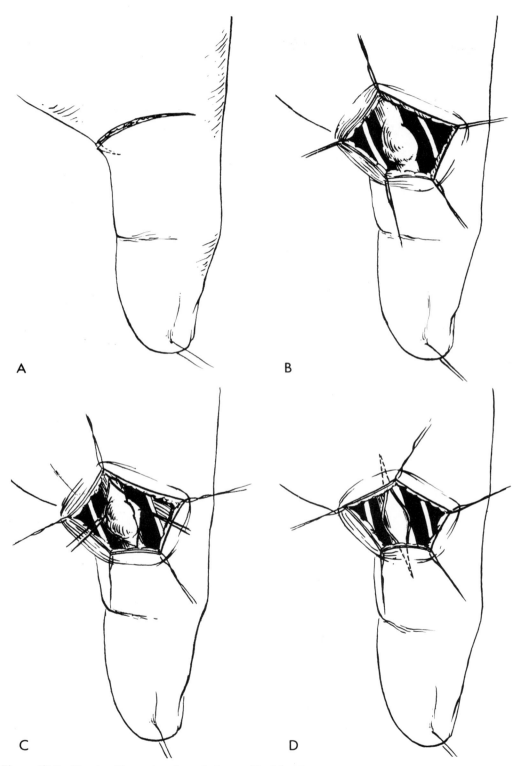

Figure 17–8 Sketches illustrating the technique utilized for the preceding two cases (Figs. 17–6 and 17–7). *A,* Incision. *B,* Exposure of the digital nerves. *C,* Exposure of the tumor. *D,* Splitting the flexor tendon sheath lengthwise and shaving the nodule on the flexor tendon of the thumb.

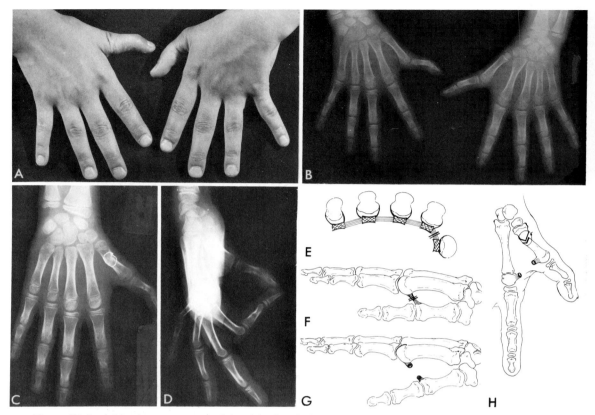

Figure 17–9 Adduction contracture of the right thumb due to anchoring of the first metacarpal by the deep transverse metacarpal ligament. *A,* Dorsal view of the hands of a 12-year-old female. *B,* Dorsopalmar roentgenograph of the hands. *C,* Postoperative roentgenograph of the right hand, showing that the first metacarpal has been subjected to abduction osteotomy. *D,* Lateral roentgenograph of the hand with the thumb and index in pulp-to-pulp opposition. *E, F,* and *G,* Sketches illustrating severance of the segment of the deep transverse metacarpal ligament tethering the first metacarpal. *H* illustrates the abduction osteotomy of the first metacarpal.

ANGULATION OF THE UNGUAL PHALANX
OF THE MIDDLE FINGER

Isolated clinodactyly involving the distal phalanx of the third digit is rare. As indicated in Chapter Four, it is occasionally seen in subjects with multiple exostoses. It is also known to occur in Klippel-Trénaunay syndrome, which will be taken up in Chapter Nineteen. The condition is corrected by subcapital osteotomy of the middle phalanx or by fusion of the distal interphalangeal joint (Fig. 17–10).

FLEXION DEFORMITY OF THE MIDDLE
FINGER

This is rarely an isolated entity. Fixed flexion contracture at the first interphalangeal joint of the third digit is occasionally seen in association with absent or rudimentary ungual phalanx (Fig. 17–11).

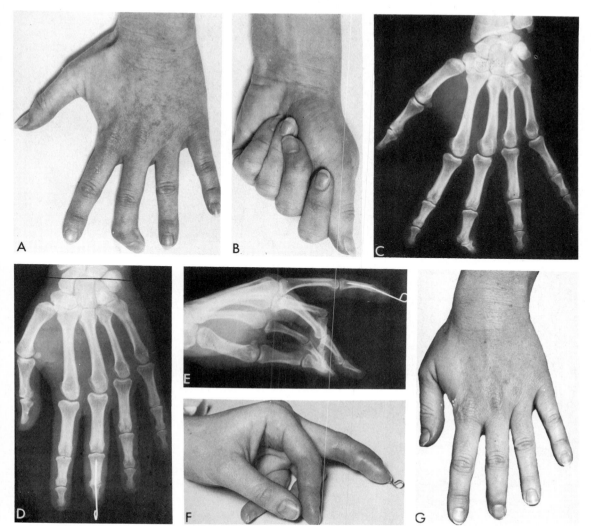

Figure 17–10 Angulated dwarf ungual phalanx of the left middle finger treated by interphalangeal fusion. *A* and *B*, Preoperative dorsal views of the affected digit. *C*, Preoperative dorsopalmar roentgenograph of the hand. *D*, Postoperative roentgenograph showing fixation of the phalanges by a K-wire. *E*, Lateral roentgenograph. *F*, Radial view of the hand. *G*, Dorsal view showing the final postoperative result.

FLEXION DEFORMITY OF THE RING FINGER DUE TO CONGENITAL ABSENCE OF THE THIRD LUMBRICAL AND ABDUCTION CONTRACTURE OF THE LITTLE FINGER

An 11-year-old boy came under the author's care and the parents attested that ever since birth the boy had a bent right ring finger and abducted little finger. Examination showed a shorter and thinner right thumb and sunken first intermetacarpal space. The ring finger was extended at the metacarpophalangeal juncture and flexed at both interphalangeal joints. The little finger was abducted. The palm was explored surgically; the third lumbrical was found

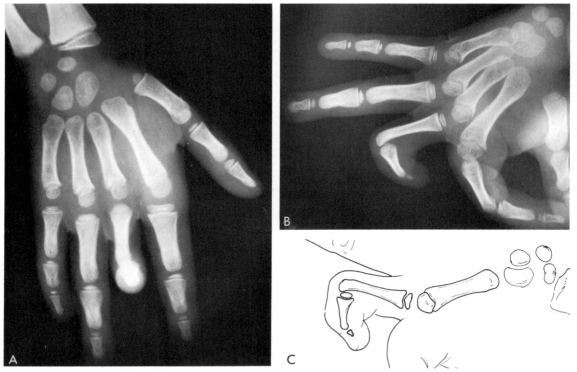

Figure 17–11 Flexion contracture of the middle finger at the first interphalangeal joint associated with vestigial ungual phalanx. *A*, Dorsopalmar roentgenograph of the right hand of a four-year-old boy. *B*, Oblique roentgenograph. *C*, Sketch illustrating the skeletal elements of the affected middle finger.

wanting. The fourth lumbrical was thin, and the abductor of the little finger was taut. The sublimis of the ring finger was transferred to its extensor expansion and the abductor digiti minimi was tenotomized (Figs. 17–12 to 17–14).

FLEXION DEFORMITY OF THE LITTLE FINGER AT THE FIRST INTERPHALANGEAL JOINT (Crooked Little Finger; Camptodactyly of Digit V; Streblomicrodactyly)

Lucas (1892), Little (1894), and Fantham (1924) said all that need be said about this anomaly; namely, that the postural change starts at the first interphalangeal joint, that the condition is hereditary and can be traced through several generations, and that the deformity is at times very severe and disabling. More recent authors have meandered into the domain of theoretical speculations concerning the cause of this anomaly. Some have placed the blame upon

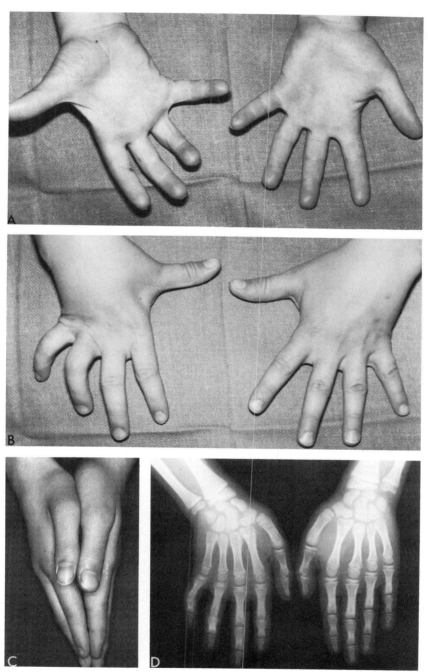

Figure 17–12 Flexion deformity of the ring finger due to congenital absence of the third lumbrical and abduction contracture of the little finger—treated by transfer of the sublimis of the ring finger to its extensor expansion and tenotomy of the abductor digiti minimi. *A,* Palmar view of the right (affected) and left hands of an 11-year-old male. *B,* Dorsal view of the same: the first inter-metacarpal space of the right hand is sunken, indicating aplasia or hypoplasia of the underlying dorsal interosseus muscle. *C,* Radial view of opposed right and left hands: the right thumb is thinner. *D,* Dorsopalmar roentgenograph of the hands: the second phalanges of the right ring and little fingers are short.

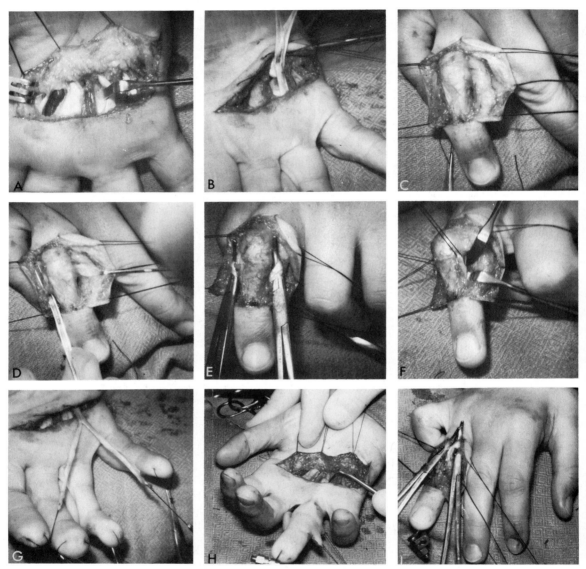

Figure 17–13 Transfer of the sublimis for correction of deformity due to absent third lumbrical. *A*, Exposure of the right palm of the 11-year-old boy featured in Figure 17–12: the bipinnate lumbrical arising from the adjacent sides of the deep flexor tendons of the middle and ring fingers was found missing; the fourth lumbrical going to the little finger was puny. *B*, Lifting the sublimis tendon of the ring finger. *C*, Exposure of the dorsal expansion of the ring finger. *D*, Isolation of Cleland's ligament, which was cut. *E*, Isolation of sublimis tendons near their insertions. *F* shows that the radial limb of the bifurcated sublimis has been cut. *G*, Delivery of the sublimis tendon, which was rethreaded through a dorsal plane to the back of the first interphalangeal joint of the ring finger. *H* shows that percutaneous wire had been inserted to hold the finger in extended position. *I*, The limbs of the sublimis tendon have been crossed and sutured to the extensor expansion of the ring finger.

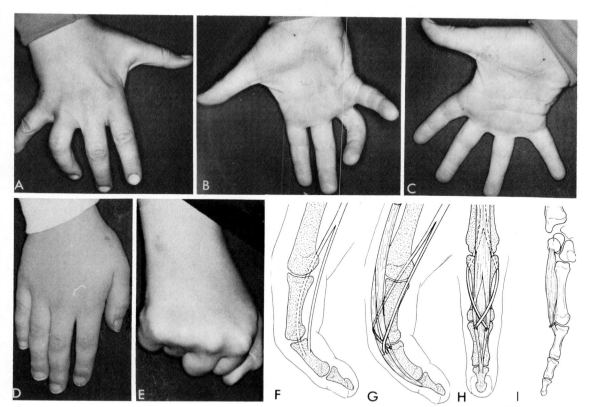

Figure 17–14 The outcome of the treatment of the right hand of the 11-year-old boy featured in Figures 17–12 and 17–13. *A*, Preoperative dorsal view of the hand. *B*, Preoperative palmar view. *C*, Postoperative palmar view. *D*, Postoperative dorsal view. *E*, Postoperative clenched fist. *F*, *G*, and *H* illustrate transfer of the sublimis slips of the ring finger to its extensor expansion. *I*, Sketch shows tenotomy of abductor of the little finger.

the congenitally contracted flexor sublimis; others relate the deformity to abnormalities of the expansion on the back of the first interphalangeal joint. Several authors have put the onus on the volar tilt of the distal portion of the proximal phalanx, and there are those who contend that the anterior capsule of the joint is contracted. No author seems to have proved his point by surgical exploration or by anatomical study of the hand of an affected infant. The author of this book has explored a number of affected adolescents and has found both slips of the flexor sublimis contracted. This contracture may well be consequential rather than causative. In many cases of camptodactyly of the little finger, the ring finger is similarly affected (Figs. 17–15 to 17–20).

Subclinical flexion deformity of the little finger is very common and does not require any treatment—least of all surgical intervention. In moderate deformities, one may attempt Z-plasty of the palmar skin and supplement this procedure with anterior capsulotomy of the first interphalangeal joint. In more severe angulations, one may choose from three alternatives: resection of the distal end of the proximal phalanx, subcapital osteotomy of the same bone, or fusion of the first interphalangeal joint, thus placing the finger in a serviceable position.

(Text continued on page 576.)

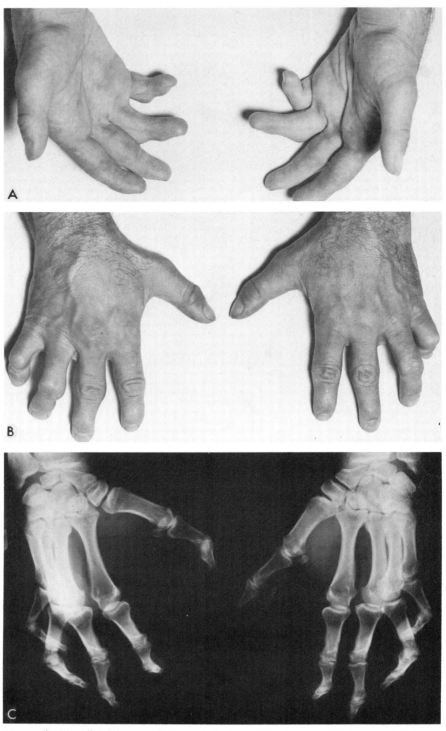

Figure 17–15 Bilateral congenital camptodactyly of the ring and little fingers. *A*, Palmar view of the hands of a 33-year-old male who had flexion contractures of the last two ulnar digits of both hands since birth. *B*, Dorsal view. *C*, Dorsopalmar roentgenograph of the hands.

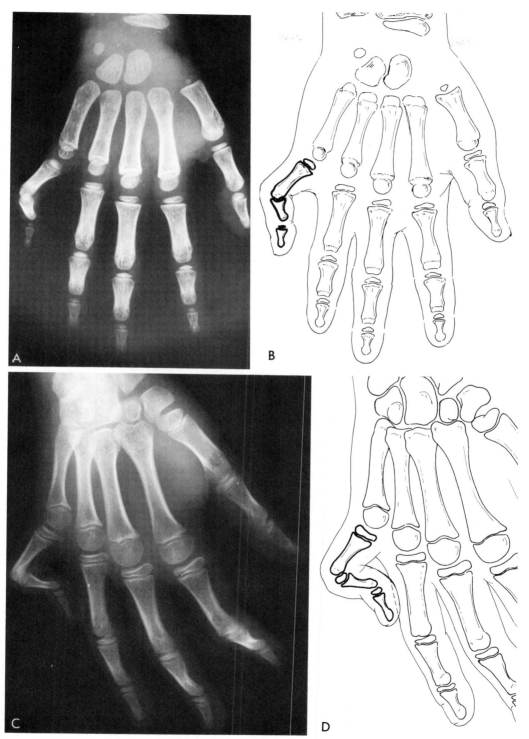

Figure 17–16 Unilateral congenital camptodactyly of the little finger. *A*, Dorsopalmar roentgenograph of the right hand of a three-year-old male. *B*, Sketch illustrating the same. *C*, Oblique roentgenograph of the right hand of another, older child. *D*, Sketch illustrating hammered little finger.

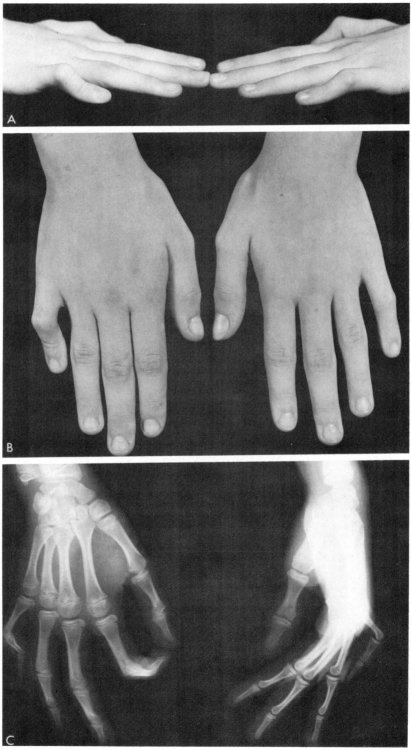

Figure 17–17   Bilateral congenital camptodactyly of the little fingers. *A*, Ulnar view of the hands of a 12-year-old female. *B*, Dorsal view. *C*, Oblique roentgenograph of the hands.

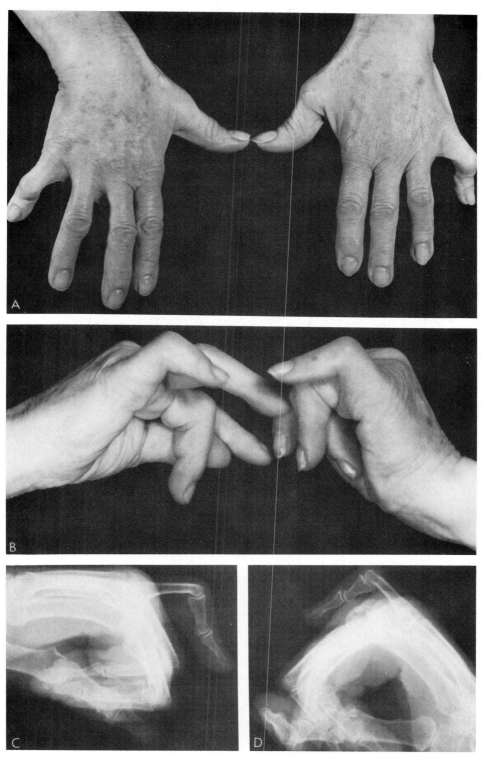

Figure 17–18 Bilateral congenital camptodactyly of the little fingers. *A*, Dorsal view of the hands. *B*, Ulnar view. *C* and *D*, Lateral roentgenographs of the right and left little fingers.

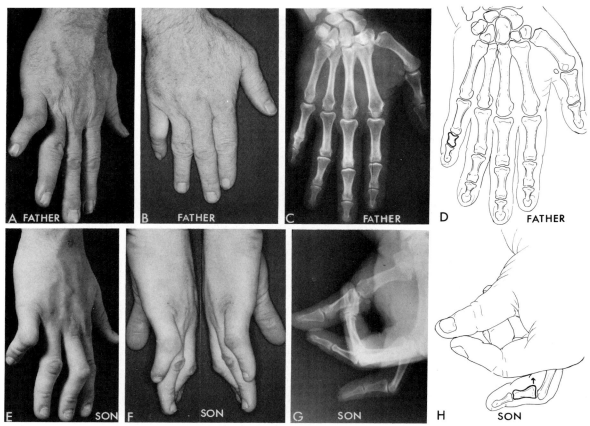

Figure 17–19 Flexion deformity of the little finger: father-to-son transmission with variable expression in the son. The father had involvement of only the right hand; the son had bilateral involvement, the deformity being more pronounced on the right side. *A*, Dorso-ulnar view of the father's right hand. *B*, Dorsal view. *C*, Dorsopalmar roentgenograph of the same: the middle phalanx of the little finger is dwarfed. *D*, Sketch illustrating the same. *E*, Dorso-ulnar view of the son's right hand. *F*, Ulnar view of the son's right and left hands. *G*, Lateral roentgenograph of the son's right hand: the middle phalanx of the little finger is of normal length. *H*, Sketch illustrating the same.

CONGENITAL DUPUYTREN'S CONTRACTURE

Greig (1917) presented a five-week-old boy whose fingers had remained flexed since birth. Greig considered this case to be one of congenital Dupuytren's contracture. Jorge (1926) described a case of bilateral flexion contracture of all fingers, and considered the basic process to be congenital retraction of the palmar aponeurosis. His patient was a three-year-old girl. Her mother had the same deformity. Zumoff (1954) traced the pedigree of a similar case through three generations, and regarded the trait as "non-sex-linked Mendelian dominant." In the cases he reported, there were no other abnormalities.

The author of this book saw a young boy with bilateral flexion contracture of the four ulnar digits at the metacarpophalangeal joints. He also had simian crease in both palms. His mother and her sister had typical Dupuytren contracture of both hands. The contracture of the fingers of the boy had been present since birth but had become progressively worse. Upon passive extension of the

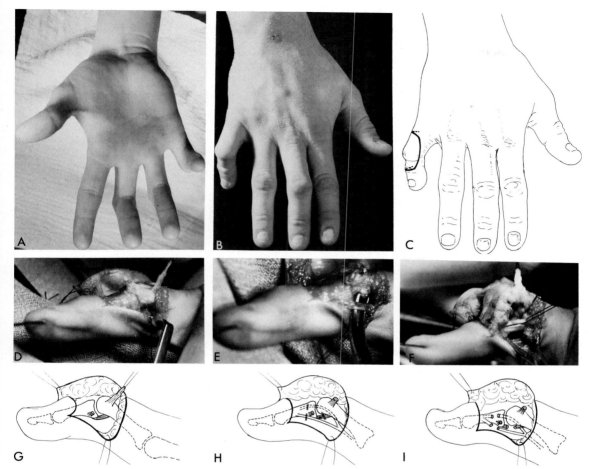

Figure 17-20 Exploration of the first interphalangeal joint of the little finger and severance of the contracted structures. *A*, Palmar view of the right hand of the son featured in Figure 17–19; his main complaint was difficulty in inserting his hand into a glove. *B*, Dorsal view. *C*, Sketch illustrating the incision for elevation of a horseshoe-shaped flap over the little finger which would afford access to both sides of the first interphalangeal joint of the little finger and at the same time expose the points of insertion of both slips of the sublimis tendon. *D*, Detachment of the radial collateral ligament from its insertion into the volar base of the second phalanx of the little finger. *E*, Isolation of the volar capsule which was severed. *F*, Isolation of the radial slip of the sublimis of the little finger which was cut. *G*, *H*, and *I* illustrate severance of both collateral ligaments and volar capsule of the first interphalangeal joint of the little finger as well as detachment of both slips of the sublimis tendon. These measures resulted in sufficient correction of the flexion deformity of the little finger to enable the patient to wear a glove. Slight residual flexion deformity remained.

fingers, taut cords overlying the palmar aponeurosis could be seen and felt. The contracted palmar fascia was extirpated in both hands (Figs. 17–21 to 17–23).

CONGENITAL ULNAR DRIFT OF THE DIGITS (La Déviation Congénitale des Doigts en Coup de Vent; Windmühlenflugelstellung; Windmill-Vane Hand)

In this anomaly, all fingers and sometimes the thumb are deviated toward the ulnar border of the hand and show varying degrees of subluxation at the

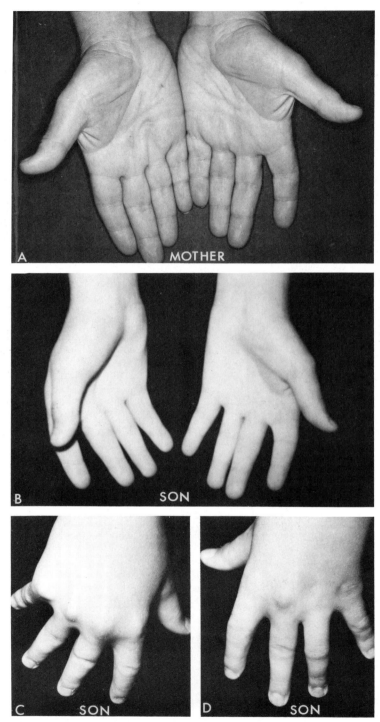

Figure 17–21 Congenital Dupuytren's contracture: mother-to-son transmission. *A,* Palmar view of the mother's hands. She had a sister who had been operated on for Dupuytren's contracture. *B,* Palmar view of the hands of her 10-year-old son who had had flexion contractures of the fingers at the metacarpophalangeal joints since birth and simian creases of the palms. *C* and *D,* Dorsal view of the son's hands.

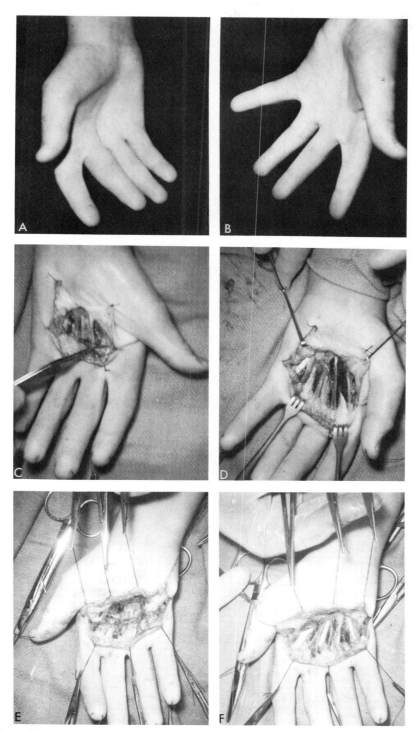

Figure 17–22 *A* and *B*, Palmar view of the hands of the boy shown in Figure 17–21 at the age of 13 years. *C*, Exposure of the palmaris fascia of the left hand. *D*, Extirpation of the palmaris fascia of the left hand. *E*, Exposure of the palmaris fascia of the right hand. *F*, Extirpation of the same.

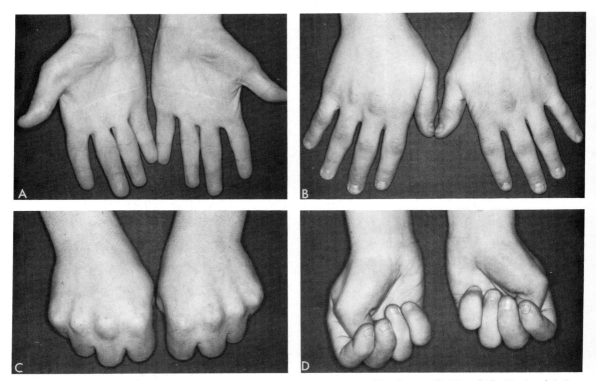

Figure 17–23   Results of the surgery on the hands of the boy featured in Figures 17–21 and 17–22. *A* and *B*, Postoperative palmar and dorsal views of the hands with fingers in extension. *C* and *D*, Dorsal and palmar views of the clenched fists.

metacarpophalangeal joints. The deformity simulates that of advanced rheumatoid arthritis, but the joints remain unaffected except in older patients. The ulnar drift of the digits is often noticed at birth but becomes progressively more pronounced as the child grows. In most reported cases, both hands are involved. The familial tendency has been recorded by Boix (1897), Lundblom (1932), and others. For correction of the deformity, the following measures are recommended: (1) corrective splints; (2) excision of ulnar capsules and collateral ligaments of the metacarpophalangeal joints; (3) tenotomy of the first lumbrical and third and fourth dorsal interossei, which, respectively, connect with the ulnar sides of the extensor expansions of the index, middle, and ring fingers, and tenotomy of the abductor of the fifth digit; (4) replacement of the displaced extensor tendons over the backs of the metacarpal heads and reconstruction of fascial retinaculae to hold these tendons in place; (5) corrective subcapital osteotomy of the metacarpal bones. Osteotomy of the proximal phalanges or metacarpals or both has given the present author the most enduring results (Figs. 17–24 to 17–26).

ASSOCIATIONS

Digital misalignments are often seen in connection with such local or regional anomalies of the hand and forearm as the following: brachydactyly,

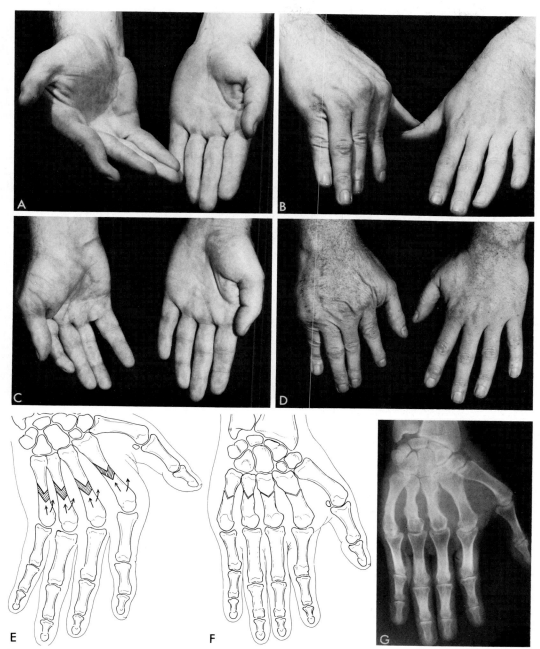

Figure 17–24 Unilateral congenital ulnar drift of the fingers with flexion contracture—treated by recession and angulation osteotomy of the metacarpals. *A*, Preoperative palmar view of the hands of a 21-year-old male who, besides the malformed right hand, had a white flock of hair on the ipsilateral aspect of the head. *B*, Preoperative dorsal view. *C* and *D*, Postoperative palmar and dorsal views. *E* and *F*, Sketches illustrating recession angulation osteotomy of ulnar four metacarpals. *G*, Dorsopalmar roentgenograph of the right hand taken a year after surgery.

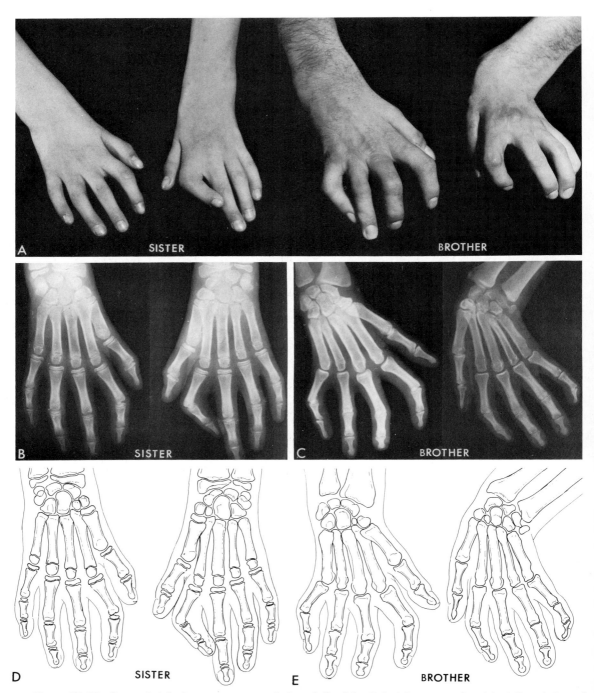

Figure 17–25 Congenital flexion contracture and ulnar drift of the digits (clinocamptodactyly). *A*, Dorsal view of the hands of an 11-year-old female juxtaposed with the same view of the hands of an older brother. *B*, Dorsopalmar roentgenograph of the sister's hands. *C*, Dorsopalmar roentgenograph of the brother's hands. *D* and *E* illustrate the roentgenograph above each. The parents were unaffected; they were not consanguineous.

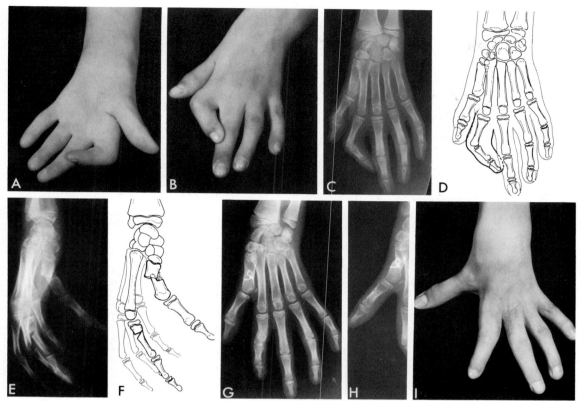

Figure 17–26 Surgical correction of the malformed left hand of the sister featured in Figure 17–25. *A* and *B*, Preoperative palmar and dorsal views of the left hand. *C*, Dorsopalmar roentgenograph. *D*, Sketch illustrating the same. *E*, Lateral roentgenograph soon after peg-and-hole osteotomy of the first metacarpal and open-wedge osteotomy of the proximal phalanx of the index finger. *F*, Sketch illustrating the same. *G*, Postoperative dorsopalmar roentgenograph showing sufficient abduction of the thumb. *H*, Dorsopalmar view of the pollical ray after an adequate abduction osteotomy of the first metacarpal. *I*, Final result after repair of partial syndactyly between the index and middle fingers.

syndactyly, polydactyly, mirror hand, hyperphalangism, split hand complex, annular grooves and acral absences, which have already been discussed, and macrodactyly, angiodysplastic deformities (Klippel-Trénaunay syndrome), and radial and ulnar defects, which will be taken up in subsequent chapters. Mention has already been made of the proximal placement of the thumb in DeLange dwarfs, hitchhiker's thumb in craniosynostosis (Pfeiffer syndrome), diastrophic dwarfism, achondroplasia, and axial deviation of one of the central digits in multiple exostoses. The ensuing sections are devoted to other syndromes in which the digits assume anomalous postures.

ABSENT TIBIA AND CAMPTODACTYLY

A female child with total absence of one tibia and flexion contracture of the digits of both hands came under the author's care. As she grew, she developed a tilted pelvis and lumbar scoliosis, which may have been due to the marked discrepancy of length between the normal and defective lower limbs. Her family history was not revealing (Fig. 17–27).

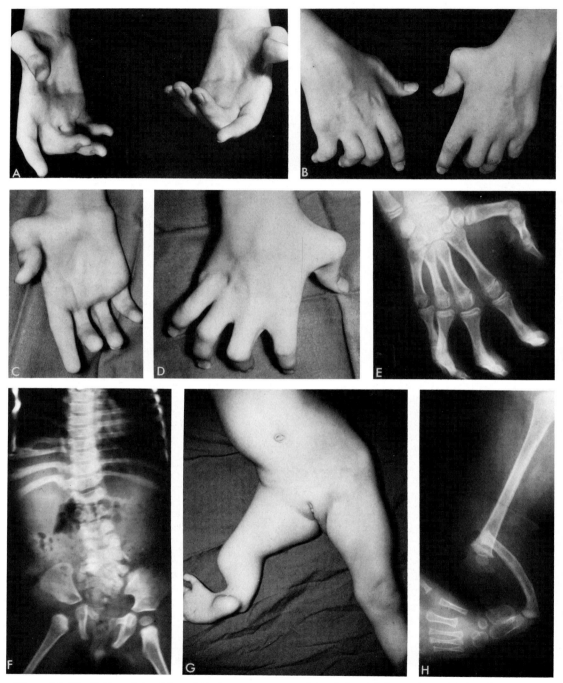

Figure 17–27   Defect of the tibia and flexion contractures of the digits. *A*, Palmar view of the hands of an 11-year-old female with absent right tibia: note the subluxation of the thumbs at the metacarpophalangeal joints. *B*, Dorsal view of the same. *C*, Palmar view of the right hand — enlarged. *D*, Dorsal view of the same. *E*, Dorsopalmar roentgenograph of the right hand. *F*, Anteroposterior roentgenograph of the spine and pelvis shows agenesis of femoral head on the right side, scoliosis, and spina bifida of the lumbar vertebrae. *G*, Frontal view of the affected right lower limb. *H*, Roentgenograph of the right lower limb.

ABDUCTION DEFORMITY OF THE THUMBS ASSOCIATED WITH BILATERAL HALLUX VARUS

Christian et al (1972) reported a family in which eight members of four generations had short thumbs and short toes with abduction deformity of these digits. The pre-axial brachydactyly was due mainly to the shortness of the first metacarpals and first metatarsals. The ungual phalanges were also dwarfed. The proximal phalanges were normal. The trait was transmitted as an autosomal dominant.

AMINOACIDURIA AND TAURINURIA CUM CAMPTODACTYLY

Parish et al (1963) described a family in which 10 females in three generations manifested aminoaciduria and had flexion contractures ("streblodactyly") of the fingers. Nevin et al (1966) noted the association of taurinuria and flexion contracture of the fingers.

ARTHROGRYPOSIS MULTIPLEX CONGENITA (Amyoplasia Congenita; Pterygomyodysplasia; Myodystrophia Fetalis; Multiple Congenital Articular Rigidity)

This disorder shows distinct predilection for the extremities. It may involve one, two, or all four limbs. Muscles are either absent or replaced by fibrous tissue; the joints are stiff; the bones are thin and misaligned. Derangement of the muscles is regarded as primary and deformities as secondary.

Arthrogryposis has been identified antepartum by Sheldon (1932) and more recently by Epstein (1961). It is apparent at birth. Although familial cases and occurrences in monozygotic twins have been reported, the genetic background remains obscure. Swinyard and Magora (1962) reported a kindred in which arthrogryposis was transmitted as a dominant trait. Weissman et al. (1963) described an Arab family with six affected members of both sexes. In this kinship consanguineous marriages were very common, and Weissman and colleagues thought the trait was inherited by a simple recessive gene. Wright and Aase (1969) reported an autosomal dominant form of arthrogryposis in an Alaskan Eskimo family. Most reported cases of arthrogryposis have been sporadic. Drachman and Banker (1961) conducted necropsy study of a case, and noted degeneration and loss of motor neurons with reduction in the spinal cord size and mild increases in glial elements in the anterior horns.

In the upper extremity, the following abnormalities have been reported: webbing of the axilla and antecubital area; stiff, unbending elbows; dislocation of the radial head; and anomalous posture of the digits. The thumb helplessly

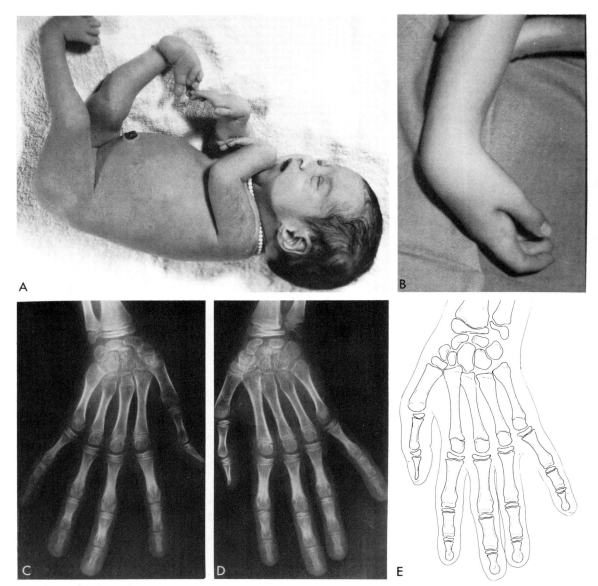

Figure 17–28   Arthrogryposis. *A*, Left profile view of a newborn female infant. *B*, Radial view of the right wrist and hand, showing persistent contracture after six years of intermittent splintage. *C* and *D*, Dorsopalmar roentgenographs of the hands taken at the age of 11 years; the tubular bones, especially the proximal phalanges, have constricted shafts and bulbous articular ends; the radial epiphysis is flat. *E*, Sketch illustrating the roentgenograph of the left hand.

drops into the palm, and it cannot voluntarily be abducted or extended. On surgical exploration, one often finds the extensors and long abductor of the thumb missing; the extensors of the wrist are represented by attenuated fibrous bands. The carpal bones become fused in due course of time (Figs. 17–28 to 17–31).

    The treatment in the early stages of arthrogryposis consists of manipulation of the thumb and wrist followed by retentive night splint. The first webspace

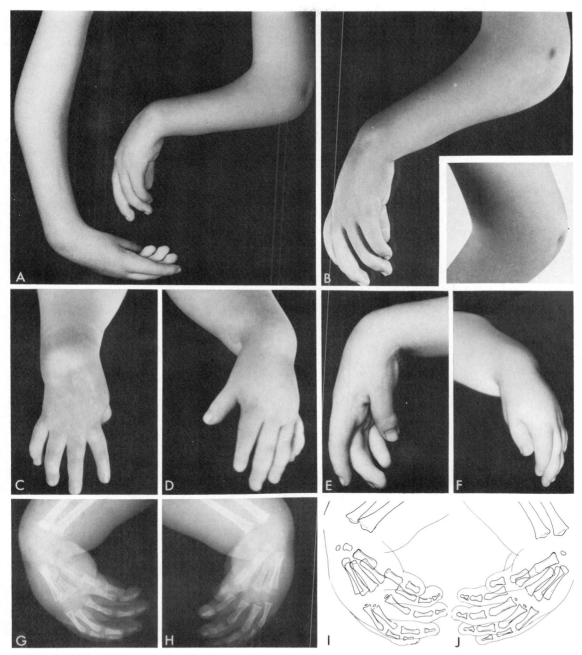

Figure 17–29   Arthrogryposis with pterygium anticubiti, dimple over the ulnar aspect of the left elbow, flexion contracture of both wrists, flexed, adducted thumbs, and flexed fingers. *A*, Ulnar view of the upper limbs of a six-month-old male. *B*, Dimple on the ulnar aspect of the left elbow. *C* and *D*, Dorsal views of the right and left hands. *E* and *F*, Radial views of the right and left hands. *G* and *H*, Lateral roentgenographs of the right and left hands. *I* and *J*, Sketch illustrating the same.

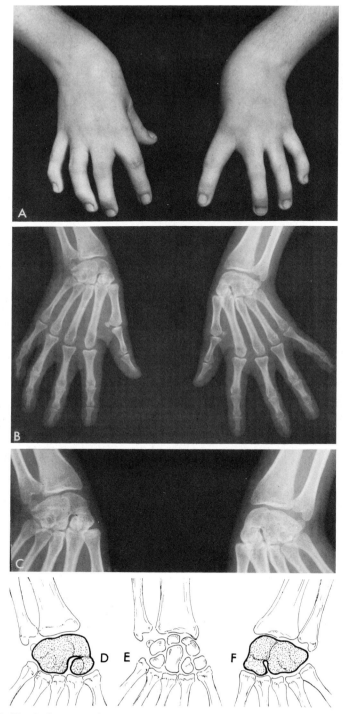

Figure 17–30   Arthrogryposis associated with massive carpal coalescence. *A*, Dorsal view of the hands of a 17-year-old female. *B*, Dorsopalmar roentgenograph of the same. *C*, Enlarged roentgenograph of the wrists, showing massive fusion of all carpal ossicles. *D* and *F* illustrate roentgenograph above each. *E*, Sketch illustrating carpal ossicles of the right wrist of a normal female of the same age—used here for contrast.

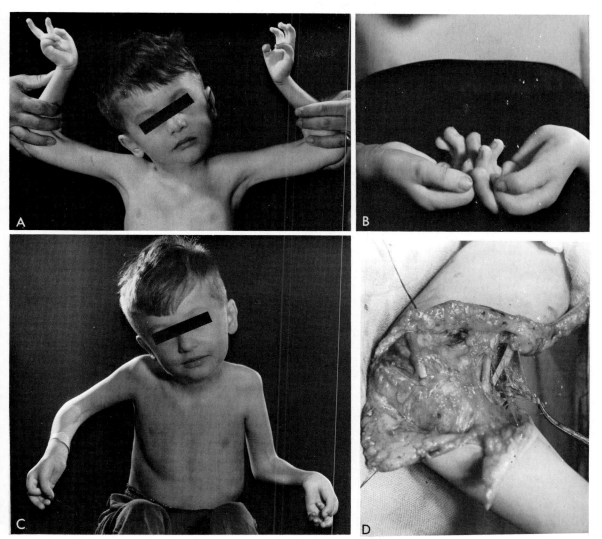

Figure 17–31 Arthrogryposis with pterygium anticubiti and digital contractures. *A*, Frontal view of a four-year-old male: the elbows could not be extended, even passively. *B*, Radial view of the hands. *C*, Frontal view after Z-plasty of the right cubital fossa and anterior capsulotomy of the elbow. *D*, Surgical exposure of the cubital fossa showing stringy adhesions around the median and ulnar nerves and also around the tendon of the biceps muscle.

may be widened by either Z-plasty or flap graft; tendon transplants have been attempted and found useless. Osteotomy of the first metacarpal and distal radius is at times indicated. After osteotomy, the thumb and the wrist are placed in functional position. At about the age of 12, the patient's thumb may be stabilized either by carpometacarpal fusion or with the aid of an intermetacarpal bone block. When both elbows are fused in extension, one of them may have to be resected and placed in flexion to enable the patient to feed himself. Arthrodesis of the wrist joint is delayed until the closure of the distal radial epiphysis (Figs. 17–32 to 17–34).

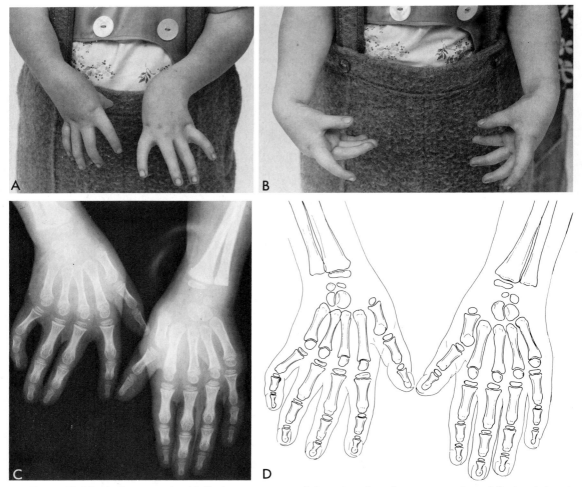

Figure 17–32   Arthrogryposis with flexion contracture of the wrists, short first metacarpals, and flexion deformity of the digits. *A*, Dorsal view of the forearms and wrists of a four-year-old female. *B*, Radial view of the same. *C*, Dorsopalmar roentgenograph of the right and left hands. *D*, Sketch illustrating the same.

CHONDRODYSTROPHIA CALCIFICANS
CONGENITA (Dysplasia Epiphysealis Punctata; Conradi's Disease; Conradi-Hunermann Syndrome; Stippled Epiphyses; CCC)

Conradi (1914) identified this disorder roentgenographically. Hunermann (1931) gave it its present name. Fairbank (1951) likened the roentgenographic appearance of affected epiphyses to the "flicking of paint from a brush onto a clean surface." These spots are interpreted as nests of degenerated cartilage cells which have become impregnated with calcium; they lack trabecular pattern and disappear within two or three years if the infant survives. Very few subjects have survived and reached the age of maturity. The surviving child becomes a short-limbed dwarf with congenital cataract, saddle nose, whorls of hyperemic keratosis of the skin, and early flexion contracture of joints, including the elbows, wrists, and joints of the hands.

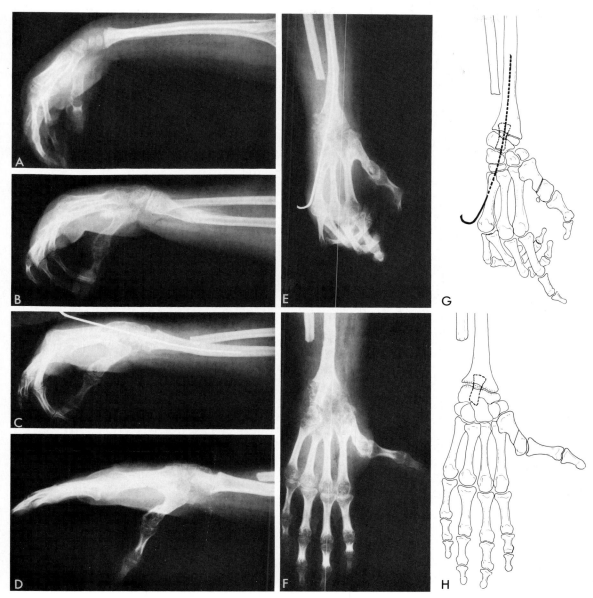

Figure 17–33 Procedures utilized for the correction of the deformity of the wrists and hands of the female arthrogrypotic featured in Figure 17–32. *A*, Radial roentgenograph of the right forearm and the hand taken at the age of four. *B*, Osteotomy of the distal radius after attempt at dorsal wedge resection of the carpus failed to correct the deformity. *C*, At the age of eight, the first metacarpal was subjected to extension-abduction osteotomy; at 12 years of age, fusion of the first carpometacarpal joint was performed and at 14 the wrist was fused. *D*, Postoperative lateral roentgenograph. *E*, Oblique view showing K-wire passing through the fourth metacarpal, through the bone graft (which was taken from the distal ulna and doweled into the radius and then into the carpus), into the radial shaft. *F*, Postoperative dorsopalmar roentgenograph. *G* and *H* illustrate the roentgenograph adjacent to each. The left wrist was similarly treated except that the thumb was not fused; instead, the flexor carpi ulnaris was utilized to reinforce the weak extensors and long abductor of the left thumb; this did not help much; finally, the first carpometacarpal joint of this hand was fused.

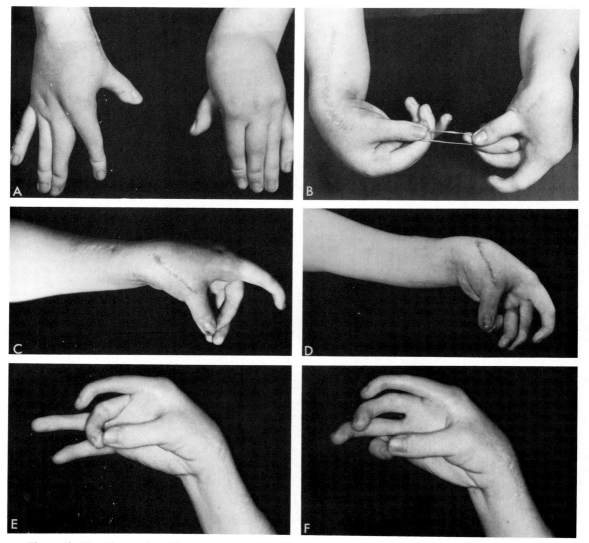

Figure 17–34   The results of the procedures utilized for the treatment of arthrogrypotic wrists and hands. *A*, Dorsal view of the hands after osteotomy of the distal radius, osteotomy of the first metacarpal, fusion of the first metacarpophalangeal joint of the right hand, and osteotomy of the left radius. *B*, Radial view after attempted reinforcement of extensors and long abductor of the left thumb with transferred flexor carpi ulnaris. *C* and *D*, Radial views of the left wrist and hand after fusion of the first carpometacarpal joint. *E* and *F*, Radiovolar views of the right wrist and hand after fusion of the radiocarpal joint.

CHROMOSOMAL ABERRATIONS

In trisomy 13-15 or D, described by Patau et al (1960), the affected child held both of the thumbs flexed and, upon passive extension, two "small clicks" were felt on the volar aspect of the metacarpophalangeal joint. In trisomy 16-18 or E, described by Edwards .et al (1960), there was flexion contracture and overlapping of the fingers. The patient with trisomy 17-18 reported by Wender et al (1965) had "retroflexed" thumb. Lindenbaum and Butler (1971) described a male neonate with group B (4-5) long arm deletion and multiple congenital anomalies, including short arms, ulnar angulation of the wrists, and grossly deviated little fingers.

CONGENITAL ANALGESIA

In this syndrome, partly described in previous chapters, there is insensitivity to pain, and the joints, including those of the forearm and the hand, often undergo neuropathic distortions. The metacarpophalangeal joints of the fingers often become swollen, allowing limited flexion; the distal joints are hyperextensible. When extended and spread out, the fingers simulate swan-neck deformity (Fig. 17–35).

CONGENITAL CONTRACTURAL ARACHNODACTYLY

Under this heading, Beals and Hecht (1971) described a female whose fingers and toes were long, thin, and incurving; her external ears had a crumpled appearance. These anomalies had been present since birth. At twenty-two months, her fingers became definitely flexed and her thumb tended to stay in the palm. She did not have ectopia lentis or any of the cardiovascular insignia of Marfan s arachnodactyly.

CRANIOCARPOTARSAL DYSTROPHY
(Freeman-Sheldon Syndrome; Whistling Face Syndrome; Cheiro-Cheilo-Podac Syndrome; Whistling Face-Windmill Vane Syndrome)

Freeman and Sheldon (1938) described two children—a male and a female. The probands were not related but came from the same town. Both children were firstborn in their respective families; they were born prematurely—one at seven and a half months and the other at eight months. Both were underweight at birth. Each child possessed prominent frontal bones, eyes that were sunken and widely separated, a narrow nose, and a small, puckered mouth. The hands were deviated in the ulnar direction; the feet were clubbed. Otto (1953) described a small girl with the same facial characteristics and flexion contracture of the fingers.

Burian (1963) reported four youngsters with what he called "whistling face." Each boy or girl had deeply set eyes, convergent squint, a small nose, and a small oral aperture. The upper extremities were lean and had flabby musculature; joint motion was restricted. The photograph of a pair of hands showed ulnar deviation of the fingers at the metacarpophalangeal joints and flexion contracture at the interphalangeal articulations. Analogous cases have been described by Rintala (1968), Walker (1969), Pitanguy and Bosaggio (1969), Weinstein and Gorlin (1969), Cervenka et al (1969, 1970), Sharma and Tandon (1970), Fraser et al (1970), and Gross-Kieselstein et al (1971). The trait is transmitted as an autosomal dominant. A young boy came under the author's care with characteristic facial features (flattened face, sunken eyes, hypertelorism, narrow nostrils, long filtrum, and small mouth) and flexion contracture of the wrists and digits (Fig. 17–36).

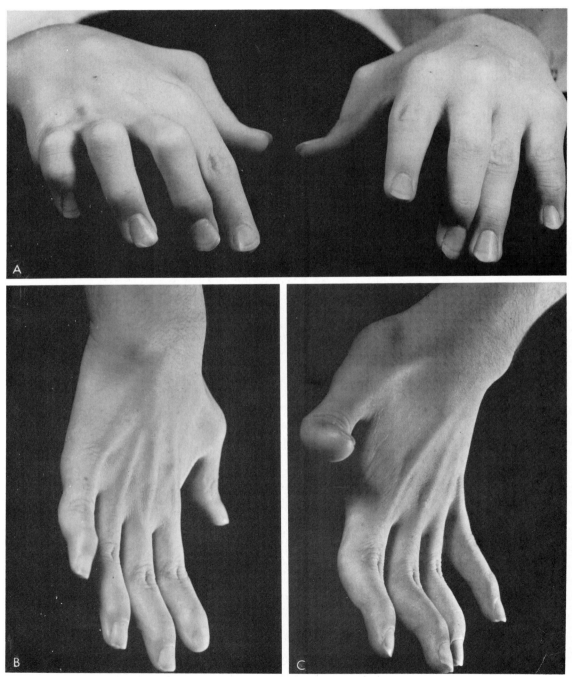

Figure 17–35 Anomalies of digital posture consequential to congenital analgesia for pain. *A*, Dorsal view of the hands of a male adolescent, born of a first cousin marriage. *B* and *C*, Swan-neck deformity.

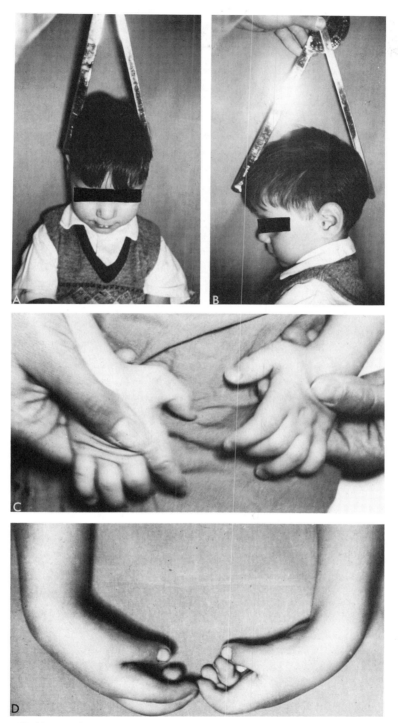

Figure 17–36 Craniocarpotarsal dystrophy. *A*, Frontal view of the head, showing diminished bitemporal span of the skull and "whistling face" of a six-year-old boy. *B*, Profile: the fronto-occipital span of the calvarium is proportionately long. *C*, Dorsal view of the hands with flexion contracture of the wrists and the digits. *D*, Radial view of the wrists and the hands.

DIGITO-TALAR DYSMORPHISM

Sallis and Beighton (1972) described a kindred, the affected members of which presented the following features: flexion deformities, narrowing and ulnar deviation of the fingers, and rocker-bottom feet due to vertical talus. In some cases, the thumb was rotated in an ulnar direction and its movements were limited by a "fleshy web." The trait was transmitted as an autosomal dominant.

EMERY-NELSON SYNDROME

Emery and Nelson (1970) described a mother and daughter with short stature, characteristic facies (high forehead, depressed nasal bridge, long filtrum, flattened malar region), small hands, flexion deformity of the first three metacarpophalangeal joints, and extension at the interphalangeal articulation of the thumbs.

FACULTATIVE CAMPTODACTYLY

Hecht and Beals (1969) presented a father and his six children who were moderate dwarfs and could not open their mouths fully. They also had facultative camptodactyly (the fingers remained flexed when the wrist was extended and they could only be extended when the wrist was flexed). Hecht and Beals ascribed this phenomenon to the short flexors in the forearm.

HYDROCEPHALUS AND IRREDUCIBLE FLEXION-ADDUCTION DEFORMITY OF THE THUMB

Gilly et al (1971) described a family in which five boys had congenital hydrocephalus and bilateral flexion-adduction contracture of the thumb. These authors reviewed 16 other families with 69 affected males which had been reported in the literature. The trait is transmitted as an X-linked recessive.

KLIPPEL-FEIL SYNDROME

The basic disturbance in this well-known complex consists of anomalous segmentation of the thoracocervical vertebral column—two or more vertebrae are fused together. There is low implantation of the hairline of the nape; the neck is short, giving the impression that the head is directly connected with the trunk. Bauman's (1932) patient with Klippel-Feil syndrome manifested "marked mirror movements in the hands." The patient reported by Erskine (1946) presented "bimanual synkinesia." A similar case came under the author's care. Another patient, a teenage female, did not show mirror movements of the hands but had flexion contracture of the left little finger which, according to the parents, had been present since birth (Figs. 17–37 and 17–38).

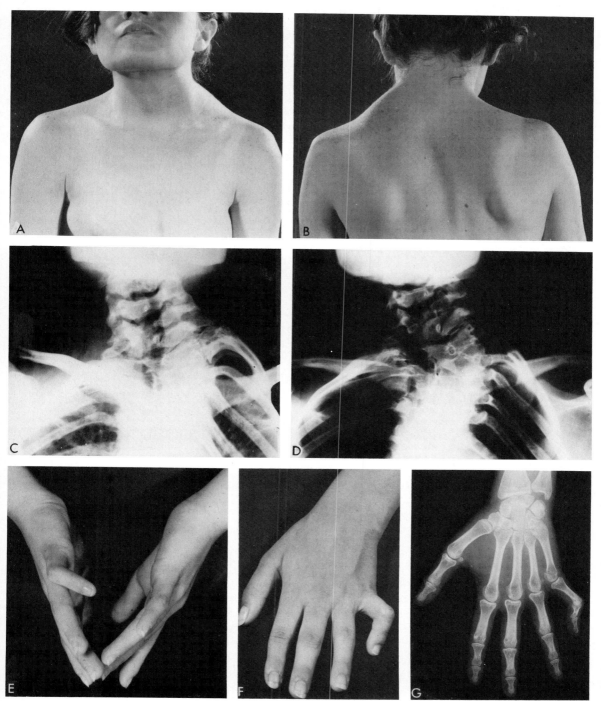

Figure 17–37 Klippel-Feil syndrome with high-riding left first rib and flexion contracture of the left little finger at the first interphalangeal joint. *A*, Frontal view of the neck of a 13-year-old female. *B*, Dorsal view. *C*, Preoperative anteroposterior roentgenograph of the cervicothoracic region. *D*, The same after excision of the medial, domed portion of the first rib. *E*, Ulnar view of both hands. *F*, Dorsal view of the left hand. *G*, Dorsopalmar roentgenograph of the same.

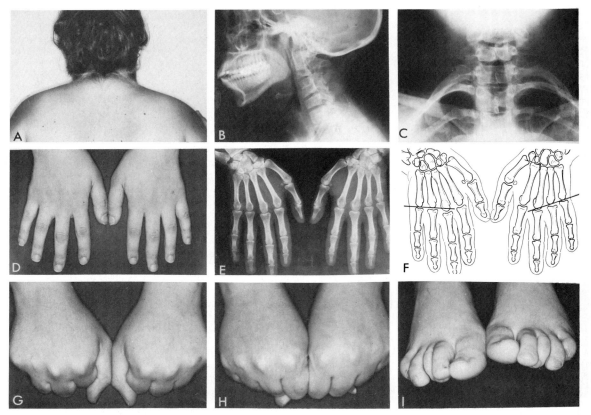

Figure 17–38   Klippel-Feil syndrome with mirror image movements of the digits. *A*, View of the nape. *B*, Lateral roentgenograph of the cervical spine, showing fusion of the upper cervical vertebrae. *C*, Anteroposterior roentgenograph of the neck, showing spina bifida of the lower cervical vertebrae. *D*, Dorsal view of the hands with extended digits. *E*, Dorsopalmar roentgenograph showing discernibly dwarfed fourth and fifth metacarpals of both hands. *F*, Sketch illustrating the same. *G* and *H*, Mirror image effect produced by clenched fists. *I*, Bilateral curling of the third toes.

LERI'S PLEONOSTEOSIS

In compounding this term, Léri (1921) made use of the Greek root *pleon* which means *plenty*. The patient he reported was a middle-aged man. He had two children — a daughter and a son, aged four and three years, respectively. The father was short in stature and had dwarfed spadelike hands with thick palmar pads and accentuated flexion creases. His thumbs were massive, knobby; his fingers were short and thick and flexed to almost 90 degrees at the interphalangeal joints. The movements of the wrists were slightly limited; the forearms were pronated, and the elbows could not be fully extended. X-rays of the father's and daughter's hands showed thickening of all bones and lack of construction of metacarpal and phalangeal midshafts. Léri (1922, 1924) singled out the following as the main features of this syndrome: short stature; short, thick hands; broad thumbs; flexion contractures of the fingers; and generalized limitation of joint motion. He considered this complex to be a systemic, congenital, hereditary disorder. The contractural aspect of this disorder was emphasized again by Léri (1926).

MARFAN'S ARACHNODACTYLY
(Dolichostomely; Dystrophia Mesodermalis Typus Marfanis; Hyperchondrodysplasia)

Full-fledged Marfan syndrome presents the following features: long, thin skeletal framework involving especially the bones of the limbs; lax joints and underdeveloped, feeble musculature; scant subcutaneous fat; cardiovascular abnormalities, consisting of patent foramen ovale, dilatation of the heart, diffuse or dissecting aneurysm involving, in particular, the ascending aorta; dislocation of the lenses; and preponderance in females, with autosomal dominant inheritance and high grade penetrance. As in other genetically determined traits, the manifestations of Marfan syndrome vary in extent and intensity. Formes frustes have been reported within the same family. In a number of reported cases, the digits have been described as having assumed anomalous postures not unlike those seen in arthrogryposis.

The fingers of patients with Marfan syndrome, besides being slender and long, are deficient in muscular power. In the original case described by Marfan (1896), there was a flexion contracture of the fingers. Later authors have ascribed this deformity to the comparative weakness of the extensors; the fingers may eventually undergo fixed contractures. In the case reported by Thomas (1914), the thumbs could not be actively abducted. The child described by Thursfield (1917) was unable to effect extension of the thumb. Kingsley-Pillers (1946) reported a case in which stiff, contracted joints coexisted with long, slender fingers. Reeve et al (1960) described an infant with findings of both Marfan syndrome and arthrogryposis. Analogous cases have also been reported by Udani (1955) and Grenier et al (1969). Bercu (1966) reported a patient with dislocation of the thumb at the carpometacarpal joint (Fig. 17–39).

MUCOPOLYSACCHARIDOSES

In various forms of mucopolysaccharide storage disorders—described by Hunter (1917), Hurler (1919), Morquio (1929), Brailsford (1929), Scheie et al (1962), Sanfilippo et al (1963), and Maroteaux and Lamy (1965)—the digits undergo varying degrees of contractural changes. In one of the cases presented by Scheie et al, there was a fusiform swelling and ankylosis in flexion position of the middle and distal interphalangeal joints of the hands, synovial thickening of the wrists, atrophy of the thenar eminence on both sides, and limited adduction of the thumbs; the radii were short and the skin over the hands was bound to the underlying structure. In another case, roentgenographic examination of the hands showed soft-tissue swelling around the interphalangeal joints; the radius was defective at its carpal end, and the metacarpals appeared hypoplastic. Winchester et al (1969) described two siblings with mucopolysaccharidosis. The younger sibling presented marked destructive changes in the joints of the hands and the wrists, and the older child's hands revealed "relentless progression of the process" resembling changes caused by fulminant rheumatoid arthritis. The cases reported by Lyon et al (1971) had flexion contracture of the fingers and resembled Scheie mucopolysaccharidosis.

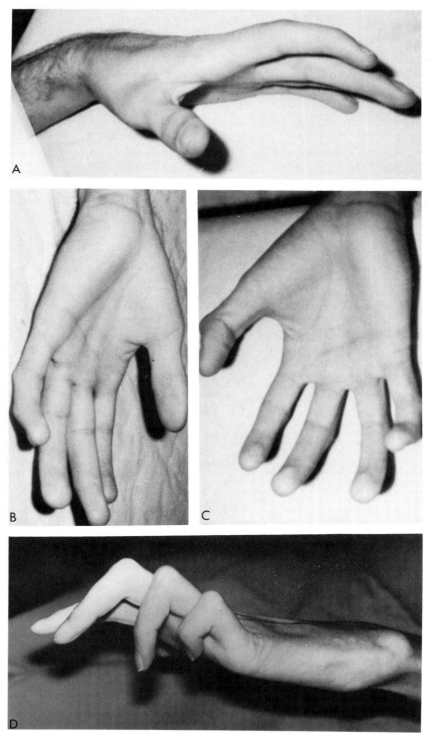

Figure 17–39   Marfan's syndrome with contractural arachnodactyly. *A*, Radial view of the left hand of an adult male. *B*, Palmar view of the same. *C*, Palmar view of the right hand. *D*, Ulnar view of the left hand of a 16-year-old female with contractural arachnodactyly incident to Marfan's syndrome.

MULTIFOCAL FIBROSCLEROSIS

Cumings et al (1967) described two male siblings with mediastinal and retroperitoneal fibrosis, sclerosing cholangitis, and sclerosing thyroiditis. One sibling had fibrotic contractures of the fingers. The parents were first cousins. The trait is regarded as an autosomal recessive.

OCULODIGITAL COMPLEXES

Koby (1923) reported a man with camptodactyly of the left little finger. His daughter and her child were affected by cataracts. Lowry et al (1971) reported two siblings with the following abnormalities: cataract, microcephaly, kyphosis, and congenital clasped thumb. The photograph of one child showed "persistent fisting with adduction of the thumb."

Lenz (1955) reported a boy with unilateral microphthalmia and ulnar deviation of the little finger. Betetto's (1958) patient with bilateral microphthalmia had camptodactyly of the right hand, "perodactyly," and syndactyly of the left hand.

Oculo-dento-digital dysplasia has already been discussed in Chapter Twelve. It is manifested as microphthalmos, missing teeth or small teeth with defective enamel, camptodactyly of the little finger, or syndactyly of the fourth and fifth digits, in which instance the longer ring finger is pulled in an ulnar direction by the short little finger.

ORO-DIGITAL COMPLEX

Juberg and Hayward (1969) described a complex consisting of cleft lip-palate together with microphthalmos and an underdeveloped, distally positioned thumb. The affected thumbs were hypoplastic and lacked muscular control, failing to effect flexion at the interphalangeal joints. Gordon et al (1969) noted the association of camptodactyly, club foot, and cleft palate.

OTODIGITAL COMPLEX

Stewart and Bergstrom (1971) described a family in which "arthrogryposis-like" contracture of the digits has been transmitted through seven generations as an autosomal dominant trait with penetrance and variable expressivity. Seven out of twelve affected individuals had sensorineural deafness.

RUBENSTEIN-TAYBI SYNDROME

Sinnette and Odeku (1968) described an African child with broad thumb–big toe complex. The thumbs were abducted and extended, simulating hitchhiker's position (Fig. 17–40).

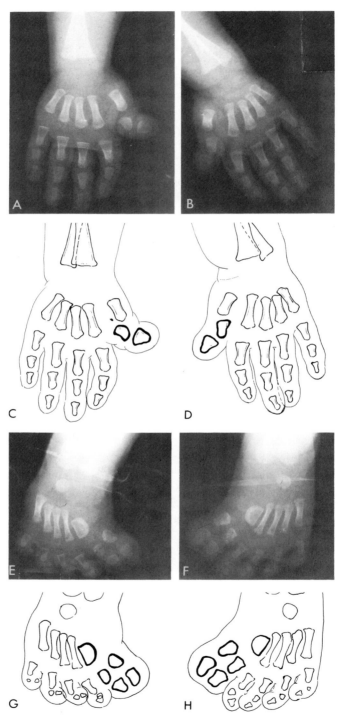

Figure 17–40   Rubinstein-Taybi syndrome. *A* and *B*, Dorsopalmar roentgenographs of the right and left hands of a neonate with hitchhiker's thumb. *C* and *D* illustrate the roentgenograph above each. *E* and *F*, Dorsoplantar roentgenographs of the right and left feet. *G* and *H* illustrate roentgenograph above each.

SUBLUXATION OF THE KNEE AND CAMPTODACTYLY

Murphy (1926) studied a family in which many members of five generations had flexion contracture of the fingers. Eleven of the affected individuals had recurrent subluxation of the knee.

SUMMARY

The marginal digits—the thumb and the little finger, the latter more commonly than the former—assume anomalous postures most often. Of the central digits, the index is affected more often than the ring finger; the middle or axial finger is rarely involved by itself. Adduction-flexion deformity of the thumb occurs as an isolated entity. It is also seen in cases of arthrogryposis, in association with congenital cataract, in Marfan's arachnodactyly, and in chromosomal aberrations. Hitchhiker's thumb occurs as an isolated entity and in cases of triphalangeal thumb when an extra bone has a broad ulnar base; it is also known to occur in craniosynostosis (Pfeiffer syndrome), diastrophic dwarfism, Rubenstein-Taybi syndrome, and in association with hallux varus.

The thumb is proximally placed in de Lange degeneration, and it is distally positioned in Juberg-Hayward orodigital complex. Flexion contracture of the fingers is a feature of absent tibia–camptodactyly complex, arthrogryposis, congenital contractural arachnodactyly, cranio-carpo-tarsal dystrophy, and facultative camptodactyly complex. It is also seen in connection with congenital cataract, mucopolysaccharidoses, and trisomy 16-18.

Misalignments of the little finger only occasionally necessitate surgical interference. The converse holds true for the anomalous postures of the thumb. Postural anomalies of the digits due to skeletal abnormalities are treated by surgery on bones, usually corrective osteotomy, while those resulting from soft-tissue derangement are redressed by appropriate procedures on muscles, tendons, fascial bands, and the skin. In many instances, one needs to combine surgery on soft tissues with operations on bones.

References

Adams, W.: On congenital contraction of the fingers and its association with "hammer toe," its pathology and treatment. *Lancet, 2*:165–168, 1891.

Allan, W.: Inheritance of short finger tendons. *J. Hered., 30*:218, 1939.

Allaria, A.: Assenza congenita bilaterale dell' estensione del pollice. *Chir. Organi. Mov., 43*:423–426, 1956.

Anderson, W.: Contractions of fingers and toes; their varieties, pathology and treatment. *Lancet, 2*:107–111, 161–163, 213–215, 279–282, 1891.

Anderson, W. E.: Camptodactylia (Landouzy) with other naevi. *Br. J. Dermatol., 65*:410–411, 1953.

Ashley, L. M.: Inheritance of streblomicrodactyly. *J. Hered., 38*:93–96, 1947.

Avendano, A., and Fanta, E.: Aracnodactilia y artrogriposis. Relato de un caso en un lactante con asociacion de ambas enfermedades. *Pediatria* (Santiago), *6*:47–54, 1963.

Babonneix, L.: Flexion permanente des doigts chex une enfant de 14 ans. *Bull. Soc. Pediatr.* (Paris), *9*:194, 1907.

Barinka, L.: Kamptodactylia. *Acta Chir. Orthop. Traum.* (Praha), *28*:279–289, 1961.

Barinka, L.: Camptodactylia (a preliminary communication). *Acta Chir. Plast.* (Praha), *6*:54–60, 1964.

Barinka, L.: Notes on camptodactylia (second communication). *Acta Chir. Plast.* (Praha), *6*:154–161, 1964.

Barletta, P. P. A.: Campilodactilia. *La Prensa Med.* (Argentina), *46*:758–760, 1959.

Bauman, G. I.: Absence of the cervical spine. Klippel-Feil syndrome. *J.A.M.A., 98*:129–132, 1932.

Beals, R. K., and Hecht, F.: Congenital contractural arachnodactyly. *J. Bone Joint Surg., 53A*:987–993, 1971.

Beck, W.: Die Angeborene Daumenkontraktur. *Arch. Orthop. Unfallchir., 40*:318–325, 1940.

Bercu, G.: Erblichkeitsfaktor beim Marfan-syndrom. *Fortschr. Röntgenstr., 104*:820–825, 1966.

Betetto, G.: Microftalmia e malformazioni della ditta. *Ann. Oftal., 84*:368–381, 1958.

Birnhacher, G.: *Drei Beobachtungen über Verkummerung der oberon Extremitäten.* Inaug. Diss. Konigsberg, R. Loupold, pp. 1–29, 1891.

Boerema, I.: Über die angeborene "Windmühlenflügelstellung" der Finger ("deviation des doigts en coup de vent"). *A. Orthop. Chir., 55*:241–249, 1931.

Boix, E.: Déviation des doigts en coup de vent et insuffisance de l'aponévrose palmaire d'origine congénitale. *N. Iconog. Salp., 10*:180–194; pl. XX, 1897.

Boppe, M., and Faugeron, P.: La deviation congénitale des doigts "en coup de vent." *Rev. d'Orthop., 26*:547–557, 1939.

Brailsford, J. F.: Chondro-osteo-dystrophy. Roentgenographic and clinical features of a child with dislocation of vertebrae. *Am. J. Surg., 7*:404–410, 1929.

Broadbent, T. R., and Woolf, R. M.: Flexion-adduction deformity of the thumb—congenital clasped thumb. *Plast. Reconstr. Surg., 34*:612–616, 1964.

Burian, F.: The "whistling face" characteristic in a compound cranio-facio-corporal syndrome. *Br. J. Plast. Surg., 16*:140–143, 1963.

Casacci, A.: Sul quadro istopatalogica della malattie di Notta. *Clin. Orthop., 1*:452–459, 1949.

Cervenka, J., Figalova, P., and Gorlin, R. J.: Cranio-carpo-tarsal dysplasia or the whistling face syndrome. II. Oral intercommissural distance in children. *Am. J. Dis. Child., 117*:434–435, 1969.

Cervenka, J., Gorlin, K. J., Givalova, P., and Farkasova, J.: Cranio-carpo-tarsal dysplasia or whistling face syndrome. *Arch. Otolaryngol., 91*:183–187, 1970.

Christian, J. C., Cho, K. S., Franken, E. A., and Thompson, B. H.: Dominant preaxial brachydactyly with hallux varus and thumb abduction. *Am. J. Genet., 24*:694–701, 1972.

Chureau, H., and Detouillon, M.: Flexion permanente de deux pouces chez un enfant. *Bull. Mém. Soc. Chir., 61*:285–286, 1935.

Condon, E. D.: Anomalous fibrous cords in the hand and the phylogeny of the flexor digitorum sublimis tendon. *Anat. Rec., 19*:159–163, 1920.

Conradi, E.: Vorzeitiges Auftreten von Knochen—und eigenartigen Verkalkungskernen bei Chondrodystrophia fötalis hypoplastica: Histologische und Röntgenuntersuchungen. *Jb. Kinderheilkd., 80*:86–97, 1914.

Coudray: Traitement de la flexion congénitale du petit doigt par la resection. *Sem. Méd., 15*:372, 1895.

Courtemanche, A. D.: Campylodactyly: etiology and management. *Plast. Reconstr. Surg., 44*:451–454, 1969.

Crawford, H. H., Horton, C. E., and Adamson, J. E.: Congenital aplasia or hypoplasia of the thumb and finger extensor tendons. *J. Bone Joint Surg., 48A*:82–91, 1966.

Creig, D.: A case of congenital Dupuytren's contraction of the fingers. *Edinburgh Med. J., 19*:384–386, 1917.

Cumings, D. E., Skubi, K., Van Eyes, J., and Motulsky, A. G.: Familial multifocal fibrosclerosis. Findings suggesting that retroperitoneal fibrosis, mediastinal fibrosis, sclerosing cholangitis, Liedel's thyroiditis and pseudotumor of the orbit may be different manifestations of a single disease. *Ann. Intern. Med., 66*:884–892, 1967.

Currarino, G., and Waldman, I.: Camptodactyly. *Am. J. Roentgenol., 92*:1312–1321, 1964.

DeHaas, W. H. D.: Camptodactylie. *Ned. T. Geneesk., 101*:2121–2124, 1957.

Delitala, F.: Un caso di pollice flesso addato bilateral congenito. *G. Veneto Sci. Mediche, 12*:60, 1938.

Derscheid-Delcourt, M.: Un cas de doigt varus double congénital et héréditaire. *J. Méd. Bruxelles, 8*:33–36, 1903.

Dittrich, H.: Die Ulnarabduktionsstellung von Hand und Fingern. *25 Kongr. Dtsch. Orthop. Ges.* (Heidelberg, 1930), *25*:193–196, 1931.

Drachman, D. B., and Banker, B. Q.: Arthrogryposis multiplex congenita. Case due to disease of anterior horn cells. *Arch. Neurol., 5*:77–93, 1961.

Dreyfus, J. R.: Die Kamptodaktylie im Kinderalter. *Jb. Kinderheilkd., 148*:336–345, 1937.

Dreyfus, J. R.: La camptodactylie chez les enfants. *Rev. d'Orthop., 25*:35–41, 1938.

Dreyfuss, M.: Beitrag zum Bilde der angeborenen Windmühlenflügelstellung. (Deviation des doigts en coup de vent). *Z. Orthop. Chir., 65*:205–226, 1936.

Dubois, H., and Mullier, J. C.: Knipdium of stenoserende tendovaginitis van der flexor pollicis longus bij Kinderen. Studie von tweeedertig gevallen. *Acta Orthop. Belg., 35*:506–514, 1969.

Dubreuil-Chambardel, L.: Des deviations latérales des doigts (l'index varus). *Bull. Mém. Soc. d'Anthrop.* (Paris), *7*:143–147, 1906.

Dubreuil-Chambardel, L.: L'index varus et les deviations latérales des doigts. *Gaz. Méd. Centre* (Tours), *9*:55–59, 1906.

Dubreuil-Chambardel, L.: *Les Clinodactylies.* Paris, Vigot Frères, pp. 1–54, 1908.

Edwards, J. H., Harden, D. G., Cameron, A. H., Grosse, V. M., and Wolff, O. H.: A new trisomic syndrome. *Lancet, 1*:787–790, 1960.

Egawa, T., Minamide, H., Kawamura, J., Katagiri, K., and Sumiyoshi, S.: Congenital flexion contracture of the fingers. (Japanese). *Seikeigeka, 16*:855–860, 1965.

Ehalt, W.: Defekt an einem Fingerknochen. *Röntgenpraxis, 7*:359, Abb 2, 1935.

Elliot, W. A.: Congenital malformations and contractions of the hand and fingers arising from various causes. *Dublin J. Med. Sci., 88*:193–206, 1899.

Emery, A. E. H., and Nelson, M.: A familial syndrome of short stature, deformities of the hands and feet and unusual facies. *J. Med. Genet., 7*:379–382, 1970.

Epstein, B. A.: Radiographic identification of arthrogryposis multiplex congenita in utero. *Radiology, 77*:108–110, 1961.

Erskine, C. A.: An analysis of the Klippel-Feil syndrome. *Arch. Pathol., 41*:269–281, 1946.

Fairbank, H. A. T.: *An Atlas of General Affections of the Skeleton,* Edinburgh, L. S. Livingston, LTD., pp. 102–110, 1951.

Falk, E.: Über den Schnellende Dauman bei Kindern. *Beit. Klin. Chir., 153*:559–569, 1931.

Fantham, H. B.: Heredity in man: its importance both biologically and educationally. *S. Afr. J. Sci., 21*:298–527; fig. 4, 1924.

Féré, C.: Note sur une anomalie des doigts en particulier de petit doigt devié. *Rev. Chir.* (Paris), *33*:185–187, 1906.

Féré, C., and Perrin, J.: Note sur des anomalies des doigts et en particulier du petit doigt valgus. *Rev. Chir., 31*:66–70, 1905.

Fèvre, M.: Camptodactylie. (Lesion anatomique d'un doigt surnuméraire atteint camptodactylie). *Ann. Anat. Pathol., 13*:1018–1023, 1936.

Forral, G.: Gehauftes Verkommen von Kamptodaktylia und Leinersher Krankheit in derselben Familie. *Wien. Klin. Wochenschr., 77*:259–260, 1965.

Fraser, F. C., Pashayan, H., and Kadish, M. E.: Cranio-carpo-tarsal dysplasia. Report of a case in the father and son. *J.A.M.A., 211*:1374–1376, 1970.

Freeman, E. A., and Sheldon, J. H.: Cranio-carpo-tarsal dystrophy. An underscribed congenital malformation. *Arch. Dis. Child., 13*:277–283, 1938.

Freese, C. de: Über angeboren Digiti vari und valgi. *Z. Arztl. Fortbildg., 18*:312–316, 1921.

Gasne, E.: Malformations symétriques des extrémites et particulièrement des pouces: déviation latérale des pouces. *Rev. d'Orthop.,* (3 s.), *8*:299–302, 1907.

Gassul, R.: Eine durch Generationen prävalierende symmetrische Fingerkontraktur. *Dtsch. Med. Wochenschr., 44*:1196–1197, 1918.

Gellis, S. S., Feingold, M., and Forlin, R.: Picture of the month. Oral-facial-digital syndrome. *Am. J. Dis. Child., 120*:241–242, 1970.

Gilly, R., Cotton, J., Farouz, S., Moiret, A., and Maclet, M.: Hydrocéphalie congénital et anomalie bilatérale des pouces syndrome malformatif lié au chromosome "X". *Pédiatrie, 26*:365–378, 1971.

Giordani, C.: Contributo clinico allo studio del pollice flesso addatto. *Chir. Organi. Mov., 40*:513–517, 1954.

Glass, L. C., and Magee, E.: The inheritance of crooked little finger. *J. Hered., 26*:490, 1935.

Göb, A.: Zur Aetiologie der angeboren ulnaren Deviation des Finger in den Grundgelenken. *Z. Orthop., 88*:219–225, 1956.

Gold, A. M., and Perlman, R. D.: Congenital clasped thumb deformity. *Bull. Hosp. Joint. Dis., 29*:255–258, 1968.

Gordon, H., Davies, D., and Berman, M.: Camptodactyly, cleft palate, and club foot. A syndrome showing the autosomal dominant pattern of inheritance. *J. Med. Genet., 6*:266–274, 1969.

Greig, D. M.: A case of congenital Dupuytren's contracture of the fingers. *Edinburgh Med. J.,* (n.s.), *19*:384–386, 1917.

Grenier, B., Laugier, J., Soutoul, J., and Desbuquois, G.: Maladie de Marfan et arthrogrypose. Á propos d'un cas chez un nouvenauné. *Ann. Pédiatr.*, *45*:182–186, 1969.

Grob, M., and Stockmann, M.: Über Tendovaginosis stenosans, eine typisch Affektion des Kleinkindes. "Stenosing tenovaginitis, a typical affection of early childhood." *Helvet. Paediatr. Acta*, *6*:112–118, 1951.

Gross-Kieselstein, E., Abrahamov, A., and Ben-Hur, N.: Familial occurrence of the Freeman-Sheldon syndrome: cranio-carpo-tarsal dysplasia. *Pediatrics*, *47*:1064–1067, 1971.

Gruca, A.: Un cas de main bote cubito-palmaire congénitale avec subluxation des phalanges. *Rev. d'Orthop.*, (3 s.), *14*:407–412, 1927.

Haas, W. H. D. de: Camptodactyly. *Ned. T. Geneesk.*, *101*:2121–2124, 1957.

Harrenstein, R. J.: De "veerende vinger" bij jonge Kindern. *Ned. T. Geneesk.*, *81*:1237–1241, 1937.

Hässler: Kamptodaktylie-Krummfingerkeit. *Münch. Med. Wochenschr.*, *89*(2):694, 1942.

Hecht, F., and Beals, R. K.: Inability to open mouth fully: an autosomal dominant phenotype with facultative camptodactyly and short stature. Preliminary note. *In* Bergsma, D., (ed.): *Birth Defects—Original Article Series*. Vol. V. No. 3:96–98, 1969.

Hefner, R. A.: Inherited abnormalities of fingers. III. Subterminal articulation in proximal joint of the little finger. *J. Hered.*, *15*:481–483, 1924.

Hefner, R. A.: Inheritance of crooked little fingers (streblomicrodactyly). *J. Hered.*, *20*:395–398, 1929.

Hefner, R. A.: Crooked little finger: (minor streblomicrodactyly). *J. Hered.*, *32*:37–38, 1941.

Hennenberg: Kasuistischer Beitrag zur kongenitalen familiären, dermatogenen Kontraktur der Fingergelenke. *Dtsch. Med. Wochenschr.*, *34*(2):1804–1805, 1908.

Herbert, H.: *Etude sur la Camptodactylie*. Thèse. Paris, H. Jouvé, pp. 9–47, 1898.

Herbert, H.: La camptodactylie. *Gaz. Hebd. Méd. Paris.*, (n.s.), *3*:771–773, 1898.

Heron, R.: *Les Clinodactylies Latérales Congénitales*. Thèse. Bordeau, Imp. Commerciale et Industrielle, pp. 1–55, 1906.

Herzog, W.: Ueber angeborenen Deviationen der Fingerphalangen (Klinodaktylie). *Münch. Med. Wochenschr.*, *39*:344–345, 1892.

Hester, J. T.: On congenital contractions of fingers and nerve operation for their relief, and for cure of deformities arising from contraction of cicatrices. *Med. Times* (London), *23*:315–316, 1851.

Hunermann, C.: Chondrodystrophia calcificans congenita als abortive Form der Chondrodystrophia. *Z. Kinderheilkd.*, *51*:1–19, 1931.

Hunter, C.: A rare disease in two brothers. *Proc. R. Soc. Med.* (Sect. Study Dis. Child.), *10*:104–116, 1917.

Hurler, G.: Über einen Typ multipler abartungen, vorweighend am Skelettsystem. *Z. Kinderheilkd.*, *24*:220–234, 1919.

Hyden, H.: Mitteilung eines Falles von angeborener, symmetrischer Windmühlenflügelstellung der Finger. *Zentralbl. Chir.*, *79*:413–417, 1954.

Iselin, F., Levame, J., and Afanassief, A.: Les camptodactylies congénitales (Soc. Mèd. Chir. des Hôpitaux libres de Fourier, 1966). *Arch. Hôp.*, No. 5:1–4, 1966.

Jacquemain, B.: Die angeborene Windmühlenflügelstellung als erbliche Kombinationsmissbildung. *Z. Orthop.*, *102*:146–154, 1966.

Jeanin, G.: *Pathogénie et Traitement du Doigts a Rassort*. Thèse. Paris. G. Steinheil. Editeur. pp. 5–109, 1895.

Jerusalem, M.: Kamptodaktylie. *Wien. Med. Wochenschr.*, *78*:611, 1928.

Joachimsthal, G.: Über angeborene seitliche Deviationen der Fingerphalangen. *Z. Orthop. Chir.*, *2*:265–271, 1893.

Joachimsthal, G.: Über Kongenitale Fingeranomalien. *Z. Orthop. Chir.*, *2*:441–447; fig. 1, 1893.

Jorge, J. M.: Retraction palmaire congénitale. *Rev. d'Orthop.*, (3 s.), *13*:97–109, 1926.

Juberg, R. C., and Hayward, J. R.: A new familial syndrome of oral, cranial, and digital anomalies. *J. Pediatr.*, *44*:755–762, 1969.

Kartik, I.: Kamptodaktylie (Hungarian). *Orvosi Hetilip.*, *99*:1652–1655, 1958.

Katz, G.: A pedigree of anomalies of the little finger in five generations and seventeen individuals. *J. Bone Joint Surg.*, *52A*:717–720, 1970.

Kingsley-Pillers, E. M.: Arachnodactyly with amyoplasia congenita. *Proc. R. Soc. Med.*, London (Sect. Study Dis. Child.), *39*:696–697, 1946.

Kirmission, E.: *In Traité des Maladies Chirurgicales d'Origine Congénitale*. Paris, Masson et Cie., pp. 417–485; 732–747, 1898.

Koby, F. E.: Cataract familiale d'un type particulier, se transmettant apparement suivant le mode dominant. *Arch. Ophthalmol.*, *40*:492–503, 1923.

Krukenberg: Über (angeborenen) Schnellender Finger bei Kleinen Kindern. *Zentralbl. Chir.*, *56*:2406–2407, 1929.

Külz, J.: Das Freeman-Sheldon-Syndrome. *Med. Bild.*, *4*:79–81, 1961.

Landouzy, L.: Camptodactylie: stigmate organique précocé du neuro-arthritisme. *Presse Méd.*, *14*:251–253, 1906.

LeJemtel, M.: Flexion permanente de deux pouces chez un enfant. *Bull. Mém. Soc. Chir.*, *61*:905–907, 1935.

Lenz, W.: Rezessive-geschlechtsgebundene Mikrophthalmie mit multiplen Missbildungen. *Z. Kinderheilkd.*, *77*:384–390, 1955.

Léri, A.: Une maladie congénitale et héréditaire de l'ossification: la pléonostéose familiale. *Bull. Mém. Soc. Méd. Hôp. Paris, 45*:1228–1230, 1921.

Léri, A.: Dystrophie osseus généralisée congénitale et hereditaire: la pléonostéose familiale. *Presse Méd., 30*:13–16, 1922.

Léri, A.: Sur la pléonostéose familiale. *Bull. Mém. Soc. Méd. Hôp. Paris, 48*:216–220, 1924.

Léri, A.: *Études sur les Affections des Os et des Articulations.* Colonne vertébrale exceptée. Paris, Masson et Cie, pp. 5–34, 1926.

Ligorio, E.: Deviazione laterale della terza falange del mignolo in piu membri di una familia. *La Clinica Moderna, 10*:18–19, 1904. Also in *Med. Ital., Napoli, 2*:143, 1904.

Lindenbaum, R. H., and Butler, L. J.: Child with multiple anomalies and a group B(4–5) long arm deletion (Bg-). *Arch. Dis. Child., 46*:99–101, 1971.

Little, E. M.: Remarks on congenital contractions of the fingers and their treatment by forcible extension. *Internat. Med. Mag., 3*:241–244, 1894.

Littman, A., Yates, J. W., and Treger, A.: Camptodactyly—a kindred study. *J.A.M.A., 206*:1565–1567, 1968.

Lombard, P.: Les anomalies congénitales de l'attitude des membres par troubles du tonus musculaire. *Rev. d'Orthop., 31*:89–103, 1945.

Loomis, L. K.: Flexion deformity of the infant thumb. *South. Med. J., 502*:1259–1261, 1957.

Lowry, R. B., MacLean, R., MacLean, D. M., and Tischler, B.: Cataract, microcephaly, kyphosis and limited joint movements in two siblings: a new syndrome. *J. Pediatr., 79*:282–284, 1971.

Lucas, R. C.: On a case of hereditary suppression of fingers and the relation of this kind of defect to the crooked little finger, with remarks on disappearing little toe. *Lancet, 1*:462–464, 1892.

Lundblom, A.: On congenital ulnar deviation of the fingers of familial occurrence. ("deviation des doigts en coup de vent"). *Acta Orthop. Scand., 2*:393–404, 1932.

Lyon, G., Rosemberg, S., and Thieffrey, St.: Une forme rare de mucopolysaccharidose chez l'enfant. A rapprocher du "Hurler tardif" et du "syndrome de Scheie." *Arch. Franc., 28*:83–94, 1971.

Magnusson, R.: La camptodactylie. *Acta Chir. Scand., 87*:236–242, 1942.

Mangini, U.: La tendovaginite stenosante del flessore lungo de pollice nei bambini. *Arch. Putti, 8*:205–215, 1957.

Marfan, A. B.: Un cas de déformation congénitale des quatre mémbres, plus prononcée aux extremités, characterisée par l'allongement des os avec un certain degré d'amincissement. *Bull. Mém. Soc. Med. Hop. Paris, 13*:220–227, 1896.

Maroteaux, P., and Lamy, M.: Hurler's disease, Morquio's disease and related mucopolysaccharidoses. *J. Pediatr., 67*:312–323, 1965.

Marriot, F. P. S., and Basu, S.: Trigger thumb in infancy and childhood. *Ulster Med. J., 36*:53–61, 1967.

Marton, R., and Steinbrocker, O.: Congenital contracture of the fifth finger. *N.Y. State J. Med., 49*:1064–1066, 1949.

Maurer, G.: Die Kamptodaktylie. *Arch. Orthop. Unfallchir., 39*:365–374, 1938.

Melnick, J. C.: Chondrodystrophia calcificans congenita, chondrodystrophia epiphysialis punctata, stippled epiphyses. *Am. J. Dis. Child., 110*:218–225, 1965.

Michail, J.: Pollex varus rigidus et hallux valgus chez un jeune. *Rev. d'Orthop., 35*:461–464, 1949.

Middleton, D. S.: Myodystrophia foetalis deformans. *Edinburgh Med. J., 61*:421–442, 1936.

Miller, J. W.: Pollex varus: a report of two cases. *Univ. Hosp. Bull. Ann Arbor, 10*:10–11, 1943.

Mills, A.: A propos d'un cas de pouce bot double (pollex varus). *Vingtième Cong. de Chir., 20*:693–695, 1907.

Monnier, L.: Malformation rare de la main (pouce bot.).—Opération—Guèrison. *France Méd. Paris Méd., 35*:465–473, 1891.

Montagu, M. F. A.: The inheritance of streblomicrodactyly. *J. Hered., 38*:93–96, 1947.

Moore, W. G., and Messina, P.: Camptodactylism and its variable expression. *J. Hered., 27*:28–30, 1936.

Morquio, L.: Sur une forme de dystrophie osseuse familiale. *Bull. Soc. Pédiatr., 27*:145–152, 1929. Also: *Arch. Méd., 32*:129–140, 1929.

Mundorff, G. T.: Hereditary abnormality of the little finger. *N.Y. State Med. J., 80*:642–643, 1904.

Murphy, D. P.: Familial finger contracture and association familial knee-joint subluxation. *J.A.M.A., 86*:395–397, 1926.

Muskat: Angebornen familiare kontraktur des kleinen Finger. *Med. Klin., 5*:1478–1480, 1909.

Maumann, P.: Weiterer Beitrag zur angeborenen symmetrische Ulnar-abduktion der Finger (Windmühlenflügelfinger). *Zentralbl. Chir., 79*:1447–1450, 1954.

Namba, K., Muda, G., and Hachiguchi, I.: Congenital clasped thumb. *Orthop. Surg. (Tokyo), 16*:1031–1035, 1965.

Neuhof, H., and Oppenheimer, E. D.: Congenital contractures of the fingers with a report of case of familial type. *Surg. Gynecol. Obstet., 19*:193–198, 1914.

Nevin, N. C., Hurwitz, L. J., and Neill, D. W.: Familial camptodactyly with taurinuria. *J. Med. Genet., 3*:365–368, 1966.

Notta, A.: Recherches sur une affection particulière des gaines tendineuses de la main, caracterisée par le développement d'une nodosite sur le trajet des tendons fléchisseurs des doigts et par l'empechement de leurs mouvements. *Arch. Gén. Méd.,* (4 s.), *24*:142–161, 1850.

Notta, A.: Tumeur fibreuse de la paume de la main développée dans le gaine des tendons—Difficultés du diagnostic—Guérison. *Bull. Mém. Soc. Chir. Paris*, 3:664–666, 1877.

Nowak, H.: Drei Stammbäume von Klinodaktylie. *Dtsch. Med. Wochenschr.*, 60:2001, 1934.

Oldfield, M. C.: Camptodactyly: flexion contracture of the fingers in young girls. *Br. J. Plast. Surg.*, 8:312–317, 1956.

Otto, F. M.: Die "Cranio-carpo-tarsal Dystrophie" (Freeman und Sheldon). Ein Kasuistischer Beitrag. *Z. Kinderheilkd.*, 73:240–250, 1953.

Parish, J. G., Horn, D. B., and Thompson, M.: Familial streblodactyly with aminoaciduria. *Br. Med. J.*, 2:1247–1250, 1963.

Patau, K., Therman, E., Smith, D. W., Inhorn, S. L., and Wagner, H. P.: Multiple congenital anomalies by an extra autosome. *Lancet*, 1:790–793, 1960.

Pauly, R.: Doigts en valgus. *Rev. Méd., Paris*, 22:1078–1081, 1902.

Pausa Trujillo, J.: Tenosinovitis estenosante congenita del flexor proprio del pulgar et el nino. *Cir. Ortop. Traum.*, 20:66–71, 1956.

Peregalli, P. F.: Assenza familiare del profondo dell'indice. *Arch. Ortop.*, 63:87–91, 1955.

Pitanguy, T., and Bisaggio, S.: A cheiro-cheilo-podalic syndrome. *Br. J. Plast. Surg.*, 22:79–85, 1969.

Poli, A.: Contributo allo studio dell assenze muscular congenita. *Arch. Ortop.*, 45:775, 1922.

Poncelet, F. A.: Pouce à ressort et pouce bot flexus. *Bull. Soc. Belge Ortop. Chir. App. Mot.*, 10:164–172, 1938.

Pouvreau, G.: *Contribution à l'Étude de la Camptodactylie*. Thèse. Bordeaux, 1909.

Poznanski, A. K., Pratt, G. B., Manson, G., and Weiss, L.: Clinodactyly, camptodactyly, Kirner's deformity and other crooked fingers. *Radiology*, 93:573–582, 1969.

Reeve, R., Silver, H. K., and Ferrier, P.: Marfan's syndrome (arachnodactyly) with arthrogryposis (amyoplasia congenita). *A.M.A.J. Dis. Child.*, 99:101–106, 1960.

Regele, H.: Die angeborene beidseitige Brugkontraktur des Daumengliedes beim Kindern (Schnellender Finger). *Münch. Med. Wochenschr.*, 83:391–392, 1936.

Rintala, A. E.: Freeman-Sheldon's syndrome. Cranio-carpo-tarsal dystrophy. *Acta Paediatr. Scand.*, 57:553–556, 1968.

Ritterskamp, P.: Eine Familie mit Kamptodaktylie. *Münch. Med. Wochenschr.*, 83:724–725, 1936.

Rocher, H. L., and Roudil, G.: Deux observations des pouces bots flexus. *Rev. d'Orthop.*, 21:37–41, 1934.

Rose, T. F.: Bilateral trigger thumb in infants. *Med. J. Australia*, 1:18–20, 1946.

Ruschemberg, E.: Die Beuge-Kontrakturen des Daumens bei kleinen Kindern ein typisches Krankheitsbild. *Z. Orthop. Chir.*, 68:172–178, 1938.

Rutt, A.: Die angeboren Windmühlenflügelstellung der Finger. *Arch. Orthop. Unfallchir.*, 49:387–391, 1957.

Sallis, J. G., and Beighton, J. G.: Dominantly inherited digito-talar dysmorphism. *J. Bone Joint Surg.*, 54B:509–515, 1972.

Samouilovitch, M.: *De la Gampsodactylie*. Thèse. Paris, Jouvé, pp. 4–48, 1896.

Sanfilippo, S. J., Podosin, R., Langer, L., and Good, R. A.: Mental retardation associated with acid mucopolysaccharisuria (heparitin sulfate type). *J. Pediatr.*, 63:837–838, 1963.

Schaff, B., and Schafer, P. W.: Camptodactyly. *Arch. Surg.*, 57:633–636, 1948.

Scheie, H. G., Hamrick, G. W., Jr., and Barness, L. A.: A newly recognized forme fruste of Hurler's disease (gargoylism). *Am. J. Ophthalmol.*, 53:753–769, 1962.

Schmidt, L. V.: Die Streckung Krummer Finger. *Dtsch. Med. Wochenschr.*, 47:564–565, 1921.

Schultze, E.: Angeborene familiäre Kontraktur der Gelenke des kleinen Fingers. *Cbl. Grenzgel Med. Chir.*, 16:608–621, 1913.

Scott, J.: Hammer-finger, with notes on seven cases occurring in one family. *Glascow Med. J.*, 60:335–344, 1903.

Secheyren, L., and Desforges-Mériel: Les doigts en marteau ou la fixation dite congénitale du petits doigts. *Arch. Med. Toulouse*, 3:167–171; 182–189, 1897.

Sedel, L., and Masse, P.: Orthopédie le l'arthrogrypose. *Rev. Chir. Orthop. Rep. App. Mot.*, 56:537–552, 1970.

Selander, P.: Über kongenitale doppelseitige Beugestellung der Daumen. *Kinder Arzt. Praxis 13 jhr.* (Heft), 11:286–288, 1942.

Sengupta, A.: Multiple congenital contracture of fingers. *J. Indian Med. Assoc.*, 43:285–286, 1964.

Sharma, R. N., and Tandon, S. N.: "Whistling face" deformity in compound cranio-facio-corporal syndrome. *Br. Med. J.*, 4:33, 1970.

Shattock, S. G.: On a case of arrested development and growth of the right upper limb in man. *Trans. Pathol. Soc. London*, 32:276–279, 1881.

Sheldon, W.: Amyoplasia congenita (multiple congenital articular rigidity: arthrogryposis multiplex congenital). *Arch. Dis. Child.*, 7:117–136, 1932.

Sinnette, C., and Odeku, E. L.: Rubenstein-Taybi syndrome. The first case in an African child and the first case recognized at birth. *Clin. Pediatr.*, 7:488–492, 1968.

Smith, R. J., and Kaplan, E. B.: Camptodactyly and similar atraumatic flexion deformities of the proximal interphalangeal joints of the fingers. *J. Bone Joint Surg.*, 50A:1187–1203; 1249, 1968.

Sorrel, E., and Benoit, H.: Flexion permanente du pouce chez un enfant (camptodactylies et pouces à ressort). *Bull. Soc. Nat. Chir.*, 40:703–709, 1934.

Sorrel, E.: Un cas de camptodactyly de deux pouces. *Mém. Acad. Chir., 64*:628–632, 1938.

Spear, G. S.: The inheritance of flexed fingers. *J. Hered., 37*:189–192, 1946.

Sprecher, E. E.: Trigger thumb in infants. *J. Bone Joint Surg., 31A*:672–674, 1949.

Stewart, J. M., and Bergstrom, L.: Familial hand abnormality and sensori-neural deafness: a new syndrome. *J. Pediatr., 78*:102–110, 1971.

Stiles, K. A., and Schalck, J.: A pedigree of curved forefingers. *J. Hered., 36*:211–216, 1945.

Stoddard, S. E.: Nomenclature of hereditary crooked fingers. *J. Hered., 30*:511–512, 1939.

Sutro, C. J.: Pollex valgus (A bunion-like deformity of the thumb corrected by surgical intervention). *Bull. Hosp. Joint Dis., 18*:135–139, 1957.

Swinyard, C. A., and Magora, A.: Multiple congenital contractures (arthrogryposis): an electromyographic study. *Arch. Phys. Med., 43*:36–41, 1962.

Tamplin, R. W.: *Lectures on the Nature and Treatment of Deformities.* London, Longman, Brown, Green, and Longman, pp. 256–267, 1846.

Thomas, E.: Ein Fall von Arachnodaktylie mit Schwimmhautbildung und einer eigenartigen Ohrmuscheldeformität. *Z. Kinderheilkd., 10*:109–115, 1914.

Thomas, L. C.: Bent little finger on right hand. *Eugenical News, 11*:158–159; fig. 7, 1926.

Thursfield, H.: Arachnodactyly. *St. Bartholomew Hosp. Rep., 53*:35–40, 1917.

Todd, A. H.: A case of hereditary contracture of little finger (kamptodactyly). *Lancet, 2*:1088–1090, 1929.

Tomesku, I.: Kongenitale Deviationen der Phalangen. (Angeborene Contrakturen der Finger und Klinodaktylien). *Arch. Orthop. Unfallchir., 26*:126–137, 1928.

Tupper, J. W.: Pollex abductus due to congenital malposition of flexor pollicis longus. *J. Bone Joint Surg., 49A*:575–576, 1967.

Udani, P. M.: Arachnodactyly with arthrogryposis. Marfan's syndrome (A case report with a review). *Indian J. Child. Health, 4*:623–630, 1955.

Van Neck, M.: Nodules congenitaux des tendons. Etiologie des pouce à ressort. *Arch. Franc. Belg. Chir., 29*:924–927, 1936.

Verneuil: Déviation particuliére de doigt annulaire. *Bull. Soc. Anat.* (Paris), *26*:223, 1851.

Walker, B. A.: Whistling face-windmill vane hand syndrome (cranio-carpo-tarsal dystrophy; Freeman-Sheldon syndrome). *In* Bergsma, D., (ed.): *Birth Defects. Original Article Series.* New York: National Foundation—March of Dimes. Vol. V., No. 2:228–230, 1969.

Weckesser, E. C.: Congenital flexion-adduction deformity of the thumb (congenital "clasped thumb"). *J. Bone Joint Surg., 37A*:977–983, 1955.

Weckesser, E. C., Reed, J. R., and Heiple, K. G.: Congenital clasped thumb (congenital flexion-adduction deformity of the thumb). *J. Bone Joint Surg., 50A*:1417–1428; 1436, 1968.

Weeks, P. M.: Surgical correction of arthrogrypotic deformities of the upper extremity. *J. Bone Joint Surg., 49A*:579–580, 1967.

Weinstein, S., and Gorlin, R. J.: Cranio-carpo-tarsal dysplasia or the whistling face syndrome. I. Clinical considerations. *Am. J. Dis. Child., 117*:427–433, 1969.

Weisenbach, R. J., and Faulong, L.: Camptodactylie par retraction des tendons flechisseurs. *Rev. Rheum., 15*:52–53, 1948.

Weissman, S. L., Khermosch, C., and Adam, A.: Arthrogryposis in an Arab family. *In* Goldschmidt, E., (ed.): *Genetics of Migrant and Isolate Populations.* Baltimore, Williams & Wilkins, p. 313, 1963.

Welch, J. P., and Temtamy, S. A.: Hereditary contractures of the fingers. (Camptodactyly). *J. Med. Genet., 3*:104–113, 1966.

Wender, M., Kosowicz, J., Steefen, J., and Zgorzalewicz, R.: Familial occurrence of trisomy 17–18. *J. Med. Genet., 2*:200–204; fig. 4, 1965.

White, J. W., and Jensen, W. E.: The infant's persistent thumb-clutched hand. *J. Bone Joint Surg., 34A*:680–688, 1952.

White, J. W., and Jensen, W. E.: Trigger thumb in infants. *A.M.A. Am. J. Dis. Child., 85*:141–145, 1953.

Wildervanck, L. S.: Erbliche Klinodaktylie. *Ned. T. Geneesk., 92*:3491, 1948.

Winchester, P., Grossman, H., Lim, V. N., and Danes, B. S.: A new acid mucopolysaccharidosis with skeletal deformities simulating rheumatoid arthritis. *Am. J. Roentgenol., 106*:121–128, 1969.

Wright, D. D., and Aase, J.: The kuskokwin syndrome: an inherited form of arthrogryposis in the Alaskan Eskimo. *In* Bergsma, D., (ed.): *Birth Defects. Original Article Series.* New York, National Foundation—March of Dimes, Vol. V, No. 3:91–95, 1969.

Zadek, I.: Congenital absence of the extensor pollicis longus of both thumbs; operation and cure. *J. Bone Joint Surg., 16*:432–434, 1934.

Zadek, I.: Stenosing tenovaginitis of the thumb in infants. *J. Bone Joint Surg., 24*:326–328, 1942.

Zumoff, B.: Congenital symmetrical finger contractures: report of a case. *J.A.M.A., 155*:437–440, 1954.

Chapter Eighteen

MACRODACTYLY

Disproportionate enlargement of one or more digits present at birth has been given a variety of names: hypertrophy, giant growth, hyperplasia, partial acromegaly, macrosomia, elephantiasis, hamartoma, megalodigity, macrodystrophia lipomatosa, dactylomegaly, and macrodactyly. In most instances, more than one digit is involved; occasionally, the entire limb is overgrown. At times, half of the body is affected. When confined to the hand, the tumefaction extends beyond the base of the enlarged digit and involves the corresponding portion of the palm. For this reason, perhaps, the name *macrocheir*, meaning oversized hand, would seem more appropriate. In fact, this was the term which first appeared in the literature. As will be pointed out in Chapter Twenty-nine, at least one nonmedical author used the designation macrocheir in describing the oversized hand of an ancient Persian king.

Medical writers today seldom use the term macrocheir. Observers in this field may be likened to the man who sees a tree and forgets the forest. The striking bulk of the affected finger seems to have snared their attention; the involvement of the palm is often overlooked. Hence, the literature demonstrates the almost universal employment of the term *macrodactyly* or one of its synonyms.

RECORDED CASES

There are sixteen or more collective reviews of macrodactyly. Some of these documents contain names of authors who do not seem to have left written records of cases credited to them. A few compilers list cases which are erroneously interpreted as macrodactyly. More recent authors have copied earlier ones—in particular Busch (1866), Wittelshöfer (1879), and Pollailon (1884)—and perpetuated some of their errors. Barsky (1967) appears to have gotten his information about earlier reported cases of macrodactyly from Pollailon's tabulation, which is very inaccurate. Barsky (1967) claimed he could find only 64 authenticated cases of macrodactyly prior to the publication of his own paper. There are at least six times as many cases reported in the literature.

Tuli et al (1969) complained that the literature on macrodactyly is scarce. As attested by the bibliography at the end of this chapter, the literature on macrodactyly is voluminous. Authors who seek and study original communications are scarce.

The first authenticated case of macrodactyly was described by Klein (1824). He was followed by Beck (1836), Power (1840), Reid (1843), and Curling (1845). Klein's patient was a female with an oversized left index finger. Beck's patient was a male who had an overgrown right thumb and right index finger. Power reported two cases: one of his own, a living patient, and one represented by a plaster model in the museum of King's College, London. Power's own patient was a female child whose right middle finger was "enlarged to the size it would be in a fully grown, very corpulent person"; her right index and ring fingers were only slightly enlarged. The museum model featured the left hand of an adult male with an enormous middle finger. Reid's (1843) patient, a boy, had an oversized right thumb and right index finger.

Curling (1845) described a young girl with bilateral involvement: on the right hand, the index, middle, and ring fingers were enlarged, and on the left hand, the thumb, index, and middle fingers had overgrown. Curling mentioned two other cases reported to him by letters, one from Owen and another from Paget. Owen's (1845) patient, a young girl, had an oversized middle finger on each hand. Paget (1845) referred to a plaster model which, he said, represented the right hand of the governor of Luzon in the Philippines; macrodactyly affected the governor's right index and middle fingers and had been present since birth.

In a span of two decades, eight authenticated cases of macrodactyly were reported—four males and four females. There were two bilateral cases which would bring the total number of affected hands to ten. Altogether, 18 oversized digits were described; the thumb was involved in three, the index in six, the middle finger in seven, the ring finger twice, and the little finger not at all. Two or three neighboring digits were more commonly affected together than one alone. In no instance did the macrodactyly skip an adjacent digit and affect one at some distance. The index and middle fingers had the distinction of having overgrown most frequently and attained the greatest dimensions; they also tended to curve sideways, usually toward the ulnar border of the hand. In most instances, the oversized digit was stiff and unbending—useless. In no case was the hand enlarged in its entirety; some parts escaped involvement. There was no numerical difference between affected males and females, and the right and left hands were implicated almost equally.

The pattern established by the above earlier reported cases remains unchanged. Macrodactylies of the middle and index fingers continue to maintain their overwhelming majority; in most cases, the area of involvement corresponds to the territory supplied by the sensory branches of the median nerve. The volar surfaces of the thumb, index, and middle fingers are supplied exclusively by the median nerve: these digits are affected most often. The median nerve sends sensory twigs to supply the dorsal aspects of the last two phalanges of the index and middle fingers. Curiously these segments are often bulkier than the proximal ones which receive their dorsal sensory supply from the radial nerve. The median nerve also supplies the radial half of the volar and dorsal surface of the ring finger; this digit is enlarged only occasionally. The little finger does not receive any contribution from the median nerve: this digit is affected least frequently and rarely by itself (Fig. 18-1).

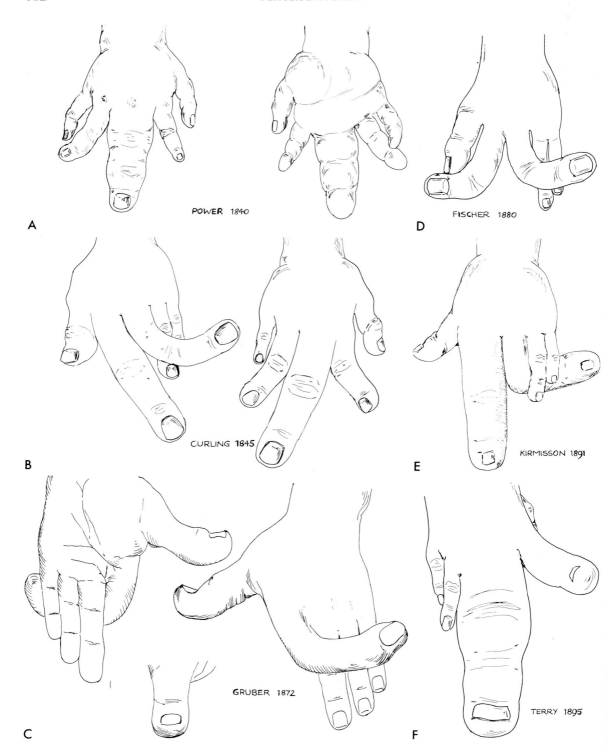

Figure 18–1 Samples of macrodactyly reported with drawings prior to the advent of roentgenography. *A*, The first reported case in English. *B*, The first reported bilateral case. *C*, *D*, and *E*, Cases with clinodactyly. *F*, Inordinate gigantism of the middle finger.

SEARCH FOR IDENTIFICATION

Holmes (1869) distinguished two classes of macrodactyly and qualified them with the adjectives *symmetrical* and *asymmetrical*, respectively. In the symmetrical type, all elements of the digit—bones, tendons, vessels—are said to be proportionately enlarged; in the asymmetrical variety, "the parts are variously deformed by large fatty excrescences, and by overdevelopment of joint ends of the bones leading to unnatural position." Richardière (1891) considered the adjectives *true* and *false* as being more appropriate, but most French authors favored the epithets *regular* and *irregular*. Froelich (1908) equated the adjective *true* with regular and *false* with irregular, and evolved the following classification: (1) congenital gigantism or true hypertrophy; (2) false hypertrophy or elephantiasis; (3) hypertrophy due to superimposed tumors.

For some years the adjectives *true* and *false* disappeared from the literature on macrodactyly, to be revived again by Kanavel (1932) and Barsky et al (1964). Kanavel distinguished two types of macrodactyly: "that due to bone growth alone. . . and that due to neurofibromatous and lymphatic overgrowth." Kanavel used the adjective *spurious* to characterize digital enlargements "due to neurofibromatous tissue." Barsky et al accorded the same definition to true macrodactyly as had been given to symmetrical hypertrophy by Holmes (1869) almost a century earlier, namely, "hypertrophy of all elements including bones, tendons, and vessels." Barsky et al insisted that "true macrodactyly should be distinguished from neurofibromatosis in which neoplastic growth is responsible for the enlargement."

Authors in the past and some even now tend to oversimplify the problem and conjecture a single process to account for all types of digital overgrowth. Some relate the dimensional discrepancies to vasomotor disturbances; others, to endocrine aberrations. There are those who regard macrodactyly as a form of elephantiasis. Osteoplastic changes have received their share of blame. In a number of cases, the onus is placed on tumors, and neurotrophic and metameric influences have also been incriminated. All these ideas have had their respective periods of popularity. Currently, two concepts dominate: (1) that the basic process in macrodactyly is lipomatous degeneration; (2) that macrodactyly is one of the many manifestations of multiple neurofibromatoses or Recklinghausen's disease. Curiously, adherents of the second theory base their conclusion on cases which are similar to those designated by earlier authors as true macrodactyly, which Kanavel and Barsky et al insisted should not be confused with the spurious form of enlargements caused by Recklinghausen's disease.

THE CONCEPT OF LIPOMATOUS MACRODYSTROPHY

Surgeons in the past were cautious about amputating oversized fingers, but they did not hesitate to dispose of gigantic toes which as a consequence, provided the main material for tissue studies. Excessive accumulation of fat is the most striking feature of pedal macrodactyly. Feriz (1925), who described a number of cases of oversized toes, coined the designation macrodystrophia lipomatosa progressiva. Werthemann (1952) and, after him, Golding (1960), Mikhail (1964) and Ranawat et al (1968) adopted this term in describing cases of macrodactyly of the hand. These authors considered the basic lesion in macrodactyly to be overgrowth of fibro-fatty tissue. It is true that in some cases of manual macrodactyly one meets with an excessive amount of subcutaneous fat, but one is struck more by the tumefaction of palmar nerves, the median nerve in particular, and the tortuosity of their digital branches. One hardly ever sees tumor-bearing plantar nerves, nor thick tortuous digital branches in pedal macrodactyly.

LINK WITH NEUROFIBROMATOSIS

Medicine attained its nineteenth century renaissance first in one European country, then in another. It reached one of its periodic peaks in Ireland around the time when Power (1840) of Dublin wrote the first knowledgeable article in English on macrodactyly. Power's contemporaries were such notables as Stokes, Adams, Colles, and Smith. It is ironic that Smith is now remembered in connection with one of his minor contributions, Smith's fracture, while his major work on neurofibromatosis has passed practically unnoticed. Nine years after the appearance of Power's paper on macrodactyly, Smith (1849) published his treatise. It is one of the most erudite monographs in medicine and is a classic on the subject of multiple neurofibromatoses, the disease which bears Recklinghausen's name, though Recklinghausen did not write on the subject until 33 years later. One of Smith's lithographs featured the dissected specimen of a hand showing a tumor arising from the digital branch of the median nerve.

Smith referred to Naegele's (1827) patient who was "laboring under elephantiasis. . . . The nerve of the affected limb was larger than usual; it was studded with numerous small cysts, both on its surface and in its interior. . . . The increase of size . . . is not to be ascribed to hypertrophy of the nervous structure, but should rather be considered as an effect of irritation established in neurolemma," Smith wrote. In view of the clarity of Smith's statement, it is hard to understand how, 99 years later, Holt and Wright (1948) arrived at the conclusion that Smith failed to recognize the nervesheath origin of neurofibromas.

During the decades following the publication of Smith's monograph, tortuous nerves studded with nodular tumors acquired the name plexiform neurofibroma. Puckering of the skin, caused by bulbous terminals of such nerves, was called molluscum fibrosum. When there was also an overgrowth of the part supplied by the affected nerve, the condition was given the name elephantiasis neuromatodes to distinguish it from elephantiasis telangiectodes, in which all the blood vessels were enlarged.

Recklinghausen (1882) described mainly skin and subcutaneous tumors. Such well-known stigmata of multiple neurofibromatoses as patches of pigmentation of the skin, or *café-au-lait* spots, were added by later authors who also advanced the view that Recklinghausen's neurofibromatosis was not merely a disorder of the skin and peripheral nerves but that it also affected the central nervous system, the viscera, the bones and joints—in fact, almost any organ or part of the body. It was also pointed out that Recklinghausen's disease might deviate from its classic manifestations and reveal itself with bizarre symptoms or pass unnoticed as *forme fruste*.

Guersant (1857) had described fullness of the palm in a case of macrodactyly. The year after the publication of Recklinghausen's (1882) paper, Halderman (1883) noted that in macrodactyly the area of overgrowth corresponded to the territory supplied by one of the volar nerves. Humme (1884) presented a patient with an overgrown index finger, which was amputated and carefully dissected. The volar digital branches of the median nerve going to the amputated finger were found to be inordinately enlarged. After microscopic examination, Humme concluded that the enlargement of the digital nerves was due to fibrous tissues deposited on the perineurium. Köhler (1888) reported a case of macrodactyly of the middle finger; in the same hand a tumor bulged from the corresponding portion of the palm in the area overlying the main trunk of the median nerve before it splits into digital branches.

Under the heading of plexiform neuroma, Bell and Inglis (1925) described a patient who had been born with macrodactyly of the left middle finger, which was amputated soon after birth. Subsequently, the left index finger progressively gained disproportionate dimensions and a mass developed in the corresponding part of the palm. On surgical exploration, the mass was found to be a tumor of the median nerve. Rogers (1929) described a little girl who was born with macrodactyly of the right thumb and index finger. When the girl was eight years old, Rogers removed a sizable tumor from her overgrown thumb. It was examined microscopically and diagnosed as neurofibroma. Rogers concluded that in the case he reported, the macrodactyly was "produced by neurofibromatosis." This conclusion has been repeated by numerous authors in the past four decades. Posch (1956) went so far as to coin the designation "Recklinghausen's type of macrodactylism."

It is fairly well established that Recklinghausen's neurofibromatosis is frequently inherited. There are now well over 300 authenticated cases of macrodactyly on record and only three are incriminated as having hereditary antecedents. Referring to the plaster specimen in the museum of King's College, both Power (1840) and Curling (1845) attested that the patient's kindred were said to have been similarly affected, though no clue is given as to who supplied this information.

Two other cases are often mentioned as examples of hereditary macrodactylism: one was reported by Boéchat (1877, 1878) and the other by Hawkins-Ambler (1893). In both, the ring finger of each hand projected slightly ahead of the middle finger. Boéchat described his case as bilateral elongation of the ring finger. The accompanying lithographs showed the ring finger of each hand to be longer than the flanking digits, but the case bore no resemblance to macrodactylic digits reported before or since. Hawkins-Ambler described a similar case and made it clear that the ring finger was the only one that had "fully grown"—by inference, the other digits had not. Tubby (1912) appears to have misread the paper by Hawkins-Ambler, whose lithograph he reproduced and accorded the following legend: "Congenital hypertrophy of the ring finger." Both Boéchat's and Hawkins-Ambler's cases would now be classed with the type of heritable brachydactyly in which the index and middle fingers are short, and in comparison the ring finger appears elongated (Fig. 18–2).

It can safely be said that heredity does not play a role in macrodactyly. Besides the absence of an hereditary antecedent, in studying cases of macrodactyly one also misses most of the classic features of Recklinghausen's neurofibromatosis, such as multiple cutaneous and subcutaneous tumors and *café-au-lait* spots, to say nothing about scoliosis, cystic bone lesions, and congenital pseudarthrosis of the tibia or some other bone. Unless it is conceded that macrodactyly represents a very special variety of Recklinghausen's neurofibromatosis—perhaps one of the *formes frustes*—we cannot identify the two conditions

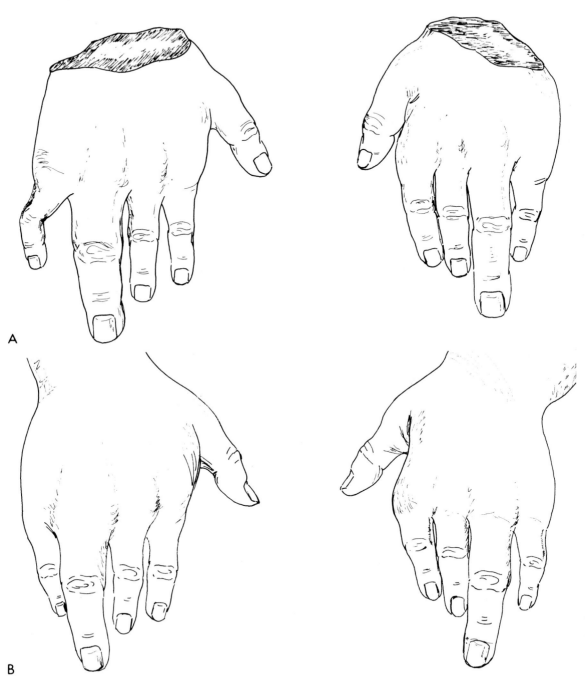

Figure 18–2   Hereditary brachydactyly involving the second and third digits erroneously interpreted as macrodactyly of the ring finger. *A*, Boéchat's case. *B*, Hawkins-Ambler's case.

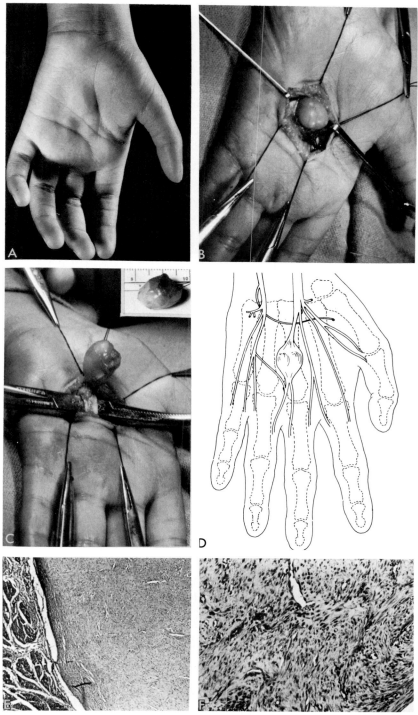

Figure 18-3 Neurofibroma of the common digital nerve of the middle and ring fingers without overgrowth of either digit. *A,* Palmar view of the left hand of an eight-year-old girl with a tumor of the common digital branch of the median nerve supplying the third and fourth digits of the left hand. *B* and *C,* Surgically exposed, encapsulated tumor. *D,* Sketch illustrating the location of the tumor. *E* and *F,* Sections of the specimen.

with each other. This is not to say that macrodactyly does not occur in generalized neurofibromatosis. Occasionally, it does.

Until more is known, it is perhaps best to eschew such presumptuous connotations as "von Recklinghausen's type of macrodactylism" and say that in the most common variety of macrodactyly the tumor of the median nerve in the proximal palm and the thickening and tortuosity of digital nerves constitute striking features. For lack of a better term, this variety should perhaps be called nerve territory oriented macrodactyly or NTOM for short. In using such an unpretentious designation, one avoids the as-yet-unfounded insinuation that the enlargement of the digit is due to the trophic influence of the tumefied nerve. Tumors are known to emanate from the main stem of the median nerve or its branches. They are not always accompanied by macrodactyly (Fig. 18–3).

STRUCTURAL ALTERATIONS IN NTOM

In the forearm, the median nerve is thick, but it bears no tumor and pursues a straight course. The tumor usually lies on the main stem of the median nerve emerging from the carpal tunnel. The volar digital nerves destined for an overgrown digit also are enlarged and studded with irregular nodules of fibroadipose tissue. These nerves are longer than the digit they supply and of necessity pursue tortuous courses, much like varicose veins. Like the latter, they occupy considerable space and contribute to the enlargement of the digit. In cases in which the overgrown digit curves toward the radial or ulnar borders of the hand, the digital nerve on the convex side is thicker and longer than the one on the concave aspect. The middle and index fingers, which are most commonly involved in macrodactyly, usually incline in an ulnar direction, and the digital nerves on their radial aspects are longer, thicker, and more tortuous than the nerves on their ulnar sides.

In NTOM, other soft tissue elements—blood vessels and tendons—are only moderately enlarged. Subcutaneous fat is overabundant; it is lumpy and held within meshes of coarse fibrous strands. The skin is glossy and pale. The phalangeal bones are broad and long. Growth from both endochondral (physeal) and membranous (periosteal) ossification is accelerated. Membranous ossification is as active as, if not more active than, enchondral deposition of bone. The nonepiphyseal or distal end of each phalanx is broader than its proximal extremity. The tuft of the ungual phalanx, which is formed by membranous ossification, is massive; this phalanx as a whole is bulkier than the middle phalanx, which in turn is bulkier than the proximal phalanx. The distal ends of the proximal phalanges are splayed and slanted, causing angulation of the phalanx next in line. In longstanding cases, the articular surfaces are interlocked and motion at the joint is nullified.

Heurtaux (1880) described a three-year-old girl with macrodactyly of the middle finger; he stated that the corresponding metacarpal was likewise overdeveloped. Metacarpal enlargement was also noted by Halderman (1883) and Streeter (1930). These observations have since been repeated by numerous authors. Kanavel (1932), Jones (1963), Iselin and Iselin (1967), and Barsky (1967) all stressed the immunity of the metacarpal bones to macrodactyly. They must have based their conclusion on cases seen in very early life, for in older children the metacarpal bone of the macrodactylous digit is thicker and projects further than its neighbors.

Numerous cases of macrodactyly detected at birth have been reported. In

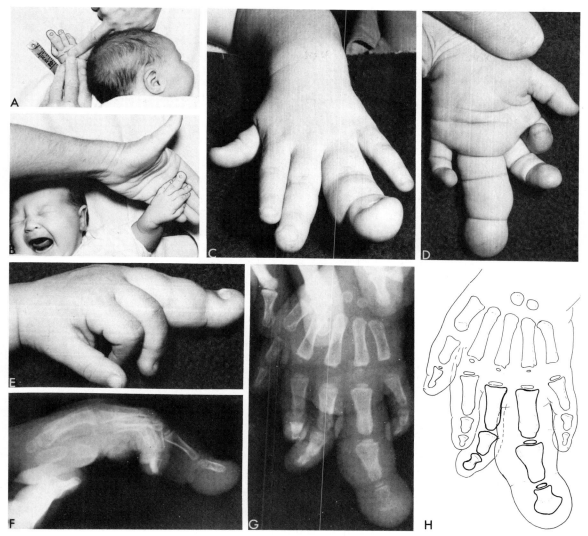

Figure 18–4 Fulminant, fast-growing macrodactyly recognized at birth. *A* and *B*, Dorsal views of the left hand of a newborn female with macrodactyly of the ring and middle fingers. *C* and *D*, Dorsal and palmar views six months later showing, besides the gigantic ring finger, an enlarged, axially deviated third digit. *E*, Radial view of the hand. *F*, Roentgenograph of the same. *G*, Dorsopalmar roentgenograph. *H*, Sketch illustrating the same.

early infancy, only one digit may appear oversized. The affected digit may not gain comparatively greater dimensions as the child grows. De Laurenzi (1962) called this variety the static type. In the progressive variety, the affected digit acquires disproportionate dimension as time goes on; in many instances, one or both flanking neighbors which appeared normal at birth will, in a few years, show signs of accelerated growth. The tempo of accelerated growth varies from case to case and even from digit to digit. The fast-growing digit—usually the index or middle finger—curves toward the ulnar border of the hand, while the macrodactylous thumb assumes a hyperextended, abducted position. The swelling in the palm, due to the tumefaction of the median nerve and its branches, usually appears three or four years after birth. The oversized digits attain their greatest dimensions by the end of puberty. Osteoarthritic changes of the interphalangeal joints intervene during adulthood (Figs. 18–4 to 18–11).

(*Text continued on page 623.*)

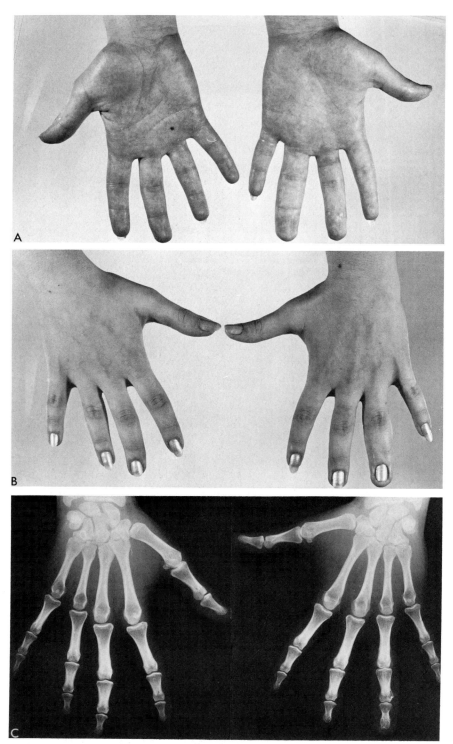

Figure 18–5 Sluggishly evolving ("static" type of) macrodactyly. *A,* Palmar view of the hands of a 23-year-old female whose left middle and ring fingers are longer and thicker than the corresponding digits of the contralateral hand. *B,* Dorsal view. *C,* Dorsopalmar roentgenograph: the affected digits, especially the left ring finger, have expanded ungual tufts.

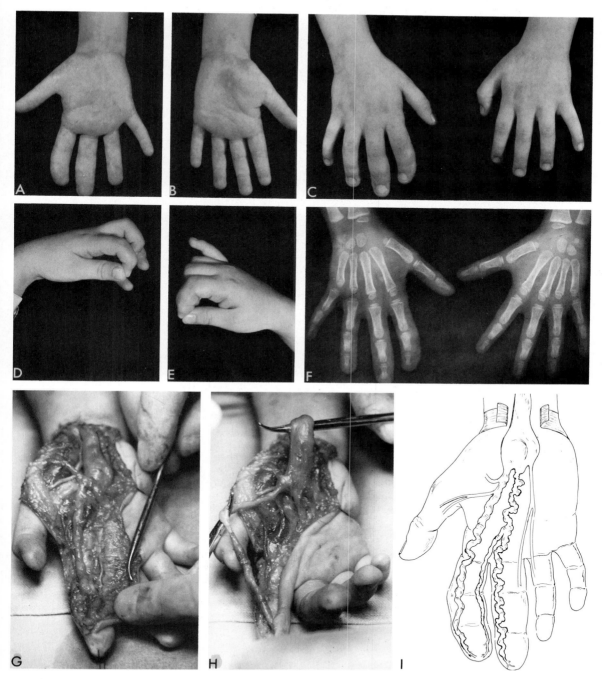

Figure 18–6 Tumefaction of the median nerve, and thickening and tortuosity of its digital branches, accompanied by macrodactyly. *A* and *B*, Palmar view of the hands of a three-year-old girl with oversized right index and middle fingers. *C*, Dorsal view. *D*, Radial view of the unaffected left hand. *E*, Radial view of the affected right hand: oversized index finger has limited flexion at the distal interphalangeal joint. *F*, Dorsopalmar roentgenograph of the hands: the phalanges of the right index and middle fingers are longer and thicker than the corresponding bones of the second and third digits of the left hand. *G*, Surgically exposed tumefied median nerve of the right hand and its thick tortuous branches going to the oversized digits. *H*, The digital nerve supplying the convex side of the curved index finger is redundant. *I*, Sketch illustrating the tumefied median nerve of the right hand and its thick tortuous branches destined to supply the oversized digits.

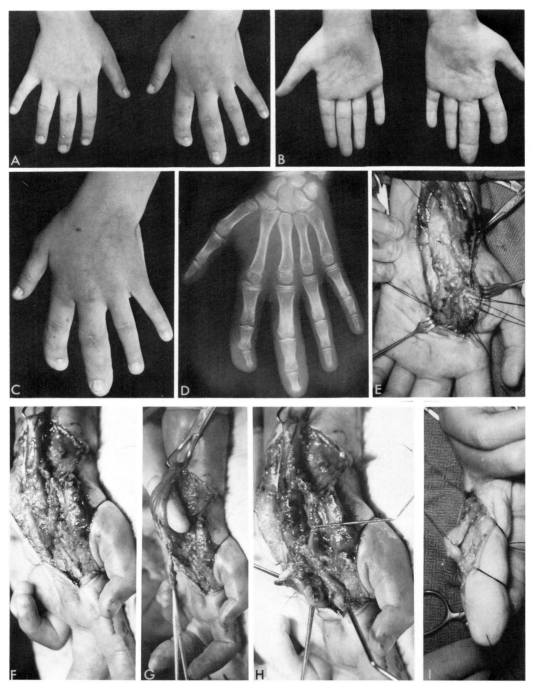

Figure 18–7   Tumefaction of the median nerve and tortuosity of the digital branches accompanied by macrodactyly. *A*, Dorsal view of the hands of a 12-year-old girl with macrodactyly of the left index and middle fingers. *B*, Palmar view: there is a definite forward bulge in the radial aspect of the left wrist and proximal palm—in line with oversized index and middle fingers. *C*, Dorsal view of the left hand—life size. *D*, Dorsopalmar roentgenograph of the left hand: when extended in the radial direction, the tangential line touching the heads of the fourth and fifth metacarpals will pass through the head of the third metacarpal, indicating that the latter is longer than it should be. *E*, Exposure of huge matted median nerve in the left proximal palm and distal forearm. *F*, Dissected nerve. *G*, Evacuation of the fatty contents of the tumefied nerve. *H*, Large intraneural cavity left after evacuation of fat globules. *I*, Thick tortuous digital nerve on the ulnar aspect of the left middle finger.

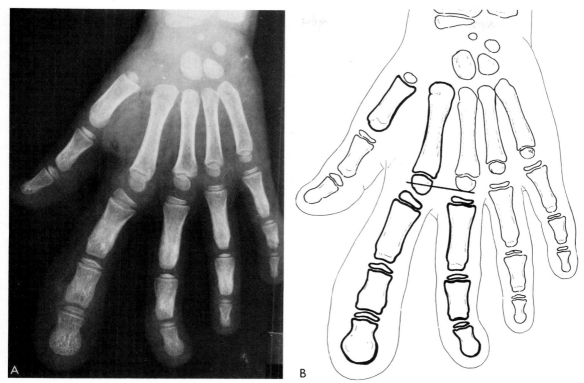

Figure 18–8 Distoproximal configuration of the digital bones in fulminant NTOM. *A*, Dorsopalmar roentgenograph of the left hand of a four-year-old girl with oversized index and, to a lesser extent, middle fingers: the ungual tuft of each affected digit is expanded; the distal phalanx is thicker than the middle bone and this in turn is thicker than the proximal phalanx which has a trapezoid epiphysis with broader radial border and slanted articular surface. The second metacarpal is longer and thicker than the third. *B*, Sketch illustrating the same.

HYPEROSTOTIC VARIETY

In a number of cases of manual macrodactyly, the median nerve and its branches are not enlarged, nor do they bear any tumors; however, the skeletal elements seem to have gone out of control. The metacarpal and phalangeal bones have attained disproportionate dimensions and undergone bizarre contortions. In some cases, one sees massive osteocartilaginous plaques around the joints. In young children, the cartilaginous component of the deposits predominates, but in time cartilage is replaced by bone. Curiously, this form of macrodactyly also favors digits which obtain their volar sensory supply from the median nerve. But here the resemblance ends. In the hyperostotic variety, the deposition of excess bone is nodular and the ungual tuft—which is characteristically massive in cases in which the median nerve is tumefied and has thick tortuous branches—is unaffected. Occasionally one also sees associated dysplasia of the radiocapitellar joint, subluxation of the radial head and osteocartilaginous loose bodies of the elbow, and even hemihypertrophy. Understandably, the hyperostotic variety of macrodactyly was not recognized until the advent of roentgenography. The first roentgenographs of macrodactylous hands were reported by Plauchu (1897). About 17 cases have since been reported. In most of them the skeletal elements of the affected digits bear cauliflower-like osteocartilaginous or osseous deposits blocking the joint motion. Killinger's (1925, 1945) patient had osteoplastic macrodactyly of both hands (Figs. 18–12 to 18–14).

(*Text continued on page 630.*)

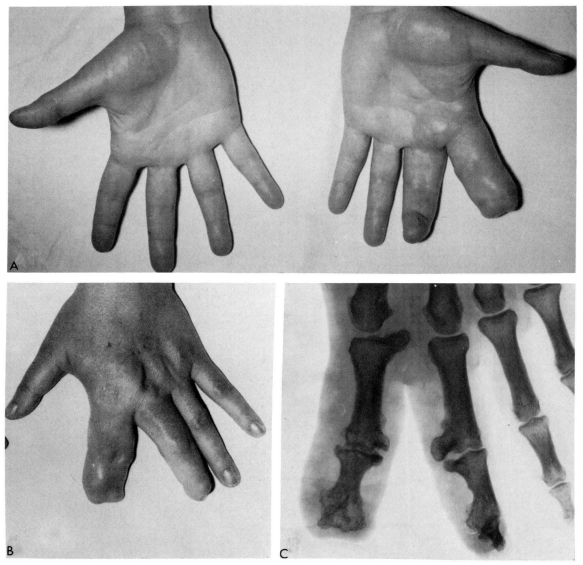

Figure 18–9 NTOM with osteoarthritic changes. *A*, Palmar view of the hands of an adult male with macrodactyly of the left index and middle fingers which had been subjected to terminal amputation, without any attempt to reduce the thickness of the affected digits. *B*, Dorsal view of the left hand. *C*, Dorsopalmar (positive) roentgenograph of the left three central digits.

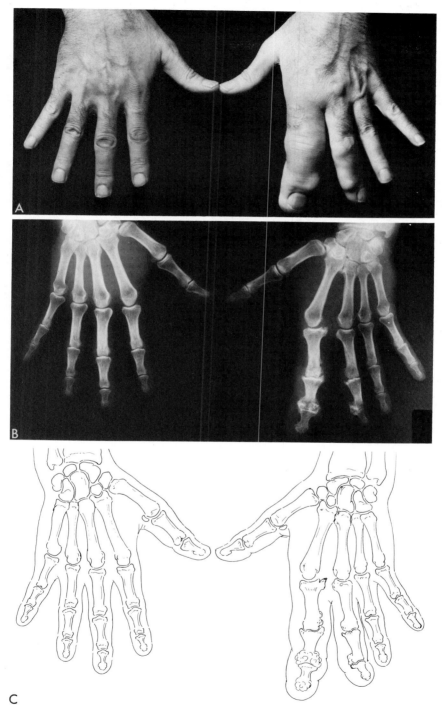

Figure 18–10 NTOM evolving into interlocking type of osteoarthritis. *A*, Dorsal view of the hands of an adult male with macrodactyly of the left index and middle fingers, but especially the former. *B*, Dorsopalmar roentgenograph: there is an osteophyte emanating from the ulnar base of the proximal phalanx of the index finger, and both interphalangeal joints of this digit are surrounded by osseous overgrowths which are more exuberant around the distal articulation; osteophytes are also seen around the interphalangeal joints of the middle finger, and here again they are more profuse around the distal than around the proximal articulations. *C*, Sketch illustrating the same.

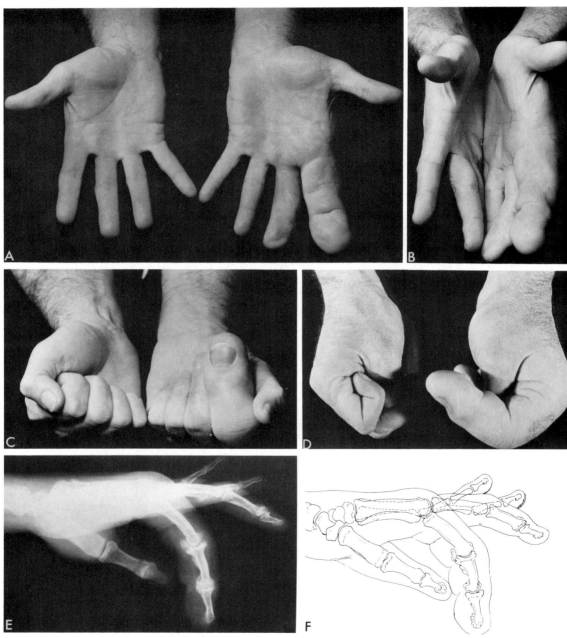

Figure 18–11 *A,* Palmar view of the hands of the adult male featured in Figure 18–10. *B,* Radial view. *C,* Frontal view of the hands in the act of making a fist: the left index and middle fingers fail to flex at the distal interphalangeal joints. *D,* Radial view of the same. *E,* Lateral roentgenograph of the left hand: articular ends of the bones entering into the proximal and distal interphalangeal joints of the middle finger have sprouted interlocking osteophytes. *F,* Sketch illustrating the same.

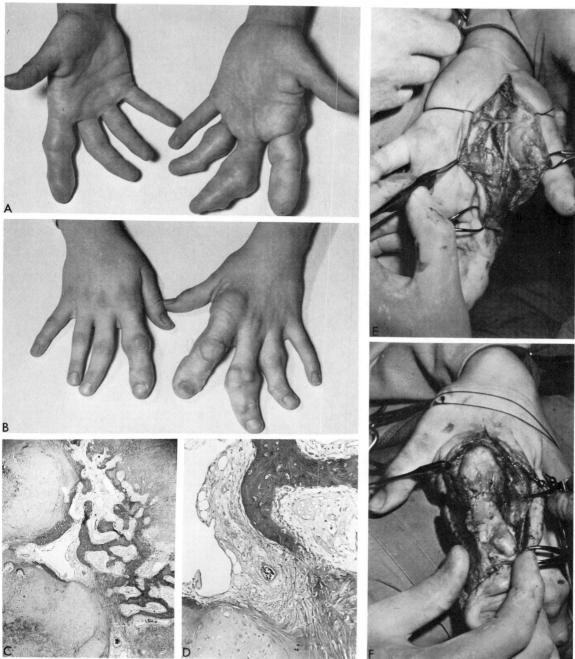

Figure 18–12 Hyperostotic macrodactyly. *A*, Palmar view of the hands of a 13-year-old female with macrodactyly of the right index and middle, and the left index, middle, and ring fingers. *B*, Dorsal view. *C* and *D*, Sections of the osteochondroma removed from the distal end of the proximal phalanx of the left index finger as shown in *F*. *E*, Surgical exposure of the left palm: the main stem of the median nerve bears no tumor and the digital branches going to the oversized fingers are neither thick nor tortuous. *F*, The left index finger seen from dorsal and radial aspect during surgical exploration: Near the joints each bone bears knobby excrescencies. This patient had a complete skeletal survey: she did not have multiple exostoses.

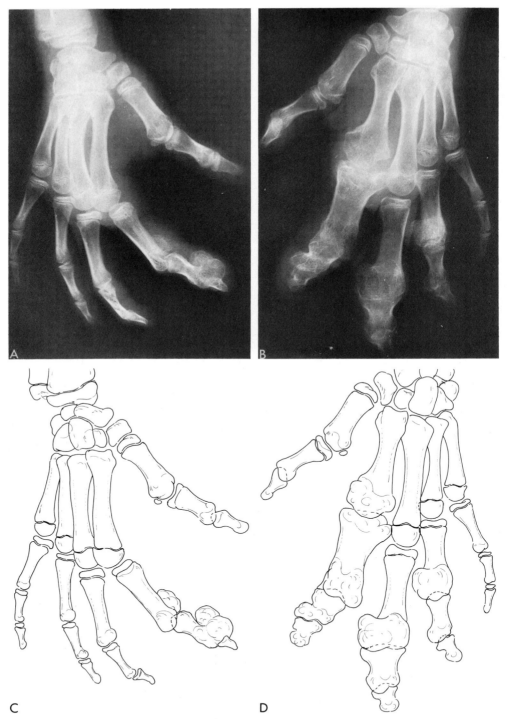

Figure 18–13 *A* and *B*, Oblique roentgenographs of the right and left hands of the 13-year-old female featured in Figure 18–12: the ungual tufts of the oversized digits are not expanded; the second metacarpal of the left hand has a bulbous head, and the third metacarpal of the same hand extends further forward than its flanking neighbors; the proximal phalanx of the left index finger is bulky; in general, the articular ends of bones entering into the interphalangeal joints are bulbous. *C* and *D* illustrate the roentgenograph above each.

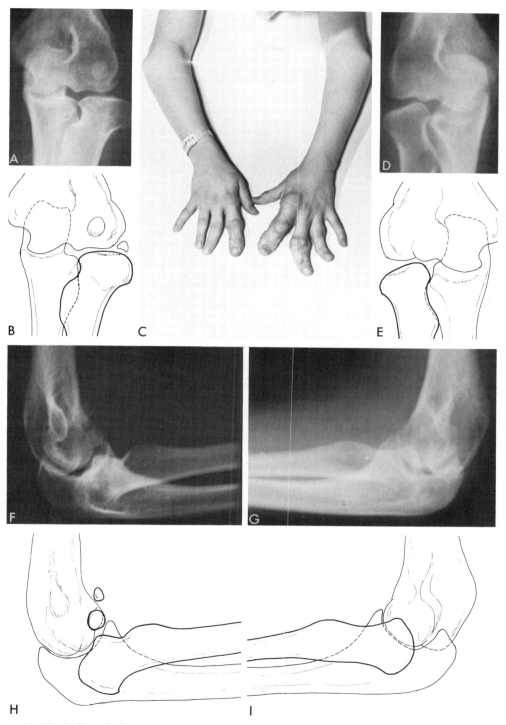

Figure 18–14 Radiocapitellar dysplasia of both elbows occurring in association with bilateral osteoplastic macrodactyly. *A*, Dorsopalmar roentgenograph of the right elbow of the 13-year-old female featured in Figures 18–12 and 18–13: the capitulum of the humerus is flat; the radial head is domed; there are two intra-articular osteocartilaginous loose bodies. *B*, Sketch illustrating the same. *C*, Elbows, forearms, and hands seen from dorsal aspect; elbows fail to extend fully. *D*, Dorsopalmar roentgenograph of the left elbow. *E*, Sketch illustrating the same. *F*, Lateral roentgenograph of the right elbow. *G*, Lateral roentgenograph of the left elbow. *H* and *I* illustrate the roentgenograph above each: both radial heads are dislocated dorsally.

ASSOCIATIONS

Bilateral macrodactyly accounts for about 5 per cent and macrosyndactyly (webbing of two neighboring oversized digits, usually of the middle and ring fingers) for 10 per cent of reported cases. Froelich's (1908) patient with macrosyndactyly had, in addition, a small supernumerary postaxial digit. Most oversized and conjoined digits and all inordinately enlarged digits have macronychia. All gigantic digits eventually turn toward one side of the hand, usually in the ulnar direction; clinodactyly is perhaps the most common accompaniment of macrodactyly. Moore (1941, 1942) described a case of macrodactyly with definite "trigger" phenomenon: the oversized digit could not be flexed or extended unimpeded until the transverse volar carpal ligament was split and the tumor-bearing median nerve permitted unhampered excursion. Carpal tunnel syndrome has been reported by several authors. Trophic changes, such as ulceration of the finger tips, are also known to occur (Fig. 18–15).

In the cases of macrodactyly described by Pool (1910), Hippe and Hähle (1937), and Schachter (1939), the enlargement extended beyond the anatomical boundary of the hand and involved parts of the forearm, upper arm, and even of the shoulder. Streeter's (1930) patient with macrodactyly of the left thumb and index finger had oversized right metacarpals, radius, and ulna, together with enlargement of the overlying soft parts. Macrodactyly is unique among congenital anomalies of the hand in that it is seldom associated with systemic disorders.

CONTRAST WITH PEDAL MACRODACTYLY

There are about 60 reported cases of pedal macrodactyly, which appears to be less common than macrodactyly of the hand. Macrosyndactyly and osteoplastic changes are relatively more common in the foot. As in the hand, the pre-axial digits—the digits supplied by the median branch of the plantar nerve—are pre-eminently affected. In macrodactyly of the foot, one hardly ever sees a tumefied median plantar nerve nor any thick and tortuous digital branches. The oversized toe owes most of its bulk to excessive fat, which is especially abundant on its plantar aspect and on its sides; accretion of fat extends into the plantar aspect of the forefoot, causing this part to bulge. The axial digit of the hand is the middle finger; in fulminant macrodactyly, this digit tends to curve sideways. The axial digit of the foot is the second toe, which is affected most commonly in pedal macrodactyly. Being supported on either side by two comparatively stable digits and possessing greater bulk on its plantar aspect, the second toe curls up in a dorsal direction (Figs. 18–16 and 18–17).

CONGENITAL TUMORS SIMULATING MACRODACTYLY

Digital enlargements due to angiodysplastic disturbances will be taken up in Chapter Nineteen. At this point, it is sufficient to say that in diffuse hemangiomas or lymphangiomas all five digits are pudgy; they are thick and

(*Text continued on page 635.*)

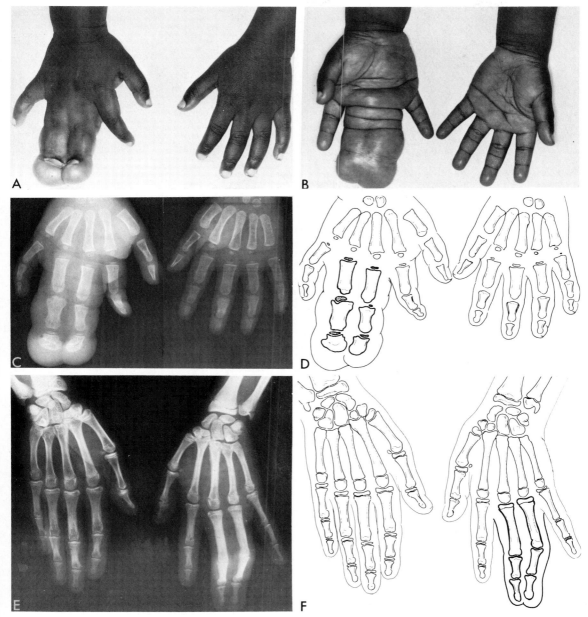

Figure 18–15 Macrosyndactyly: two different cases—one with fulminant and the other with sluggish overgrowth. *A* and *B*, Dorsal and palmar views of the hands of a nine-month-old boy with fast-growing macrosyndactyly of the right middle and ring fingers. *C*, Dorsopalmar roentgenograph: the ungual phalanges of the right middle and ring fingers are thicker than the immediate proximal bones, and these in turn are thicker than the basal phalanges; the middle and ungual phalanges of the affected digits of the right hand have acquired epiphyses precociously. *D*, Sketch illustrating the same. *E*, Dorsopalmar roentgenograph of a 15-year-old male with static macrodactyly of the left middle and ring fingers. *F*, Sketch illustrating the same.

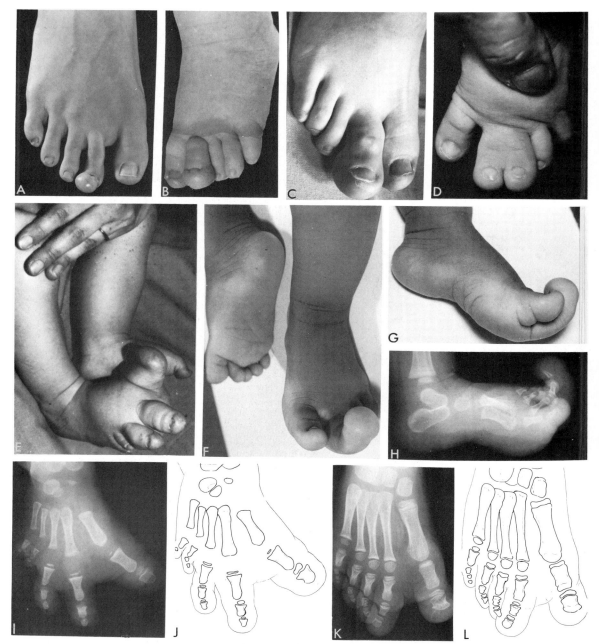

Figure 18–16 Pedal macrodactyly. *A,* Static macrodactyly involving mainly the ungual segment of the right second toe of a 12-year-old boy. *B,* Moderately progressive macrodactyly of the left second toe of an 11-month-old girl. *C,* Fulminant macrodactyly of the right second toe and moderately progressive macrodactyly of the right first toe of a three-year-old boy. *D,* Macrosyndactyly involving the left second and third toes of a two-year-old girl. *E,* Macrodactyly of the right first, second, and third toes of a two-year-old girl. *F, G,* and *H* represent the left foot of another two-year-old girl with macrodactyly of the first and second toes, with dorsal incurvation of the latter. *I,* Dorsoplantar roentgenograph of the right foot shown in *E:* interdigital accretion of fat has caused hallux varus and metatarsus primus varus. *J,* Sketch illustrating the same. *K,* Dorsoplantar roentgenograph of the right forefoot of a seven-year-old girl with macrodactyly of the first and second toes: ungual tufts of the affected toes are expanded and the distal phalanx of the great toe is as thick as, if not thicker than, the proximal phalanx. *L,* Sketch illustrating the same.

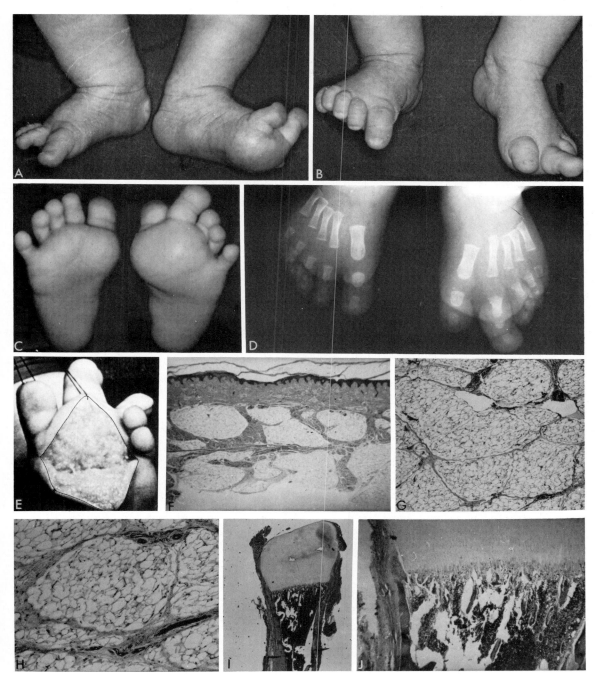

Figure 18–17 Pedal macrodactyly. *A, B,* and *C,* Sundry views of the feet of a four-week-old boy with oversized left second toe, moderately enlarged left third toe, and bulging of the area under the heads of the three tibial metatarsals. *D,* Dorsoplantar roentgenograph of the feet: the bones of the second digital ray of the left foot are longer and thicker than the corresponding elements of the right foot. *E,* Surgical exposure of the bulging area under the heads of the three tibial metatarsals. As shown in *F, G,* and *H,* biopsy sections obtained from this area and from the second toe reveal extensive fatty infiltration. *I* represents a sagittal section of the proximal half of the resected basal phalanx of the second toe, and *J* is a section through the physis.

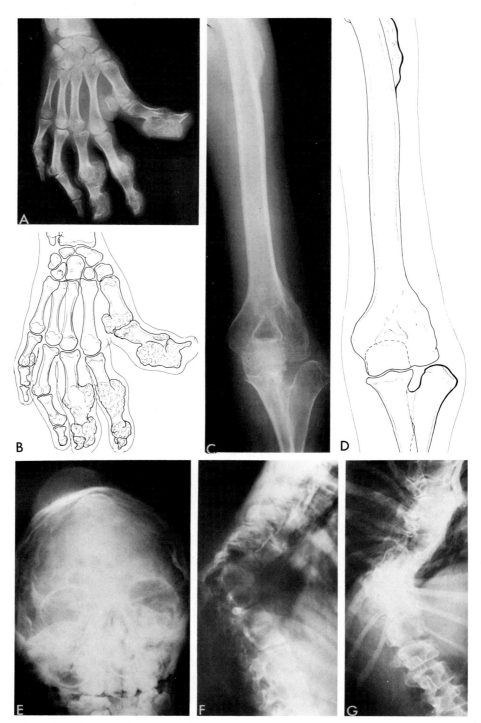

Figure 18–18 Multiple exostoses simulating osteoplastic macrodactyly and associated with so-called dislocated type (see Chapter Twenty-seven) of proximal radioulnar synostosis of the opposite arm and kyphoscoliosis. *A,* Dorsopalmar roentgenograph of the right hand of a 15-year-old female: the interphalangeal joints of the three radial digits are bridged over by massive bony overgrowth. *B* illustrates roentgenograph above it. *C,* Anteroposterior roentgenograph of the left humerus and proximal forearm: there is a sessile bony overgrowth on the lateral aspect of the proximal humerus; there is proximal radioulnar synostosis but the head of the radius is free and inclines away from the olecranon process of the ulna. *D,* Sketch illustrating the same. *E,* Exostosis emanating from the skull. *F* and *G* show kyphoscoliosis.

turgid but not too long. Selective involvement of one or two digits often occurs in Klippel-Trenaunay syndrome. In either instance, the affected digit does not attain the striking length nor the banana-like configuration of NTOM. In multiple exostoses, enchondromatosis with hemangioma (Maffucci syndrome) or without vascular tumors (Ollier's disease), the affected digits are not long but they present irregular, knobby swellings. Unlike NTOM, Ollier's enchondromatosis shows distinct predilection for the ulnar digits and yields better results after surgical intervention. Léri and Joanny (1922) described a 39-year-old female who, since the age of 10, had been aware of thick, divergent left index and middle fingers; roentgenographs revealed an irregular condensation of the humerus, radius, ulna, central carpal ossicles, and the bones of the second and third digital rays. The picture recalled the drippings of wax down the stem of a burning candle; hence, the term melorheostosis, which means flowing bone, was used. Since melorheostosis tends to involve only a single limb, the adjective monomelic applies. The involved bones, including metacarpals and phalanges of the hand, are thick but not long; the affected digit may also incline to one side as in NTOM, but outlandish axial deviations featured in Fig. 18–1 are not known to occur (Figs. 18–18 to 18–21).

TREATMENT

It was argued at one time that, since feet were made smaller by the Chinese method of binding, oversized digits could likewise be reduced in size by compression with elastic bandages. This method was tried but it failed to reduce the size of the macrodactylous digit, and in some instances it was followed by disastrous consequences. It was also hoped that curtailing the blood supply of a gigantic digit would reduce its size. Ligation of the artery of the oversized finger likewise enjoyed a temporary vogue and was eventually given up. However, the following procedures are still in use: excision of soft-tissue mass, growth arrest and attenuation of thick phalanges, angulation osteotomy, recession osteotomy, resection of articular ends followed by fusion or arthroplasty, and amputation. In the fulminant, fast-growing type of macrodactyly, several of these measures are dovetailed.

The incision for resection of excessive soft tissue is longitudinally disposed and is elliptical. It is carried out on one side of the oversized digit at a time. Usually, the convex side of the digit is attacked first. The skin and the subcutaneous tissue are removed. In the fast-growing, fulminant type of macrodactyly, the redundant segment of the volar digital nerve is included in the resected soft-tissue mass. Volar digital branches send twigs to supply the skin on the back of the distal two phalanges. Each dorsal twig splits away from the corresponding digital branch before the latter reaches the level of the first interphalangeal joint. A segment of the redundant volar digital nerve distal to this point is removed and the remaining ends are sutured together. In six out of seven digits operated on by this method, sensation returned within three months. In one case, the index finger remained anesthetic; sensation was restored by transferring a neurovascular island-graft from the ulnar side of the ring finger to the radial and volar aspect of the index finger. In the proximal palm, an elliptical segment

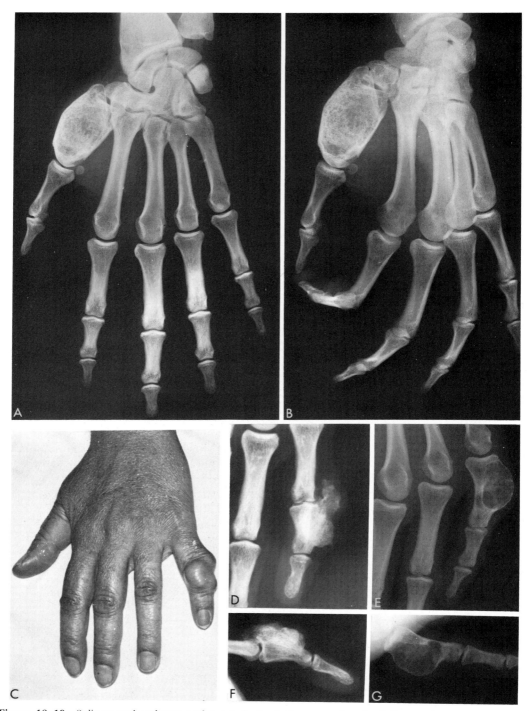

Figure 18–19   Solitary enchondroma and exostosis simulating macrodactyly. *A*, Dorsopalmar roentgenograph of the left hand of an adult male with ossifying enchondroma of the first metacarpal. *B*, Oblique view of the same. *C*, Dorsal view of the left hand of an adult female with a massive exostosis emanating from the ulnar and dorsal aspect of the middle phalanx of the little finger. *D*, Dorsopalmar roentgenograph of the little finger of the same patient. *E*, Lateral roentgenograph of the same. *F*, Dorsopalmar roentgenograph of the left little finger of another patient with expanding enchondroma of the proximal phalanx. *G*, Lateral roentgenograph of the same.

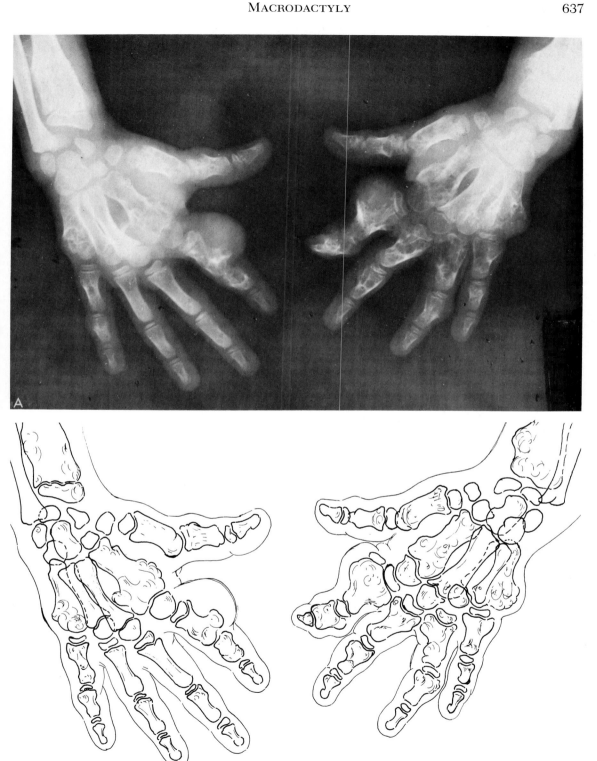

Figure 18–20   Multiple enchondromatosis of the hands simulating macrodactyly. *A*, Dorsopalmar view of the hands of a seven-year-old boy with thick but not long digits: characteristically, ungual tufts which are formed in membrane are not affected in this disease. *B*, Sketch illustrating the same.

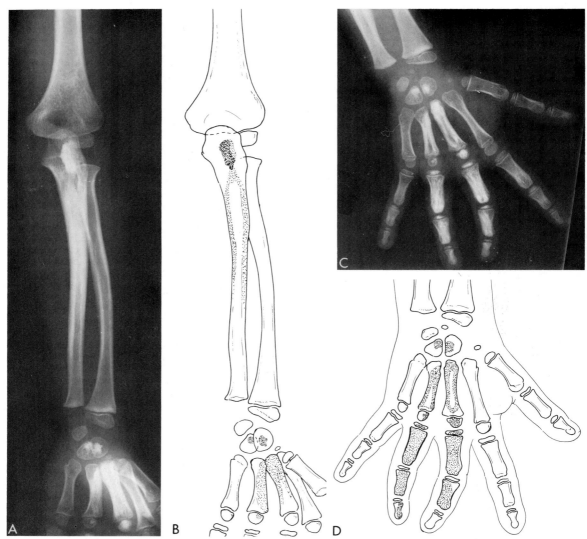

Figure 18–21   Léri's melorheostosis. *A,* Dorsovolar roentgenograph of a three-year-old girl who was brought for consultation for axially deviated right middle and ring fingers: hyperostosis involved the ulna, the capitate and hamate bones, and the third and fourth digital rays of the right upper limb. *B,* Sketch illustrating flowing hyperostosis of the ulna, capitate, hamate, and third and fourth metacarpals of the right upper limb. *C,* Dorsopalmar roentgenograph of the hand. *D,* Sketch illustrating the same.

of the sheath enveloping the tumor of the median nerve is resected, the interfibrillar globules of fat are evacuated, and the edges of the sheath are sutured together. In subjects with carpal tunnel syndrome or "trigger" phenomenon, the volar carpal ligament is slit open.

    Surgical arrest of the growth of the skeletal elements of the macrodactylous digit was advocated long ago by Massonnaud (1874), who recommended destruction of the growth cartilage plate of each phalanx. Sicard and associates (1916) advised excision of the metacarpal epiphysis. Sorrel et al (1934) recommended resection of the "fertile cartilage," meaning the physes. Clifford (1959) destroyed the growth plate with a motorized drill. Jones (1963) considered the

(*Text continued on page 642.*)

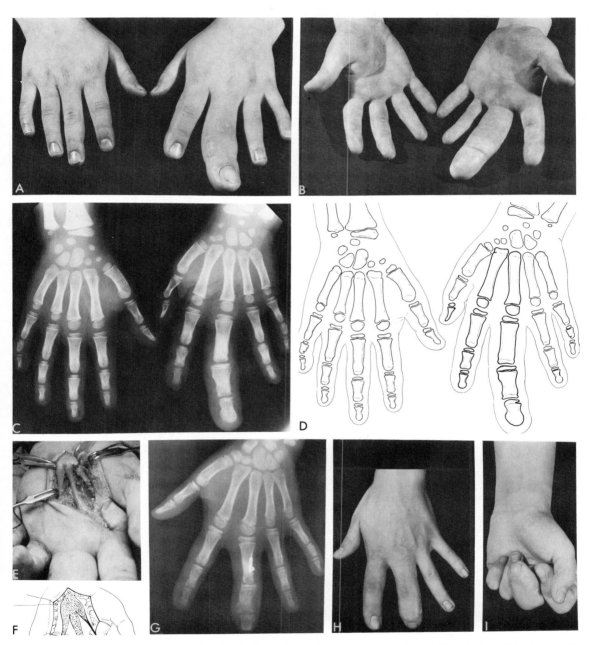

Figure 18–22 Macrodactyly associated with signs of carpal tunnel compression. *A*, Dorsal view of the hands of a six-year-old boy with macrodactyly of the left index, but mainly of the left middle, finger which had been subjected to elliptical excision of excess soft tissue from its radial aspect. Subsequent surgery consisted of releasing the tumor-bearing median nerve from under the deep transverse carpal ligament, epiphysiodesis of the proximal two phalanges of the middle finger, amputation of its splayed ungual tuft and thinning of the diaphysis, as well as closed wedge osteotomy of the second phalanx. *B*, Palmar view: note the comparatively flat thenar eminence of the left hand. *C*, Dorsopalmar roentgenograph of the hands: the metacarpals of the affected digits of the left hand are longer and thicker. *D*, Sketch illustrating the same. *E*, Part of the tumor of the median nerve protruded from under the transverse carpal ligament which necessitated extension of the incision proximally as illustrated in *F*. *G*, Postoperative roentgenograph of the left hand taken four years after surgery at the age of 14. *H* and *I*, Results. The second interphalangeal joint of the middle finger was stiff, as was the corresponding joint of the index finger, which was not operated upon.

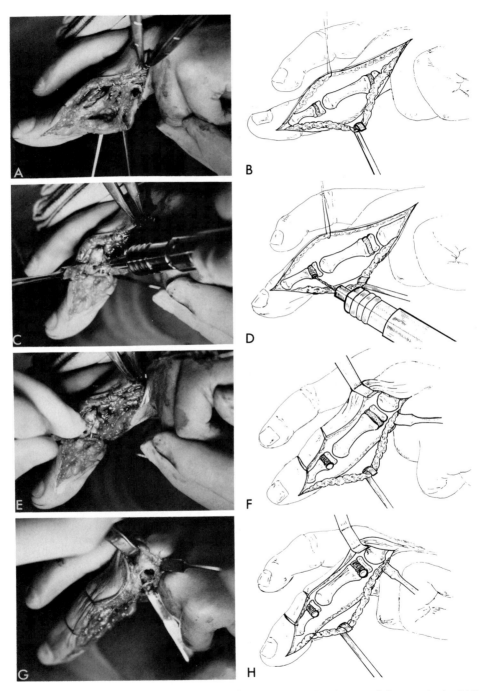

Figure 18–23   Epiphysiodesis. *A* and *B*, Exposure of the ulnar aspect of the oversized middle finger of the left hand of the boy featured in Figure 18–22. *C* and *D*, Destruction of the physis of the middle phalanx by a motorized drill. *E*, *F*, *G*, and *H*, The holes across the physes of both phalanges.

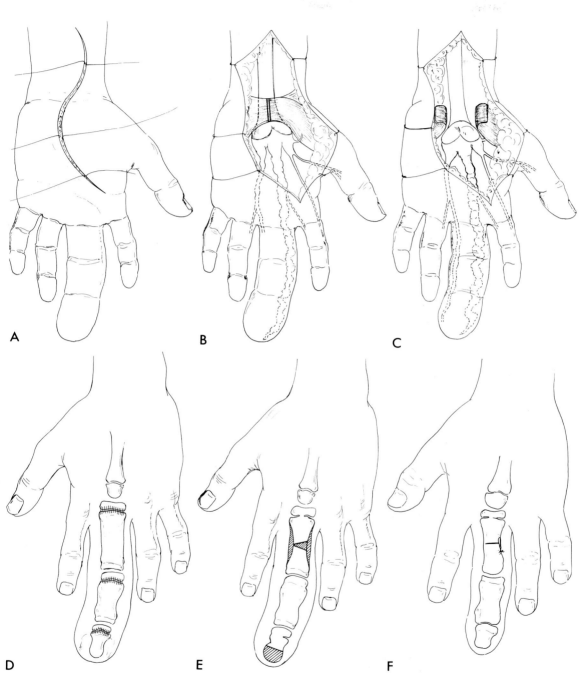

A

B

C

D

E

F

Figure 18–24 Sketches illustrating sundry procedures utilized for relieving carpal tunnel syndrome and for shortening an oversized ulnarly deviated middle finger of the boy featured in Figures 18–22 and 18–23. *A*, Incision. *B*, Severance of transverse carpal ligament. *C*, Tumefied median nerve freed from its entrapment. *D*, Epiphysiodesis of the phalanges. *E*, Corrective osteotomy combined with attenuation of the proximal phalanx. *F*, Holding the fragments of osteotomized phalanx together with a stainless steel wire suture.

surgeon fortunate if he saw a patient with macrodactyly at an early age. He thought that epiphyseal arrest "would lessen the final disparity and would at the same time preserve the function of abnormally growing digits."

One wishes that the problem were as simple as implied. Growth in length is only one aspect of macrodactyly. Not only are the bones long but they are also inordinately thick. The affected digit is voluminous and, in many instances, curved. In the sluggishly growing type of macrodactyly, it is feasible to obtain satisfactory results by epiphysiodesis of two or more phalanges and by longitudinal wedge resection of soft tissue from the sides of the digit. In the fast-growing, fulminant variety, epiphysiodesis of the phalanges may arrest their growth in length, but it will not reduce their bulk. Following destruction of the growth cartilage, the phalanges continue to gain girth owing to the continued addition of bone by periosteum. In macrodactyly of young, growing children, epiphysiodesis is supplemented by stripping the periosteum of the thickened phalanx. When the periosteum is stripped, the osteogenic layer remains with the shaft of the bone. It is necessary to shave slivers from the cortex of the shaft and cauterize the remaining surface. Even such a drastic measure may fail to destroy the bone-producing cambium layer of the periosteum. The stripped and cauterized phalangeal bone may continue to thicken, though, one hopes, not as vigorously. In older children and adults, the thickened phalanx is surgically attenuated.

Angulation osteotomy of one of the phalanges—usually of the middle phalanx—is often employed to correct the axial deviation of the digit. To reduce the length of the digit, a segment of bone is removed from the midshaft of the phalanx and the remaining fragments are connected together. This procedure is called recession osteotomy. It is carried out on one phalanx at a time. By resecting an appropriate piece of bone, one may shorten the long finger and correct its deviation at the same time.

Recession osteotomy may include one of the interphalangeal joints, the ultimate result being that of arthrodesis. Unfortunately, sufficient bone cannot be excised from the basal portion of the terminal phalanx without disturbing the nail matrix. If a large segment is removed from the middle phalanx and the terminal bone is pushed back toward it, excessive soft tissue bulges sideways at this juncture.

Arthrodesis of the first metacarpophalangeal joint of the thumb is justifiable in macrodactyly of this digit. Sufficient bone is removed from both sides of this joint; the thumb is shortened and stabilized in a serviceable position. The bulk of the thenar eminence is reduced by removing the skin, subcutaneous fat, and, if necessary, a segment of the tortuous digital nerve and suturing the remaining ends.

Amputation would seem to offer a logical solution for isolated macrodactyly of one of the lesser digits. It has been noted time and again, however, that in the wake of the amputation of a single macrodactylous member, the digit next to it, which merely looked pudgy before, soon demonstrates accelerated growth. Almost invariably, the concavity of the palm disappears and a tumor begins to bulge in the area overlying the main trunk of the median nerve. It is now generally agreed that most cases of macrodactyly are progressive. What appears as a plump digit in a newborn may in a year or two acquire gigantic proportions; the tumor of the median nerve, seldom suspected at birth, grows insidiously. Amputation of the spatulate, sprawling ungual tuft or even of the entire distal phalanx is often indicated. Dufourmentel and Mouly (1959) and Mouly and Debeyre (1961) supplemented terminal amputation of the digit by free graft of the nail.

(*Text continued on page 650.*)

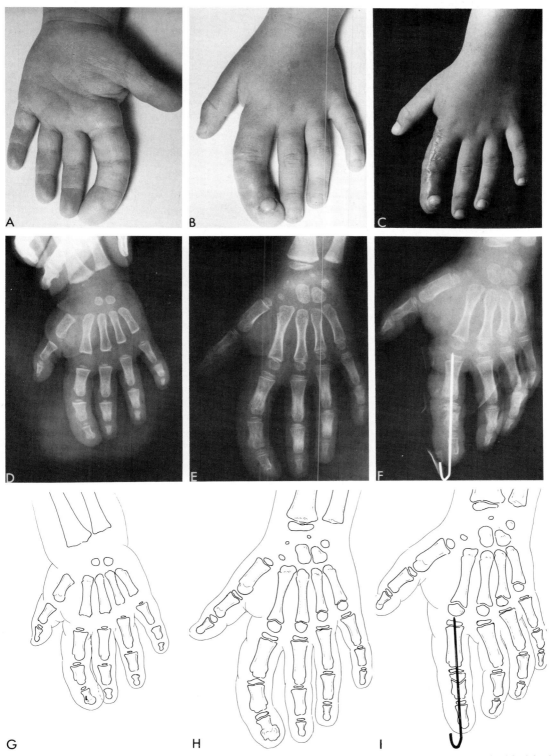

Figure 18–25 Sluggishly evolving macrodactyly. *A*, Palmar view of the left hand of a five-month-old girl with moderately enlarged index finger. *B*, Dorsal view. *C*, The same four years after surgery. *D*, Dorsopalmar roentgenograph prior to surgery. *E*, Dorsopalmar roentgenograph four years after surgery. *F*, Site of osteotomy and fixation of fragments with transosseous K-wire. *G*, *H*, and *I* illustrate the roentgenograph above each.

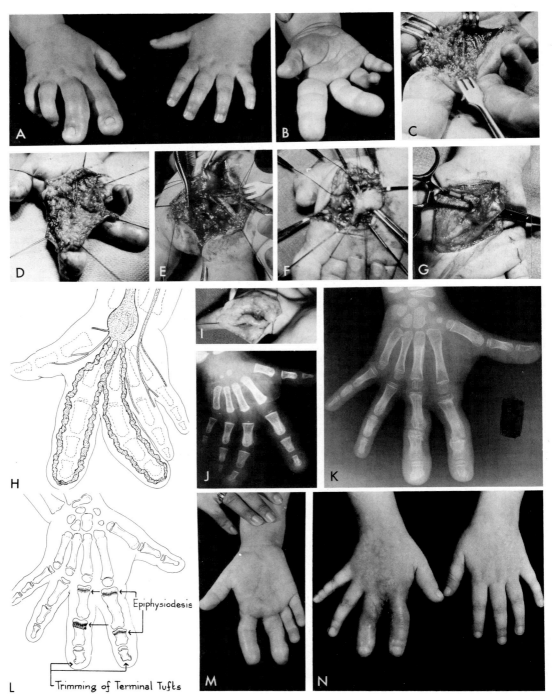

Figure 18–26 Fulminant macrodactyly of the right index and middle fingers with sluggish overgrowth of the thumb—treated by removal of fibroadipose tissue from inside the tumefied median nerve, elliptical excision of excess soft tissue from the sides of affected digits, attenuation of diaphysis and epiphysiodesis of the proximal two phalanges, and amputation of ungual tufts. *A*, Dorsal view of the hands of a five-month-old girl with macrodactyly of the right thumb and index and middle fingers. *B*, Palmar view of the right hand. *C*, Exploration of the palm: digital nerves going to the index and middle fingers are thick. *D*, Extension of the incision along the ulnar aspect of the index finger, showing over-abundance of subcutaneous fibroadipose tissue, which was extirpated. *E*, At a later date, the proximal palm was explored, revealing a globular tumor on the main stem of the median nerve. *F*, The tumor after it was cleared of the overlying and surrounding fibroadipose tissue. *G*, Excision of an elliptical segment of the nerve sheath and evacuation of intrathecal fat globules. *H*, Sketch illustrating the tumefied median nerve and its thick tortuous branches supplying the oversized index and middle fingers. *I*, Tortuous digital nerve passing along the convex radial aspect of the middle finger. *J*, Preoperative dorsopalmar roentgenograph taken at the age of five months. *K*, Postoperative dorsopalmar roentgenograph taken at

Legend continued on opposite page.

644

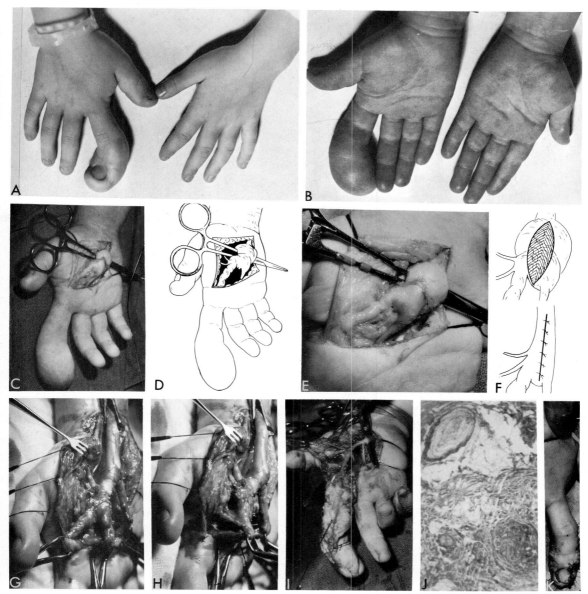

Figure 18–27 Fulminant macrodactyly. *A*, Dorsal view of the hands of a five-year-old girl with macrodactyly of the right thumb and right index finger. *B*, Palmar view. *C*, Exposure of the tumefied median nerve in the proximal palm of the right hand. *D*, Sketch illustrating the same. *E*, Enlarged photograph of the tumor of the median nerve. *F*, Sketch illustrating the elliptical incision of the nerve sheath for evacuation of interstitial fat globules and closure of the sheath. *G* and *H*, The repaired nerve sheath. *I*, The incision has been extended along the radial aspect of the index finger for resection of the redundant segment of the digital nerve. *J*, Section of the resected digital nerve which was interpreted as fibrosis of the nerve sheath in fibroadipose tissue. *K*, Dorsal view of the operated index finger immediately after closure of the surgical wound: only a small portion of the nail survived. At a later date the size of the right thumb was reduced by elliptical excision of soft tissues from its ulnar aspect.

Figure 18–26 *(Continued)*

the age of five years—after epiphysiodesis of the proximal and middle phalanges and amputation of the ungual tufts of the oversized digits were performed; resection of the physis of the middle phalanx of the curved third digit included a wedge of the metaphysis to correct the ulnar deviation of the distal segments. *L*, Sketch illustrating epiphysiodesis and amputation of the ungual tufts of the affected digits. *M*, Postoperative palmar view of the right hand. *N*, Postoperative dorsal view of both hands. The last two photographs were taken at the age of five and have been reduced in order to be fitted into the available space in this montage.

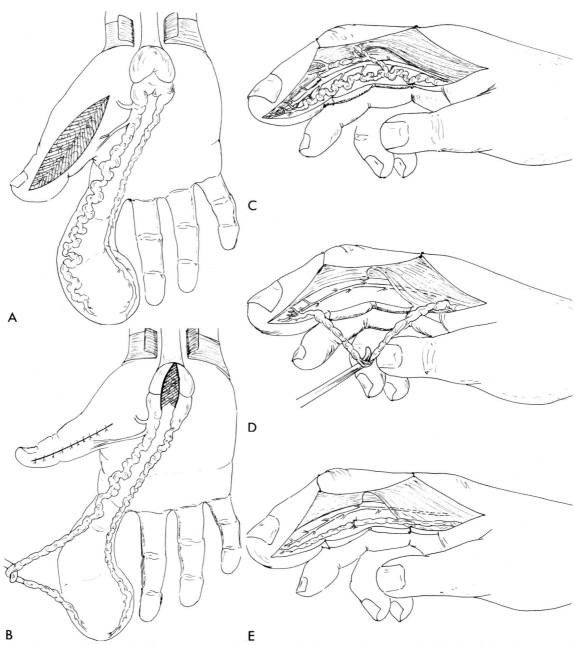

Figure 18–28   Sketches illustrating operative work on soft tissues carried out on the right hand of the five-year-old girl featured in Figure 18–27. *A*, Elliptical incision on the ulnar aspect of the thumb, tumor of the median nerve in the proximal palm, and the tortuous distal nerve on the radial aspect of the index finger. *B*, Closure of the incision on the thumb, and elliptical excision of the sheath enveloping the median nerve tumor and redundant digital nerve. *C*, Tortuous digital nerve in relation to the artery. *D*, Redundant segment of the digital nerve which was resected. *E*, Suturing the remainder of the digital nerves.

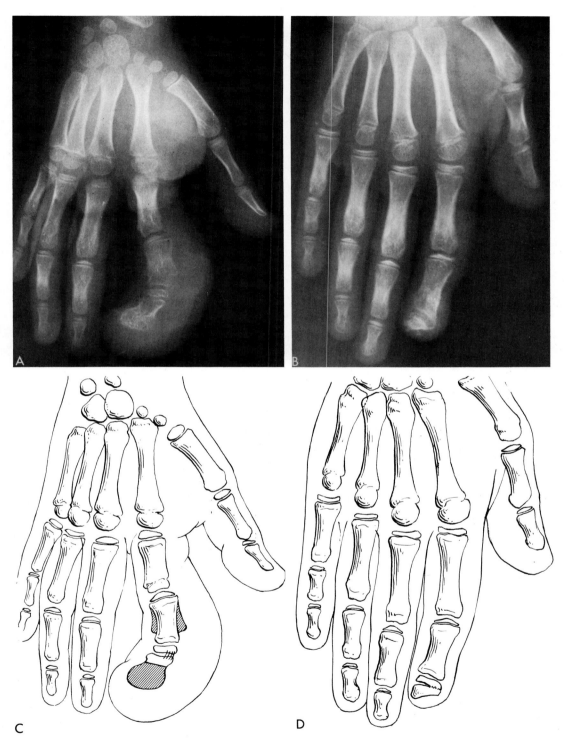

Figure 18–29 Resection of the ungual tuft, attenuation of the shaft of the middle phalanx, and partial epiphysiodesis of the ungual phalanx. *A*, Preoperative dorsopalmar roentgenograph of the right hand of the five-year-old girl featured in Figure 18–28. *B*, Postoperative dorsopalmar roentgenograph. *C*, Sketch illustrating amputation of the ungual tuft, attenuation of the shaft of the middle phalanx, and epiphysiodesis of the radial sector of the epiphysis of the ungual phalanx of the right index finger. *D*, Sketch illustrating postoperative roentgenograph.

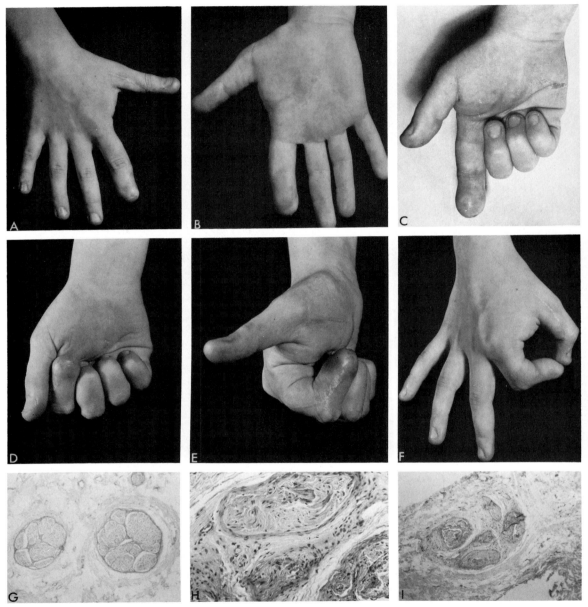

Figure 18–30   The outcome. *A*, Postoperative dorsal view of the right hand of the five-year-old girl featured in Figures 18–27 to 18–29. *B*, Palmar view. *C, D, E,* and *F*, Postoperative functional ability. *G, H,* and *I*, Biopsy sections which were interpreted as fibrosis of digital nerves and surrounding fibroadipose tissue.

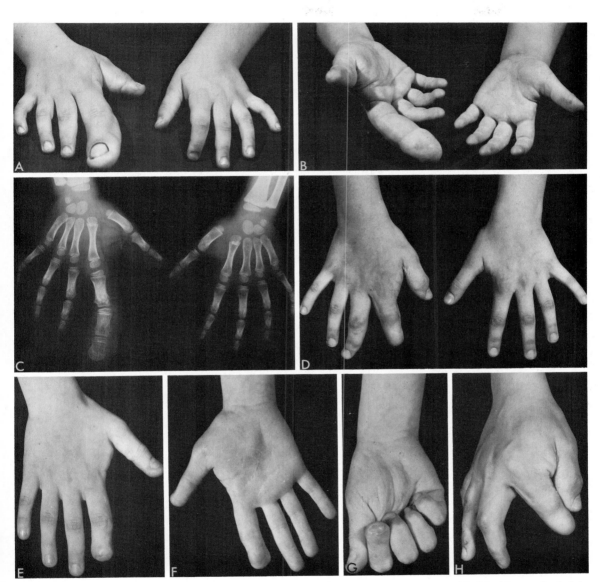

Figure 18–31 Fulminant macrodactyly. *A*, Dorsal view of the hands of a three-year-old girl with oversized right thumb and index and middle fingers. *B*, Palmar view. *C*, Dorsopalmar roentgenograph of the right and left hands. *D*, Dorsal view of the hands eight years after surgery, which included: excision of an elliptical segment of skin and subcutaneous tissue from the ulnar aspect of the right thumb and radial side of the index finger; shortening of the digital nerve on the ulnar aspect of the thumb and the radial side of the index finger; terminal amputation of the index finger; trimming of the middle phalangeal shaft; and epiphysiodesis of its proximal two phalanges. Subsequently, osteotomy of the second phalanx of the right middle finger was performed to correct the ulnar deviation of its ungual segment. By this time, she had stiffness in the proximal interphalangeal joint of the right index finger and radial inclination of its distal segment; this was corrected by wedge arthrectomy and fusion. *E, F*, and *G*, Results after the first series of operations. *H*, Final outcome.

    The author has seen two patients with macrosyndactyly, and both declined surgery. Another pair of patients with hyperostotic macrodactyly came to the author's attention. Surgical exploration of the hands of both patients failed to reveal any enlargement of the median nerve. In both cases, the metacarpal heads of the affected digits were large. The phalanges were massive, especially at their distal ends. The metacarpal head as well as the distal articular ends of the proximal two phalanges of the affected digits were resected. The digits were thus shortened, but they remained stiff. An attempt at arthroplasty was made on one digit with the aid of silicone rubber-dacron endoprosthesis. Only a negligible degree of active joint mobility was obtained (Figs. 18–22 to 18–33).

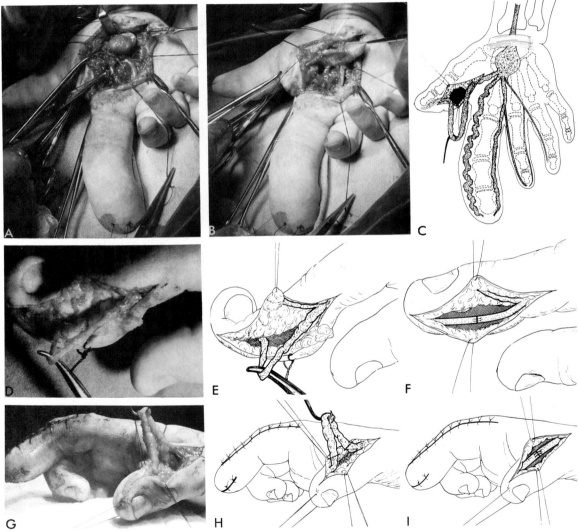

Figure 18–32   Defatting the median nerve tumor in the palm and shortening the digital nerve on the radial aspect of the index finger and ulnar side of the thumb. *A*, Exposure of the median nerve tumor in the proximal palm of the right hand of the three-year-old girl featured in Figure 18–31. *B*, The tumor is pulled toward the ulnar border of the hand, bringing into view the digital branches destined for the oversized thumb and index finger. *C*, Sketch illustrating the redundant digital branch on the ulnar aspect of the thumb and the tortuous thick nerve passing along the radial side of the index finger. *D*, The redundant segment of the index digital nerve. *E*, Sketch illustrating the same. *F*, Nerve suture after resection of the redundant segment. *G*, Redundant segment of the pollical digital nerve. *H*, Sketch illustrating the same. *I*, Suturing the ends of the nerve after resection of the redundant segment.

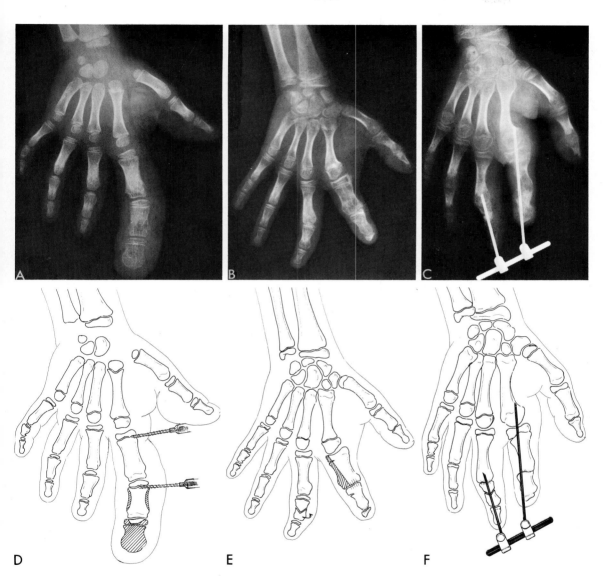

Figure 18–33 Terminal amputation, epiphysiodesis, and attenuation of the second phalanx of the index finger and angulation osteotomy of the second phalanx of the middle finger. *A,* Preoperative dorsopalmar roentgenograph of the three-year-old girl featured in Figures 18–31 and 18–32. *B,* The same, six years after terminal amputation, epiphysiodesis, and attenuation of the second phalanx of the index finger: note the increased ulnar inclination of the last two phalanges of the middle finger. *C,* Four years later at the age of 13, angulation osteotomy was performed through the second phalanx of the middle finger, and the two remaining phalanges of the index finger were fused. *D, E,* and *F* illustrate the roentgenograph above each.

SUMMARY

Nerve territory–oriented macrodactyly is a distinct clinical entity. It is characterized by excessive gain in length and girth of one or more digits which receive their palmar sensory supply either from the median or ulnar nerves—by far the great majority of cases receive their supply from the former. In no reported case of NTOM have all five digits been involved simultaneously, nor has there been a case in which overgrowth affected one digit, skipped its immediate neighbor, and involved a distant member. NTOM is a progressive, dynamic disorder; the affected digit continues to gain in length and girth as long as the child grows. In some instances, the pace of overgrowth is slow; in others, it is accelerated. The rapidly growing digit tends to undergo axial deviation, turning toward the radial or ulnar border of the hand, usually the latter. In time, a tumefaction appears in the region of the palm, in the area corresponding to the main stem of the median nerve. Occasionally, the opposite hand is involved, and at times two neighboring macrodactylous digits are enclosed within the same sleeve of skin. In some instances, the skeletal elements seem to have gone out of control early in life, and the enlarged bones crowd out the soft tissues. In time, the articular ends of the phalanges of all macrodactylous digits undergo hyperostotic changes, causing interlocking of the joints and rendering the affected member functionally defunct. The treatment is directed toward arresting the growth of the macrodactylous digit. In the slow-growing variety, epiphysiodesis of the two proximal phalanges may suffice. In the fast-growing type, no single procedure or combination of procedures preserves the function of the gigantic digit. The best one can hope for is a digit with diminished disparity of dimension, with ability to flex and extend at the metacarpophalangeal joint, and with some degree of tactile sensation at its tip. Quite often, periodic intervention becomes necessary. One is forced, at times, to amputate a gigantic finger. The thumb should never be amputated; it may be shortened by arthrectomy and fusion of the first metacarpophalangeal joint.

References

Abbe, R.: Hypertrophy of the fingers. *In The Surgery of the Hand.* Wesley M. Carpenter Lecture delivered on November 20, 1893. *Trans. N.Y. Acad. Med.* (2 s.), *10*:639–662, 1894. Also in *N.Y. State Med. J.,* *59*:33–40, fig. 7, 1894.

Abramovics, H.: Ein Fall von Megalosyndaktylie. *Münch. Med. Wochenschr.,* 76:921, 1929.

Adams, J.: Cases of hypertrophied fingers and toes. *Monthly J. Med.* (London and Edinburgh), *20*:170–173, 1855.

Adams, R.: Case of congenital hypertrophy of the index and middle fingers. *Dublin Hosp. Gaz.,* *1*:260–262, 1854–1855.

Adda, M.: Dystrophies gigantiques sans acromégalie. *N. Iconog. Salp.,* *27*:90–93, 1914. pl. XXIII, 1914.

Albert, E.: Fälle von Macrodactylie (mit Nachtrag). *Wien Med. Presse,* *13*:10, 71, 1872.

Allende, B. T.: Macrodactyly with enlarged median nerve associated with carpal tunnel syndrome. *Plast. Reconst. Surg.,* *39*:578–582, 1967.

Aloi, V.: Per la patogenesi d'un dito gigante. *Riforma Med.,* *43*:79–80, 1927.

Alosio, S., and Novellino, L.: Due casi di gigantismo parziale congenito. *Acta Ortop. Ital.,* 7:245–253, figs. 4–6, 1961.

Anderson, W.: *The Deformities of the Fingers and Toes.* London, J. & A. Church, pp. 128–144, 1897.

Annandale, T.: *The Malformations, Diseases, and Injuries of the Fingers and Toes and Their Surgical Treatment.* Philadelphia, J. B. Lippincott Co., pp. 3–10; pl. I; figs. 1,2,4, 1866.

Annecchino, A.: Su di caso di macrodattilia. *Pediatria,* *49*:162–166; figs. 1–3, 1941.

Baldazzi, G.: L'ipertrofia parziale congenita. *Riv. Clin. Pediatr.* (Firenze), *22*:729–754, 1924.

Baraldi, A.: Megalosindactylia. *Rev. Med. Rosario,* *19*:407–409; figs. 1–5, 1929.

Baraldi, A., and Ruiz, F. R.: Megaloquiria distrofica parcial secundaria a neurinoma del mediano. *Rev. Med. Rosario,* *24*:1243–1252, 1934.

Barsky, A. J.: Macrodactyly. *J. Bone Joint Surg.,* *49A*:1255–1266, 1967.

Barsky, A. J., Kahn, S., and Simon, B. E.: Macrodactyly. *In* Converse, J. M., and Littler, J. W., (eds.): *Reconstructive Plastic Surgery.* Philadelphia, W. B. Saunders Co. Vol. 4, pp. 1721–1722, 1964.

Bartholome, R.: Demonstration eines Patienten, bei dem seit der Jugend ein partieller Riesenwuchs der rechten Hand beider Daumen und der rechten Zehe mit hochgradigen Venektasien an den unteren Extremitäten bestand. *Klin. Wochenschr.,* *5*:1950, 1926.

Battelli, L.: Rilievi patogenitici e clinici sulle macrosomie parziali. *Chir. Organi Mov.,* *55*:138–148; figs. 1,2,7,8, 1966.

Battersby, F.: Congenital hypertrophy of the fingers and toes. *Dublin Med. Press,* *23*:289–290, 1850.

Bean, W. B., and Peterson, P. K.: Note on a monstrous finger. *Arch. Intern. Med.,* *104*:433–438; figs. 1–4, 1959.

Beck, G. H.: Abnorme Grösse des Daumens und des Zeigefingers der rechten Hand bei vergrössertem Umfange der ganzen oberen Extremität der rechten Seite. *Med. Annalen Heidelberg,2*:89–93, 1836.

Bégouin, P., and Sabrazès, J.: Macrodactylie et microdactylie. *N. Iconog. Salp.,* *14*:305–315, 1901.

Bell, G., and Inglis, K.: Plexiform neuroma. *Med. J. Aust.,* *2*:423–426 and supplement, 1925.

Bell, G., and Inglis, K.: Congenital tumor of the left upper limb. *Med. J. Aust.,2*:427–428; fig. 1, 1925.

Ben-Bassat, M., Casper, J., Kaplan, I., and Laron, Z.: Congenital macrodactyly: a case report with a three-year follow-up. *J. Bone Joint Surg.,* *48B*:359–364, 1966.

Berend, N.: Ein 3 Monate altes Kind mit einseitiger partieller Makrosomie. *Wien Med. Wochenschr.,* *35*:1625, 1897.

Bernoulli, P.: Ein Fall von partiellem Riesenwuchs (Macrodactylia simplex congenita). *Anat. Anz.,* *95*:372–395,; figs. 1–3, 1944.

Bibergeil, E.: Beitrag zur Histologie des kongenitalen Riesenwuchses. *Z. Orthop. Chir.,* *24*:530–537, 1909.

Bibergeil, E.: Ueber partiellem Riesenwuchs. *Berl. Klin. Wochenschr.,* *46*(1):564–566, 1909.

Bibergeil, E.: Zur Kasuistik des angeborenen partiellen Riesenwuchses. *Charité-Annalen,33*:744–754, 1909.

Bigelow, H. J.: Congenital hypertrophy of the middle finger. *Boston Med. Surg. J.,* *43*:341, 1851. See also Jackson, J. B. S., (ed.): *A Descriptive Catalogue of the Warren Anatomical Museum.* Harvard University, entry 921, p. 138, 1870.

Bilhaut, M.: Observation de mégalo-dactylie. *Ann. d'Orthop.,* *8*:65–69, 1895.

Bloom, J. D.: Macrodactylism. *New Orleans Med. Surg. J.,* *90*:29–30, 1937.

Boéchat: Anomalie symétrique héréditaire des deux mains. *Gaz. Hebd. Méd. Chir.,* (2 s.), *14*:639, 1877. Also in *Congrès Périodique Internationale des Sciences Médicales.* Section de Biologie (5 s.). Génève. H. George, Librairie de l'Université, pp. 691–697, 1878.

Boehm, T.: *Ueber Macrodactylie.* Inaug. Diss. Giessen, M. Merck, pp. 1–14, 1856.

Boinet: De la macrodactylie congénitale *Presse Méd.,* *71*:117–118, 1901.

Bonnet, M. P.: Hypertrophie congénitale des extrémités. *Lyon Méd.,* *69*:363–365, 1892.

Booher, R. J.: Lipoblastic tumors of the hands and feet, review of the literature and report of 33 cases. *J. Bone Joint Surg.,* *47A*:727–740; fig. 3, 1965.

Borst, W.: Über partiellem Riesenwuchs. *Fortschr. Röntgenstr., 58*:121–124.

Bricage, R. E.: *Contribution à l'Étude des Hypertrophies Congénitales des Doigts.* Thèse. Paris, Imprimérie Richard, pp. 9–44; figs. 1–8, 1935.

Brinitzer, W.: Dactylomegaly: a case note. *Indian Med. Gaz.,* 76:286–287, 1941.

Broca, P.: Elephantiasis congénital d'un doigt. *Gaz. Hôp.,* 52:583–584, 1856.

Brunelli, G.: Lipoma interfibrillare del nervo mediano con sindrome da compressione del canale del carpo. *Minerva Ortop.,* 15:211–217, 1964.

Busch, W.: Beitrag zur Kenntniss der angeborenen Hypertrophie der Extremitäten. *Arch. Klin. Chir.,* 7:174–198, 1866.

Byrne, J. J.: Megalodactylism. *In* Hand Surgery. *Am. J. Surg.,* 88:470, 1954. Also in *The Hand: Its Anatomy and Diseases.* Springfield, Illinois: Charles C Thomas, pp. 275–276; fig. 139, 1959.

Caffey, J., and Silverman, F. N.: *Pediatric X-ray Diagnosis.* Chicago, Year Book Medical Publishers, Inc., pp. 709–808; fig. 1230, 1967.

Callison, J. R., Thomas, O. J., and White, W. L.: Fibro-fatty proliferation of the median nerve. *Plast. Reconstr. Surg.,* 42:403–413, 1968.

Capel, E.: Macrodactyly, with a report of a case. *J. Anat.,* 69:528–529, 1935.

Cayla: Macrodactylie. *N. Iconog. Salp.,* 16:41; pl. IX, 1903.

Cazin: Macrodactylie éléphantiasique. *Bull. Mém. Soc. Chir.* (Paris), 7:147–148, 1881.

Cestan, R.: Hypertrophie congénitale des doigts médius et index de la main gauche. *N. Iconog. Salp.,* 10:339–403, 1897.

Chandler, F. A.: Local overgrowth. *J.A.M.A.,* 109:1411–1414; fig. 5, 1937.

Charters, A. D.: Local gigantism. *J. Bone Joint Surg.,* 39B:542–547, 1957.

Chassel: Riesenwuchs der rechten Hand. *Berl. Klin. Wochenschr.,* 46(1):282, 1909.

Chiarolanza, P.: Gigantismo congenito parziale. *Riforma Med.,* 73:917–918, 1959.

Clifford, R. H.: The treatment of macrodactylism: a case report. *Plast. Reconstr. Surg.,* 23:245–248, 1959.

Cocchi, U.: Congenital partial gigantism. Heredity diseases with bone changes. *In* Schinz, H. R., Baensch, W. E., Friedl, E., and Uehlinger, E., (eds.): *Roentgen-Diagnostics.* First American edition based on fifth German edition. English translation arranged and edited by J. T. Case. New York, Grune & Stratton, Vol. I, Part I (Skeleton), pp. 807–810; fig. 1149, 1951.

Cockshott, W. P., and Evans, K. T.: The place of soft tissue angiography. *Br. J. Radiol.,* 37:367–375; fig. 5, 1964.

Coninck, A. de: Mégalodactylie. *Ann. Chir. Plast.,* 10:45–48, 1965.

Costelo, M. J., and Gibbs, R. C.: *The Palms and Soles in Medicine.* Springfield, Illinois, Charles C Thomas, pp. 185–186, 1967.

Coutagne, H.: Hypertrophie congénitale des doigts médius et annulaire de la main gauche. *Gaz. Méd. Lyon, 19*:112, 1867.

Curling, T. B.: Case of remarkable hypertrophy of the fingers, in a girl, with a notice of some similar cases. *Med. Chir. Tr.,* 28:337–344; Pl. 2, 3, 1845.

Cusson, P.: *Contribution a l'Étude de l'Hypertrophie Congénitale.* Thèse. Paris. J. B. Baillière et Fils, pp. 8–103, 1905.

Dal Monte, A., and Negri, L.: La macrodattilia *Atti S.E.R.O.T.* (Atti della Societa Emiliana Romaglona-Trivenita di Ortopedia), Bologna, 3:381–593, 1958.

Dambrin, L.: Les macrodactylies. *Rev. d'Orthop.,* 23:215–229, 1936.

De Laurenzi, V.: Macrodattilia del medio. *G. Med. Mil.,* 112:401–405, 1962.

Delplanque, E.: Brachydactylie et mégalodactylie. *Bull. Sci. Dept. Nord,* 5:118–122, 1878.

Del Torto, P.: Sopra due casi macrosomia parziale congenita. *Arch. Ortop.,* 41:470–472, 1925.

Dennison, W. M.: *Surgery in Infancy and Childhood.* Second edition. Edinburgh, E. S. Livingston Ltd, pp. 508–510; fig. 283, 1967.

Despin, J. B.: *Contribution a l'Étude de l'Hypertrophie Congénitale des Membres.* Thèse. Bordeaux, Imprimérie Barthelemy et Cledes. pp. 1–64, 1914.

Dombrowski, A.: Ein Fall von Megalosyndaktylie. *Münch. Med. Wochenschr.,* 75(2):1503, Abb. 1–2, 1928.

Dreifuss, A.: Ein Fall von angeborenem Riesenwuchs des Zeigefingers. *Z. Orthop. Chir.,* 24:538–540, 1909.

Düben, W.: Doppelseitiger Riesenwuchs bei 7 Jährigen. *In* Helner, H., Nissen, R., and Vesschulte, K., (eds.): *Lehrbuch der Chirurgie.* Stuttgart, G. Thieme, pp. 927–928; fig. 469, 1962.

Dufourmentel, C., and Mouly, R.: *Chirurgie Plastique.* Éditions Médicales. Paris, Flammarion, pp. 461–462; figs. 288–289, 1959.

Elkeles, A.: Local gigantism involving second and third fingers associated with lymphangioctatic condition of right palm. *Proc. R. Soc. Med.* (Clinical section), 44:918–919; figs. 1–3; Case II (Parkes Weber pronounced this case one of true gigantism of fingers as opposed to haemangiocatatic hypertrophy), 1951.

Ellis, R. W. B., and Mitchell, R. Q.: *Diseases in Infancy and Childhood.* Sixth edition. Edinburgh, E. & S. Livingston, pp. 199–200, fig. 92, 1968.

Emmett, A. J. J.: Lipomatous hamartoma of the median nerve in the palm. *Br. J. Plast. Surg.,* 18:208–213, 1965.

Estevez: Localized gigantism: roentgen study of macrodactylia of the right hand. *Rev. Med. Chile*, 67:801–804, 1939.

Eve, F. S.: Two specimens of congenital hypertrophy of giant-growth of limbs. *Trans. Path. Soc.* (London), 34:298–304, 1883.

Ewald, A.: Angeborene und fortschreitende Hypertrophie der linken Hand. *Arch. Pathol. Anat. Physiol.*, 56:421–422, 1872.

Feriz, H.: Makrodystrophia lipomatosa progressiva. *Arch. Pathol. Anat. Physiol.*, 260:308–368, 1925.

Ferreira de Magalhäes, A.: Megaloclinodactylia vara. *Brasil-Medico*, 33:347, 1919. See also 34:3, 1920.

Fèvre, M., and Bricage, R.: Hypertrophie congénitale irrégulière des doigts. *Ann. Anat. Pathol.*, 13:337–341, 1936.

Fèvre, M., and Huguenin, R.: Hypertrophie congénitale irrégulière de l'index droit de cause exceptionelle. *Ann. Anat. Pathol.*, 13:343–345, 1936.

Fielder: Zwei Fälle von Makrodactylie. *Arch. Heilkunde* (Leipzig), 7:316–321, 1866.

Filippucci: Dactylomégalie congénitale de l'index droit observée chez une demoiselle âgée de 20 ans revolus. *J. Pract. Rév. Clin. Thérap.*, 20:120, 1906.

Fischer, H.: Der Riesenwuchs. *Dtsch. Z. Chir.*, 12:1–59; Taf. II, III, 1880.

Fliegel, O.: Zur Aetiologie des angeborenen partiellen Riesenwuchses. *Dtsch. Z. Chir.*, 206:198, 1927.

Flinker, A.: Ueber eine seltene Makrodaktylie. *Wien. Klin. Wochenschr.*, 21:1241–1243, 1908.

Folier, C.: Sulla ipertrofia congenita delle membra. *Bull. Sci. Mediche*, (s. b.), 9:19–38; 76–91, 1882.

Fontana, A. M., Vinay, L., and Verga, G.: La macrodattilia. Ethiopathogenesi e trattamento chirurgico riparatore. *Bull. Soc. Piedmont. Chir.*, 34:447–473, 1964.

Foucher, M.: Hypertrophie congénitale du membre thoracique gauche et peutêtre du membre abdominal du même coté; développement anormal de l'index et du médius de la main gauche. *Bull. Soc. Anat. Paris*, 25:108, 1850.

Friedberg, H.: Riesenwuchs des rechten Beines. *Arch. Pathol Anat. Physiol.*, 40:353–379; Taf. IV-VI, 1867.

Fritsche, H.: Zur symptomatik und Therapie des partiellen Riesenwuchses. *Zentralbl. Chir.*, 80:1200–1210; Abb. 1–11, 1955.

Froelich, M.: Quelques types d'hypertrophie congénitale des membres. *Rev. d'Orthop.*, (2 s.), 9:193–200, figs. 1 and 2, 1908.

Fumarola, G.: Contribution a l'étude des difformités congénitales associées des mains. *N. Iconog. Salp.*, 24:329–334, 1911.

Gaisford, J. C.: Tumors of the hand. *Surg. Clin. North Am.*, 40:549–566; fig. 15c, 1960.

Gallard, J. S., and Llado, A. C.: Consideraciones sobre un raro caso de macroniquia por macrodactylia del pulgas izquierdo (gigantism parcial unilateral). *Acta Dermo-Sif.*, 32:18–25, 1940.

Galvani: Macrodactylie du membre supérieur droit. (Présentation des malades). *Bull. Soc. Chir* (Paris), 19:619–620, 1893.

Galvani: Deux cas d'hypertrophie congénitale des membres. *Rev. d'Orthop.*, (1 s.), 9:421–424, 1898.

Geipel, G., and Grebe, H.: Tastleistungsbefunde bei Gliedmassenmissbildungen. *Folia Hered. Pathol.*, 3:205–234; Taf. XIX, 1954.

Golding, F. C.: Localized gigantism. *In* McLaren, J. E., (ed.): *Modern Trends in Diagnostic Radiology*. Third edition. New York, P. B. Hooker, Inc., pp. 160–163; fig. 137, 1960.

Gould, G. M., and Pyle, W. L.: *Anomalies and Curiosities of Medicine*. Philadelphia, W. B. Saunders Co., p. 276, 1897.

Gray, T.: A case of gigantism of index and second fingers. *West London Med. J.*, 23:34–35, 1918.

Grebe, H.: Kasuistischer Beitrag zur Atiologie der konstitutionellen Vergrösserung unscheberner Körperabschnitte. *Z. menschl. Vererb. Konstitutionslehre*, 30:393–433; Abb. 6, 1952.

Gruber, G. B., and Kuss, O. E.: Der angeborene örtliche Riesenwuchs. *In* Schwalbe, E., and Gruber, G. B., (eds.): *Die Morphologie der Missbildungen in Menschen und der Tiere*. Jena, G. Fischer, 3T., 17 Lief, 1 Abt., 7 Kap. 1 Halfte, pp. 423–454, 1937.

Gruber, W.: Ueber einen Fall von Macrodactylie bei einem Lebenden. *Arch. Pathol. Anat. Physiol.*, 56:416–419; Taf. IX, 1872.

Guadagno, N.: Macrosomia parziale del nevrofibromatosi. *Arch. Ital. Anat. Inst. Pat.*, VII Suppl., pp. 169–176, 1936.

Guadagno, N., and Mungo, A.: Sulle malformazioni congenite del estremita. *Atti S.O.T.I.M.I.*, 7:248–252, 1962.

Guersant: Hypertrophie éléphantiasique de l'auriculaire et de l'annulaire de la main droite. *Gaz. Hôp.*, 53:463, 1857.

Guerzoni, P. L.: (Parla ancho a nome del Socio Prof. Francesco Ruggeri): Macrodattilie congenite da neurinoma plessiforme del mediano. *Bull. Sci. Mediche*, 139:336–348, 1967.

Halderman, D.: Monstrosity of a hand. *Med. Rec.*, 23:320–321, 1883.

Hart, D.: *Lewis' Practice of Surgery*. Hagerstown, W. F. Prior, Vol. V, pp. 287–288; figs. 279, 280, 1951.

Hawkins-Ambler, G. A.: Case of unequal growth of fingers. *Lancet*, 1:244, 1893.

Heiple, K. G., and Elmer, R. M.: Chondromatous hamartoma arising from the volar digital plates. *J. Bone Joint Surg.*, 54A:393–398, 1972.

Hellmann, K.: Ueber die Behandlung der Makrodaktylies. *Ann. Chir. Plast.*, 9:184–187, 1964.

Henschen, C.: Plastische Wiederherstellung riesenwüchsiger Finger durch phalangeale Umkippplastik, Verküerzungsexcision und Weichteilexcisionen. *Helvet. Med. Acta.*, 3:166–176, 1939.

Herget, R.: Die Makrodystrophia fibromatosa progressiva. *Beitr. Klin. Chir.*, *168*:189–192, 1938.

Heurtaux: Macrodactylie. *Bull. Soc. Anat.* (Nantes), *4*:62, 1880.

Higginbotham: Ein Fall von Makroplasie der linken oberen Extremität. *St. Petersburg Med. Z.*, *4*:205–207, 1863.

Hinterstoisser, H.: Ueber einen Fall von angeborenem partiellem Riesenwuchs. *Arch. Klin. Chir.*, *103*:297–304; figs. 1–3, 1913.

Hippe, H., and Hähle, K.: Angeborener partieller Riesenwuchs, *Röntgenpraxis*, *9*:116–118; Abb. 1–4, 1937.

Hoche, O.: Partieller Riesenwuchs von seltener Form bei gleichzeitiger Erkrankung der Weichteile des Knochensystems. *Arch. Klin. Chir.*, *185*:633–641, 1936.

Hohmann, M.: Zur Pathologie des angeborenen, partiellen Riesenwuchses. *Beit Klin. Chir.*, *48*:391–424, 1906.

Holmes, R.: *The Surgical Treatment of the Diseases of Infancy and Childhood*. Second edition. Philadelphia, Lindsay & Blakiston, pp. 207–221, 1869.

Holt, J. F., and Wright, E. M.: The radiologic features of neurofibromatosis. *Radiology*, *51*:647–663, 1948.

Hopf, A.: Der angeborene oertliche Riesenwuchs im Bereich der Hand. *In* Hohmann, G., Hackenbroch, M., and Lindemann, K., (eds.): *Handbuch der Orthopaedie*. Stuttgart, G. Thieme Verlag. Vol. III, pp. 486–488, 1959.

Horz: Verhandlungen ärztli cher Gesellschaften – Partieller Riesenwuchs. *Berl. Klin. Wochenschr.*, *48*(2):1700, 1911.

Houel: (Viardin's case). Moule en platre d'une main gauche avec syndactylie et lipome volumineux. *Bull. Soc. Chir.* (Paris), *6*:498–499, 1880.

Huber, F.: Congenital hypertrophy of the fingers. *Arch. Pediatr.*, *11*:592–594, 1894.

Huesch, K.: Über die Beziehungen des Sympathiens zur Neurofibromatose und dem partiellem Riesenwuchs. *Arch. Pathol. Anat. Physiol.*, *255*:71–106; Abb. 4, 6, 1925.

Humme, C. T.: *Een Geval von Makrodactylie*. Leiden, S. C. Van. Doesburgh, pp. 1–47, 1884.

Hurley, T. W.: Hypertrophy and elongation of the thumb, index, and middle fingers of the right hand from congenital occlusion of lymph channels. *Am. Med. Bi-Weekly*, *9*:49–50, 1878.

Inglis, K.: Local gigantism (a manifestation of neurofibromatosis): its relation to general gigantism and to acromegaly illustrating the influence of intrinsic factors in disease when development of the body is abnormal. *Am. J. Pathol.*, *26*:1059–1076, Case 2, fig. 10, 1950.

Iselin, M., and Iselin, F.: *Traité de Chirurgie de la Main*. Paris, Editions Médicales Flammarion, pp. 295–299; figs. 280–282, 1967.

Jager, M.: Der angeborene umschriebene Riesenwuchs der Hand und des Fusses. Differentialdiagnose, Kasuistik, operative Therapie. *Arch. Orthop. Unfallchir.*, *61*:151–163, Abb. 6–10, 1967.

Jones, K. G.: Megalodactylism: case report of a child treated by epiphyseal resection. *J. Bone Joint Surg.*, *45A*:1704–1708, 1963.

Jones, R.: Chronic hypertrophy of the fingers. *Provincial Med. J.*, p. 575, 1895.

Jones, R.: Macrodactyly due to diffuse lipoma. *Trans. Path. Soc. London*, *69*:203; 1 pl., 1897–1898.

Jouon, E.: Hypertrophie congénitale monstrueuse de la main droite ayant nécessité l'ablation de la main chez un enfant de 4 mois. *Rev. d'Orthop.*, (3 s.), *8*:305–307, 1921.

Jovino, F.: Contributo allo studio della macrosomia parziale congenita. *Atti S.T.O.T.*, *28*:226–227, 1843.

Kanavel, A. B.: Hypertrophy. *In* Congenital malformations of the hands. *Arch. Surg.*, *25*:317–318; figs. 47, 48, 1932.

Kaplan, E. B.: Congenital giant thumb. *Bull. Hosp. Joint Dis.*, *8*:38–44; figs. 1–3, 1947.

Kappeler, O.: *Chirurgische Beobachtungen aus dem Thurgauischen Kantonsspital Muensterlinger: Waehrend der Jahre (1865–1870)*. Frauenfeld, J. Huber's Buchdruckerei, pp. 246–248, 1874.

Karewski, F.: *Die chirurgischen Krankheiten des Kindesalters*. Stuttgart, F. Enke. pp. 571–572, 1894.

Kastein, W.: Kongenitale Hypertrophie. *Münch. Med. Wochenschr.*, *88*:273–276, 1941.

Katayama, K.: Uber einen Fall von kongenitalem Riesenwuchs. *Arch. Orthop. Mech. Unfallchir.*, *13*:53–55; figs. 1, 2, 1914.

Kaufmann, M.: Über partiellen Riesenwuchs. *Med. Klin.*, *25*:907–908; Bild 1, 2, 1929.

Keskineff, G.: *Hypertrophies Congénitales des Membres*. Thèse. Nancy, A. Grépin-Leblond, pp. 7–99, 1900.

Killinger, R. R.: Dactylomegaly: a bilateral affection. The only case reported. *J. Fla. Med. Assoc.*, *12*:6–10, 1925.

Killinger, R. R.: Bilateral dactylomegaly. *J. Fla. Med. Assoc.*, *31*:471–475, 1945.

Kirmisson, E.: Macrodactylie de la main gauche. *Bull. Mém. Soc. Chir. Paris*, *17*:367–368, 1891.

Kirmisson, E.: *Précis de Chirurgie Infantile*. Paris, Masson et Cie. pp. 781–786; fig. 460, 1906.

Kitaigorodskaja, O. D.: Angeborene Hypertrophie im Kindesalter. *Jb. Kinderheilkd.*, *125*:38–89; figs. 5, 15, 17, 20, 21, 22, 1929.

Klein, V.: Ausschälung eines ungewöhnlich grossen Fingers aus dem Gelenk. *Graefe und von Walther J. der Chir.*, *6*:379–382, 1824.

Köhler, A.: Angeborener Riesenwuchs des linken Mittelfingers mit Polysarcie an Finger und Hohlhand. *Berl. Klin. Wochenschr.*, *25*:216, 1888.

Krakenberger, A.: *Über Makrodaktylie*. Inaug. Diss. Würzburg. F. Scheiner Buchdruckerei, pp. 7–33; figs. I-IV, 1894.

Kratochvil, K.: Über partiellen Riesenwuchs vereint mit degenerativen Veränderungen am Augenhintergrund. *Arch. Klin. Chir.*, *190*:802–809; Abb. 1–3, 1937.

Kulbs: Demonstration eines Patienten mit partiellem Riesenwuchs. *Berl. Klin. Wochenschr.*, *48*(1):132–133, 1911.

Kuss, G., and Jouon, E.: Sur deux cas d'hypertrophie congénitale des membres. De la nécessité d'une classification nouvelle des faits d'hypertrophie congénitale. *Rev. d'Orthop.*, (1 s.), *10*:444–465, 1899.

Kuss, O. E.: *Über den angeborenen partiellen Riesenwuchs.* Inaug. Diss. Göttingen, Buchdruckerei F. Pieper, pp. 1–33, 1938.

Laignel-Lavastine, and Viard, M.: Macrodactylie (Présentation du sujet). *Bull. Mém. Hôp.* (Paris), (3 s.), *42*:1031–1035, 1918.

Lane, A.: Congenital hypertrophy of fingers. Reported by P. T. *Guys Hosp. Gaz.*, (n.s.), *12*:336–338, 1898.

Lange, F.: *Lehrbuch der Orthopädie.* Jena, G. Fischer, pp. 103; 105–106; fig. 9, 1954.

Langsteiner, F., and Stiefler, G.: Über die kongenitalen Hypertrophien (Hyperplasien). *Dtsch. Z. Nervenheilkd.*, *138*:274–307; figs. 8, 9, 11, 12, 1935.

Lannelongue: Macrodactylie éléphantiasique. *Bull. Mém. Soc. Chir.* (Paris), *6*:710–711, 1880.

Lannelongue: L'hypertrophie congénitale, *Arch. Méd. Enfants*, *2*:319–320, 1899.

Lasserre, C.: Hypertrophie congénitale de la main avec clinodactylie. *J. Méd. Bordeaux*, *56*:841, 1926.

Learmonth, J.: A propos de certaines augmentations de volume des membres. *Lyons Chir.*, *53*:801–812; fig. 8, 1957.

Leblanc, E.: *Contribution è l'Etude de l'Hypertrophie Congénitale, Unilatérale, Partiale ou Complète.* Thèse. Paris, H. Jouve, pp. 5–70, 1897.

Legal: Angeborener Riesenwuchs des linken Zeige u. Mittel-fingers bei einer 25 Jährigen. *Zentralbl. Chir.*, 55 Jhrg:605–606, 1928.

Legendre: Diffomité congénitale des doigts annulaire et auriculaire droits et de la moitié correspondante de la paume de la main. *Union Méd.*, *9*:196, 1855.

Lejars, F.: Un fait de macrodactylie. *N. Iconog. Salp.*, *16*:37–40, 1903.

Lerch, H.: Zum Problem des angeborenen, umschriebenen Riesenwuchses *Z. Orthop. Chir.*, *96*:290–298, Abb. 4, Fall 6, 1962.

Léri, A., and Joanny: Une affection non décrite des os: hyperostéose "en coulée" sur toute la longeur d'un membre ou "mélorhéostose." *Bull. Mém. Soc. Méd. Hôp. Paris*, *46*:1141–1145, 1922.

Levi, D.: Local gigantism involving webbed fingers. *Proc. Roy. Soc. Med. London* (Sect. Dis. Child.), *31*:764–765, 1938.

Lolli: Su di caso di ipertrophia parziale dell arto superiore desto. *Pediatr. Prat.*, *5*:141, 1929.

Lombard, P.: Un cas de macrodactylie. *Afrique Franc. Chir.*, *11*:338–340, 1953.

Longhi, L.: Malformazioni congenite delle mani. *Arch. Orthop.*, *55*:183–212; figs. 30–32, 1939.

Lopez, R. V.: Sobre gigantismo parcial congénito. Megalodactilia. *Prog. Clin.*, *42*:96–99, 1934.

Lunardo, C.: Sulla anomalie congenite di volume delgi arti. *Atti Soc. Emil. Orthop. Traum.*, *3*:251–260, 1958.

Lund, F. B.: Congenital anomalies of the phalanges, with report of cases studied by Skiagraphy, *Med. Surg. Rep. Boston City Hosp.*, (13 s.), pp. 1–21, figs. 10–11, 1902.

Macedo, O.: Gigantismo local. *Brazil Med.*, *70*:69–73, 1956.

MacGillivray, P. H.: On a case of congenital hypertrophy of the hand and arm. *Aust. Med. J.*, *17*:9–11, 1872.

Magni, L.: Ipertrofia parziale congenita. *Riv. Clin. Pediatr.*, *28*:688–697, 1930.

Makowski, H.: Ein Fall von angeborenen partiellen Riesenwuchses ("Hyperplasia partialis congenita"). *Z. Orthop.*, *69*:127–135, 1939.

Markoff, S. I.: Sluchai pseudo-macrodactili. (Russian). *Laitop. Khirurg. Obsh. Mosk.*, *6*:168–173, 1883–1884.

Martinez, E. A.: Consideraciones sobre la mega-dolicodactilia. *Rev. Med. Peruna*, *13*:689–696, 1941.

Martinez-Fortun, O.: Macromelia: un caso de macrodactilia. *Rev. Med. Cir.* (Habana), *32*:178–179, 1927.

Martinová, M., and Kubáçek, V.: Gigantodaktylie. (Czech). *Acta Chir. Orthop. Traum. Ceck.*, *33*:292–296, 1966.

Marziani, R.: Macrosomia parziale da nevrofibromatosi. *Arch. Ital. Anat. Istol. Pat.*, *6*(VI Suppl.):169–176, figs. 1 and 2, 1936.

Masmejean, J.: *Des Hypertrophies Latérales du Corps. Totales ou Partielles.* Thèse. Montpellier, Imprimérie Serré et Ricome, pp. 1–109, 1888.

Massonnaud, A.: *Essai sur la Pathogogénie de l'Hypertrophie Unilatérale Partielle ou Totale du Corps.* Thèse. Paris, A. Parent, pp. 5–34, 1874.

Matas, R.: Macrodactilie congénitale. See G. Potel: Hypertrophie des doigts et des orteils. *Rev. Chir.*, *49*:646–648; fig. 16, 1914.

Mauclaire, M.: Macrodactylie congénitale du médius. *Bull. Mém. Soc. Anat.* (Paris), *92*:342–343, 1922.

McCarroll, H. R.: Clinical manifestations of congenital neurofibromatosis. *J. Bone Joint Surg.*, *32A*:601–617; figs. 3a–4c, 1950.

McCarroll, H. R.: Soft-tissue neoplasms associated with congenital neurofibromatosis. *J. Bone Joint Surg.*, *38A*:717–731; 900, 1956.

McCarthy, A. M., Dorr, C. A., and Mackintosh, C. E.: Unilateral gigantism of the extremities associated with lipomatosis, arthropathy and psoriasis. *J. Bone Joint Surg., 51B*:348–353, 1969.

Meyerding, H. W., and Dickson, D. D.: Correction of congenital deformities of the hand. *Am. J. Surg.,* (n.s.), *44*:218–231; fig. 6, 1939.

Mikhail, I. K.: Median nerve lipoma in the hand. *J. Bone Joint Surg., 46B*:726–730; fig. 1, 1964.

Millesi, H.: Korrektur der Makrodaktylie bei Erwa chsenen durch multiple Osteotomie. *Zentralbl. Chir., 91*(2):1472–1475, 1966.

Minkowitz, S., and Minkowitz, F.: A morphological study of macrodactylism: a case report. *J. Pathol. Bacteriol., 90*:323–328, figs. 1 and 2, 1965.

Monod, M.: Éléphantiasis cutané de l'index et de la face latérale du médius de la main droite. *Bull. Soc. Anat.,* (3 s.), *2*:564, 1872.

Moore, B. H.: Some orthopedic relationships of neurofibromatosis. *J. Bone Joint Surg.,* (n.s.), *23*:109–140, Case 1, fig. 1, 1941.

Moore, B. H.: Macrodactyly and associated peripheral nerve changes. *J. Bone Joint Surg., 24*:617–631, fig. 1, 1942.

Moore, B. H.: Peripheral nerve-changes associated with congenital deformities. *J. Bone Joint Surg., 26*:282–288, 1944.

Moraza, M.: Dos casos de gigantismo parcial. *Med. Iberia, 2*:630–633, Caso primero, 1930.

Morestin, H. M.: Lipome congénital de la main. *Bull. Soc. Anat.,* (6 s.), *15*:467–470, 1913.

Morley, G. H.: Intramural lipoma of the median nerve in the carpal tunnel. *J. Bone Joint Surg., 46B*:734–735, 1964.

Morton, T. S. K.: Two cases of congenital hypertrophy of the fingers. *Med. News, 64*:294–296, Case 1, 1894.

Mouchet, A.: Sur un cas de doigts géants congénitaux (Katayama's case). *J. Chir., 12*:132, 1914.

Mouly, R., and Debeyre, J.: Le gigantisme digital. Étiologie et traitement. A propose d'un cas. *Ann. Chir. Plast., 6*:187–194, 1961.

Mouriguand, G., and Buche: Sur un cas de macrodactylie congénitale. *Lyon Med., 130*:110–112, 1921.

Moutier, F.: Maladie de Recklinghausen avec nevrome plexiforme du dos de la main. *Rev. Neurol., 14*:1081–1082, 1906.

Muller, W.: *Die angeborenen Fehlbildungen der menschlichen Hand.* Leipzig, G. Thieme, pp. 127–133; figs. 96–97, 1937.

Naegele: Amputation de la jambe dans un cas d'éléphantiasis, pratiquée avec succés au milieu des tissue dégénerés. *Arch. Gen. Med., 13*:426–432, 1827.

Neurath, R.: Zwei Fälle von angeborenen Riesenwuchs. *Wien Klin. Wochenschr., 26*:2015, 1913.

Nolda, A.: Ein Fall von kongenitalem Riesenwuchs des rechten Daumens. *Arch. Pathol. Anat. Physiol., 178*:504–507, 1904.

Nozarova, P.: Congenital defects of the hand and fingers and their treatment (Czech). *Pediatr. Listy, 5*:275–281; fig. 11, 1951.

Ollive, M.: Macrodactylie. *In Bull. Soc. Anat.* (Nantes). Recueillis par A. Malherbe. Paris, A. Delahage, pp. 92–93, 1879.

Oprandi, C.: Sul gigantismo parziale congenito. *Arch. Orthop., 81*:11–118, 1968.

Owen: Letter to Curling. *Med. Chir. Tr., 28*:341–342, 1845.

Paci, A.: Considerazioni sulla macrodattilia. *Boll. Med.* (Trentino), *17*:135–145, 1898.

Paget: Letter to Curling. *Med. Chir. Tr., 28*:341–342, 1845.

Peiser, E.: Über angeborenen partiellen Riesenwuchs. *Dtsch. Z. Chir., 137*:189–221, 1916.

Peltier, L. F.: *Joseph Brenneman's Practice of Pediatrics.* Hagerstown, Md., W. F. Prior Co., Inc., Vol. IV, pp. 2–4; fig. 2, 1964.

Pernet, A.: Megalodactilia do IV e V de dos—megalodactyly of ring and little fingers. *In* Anomalias congenitas das maos. *Rev. Lat. Amer. Cir. Plast., 6*:377–404; fig. 7A and 7B, 1962.

Petit, P., and Bedouelle, J.: *Malformations Congénitales des Membres.* Encyc. Med. Chir. Paris. Vol. III, Appareil Moteur, No. 15200, pp. 1–6; figs. 3–5, 1955.

Petit, P., and Bedouelle, J.: *Malformations Congénitales des Membres.* Encyc. Med. Chir. Paris. Vol. III, Appareil Moteur, No. 15202, pp. 3–4; figs. 6–8, 1957.

Plauchu, E.: Un cas de macrodactylie. *Lyon Med., 84*:372–375, 1897.

Pollailon: Doigt.: *In* Dechambre, A., (ed.): *Dictionnaire Encyclopédique des Sciences Medicales.* Paris, G. Masson et P. Asselin et Cie, *30*:115–353, in particular pp. 143–160, 1884.

Pool: Congenital macrodactylia. *Ann. Surg., 52*:562–563; fig. 3, 1910.

Posch, J. L.: Soft tissue tumors of the hand. *In* Flynn, J. E., (ed.): *Hand Surgery.* Baltimore, Williams and Wilkins Co., pp. 99–1027, 1956.

Power, R. F.: Cases with observations. Case II—Peculiar congenital malformation of the middle finger. *Dublin J. Med. Sci., 17*:243–257, 1840.

Preiser: Partieller Riesenwuchs (Makrodaktylie). *Münch. Med. Wochenschr., 54*(2):2617, 1907.

P. T.: See Lane (1898).

Pulvertaft, R. G.: Unusual tumors of the median nerve. Report of two cases. *J. Bone Joint Surg., 46B*:731–733, 1964.

Quillon, E.: *Formes et Pathogénie de l'Hypertrophie Congénitale des Membres.* Thèse. Paris, L. Roux, pp. 7–79, 1901.

Rach: Fall von symmetrischer Makrodaktylie an den Händen. *Mitt. Gessellsch. Med. Kinderheilkd.* (Wien), *5*:165, 1906.

Ranawat, C. S., Arora, M. M., and Singh, R. G.: Macrodystrophia lipomatosa with carpal-tunnel syndrome. A case report. *J. Bone Joint Surg., 50A*:1342–1344, 1968.

Ranke, H.: Ueber Lipome an der Volarseite der Finger. *Arch. Klin. Chir., 20*:379–385, 1876–1877.

Rechnagel, K.: Megalodactylism: report of 7 cases. *Acta Orthop. Scand., 38*:57–66, 1967.

Recklinghausen, F.: *Ueber die multiplen Fibroma der Haut und ihre Beziehung zu den multiplen Neuromen.* Berlin, A. Hirschwald, pp. 1–138, 1882.

Redard, P.: De l'hypertrophie congénitale partielle. *Arch. Gén. Méd., 1*:31–52, 1890.

Reid, J.: Three cases of partial hypertrophy of a portion of the organs of voluntary motion. (London and Edinburgh), *Monthly J. Med. Sci., 3*:198–201, 1843.

Ribeiro, A. L.: Lobster claw hands. *Br. Med. J., 1*:1209, 1954.

Richardière: Hypertrophie congénitale de la main. *Sem. Méd., 11*:125, 1891.

Riedinger, J.: Riesenwuchs (Malrosomia). *In* Lange, F., (ed.): *Lehrbuch der Orthopädie.* G. Fischer, pp. 103–106; fig. 9, 1914.

Rocher, H. L., Secousse, and Pouyanne, L.: Hypertrophie congénitale de deux doigts (I et II) et de l'éminence thenar. *J. Méd. Bordeaux, 112*:395–396, 1935.

Rochlin, D. G., and Zeitler, E.: Makrodaktylie. *In* Diethelm, L., (ed.): *Skeletanatomie (Röntgendiagnostik).* Teil 2. Berlin, Springer, pp. 83–85, 1968.

Rogers, L.: Macrodactylia in a child, due to neurofibromatosis (elephantiasis neuromatosa). *Br. J. Surg, 16*:684–686, 1929.

Rosenfeld, E.: Angeborene abnorme Grösse des Daumens und Zeigefingers der rechten Hand. *Aerztl. Mittheilungen aus Baaden, 55*:366–367, 1858.

Roubinovitch, and Soudière, R.: Deux cas de neurofibromatose familiale dont un avec cheiromégalie unilatérale. *N. Iconog. Salp., 27*:327–332, 1914–1915.

Rowe, E. W.: Local gigantism. *Radiog. Clin. Photog., 20*:20–21; fig. 4, 1944.

Rowland, S.: Lipofibroma of the median nerve. *J. Bone Joint Surg., 49A*:581, 1967.

Ruggiero, C.: Un caso raro di macrosomia. *Med. Ital.* (Napoli), *9*:227–246, 1911.

Salvadore-Gallardo, J., and Cortez Llado, A.: Consideraciones sobre un raro caso de macroniquia por macrodactylia del pulgar izquierdo (gigantismo parcial unilateral) *Acta Dermo-Sif., 32*:18–25, 1940.

Sarnecka-Stefanowicz, D., and Serafin, J.: An attempt at the management of gigantism of the upper limb. (Polish). *Chir. Narzadow Ruchu, 32*:205–211, 1967.

Schachter, M.: Les mégalosomies ou hypertrophies localisées d'origine congénitale. *Rev. Franc. Pédiatr., 15*:268–273, 1939.

Schoch, J.: Zur Symptomatologie und Ätiopathogenese der angeborenen partiellen Riesenwüchse. *Med. Welt., 16*:845–852, 1960.

Seghini, G.: Macrosomie parziali da neurofibrolipomatosi. *Arch. Chir. Ortop. Med., 20*:173–194, fig. 1, 1955.

Shima, Y., Kasahara, K., and Nakeseko, T.: Experiences in the treatment of macrodactylia (Japanese). *Orthop. Surg.* (Tokyo), *18*:292–293, 1967.

Sicard, J. A., Naudin, L., and Cantaloube, P.: Macrodactylie chez un blessé de guerre. *N. Iconog. Salp., 28*:144–146, 1916.

Smith, R. W.: *A Treatise on the Pathology, Diagnosis, and Treatment of Neuroma.* New Sydenham Society, London, pp. 5–38, 1898. Orginally published in 1849.

Sorrel, Benoit, and Dastuque: Un cas de macrodactylie. *Bull. Soc. Pédiatr.,* (Paris), *32*:174–178, 1934.

Souligoux, and David, C.: Macrodactylie. *Bull Soc. Anat.* (Paris), *8*:466, 1906.

Southam: A case of extreme hypertrophy of fingers (congenital). *Illustrated Med. News* (London), *2*:269, 1889.

Spreitzer, O. H.: Über agneborenen Riensenwuchs. *Z. Orthop. Chir., 58*:423–431, 1933.

Steffes, W.: Über echten partiellen Riensenwuchs. *Z. menschl. Vererb. Konstitutionslehre., 20*:246–253, 1937.

Steindle, H.: Über einen Fall von echtem, partiellem Riesenwuchs. *Dtsch. Z. Chir., 185*:356–367, 1924.

Streeter, G. L.: Focal deficiencies in fetal tissues and their relation to intrauterine amputation. *Carnegie Inst.* Washington, Publ. #414, *22*:18–19; figs. 99–101, 1930.

Szelei, B.: Congenital partial gigantism: macrodactyly of II–IV digits. (Hungarian). *Magyar Radiol., 9*:123–124, 1957.

Tachard, E.: Sur une observation de mégalodactylie congenitale de l'annulaire droit. *Courrier Med.,* (Paris), *39*:221–222, 1889.

Tagliabue, D., and Spina, G. M.: Le macrodattilie. *Arch. Orthop., 73*:792–804, 1960.

Tailhefer, A.: Un cas de macrodactylie. *Bull. Mém. Soc. Anat.,* (6 s.), *22*:284, 1925.

Taruffi, C.: Della macrosomia. *Ann. Univ. Med. Chir. Milano, 249*:45–80, 1879.

Taruffi, C.: Sulla ipertrofia congenita dell membra. *Riv. Clin. Bologna,* (2 A.), *9*:43–52, 1879.

Tatafiore, E.: Un caso di macrosomia parziale congenita (macrodactyly of right index and middle fingers). *La Pediatria, 42*:405–409, 1934.

Taylor, F. A.: Congenital asymmetry of index finger. (Macrodactyly). *Arch. Pediatr., 21*:29, 1904.

Taylor, F. L.: A case of congenital macrodactylism. *Pediatrics, 8*:488–501, 1899.

Temel, T.: Sur un case rare de malformation congénitale de la main. *Bull. Mém. Soc. Radiol. Méd. France, 18*:109–111; figs. 1 & 2, 1930.

Terry, T. L.: Case of congenital elephantiasis arabum. *New Orleans Med. Surg. J., 23*:20–21; figs. 1 and 2, 1895.

Thorne, F. L., Posch, J. L., and Mladick, R. A.: Megalodactyly. *Plast. Reconstr. Surg., 41*:232–239, 1968.

Timoney, F. X.: Macrodactyly: case report. *Ann. Surg., 119*:144–147, 1944.

Trélat, U., and Monod, A.: De l'hypertrophie unilatérale partielle ou totale du corps. *Arch. Gén. Méd.,* (6 s.), *13*:536–559; 676–705, 1869.

Tridon, P.: Hypertrophie congénitale du pouce gauche. *Rev. d'Orthop.,* (3 s.), *4*:475–477, 1913.

Trivelli, L.: Contributo allo studio della macrosomia parziale congenita. *Ann. Ital. Chir. 21*:92–104; figs. 1 and 2, 1942.

Truc, H., and Masmejean, J.: Des hypertrophies du corps latérales totales ou partielles. *Montpellier Méd., 10*:257–276, 1888.

Tsuge, K.: Treatment of macrodactyly. *Plast. Reconstr. Surg., 39*:590–599, 1967.

Tubby, A. H.: *Deformities Including Diseases of the Bones and Joints: A Text-Book in Orthopaedic Surgery.* Second edition. London, Macmillan & Co. Ltd., Vol. I, pp. 106–107, 1912.

Tuli, S. M., Khanna, N. N., and Sinha, G. P.: Congenital macrodactyly. *Br. J. Plast. Surg., 12*:237–243, 1969.

Ueblin, F.: Beitrag zur Kasuistik des angeborenen partiellen Riesenwuchses. *Jb. Kinderheilkd.,* 91, 3. Folge, *41*:134–150, 1920.

Van Neck, M.: Macrodactylie des quatrièmes et cinquièmes doigts. *Arch. Franco-Belge Chir., 26*:895–898, 1923.

Vogt, P.: *Die Chirurgischen Krankheiten der oberen Extremitäten.* Stuttgart, F. Enke, pp. 4–9, 1881.

Voinich-Syanozhentski, A.: Poly- et macrodactylia congenita. *Chir. Laitop. Mosk.* (Russian), *3*:952–954, 1893.

Wagner, P.: Zur Casuistik angeborenen und erworbenen Riesenwuchs. *Dtsch. Z. Chir., 26*:281–306; fig. 4, 1887.

Wahl, L.: Un cas de macrodactylie congénitale chez une aliénée dégénerée. *C. R. Hebd. Soc. Biol., 55*:595–597, 1903.

Wakeley, C. P. G., and Hunter, J. B.: *Rose and Carless Manual of Surgery.* 15th edition. London, Bailliere, Tindall & Cox, Vol. I, pp. 500–501; fig. 218, 1937.

Walsh, R. W.: See Southam (1889).

Warner, E. C.: Megalodactyly. ? cause. *Proc. R. Soc. Med.* (Section Dis. Child.), *26*:1373–1374, 1933.

Weissenbach, R. J., Ravina, A., and Lievre, J. A.: Hypertrophie congénitale des doigts, osteo-arthrite hypertrophique dégénerative. *Bull. Mém. Soc. Med. Hôp.* (Paris), *2*:1303–1308, 1935.

Werthemann, A.: *Handbuch der speziellen pathologischen Anatomie und Histologie.* Berlin, Springer Verlag, Vol. IX, Section VI, pp. 377–393; figs. 249–252, 1952.

Wieland, E.: Zur Pathologie der dystrophischen Form des angeborenen partiellen Riesenwuches. *Jb. Kinderheilkd., 65*:519–584; figs. 1–5, 1907.

Williams, C.: Macrodactylie. *Ann. Soc. Belge Chir.* (Bruxelles), *6*:224–226, 1898–1899.

Wilms: Missbildungen der Extremitäten. *In* Wullstein, (ed.): *Lehrbuch der Chirurgie.* Vol. II, pp. 193–200; figs. 12 and 13, 1909.

Winckler, E.: Ein Fall von Makrodactylie. *Wien. Med. Wochenschr., 42*:1149–1152; 1191–1193, 1892.

Witt, A. N., Cotta, J., and Jager, M.: *Die angeborenen Fehlbildungen der Hand und ihre operative Behandlung.* Stuttgart, G. Thieme, pp. 20–21; 155–157, 1966.

Wittelshöfer, R.: Ueber angeborenen Riesenwuchs der oberen und unteren Extremitäten. *Arch. Klin. Chir., 24*:57–70, 1879.

Wulff, F.: Über Makrodaktylie. *St. Petersburg Med. Z., 1*:281–295, 1861.

Yeoman, P. M.: Fatty infiltration of the median nerve. *J. Bone Joint Surg., 46B*:737–739, 1964.

Ymaz, J. T.: Una ovservacion de macrodactilia. *Hosp. Argent., 3*:1100–1103, 1933.

Zerenin, V.: Macrosyndactylia. (Russian). *Laitop. Khirurg. Obsh. Mosk., 15*:101–105, 1896.

Zerenin, V.: Demonstration of a patient with macrodactylia after plastic formation of a finger with normal measurement. (Russian). *Tradi Obsh. Russk vrach Mosk., 6*:243–245; 1 pl., 1897.

Chapter Nineteen

ANGIODYSPLASTIC DEFORMITIES

Most compilers of the literature on macrodactyly include Wagner's name on their list. They credit him with treating a gigantic finger. Wagner (1839) spoke of disarticulating the right index finger of a boy because of a bleeding, ponderous tumor — probably a hemangioma. This tumor weighed five "European pounds." The illustration accompanying Wagner's article shows a large tumor surrounding the index finger. The tumor is overlaid with dilated, tortuous vessels (Fig. 19–1).

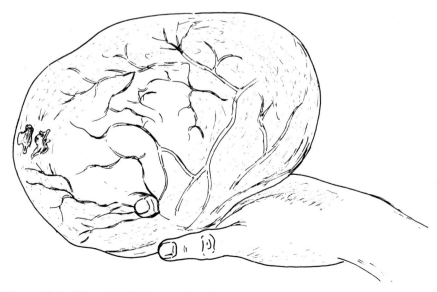

Figure 19–1 Wagner's (1839) case of angiomatous tumor of the right index finger, which has been classed with macrodactyly by many compilers of the literature on that anomaly.

Smith (1882) presented a 25-year-old female who, according to her mother, had begun to show signs of dilated vessels on her left hand at the age of one and a half years. The affected hand was much larger than the opposite; its temperature was higher and the subcutaneous tissue of the whole hand was occupied by dilated and tortuous veins. Smith's article contains a photograph of the involved left hand, showing prominent tortuous veins on its back. One of these veins extends over the index finger, which is almost twice as thick as its immediate ulnar neighbor. Smith attested that when the hand was lightly grasped, a purring thrill could be felt; he suspected arteriovenous communications.

Eve (1883) reported a case of congenital hypertrophy of the left hand and forearm. The fingers were proportionately enlarged. The affected digit gradually tapered from a thick base toward the tip. Over the hand and forearm, lymphatic vessels could be traced as knotted cords. A colored fluid was injected and it was seen to pass freely into the superficial lymphatics. These vessels were distinctly dilated and unusually numerous.

Lymphatic stasis only causes tumefaction of soft tissues. Paget (1866) pointed out that prolonged venous congestion in young children would cause overgrowth of parts. Duzea (1886) considered the excessive circulation incident to hemangiomas to be the cause of accelerated growth of bone. "Arteriovenous aneurysms are usually congenital in origin . . . . In young individuals an increase in the growth of the involved finger may occur," Posch (1956) wrote. Weisman (1959) said that, prior to the closure of epiphyses, arteriovenous aneurysm may contribute to the added gain of bone length.

SEMANTIC CONFUSION

The multiplicity of names used for vascular lesions causing enlargement of parts, including digits, betrays what Weisman (1959) aptly phrased "a state of semantic confusion." Devilliers (1876) described a seven-year-old child with tumefaction of the thumb and fingers; he used the designation "angioma with fibrous hypertrophy and dilation of the lymphatics." Under the heading "Cavernous angiolipoma of the hand," Terrier (1887) reported a tumor which had been resected from the little finger and the adjoining dorsal aspect of the hand. Morton (1894) presented a young female with "cavernous angioma affecting the fingers and thumb." Comby (1889) spoke of a congested left hand and called it "silent angiomatous tumor." Fowler (1907) featured the photographs of a hand with tumescent index, ring, and little fingers and a gigantic middle digit. The legend under the photographs reads: "Congenital cavernous nevus in the right hand." Stolz (1923) used the title "Cirsoid aneurysm of the finger"—the ring finger to be exact. Steinsleger (1923) described a one-month-old female with a voluminous right arm and hand, which he diagnosed as "diffuse subcutaneous angiocavernous tumor." Middleton (1932) employed the title "Congenital lymphangiectatic fibrous hypertrophy" and equated it with "elephantiasis congenita fibrosa lymphangiectatica" when he reported a 10-month-old child with a swollen distal forearm and completely functionless hand. In Bucher's (1934) case, both upper extremities were involved and his diagnosis was "lymphangioma cysticum congenitum."

Singleton (1937) included in his series of congenital lymphangiomas an enlarged right hand and arm; the legend under the accompanying photograph reads, "Cavernous and cystic lymphangioma . . . ." Matas (1940) used the title "Congenital arteriovenous angioma of the arm." Ravitch (1951) employed the terms "massive mixed angioma" and "hemolymphangioma" interchangeably when he described a case of congenital enlargement of the upper extremity.

In their series of hemangiomas, Brown and Fryer (1952) included a patient with "huge cystic hygroma throughout the arm." MacCollum and Martin (1956) described a "capillary hemangioma of the hand." Weisman (1959) used the following designations: "port wine stain of the right hand and arm, hemangioma of the hand, cavernous hemangioma" causing swelling of the left ring finger, "diffuse hemangiomatosis of right arm and hand," and "pulsating arteriovenous aneurysm" of the left middle finger. In his article entitled "Congenitally deformed hand," Matthews (1964) included a case of "gigantism associated with hemangioma."

There are two syndromes which implicate the hand and include, among other features, dilated blood vessels. Klippel-Trénaunay syndrome consists of congenital varices of the skin, nevus flammeus, and asymmetrical enlargement of parts, including fingers. In Maffucci's syndrome, diffuse hemangiomas and widespread phlebectasias coexist with irregularly distributed nests of unossified cartilage within the metaphyses and diaphyses of long bones, including the metacarpals and phalanges of the hand.

THE ORIGIN AND DEVELOPMENT OF VASCULAR CHANNELS

The semantic confusion about vascular tumefactions may perhaps be clarified in part if some of the pertinent points regarding the origin and development of lymphatics, veins, and arteries are reviewed.

In the embryo, all these vessels are developed alike as tissue spaces, which afterward become confluent and form a connected system of channels. These channels ramify, communicating freely among themselves. During this plexiform stage, channels which are destined to become lymphatics or veins may function as arteries, and arterial pathways convey constituents which are ordinarily transported by veins or lymphatics. As development proceeds, lymphatics, veins, and arteries insulate themselves into separate systems. Lymphatics precede the others in establishing a closed system. Even though they eventually empty into some central vein, lymphatic terminals do not communicate with terminal veins as do the capillaries of veins and arteries with each other. Red corpuscles, which may travel from the arteries into veins, are debarred from finding entrance into lymphatic terminals. Each large lymphatic vessel presents a beaded appearance; it consists of dilatations and constrictions. Dilatations occur immediately proximal to each pair of valves.

Persistence of various patterns of embryonic vascular channels results in lymphangiomas, hemangiomas, lymphangiohemangiomas, congenital varicosities, arteriovenous fistulas, and consequent aneurysmal dilatation of vessels. In the more pervasive cavernous hemangiomas, one must suspect persisting embry-

onic communications between the veins and arteries. Unlike traumatic arteriovenous fistula, which is usually single and sizable, congenital communicating vessels are small in caliber and are multiple. Enlargements due to abnormal
arteriovenous communications are variously called arteriovenous aneurysm, cirsoid aneurysm, racemose aneurysm, and pulsating angioma. Pulsation and bruit
are common signs of acquired arteriovenous communications. They are seldom
detected in congenital arteriovenous fistulas of the arms and hands.

LYMPHANGIOMA

Lymphangiohemangioma is a name given to tumors which consist of dilated
lymphatic channels and engorged varicose veins. In these mixed tumors, there
does not seem to be intercommunication between the two systems; the content of
the lymph spaces remains clear and untainted by venous blood. Large, loculated,
thin-walled dilations are called lymphatic cysts or cystic hygromas; these are
more common in the neck. In the arm, both lymphangiomas and lymphangiohemangiomas are usually diffuse, involving the entire extremity, including the
hand. These tumors do not pervade the deeper structures and can be removed
surgically. Diffuse variants are excised in repeated sessions. Sometimes it becomes expedient to utilize long incisions which may heal with contracting scars.
The latter are resected, and the new surgical wound is closed by Z-plasty technique (Figs. 19–2 to 19–4).

HEMANGIOMA

Congenital tumefaction, composed either of veins or arteries or both, is
called hemangioma. Depending upon the size of component channels,
hemangiomas are qualified as being capillary or cavernous. Either type may be
localized or diffuse. Capillary hemangioma is usually superficial and is known to
regress spontaneously. Cavernous hemangioma tends to invade deeper structures, including the muscles and bones. Localized hemangiomas may be excised,
and the surgical wound closed by Z-plasty or skin grafting. Multiple excisions are
required for more extensive tumors. When only a segment of such a bone as the
metacarpal is involved, the part may be resected and replaced by bone graft.
Curtis (1953) advocated arteriography to ascertain the location of intercommunicating vessels. Julian and Dye (1955) considered arteriography of the arm
and hand hazardous. Weisman (1959) regarded arteriography as usually unnecessary. More reliable information is obtained by surgical exploration, which is
carried out in successive sessions. The feeders are identified, doubly ligated, and
severed between ligatures. Tortuous, dilated venous channels are dissected out.
Muscles which have been extensively involved are extirpated. When a single
bone is invaded, the involved segment may be resected. In more extensive in-
vasions by large vascular channels, one has no other recourse except amputation
(Figs. 19–5 to 19–15).

(Text continued on page 668.)

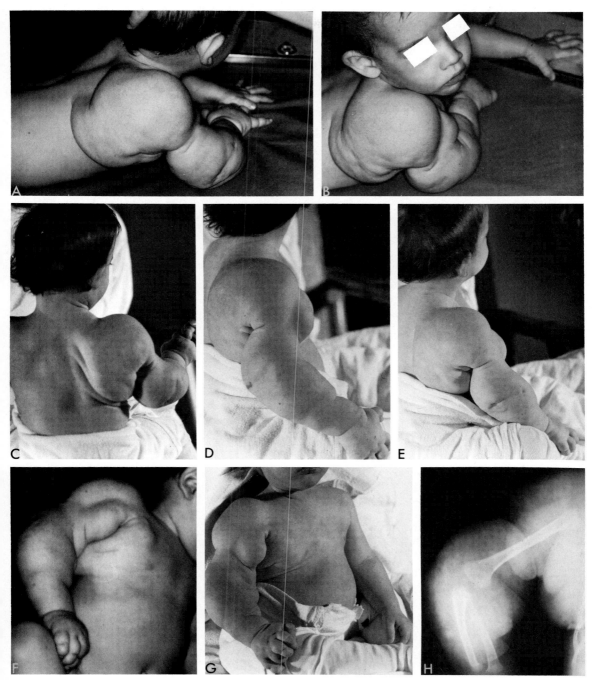

Figure 19–2 Lymphangiohemangioma. *A* to *G*, Sundry views of an 11-month-old male infant with oversized turgid soft-tissue swelling of the right upper chest, pectoral region, forearm, and fingers, which were held in flexion except when pressed against a flat surface as shown in *A* and *C. H*, Anteroposterior roentgenograph of the right pectoral region, upper arm, and forearm, showing extensive soft-tissue swelling.

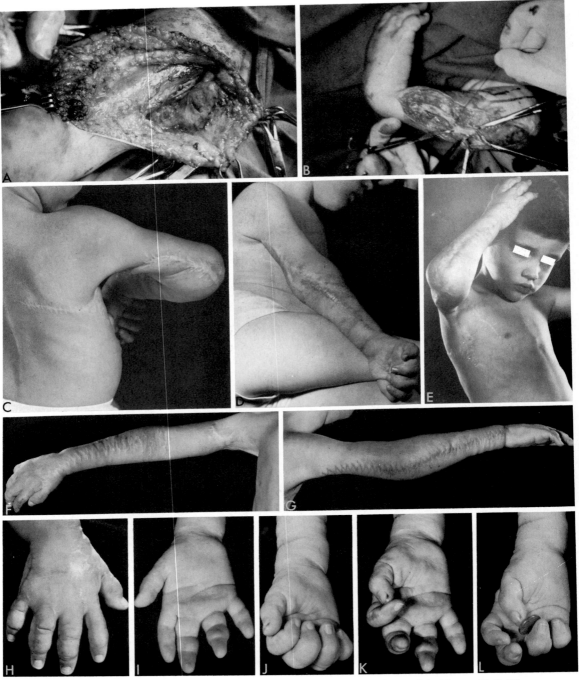

Figure 19–3 *A*, Exposure of the right axilla of the 11-month-old boy featured in Figure 19–2. There were a number of large intercommunicating lacunae filled with clear yellowish fluid. *B*, Exposure of an oversized tortuous vein on the ulnar aspect of the right forearm. *C, D,* and *E,* Keloid formation after resection of the hemangioma, excision of which was carried out in several sessions, at varying intervals. *F* and *G,* Elimination of keloids by Z-plasty. *H* to *L,* Postoperative appearance and function of the right hand.

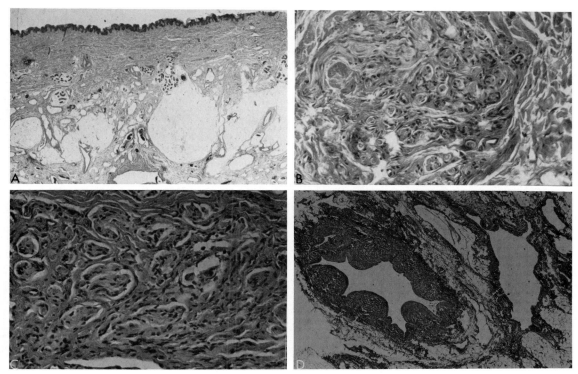

Figure 19–4 Biopsy specimens obtained from the 11-month-old boy featured in Figures 19–2 and 19–3. *A,* Large lymphatic lacunae under the skin. *B* and *C,* Fibrosis and cellular infiltration of the surrounding tissues. *D,* Large vein with thick sclerosed wall next to a sizable lymphatic lacuna.

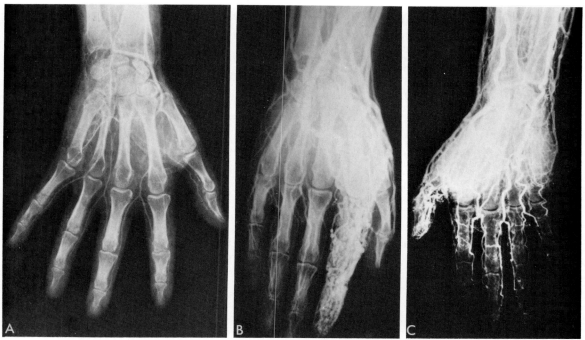

Figure 19–5 Arteriography of the hand. *A,* Arteriograph of the right hand of a normal young adult. *B,* Arteriograph of another young adult with congenital hemangioma of the right index finger. *C,* Arteriograph of an older individual with numerous intercommunicating vessels of the thumb.

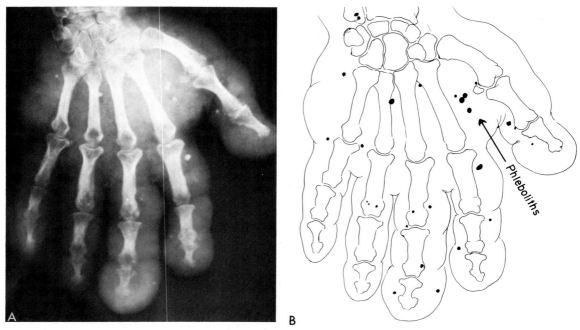

Figure 19–6   Phleboliths and soft-tissue thickness. *A*, Dorsopalmar roentgenograph of an adult male with congenital hemangioma of the right hand with thick, turgid but not long digits and numerous phleboliths. *B*, Sketch illustrating the same.

KLIPPEL-TRÉNAUNAY SYNDROME (Parkes-Weber Syndrome; Angioosteohypertrophic Syndrome; Hemangiectatic Enlargement; Angiodysplastic Hypertrophy; Nevus Osteohypertrophicus; Nevus-Varicosus Osteohypertrophicus; Osteohypertrophic Varicose Nevus Syndrome)

In describing the symptom complex which bears their hyphenated names, Klippel and Trénaunay (1900) insisted upon the presence of the following triad: (1) nevi with metameric distribution, (2) precocious varicosities confined to one side of the body and dating from infancy or already evident at birth, and (3) hypertrophy of the underlying tissues, particularly of the bones which become longer and thicker. Weber (1907) described a 12-year-old girl with diffuse cutaneous hemangioma involving the left side of the body; the left upper and lower limbs were decidedly bulkier than the extremities on the right side. In a later communication, Weber (1918) drew attention to the fact that, in hemangiectatic hypertrophy, enlargement of the fingers is not as great as that seen in "true. . .giant growth," meaning nerve territory–oriented macrodactyly.

As part of the Klippel-Trénaunay syndrome, one of the fingers is usually larger and longer and, at times, is bent sideways. A number of such moderately macrodactylic digits of the hand have been reported in the literature. In the dis-

(Text continued on page 676.)

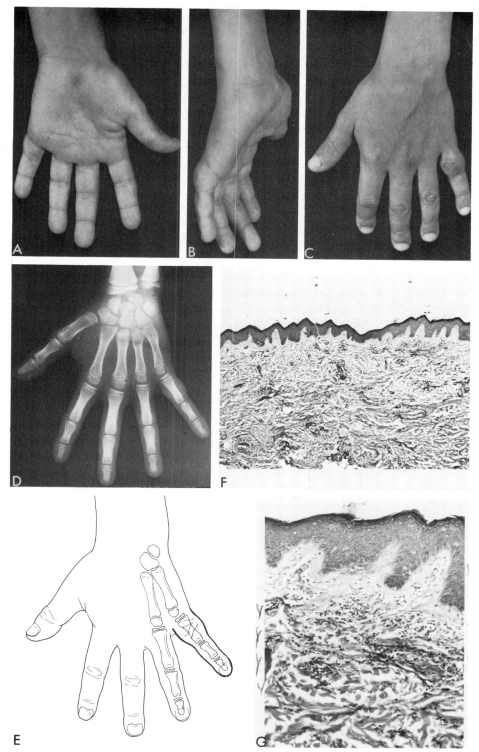

Figure 19–7 Localized hemangioma of the little finger associated with a pigmented patch at the base of the palm. *A, B,* and *C,* Sundry views of the left hand of a nine-year-old boy who, since birth, has had a vascular tumor behind the proximal phalanx of the little finger which had repeatedly been operated upon but had recurred. *D,* Dorsopalmar roentgenograph of the left hand, showing soft-tissue bulge around the proximal phalanx of the little finger. *E,* Sketch illustrating the same. *F* and *G,* Sections of the excised specimen. There has been no recurrence since the last resection of the tumor eight years ago.

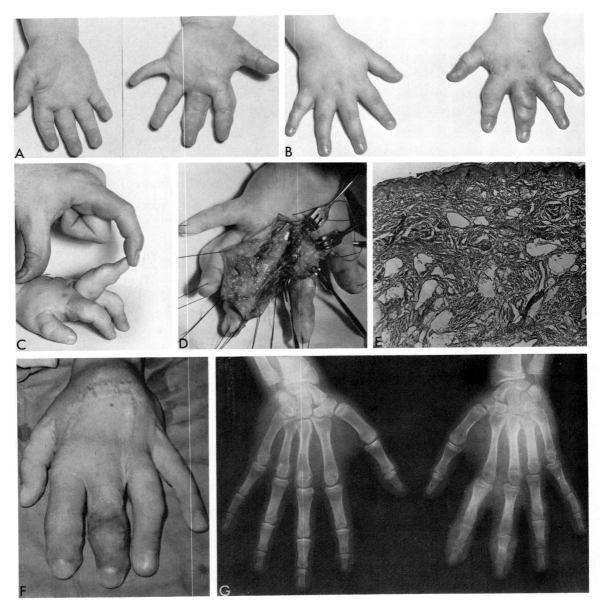

Figure 19–8   Localized hemangioma of the hand. *A, B,* and *C,* Sundry views of the hands of a four-year-old boy born with hemangioma of the left hand, involving mainly the three central digits; the index and ring fingers had previously been operated on. *D,* Surgical exposure of the volar aspect of the left middle finger and the corresponding portion of the distal palm showing tortuous, intercommunicating vessels. *E,* Section of the extirpated tissue. *F,* Dorsal view of the left hand 10 years after three surgical attempts at extirpation of the hemangioma, showing recurrence on the back of the distal phalanx of the left middle finger. *G,* Dorsopalmar roentgenograph of the hands: the second and third phalanges of the left index and middle fingers show premature closure of physes; the left middle finger is shorter than the third digit of the right hand.

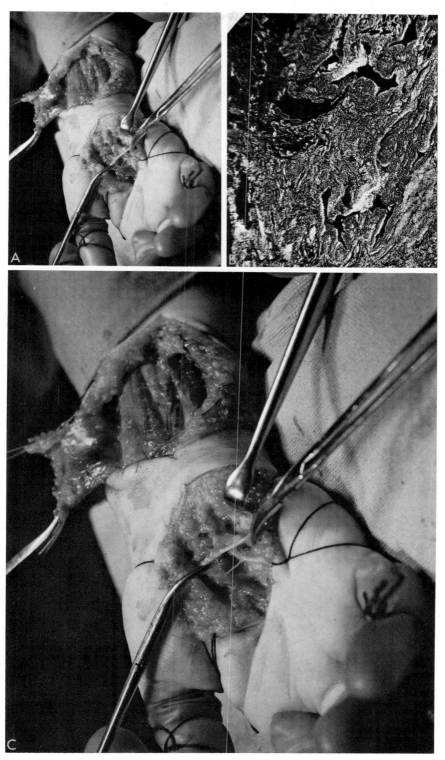

Figure 19–9 Aberrant congenital venous plexus of the distal forearm and proximal palm. *A*, Surgical exposure of the tumor in the distal forearm and palm of a six-year-old boy. *B*, Section of the biopsy specimen, showing large intercommunicating vessels. *C*, Enlarged portion of *A*, demonstrating transversely disposed large vessels, one of which is held by a pair of hemostats.

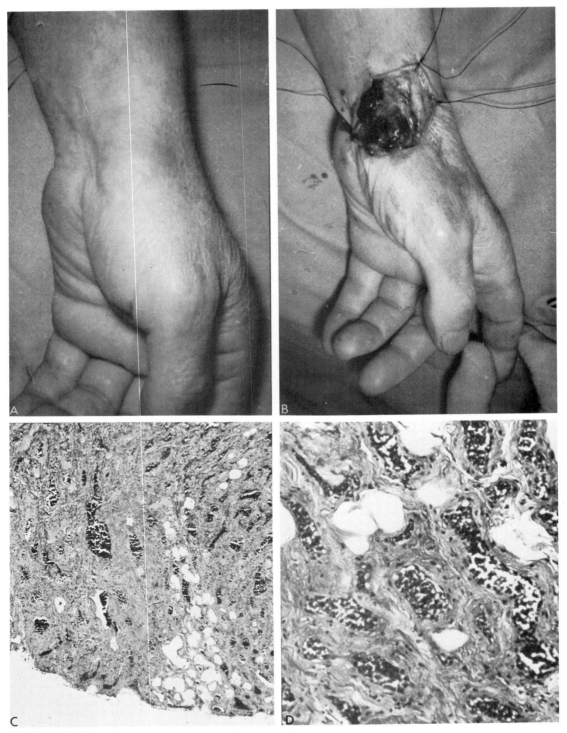

Figure 19–10   Localized hemangioma. *A,* Oblique view of the wrist of an adult man who, as long as he could remember, had had a swelling on the radial and volar aspect of the left wrist which had been diagnosed as ganglion. *B,* Surgically exposed vascular tumor. *C* and *D,* Biopsy sections, interpreted as sclerosing hemangioma.

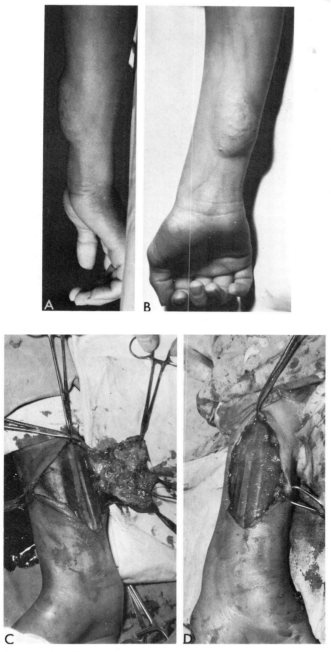

Figure 19–11 Localized hemangioma. *A*, Ulnar view of the right forearm of a five-year-old boy. *B*, Volar view. *C*, Surgically dissected tumor: a large aberrant vein pinched proximally by two hemostats ramified into an irregular plexus. *D*, The area left after extirpation of the tumor, which was surfaced by full-thickness free graft.

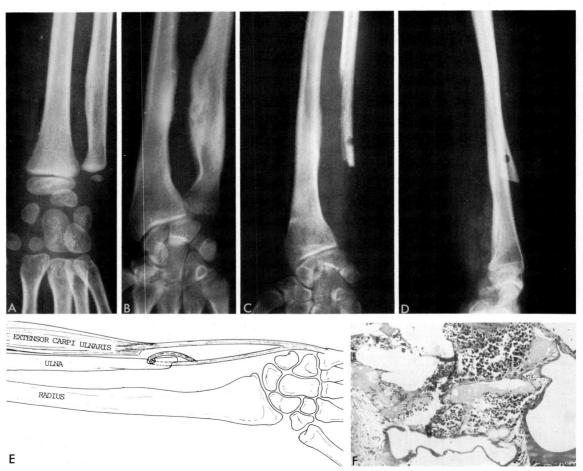

Figure 19–12   Hemangioma involving bone. *A*, Dorsovolar roentgenograph of the left distal forearm and wrist of a seven-year-old girl who had complained since infancy of pain in the region of the distal ulna; note the thickening of the cortex on the radial aspect of the distal ulna. *B*, Preoperative dorsovolar roentgenograph of the same, taken at the age of 17 years. The head of the ulna and its tumor-bearing radial cortex were resected and the split half of the extensor carpi ulnaris was utilized to reconstruct an ulnar collateral ligament. *C* and *D*, Postoperative dorsopalmar and lateral roentgenographs of the distal forearm and wrist. *E*, Sketch illustrating excision of the tumor-bearing portion of the distal ulna and also of the ulnar head and establishment of an ulnar collateral ligament by utilizing the split half of the extensor carpi ulnaris. *F*, Section of the tumor.

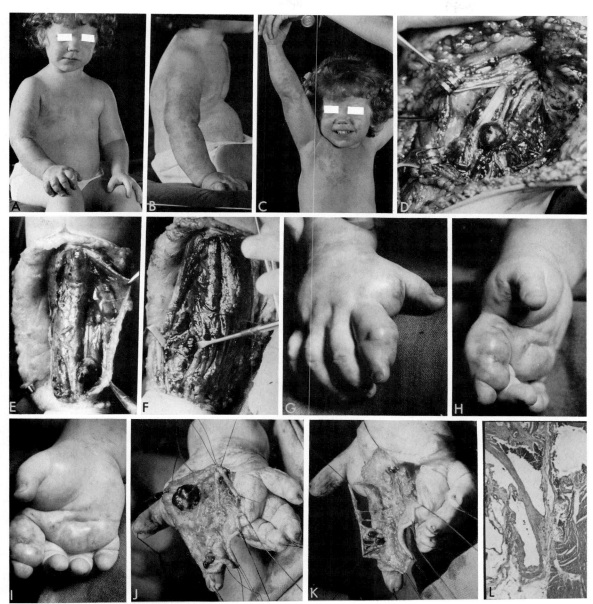

Figure 19–13   Diffuse cavernous hemangioma. *A*, Frontal view of the upper limbs of a three-year-old girl with hemangioma of the right lateral chest wall and upper limb. *B*, Profile view of the right chest and upper limb. *C*, Axillary view: on elevation, the arm shrinks. *D*, Exploration of the right axilla showing segmental dilatation of deeper veins. *E*, Exploration of the right forearm: the flexor carpi radialis is invaded with dilated vessels replacing muscular elements. *F*, Dilated vessels between the deeper muscles and tendons of the forearm. *G*, *H*, and *I*, Sundry views of the right hand. *J*, Exploration of the palm and volar aspect of the index finger, showing thick tortuous vessels and aneurysmal dilatations. *K*, Dissection showing the deep vein (retracted by black silk) communicating with the digital artery by way of numerous vessels, some of which bear large varices. *L*, Section of biopsy specimen.

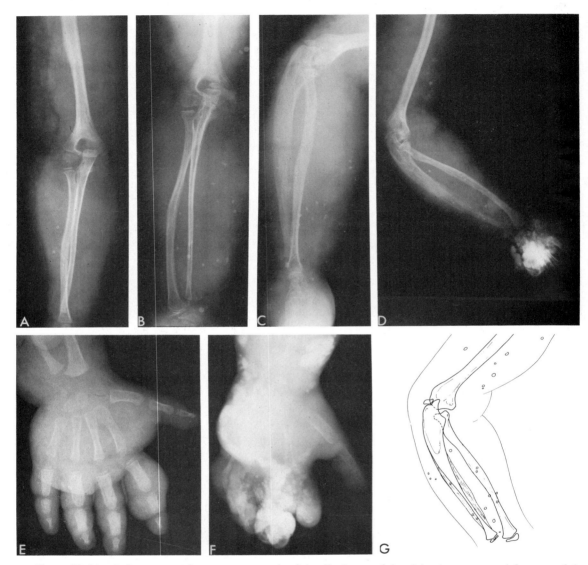

Figure 19–14 *A*, Anteroposterior roentgenograph of the distal part of the right upper arm and forearm of the three-year-old girl featured in Figure 19–13 taken at the age of six years and showing very few phleboliths. *B* and *C*, anteroposterior and lateral roentgenographs of the right forearm taken two years later, showing numerous phleboliths. *D*, Lateral roentgenograph of distal right upper arm and right forearm taken at the age of 13, showing lamellar thickening of the ulna. *E*, Dorsopalmar roentgenograph of the right hand taken at the age of three. *F*, The same, following arteriography. *G*, Sketch illustrating the roentgenograph above it.

cussion which followed Apert's (1931) paper, Huc suggested arresting the growth of the enlarged bone—which in the hand would involve the phalanges of the overgrown digit—by destroying the physeal cartilage plate. The author of this book has seen a number of cases of Klippel-Trénaunay syndrome implicating the hand and associated with moderately enlarged deviated digits and, in one instance, with dislocation of the radial head. The digital overgrowth or deformity was not severe enough to necessitate surgical interference. Klippel-Trénaunay syndrome is transmitted as an autosomal dominant trait (Figs. 19–16 to 19–23).

(Text continued on page 682.)

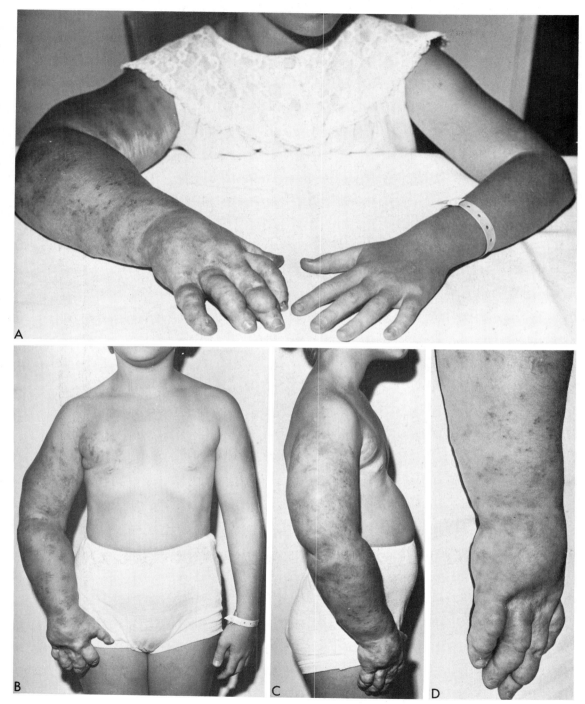

Figure 19–15 *A* and *B*, Various views of the upper limbs of the child featured in Figures 19–13 and 19–14, taken at the age of 13—after a number of segmental resections of angiomas. In 10 years there was no discrepancy between the length of the two arms; the thickening of the right upper limb was mainly due to dilated vessels. *C*, Profile view of the right upper limb. *D*, Ulnar view of the right forearm and hand.

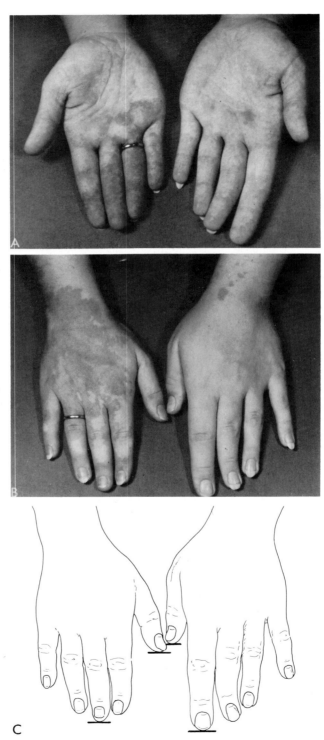

Figure 19–16   Klippel-Trénaunay syndrome. *A*, Palmar view of the hands of a 19-year-old woman who since birth has had blotchy spots on both hands, especially on the right hand. *B*, Dorsal view of the hands: the right thumb is longer than the left; the left index is thicker and longer than the right; the distal phalanx of the left middle finger inclines in the ulnar direction. *C*, Sketch illustrating the same.

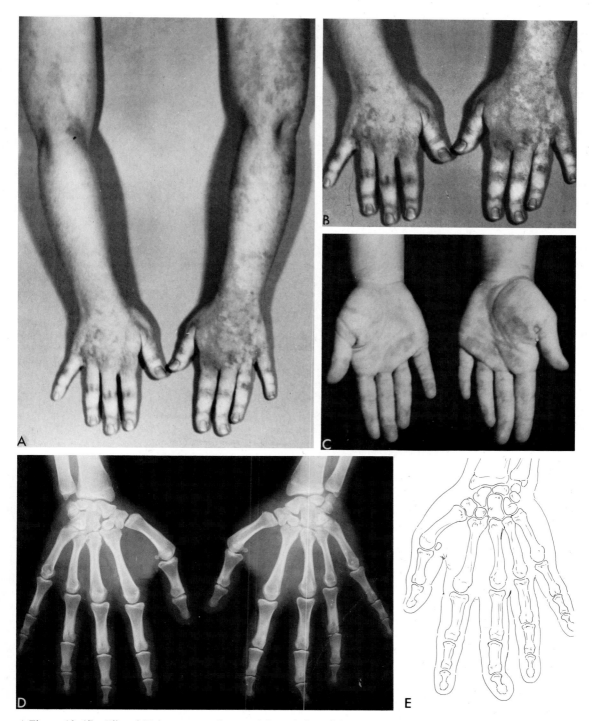

Figure 19–17 Klippel-Trénaunay syndrome. *A*, Dorsal view of the upper limbs of a 14-year-old girl with extensive subcutaneous varicosities which have been present since birth, being more marked in the back of the left forearm and hand: the ungual phalanx of the left middle finger inclines in the ulnar direction, as in the case featured in Figure 19–16. *B*, Dorsal view of the hands. *C*, Palmar view. *D*, Dorsopalmar roentgenograph. *E*, Sketch illustrating the roentgenograph of the left hand.

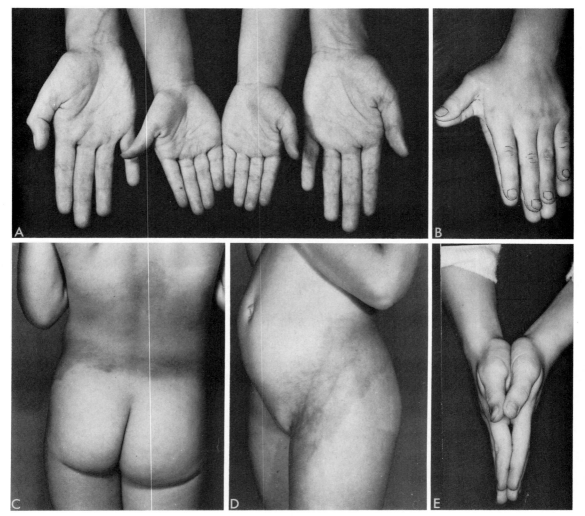

Figure 19–18   Klippel-Trénaunay syndrome: mother-to-daughter transmission with accentuated expression in the progeny. *A*, Palmar view of the hands of a six-year-old girl flanked by the hands of her mother: all four palms present patches of visible subcutaneous venules which are seen more distinctly in the enlarged photograph of the daughter's hands featured in Figure 19–19; the daughter's right index finger has a pigmented mole, and her right little finger is longer and thicker than her left fifth digit. *B*, Dorsal view of the left hand superimposed on the right hand which has longer fingers. *C*, Dorsal view of the torso, showing extensive pigmentation of the lumbar spine and tilted pelvis with a higher left iliac crest. *D* shows extension of the pigmentation down into the left thigh which is thicker and longer. *E*, Radial view of the opposed hand, showing longer right index and middle fingers.

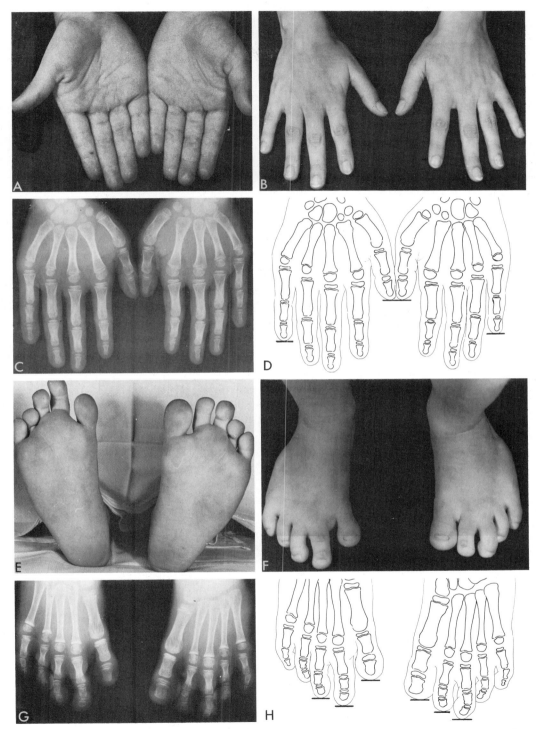

Figure 19–19 *A,* Palmar view of the hands of the six-year-old daughter featured in Figure 19–18: note the visibly congested subcutaneous veins. *B,* Dorsal view. *C,* Dorsopalmar roentgenograph of the hands: the right little finger is longer. *D,* Sketch illustrating the same. *E,* Plantar view of the feet: the right second toe is longer, but the right great toe is shorter and thinner. *F,* Dorsal view of the same. *G,* Dorsoplantar roentgenograph of the feet. *H,* Sketch illustrating the same.

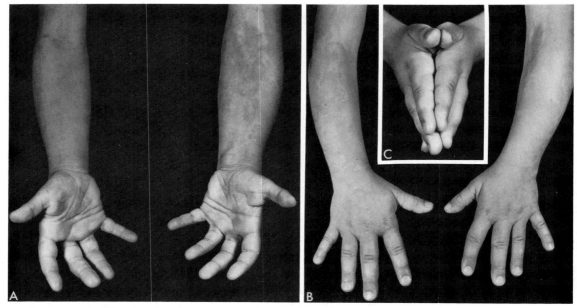

Figure 19–20   Klippel-Trénaunay syndrome. *A*, Volar view of the forearms and hands of an 18-year-old woman with numerous visible subcutaneous venules on both sides, but especially on the left forearm: note the bulge in front of the wrist on the ulnar aspect of the left palmaris longus tendon; the left forearm is thicker. *B* and *C*, Dorsal and radial view: the fingers are longer than the corresponding digits of the left hand.

MAFFUCCI SYNDROME (Angiodysplastic Enchondromatoses; Dyschondroplasia with Hemangiomas; Chondrodystrophy with Vascular Hamartoma; Kast Syndrome; Maffucci-Kast Syndrome)

Maffucci (1881) appears to have been the first to describe ever-expanding multiple nests of cartilage in bones associated with hemangiomas. Kast (1889) and Steudel (1891) featured patients with enormous cauliflower-like enlargement of digits (Fig. 19–24).

In Maffucci's disease, hemangiomas are widely distributed and form blue or reddish blue tumors which are soft, compressible, and sometimes tender to pressure. Thrombi form in these vascular tumors, and calcified thrombi or phleboliths produce a striking roentgenographic picture in the soft tissues. Phlebectasia is common and may affect large groups of veins or be confined to a few local areas in a vein, causing beadlike swelling. The enchondromas are multiple; they are predominantly unilateral, and they favor the growing ends of the bones. The involved bone is short, thick, and bowed. The phalanges and metacarpals of the hand are often affected and may undergo pathologic fractures. The complex appears to be more common in males. It is not hereditary or familial, and sarcomatous degeneration, malignant tumors of the brain, and lipomas of the muscles have been reported. The surgery is palliative and mutilating; it consists of amputation of the tumefied, useless, painful digit. Prognosis is grave (Fig. 19–25).

(*Text continued on page 688.*)

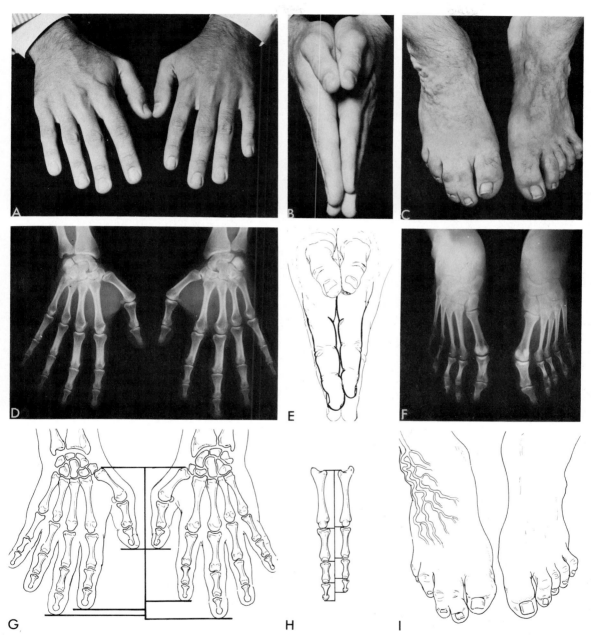

Figure 19–21   Klippel-Trénaunay syndrome associated with longer right index and left middle fingers and webbed second and third right toes. *A*, Dorsal view of the hands of a 24-year-old man who has had varicosities on the fibular side of the right ankle and foot since birth. *B*, Radial view of the hands. *C*, Dorsal view of the feet. *D*, Dorsopalmar roentgenograph of the hands. *E*, Sketch illustrating the photograph above it. *F*, Dorsoplantar roentgenograph of the feet. *G*, Sketch illustrating the roentgenograph above it. *H*, Sketch showing the juxtaposed skeletal components of the right and left second digital rays. *I*, Sketch illustrating *C*.

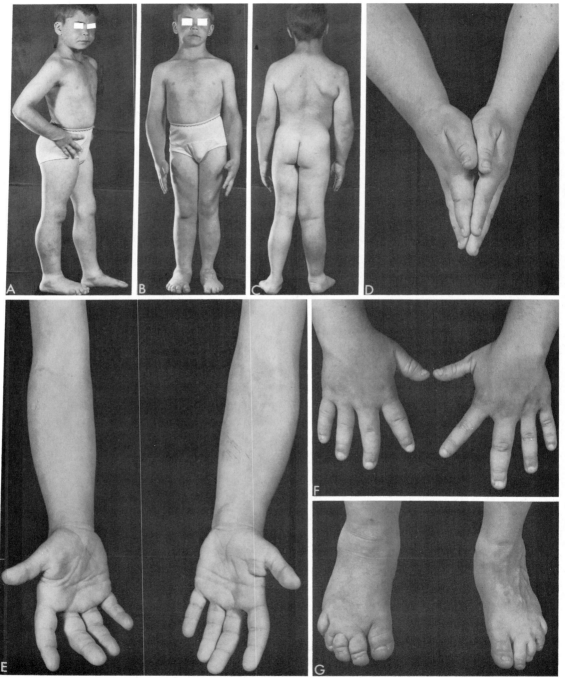

Figure 19–22   Klippel-Trénaunay syndrome associated with asymmetry between the two halves of the body and dislocation of the radial head. *A, B,* and *C,* A seven-year-old boy with thicker right lower limb and longer left upper and lower extremities; the right elbow does not fully extend because of a posteriorly dislocated radial head; the pelvis is tilted, the left iliac crest being higher. *D,* Radial view of juxtaposed hands: the right thumb is thicker; the left thumb and middle fingers are longer. *E,* Volar view of the distal portions of the upper limbs: there are numerous visible venules on the volar aspect of the left forearm, and a sizable dilated vein is seen bulging in front of the distal ulna. *F,* Dorsal view of the hands, showing thicker right thumb and longer left thumb and middle finger. *G,* Dorsal view of the feet: the right first and second toes are thicker but shorter than the corresponding digits of the left foot, which has patchy pigmentations and visible varices.

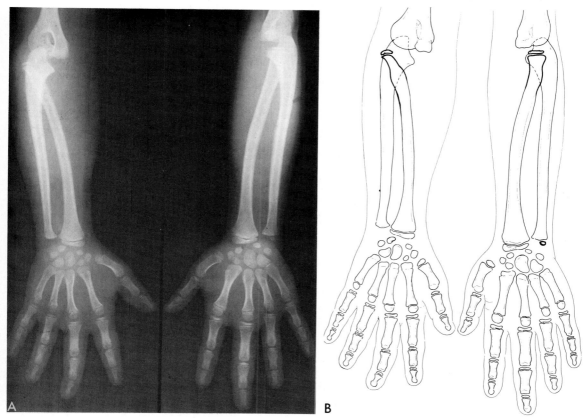

Figure 19–23 *A*, Dorsovolar roentgenograph of the forearms and hands of the seven-year-old boy featured in Figure 19–22: the right radial head is dislocated posteriorly; the distal epiphyses of the right ulna has not ossified as yet; the bones of the left forearm are longer and thicker; the skeletal components of the left third ray are longer and thicker than the corresponding elements on the right side. *B*, Sketch illustrating the same.

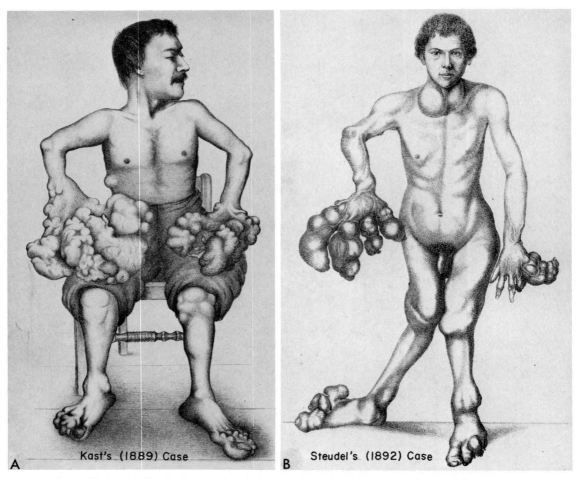

Figure 19–24 Maffucci's disease: historical cases. *A*, Kast's (1888) patient. *B*, Steudel's (1892) case.

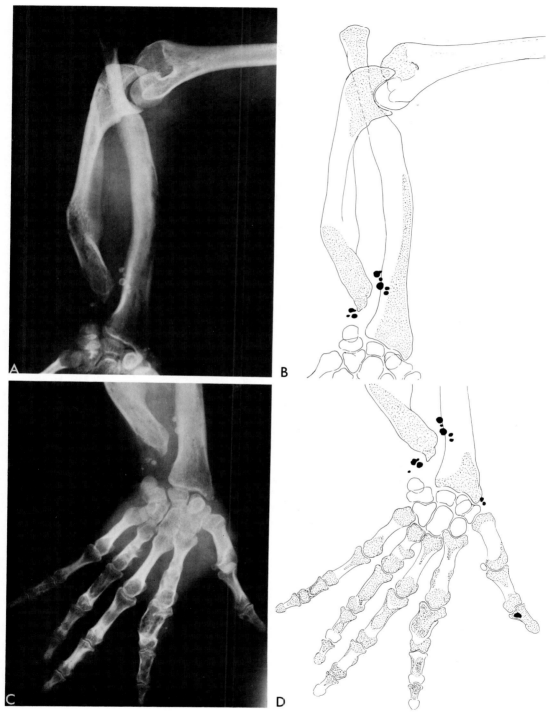

Figure 19–25 Multiple enchondromatosis with hemangioma—Maffucci's syndrome. *A*, Dorsovolar roentgenograph of the right forearm of an adult man: the head of the radius is dislocated; the ulna is short; both forearm bones bear irregular translucent areas, and there are extraskeletal circular densities indicative of phleboliths. *B*, Sketch illustrating the same. *C*, Dorsopalmar roentgenograph of the right wrist and hand: practically all digital rays show irregularly shaped intraosseous translucent areas which are more abundant as one approaches the ulnar border of the hand; there are many phleboliths. *D*, Sketch illustrating the same.

SUMMARY

Vascular tumors are regarded as persisting patterns of embryonic channels. They are categorized as lymphangiomas and hemangiomas. In most instances these tumors are mixed; they consist of dilated lymphatics and veins, or dilated veins which are being fed by the arteries via multiple communicating branches. The affected parts are enlarged. The enlargement involves mainly the soft tissue and, only rarely, the bones. In the hand, the digits are thick and pudgy. As a rule, one extremity only is affected, and a given digit on the affected side may be slightly longer than the corresponding member on the opposite side. The elongated digit fails to attain the dimension seen by nerve territory–oriented macrodactyly. Numerous methods, such as compression, injection of sclerosing solutions, radiotherapy, and amputation, have been tried in the treatment of vascular tumors. Except in cases of extensive involvement of bones, these tumors are amenable to periodic segmental resection. Two complexes, Maffucci disease and Klippel-Trénaunay syndrome, belong to the category of angiodysplastic enlargement.

References

Akerman, A. J., and Hart, M. S.: Multiple primary hemangioma of bones of the extremities. *Am. J. Roentgenol., 48*:47–52, 1952.

Andrews, G. C., Demonkos, A. N., and Post, C. G.: Treatment of angiomas; summary of twenty years experience at Columbia Presbyterian Medical Center. *Am. J. Roentgenol., 67*:273–285, 1952.

Apert, M. E.: Noevus variqueux ostéo-hypertrophique de Klippel et Trénaunay à extension précocé et rapide. *Bull. Soc. Pédiatr., 29*:206–210, 1931.

Atkins, H. L., Wolff, J. A., and Sitarz, A.: Giant hemangioma in infancy with secondary thrombocytopenia purpura. *Am. J. Roentgenol., 89*:1062–1066, 1963.

Beckmann, R., and Koch, F.: Zur Kongenitalen dystrophischen Angiektasie. *Mschr. Kinderheilkd., 104*:384–387, 1956.

Bedford, D. E.: Coarctation of the aorta and congenital phlebarterectasis of the left arm. *Proc. R. Soc. Med.* (Clinical section), *31*:557–558, 1937.

Benassi, E.: Evoluzione delle fistole artero-venose congenite delgi arti (Osservazione di un caso) *Chir. Triven., 8*:846–857, 1968.

Benassi, E., Garusi, G. F., and Scappini, G.: Fistole arterio-venose congenite degli arti (Multiformita degli aspeti clinico-radiologici et rapporti con l'alterato sviluppo somatico) *Chir. Triven., 9*:175–269, 1969.

Blackfield, H. M., Torrey, F. A., Morris, W. J., and Low-Beer, B. V. A.: The management of visible hemangiomas. *Am. J. Surg., 94*:313–320, 1957.

Bourde, C.: Les fistules artério-veineuses congénitales des membres. *J. Chir., 69*:728–748, 1953.

Bourde, C., and Jouve, A.: Problèmes diagnostiques et nosologiques posés par les fistules artério-veineuses congénitales des membres. *Pédiatrie, 12*:81–84, 1957.

Braun, H.: Ein Fall von Phlebarteriektasia der rechten oberen Extremität. *Münch. Med. Wochenschr., 49*:163–165, 1902.

Brown, J., and Fryer, M. P.: Hemangiomas. Treatment and repair of defects: report of minimal radiation dosage and of multiple suture procedure. *Surg. Gynecol. Obstet., 95*:33–44, 1952.

Brown, J. B., and Fryer, M. P.: Treatment of hemangiomas. *A.M.A. Arch. Surg., 65*:417–421, 1952.

Bucher, R.: Ein seltener Fall eines Lymphangioma cysticum congenitum. *Dtsch. Z. Chir., 243*:161–176, 1934.

Buchtala, V.: Phlebolithen und Hämangiome. *Röntgenpraxis, 13*:45–52; Abb 3–5, 1941.

Byers, L. T.: The "malignant" hemangioma. *Surg. Gynecol. Obstet., 77*:193–198, 1943.

Carpenter, F. B., and Strawn, L. M.: Hemangiomatosis of the ulna and flexor muscles of the forearm with secondary flexion contracture of the wrist and hand. *J. Bone Joint Surg., 45A*:1472–1478, 1963.

Chamberlain, R. H., and Pendergrass, E. P.: Some considerations regarding the treatment of hemangiomas. *Penn. Med. J., 51*:867–869, 1948.

Chassaignac: Hypertrophie congénitale des deux membres droits. — Taches sanguines multiples: Varices, etc. *Gaz. Hôp., 54*:215, 1858.

Comby, J.: Deux observations d'hypertrophie congénitale. *Arch. Méd. Enfants.* (l.s.), *2*:271–275, 1899.

Copperstock, M.: Congenital enlargement of the extremities. *Am. J. Dis. Child., 57*:309–321, 1939.

Curtis, R. N.: Congenital arteriovenous fistulae of the hand. *J. Bone Joint Surg., 35A*:917–928, 1953.

D'Allaines, C., and Maillet, R.: Fistules artério-veineuses congénitales des membres. *Arch. Mal. Coeur Vars., 55*:856–870, 1962.

Da Silva, M. V., and Neves, H.: Über einen Fall von Klippel-Trenaunayschem Symptomenkomplex, der erfolgreich mit Röntgenstrahlen behandelt wurde. *Fortschr. Röntgenstr., 90*:475–482, 1959.

Devilliers: Tumeur de la main. (Angiome avec hypertrophie fibreuse et dilatations lymphatiques). *Bull. Soc. Anat. Paris,* (4 s.), *1*:215–217, 1876.

Downing, J. G.: Osteohypertrophic varicose nevus. *Arch. Derm. Syph., 35*:740–741, 1937.

Duzea, R.: *Sur Quelques Troubles de Développement du Squélette du a des Angiomes Superficiels.* Thèse. Lyon, Imprimérie Typographique Bellon, pp. 1–97, 1886.

Elkeles, A.: Local gigantism of right third and fourth fingers associated with multiple haemangiomata of right chest wall. *Proc. R. Soc. Med.* (Clinical section), *44*:917–918, 1951.

Elkeles, A.: Local gigantism involving second and third fingers associated with lymphangiostatic condition of the right palm. *Proc. R. Soc. Med.* (Clinical section), *44*:918–919, 1951.

Elkin, D. C., and Cooper, F. W., Jr.: Extensive hemangioma. Report of cases. *Surg. Gynecol. Obstet., 71*:569–588, 1940.

Eve, F. S.: Two specimens of congenital hypertrophy or giant-growth of limbs. *Trans. Path. Soc. London, 34*:298–304, 1883.

Fayos, J., and Lampe, I.: Le traitement des angiomes chez les enfants. *Ann. Radiol., 8*:53–59, 1965.

Finlayson, J.: On the case of a child affected with congenital unilateral hypertrophy and patches of cutaneous congestion. *Glascow Med. J., 22*:327–337, 1884.

Fowler, G. R.: *A Treatise on Surgery.* Philadelphia, W. B. Saunders Co., Vol. 2, p. 487; fig. 741, 1907.

Fox, T. C.: Cases of lymphangiectasis of the hands and feet in children. *Illust. Med. News., 4*:73–75, 1889.

Garuci, G. F., Noto, L., and Castellarin, T.: Richerche angiografiche sulla mano. *Chir. Triven.*, 7:459–487, 1967.

Glanz, S.: The surgical treatment of cavernous haemangiomas of the hand. *Br. J. Plast. Surg.*, 22:293–301, 1969.

Goidanich, I. F., and Venturi, R.: Contributo alla conoscenza del neurinoma plessiforme; varieta lipo-angiomatosa. *Chir. Organi Mov.*, 42:15–35, 1955.

Gold, H., Cattell, M., Wilder, J. R., and Michaels, G. L.: Current status of vascular surgery. *Am. J. Med. Sci.*, 245:102–111, 1963.

Gottschalk, M.: Zur Ätiologie, Klinik und Therapie der Lymphangiome. *Beitr. Klin. Chir.*, 216:673–686; Abb 7, 8, 10a, 1968.

Halsted, W. S.: Congenital arteriovenous and lymphaticovenous fistulae; unique clinical and experimental observations. *Trans. Am. Surg. Assoc.*, 37:262–272, 1919.

Harris, K. E., and Wright, G. P.: A case of hemangiectatic hypertrophy of a limb and observation upon rate of growth in the presence of increased blood supply. *Heart*, 15:141–149, 1930.

Harrison, S. H.: Haemangioma of the flexor sublimis. *Br. J. Plast. Surg.*, 7:353–356, 1955.

Henssge, J., and Werner, H.: Zur Diagnostik und Therapie des umschriebenen Riesenwuchses vom Typ *Klippel-Trenaunay. Z. Orthop.*, 94:83–88, 1961.

Hewett, P.: A case of congenital aneurysmal varix. *Lancet*, 1:146–147, 1867.

Heymann, E.: Die chirurgische Behandlung der Angiome. *Rev. Chir. Plastique*, 1:253–263, 1931.

Hitzrot, J. M.: Hemangioma cavernosum of bone. *Ann. Surg.*, 65:476–482, 1917.

Holman, E.: The physiology of an arteriovenous fistula. *Arch. Surg.*, 7:64–82, 1923.

Homans, J.: Lymphedema of the limbs. *Arch. Surg.*, 40:232–252, 1940.

Homorodeanu, J., and Berçu, G.: A propos d'un cas clinique de syndrome de Radulerçu (gigantism partiel congénital associé a naevus flemmeus). *Ann. Chir. Inf.*, 9:257–259, 1968.

Horton, B. T.: Hemihypertrophy of extremities associated with arterio-venous fistula. *Proc. Mayo Clin.*, 6:316–319, 1931.

Horton, B. T.: Hemihypertrophy of extremities associated with congenital arteriovenous fistula. *J.A.M.A.*, 98:373–379, 1932.

Horton, B. T., and Ghormeley, R. H.: Congenital arteriovenous fistula. *Proc. Staff Meet. Mayo Clin.*, 8:773–776, 1933.

Hurwitt, E. S., and Johnston, A.: Interscapulothoracio amputation for diffuse angiomatous malformation. *Ann. Surg.*, 142:115–120, 1955.

Jenkins, H. P., and Delaney, P. A.: Benign angiomatous tumors of skeletal muscles. *Surg. Gynecol. Obstet.*, 55:464–480, 1932.

Jouve, A., and Bourde, C.: Syndrome de Klippel-Trénaunay et shunt artério-veineux. *Arch. Mal. Coer.*, 4:649–650, 1952.

Jouve, A., Bourdoncle, E., and Bourde, C.: Fistules arterio-veineuses congénitales des membres et syndrome de Klippel-Trénaunay. *Sem. Hôp.*, 28:2674–2688, 1952.

Julian, O. C., and Dye, W. S.: Symposium on techniques and procedures in surgery: arteriography. *Surg. Clin. North Am.*, 35:275–284, 1955.

Kast: Ein Fall von Enchondromen mit ungewöhnlicher Multiplication. I. Klinische Beobachtung. II. Multiple Enchondrome der Knochen in Verbindung mit multiplen phlegmon covernösen Angiomen bedeckenden Weichtheil (Anatomisch beschrieben von Prof. v. Recklinghausen). *Arch. Pathol. Anat. Physiol.*, 118:1–18; Hierzu Taf. I, 1889.

Klippel, M., and Trénaunay, P.: Du noevus variqueux ostéo-hypertrophique. *Arch. Gén. Méd. Paris*, 77:641–672, 1900.

Klippel, M., and Trénaunay, P.: Noevus variqueux ostéo-hypertrophique. *J. Practiciens*, 14:65–70, 1900.

Lampe, I., and Latourette, H. B.: The management of cavernous hemangiomas in infants. *Postgrad. Med.*, 19:262–270, 1956.

Läwen: Über die genuine diffuse Phlebarteriektasie an der oberen Extremität. *Dtsch. Z. Chir.*, 68:364–390, 190 .

Leriche, R.: A propos de 12 cas d'aneurysme cirosoide. *Lyon Chir.*, 46:5–24, 1951.

Lewis, D. D.: Congenital arteriovenous fistula. *Lancet*, 2:621–628, 682–686, 1930.

Lunardo, C.: Sulle anomalie congenite di volume degli arti. *Atti. D.S.R.T. Ortop. Traum.*, 3:251–260, 1958.

MacCollum, D. W., and Martin, L. W.: Hemangiomas in infancy and childhood; a report based on 6,479 cases. *Surg. Clin. North Am., Nationwide Nr.*, 1647–1663, 1956.

Madelaine: Petit angioma de la paume de la main. Processus de cicatrisation profonde tendant a l'isoler du tissue cellulaire sous-cutane. *Bull. Mem. Soc. Anat.* (Paris), 65:250–251, 1911.

Maffucci, A.: Di un caso enchondroma e angioma multiple. *Mov. Med. Chir.*, 3:399–412; figs. 1–5; 2 tables, 1881.

Malan, E., and Puglionisi, A.: Congenital angiodysplasias of the extremities (Note I: Generalities and classification: venous dysplasias). *J. Cardiovasc. Surg.*, 5:87–130, 1964.

Matas, R.: Congenital arteriovenous angioma of the arm: Metastases eleven years after amputation. *Ann. Surg.*, 111:1021–1045, 1940.

Matthews, D. N.: Treatment of hemangiomata. *Br. J. Plast. Surg.*, 6:83–98, 1953.

Matthews, D.: The congenitally deformed hand. *Br. J. Plast. Surg.*, *17*:366–375; fig. 7, 1964.

Middleton, D. S.: Congenital lymphangiectatic fibrous hypertrophy (Elephantiasis congenita fibrosa lymphangiectatica). *Br. J. Surg.*, *19*:356–361; fig. 274, 1932.

Monod, E.: Fibroma vasculaire du doigt. *Bull. Soc. Anat. Paris*, (4 s.), *1*:235–236, 1876.

Morton, T. S. K.: Two cases of congenital hypertrophy of the fingers. *Med. News*, *64*:294–296; cas II, 1894.

Murphy, T. O., and Margulis, A. R.: Roentgenographic manifestations of congenital peripheral arterio-venous communications. *Radiology*, *67*:26–33, 1956.

Nicoladeni, C.: Phlebarterectasie der linken oberen Extremität. *Arch. Klin. Chir.*, *20*:146–165; Taff. III; fig. 1, 1877.

Owens, N., and Stephenson, K. L.: Hemangioma: an evaluation of treatment by injection and surgery. *Plast. Reconstr. Surg.*, *3*:109–123, 1948.

Packard, M., and Barrie, G.: Gigantism with hemorrhagic osteomyelitis of metacarpal bone. *J.A.M.A.*, *78*:8–10, 1922.

Paget, J.: On gouty and some other forms of phlebitis. *St. Barth. Hosp. Reports*, *2*:82–92, 1866.

Paschke, K. G., Huring, H., Schoop, W., and Zeitler, E.: Untersuchungen zur Angioszintigraphie der Hände und Füsse. *Fortschr. Röntgenstr.*, *115*:333–339; Abb 8a, b, c, 1971.

Paterson, D., and Wyllie, W. G.: Hypertrophy of the bones in a limb due to a naevus. *Br. J. Child. Dis.*, *22*:36–39, 1925.

Pemberton, J. de J., and Saint, J. H.: Congenital arteriovenous communications. *Surg. Gynecol. Obstet.*, *46*:470–483, 1928.

Petschelt, E.: Zur Klinik, Symptomologie, Lokalisation Alters-und Geschlechtsverteilung des Naevus vasculosus osteohypertrophicus. *Arch. Dermot. Syph.*, *196*:155–169, 1953.

Posch, J. L.: Tumors of the hand. *J. Bone Joint Surg.*, *38A*:517–540; 562, 1956.

Ravitch, M. M.: Radical treatment of massive mixed angiomas (hemolymph angiomas) in infants and children. *Ann. Surg.*, *134*:228–243, 1951.

Reid, M. R.: Abnormal arteriovenous communications, acquired and congenital. *Arch. Surg.*, *11*:237–253, 1925.

Reid, M. R.: Studies on abnormal arteriovenous communications, acquired and congenital. *Arch. Surg.*, *10*:601–638, 1925.

Reus, H. D. de, and Vink, H.: Kongenitale dystrophische Angiektasie. *Fortschr. Röntgenstr.*, *83*:690–702, 1955.

Rienhoff, W. F., Jr.: Congenital arteriovenous fistula: an embryological study, with report of a case. *Bull. Johns Hopkins Hosp.*, *35*:271–284, 1924.

Rowlands, R. P.: Two cases of cirsoid aneurysm. *Proc. R. Soc. Med. London* (Clinical section), *13*:23–26, 1919.

Schönenberg, H.: Ueber die Beziehungen des Klippel-Trénaunay-Weber-Syndroms zum "umschriebenen Riesenwuchs." *Z. Kinderheilkd.*, *77*:636–652, 1955.

Schönenberg, H.: Klippel-Trénaunay-Weber-Syndrom. Die Pathogenese des Klippel-Trénaunay-Weber-Syndroms. *In Missbildungen der Extremitäten*. Bibliotheca Paediatrica Fase 80. Basel (Schweiz)-New York, S. Karger, pp. 90–104, 1962.

Simpson, S. S.: A case of unilateral hypertrophy ("Extensive varices . . . cavernous venous angioma . . ."). *Edinburgh Med. J.*, *33*:623–626, 1926.

Singleton, A. O.: Congenital lymphatic diseases—lymphangiomata. *Ann. Surg.*, *105*:952–968, 1937.

Smith, T.: Angiectasia of hand and fingers. *Trans. Clin. Soc.* (London), *15*:195–199, 1882.

Souquer, A., and Gasne, G.: Un cas d'hypertrophie des pieds et des mains avec trouble vasomoteur des extrémites chez un hystérique. *N. Iconog. Salp.*, *5*:281–285, 1892.

Steinsleger, M.: Hiportrofia congenita de membros. *Rev. Med. Rosario*, *13*:265–272, 1923. Review in *Arch. Med. Enfants*, *29*:304–305, 1926.

Steudel: Multiple Enchondrome der Knochen in Verbindung mit venosen Angiomen der Weichteile. *Beitr. Klin. Chir.*, *8*:503–521; Taf. XI, 1891.

Stojamov, P.: Klippel-Trénaunay syndrome. *Lancet*, *2*:1331–1332, 1962.

Stolz: Aneurysme cirsoide du doigt. *Bull. Mem. Soc. Anat.*, (6 s.), *20*:612–613, 1923.

Strang, C., and Rannie, I.: Dyschondroplasia with hemangiomata (Maffucci's syndrome). *J. Bone Joint Surg.*, *32B*:376–383, 1950.

Szilagi, D. E., Elliot, G. P., De Russo, F. S., and Smith, R. F.: Peripheral congenital arterio-venous fistulas. *Surgery*, *57*:61–81, 1965.

Telford, E. D.: Hemihypertrophy of the body with nevus and varicose veins. *Lancet*, *2*:1291, 1912.

Terrier: Angio-limpome caverneux de la main: Opération et guérison par le Dr. H. Bousquet. *Bull. Soc. Chir. Paris*, *13*:419–422, 1887.

Verdan, C.: Traitement chirurgical des hemangiomes des membres et aspects particuliers de leur localization à la main. *Ann. Chir. Plast.*, *9*:304–316, 1964.

Vollmar, J.: Sonderformen des umschriebenen Riesenwuchses (Klippel-Trénaunay, Parkes-Weber u. Sturge-Weber Syndrom). Diagnostik, Terminologie und therapeutische Fragestellungen. *Ergb. Chir. Orthop.*, *42*:242–255, 1959.

Wagner: Fall einer Exarticulation des rechten Zeigefingers. *Med. Jahrb. oesterr. Staates (Wien)*, *29*:565–567, 1839.

Wakefield, E. G.: Hypertrophy, congenital, of the left shoulder girdle, arm and hand with navus and varicose veins. *Am. J. Med. Sci., 171*:569–575, 1926.

Ward, C. F., and Horton, B. T.: Congenital arterio-venous fistulas in children. *J. Pediatr., 16*:746–766; fig. 2, 1940.

Watson, W. L., and McCarthy, W. D.: Blood and lymph vessel tumors. *Surg. Gynecol. Obstet., 71*:569–588, 1940.

Weber, F. P.: Angioma-formation in connection with hypertrophy of limbs and hemihypertrophy. *Br. J. Dermatol., 19*:231–235, 1907.

Weber, F. P.: Haemangiectitic hypertrophy of limbs—congenital phlebarteriectasis and so-called "congenital varicose veins." *Br. J. Dis. Child., 15*:13–18, 1918.

Weber, J.: Der umschriebene Riesenwuchs, Typ Parkes-Weber. (Beitrag zur Diskussion des Klippel-Trénaunay-Weber Syndroms). *Fortschr. Röntgenstr., 113*:734–739; Abb, 1a, 1b, 2–6, 1970.

Weisman, P. A.: Blood vessel tumors of the hand. *Plast. Reconstr. Surg., 23*:175–186, 1959.

Chapter Twenty

OTHER STATES OF ASYMMETRY

In more diffuse enlargements discussed in Chapter Nineteen, the affected segments of the upper extremity are larger than the corresponding parts of the opposite limb. In locally confined unilateral augmentation anomalies of the hand (for example, polydactyly, mirror hand, and macrodactyly), the affected segments are larger than their counterparts; conversely, in unilateral diminution anomalies (terminal and intercalary defects), the affected segments are smaller than the corresponding parts of the contralateral limb.

Mouchet (1902) reported a five-year-old boy who was born with diminutive right thumb and right little finger. The two ulnar metacarpals had affected side-to-side bony union. Mouchet used the title "Congenital atrophy of the right hand." In the absence of skeletal abnormalities, atrophy of the hand is to be regarded as consequential to paralytic states. In neurogenic hemiatrophy, the muscles of the affected limb waste away and the joints eventually undergo contractures, but parts are not missing—there is no absence abnormality. Bizarre forms of asymmetry between opposite extremities are also known to occur in connection with a number of well-defined syndromes. Some of these—multiple exostoses, Klippel-Trénaunay syndrome, and Maffucci's enchondromatosis—have already been discussed. Others will be taken up later in this chapter.

The most perplexing form of asymmetry is the one which, for want of a more specific designation, is called hemihypertrophy—a condition in which the affected side, limb, or segment is larger than the corresponding part on the opposite side. There is, however, no drastic disturbance of contour or alignment. Many authors regard hemihypertrophy as an exaggerated form of the discrepancy which accompanies handedness; conversely, handedness is considered to be a mild form of hemihypertrophy.

HANDEDNESS

A barely discernible degree of asymmetry between the two sides of the body—between the right and left hands in particular—is the rule, and handedness is considered as the main cause of such slight inequalities. Since most individuals are right handed, the right hand is better developed than the left. Dwight (1891) wrote: "The right arm is the most used and is stronger and larger. . . . The skill, the ease, the readiness, the dexterity . . . which is an essential characteristic of the favorite side, though usually associated with greater development is yet distinct from it." Faure (1902) pointed out that the right upper limbs of right-handed subjects or dextrals possessed larger vessels, muscles, and bones than the left upper extremities of the same individuals; conversely, the left upper limbs of sinistrals had larger vessels, muscles, and bones. Faure considered two factors responsible for the structural disparity between opposite limbs, hands in particular: heredity and training. By implication, the right-handed individual is born with a larger right hand which gains an additional increment of dimension by greater use. After studying her own child, Wooley (1910) conceded that right-handedness could not be explained fully on the basis of training alone and was determined by heredity.

Cunningham (1902) explained the preponderance of right-handedness on

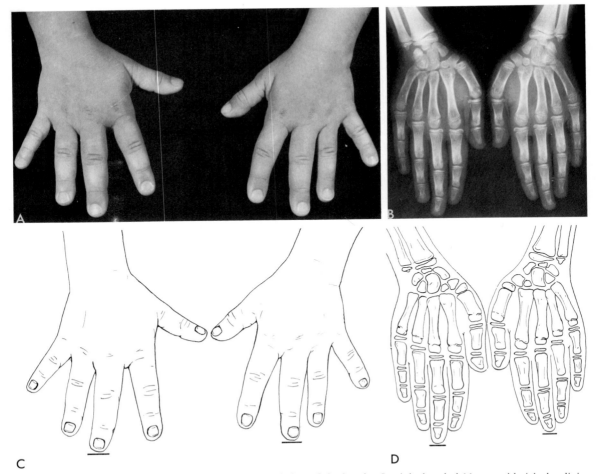

Figure 20–1   Asymmetry of handedness. *A*, Dorsal view of the hands of a right-handed 11-year-old girl: the digits of the right hand are discernibly thicker and longer than those of the left. *B*, Dorsopalmar roentgenograph of the hands. *C* illustrates the photograph and *D*, the roentgenograph above.

the basis of evolution and natural selection. He argued that from the earliest times, even though unjustifiably, dextrality had been identified with dexterity, and sinistrality was equated with clumsiness. Right-handed males were preferred, and dextrals outnumbered sinistrals. "Right-handedness," Cunningham wrote, "is due to a transmitted functional preeminence of the left brain. . . . Left-brainedness or the functional preeminence of the left brain is not the result, but, through evolution, it has become the cause of right-handedness." Cunningham thought that the functional superiority of the left brain rested upon "some structural foundation which is transmitted from parent to child."

The role of heredity in the structural as well as in the functional superiority of the left cerebral hemisphere in right-handed individuals, or of the right cerebral hemisphere is left-handed persons, has been expatiated upon by numerous authors and almost all of them condemn the persisting attempts at conversion of sinistrals into dextrals. The left hand of the converted sinistral is called upon to act in accordance with the dictates issuing from the biologically nondirective left cerebral lobe. The primary impulse goes to the right cerebral lobe, and from there it must be redirected to the left hemisphere. This rerouting of impulses not only retards the effective response, but also counteracts coordination. Confusion and consequent tension are inevitable. In the brain, moreover, the areas of speech, ocular movements, and movements of the hand lie close to one another; their responses to the rerouted impulses become entangled. Sinistrals who have been forced to become dextrals often stutter, lack visual coordination, write poorly, and are subject to psychological disturbances (Fig. 20–1).

HEMIHYPERTROPHY (Curtius I Syndrome; Congenital Hemimegalosomia; Hemimacrosomia; Hemiacromegaly; Hemigigantism)

Occasionally, one runs across an infant in whom the smaller hand is commensurate with the child's age while the opposite member has the dimensions of an individual several years older. In many such cases, the homolateral arm, forearm, and pectoral girdle are oversized; in some, the contralateral lower limb is similarly affected, and in a few, the entire half of the body is enlarged. Disparity between the two sides of the body which is striking enough to suggest that the opposite halves belong to two different individuals is considered pathologic. The uncomplicated form of such gross asymmetry has come to be known as hemihypertrophy, which is qualified as being total or partial. In total hemihypertrophy, which is comparatively rare, the entire half of the body from head to toe is affected. In the more common partial hemihypertrophy, there is uniform overdevelopment of one or more segments. Partial hemihypertrophy may be crossed, affecting a portion of one side of the body and a part of the opposite side at a different level. Occasionally, only a single extremity is overdeveloped; the hypertrophy is then said to be monomelic. Variability is perhaps the most constant feature of the more extensive enlargements which, when they involve one of the upper extremities, also affect the hand and the digits. The term segmental hypertrophy is used by some authors for macrodactyly, described in Chapter Eighteen.

In comparatively few reported cases of congenital hemihypertrophy and monomelic hyperplasia is the enlargement of the hands or fingers specified. The patient reported by Devouges (1856) had three oversized radial digits on the affected side. Osler (1879) presented a young girl whose right upper extremity afforded striking contrast to the childlike aspect of the left arm: the wrist was thick; the hand was "square" and had prominent knuckles; the palm was filled with a thick pad of fat; and the ball of the thumb was large. Langlet's (1882) patient had a longer right arm, and the right middle finger extended beyond the third digit of the left hand. The circumference of the right hand of Coston's (1920) patient measured one-half inch more than that of the left. Gesell's (1927) patient had a longer and larger right arm and hand.

Ducroquet's (1928) patient had hemihypertrophy on the left side; the left upper extremity was considerably longer than the right. Hemihypertrophy involved the entire right side of McFarland's (1928) patient, a young boy, whose right arm and hand were bigger than his left. Halperin's (1931) patient with hemihypertrophy of the left side showed "gigantic proportions" of the left hand. A patient with hemihypertrophy reported by Guillain and Bize (1934) had three large fingers on the left side. In the case described by Huse (1944), the bones of the left hand were larger than those of the right hand. One of the patients reported by Johnston and Penrose (1966) had an abnormally thick right middle finger.

Meckel (1822) is said to be the first clinician to have demonstrated the presence of asymmetry and hemihypertrophy in a cadaver. Wagner (1839) described a living subject, a woman with an enlarged right chest and right upper extremity and four turgid, swollen ulnar digits on the right side. The right hand became red and congested when in a dependent position; it weighed twelve European pounds and resembled a blood-soaked sponge—*Blutschwamm.* It might well have been the seat of cavernous hemangioma. Notwithstanding, numerous authors—Fortescue-Brickdale (1915), Wakefield (1926), Ward and Lerner (1947), Sabanas and Chatterton (1955), and Lall and Dayal (1967) among more recent ones—list Wagner's case with congenital hemihypertrophy.

The cause of congenital hemihypertrophy remains obscure. Numerous theories have been advanced; namely, that it is due to vasomotor paralysis, vasoconstriction, or trophoneurotic or hormonal influence, that it results from disturbed epiphyseal and periosteal growth, and that it is a sort of perverted twinning process. Noé and Berman (1962) reviewed these concepts and found them untenable. In their turn, they proposed a theory of their own which is far from being clear. They classified hemihypertrophy as a form of mesodermosis which might be of the same origin as the ectodermosis, the pathogenesis of both being "a process of pleonastic regeneration initiated by mitochondria which in the course of over-ripening of ovum has been damaged."

It is generally agreed that asymmetry begins during early embryonic development. Phisalix (1888) described a 10-mm. embryo which lacked symmetry. Johnston and Penrose (1966) studied nine patients with congenital asymmetry. Dermoglyphic studies suggested that the asymmetrical disturbance of growth might have taken place before the eighth week of pregnancy, since in some cases the dermal patterns were abnormal. Some authors consider hemihypertrophy to be more common in males than in females. Negroes are said to be comparatively immune.

Stier (1912) advanced the view that hemihypertrophy and supernumerary parts occur more often on the side of the body enervated by the dominant hemi-

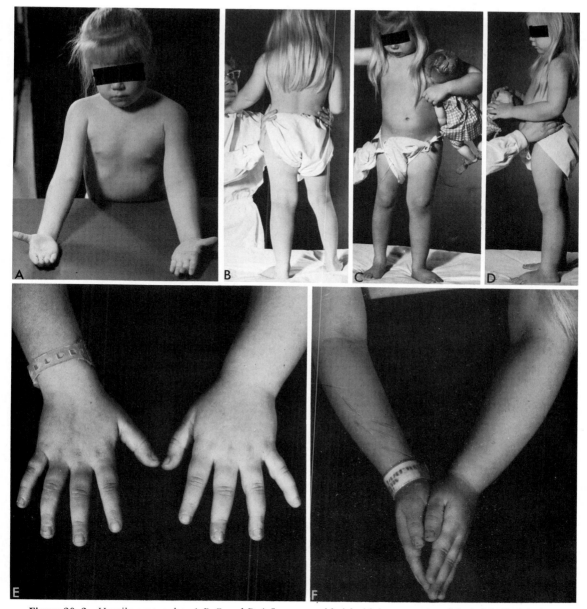

Figure 20–2 Hemihypertrophy. *A, B, C,* and *D,* A four-year-old girl with hypertrophy of the left half of the body. *E,* Dorsal view of the distal forearms and hands. *F,* Radial view of the forearms and hands: the left forearm and hand are pudgier. The skeletal structures are equal on both sides. Thickening was due to soft-tissue hypertrophy only.

sphere of the brain. Speese (1914) said that hypertrophy is encountered more often on the right side. Gesell (1927) reviewed the literature and found 53 cases of hemihypertrophy, 35 of which occurred on the right side. Schwartzman et al (1942) cited 102 cases of congenital hemihypertrophy. Sabanas and Chatterton (1955) found 10 additional cases, added one of their own, and disagreed with the previous authors concerning the more frequent involvement of the right side.

Gesell (1921) reported a case of hemihypertrophy associated with mental defect and suggested that "hemihypertrophy should be added to the list of de-

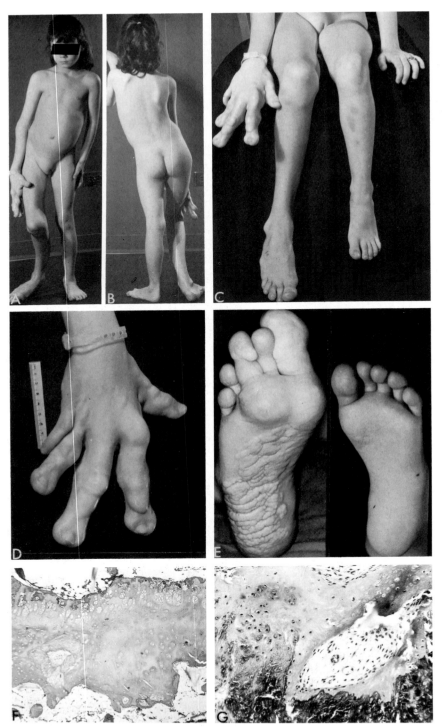

Figure 20–3 Hemihypertrophy which presents some of the features of nerve territory–oriented macrodactyly (NTOM), especially the osteoplastic variety, and a few insignia of Reckling-hausen's disease, yet it is distinct from both. *A, B,* and *C,* A six-year-old girl with no hereditary antecedent, no subcutaneous neurofibromas and no *café-au-lait* spots; she had longer and bulkier upper and lower limbs. *D,* Dorsal view of the right hand: with the exception of the little finger, all digits were oversized, bore nodular thickening, and failed to flex. *E,* Plantar view of the feet: the sole of the larger right foot is corrugating, simulating molluscum fibrosum of Recklinghausen's disease. *F* and *G,* Sections of the specimens obtained from volar digital plate of the thumb, showing hypertrophic cartilage and heterotopic bone formation.

698

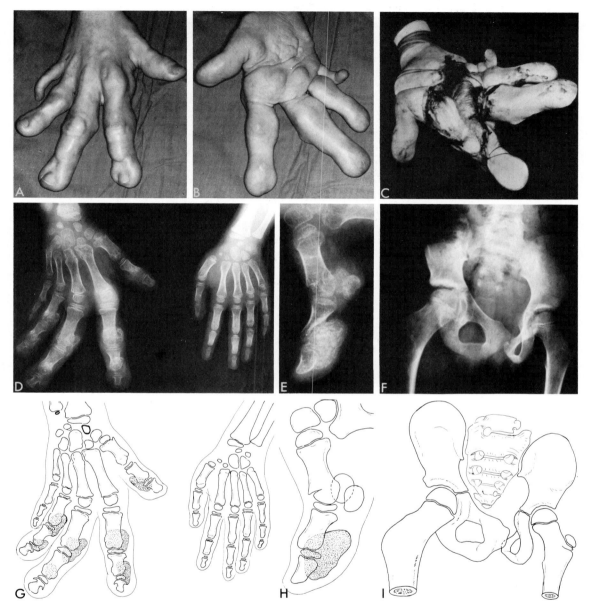

Figure 20-4   *A* and *B*, Dorsal and palmar views of the right hand of the six-year-old girl featured in Figure 20-3. *C*, Exploration of the right palm and index finger revealed no thickening of the median nerve nor tortuosity of the digital branches which are characteristic of NTOM; the palmar plate of the metacarpophalangeal and interphalangeal joints bore huge osteocartilaginous plaques which put the overlying flexor tendons under great tension. *D*, Dorsopalmar roentgenograph of the hands: the second and third metacarpals of the right hand are long and thick; the phalanges of the oversized digits of the right hand are thicker than the corresponding bones of the left hand—the apparent overexpansion of the articular ends of the enlarged bones is in part due to the superimposed shadows cast by osteocartilaginous infiltration of the volar plates; carpal bones of the right wrist are larger and more numerous than those of the left wrist; the right ulnar epiphysis is evident; the left is not; the right radial epiphysis is larger than that of the left. *E*, Lateral roentgenograph of the right thumb taken at the age of eight, showing huge sesamoids and massive osteocartilaginous tumor of the volar plates. *F*, Anteroposterior roentgenograph of the pelvis: the right pelvic bone and the right proximal femur are larger than the corresponding elements of the left side. *G, H,* and *I* illustrate the roentgenograph above each.

velopmental abnormalities which bear some lawful relation to the incidence of mental deficiency." Gesell found 53 cases of hemihypertrophy reported in the literature; in eight there was mental abnormality. "Mental defect of some degree is found with disproportionate frequency in association with hemihypertrophy," Gesell wrote. Most authors place the number of mentally defectives at 15 to 20 per cent of reported cases of hemihypertrophy. Noé and Berman (1962) found only one case of hemihypertrophy in 11,300 patients admitted to a mental institution during the past 14 years. Hemihypertrophy is also said to be associated with patches of pigmentation of the skin or even *café-au-lait* spots and subcutaneous varicosities. One wonders if these were not cases of multiple neurofibromatoses and of Klippel-Trénaunay syndrome, respectively. Association of hemihypertrophy and congenital renal tumors, mainly Wilms' tumor, has been noted by Bjorklund (1955), Benson et al (1963), Wilson and Orlin (1965), Gellis and Feingold (1966), and Fraumeni et al (1967).

Hemihypertrophy may be due to the overgrowth of soft tissues or bones or both. When it involves the hand, the osseous variety often simulates the osteoplastic type of macrodactyly affecting the digits which receive their volar sensory supply from the median nerve. Curiously, in this variety, besides the enlargement of phalanges and metacarpals, there is heterotopic osteocartilaginous invasion of the volar plates. This condition is difficult to amend. The treatment of soft tissue hemihypertrophy affecting the upper limb or the hand likewise leaves much to be desired. One attempts to reduce the thickness of the affected part by resection of longitudinally disposed elliptical segments of skin and subcutaneous fat. This is a temporizing measure only. Recurrence is inevitable, and the procedure needs to be repeated periodically (Figs. 20–2 to 20–4).

CHROMOSOMAL ABERRATIONS

Ferrier et al (1964) described a case of congenital asymmetry with diploid-triploid mosaicism and large satellites. Hook and Yunis (1965) noted the association of congenital asymmetry with trisomy 18 mosaicism.

OLLIER'S ENCHONDROMATOSIS
(Hemichondrodysplasia; Multiple Enchondromatoses without Hemangioma; Dyschondrodysplasia)

In his original communication, Ollier (1899) used the designation dyschondroplasia. Jansen (1928) related this disorder to multiple exostosis, which is predominantly hereditary, being transmitted as an autosomal dominant trait. Hunter and Wiles (1935) pointed out that in Ollier's disease there is little if any evidence of hereditary transmission. Most reported cases have been unilateral and the affected limb or segment remains smaller than its counterpart. The basic disturbance in this disorder is now considered to be a congenitally determined modeling error starting in the growth cartilage plate and extending into the metaphysis and, in more advanced cases, into the diaphysis as well. Hypertrophic

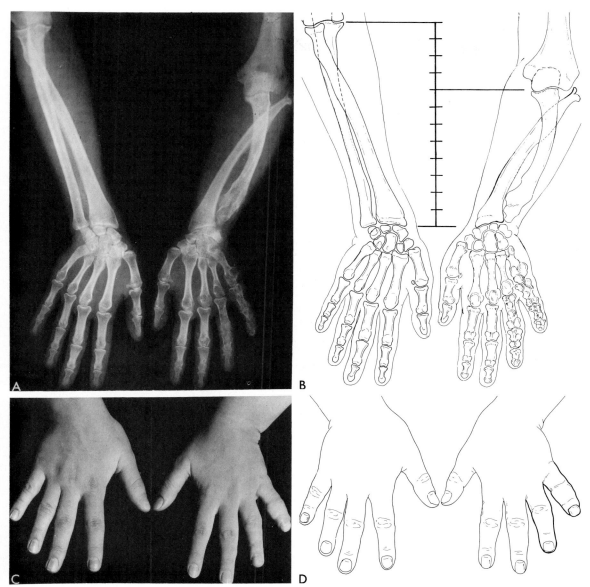

Figure 20–5   Disharmony due to multiple enchondromatoses: Ollier's disease. *A*, Dorsovolar roentgenograph of the right and left forearms and hands of a 24-year-old woman with multiple enchondromatoses involving mainly the left ulna and the last two ulnar digital rays: the left radius and ulna are considerably shorter than the corresponding bones of the right forearm; the left radial head is dislocated. *B*, Sketch illustrating the same. *C*, Dorsal view of the hands: the left ring and little fingers are thicker than the fourth and fifth digits of the right hand. *D*, Sketch illustrating the same.

cartilage cells produced by the growth plate fail to be converted into bone; they undergo rapid proliferation and form tumors within the cortical confines of tubular bones. The most rapidly growing ends of these bones constitute favored sites. The affected bone remains short but gains in girth—it becomes broad in parts and bowed. The carpal ends of the radius and ulna are common locations; these bones may be involved alone or together. Ollier's disease shows distinct predilection for the ulna and ulnar digits. The affected ulna remains short, caus-

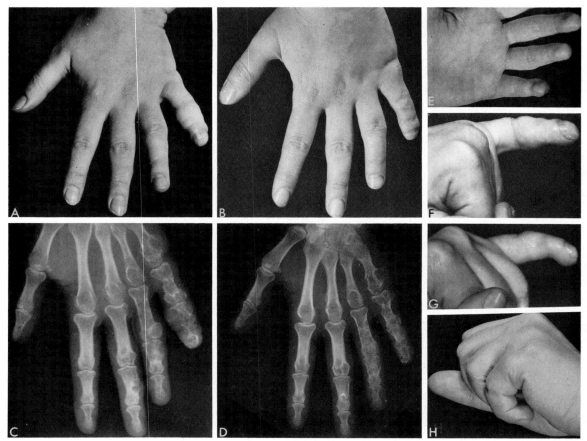

Figure 20–6   *A*, Preoperative dorsal view of the left hand of the 24-year-old woman featured in Figure 20–5: note the nodular thickening of the little finger. *B*, Postoperative dorsal view: the little finger is thinner and has attained regularity of contour. *C*, Preoperative dorsopalmar roentgenograph of the left hand. *D*, Postoperative roentgenograph showing attenuated left little finger. *E*, Palmar view of the left little finger six months after surgery. *F*, Preoperative radial view of the little finger. *G*, Postoperative radial view. *H*, Postoperative ulnar view of the left fist: in spite of extensive surgery, shown in Figure 20–7, the little finger could fully flex and extend.

ing dislocation of the radius at the elbow. Ollier's disease also appears to favor the ulnar digits. Enchondromas often cause expansion of the cortex. In the hand, the phalanges are affected more often and extensively than the metacarpals, causing the involved finger to become knobby. The cartilaginous content of the tumefied phalanges is surgically evacuated and the cavity thus created is packed with cancellous bone chips. The functional and cosmetic results are usually gratifying (Figs. 20–5 to 20–7).

RECKLINGHAUSEN'S
NEUROFIBROMATOSIS

This complex has already been discussed in Chapter Eighteen. Briefly, it consists of multiple cutaneous and subcutaneous neurofibromas and *café-au-lait*

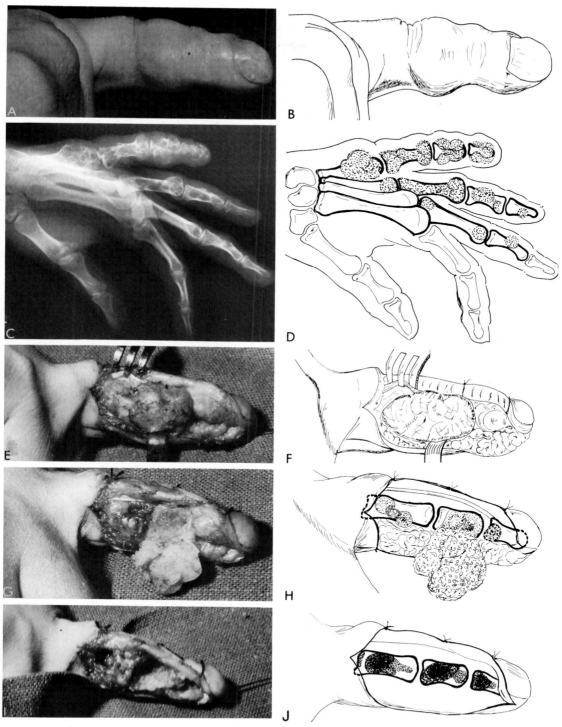

Figure 20–7 Procedure utilized for thinning out and restoring the contours of the left little finger with nodular thickening and irregularity of contour due to multiple enchondromatoses. *A,* Preoperative radial view of the left little finger of the 24-year-old woman featured in Figures 20–5 and 20–6. *B,* Sketch of the same. *C* and *D,* Lateral roentgenograph and sketch of the left hand. *E* and *F,* Exposure of the enchondromas bulging out of the phalanges of the left little finger. *G, H, I,* and *J,* Evacuating the cartilaginous contents of the phalanges and packing the cavities with cancellous bones.

spots and, in about 50 per cent of cases, hereditary transmission. Asymmetry between two sides of the body has been reported by many authors—in particular by Winokurow (1926), Anzinger (1931), and Schlenzka (1955).

SILVER-RUSSELL DWARFISM

Silver et al (1953) described two unrelated children with congenital asymmetry, shortness of stature, and elevated urinary gonadotropins. Russell (1954) reported five children whose dwarfism was "already recognizable at birth and two of them manifested congenital asymmetry." Many cases of Silver-Russell dwarfism have since been reported. The complex consists of congenital asymmetry, intrauterine growth retardation, genital malformation, triangular face with down-curving of the mouth, syndactylism of the second and third toes, and clubbing of the fingers in the absence of heart and lung diseases. Rimoin (1969) described two monozygotic male twins with this constellation (Fig. 20–8).

STURGE-WEBER SYNDROME

Warkany (1971) gives the following as the components of the complete form of this complex: (1) cutaneous angioma, (2) seizures, (3) hemiparesis, (4) characteristic intracranial calcifications, (5) mental retardation, and (6) glaucoma. The condition is ascribed to congenital angiomas of the leptomeninges; telangiectasia affects ipsilateral acral parts, including the upper portion of the face, while hemiplegia and atrophy involve contralateral structures (Fig. 20–9).

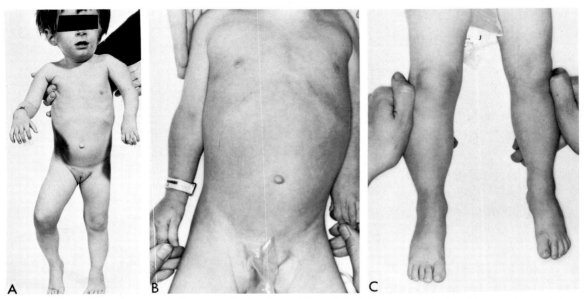

Figure 20–8 Asymmetry of Silver-Russell dwarfism. *A, B,* and *C.* A three-year-old girl with mental retardation, microcephaly, and asymmetry between the two halves of the body.

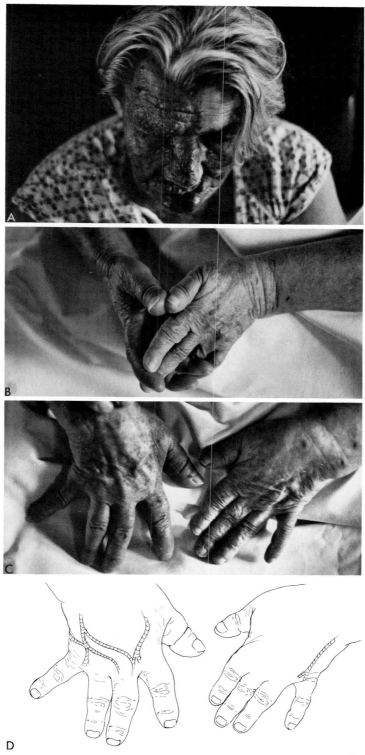

Figure 20–9 Asymmetry of Sturge-Weber syndrome. *A*, The face of a mentally retarded adult woman with an extensive port-wine nevus mainly on the right side. *B* and *C*, Two views of the hands: the right hand, which has more abundant subcutaneous veins, is larger. *D*, Sketch illustrating the same.

SUMMARY

Handedness is considered to be the cause of barely discernible asymmetry. More gross forms of disparity between the two sides of the body are comparatively rare. Hemihypertrophy is categorized as either total, or partial; to the latter category belong monomelic and crossed congenital hypertrophies. Two abnormalities are known to occur in association with hemihypertrophy—defective mentality and Wilms' tumor. Congenital asymmetry between the two sides of the body—in particular between the contralateral forearms and hands—has been reported in cases of chromosomal mosaicism, Léri's melorheostosis, Ollier's disease, Recklinghausen's neurofibromatosis, Silver-Russell dwarfism, and Sturge-Weber syndrome. In the lower limb, when there is marked discrepancy of the leg length, one may consider a growth arrest operation on the longer extremity. In the upper extremity, this procedure is rarely ever indicated. For cosmetic reasons, an attempt is sometimes made to reduce the bulk of the forearm and the hand. Longitudinally disposed elliptical incisions are used for this purpose and sizable segments of skin and subcutaneous tissue—mainly fat—are resected.

References

Ajurianguerra, J. de, and Diatkine, R.: Problèmes théoriques et practique posé par la gaucherie infantile. *Presse Méd., 64*:1905–1908, 1856.

Annett, M.: Model of inheritance of handedness and cerebral dominance. *Nature, 204*:59–60, 1964.

Anzinger, F. P.: Congenital plexiform neuro-fibromas and elephantiasis neuromatosa of the right arm and neck (von Recklinghausen's disease): supplementary report. *J.A.M.A., 96*:1381–1382, 1931.

Arnheim, G.: Über einen Fall von congenitaler halbseitiger Hypertrophie mit angeborenen Bronchiektasien. *Arch. Pathol. Anat. Physiol., 154*:300–320; Taf. VIII, 1898.

Arnold, E. B.: Case of hemiacromegaly. *Int. J. Orthod., 22*:1228–1233, 1936.

Babonneix, and Buizard: Hemihypertrophie congenitale. *Bull. Soc. Pediatr., 20*:283–285, 1922.

Bakwin, H.: Lateral dominance. Right and left handedness. *J. Pediatr., 36*:385–391, 1950.

Baldazzi, G.: L'ipertrofia parziale congenita. *Riv. Clin. Pediatr., 22*:729–754, 1924.

Bankart, A. S. B.: Case of hypertrophy of the right side of the face, right half of the tongue, left upper extremity and right lower extremity; hemihypertrophy? *Proc. R. Soc. Med.* (Sec. Dis. Child.), *9*:77–79, 1915–1916.

Bardeleben, K. V.: Über bilaterale Asymmetrie beim Menschen und bei höheren Tieren. *Anat. Anz., 34*:2–72, 1909.

Bassoe, P.: Unilateral hypertrophy involving the entire left side of the body. *Am. J. Insan., 69*:91–96, 1912.

Bassoe, P.: Left hemihypertrophy: re-examination after twenty years. *Arch. Neurol. Psychiat., 26*:881–884, 1931.

Benson, P., Vulliamy, D. G., and Taubman, J. O.: Congenital hemihypertrophy and malignancy. *Lancet, 1*:648–649, 1963.

Benton, A. L., Meyers, R., and Polder, G. J.: Some aspects of handedness. *Psychiatr. Neurol.* (Basel), *144*:321–337, 1962.

Berend, N.: Ein 3 Monate altes Kind mit einseitiger partieller Makrosomie. *Wien. Med. Wochenschr., 47*:1625, 1897.

Bihler, K.: Ein Fall von angeborener totaler Hemihypertrophie. *Zentralbl. Gynäkol., 57*:253–257, 1933.

Bjorklund, S. I.: Hemihypertrophy and Wilms' tumor. *Acta Paediatr., 44*:287–292, 1955.

Blau, A.: *The Master Hand.* A study of origins and meaning of right and left sidedness and its relation to personality and language: Research Monograph No. 5: New York, *American Orthopsychiatric Association Inc.,* pp. 1–206, 1946.

Bosio, P.: Contributo clinico allo studio dello ipertrofie (sopra un caso di emiipertrofia). *Clin. Ig. Infant, 6*:219–232, 1930.

Bousquet, P.: Hypertrophie congénitate. *Gaz. Hebd. Sci. Méd.* (Bordeaux), *42*:500, 1921.

Bowers, D.: Congenital hemihypertrophy and hemihypoplasia. *Minn. Med., 39*:461–466, 1956.

Brain, W. R.: Speech and handedness. *Lancet, 2*:837–841, 1945.

Broca, P.: Inegalité congénitale de deux moities du corpe. *J. Physiol. Hommes Animaux, 2*:70–74, 1859.

Broda, T., and Barbet, F.: Hypertrophie congénitale de toute la moitié droite du corps. *Rev. d'Orthop., 9*:467–470, 1908.

Brüning, H.: Über angeborenen, halbseitigen Riesenwuchs. *Münch. Med. Wochenschr., 51*(1):385–387, 1904.

Bryan, R. S., Liscomb, P. R., and Chatterton, C. C.: Orthopedic aspects of congenital hypertrophy. *Am. J. Surg., 96*:654–659, 1958.

Busch: Ein Mann mit asymmetrischen Riesenwuchs der linken Hälfte des Unterkiefers. *Klin. Wochenschr.* (Berlin), *17*:127, 1880.

Byrom, E. T.: The left dominant child. *Tex. St. J. Med., 43*:782–785, 1948.

Cagiati, L.: Klinischer und pathologischer Beitrag zum Studium der halbseitigen Hypertrophie. *Dtsch. Z. Nervenheilkd., 32*:282–293, 1907.

Carpenter, G., and Mummary, L.: A case of hemihypertrophy. *Rep. Soc. Study Dis. Child.* (London), *6*:1532, 1907.

Carron, R.: L'hémihypertrophie congénitale. *Pédiatrie, 6*:969–983, 1951.

Carter, F. S., and Dockery, M. C.: A case of congenital hemihypertrophy showing variations in bone age and development. *Arch. Dis. Child., 28*:321–324, 1953.

Chamberlain, H. B.: The inheritance of left-handedness. *J. Hered., 19*:557–559, 1928.

Charocopos, S., and Coccolis, J.: Sur la pathogénie de l'hémihypertrophie congénitale (perturbation de la function morphologique de l'hipothalamus). *Pédiatrie, 10*:709–713, 1955.

Coccheri, P.: Emiipertrofia totale congenite e reazioni adrenaliniche sotto epiedermiche. *Lattante, 2*:239–258, 1931.

Cohen, H.: A case of hemihypertrophy with increased sugar tolerance. *J.A.M.A., 69*:463–464, 1917.

Collins, R. L.: On the inheritance of handedness. *J. Hered., 59*:9–12, 1968.

Compton, R. H.: A further contribution to the study of right- and lefthandedness. *J. Genet., 2*:53–70, 1912.

Conrad, K.: Über aphasische Sprachstörungen bei hirnverletzten Linkshändern. *Nervenarzt, 20*:148–154, 1959.

Cortes, F. F.: Las hipertrofias unilaterales congenitas genuinas. *Med. Clin.* (Barcelona), *9*:301–307, 1947.

Coston, H. R.: A case of congenital hemi-hypertrophia totalis. *Med. Rec.*, *97*:222–223, 1920.

Cox, W. C.: On the want of symmetry in the length of opposite sides of persons who have never been subject of disease or injury to their lower extremities. *Am. J. Med. Sci.*, *69*:438–439, 1875.

Cozzolino, O.: Emiipertrofia congenita lattante. *Pediatria* (Napoli), *31*:521–531, 1923.

Crosby, E. H.: Hemihypertrophy totalis. *J. Bone Joint Surg.*, *17*:1025–1026, 1935.

Crouzon, O., and Villaret, G.: Hemihypertrophie congénitale. *Rev. Neurol.* (Paris), *15*:406–408, 1907.

Cunningham, D. J.: Right-handedness and left-brainedness. *J. Anthrop. Inst. G. Br. Ir.*, *32*:273–296, pl. XXI–XXII, 1902.

Curtius, F.: Kongenitaler, partieller Riesenwuchs mit endokrinen Störungen. *Dtsch. Arch. Klin. Med.*, *147*:310–319, 1925.

Danforth, C. H.: The heredity of unilateral variations in man. *Genetics*, *9*:199–211, 1924.

Dardani: Per un caso di emi-ipertrofia congenita. *Pediatria*, *37*:535–549, 1929.

Davidson, A. J.: A case of true congenital unilateral hypertrophy. *Med. Rec.*, *80*:420–421, 1911.

Davidson, W.: Elephantiasis of forearm and hand: amputation of the arm. *Edinburgh Med. Surg. J.*, *49*:54–55, 1838.

Davidson, W. C.: Partial hemihypertrophy. *Proc. R. Soc. Med.* (London), *24*:1340, 1930.

Devouges: Prédominance de developpement du côté droit sur le côté gauche; developpement hypertrophique des trois premiers doigts de la main et du pieds droits. *Bull. Soc. Anat.*, (2 s.), *1*:540–548, 1856.

Dietlein, M.: Ein Fall von halbseitigem Riesenwuchs. *Münch. Med. Wochenschr.*, *61*(1):130–132, 1914.

Ducroquet, M. R.: Hémihypertrophie gauche. *Bull. Soc. Pédiatr.*, (Paris), *26*:19–20, 1928.

Dunlop, G. H. M.: Hemihypertrophy, *Trans. Med. Chir. Soc.* (Edinburgh), *21*:245, 1901–1902.

Duplay: Hémihypertrophie partielle. *Gaz. Hebd. Méd. Chir.*, (n.s.), *2*:529–532, 1897.

Dwight, T.: What is right-handedness? *Scribner's Mag.*, *9*:464–476, 1891.

Eames, T. H.: Frequency of cerebral lateral dominance variations among school children of premature and full-term birth. *J. Pediatr.*, *51*:300–302, 1957.

Eaton, J.: A case of congenital asymmetry. *Br. Med. J.*, *1*:157–158, 1886.

England, W. S.: Hemihypertrophy with multiple neurofibromata. *Montreal Med. J.*, *31*:855–862, 1902.

Esau: Die angeborene Hemihypertrophia totalis des Körpers. *Med. Klin.*, *27*:1861–1863, 1931.

Eustis, R. S.: Right- or lefthandedness. *N. Engl. J. Med.*, *240*:249–253, 1949.

Falek, A.: Handedness: a family study. *Am. J. Hum. Genet.*, *1*:52–62, 1958.

Faure, L.: *Essai d'Etude Comparative de l'Homme Droit et de l'Homme Gauche.* Thèse. Lyon, A. Storck & Cie, pp. 1–99, 1902.

Ferri, U.: Un caso di emi-ipertrofia in un lattante. *Clin. Ig. Infant*, *2*:18–24, 1927.

Ferrier, P., Ferrier, S., Buhler, E., Bamatter, F., and Klein, D.: Congenital asymmetry associated with diploid-triploid mosaicism and large satellites. *Lancet*, *1*:80–82, 1964.

Finesilver, B., and Rostow, H. M.: Total hemiatropy. *J.A.M.A.*, *110*:366–368, 1938.

Finlayson, J.: On the case of a child affected with congenital unilateral hypertrophy and patches of cutaneous congestion. *Glasgow Med. J.*, *22*:327–337, 1884.

Fordyce, A. D.: Hemi-hypertrophie alterne. *Arch. Dis. Child.*, *3*:300–309, 1928.

Forrai, G., and Bankövi, G.: Relation of hand clasping and arm folding to handedness in Hungarian children. *Acta Genet. Med. Gemellol.* (Roma), *18*:166–174, 1969.

Fortescue-Brickdale, J. M.: A case of congenital hemihypertrophy. *Lancet*, *2*:10–13, 1915.

Fraumeni, J. F., Jr., and Miller, R. W.: Adrenocortical neoplasms with hemihypertrophy, brain tumors and other disorders. *J. Pediatr.*, *70*:129–138, 1967.

Fraumeni, J. F., Jr., Geiser, C. F., and Manning, M. D.: Wilms tumor and congenital hemihypertrophy. *Pediatrics*, *40*:886–899, 1967.

Friedberg, H.: Riesenwuchs des rechten Beines. *Arch. Pathol. Anat. Physiol.*, *28*:474–481, 1863.

Geiser, C. F., Baez, A., Schindler, A. M., and Shih, V. E.: Epithelial hepatoblastoma associated with congenital hemihypertrophy and cystathioni nuria: presentation of a case. *Pediatrics*, *46*:66–73, fig. 1, 1970.

Gellis, S. S., and Feingold, M.: Picture of the month: congenital hemihypertrophy and adrenal carcinoma. *Am. J. Dis. Child.*, *111*:419–420, 1966.

Gerloczy, F., and Pap, D.: Contribution à l'étude de l'hemihypertrophie (A propos de dix observations d'hemihypertrophie vraie). *Acta Méd. Acad. Sci. Hung.*, *15*:145, 1960.

Gesell, A.: Hemihypertrophy and mental defect. *Arch. Neurol. Psychiatr.*, *6*:400–423, 1921.

Gesell, A.: Hemihypertrophy and twinning. A further study of the nature of hemihypertrophy with report of a new case. *Am. J. Med. Sci.*, *173*:542–555, 1927.

Gesell, A., and Ames, L. B.: Development of handedness. *J. Genet. Psychol.*, *70*:155–175, 1947.

Ghio, A.: Su un caso di empiipertrofia congenita total. *Lattante*, *3*:32–42, 1932.

Giesecke, M.: *Genesis of Hand Preference.* Monographs, Society for Research in Child Development. Vol. I, No. 5, 102. Washington, D.C., National Research Council, 1936.

Glanzer, J.: Total unilateral hypertrophy. *Am. J. Dis. Child.*, *45*:1056–1063, 1933.

Gordinier, H. C.: A case of unilateral hypertrophy of the whole left side with autopsy. *Albany Med. Ann.*, *39*:47–57, 1918.

Gordon, A.: Family stock betterment with response to lefthandedness. *Eugen. News, 17:87–88, 1932.*

Gorlin, R. J., and Meskin, L. H.: Congenital hemihypertrophy. *J. Pediatr., 61:870–879, 1962.*

Graetz, I.: Über einen Fall von sogenannter "totaler halbseitiger Körperhypertrophie." *Z. Kinderheilkd., 45:381–403; figs. 1, 4a, 4c, 1928.*

Greig, D. M.: Unilateral hypertrophy. *Edinburgh Hosp. Rep., 5:212–236, 1898.*

Guillain, G., and Bize, P. R.: Hémihypertrophie corps, du type congénitale, total pur, associée à un dolicocolon. *Rev. Neurol., 1:76–84; fig. 3, 1934.*

Hahn, E.: Über den reinen partiellen Riesenwuchs. *Cent. Grenzgbt. Med. Chir., 16:19–31, 1913.*

Hall, E. G.: A case of hemihypertrophy. *Br. J. Child. Dis., 18:21–24, 1921.*

Halperin: Normal asymmetry and unilateral hypertrophy. *Arch. Intern. Med., 48:676–682, 1931.*

Haridas, G., and Gek, L.: Right segmental hypertrophy and adrenogenital syndrome. *Proc. Alumni A. King Edward VII Coll. Med., 3:36–42, 1950.*

Harwood, J.: Right hemihypertrophy and pubertas praecox. *Proc. R. Soc. Med. London* (Sec. Dis. Child.), 25:951–954, 1932.

Hecaen, H., and Ajuriaguerea, J. de.: *Les Gauchers.* Paris, Edit. Presses, Université de France, 1963.

Hermanides, S. R.: Een geval hemihypertrophia congenital. *Psychiatr. Neurol Bl.* (Amsterdam), 3:109–121, 1899.

Hertz, R.: La prééminence de la main droite. Étude sur la polarité religieuse. *Rev. Philos. France Etranger, 68:553–580, 1909.*

Hofmann, M.: Zur Pathologie des angeborenen partiellen Riesenwuches. *Beitr. Klin. Chir., 48:391–424, 1906.*

Holden, J. D.: Russell-Silver dwarfs. *Develop. Med. Child. Neurol., 9:457–459, 1967.*

Hollis: Lopsided generations. *J. Anat. Physiol., 9:263–271, 1875.*

Hook, E. B., and Yunis, J. J.: Congenital asymmetry associated with trisomy 18 mosaicism. *A.M.A.J. Dis. Child., 110:551–555, 1965.*

Hornstein, S.: Ein Fall von halbseitigem Riesenwuchs. *Arch. Pathol. Anat. Physiol., 133:440–463, 1893.*

Horwitt, S.: Congenital macropomia. *Arch. Pediatr., 43:67–71, 1926.*

Hrach, P.: Über einen Fall von angeborener neuratischer Hemiatrophie. *Wien. Med. Wochenschr., 54:343–346, 1904.*

Humphrey, M. E.: Consistency of hand usage. *Br. J. Educ. Psychol., 21:214–225, 1951.*

Humphry: Asymmetry of the two halves of the body. *J. Anat. Physiol., (2 s.), 4:226–229, 1869.*

Hunter, D., and Wiles, P.: Dyschondroplasia (Ollier's disease) with report of a case. *Br. J. Surg., 22:507–519, 1935.*

Huse, A.: A case of partial congenital hemi-hypertrophy. *J. Neurol. Psychiatr., 7:30–32; fig. 2, 1944.*

Hutchinson, R.: Hypertrophy of the left side of the body in an infant. *Rep. Soc. Study Dis. Child.* (London), 3:194, 1902–1903.

Hutchison, R.: A case of hemihypertrophy in which the internal organs were affected. *Rep. Soc. Study Dis. Child.* (London), 4:145–148, 1903–1904. See also *Br. J. Dis. Child., 1:258–260, 1904.*

Hutchison, R.: Report on a case of hemihypertrophy with post-mortem examination. *Proc. R. Soc. Med. London* (Sec. Dis. Child.), 9:66–68, 1915–1916. See also *Br. J. Child. Dis., 13:233–237, 1916.*

Ingalls, N. W.: On right-handedness. *Sci. Monthly, 27:307–321, 1928.*

Jansen, M.: *In The Robert Jones Birthday Volume.* Oxford, Med. Publications, pp. 43–72, 1928.

Jenkins, M. E., Eisen, J., and Sequin, F.: Congenital asymmetry and diploid-triploid mosaicism. *Am. J. Dis. Child., 122:80–84, 1971.*

Johnston, A. W., and Penrose, L. S.: Congenital asymmetry. *J. Med. Genet., 3:77–85, 1966.*

Jordan, H. E.: The inheritance of left-handedness. *Am. Breeders Mag., 2:19–29, 1911.*

Jordan, H. E.: Hereditary left-handedness with a note on twinning. *J. Genet., 4:67–81, 1914.*

Kartein, W.: Kongenitale Hypertrophie. *Münch. Med. Wochenschr., 88:273–276, 1941.*

Kneer, M.: Halbseitiger Riesenwuchs. *Zentralbl., Gynäkol., 63(3):2409–2416, 1939.*

Kohlmann, T.: Zum psychol. und paedagogischen Problem der Linkshändigkeit. *Wien. Z. Nervenheilkd., 3:89–100, 1950.*

Korting, G. W., and Ruther, H.: Zur nervalen Genese von Hemihyperund Hemiatrophie. *Arch. Derm. Syph., 198:384–395, 1954.*

Kourilsky, R., and Grapin, R.: *Main droite et main gauche.* Paris, Edition Press, Université de France, 1968.

Lall, J. C., and Dayal, R. S.: Hemihypertrophy. Report of a case and a brief review of the literature. *Indian J. Pediatr., 34:179–182, 1967.*

Landauer, W.: Supernumerary nipples, congenital hemihypertrophy and congenital hemiatrophy. *Hum. Biol., 11:447–472, 1939.*

Lange, W.: Zwei Fälle von Hemihypertrophie. *Med. Welt, 2:1231, 1928.*

Langlet: Hypertrophie congénitale de la moitié droit du corps. *Union Méd. Sci. Nord-Est, 6:276–278, 1882.*

Laufer, M.: Contribution to the problem of congenital hemihypertrophy. (Czech) *Acta Chir. Orthop. Traum. Cechoslovaca, 19:217–219, 1952.*

Lausecker, H.: Uber halbseiten Reisenwuchs. *Dermatologica, 100:98–101, 1950.*

Leche, S. M.: Handedness and bimanual dermatoglyphic differences. *Am. J. Anat., 53:1–53, 1933.*

LeCoute, J.: Right-sidedness. *Nature, 29:452, 1884.*

LeFevre, A. B.: Hemi-hipertrofia corporal congenita. *Arq. Neuro. Psiquiat.* (Sao Paulo), 5:359–362, 1947.

Leibreich, R.: *Die Asymmetrie des Gesichtes und ihre Entstehung.* München, J. F. Bergmann, 1908.

Lelong, M., Canlorbe, P., Mathieu; Berkmann, and Drouet: Un cas d'hémihypertrophie congénitale avec anomalies du développement osseux. *Arch. Franc. Pediatr., 13*:301–303, 1956.

Lenstrup, E.: Eight cases of hemi-hypertrophy. *Acta Paediatr., 6*:205–213, 1926.

Lereboullet, P., and Ectors, M. L.: Un cas d'hémi-hypertrophie craniofaciale. *Arch. Méd. Enfants, 39*:37–39, 1936.

Levy, J., and Nagylaki, T.: A model for the genetics of handedness. *Genetics, 72*:117–128, 1972.

Liebmann, L.: Diskordantes Auftreten von partiellem Riesenwuchs bei einem eineiigen Zwillingspaar. *Z. menschl. Vererb. Konstitutionslehre, 22*:374–389, 1938.

Lisser, H.: Congenital total hemihypertrophy. *J.A.M.A., 82*:1046, 1924.

Lockhart-Mummery, J. P.: Case of hemi-hypertrophy, traced for eighteen and a half years. *Proc. R. Soc. Med.* (Sect. Dis. Child.), *17*:1–2, 1923.

Logan, S.: Hypertrophy of the right half of the body in a child aged four years, first noticed shortly after birth. *New Orleans J. Med., 21*:733, 1868.

Lombrosa, C.: Left-sidedness. *N. Am. Rev., 177*:440, 1903.

MacEwen, G. D., and Case, J. L.: Congenital hemihypertrophy. *Clin. Orthop., 50*:147–150, 1967.

MacGillivray, P. H.: On a case of congenital hypertrophy of the hand and arm. *Aust. Med. J., 17*:9–24, 1872.

Makida, T.: A case of hemimacrosomia. (Japanese). *Chingai Iji Shimpo* (Tokyo), *25*:367–375, 1904.

Mann, T. P.: Hemihypertrophy left side of the body. Congenital lymphatic oedema of left arm. Radiological enlargement of heart shadow. *Proc. R. Soc. Med.* (Sect. Pediatrics), *48*:330–331; fig. 2, 1955.

Mayers, L. H.: Hemihypertrophy. *Surg. Gynecol. Obstet., 43*:746–749, 1926.

McFarland, B. L.: Hemihypertrophy. *Br. Med. J., 1*:345–346, 1928.

McGregor, A. N.: A remarkable case of unilateral hypertrophy in a child. *Glasgow Med. J., 41*:189–196, 1894.

Meckel, J. F.: *Anatomische Physiologische Beobachtungen und Untersuchungen.* Halle, Renger, p. 147, 1822.

Merrel, D. J.: Dominance of eye and hand. *Hum. Biol., 29*:314–328, 1957.

Messer, E.: Consid. sul manchinismo latente nell 'infanzia. *Agg. Pediatr.* (Roma), *20*:1, 1969.

Miller, R. W., Fraumeni, J. F., and Manning, M. A.: Association of Wilms tumor with aniridia, hemihypertrophy and other congenital malformations. *N. Engl. J. Med., 270*:922–927, 1964.

Milne, J. B.: Congenital asymmetry in a female child. *Lancet, 1*:752–753, 1895.

Möbius, J. P. Über Hemihypertrophie, *Münch Med. Wochenschr., 37*:751–752, 1890.

Mohr, G. J.: Complete left hemihypertrophy. *Arch. Pediatr., 42*:339–341, 1925.

Moore, J. J., and deLorimer, A. A.: Melorheostosis Léri. Review of literature and report of case. *Am. J. Roentgenol., 29*:161–171, 1933.

More, J.: Righthandedness and leftbrainedness. *Lancet, 1*:200, 1903.

Morris, J. V., and MacGillivray, R. C.: Mental defect and hemihypertrophy. *Am. J. Ment. Defic., 59*:645–651, 1955.

Moseley, J. B., Moloshok, R., and Freiberger, R. H.: The Silver syndrome: congenital asymmetry, short stature and variations in sexual development. *Am. J. Roentgenol., 97*:74–81, 1966.

Mouchet, A.: Atrophie congénitale de la main droite avec brachydactylie du pouce du petit doigts fusion des deux derniers métacarpiens. *Rev. d'Orthop.,* (3 s.), *3*:53–55, 1902.

Mummery, P. L.: A case of hemihypertrophy. *Proc. R. Soc. Med.* (Clinical section), *1*:61–62, 1908.

Muschlitz, C. H.: Congenital unilateral hypertrophy. Report of a case. *Month. Cycl. Med. Bull.* (Philadelphia), *13*:16, 1909.

Neimann, H., Pierson, M., Lascombes, G., and Manciaux, M.: Hémihypertrophie congénitale associée à une atrophie cérébrale homolatérale. *Ann. Méd. Nancy, 82*:487, 1957.

Neimark, E. Z., and Panchenko, E. N.: Hemihypertrophy. (Russian). *Pediatriia, 43*:34–35, 1964.

Newman, H. H.: *Physiology of Twinning.* Chicago, University of Chicago Press, p. 159, 1923.

Noé, O., and Berman, H. H.: The etiology of congenital hemihypertrophy and one case report. *Arch. Pediatr., 79*:278–288, 1962.

Ollier, M.: De la dyschondroplasie. *Bull. Soc. Chir.* (Lyon), *3*:22–27, 1899.

Ord, W.: Complete unilateral arrest of development. *Br. Med. J., 1*:587, 1895.

Osler, W.: Case of congenital and progressive hypertrophy of the right upper extremity. *J. Anat. Physiol., 14*:10–12, 1879.

Ougrelidze, M.: Hémihypertrophie congénitale droite stridor laryngé congénitale. *Nourison, 16*:40–45, 1928.

Overstreet, R.: An investigation of prenatal position and handedness. *Psychol. Bull., 35*:520–521, 1938.

Paget, J. P.: Imperfect symmetry. *Am. J. Med. Sci., 91*:41–44, 1886.

Panday, S. R., Kelkar, M. D., Parulekar, G. B., and Sen, P. K.: Congenital hemihypertrophy. Report of two cases and review of the literature. *J. Postgrad. Med., 12*:79–87, 1966.

Passauer, O.: Angeborene Hyperplasie der linken Gesichtshälfte. *Arch. Pathol. Anat. Physiol., 37*:410–411, 1866.

Paterson, D., and Reynolds, F. N.: Two cases of congenital hemihypertrophy. *Lancet, 1*:237, 1923.

Peabody, C. W.: Hemihypertrophy and hemiatrophy: congenital total unilateral somatic asymmetry. *J. Bone Joint Surg.*, *18*:466–474, 1936.

Peterson, G. M.: Inheritance of left-handedness. *Am. Naturalist*, *47*:730–738, 1934.

Petre, A., Schere, S., and Pellerano, J. C.: Disarmomias hemicorporales congenitas; hemiatrofias o hemihypertrofias. *Arch. Argent. Pediatr.*, *10*:294–300, 1939.

Phisalix, C.: Étude d'un embryon humain. *Arch. Zool. Exp. Gen.*, *6*:279, 1888.

Piazza, A.: Ein Fall von erworbener, totaler, rechtsseitiger Hypertrophie des Körpers. *Mschr. Psychiat. Neurol.* (Berlin), *25*:497–511, 1909.

Ramaley, F.: Inheritance of left-handedness. *Am. Naturalist*, *47*:730–738, 1913.

Rebez, P.: Un caso di emipertrofia congenita. *Gior. Veneto Sc. Med.*, *8*:43–55, 1934.

Redard, P.: L'hypertrophie congénitale partielle. *Arch. Gén. Méd.*, (7 s.), *1*:31–51, 1890.

Reed, A. C.: Congenital hemihypertrophy. *N.Y. Med. J.*, *118*:483–484, 1923.

Reed, E. A.: Congenital total hemihypertrophy. *Arch. Neurol. Psychiatr.*, *14*:824–827, 1925.

Reissmann: Un cas de gigantism unilateral avec hypertrophy de l'hémisphere cérébral du coté opposé. *Ann. Med. Chir. Inf.* (Paris), *6*:793–795, 1902.

Reissmann, C.: A case of complete one-sided gigantism with enlargement of the opposite side of the brain. *Aust. Med. Gaz.*, *21*:280, 1904.

Reissmann, C.: Further note on a case of unilateral gigantism. *Aust. Med. Gaz.*, *23*:280, 1904.

Reissmann, C.: Über angeborenen, halbseitigen Riesenwuchs; Nachwort zu meiner Veröffentlichung in No. 9 der *Münch. Med. Wochenschr.*, *51*:930, 1904.

Riedel, H. A.: Adrenogenital syndrome in male child due to adrenocortical tumor: report of case with hemihypertrophy and subsequent development of embryoma (Wilms' tumor). *Pediatrics*, *10*:19–27, 1952.

Rife, D. C.: Handedness with a special reference to twins. *Genetics*, *25*:176–186, 1940.

Rife, D. C.: Handedness and dermatoglyphics in twins. *Hum. Biol.*, *15*:46–54, 1943.

Rife, D. C.: Hand prints and handedness. *Am. J. Hum. Genet.*, *7*:170–179, 1955.

Rimoin, D. L.: Silver syndrome in twins. *In* Bergsma, D., (ed.): *Birth Defects: Original Article Series.* New York, National Foundation – March of Dimes. Vol. V., pp. 183–187, 1969.

Ringrose, R. E., Jabbour, J. T., and Keele, D. K.: Hemihypertrophy. *Pediatrics*, *36*:434–448, 1965.

Roget, J., Beaudoing, A., and Guilhot, J.: Un cas de'hémihypertrophie congénitale avec aspect normal des citernes de la base du crane. *Pédiatrie*, *10*:195–197, 1955.

Roudinesco, J., and Thyss, J.: L'enfant gaucher. *Enfance* (Paris), *8*:28, 126–141, 195–197, 1948.

Rugel, S. J.: Congenital hemihypertrophy. Report of a case with postmortem observation. *Am. J. Dis. Child.*, *71*:530–536, 1946.

Russell, A.: A syndrome of "intrauterine" dwarfism recognizable at birth with cranio-facial dysostosis, disproportionately short arms and other anomalies (5 examples). *Proc. R. Soc. Med. London.* (Sect. of Pediatrics), *47*:1040–1044, 1954.

Sabanas, A. O., and Chatterton, C. C.: Crossed congenital hemihypertrophy. *J. Bone Joint Surg.*, *37A*:871–874, 1955.

Sabie, J.: Sur un cas d'hémihypertrophie droite totale du corps, d'origine congénitale avec hydrocephalie. *J. Sci. Med.* (Lille), *1*:302–310, 1909.

Salle, V.: Über einen Fall von angeborener abnormer Grösse der Extremitäten mit einem an Akromegalie erinnernden Symptomenkomplex. *Jb. Kinderheilkd.*, *25*:540–550, 1913.

Sayer, A., and Fatherree, T. J.: Congenital hemihypertrophy. Report of a case. *U.S. Nav. Med. Bull.*, *44*:142–147, 1945.

Scarabicchi, S., Massimo, L., and Tortorolo, G.: L'emiipertrofia e il tumore d. Wilms. *Minerva Pediatr.*, *12*:1368–1371, 1960.

Schachter, M.: Les megalosomies ou hypertrophie localisées d'origine congénitales. *Rev. Franc. Pédiatr.*, *15*:268–273, 1939.

Schachter, M.: La gaucherie infantile: Hypothèses et faits. *Neurone*, *3*:39, 1955.

Schachter, M.: Gauchers et droitiers: contribution à l'étude de la gaucherie scolaire dans la perspective pédo-psychiatrique. *Pédiatrie*, *25*:499–509, 1970.

Schachter, M., and Cotto, S.: Recherches sur la gaucherie infantile. *Praxis*, *40*:195–197, 1951.

Schaeffer, E.: Halbseitenriesenwuchs und Wilms Tumor. *Mschr. Kinderheilkd.*, *108*:504–507, 1960.

Schaeffer, M.: Die Linkshänder in den Berliner Gemeindeschulen. *Berlin. Klin. Wochenschr.*, *48*:295–300, 1911.

Schiller, M.: Totale Hypertrophie einer Körperhälfte. *Berl. Klin. Wochenschr.*, *47*:366, 1910.

Schiller, M.: The problems in left handedness, with investigation on Stuttgart children. *Z. Ges. Neurol. Psychol.*, *140*:496, 1932. Abstract in *Arch. Neurol. Psychiat.*, *29*:1340–1342, 1933.

Schlenzka, W.: Über einen Krankheitsfall einer Recklinghausenschen Neurofibromatosis. *Z. Orthop.*, *87*:84–89, 1955.

Schwartzman, J., Grossman, L., and Dratgutsky, D.: True total hemihypertrophy. Case report. *Arch. Pediatr.*, *59*:637–645, 1942.

Scott, A. J.: Hemihypertrophy: report of four cases. *J. Pediatr.*, *6*:650–656, 1935.

Seldowitz, M., and Berman, A. B.: Crossed laterality in children. *Am. J. Dis. Child.*, *85*:2–33, 1953.

Sequelto: A remarkable case of unilateral hypertrophy in a child. *Trans. Med. Chir. Soc.* (Glasgow), *1*:130–132, 1895–1897.

Shukoyski, V. P.: Hemihypertrophia sinistra in an 11-year-old boy. (Polish). *Arch. Psychiatr.* (Varshava), *26*:1–20, 1895.

Silver, H. K.: Congenital asymmetry, short stature and elevated urinary gonadotropin. *A.M.A.J. Dis. Child.*, *9*:768–773, 1959.

Silver, H. K.: Asymmetry, short stature, and variations in sexual development. *Am. J. Dis. Child.*, *107*:495–515, 1964.

Silver, H. K., and Grusaky, F. L.: Syndrome of congenital hemihypertrophy and elevated urinary gonadotropins: occurrence in a seventeen-year-old boy. *A.M.A.J. Dis. Child.*, *93*:559, 1957.

Silver, H. K., Kiyasu, W., George, J., and Deamer, W. C.: Syndrome of congenital hemihypertrophy, shortness of stature, and elevated gonadotropins. *Pediatrics*, *12*:368–376, 1953.

Simian, J., and Schachter-Nancy, M.: Un cas d'hémi-hypertrophie congénitale chez un nourisson. *Rev. Franc. Pediatr.*, *13*:187–191, 1937.

Simpson, B. S.: A case of unilateral hypertrophy. *Edinburgh Med. J.*, *33*:623–626, 1926.

Slaughter, W. H.: A case of abnormal growth of the upper extremity. *J.A.M.A.*, *78*:426–427; figs. 1 and 2, 1922.

Speese, J.: Unilateral congenital hypertrophy. *Arch. Pediatr.*, *31*:278–284, 1914.

Stanton, I. N., and Tuft, L.: Congenital total hemihypertrophy. *J.A.M.A.*, *80*:1432–1434, 1923.

Steffen, W.: Angeborene Hypertrophie der einen Körperhälfte. *Jb. Kinderheilkd.*, *38*:379–384, 1894.

Steffen, W.: Über echten partiellen Riesenwuchs. *Z. menschl. Vererb. Konstitutionslehre*, *20*:246–253, 1937.

Steinsleger, M.: Hipertrofia congenita de membros. *Riv. Med.* (Rosario), *13*:265–272, 1923.

Stembo, L.: Ein Fall von Hypertrophie lateralis superior. *St. Petersburg Med. Wochenschr. F.*, *13*:245, 1896.

Stier, E.: Über Hemiatrophie und Hemihypertrophie nebst einigen Bemerkungen über ihre laterale Lokalisation. *Dtsch. Z. Nervenheilkd.*, *24*:21–64, 1912.

Stoesser, A. V.: Hypertrophies of infancy and childhood. *Am. J. Dis. Child.*, *35*:885–893, 1928.

Sturge, W. A.: A case of partial epilepsy apparently due to a lesion of one of the vasomotor centers of the brain. *Clin. Soc. Tr.*, *12*:162, 1879.

Subirana, A.: La droiterie (Die Rechtshandigkeit — righthandedness). *Schweiz. Arch. Neurol. Psychiatr.*, *69*:321–359, 1952.

Sumner, F. B., and Huestis, R. R.: Bilateral asymmetry and its relation to certain problems of genetics. *Genetics*, *6*:445–485, 1921.

Thifors, J.: Fall of kongenital hemi-hypertrofi och macroglossi. *Hygiea* (Stockholm), *9*:62–75, 1909.

Tietz, H.: Über konnatalen partiellen Riesenwuchs. *Z. menschl. Vererb. Konstitutionslehre*, *34*:555–562, 1958.

Tilanus, C. G.: Uber einen Fall von hemihypertrophia dextra. *Münch. Med. Wochenschr.*, *40*:65–66, 1893.

Tobias, N.: Congenital hemiatrophy associated with linear nevus: report of a case. *Arch. Pediatr.*, *45*:673–680, 1928.

Tuckerman, F.: Some observations in reference to bilateral asymmetry of form and function. *J. Anat. Physiol.*, *19*:307, 1885.

Verschueren, F.: Hémihypertrophie alterne cranio-acrale avec imbécilité (Étude clinique et encéphalographique). *J. Belg. Neurol. Psychiat.*, *38*:431–441, 1938.

Vestermark, S.: Silver's syndrome. *Acta Paediatr. Scand.*, *59*:435–439, 1970.

Volz, W.: Ein Fall bilateralem symmetrischen Riesenwuchs der Extremitäten des Schulter-und Beckengürtels in Verbindung mit Kryptorchismus. *Z. Orthop. Chir.*, *12*:801–813, 1904.

Vonderweidt: Un cas d'hémihypertrophie congénitale. *Med. Inf.* (Paris), *28*:317–320, 1922.

Wachsner, F.: Zur Kenntnis der bilateralen Asymmetrie des menschlichen Körpers. *Berl. Klin. Wochenschr.*, *51*:1953, 1914.

Wagner, H.: Hypertrophie der rechten Brust und der rechten oberen Extremität besonders der Hand und der Finger. *Med. Jb. D.K.K. Österreichischen Staats*, *19*:378–381, 1839. Also in *Schmidt's Jb.*, *37*:226, 1842.

Wagner, R., and Kottmeir, H. L.: Über Hemihypertrophia und Hemiatrophia Corporis totalis nebst spontaner Extremitätgengangräne bei Säuglingen im Anschluss zu einem ungewöhnlichen Fall. *Acta Paediatr.*, *20*:531–543, 1938.

Wakefield, E. G.: Hypertrophy, congenital, of the left shoulder girdle, arm and head, with naevus and varicose veins. *Am. J. Med. Sci.*, *171*:569–575, 1926.

Wakefield, E. G.: Unilateral, congenital hypertrophy, involving the right side of a female aged six. *Ann. Intern. Med.*, *1*:219–221, 1927.

Wakefield, E. G., and Hines, E. A.: Congenital hemihypertrophy; report of eight cases. *Am. J. Med. Sci.*, *185*:493–500, 1932.

Wallin, J.: Ein Fall von kongenitaler, unilateraler Hypertrophie. *Acta Paediatr.*, *18*:503–510, 1936.

Ward, J., and Lerner, H. H.: A review of the subject of congenital hemihypertrophy and complete case report. *J. Pediatr.*, *31*:403–414, 1947.

Warkany, J.: *Congenital Malformations.* Chicago, Year Book Medical Publishers, Inc., pp. 349–352, 1971.

Weber, F.: Right sided hemihypertrophy from right sided congenital spastic hemiplegia with morbid condition of the left side of the brain, revealed by radiogram. *N. Neuro. Psychopat.* (London), *37*:301–311, 1922.

Wegener, H.: Zur Psychologie der Linkshändigkeit. *Praxis Kinderpsychol., 1*:257–265, 1952.

Widemann: Ein Fall von halbseitigem Riesenwuchs. *Berl. Klin. Wochenschr., 38*:145–146, 1901.

Wieland, E.: Zur Pathologie der dystrophischen Form des angeborenen partiellen Riesenwuches. *Jb. Kinderheilkd., 65*:519–584, 1907.

Wiesberg, M.: An unusual case of hemigigantism. *Can. Med. J., 25*:590–593, 1931.

Wile, T. S.: *Handedness. Right and Left.* Boston, Lothrop, Lee and Shepard Co., pp. 3–409, 1934.

Wilks, S.: Righthandedness and left-brainedness. *Lancet, 2*:1658–1659, 1902. Also *Lancet, 2*:266, 1903.

Williams, J. A.: Congenital hemihypertrophy with lymphangioma. *Arch. Dis. Child., 26*:158–161, 1951.

Wilson, F. C., Jr., and Orlin, H.: Crossed congenital hemihypertrophy associated with a Wilms' tumor. Report of a case. *J. Bone Joint Surg., 47A*:1609–1614, 1965.

Wilson, M. O., and Dolan, L. B.: Handedness and ability. *Am. J. Psychol., 43*:261–268, 1931.

Winokurow, E.: Kongenitaler Riesenwuchs mit Neurofibromatose. *Verh. Dtsch. Orthop. Ges., 47*:386–390, 1926.

Wiseberg, M.: An unusual case of hemigigantism. *Can. Med. Assoc. J., 25*:591–593, 1931.

Woo, T. L., and Pearson, K.: Dextrality and sinistrality of hand and eye. *Biometrika, 9*:169, 1927.

Wooley, H. T.: The development of right-handedness in a normal infant. *Psychol. Rev., 17*:40–41, 1910.

Wurtz: Note sur un cas d'hypertrophie congénitale du membre supérieur. *Rev. Méd. Hygiene Trop., 6*:17–19, 1909.

Chapter Twenty-One

ANOMALIES OF CARPAL BONES

At birth, the carpus is entirely cartilaginous. The appearance of bone in cartilaginous anlagen is subject to variations. These variations are genetically determined and are also dependent upon the ethnic origin, health, nutritional status, endocrine state, exposure to irradiation, intercurrent illness, and the sexual development of the child. Females are more precocious.

The osseous nucleus of the capitate may become visible six weeks after birth; it is usually present during the third or fourth month when it is accompanied by the smaller kernel of the hamate bone. The osseous nucleus of the triquetrum is seen as early as the seventh month and as late as the twenty-fourth month. The lunate becomes roentgenographically visible between the third and fourth years. The trapezium, the trapezoid, and the scaphoid acquire their ossific nuclei between the ages of three and six years. In most cases the trapezium ossifies first, the trapezoid next, and the scaphoid last. The pisiform becomes visible between the ages of 8 and 12 years. Normally all these bones attain full maturity between the fourteenth and eighteenth postnatal year. Roentgenographic diagnosis of congenital anomalies of the carpal bones—disorderly and disharmonious development, deletion, duplication, fusion, and articular incongruities—cannot be established definitely until years after birth. Many anomalies of the carpal bones are bilateral. Some are hereditary and are occasionally associated with comparable abnormalities of the tarsus. They are often seen in connection with other anomalies of the hand and forearm. Anomalies of the carpal bones also occur in a number of syndromes (Figs. 21–1 to 21–6).

DISORDERLY AND DISHARMONIOUS DEVELOPMENT

The sequence of ossification of the capitate, hamate, triquetrum, and lunate is in the order given. In an occasional instance the kernel of the lunate will precede that of the triquetrum. The sequence of ossification of the trapezium, trapezoid, and scaphoid is often irregular. In a considerable number of cases, even in right-handed children, the bones of the left carpus seem to develop ear-

714

(Text continued on page 718.)

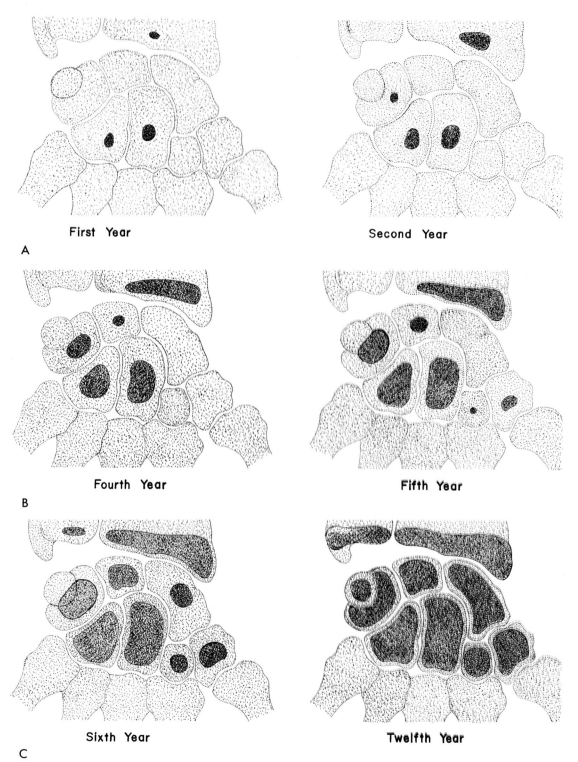

First Year

Second Year

A

Fourth Year

Fifth Year

B

Sixth Year

Twelfth Year

C

Figure 21-1 Sketches showing textbook estimation of the time of appearance of ossific centers of the various carpal bones in males.

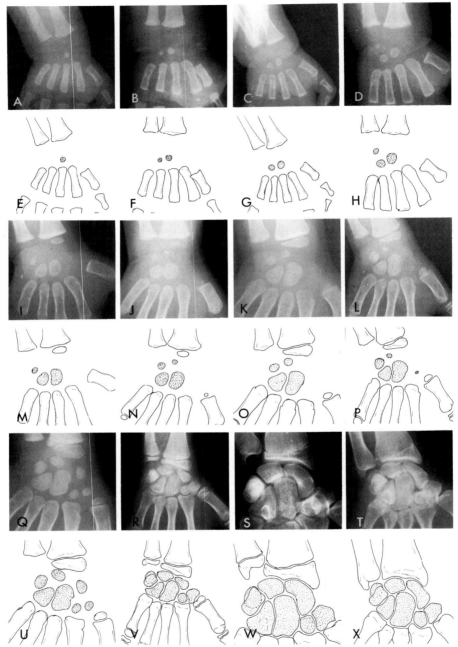

Figure 21–2   Carpal bones. *A*, Dorsovolar roentgenograph of the right wrist of a six-week-old boy: the nucleus of the capitate is visible. *B*, Four-month-old girl: the hamate is seen as a small ossicle next to the capitate. *C*, Five-month-old girl: the nuclei of the hamate and the capitate have become rounded. *D*, Seven-month-old girl: triquetrum has appeared rather precociously. *E*, *F*, *G*, and *H* illustrate the roentgenographs above each. *I*, Boy, twentieth month: triquetrum is seen as a rounded ossicle. *J*, Boy, three years old: lunate is seen as a small seed. *K*, Boy, four years old: lunate is clearly delineated. *L*, Girl, four and one half years old: trapezium is seen as a small seed. *M*, *N*, *O*, and *P* illustrate the roentgenographs above each. *Q*, Girl, five and one half years old: all carpal bones except pisiform have become ossified. *R*, Girl, seven and one half years old: pisiform is seen as a small seed. *S*, Girl, eight years old: all carpal bones have gained bulk. *T*, Girl 15 years old: maturation. *U*, *V*, *W* and *X* illustrate the roentgenograph above each.

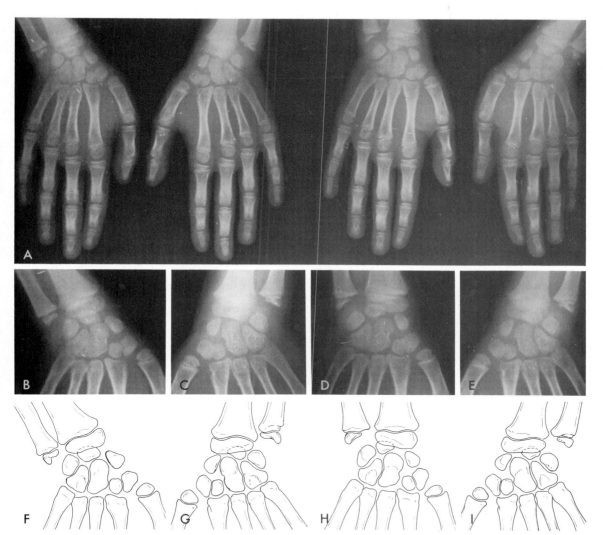

Figure 21–3 Carpal development of homozygotic twins born at full term. *A*, Dorsopalmar roentgenograph of the wrists and hands of seven-year-old female identical twins: with the exception of slight dissimilarity of ulnar epiphyses, all bones are symmetrically developed. *B* and *C*, Enlarged roentgenographs of the right and left wrists of one sister. *D* and *E*, Enlarged roentgenographs of the wrist of the other sister. *F*, *G*, *H*, and *I* represent the roentgenograph above each.

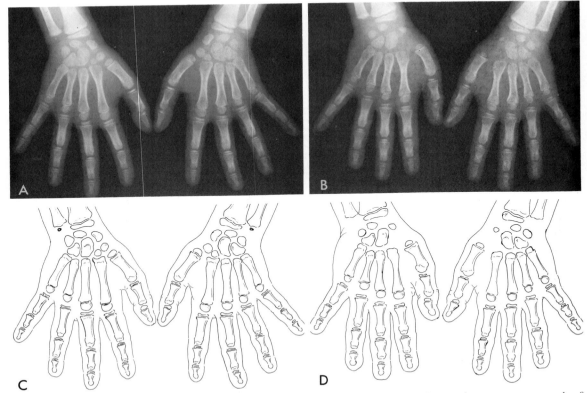

Figure 21–4 Carpal development in heterozygous, prematurely born twins. *A*, Dorsopalmar roentgenograph of an eight-year-old girl born after a seven-and-one-half-month pregnancy, weighing 3 pounds 10 ¾ ounces. All carpal ossicles except the pisiform are manifest, as are the carpal epiphyses of the radius and ulna. *B*, Dorsopalmar roentgenograph of the wrists and hands of her twin brother whose birth weight was 3 pounds 10 ounces. The epiphysis of the ulna is not evident, nor are the nuclei of the trapezium and trapezoid. *C* and *D* illustrate the roentgenograph above each.

lier. Disharmony of skeletal maturation of carpal ossicles is known to occur in bird-headed dwarfism, and in various types of mucopolysaccharidoses. In homocystinuria, a carpal bone, usually the lunate, may remain diminutive and another, as a rule the capitate, is found disproportionately enlarged. Early maturation of carpal ossicles has also been reported in children with homocystinuria (Figs. 21–7 and 21–8).

Hemimelic epiphyseal dysplasia is characterized by asymmetrical cartilaginous overgrowth of tarsal or carpal bones—more commonly the former—and failure of one half of the epiphysis of a limb bone to keep pace with the other half; in consequence, the shaft of the affected bones becomes bowed on the side of the greater growth. Saxton and Wilkinson (1964) reported a three-and-one-half-year-old child who, in addition to a longer, bowed left leg had a longer left arm with exaggerated carrying angle at the elbow. In the right wrist, only the four bones (capitate, hamate, triquetrum, and lunate) were visualized, and the epiphysis of the first metacarpal had not ossified. In the left wrist, in addition to the ossicles mentioned, there were two large bones representing the scaphoid and the trapezium, respectively, and the epiphysis of the first metacarpal was manifest; the scaphoid and the trapezium were almost three times as large as the lunate and the triquetral of this on the opposite wrist. Hemimelic epiphyseal dysplasia is said to be three times more common in males than in females.

(*Text continued on page 723.*)

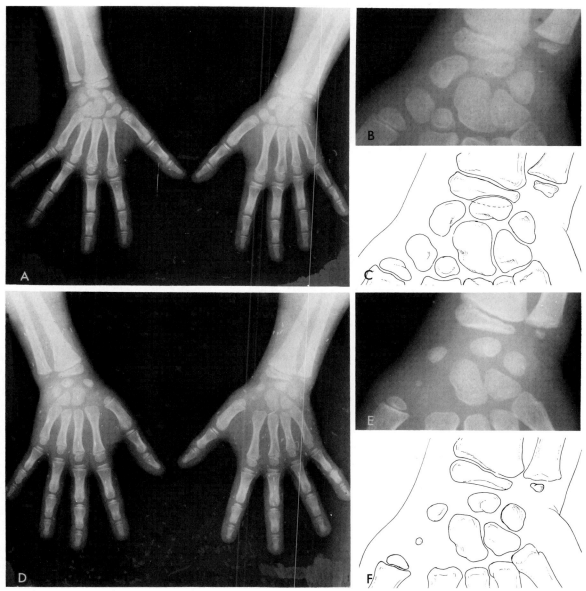

Figure 21-5 The same twins (Fig. 21-4) a year later. *A*, Dorsopalmar roentgenograph of the wrists and hands of the sister. *B*, Enlarged roentgenograph showing the ossified nuclei of the following carpal bones: scaphoid, lunate, triquetrum, trapezium, trapezoid, capitate, and hamate. *C*, Sketch illustrating the same. *D*, Dorsopalmar roentgenograph of the brother's hands. *E*, Enlarged roentgenograph of the left wrist: the trapezoid has not appeared as yet and the nuclei of the other bones are comparatively small. *F*, Sketch illustrating the same.

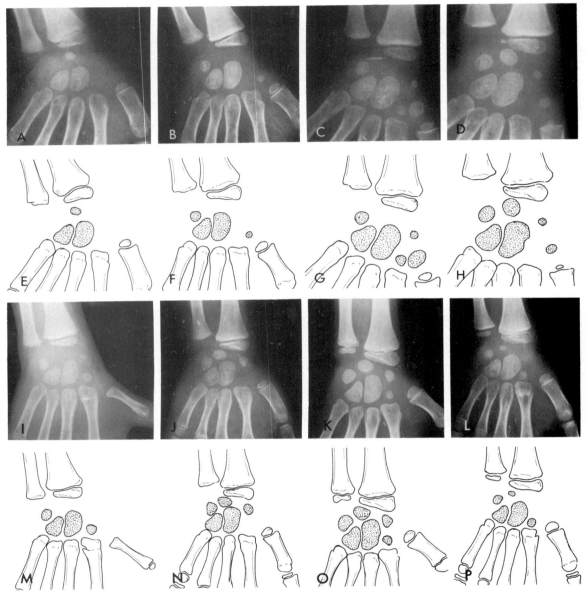

Figure 21–6 Vagaries of ossification of carpal bones as seen in dorsopalmar roentgenographs of the right wrist. *A*, Three-year-old girl: the lunate has appeared before the triquetrum. *B*, Four-year-old boy: the trapezium has appeared before the lunate. *C*, Four-and-a-half-old boy: the trapezium, trapezoid, and scaphoid have appeared before the lunate. *D*, Five-year-old boy: the trapezium and scaphoid have appeared before the trapezoid. *E*, *F*, *G*, and *H* illustrate the roentgenograph above each. *I*, Five-year-old boy: the trapezoid and scaphoid have appeared before the lunate and trapezium. *J*, Six-year-old boy: the scaphoid has appeared before the trapezium and trapezoid. *K*, Seven-year-old boy: the trapezoid and scaphoid have appeared before the trapezium. *L*, Another seven-year-old boy: the trapezoid has appeared before the trapezium and scaphoid. *M*, *N*, *O*, and *P* illustrate the roentgenograph above each.

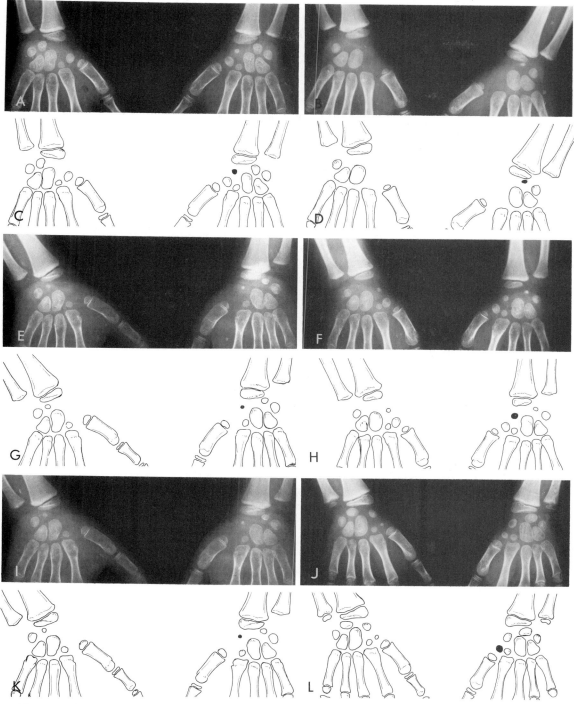

Figure 21–7 Earlier appearance of left carpal ossicles in right-handed children as seen in dorsopalmar roentgenographs. *A*, Three-year-old, normal girl with precocious ossification of carpal bones: the right wrist has six carpal bones; the left has seven. *B*, Four-year-old boy: the left lunate is visible; the right is not. *C* and *D* illustrate the roentgenograph above each. *E*, Four-year-old girl: the left scaphoid is visible; the right is not. *F*, Five-year-old boy: the left lunate is visible; the right is not; *G* and *H* illustrate the roentgenograph above each. *I*, Six-year-and 11-month-old boy: the left scaphoid is visible; the right is not. *J*, Seven-year-old boy: the carpals are more mature. *K* and *L* illustrate the roentgenograph above each.

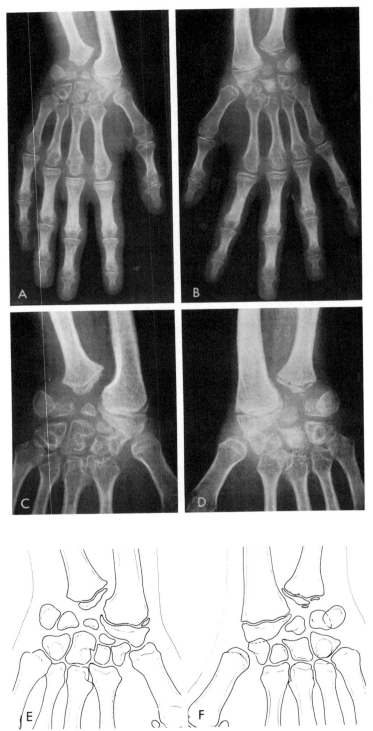

Figure 21–8   Disharmony of carpal development in Morquio's mucopolysaccharidosis. *A* and *B*, Dorsopalmar roentgenographs of the wrists and hands of a 10-year-old girl with Morquio's disease. *C*, Roentgenograph of the right wrist. *D*, Roentgenograph of the left wrist. *E* and *F* illustrate the roentgenograph above each: no two carpal bones have the same configuration in each wrist: the first metacarpal is subluxated on both sides.

ABSENCES

Isolated absences of carpal bones are rare. Behr (1911) reported a case of hypoplasia of the carpal scaphoid. Eaves and Campiche (1922) presented a 20-year-old man with hypoplasia of the scaphoid on one side and absence of it on the other. On both sides, the radial styloid process was wanting; on the side of the absent scaphoid, the thumb was diminutive. Eaves and Campiche thought their case was one of isolated absence of the scaphoid. This case would now be classified with pre-axial hemimelia and would be considered an intercalary defect of the radial ray.

Congenital absences of carpal bones are usually an associated anomaly. Stricker (1878) described a hand with only a thumb and an index finger; the triquetrum pisiform and hamate were missing. Aplasia or hypoplasia of the scaphoid has been described under a variety of misleading titles: "'Slight degree of clubhand"—by Botreau-Roussel (1922); "Congenital retardation in development of the carpal navicular, first metacarpal and styloid process of the radius"—by Hodgson (1943); "Congenital retardation in development of certain thenar muscles"—by Hanley and Conlon (1957); "Hypoplasia of the navicular"—by Neumann (1959); "Congenital hypoplasia of the carpal scaphoid bone"—by Davison (1962); and "Congenital absence of carpal scaphoid"—by Srivastava and Kochhar (1972). The cases reported by these authors all belong to the category of radial ray defect. When the ulna or the ulnar digital rays are deficient, the pisiform, hamate, and triquetrum frequently are absent. Absences of carpal bones are also known to occur in split hand and in phocomelia. In mirror hand or ulnar dimelia, radial carpal bones are absent while ulnar ossicles are duplicated. In recent years, a number of articles have appeared on the subject of carpal osteolysis, which Marie et al (1956) considered to be of congenital origin. Some of the reported cases have had hereditary antecedents. In many there is associated renal insufficiency with proteinuria which becomes manifest in early childhood (Figs. 21–9 and 21–10).

ACCESSORIA

Numerous surplus bones of the carpus have been described. They are named in accordance with shape or presumed phylogenic derivation. O'Rahilly (1953) favored a nomenclature based on the position and propinquity of the aberrant bone. The significance of these supernumerary ossicles lies in the fact that they often are confused with fractures and occasionally they cause painful swellings. The styloid process of the lunate at times develops from a separate center; it fails to unite with the main bone and is taken for the un-united fragment seen in connection with Colles' fracture. Because of its shape, this piece was at one time called os triangulare; Izquierdo (1925) called it os intermedium antibrachii, and O'Rahilly (1953) listed it as ulnastyloidium. This ossicle usually is bilateral but may appear on only one side. Os styloidium, also called metastyloidium or parastyloidium, is an accessory bone seen in relation to the styloid process of the third metacarpal base (Figs. 21–11 and 21–12).

(Text continued on page 727.)

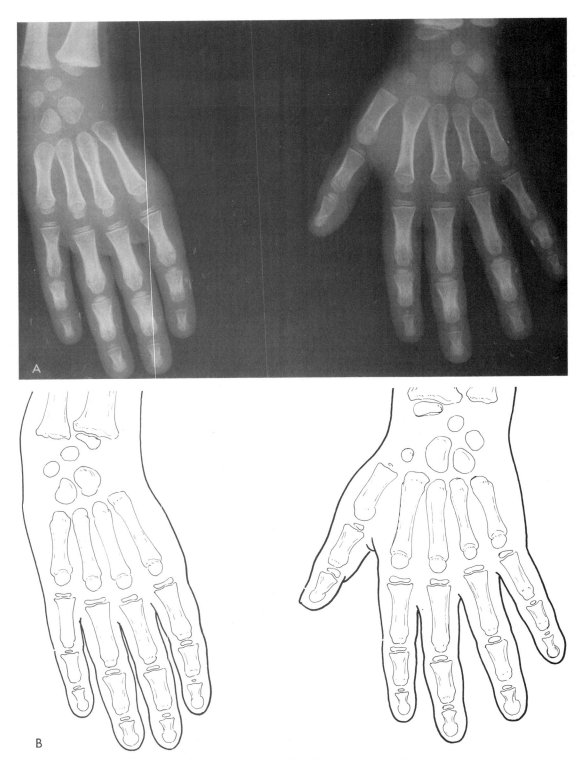

Figure 21–9 Absence of the right trapezium in a child with absent right pollical ray. *A*, Dorsopalmar roentgenograph of the wrists and hands of a five-year-old girl. *B*, Sketch illustrating the same.

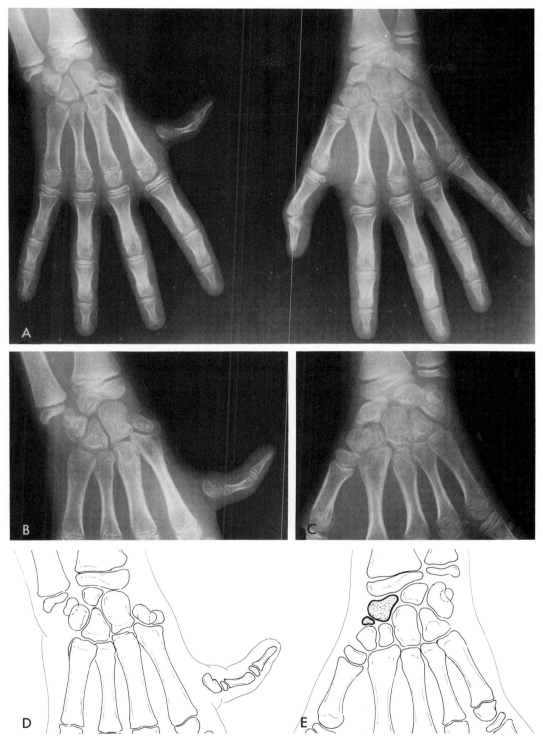

Figure 21–10   Absence of the scaphoid associated with floating thumb on the same side and accessory scaphoid bone in the opposite wrist. *A,* Dorsopalmar roentgenograph of the hands and wrists of a nine-year-old girl with intercalary defect of the right pollical ray and absent right scaphoid bone; the scaphoid of the opposite wrist is undersized and there is a small ossicle between it and the trapezoid bone. *B* and *C,* Enlarged roentgenographs, respectively. *D* and *E* illustrate the roentgenograph above each.

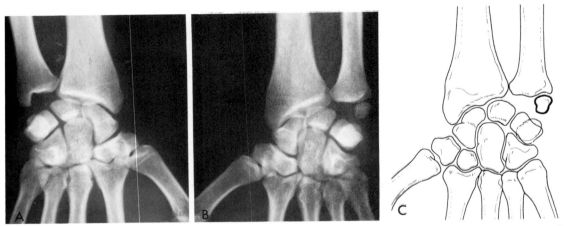

Figure 21-11 Unilateral os ulnastyloidium. *A*, Dorsopalmar roentgenograph of the right wrist of a 17-year-old boy. *B*, The left wrist: the styloid process of the ulna has developed from a separate center of ossification and has failed to unite with the main bone. *C*, Sketch illustrating the same.

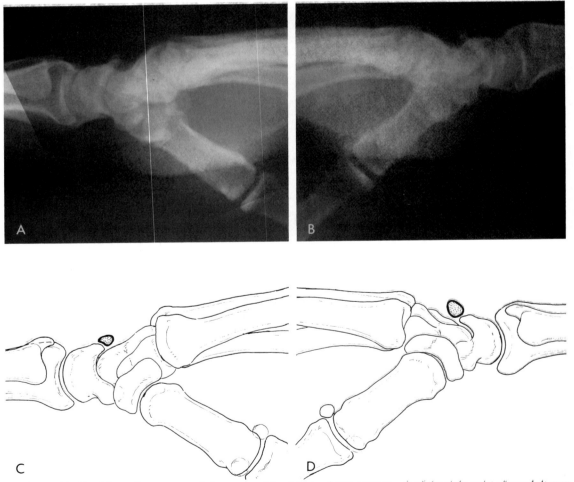

Figure 21-12 Bilateral accessory epitriquetral ossicle. *A*, Lateral roentgenograph of the right wrist of an adult man with an accessory ossicle atop the triquetral bone. *B*, Lateral roentgenograph of the left wrist showing a slightly larger epitriquetral ossicle. *C* and *D* illustrate the roentgenograph above each.

Accessory carpal bones are known to occur in the cardiomelic complex which bears the hyphenated names of Holt and Oram (1960). This is an autosomal dominant syndrome consisting of congenital heart disease and upper limb anomaly, usually nonopposable triphalangeal thumb. Pozanski et al (1970) considered the presence of extra carpal bones—remnants of the primitive central row of carpals—as the most striking melic abnormality seen in Holt-Oram syndrome. The surviving accessory ossicle may persist as a separate bone or it may become fused with one of the adjacent bones, usually with the scaphoid. Persisting os centrale has also been reported in cases of hand-foot-uterus syndrome and in subjects with otopalatodigital complex. In the latter complex, one may also encounter an extra ossicle along the distal row of carpal bones. Multiple anomalous ossification centers of the carpus is a feature of a syndrome described by Larsen and associates (1950). This syndrome has been mentioned in Chapter Eight, and it will be discussed in some detail in Chapter Twenty-seven. In Larsen's syndrome, as many as 14 ossicles per wrist have been counted.

ARTICULAR INCONGRUITIES

Carpal bossing—also called *carpe bossu*, carpal displacement, carpal kyphosis, and hunchback carpus—is a clinical entity which some authors ascribe to the prominent os styloidium of the third metacarpal and others to the "double break" or subluxation between the third metacarpal and the capitate bone. Carpal bossing is usually asymptomatic. It is more common in females. Symptomatic cases often present themselves as ganglia around the dorsum of the third metacarpal base. All ganglia surmounting the juncture of the capitate and third metacarpal base must be suspected of being caused by a spur on the dorsal rim of the capitate—resulting from recurrent subluxation of the capitate—or by an overprominent os styloidium. Recurrence after ganglionectomy is inevitable unless the dorsally protruding crest of either the third metacarpal or the capitate bone is removed (Figs. 21–13 to 21–16).

Manson (1924) described what he called a rare "congenital anomaly of hands and feet." There was cavus deformity of the feet and fibular deviation of the toes. In the hand, the fingers inclined in the ulnar direction; the first metacarpal shot out from the radial aspect of the trapezium which was closely attached, if not altogether fused, to the base of the second metacarpal bone. Rushforth's (1949) patient presented a similar malformation of the first metacarpophalangeal joint. The trapezium was long and bore an articular facet on its radial aspect for the mushroomed base of the first metacarpal. This facet was flat instead of being saddle-shaped. Each first carpometacarpal joint was deformed, osteoarthritic. There was a supernumerary ossicle in each hand; on the right side, the surplus bone was attached to the radial margin of the trapezium and seemed to form a part of its distal articular facet. Rushforth interpreted this bone as the os paratrapezium. O'Rahilly (1953) described it as "a palmar ossicle at the distal end of the crest of the trapezium." In Ehlers-Danlos syndrome, there is subluxation at the first carpometacarpal joint (Fig. 21–17).

BIPARTITION

Turner (1883) reported a case with a divided trapezoid. Buschke (1934) described a case with two bony nuclei in the lunate. Eggimann (1951) presented

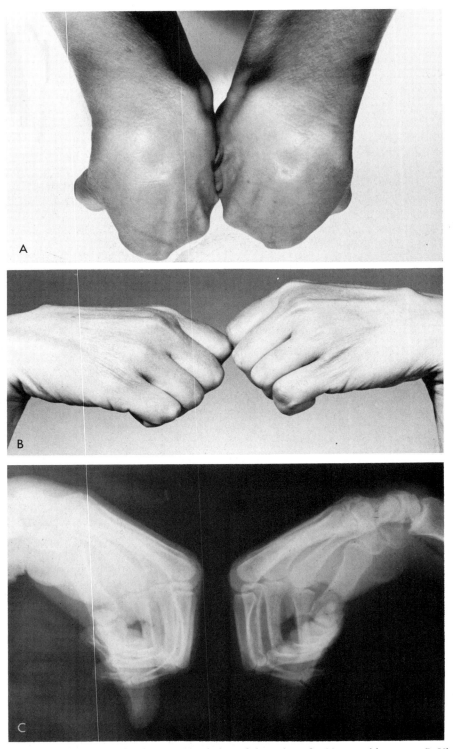

Figure 21-13   Carpal bossing. *A*, Dorsal view of the wrists of a 20-year-old woman. *B*, Ulnar view of the same. *C*, Lateral roentgenograph, showing bilateral prominence of the styloid processes of the third metacarpals.

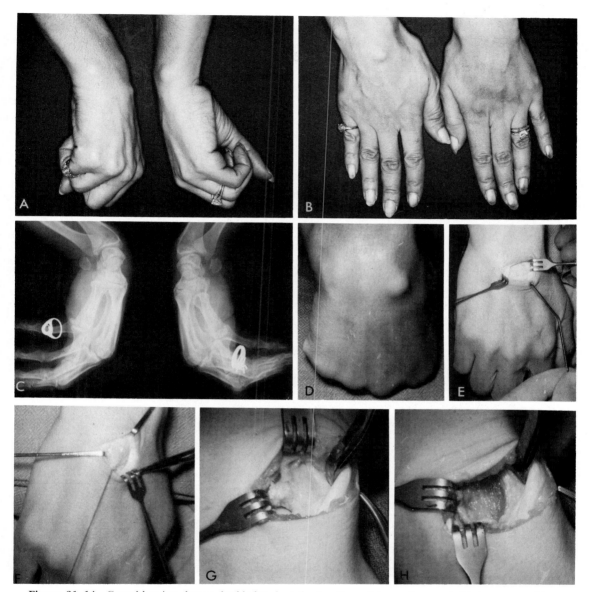

Figure 21–14 Carpal bossing due to double-break at the junction of the capitate and third metacarpal base. *A*, Ulnar view of the hands of a 24-year-old woman with a hard nodular prominence in the back of the right wrist and ever-recurring superimposed ganglion. *B*, Dorsal view. *C*, Lateral roentgenograph of both wrists, showing greater prominence at the carpometacarpal junction on the right side. *D*, Dorsal view of the flexed right wrist. *E* and *F*, Exposure of the ganglion. *G*, Exposure of underlying bony spur emanating from the capitate. *H*, Smooth surface left after resection of the dorsal osteophyte of the capitate.

a patient with bipartite lunate bones. Except for the fact that this is extremely rare, this anomaly is not of much clinical significance. However, bipartite scaphoid is accorded special importance. It is comparatively common and is often confused with fracture. Gruber (1877, 1883) reported bipartition and tripartition of the scaphoid. Bipartite carpal scaphoid has also been reported by Struthers (1874), Anderson (1883), Leboucq (1884),

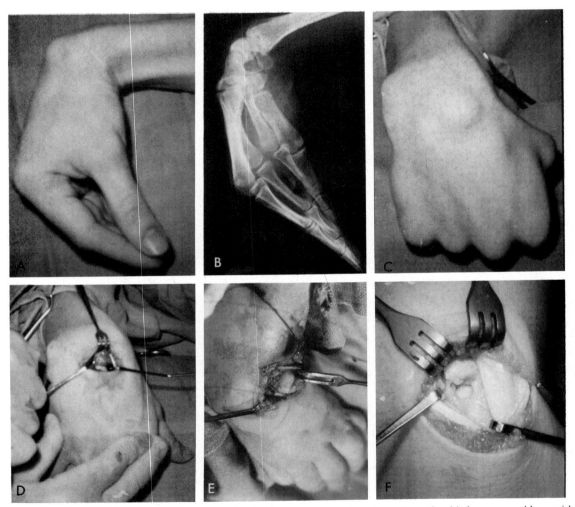

Figure 21-15   Carpal bossing due to dorsal subluxation of the capitate bone from the third metacarpal base with an overlying capsular cyst or ganglion. *A*, Radial view of the flexed right wrist of a 16-year-old girl who has had hypermobile joints since birth. *B*, Roentgenograph of the same. *C*, Dorsal view. *D* shows ganglion emanating from the dorsal joint capsule. *E*, Exposure of protruding distal dorsal margin of the capitate bone. *F*, Enlarged view of surgical exposure, showing the protruding margin of the capitate and prominent styloid process of the third metacarpal base.

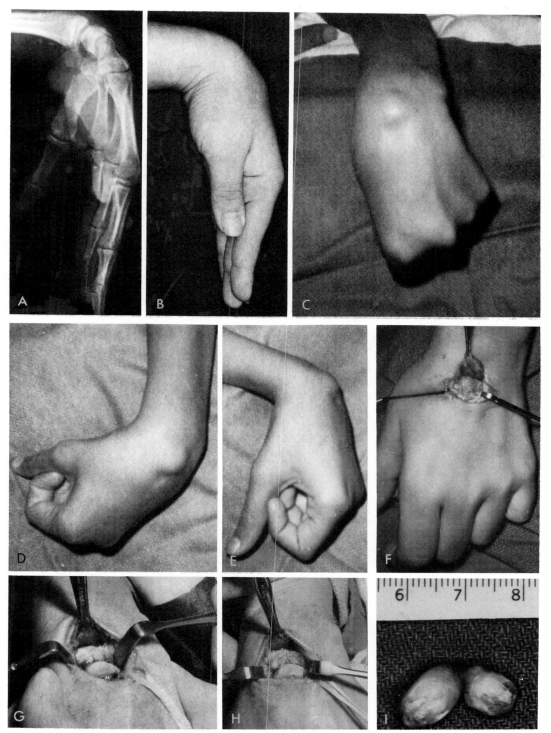

Figure 21–16 Carpal bossing due to hypermobility at the lunocapitate juncture. *A*, Lateral roentgenograph of a 17-year-old girl who complained of a constant bulge in the back of her wrist. *B, C, D*, and *E*: views of the left wrist. *F* and *G*, Exposure of the joint between the lunate and capitate bones, showing osteophytes emanating from both bones, especially the former. *H*, The osteophyte has been shaved from the distal lip of the lunate. *I*, Resected osteophytes—the scale is in centimeters.

Auvray (1898), Wolff (1903), Dwight (1906), Schulz (1909), Mouchet (1914), Blencke (1926), Faulkner (1928), Ogilvie (1930), Haehner (1932), Boyd (1933), Reich (1933), Mori (1934), Pokrovsky (1935), Volk (1937), Watkins (1937), Vaghi (1939), Lindgren (1941), Childress (1943), Marti (1944), Rose (1946), Torsten (1947), Krause (1949), Vieten (1949), Caffaratti (1950), Verö (1951), Stuart (1958), Cotta (1961), Randelli (1961), Dau (1964), Baciu et al (1966), and Sherwin et al (1971).

Dwight (1906) pointed out that the carpal scaphoid is developed from radial and ulnar elements, which normally fuse during the early cartilaginous stage. In an exceptional case, these fragments fail to fuse and the mature ossicles remain connected by fibrocartilage. "That a bone so constituted should yield to violence more easily than a normal one and that the displaced surfaces with their fibrocartilaginous covering should be ill adopted for repair is precisely in accord with clinical experience in so-called fracture of the scaphoid," Dwight wrote. Conceding as he did that a normal scaphoid could on occasion be broken, Dwight considered the great majority of un-united fractures to be "due to the in-separation of the original parts." Hardman (1928) described unfused tubercle of the navicular bone and advised studying the opposite wrist.

As seen on roentgenographs, the fragments of a bipartite scaphoid should have smooth, regular margins, a clear translucent space between them, and no arthritic changes. The opposed surface must be covered with cartilage and the fragments should show no sign of avascular necrosis; the anomaly should be bilateral and must not be preceded by trauma. O'Rahilly (1953) did not consider these criteria very illuminating. He pointed out that bipartite scaphoid may be unilateral or bilateral. It may have undergone arthritic changes; it may become fractured and one of the fragments may have undergone avascular necrosis. He also discounted the importance of trauma in a history, since both bipartite and normal scaphoid can yield to injury; the former may do so more easily than the latter.

FUSION

Carpal bones tend to coalesce with one another rather than with the radius proximally or the metacarpals distally. Radiocarpal fusion has been reported by Becker (1935), Liszka and Sik (1959), Gombert (1959), Tognolo and Poggi (1963), Girod (1964), Schacherl and Schilling (1965), and Rauterberg (1968). In some of these cases the radius had united with the lunate; in others, it had joined with the navicular. In two cases, both these carpal bones had coalesced with the radius. Schacherl and Schilling regarded the cases they presented as "inflammatory." The others claimed that theirs were of congenital origin (Fig. 21–18).

Intercarpal coalescence constitutes the most common anomaly affecting the carpal bones. There are numerous cases on record. Fusion between the lunate and triquetrum appears to be the most prevalent. Mangini and Florio (1959) surveyed 6000 radiographs of the carpus: they found one case of fusion of the

Figure 21–17 Ehlers-Danlos syndrome. *A*, Dorsopalmar roentgenograph of the wrists and hands of a 12-year-old girl. *B*, Enlarged roentgenograph of the wrist: the carpal epiphysis of the right ulna consists of several pieces and one fragment simulates os ulnastyloidium: there is bilateral subluxation at the first carpometacarpal junction. *C* illustrates roentgenograph above it.

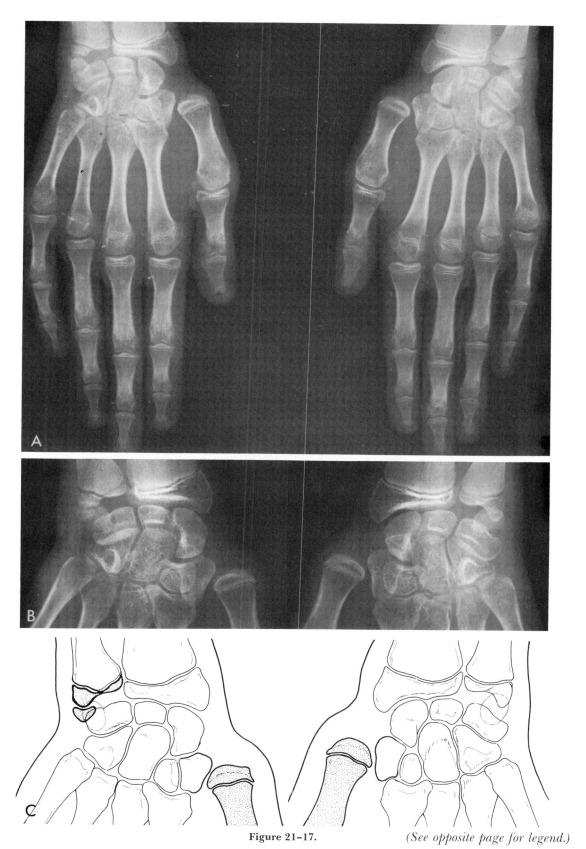

Figure 21-17. *(See opposite page for legend.)*

733

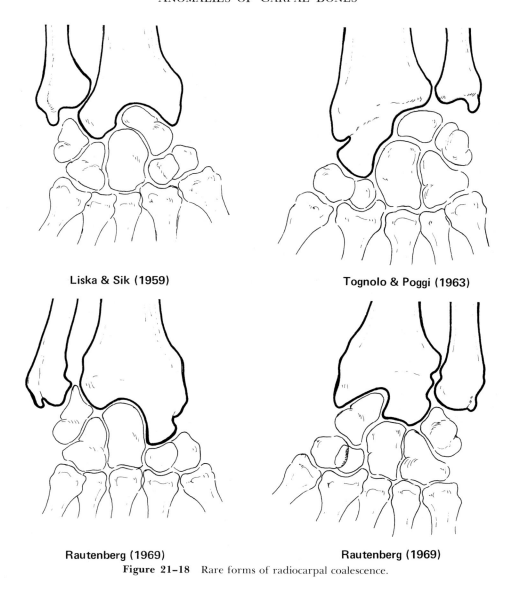

Liska & Sik (1959)

Tognolo & Poggi (1963)

Rautenberg (1969)

Rautenberg (1969)

Figure 21–18   Rare forms of radiocarpal coalescence.

triquetrum with the capitate, two cases of confluence of the capitate and hamate, one of fusion of the pisiform and hamate, and one case of the union of the capitate and third metacarpal bone. "The incidence of lunato-triquetral, capitate-hamate and pisiform-hamate fusion is . . . high in Negroes; in lunato-triquetral fusion, the incidence may be nearly a hundred times greater than in Europeans," Cockshott (1963) wrote. Garn et al (1971) found lunotriquetral fusion in 1.6 percent of 7543 subjects primarily of African origin, as compared to 0.1 percent of 11,663 persons of European extraction. Intercarpal fusion appears to be far more common in black than in white people; it occurs more often in males than in females. Carpal coalescence is often bilateral, especially in black people. Not infrequently, there is also fusion of the tarsal bones (Figs. 21–19 to 21–23).

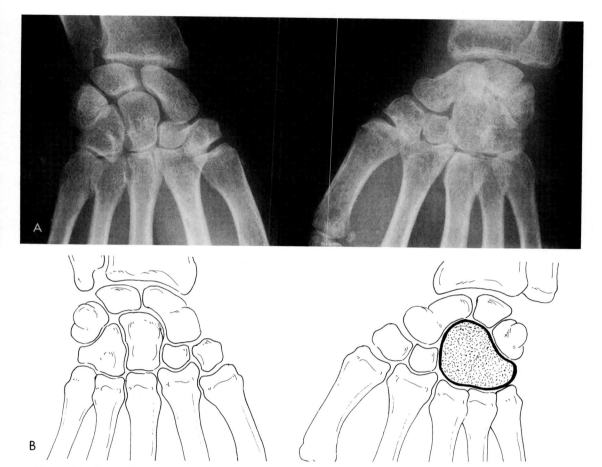

Figure 21-19 Unilateral fusion of the capitate and hamate bones associated with absence of the styloid process of the ipsilateral ulna. *A*, Dorsovolar roentgenograph of the wrist of an adult woman. *B*, Sketch illustrating the same.

Intercarpal fusion is often seen in association with regional anomalies of the hand and forearm. Algyogyi (1910) presented a case in which the same upper limb manifested coalescence of the proximal row of carpal bones, proximal radioulnar synostosis, absence of the thumb and its metacarpal, and side-to-side fusion of the two ulnar metacarpals. Campbell and Kerr (1912) featured the roentgenograph of a forearm with tortuous radius, diamond-shaped ulna, and coalescence of the carpal bones; these features were suggestive of Nievergelt's (1944) syndrome, to be discussed in Chapter Twenty-eight. Alexander and Johnson (1941) reported a case of Madelung deformity with lunotriquetral fusion.

Gordon et al (1948) reported a 13-year-old girl with bilateral dislocation of the radial heads, bilateral dislocation of the patellae, Klippel-Feil type of deformity of the cervical spine, and lunotriquetral fusion of the right wrist. Fuhrmann et al (1964–1965) described a mother and son with bilateral synostosis of the elbow, symphalangism, carpal and tarsal coalescence, short middle phalanges, and short metacarpals. Lunotriquetral fusion was reported again in the

(Text continued on page 740.)

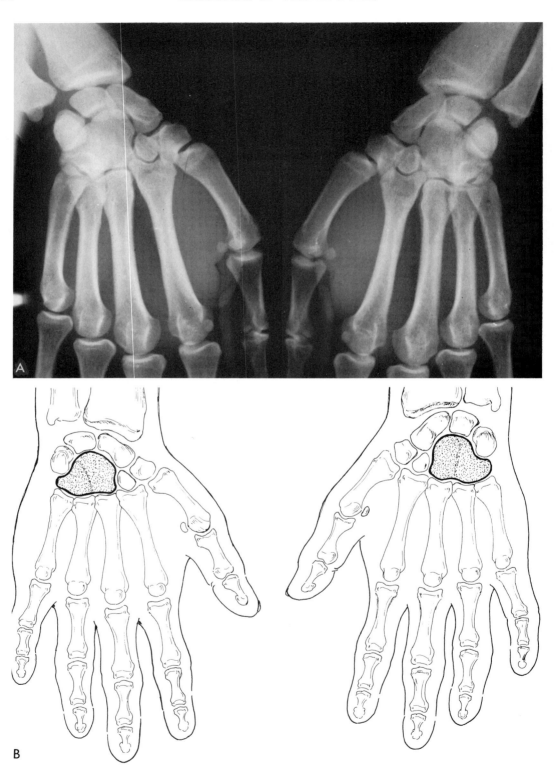

Figure 21–20   Bilateral fusion of the capitate and hamate bones. *A*, Dorsovolar roentgenograph of the wrists of a 17-year-old boy. *B*, Sketch illustrating the same.

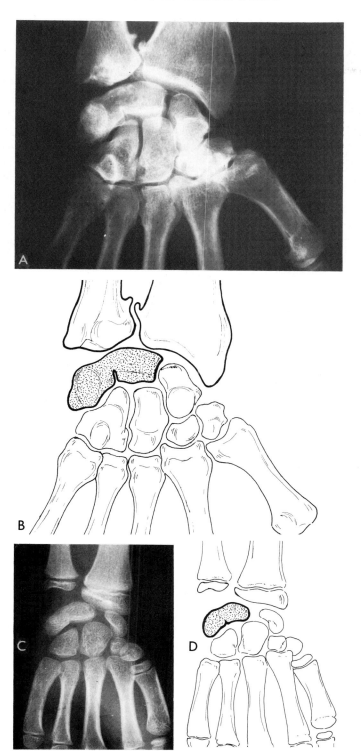

Figure 21–21 Lunotriquetral fusion. *A*, Dorsovolar roentgenograph of the left wrist of an adult man. *B*, Sketch illustrating the same. *C*, Dorsovolar roentgenograph of the left wrist of an eight-year-old girl. *D*, Sketch illustrating the same.

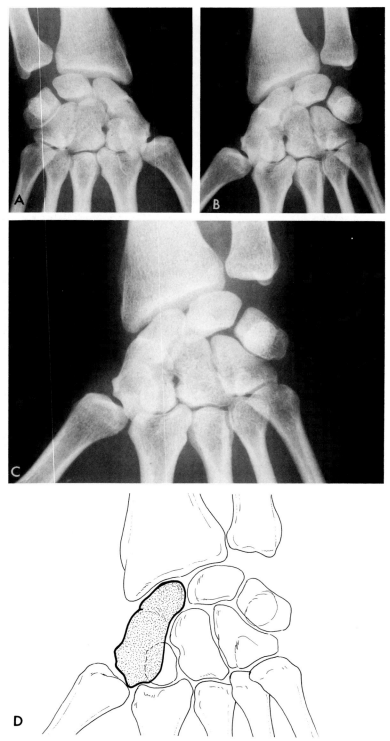

Figure 21–22 Bilateral coalescence of the scaphoid and trapezium. *A* and *B*: dorsopalmar roentgenograph of the right and left wrists of a 29-year-old woman who complained of having sprained her right wrist. *C*, Enlarged roentgenograph of the left wrist, showing that on this side also the scaphoid and trapezium had coalesced. *D*, Sketch illustrating the same.

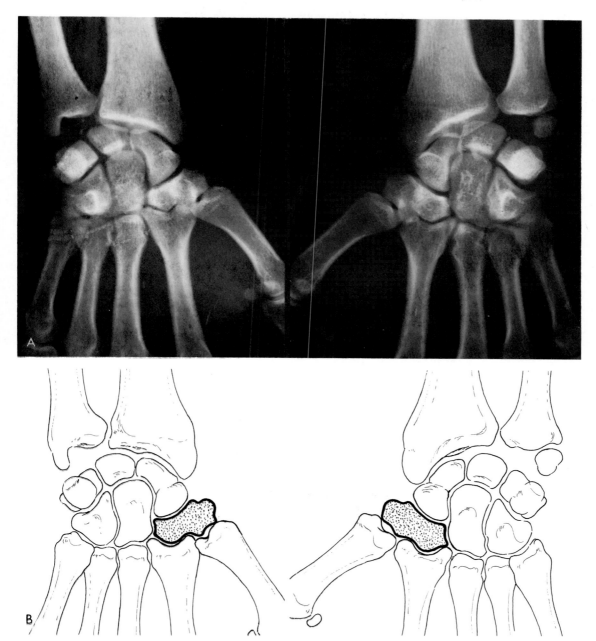

Figure 21–23   Bilateral fusion of the trapezium and trapezoid bones. *A*, Dorsovolar roentgenograph of the wrists of a 19-year-old woman. *B*, Sketch illustrating the same.

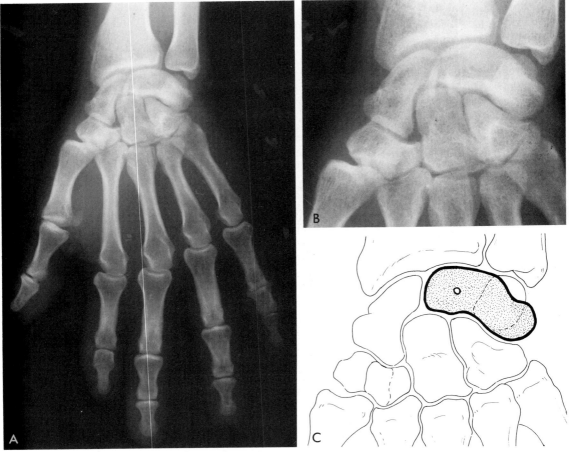

Figure 21–24 Carpal coalescence in hypophalangy. *A,* Dorsopalmar roentgenograph of the left hand of a 16-year-old boy with absent middle phalanx of the index finger and brachymesophalangy of the fifth digit. *B,* Enlarged roentgenograph of the wrist showing lunotriquetral fusion. *C,* Sketch illustrating the same.

complex described by Banki (1965) in which the carpal anomaly concurred with clinodactlyly, brachymetacarpy, and leptometacarpy or metacarpals with thin shafts. Perhaps the most common regional accompaniments of carpal coalescence are oligodactyly and brachydactyly (Figs. 21–24 to 21–28).

Carpal coalescence has also been reported in the following syndromes: acro-pector-vertebral dysplasia—by Gross et al (1969); arthrogryposis multiplex congenita—by Orlin and Alpert (1967); the complex consisting of congenital heart disease, fusion of the cervical vertebrae, and conductive deafness—by Forney et al (1966); Ellis-van Creveld chondroectodermal dysplasia—by Caffey (1952), and McKusick et al (1964); in Nievergelt syndrome—by Pearlman et al (1964); in otopalatodigital syndrome by Gorlin (1969); in bird-headed dwarfism by Seckel (1960); in hand-foot-uterus syndrome—by Stern et al (1970) and Poznanski and associates (1970, 1971). This last complex is characterized by duplication of the genital tract (in females), small feet, short great toes with spiked terminal phalanges, dwarfed thumbs due to short first metacarpals, and carpal coalescence, usually scaphoid with trapezium.

(Text continued on page 745.)

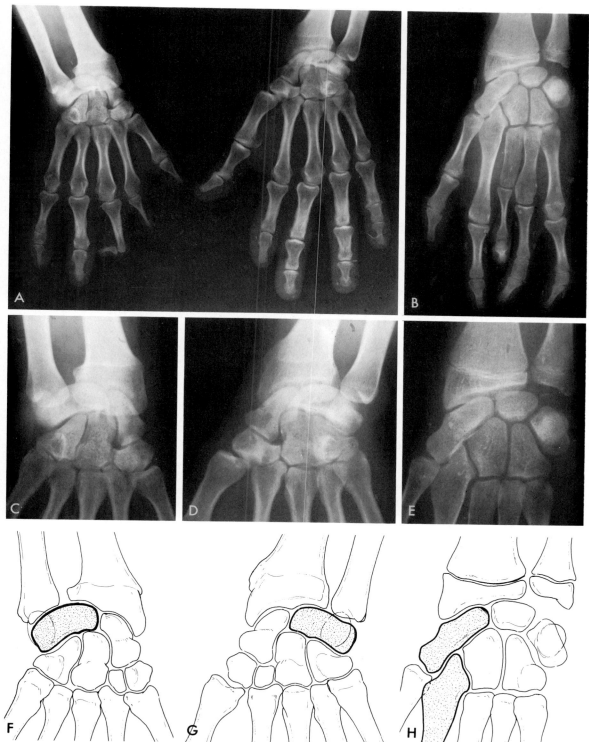

Figure 21–25 Carpal coalescence in various forms of hypophalangy. *A*, Dorsopalmar roentgenograph of the hands of an adult man with bilateral lunotriquetral fusion associated with hypophalangy. *B*, Dorsopalmar roentgenograph of the left hand of a 12-year-old girl with fusion of the scaphoid and trapezium and trapezoid with the second metacarpal. *C*, *D*, and *E*, Enlarged roentgenographs of the wrists shown in *A* and *B*. *F*, *G*, and *H* illustrate the roentgenograph above each.

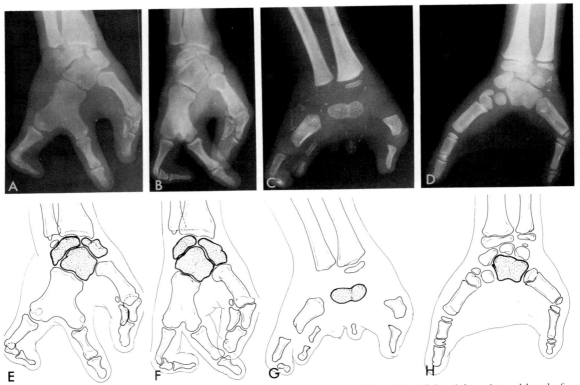

Figure 21–26 Carpal coalescence in central oligodactyly. *A*, Dorsopalmar view of the right wrist and hand of an adult man with only three massive bones in the wrist. *B*, Oblique view of the same. *C*, Dorsopalmar view of the right wrist and hand of a three-year-old boy with fused capitate and hamate bones. *D*, Dorsopalmar view of the left hand and wrist of an 11-year-old girl with a massive bone composed of capitate and hamate. *E*, *F*, *G*, and *H* illustrate the roentgenograph above each.

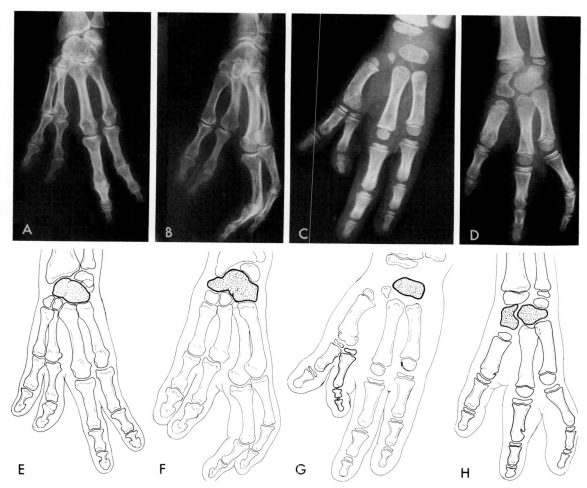

Figure 21–27 Carpal coalescence in ulnar oligodactyly. *A*, Dorsopalmar roentgenograph of the hand of a 34-year-old woman with absent ulnar styloid, two biphalangeal radial and two triphalangeal ulnar digits, and massive coalescence of the scaphoid, lunate, capitate and hamate bones. *B*, Oblique roentgenograph of the same. *C*, Dorsopalmar roentgenograph of the hand of a five-year-old boy with bifurcate thumb and two fingers and coalescence of the capitate and hamate bones. *D*, Dorsopalmar roentgenograph of the hand of an eight-year-old boy with a thumb and two fingers and fusion of the scaphoid, trapezium, and trapezoid, absent lunate, and coalescence of triquetrum, capitate, and hamate bones. *E*, *F*, *G*, and *H* illustrate the roentgenograph above each.

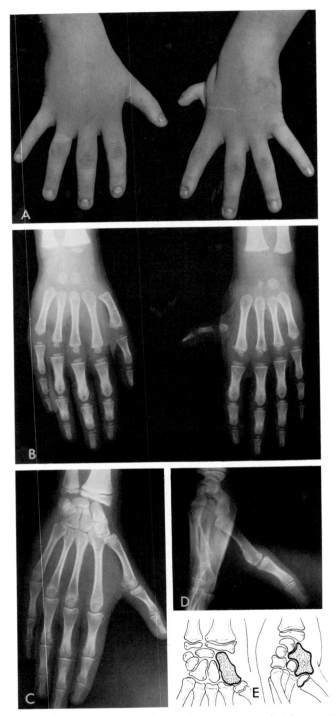

Figure 21–28 Distal intercalary defect of the radial ray associated with eventual appearance of scaphoid-trapezium coalescence of opposite carpus. *A,* Dorsal view of the hands of a 26-month-old boy with floating left thumb. *B,* Dorsopalmar roentgenograph: the carpal epiphysis of the left radius is represented by a barely discernible dot; the left ulna extends further distal than the radius; the left capitate is smaller; the left first metacarpal is defective proximally and the phalanges of the left thumb are rudimentary. *C,* Dorsopalmar roentgenograph of the right hand 10 years later, showing complete fusion of the scaphoid and trapezium. *D,* Lateral roentgenograph of the right carpus. *E,* Sketch illustrating scaphoid-trapezium fusion.

SUMMARY

Six main classes of congenital anomalies of the carpal bones are recorded: (1) disorderly and disharmonious development, (2) absences, (3) accessories, (4) articular incongruities, (5) bipartition, and (6) fusion. Absences of the carpal bones are almost always associated with defects of the radial or ulnar rays or with split hand. The most significant accessory bone of the carpus is the styloidium at the base of the third metacarpal bone. Congenital articular incongruities are comparatively rare; they seem to favor the first and third carpometacarpal joints. In the former location, they become clinically manifest as precocious osteoarthritis, and in the latter as *carpe bossu*, often surmounted by a ganglion. Bipartite scaphoid gains its importance from the fact that it may be confused with fracture. Coalescence of carpal bones is the most common congenital anomaly of the carpus and is usually associated with comparable changes of the tarsus; it often is accompanied by other synostotic states — symphalangism, radioulnar synostosis, Klippel–Feil syndrome, and stapes footplate fixation with conductive deafness. Carpal coalescence is more common in Negroes.

References

Albrecht, R.: Beitrag zum Vorkommen der Synostosen am Hand- und Fusswurzelskelett. *Z. Orthop.*, *105*:215–223, 1968.

Alexander, H.H., Jr. and Johnson, G. H.: Dyschondroplasia of the radial epiphysis (Madelung's deformity) with fusion of semilunar and triangular bones. *Am. J. Surg.*, *53*:349–351, 1941.

Algyogyi, H.: Ein seltener Fall von Missbildung einer Oberextremität. Brachydactylie mit Pero- und Ektrodaktylie. *Fortschr. Röntgenstr.*, *16*:286–290; Taf. XXII, figs. 4, 5, 1910.

Anderson, R. J.: Division of scaphoid bone of the carpus with notes on other varieties of carpal bones. *J. Anat. Physiol.*, *17*:253–255, 1883.

Arens, W.: Über die angeborene Synostose zwischen dem Os lunatum und dem Os triquetrum. *Fortschr. Röntgenstr.*, *77*:772–774, 1950.

Auvray: Scaphoïde double de la main. *Bull. Soc. Anat. (Paris)*, *12*:135–136, 1898.

Baciu, C., Gorun, N., and Roventza, N.: Le scaphoïde carpien bipartite. *Acta Orthop Belg.*, *32*:920–925, 1966.

Banki, Z.: Kombination erblicher Gelenk- und Knochenanomalien an der Hand. Zwei neue Röntgenzeichen. *Fortschr. Röntgenstr.*, *103*:598–604, 1965.

Bassöe, E., and Bassöe, H. H.: The styloid bone and carpe bossu disease. *Am. J. Roentgenol.*, *74*:886–888, 1955.

Battelli, L.: Sulle sinostosi del semilunare e piramidale. *Chir. Organi. Mov.*, *47*:506–511, 1959.

Becker, F.: Über eine ungewöhnliche Handgelenksverbindung (angeborene Radius-lunatum-Synostose). *Fortschr. Röntgenstr.*, *52*:345–349, 1935.

Behr, F.: Ein Fall von Missbildung der Handwurzel. *Fortschr. Röntgenstr.*, *18*:263–264; Taf. XVIII, Fig. b., 1911.

Behr, F.: Über eine symmetrische Synostose der Hand- und Fusswurzelknochen. *Arch. Orthop. Unfallchir.*, *32*:12–15, 1933.

Bellamy, E.: Singular malformation of the wrist and hand (coalescence of lunate, cuneiform, trapezoids, magnum and unciform; congenital dislocation of the elbow joint). *J. Anat. Physiol.*, *8*:383, 1874.

Belot, J. and Nathan, L.: Soudure du sémilunaire et du pyramidal. *Presse Méd.*, *44*:1840, 1936.

Beresowski, A., and Lundie, J. K.: Sequence in the time of ossification of the carpal bones in 705 African children from birth to 6 years of age. *South Afr. J. Sci.*, *17*:25–31, 1952.

Berthoux, F., Robert , J. M., Zech, P., Fries, D., and Traeger, J.: Acro-osteolyse essential a debut carpien et tarsien avec nephropathie. *Arch. Fr. Pediatr.*, *28*:615–630, 1971.

Bischofberger, C.: Die symmetrische angeborene Aplasie Handwurzel (angeborene Kurzhand). *Z. Orthop.*, *80*:288–294, 1951.

Blencke, H.: Ein Fall von naviculare carpi bipartitum. *Mschr. Unfallheilkd.*, *33*:75–78, 1926.

Bogart, F. B.: Variations of bones of the wrist. *Am. J. Roentgenol.*, *28*:638–646, 1932.

Boidi-Trotti, G.: Anomalia congenita dell'osso del carpo "os naviculare bipartitum." *Rev. Radiol Fisica Med.*, *4*:556–564, 1932.

Botreau-Roussel, M.: Léger degré de main bote causée par l'absence congénitale de deux scaphoïdes. *Bull. Mem. Soc. Anat.* (Paris), *92*:33–35, 1922.

Boyd, G. I.: Bipartite carpal navicular bone. *Br. J. Surg.*, *20*:455–458, 1933.

Brdiczka, G.: Vererbbare und abgeborene multiple Synostosen an zahlreichen Gelenken der oberen und unteren Extremität. *Fortschr. Röntgenstr.*, *58*:228–233, 1938.

Bugyi, B.: Über die Entwicklung der Handwurzelknochenkerne bei gesunden Schulkindern. *Kinderärztl. Prax.*, *21*:218–221, 1958.

Burckhardt, E.: Zur Klinik und zur pathologischen Histologie des Os styloideum carpi. *Röntgenpraxis*, *16*:108–115, 1944.

Buschke, F.: Doppelte Kernanlage des Lunatum carpi im Kindesalter. *Röntgenpraxis*, *6*:385–386, 1934.

Butterworth, R. D., and Daner, W. E.: A bilateral anomaly of the wrist. Report of a case. *J. Bone Joint Surg.*, *28*:385, 1946.

Bysch, K. H., Drews, J., and Gunther, D.: Synostosen zwischen Multangulum minus und Capitatum. *Fortschr. Röntgenstr.*, *115*:267–268, 1971.

Cabon, P.: A propos d'une anomalie du carpe. *J. Radiol. Electrol.*, *31*:285–286, 1950.

Caffaratti, E.: Scafoide bipartite bilateral de carpo di natura congenita. *Quad. Radiol.*, *13*:159, 1950.

Caffey, J.: Chondroechtodermal dysplasia (Ellis-van Creveld disease). Report of three cases. *Am. J. Roentgenol.*, *68*:875–882, 1952.

Campbell, W. F., and Kerr, Le G.: *The Surgical Diseases of Children.* New York, D. Appleton & Co., p. 597–598; fig. 234, 1912.

Canigiani, T.: Beiderseitige Anomalie im Bereiche der Handwurzelknochen. *Röntgenpraxis*, *8*:142–143, 1936.

Carter, R. M.: Carpal boss: a commonly overlooked deformity of the carpus. *J. Bone Joint Surg.*, *23*:935–940, 1941.

Cave, A. J. E.: Fusion of carpal elements. *J. Anat.*, *60*:460–461, 1926.

Childress, H. M.: Fracture of a bipartite carpal navicular. *J. Bone Joint Surg.*, *25*:446–447, 1943.

Clerici-Bagozzi, I.: Contributo allo studio radiologico delle ossa del carpo, III: Anomalie morfologiche et numeriche. *Rass. Prev. Soc., 29*:45–78, 1939.

Cockshott, W. P.: Carpal anomalies amongst Yorubas. *West Afr. Med. J., 8*:185–190, 1959.

Cockshott, W. P.: Carpal fusion. *Am. J. Roentgenol., 89*:1260–1271, 1963.

Cockshott, W. P.: Pisiform hamate fusion. *J. Bone Joint Surg., 51A*:778, 1969.

Conlon, P. C., and Hanley, T.: Congenital deformity of the carpus associated with maldevelopment of certain thenar muscles. *J. Bone Joint Surg., 39A*:452–462, 1957.

Cotta, H.: Ein Beitrag zur Differentialdiagnose Navicularpseudarthrose-Os naviculare bipartitum carpi. *Arch. Orthop. Unfallchir., 52*:581–589, 1961.

Curr, J. F.: Congenital fusion of lunate and triquetrum. *Br. J. Surg., 34*:99–100, 1946.

Curtis, P. H., Jr.: The hunchback carpal bone. *J. Bone Joint Surg., 43A*:392–394, 1961.

Dau, W.: Naviculare bipartitum manus. *Mschr. Unfallheilkd., 67*:74–76, 1964.

Davison, E. P.: Congenital hypoplasia of the carpal scaphoid bone. *J. Bone Joint Surg., 44B*:816–827, 1962.

Dean, R. F., and Jones, P. R.: Fusion of triquetral and lunate bones shown in serial radiographs. *Am. J. Phys. Anthropol., 17*:278–288, 1959.

Dederich, R.: Kongenitale Synostosen von Handwurzelknochen. *Mschr. Unfallheilkd., 58*:112–117, 1955.

Della Valle, L.: Contributo alla ricera di una primitiva duplicita dell' unciform del' carpo. *Boll Acad. Med. Genova, 13*:1–5, 1898.

Demoraes: Deux cas de "carpus bossum" *Rev. d'Orthop., 26*:133–135, 1953.

Dérot, M., Rathery, M., Rosselin, G., and Gatellier, C.: Acro-ostéolyse du carpe, pied creux, scoliose et strabisme chez un jeune file atteinte d'insaffisance renal. *Bull. Mém. Soc. Méd. Hop.* (Paris), *77*:223–228, 1961.

Derry, D. E.: Two cases of fusion of the semilunar and cuneiform bones in Negroes. *J. Anat. Physiol.,* (3 s), *2*:56–58, 1906.

Deutici, L.: Osso scafoide accessorio bilaterale. *Radiol. Med. Milano, 22*:1010–1012, 1935.

Dreiack, D., and Holland, C.: Synostosen im Handwurzelbereich, angeboren oder erworben? *Z. Orthop., 108*:461–468, 1970.

Drewes, J.: Die angeborenen Synostosen der Fusswurzelknochen. In: *Die Chirurgische Behandlung der angeborenen Fehlbildungen.* Herausgegeben von Priv. -Doz. Dr. K. Kremer, pp. 517–524; Abb. 2, 1961.

Drewes, J., and Günther, D.: Über angeborene Synostosen im Handwurzelbereich. *Radiologe, 6*:64–68, 1966.

Dubois, H. J.: Nievergelt-Pearlman syndrome. Synostosis in feet and hands with dysplasia of elbows. *J. Bone Joint Surg., 52B*:325–329, 1970.

Dupas, J., and Badelon, P.: La synostose pyramido-sémilunaire. *Ann. Anat. Pathol. Méd. Chir., 9*: 335–339, 1932.

Dwight, T.: The clinical significance of variations of wrist and ankle. *J.A.M.A., 47*:252–255, 1906.

Dwight, T.: *Variations of Bones of the Hand and Foot. A Clinical Atlas.* Philadelphia, J. B. Lippincott Co., pp. 1–13, 1907.

Eaves, J., and Campiche, R.: Note on malformation of the carpus. *J. Bone Joint Surg., 4*:78–80, 1922.

Eggimann, P.: Zur Bipartition des Lunatum. *Radiol. Clin., 20*:65–70, 1951.

Ellis, R. W. B., and van Creveld, S.: A syndrome characterized by ectodermal dysplasia, polydactyly, chondrodysplasia and congenital morbus cordis. *Arch. Dis. Child., 15*:65–84, 1940.

Ellsworth, H. A.: Inheritance of carpal displacement. *J. Hered., 18*:133, 1927.

Epstein, J.: Ein Fall von angeborener Anomalie der Handwurzelknochen. *Arch. Orthop. Unfallchir., 27*:266–268, 1929.

Esau, P.: Das Os triangular. *Fortschr. Röntgenstr., 37*:889–890, 1928.

Esau, P.: Angeborene Synostosen im Bereich des Carpus und Tarsus. *Röntgenpraxis, 5*:235–237, 1933.

Faulkner, D. M.: Bipartite carpal scaphoid. *J. Bone Joint Surg., 10*:284–289, 1928.

Fiolle, J., and Coudray: Dernieres observations de "carpe bossu". *Bull. Mém. Soc. Nat. Chir., 58*:545–547, 1932.

Florio, L.: L'os centrali carpi come peradigma dell' evoluzione filogenetica del carpo. *Riv. Chir. Mano., 3*:238–244, 1965.

Forney, W. R., Robinson, S. J., and Pascoe, D. J.: Congenital heart disease, deafness and skeletal malformations: a new syndrome. *J. Pediatr., 68*:14–26, 1966.

Freyer, B.: Ungewöhnliche Beobachtung doppelseitiger kongenitaler Synostosen zwischen Radius und Ulna sowie zwischen Os lunatum und Os triquetrum verbunden mit einer doppelseitigen Abortiform der Madelungschen Deformität (sog. "Hulten-plus-Variante") in der II. Generation bei doppelseitigem des equino-varus in der I. Generation. *Radiologe, 6*:235–255, 1966.

Frick, W.: Synostose zwischen Os lunatum und Os triquetrum. *Fortschr. Röntgenstr., 72*:242–243, 1949.

Fuhrmann, W. G.: Steffens, C., and Rompe, U.: Dominant erbliche doppelseitige Dysplasie and Synostose des Ellenbogengelenks. Mit symmetrischer Brachymesophalangie und Brachymetacarpie sowie Synostosen im Finger-Hand- und Fusswurelbereich. *Humangenetik, 3*:64–77, 1966.

Fuhrmann, W., Steffens, C., Schwartz, G., and Wagner, A.: Dominante erbliche Brachydaktylie mit Gelenkplasien. *Humangenetik, 1*:337–353, 1964–1965.

Garn, S. M., Frisancho, A. R., Poznanski, A. K., Schweitzer, J., and McCann, M. B.: Analysis of triquetral-lunate fusion. *Am. J. Phys. Anthropol., 34*:431–433, 1971.

Geyer, E.: Beitrag zu den Synostosbildungen der Hand- und Fusswurzel. *Z. Orthop., 90*:395–408, 1958.

Gfeller, J., and Budliger, H.: Homocystinuria and os lunatum. *Lancet, 2*:548, 1966.

Girod, E.: Beitrag zur Radius-lunatum-Synostose. *Fortschr. Röntgenstr., 100*:282–283, 1964.

Goldstein, R.: Congenital synostosis of carpal and tarsal bones and ankylosis cubiti. *Radiol. Clin., 17*:66–73, 1948.

Gollasch, W.: Die zweigeteilte Kahnbein der Hand, seine Bedeutung für die Erkennung, Behandlung und Begutachtung der Kahnbeinverletzungen. *Röntgenpraxis, 11*:564–566, 1939.

Gombert, J. H.: Rechtsseitige, kongenitale Verschmelzung des Os naviculare und lunatum mit Radiusepiphyse. *Fortschr. Röntgenstr., 91*:527–528, 1959.

Gordon, J., Schechter, N., and Perlman, A. W.: Multiple congenital malformations of the skeletal system: a case report. *Am. J. Roentgenol., 59*:533–538, 1948.

Gorham, L. W., and Stout, A. P.: Massive osteolysis (acute, spontaneous absorption of bone, phantom bone, disappearing bone); its relation to hemangiomatosis. *J. Bone Joint Surg., 37A*:985–1004, 1955.

Gorlin, R. J.: Discussion on oto-palato-digital syndrome. *In* Bergsma, D., (ed.):*Birth Defects: Original Article Series.* New York, National Foundation—March of Dimes, Vol. V, No. 3, pp. 45–47, 1969.

Graham, C. E., and Mehta, M. C.: Bilateral congenital carpal fusion in a champion golfer. *Clin. Orthop., 83*:70–72, 1972.

Grashey, R.: Handwurzelsynostose (Lunatum-Triquetrum). *Röntgenpraxis, 10*:50–51, 1938.

Greulich, W. W., and Pyle, S. J.: *Radiographic Atlas of Skeletal Development of the Hand and Wrist.* Second Edition. London, Oxford University Press, pp. 1–252, 1959.

Gross, F. R., Herrmann, J., and Opitz, J. M.: The F-form of acropectorovertebral dysplasia: The F-syndrome. *In* Bergsma, D., (ed.): *Birth Defects: Original Article Series.* New York, National Foundation—March of Dimes. Vol. V, No. 3, pp. 48–63, 1969.

Gruber, W.: Os naviculare carpi bipartitum. *Arch. Pathol. Anat. Physiol. Klin. Med., 69*:391–396, Taf. XIII, fig. 2, 1877.

Gruber, W.: Synostose des Os capitatum carpi und des Os metacarpale III. an dem Processus styloides des letzteren. *Arch. Pathol. Anat. Physiol. , 78*:100–101, 1879.

Gruber, W.: Navicularia carpi tripartita. *Arch. Pathol. Anat. Physiol. Klin. Med., 94*:343–349, Taf. VIII, figs. 1–2, 1883.

Gruber, W.: Drei neue Fälle von Os lunatum carpi bipartitum, ein Fall von Os lunatum tripartitum (vorher nicht gesehen). Verhalten des Os lunatum secundarium dorsale wie ein "Os lunatum secundarium" wie ein "Os centrale carpi medium" in einum veröffentlichtem Falle und den neuen Fällen. *Arch. Pathol. Anat. Physiol. Med., 98*:408–413, 1884.

Haehner: Doppelseitige nichttraumatische Zweiteilung des Kahnbeins. *Mschr. Unfallheilkd., 39*:210–221, 1932.

Hammond, G.: Unilateral, congenital synostosis of lunate and triangular bones. *Surgery, 22*:566–567, 1947.

Hanley, T., and Conlon, P. C.: Congenital deformity of the carpus associated with maldevelopment of certain thenar muscles. *J. Bone Joint Surg., 39b*:458–462, 1957.

Hardman, T. G., and Wigoder, S. B.: An unusual development of carpal scaphoid. *Br. J. Radiol., 1*:155–158, 1928.

Heimerzheim, A.: Über einige akzessorische Handwurzelknochen nebst ihrer chirurgischen Bedeutung. *Dtsch. Z. Chir., 190*:88–96, 1925.

Henry, M. G.: Anomalous fusion of the scaphoid and the greater multangular bones. *Arch. Surg., 50*:240–241, 1945.

Hindenach, J. C. R.: Bilateral congenital fusion of the semilunar and cuneiform bones. Report of a case. *Br. J. Surg., 35*:104–105, 1947.

Hodgson, A. R.: Congenital retardation in development of the carpal navicular, first metacarpal, and styloid process of the radius. *Br. J. Surg., 31*:95–96, 1943.

Hoffmann, D.: Einige seltenere Handwurzelverschmelzungen und andere Missbildungen des Handskeletts, *Röntgenpraxis, 12*:41–45, Abb. 1, Abb. 2, Abb. 3a, and Abb. 4, 1940.

Holl, M.: Über eine angeborene Koalition des Os lunatum und des Os triquetrum carpi. *Wien. Med. Jahrb.,* pp. 499–502, 1882.

Holland, C. T.: Two cases of rare deformity of feet and hands. *Arch. Radiol. Electrotherapy, 22*:234–239, 1918.

Holt, J. F., and Allen, R. J.: Radiologic signs in primary aminoacidurias. *Ann. Radiol., 10*;317–321, 1967.

Holt, M., and Oram, S.: Familial heart disease with skeletal malformations. *Br. Heart. J., 22*:236–242, 1960.

Hopf, A.: *Handbuch der Orthopädie.* Stuttgart, G. Thieme Bd. Ill, p. 473, 1959.

Horvath, F., and Galle, T.: Eine eigenartige Handwurzelknochenvariation. *Fortschr. Röntgenstr., 103*:500–501, 1965.

Hübner, A.: Zweiteilung des Kahnbeins der Handwurzel. *Mschr. Unfallheilkd., 56*:193, 1953.

Hudson, E.: Unusual carpal abnormality. *Radiography, 9*:81–82, 1943.

Hughes, P. C. R., and Tanner, J. M.: The development of carpal bone fusion as seen in serial radiographs. *Br. J. Radiol., 39*:943–949, 1966.

Hulten, C.: Über anatomische Variationen der Handgelenksknochen. *Acta. Radiol..* (Stockholm), *9*:155–166; Tab. IX-XXI, 1928.

Izquierdo, J.: Nouveau cas d'os intermediaire de l'avantbras. *Arch. Anat. Histol. Embryol., 4*:483–486, 1925.

Janda, J., and Stepanek, J.: Congenital confluence of the scaphoid, semilunar and radial epiphyses. (Czech) *Cesk Radiol., 22*:101–103, 1968.

Johnston, H. M.: Epilunar and hypolunar ossicles, division of scaphoid and other abnormalities in the carpal region (illustrated by drawings from specimens). *J. Anat. Physiol., 41*:59–65, 1906.

Jolly, R., Delahaye, R.P., and Kyriaco, C.: A propos des trois observations de synostose luno-pyramidale. *Rev. Rhum., 29*:288–290, 1962.

Kennedy, C., Shih, V. E., and Rowland, L. P.: Homocystinuria: report in two siblings. *Pediatrics, 36*:736–741, 1965.

Kewesch, E. L.: Über die hereditäre Verschmelzung der Hand- und Fusswurzelknochen. *Fortschr. Röntgenstr., 50*:550–556, 1934.

Klapp, B., and Gebhard, W.: Symmetrische Synostosenbildungen an Hand und Fuss. *Z. Orthop., 81*:637–640, 1952.

Kniepkamp, W.: Os capitatum secundarium und Synostose triquetr.-lunata im Röntgenbild der menschlichen Handwurzel. *Arch. Orth. Unfallchir., 28*:460–466, 1930.

Konrad, R. M.: Untersuchungen über die Beziehungen zwischen dem Stand der Ossification des Handwurzelskeletts und der geistigseelischen Reifung bei achteinhalbjährigen Knaben. *Z. Menschl. Vererb. Konstitutionslehre, 34*:171–186, 1957.

Kosowicz, J.: Carpal sign in gonadal dysgenesis. *J. Clin. Endocrinol. Metab., 22*:949–952, 1962.

Koski, K., Haataja, J., and Lappalainen, M.: Skeletal development of hand and wrist in Finnish children. *Am. J. Phys. Anthropol., 19*:373–382, 1961.

Kowalski, R.: Étude comparative de l'age osseux des enfants de race noire (Africaine) et de race blanche. *Ann. Radiol., 9*:239–250, 1966.

Krause, G. P.: Os naviculare bipartitum beider Hände. *Fortschr. Röntgenstr., 71*:359, 1949.

Kremser, K.: Kurzer Beitrag zur Bildungsanomalie der Handwurzel. *Röntgenpraxis, 6*:243–244, 1934.

Lagier, R., and Rutishauer, E.: Osteoarticular change in a case of essential osteolysis. *J. Bone Joint Surg., 47B*:339–353, 1965.

Lamphier, T. A.: Carpal bossing. *A.M.A. Arch. Surg., 81*:1013–1015, 1960.

Lange, K.: Das Naviculare bipartitum. *Röntgenpraxis, 11*:566–567, 1939.

Larson, L. J., Schottstaedt, E. R., and Bost, F. C.: Multiple congenital dislocations associated with characteristic facial abnormality. *J. Pediatr., 37*:574–581, 1950.

Larsen, R. L., Lascano, M. A., and James, J. M.: Carpal bossing, a common clinical entity. *Mayo Clinic Proc., 33*:337–343, 1958.

Leboucq, H.: Recherches sur la morphologie du carpe chez les mammifères. *Arch. Biologie, 5*:35–102, 1884.

Leger, W.: Beobachtung einer angeborenen Synostose zwischen Multangulum minus und Metacarpal. 2. *Z. Orthop., 87*:70–76, 1956.

Leni, E.: Ossa soprannumerarie, partite e sesamoide degli arti. *Arch. Ortop., 54*:347–403, 1938.

Lenz, W.: Familiäre Synostose der Hand- und Fusswurzelknochen. *Humangenetik, 2*:92, 1964.

Lewis, O. J.: Evolutionary change in the primate wrist and inferior radio-ulnar joints. *Anat. Rec., 151*:275–285, 1965.

Lewis, O. J.: The hominoid wrist joint. *Am. J. Phys. Anthropol., 30*:251–267, 1969.

Lindgren, E.: Das Naviculare bipartitum. *Acta Radiol.* (Stockholm), *22*:511–514, 1941.

Liszka, G. and Sik, J.: Der Fall einer radio-lunarischen Synostose. *Fortschr. Röntgenstr., 90*:771, 1959.

Lonnerblad, L.: Über zwei seltene Anomalien im Carpus. ("Verschmelzung"-von os lunatum und os triquetrum sowie von os multangulum minus und os capitatum. *Acta Radiol., 16*:682–690, 1935.

MacConnaill, M. A.: The mechanical anatomy of the carpus and its bearing on some surgical problems. *J. Anat., 75*:166–175, 1941.

MacKay, D. H.: Skeletal maturation in hand: study of development in East African children. *Trans. R. Soc. Trop. Med. Hyg., 46*:135–150, 1952.

MacNair, V.: Effect of dietary supplement on ossification of the bones of the wrist in institut. children. *Am. J. Dis. Child., 58*:295–319, 1939.

MacNair, V. and Roberts, J.: Effects of milk supplement in physical status of institutional children. II. Ossification of the bones of the wrist. *Am. J. Dis. Child., 56*:498–509, 1938.

Mahoudeau, D., Bubrisay, J., Elissalde, B., and Straër, C.: Osteolyse essentialle et nephrite. *Bull Mém. Soc. Med. Hôp.* (Paris), *77*:229, 1961.

Mangini, U., and Boni, V.: Gli elementi accessori delle ossa del carpo. *Arch. Putti, 12*:31–67, 1959.

Mangini, U., and Florio, L.: Sinostosi congenite delle ossa del carpo. *Arch. Putti, 11*:107–123, 1959.

Manson, J. S.: Rare congenital malformations of hands and feet. *J. Anat., 58*:250–253, 1924.

Marie, J., Salet, J., Leveque, B., and Sauvegrain, J.: Syndrome osteodystrophique de nature congenitate probable. *Presse Méd., 64*(2):2173–2176, 1956.

Marti, T.: Ein interssanter Fall von Navicular bipartitum und akzessorischen Handwurzelknochen. *Schweiz. Med. Wochenschr.*, 74:960–962, 1944.

Marti, T.: Weitere Beitrage zum Studium der Handwurzelvarietäten. *Schweiz. Med. Wochenschr.*, 77:890–891, 1947.

McConnell, A. A.: A case of fusion of semilunar and cuneiform bones. *J. Anat.*, 41:302–303, 1907.

McGoey, P.F.: Fracture-dislocation of fused triangular and lunate (congenital). Report of a case. *J. Bone Joint Surg.*, 25:928–929, 1943.

McKusick, V. A., Egeland, J. A., Eldridge, R., and Krusen, D. E.: Dwarfism in the Amish. I. The Ellis-van Creveld syndrome. *Bull. Johns Hopkins Hosp.*, 115:306–336, 1964.

Menegaux, G.: Deux cas de "carpe bossu". *Rev. d'Orthop.*, 21:231–233, 1934.

Mestern, J.: Erbliche Synostosen der Hand- und Fusswurzelknochen. Erbliches os tibiale externum. *Röntgenpraxis*, 6:594–600, 1934.

Meves, F.: Über die Synostosen der Handwurzelknochen. *Z. Orthop.*, 67:17–20, 1937.

Minaar, A. B. de V.: Congenital fusion of lunate and triquetral in South African Bantu. *J. Bone Joint Surg.*, 34B:45–48, 1959.

Morestin, H.: De l'ankylose des articulations du carpe. *Bull. Soc. Anat.*, (5 s.), 10:651, 1896.

Mori, A.: Contributo allo studio delle variazioni morphologische a delle asimetrie schletriche con speciale riguardo a quelle dello scafoide. *Atti VI. Congr. Intern. Accidents du Travail 1931.* Geneve, pp. 916–921, 1931.

Mori, A.: Della divisione dello scafoide e dell sue variazioni morfologiche in relazione alla pratica in-fortunistica. *Rass. Prev. Soc.*, 21;116–121, 1934.

Morreels, C. L., Jr., Fletcher, B. D., Weilbaecher, R. G., and Dorst, J. P.: Roentgenographic features of homosystinuria. *Radiology*, 90:1150–1158, 1968.

Mouchet, A.: Division congénitale du scaphoide carpien simulant une fracture: ("naviculare carpi bipartitum"). *Rev. d'Orthop.*, (3 s.), 5:201–211, 1914.

Müller, W.: Ein Beitrag zu den angeborenen Missbildungen der Karpelknochen (doppelseitige Hypoplasie des Mond- und Kahnbeines, angeborene Luxation des einen Os Naviculare). *Arch. Orthop. Unfallchir.*, 21:401–408, 1923.

Neiss, A.: Doppelseitige Synostose zwischen dem os multangulum und dem os capitatum. *Fortschr. Röntgenstr.*, 82:825, 1955.

Neumann, C.: Starke einseitige Hypoplasie eines os naviculare. *Fortschr. Röntgenstr.*, 91:529, 1959.

Nievergelt, K.: Positiver Vaterschaftsnachweis auf Grund erblicher Missbildungen der Extremitäten. *Arch. Julius-Klaus-Stift*, 19:157–195, 1944.

Ogilvie, W. H.: Bipartite scaphoids. *Proc. R. Soc. Med.* London (Sect. on Orthopedics), 24:40–41, 1930.

Omer, G. E., Jr., and Mossman, D. L.: Bone agenesis. A case involving the carpus and tarsus. *J. Bone Joint Surg.*, 40A:917–920, 1958.

O'Rahilly, R.: Epitriquetrum, hypotriquetrum and lunotriquetrum. *Acta Radiol.*, 39:401–408, 1953.

O'Rahilly, R.: A survey of carpal and tarsal anomalies. *J. Bone Joint Surg.*, 35A:626–639, 1953.

O'Rahilly, R.: Developmental deviations in carpus and tarsus. *Clin. Orthop.*, 10:9–18, 1957.

O'Rahilly, R., Gray, D. J., and Gardner, E.: Chondrification in the hands and feet of staged human embryo. *Contrib. Embryol. Carnegie Inst.*, 36:183–192, 1957.

Orlin, H., and Alpert, M.: Carpal coalition in arthrogryposis multiplex congenita. *Br. J. Radiol.*, 40:220–222, 1967.

Paas, R.: Doppelseitige Zweiteilung des Kahnbeins mit multiplen System der Mittelhand- und Handwurzelknochen. *Mschr. Unfallheilkd.*, 46:577, 1939.

Paterson, A. M.: Anomalies in the skeleton of a Negro. *J. Anat. Physiol.*, 27:22–24, 1893.

Pearlman, H. S., Edkin, R., and Warren, R. F.: Familial tarsal and carpal synostosis with radial head subluxation (Nievergelt's syndrome). *J. Bone Joint Surg.*, 46A:585–592, 1964.

Pellegrino, A., and Jolly, R.: Étude radiologique des malformations poignet chez l'Africain. *Bull. Soc. Med. Afr. Noire*, 4:102–105, 1959.

Pokrovsky, S. A.: Os naviculare carpi bipartitum bilaterale. (Russian). *Vestn. Rentgen.*, 12:366–369, 1935. Also in *Arch. Orthop. Unfallchir.*, 35:313–316, 1935.

Polacco, A.: Sulla carpocifusi (carpe bossu). *Atti. del XLVI Congresso Soc. Ital. Ortop. Traum.* Roma, L. Pozzi, pp. 131–138, 1961.

Politzer, W.: Über Missbildungen des Hand- und Fussskeletts und über ihre formale Genese. *Fortschr. Röntgenstr.*, 43:605–619, 1931.

Pomeranz, M. M.: Os ulnare externum. *Bull. Hosp. Joint Dis.*, 10:110–111, 1949.

Portmann, J.: Ausgedehnte Synostosen einer Handwurzel. *Fortschr. Röntgenstr.*, 98:365–366, 1963.

Poznanski, A. K., and Holt, J. F.: The carpals in congenital malformation syndromes. *Am. J. Roentgenol.*, 112:443–459, 1971.

Poznanski, A. K., Gall, J. C., Jr., and Stern, A. M.: Skeletal manifestations of the Holt-Oram syndrome. *Radiology*, 94:45–53, 1970.

Poznanski, A. K., Stern, A. M., and Gall, J. C., Jr.: Radiographic findings in hand-foot-uterus syndrome (HFUS). *Radiology*, 95:129–134, 1970.

Pryor, J. W.: Normal viariations in the ossification of bones due to genetic factors. *J. Hered.*, 30:248–255, 1939.

Pye-Smith, R. J.: Notes on a family presenting in most of its members certain deformities about the joints of both limbs. *Med. Press Circular*, 34:504–505, 1883.

Randelli, M.: Sulla bipartizione dello scafoide carpale. *Arch. Ortop.*, 74:700–706, 1961.

Rauterberg, E.: Beitrag zur Arbeit "Angeborene Synostose von Radius, Naviculare und Lunatum mit benachbarter Arthrose" von G. Reisinger und D. v. Torklus. *Arch. Orthop. Unfallchir.* 63:133–134, 1968.

Reckling, F.: Eine anlagemässige Zweiteilung des Handwurzel-Kahnbeins beiderseits. *Mschr. Unfallheilkd.*, 46:146, 1939.

Reich, B.: Ein Fall von doppelseitiger Spaltung des Naviculare der Hand durch Berufsschädigung. *Arch. Orthop. Unfallchir.*, 32:247–253, 1933.

Reisinger, G., and Torklus, D.: Angeborene Synostose von Radius, Naviculare und Lunatum mit benachbarter Arthrose. *Arch. Orthop. Unfallchir.*, 63:159–161, 1968.

Reisner, A.: Drei Fälle von os supranaviculare. *Röntgenpraxis*, 2:422–425, 1930.

Reiss, J.: Über angeborene Synostosen zwischen Lunatum und Triquetrium, *Röntgenpraxis*, 8:716–717, 1936.

Renner, E.: Entwicklung einer Synostose zwischen Lunatum und Triquetrum der rechten Hand. *Fortschr. Röntgenstr.*, 102:716–719, 1965.

Roche, A. F.: Absence of lunate. *Am. J. Roentgen.*, 100:523–525, 1967.

Rose, T. F.: Congenital bipartite carpal navicular. *Aust. N. Z. J. Surg.*, 16:149–151, 1946.

Rushforth, A. F.: A congenital abnormality of trapezium and first metacarpal bone. *J. Bone Joint Surg.*, 31B:543–546, 1949.

Saxton, H. M., and Wilkinson, J. A.: Hemimelic skeletal dysplasia. *J. Bone Joint Surg.*, 46B:608–613, 1964.

Schaaf, J., and Wagner, A.: Multiplizität von Handwurzelknochen bei drei Geschwistern mit polytoper enchondraler Dysostose. *Fortschr. Röntgenstr.*, 97:497–506, 1962.

Schacherl, M., and Schilling, F.: Zur Differentialdiagnose erworbener und abgeborener Karpalsynostosen. *Fortschr. Röntgenstr.*, 102:68–77, 1965.

Schinz, H. R.: Vererbung und Knochenbau. *Schweiz. Med. Wochenschr.*, 5:1151–1156, 1924.

Schmid, F.: Norm und Variationsbreite der Handwurzelkernentwicklung. *Z. Kinderheilkd.*, 65:646, 1948.

Schmid, F.: Die Handskelettossifikation als Indikator der Entwicklung. *Ergebn. Inn. Med. Kinderheilkd.* N. F., 1:176–246, 1949.

Schmid, F., and Halden, N.: Die postfetale Differenzierung und Grossenentwicklung der Extremitatenknochenkern. *Fortschr. Röntgenstr.*, 71:975–984, 1949.

Schmid, F., and Möll, H.: Atlas der normalen un pathologischen *Handskelettentwicklung*. Berlin, Springer-Verlag, pp. 1–109,

Schreiber, A.: Symmetrische Fuss- und Handwurzelsynostosen in 4 Generationen. *Z. Orthop.*, 104:197–202, 1967.

Schröder, W.: Über die Überähligen Handwurzelknochen, insbesondere das os styloidium. *Röntgenpraxis*, 14:190–196, 1942.

Schulin, K.: Über die Entwicklung und weitere Ausbildung der Gelenki des Menschlichen Korpers. *Arch. Anat. Entwickl.*, pp. 240–274; Taf. X, XI, 1874.

Schulte-Brinkmann, W., Konrad, R. M., Schmidt, P., and Ehlers, F.: Der heutige Entwicklungsstand des Hand- und Fusswurzelskeletts bei gesunden und herzkranken Kindern im Schulalte. *Arch. Orthop. Unfallchir.*, 62:118–133, 1967.

Schulz, O. E.: Über das os naviculare bipartitum manus. *Dtsch. Z. Chir.*, 102:141–142, 1909.

Seckel, H. P. G.: *Birdhead Dwarfs.* Springfield, Illinois, Charles C. Thomas, pp. 220–224, 1960.

Sherwin, J. M., Nagel, D. A., and Southwick, W. O.: Bipartite carpal navicular and the diagnostic problem of partition. *J. Trauma*, 11:440–443, 1971.

Silverman, F. N.: Note on os lunotriquetrum. *Am. J. Phys. Anthropol.*, 13:143–145, 1955.

Smith, G. E.: On a case of numerical reduction of carpus. *Anat. Anz.*, 23:494–495, 1903.

Smith, S. A.: A case of fusion of semilunar and cuneiform bones (os lunato-triquetrum) in an Australian aboriginal. *J. Anat.*, 42:343–346, 1908.

Smitham, J. H.: Some observations on certain congenital abnormalities of the hand in African natives. *Br. J. Radiol.*, 21:513–518, 1948.

Stepanek, J.: Congenital confluence of scaphoid, semilunar and radial epiphyses (Czech.) *Ceskosl. Radiol.*, 22:101–103, 1968.

Stern, A. M., Gall, J. C., Jr., Perry, B. L., et al: The hand-foot-uterus-syndrome. *J. Pediatr.*, 77:109–116, 1970.

Stettner, E.: Über die Beziehungen der Ossifikation des Handskeletts zu Alter und Längenwachstum bie gesunden und kranken Kindern von der Geburt bis Pubertät. *Arch. Kinderheilkd.*, 68:342–368, 1920; 69:27–62, 1921.

Stettner, E.: Ossifikationsstudien am Handskelett. *Z. Kinderheilkd.*, 51:435–458, 1931.

Stricker, G.: Grossartiger Defect an beiden Vorderarmen und Händen eines Neugeborenen. *Arch. Pathol. Anat. Physiol.*, 72:144, 1878.

Srivastava, K. K., and Kochhar, V. L.: Congenital absence of the carpal scaphoid; a case report. *J. Bone Joint Surg.*, 54A:1782, 1972.

Struthers, J.: Case of subdivision of scaphoid carpal bone. *J. Anat. Physiol.*, 8:113–114, 1874.

Stuart, C.: Bipartizione bilaterale congenita o frattura isolata bilaterale dello scafoide carpico. *Radiol.*, 14:1177–1180, 1958.

Thews, K.: Fehldeutung und-behandlung auf Grund von Varietäten der Handwurzel und Fusswurzel im Röntgenbild. *Röntgenpraxis, 11*:184–186, 1939.

Thieffry, S., and Sorrel-Déjerine, J.: Forme spéciale d'osteolyse essentielle héréditaire et familiale a stabilisation spontanée souvenant dans l'enfrance. *Presse Méd., 66*(2):1858–1861, 1958.

Tognolo, P., and Poggi, U.: Un raro caso di sinostosi congenita scaforadiale. *Arch. Putti, 18*:418–421, 1963.

Torg, J. S., and Steel, H. H.: Esssential osteolysis with nephropathy. A review of the literature and case report of an unusual syndrome. *J. Bone Joint Surg., 50A*:1629–1638, 1968.

Torge, J. S., Digeorge, A. M., Kirkpatrick, J. A., Jr., and Trujillo, M. M.: Hereditary multicentric osteolysis with recessive transmission. A new syndrome. *J. Pediatr., 75*:43–252, 1969.

Torsten, J.: Bipartite carpal scaphoid bone. *Acta Orthop. Scand., 17*:70–80, 1947.

Turner, W.: Some variations in the bones of human carpus. *J. Anat. Physiol. Norm. Pathol., 17*:244–249, 1883.

Väänänen, I., and Seppälä, P.: Dystrophia cranio-carpo-tarsalis (Freeman-Sheldon). *Duodecim., 81*:983–987, 1965.

Vaghi, A.:Scafoide bipartito e scafoide accessorio del carpo. *Arch. Orthop., 55*:50–54, 1939.

Vargha, G.: Variations in the growth centers about the wrist. *Am. Digest for. Orthop. Lit., 2*:48–50, 1970. Source: *Gyermekgyogyaszat, 19*:508–518, 1968.

Verö, G.: Über Fragen der Entstehung, Klinik und Defferentialdiagnose der Fraktur, des Überlastungsschadens und der angeborenen Zweiteilung des Os naviculare der Hand. *Zentralbl. Chir., 76*:322–330, 1951.

Vicanek, E.: Os supplementaire de la deuxieme range du carpe; analogie avec le carpe des singes. *Alger. Med., 7*:232–234, 1879.

Vieten, H.: Naviculare bipartitum oder alte, nicht erkannte, pseudoarthrotisch verheilte Navicularfraktur. *Fortschr. Röntgenstr., 71*:358, 1949.

Voldere, J. de: "A case of familial congenital synostosis in the carpal and tarsal bones." *Arch. Chir. Neerl., 12*:185–194, 1960.

Volk, C.: Zwei Fälle von os naviculare bipartitum. *Z. Orthop., 66*:396, 1937.

Watkins, W. W.: Anomalous bones of the wrist and foot in relation to injury. *J. A. M. A., 108*:270–274, 1937.

Waugh, R. L., and Sullivan, R. F.: Anomalies of the carpus. *J. Bone Joint Surg., 32A*:682–686, 1950.

Weber, B.: Multiple symmetrische Synostosen an Hand und Fuss. *Arch. Orthop. Unfallchir., 46*:277–289, 1954.

Weitzner, L.: Congenital talonavicular synostosis associated with hereditary multiple ankylosing arthropathics. *Am. J. Roentgenol., 56*:185–188; fig. 4, 1946.

Werthemann, A.: *Die Entwicklungsstörungen der Extremitäten.* Berlin, Springer-Verlag, pp. 232–340, 1952.

Wetherington, R. K.: Note on fusion of lunate and triquetral centers. *Am. J. Phys. Anthropol., 19*:251–253, 1961.

Wette, W.: Verletzungen und Anomalien im Bereich der Handwurzel. *Arch. Orthop. Unfallchir., 29*:320–341, 1931.

Wette, W.: Die röntgenologische Darstellung, die Aetiologie und die versicherungsrechtliche Bedeutung der Spaltbildungen im Kahnbein. *Arch. Orthop. Unfallchir., 33*:194–199, 1933.

Whillis, J.: The development of synovial joints. *J. Anat., 74*:277–283, pl. II. Figs. 6, 7, 1940.

White, E. H.: Bilateral congenital fusion of capitate and hamate. *Am. J. Roentgenol., 52*:406–411, 1944.

Wolff, R.: Ist das Os naviculare carpi bipartitum und tripartitum Grubers das Produkt einer Fraktur? Nebst Mitteilung eines Falles angeborener beiderseitiger Teilung des Naviculare carpi. *Dtsch. Z. Chir., 70*:254–314, Tafel IV, 1903.

Wray, J. B., and Herndon, N.: Hereditary transmission of congenital coalition of calcaneus to the navicular. *J. Bone Joint Surg., 45A*:370–372, 1963.

Zimmer, E. A.: Eine krankhafte Veränderung am os styloidium. *Fortschr. Röntgenstr., 61*:187–192, 1940.

Chapter Twenty-Two

MADELUNG DEFORMITY

In Chapter One, a number of prestigious authors were mentioned who had classed Madelung deformity with congenital anomalies. The word *congenital* appears in the title of numerous communications on this subject, and a prenatal defect of the distal radial epiphyseal anlage or of the growth cartilage plate has been incriminated by many authors. The anomaly had been discussed previously by Smith (1847), Adams (1854), Malgaigne (1855), and Jean (1875), who conducted the first anatomical study of the malformation. It remained for Madelung (1878) to give a comprehensive description of the deformity with which his name has come to be connected.

Madelung mentioned Dupuytren as being the first to recognize this condition. Many authors have since hyphenated Madelung's name with Dupuytren's, and they invariably place Dupuytren's name first, according him priority of authorship. Stetten (1909) exploded this myth. He brought forth ample evidence to prove that Dupuytren had mentioned an occupational, hence acquired, disorder. Dupuytren (1834) spoke about a form of subluxation of the wrist that he had heard described by Bégin (1825). The condition Bégin described affected laborers engaged in continuous heavy work with press levers. Madelung deformity occurs mainly in children and adolescents — more often in girls than boys — who have not yet engaged in any occupation necessitating strenuous use of their hands.

NOMENCLATURE

Many authors writing before and after Madelung used the heading "Congenital subluxation of the wrist." Madelung (1878) himself employed the title "Spontaneous forward subluxation of the hand." Duplay (1885) singled out the curvature of the distal radius as the salient feature of the deformity. In a later communication, Duplay (1891) used the designation delayed rickets; others employed the term adolescent rickets. On the basis of Duplay's earlier observation about the curvature of the radius, Delbet (1899) and Gangolphe (1899), respectively, introduced the terms carpus curvus and radius curvus. Kirmisson (1902) described a case in which the distal extremity of the radius had turned in a dorsal direction, and used the designation progressive subluxation of the wrist. In years to come, the deformity Kirmisson described became known as reversed Madelung. Ianni (1924) again drew attention to Duplay's observation and considered the curvature of the distal radius to be the basic deformity; he hyphenated Duplay's name with Madelung's and evolved the designation Madelung-Duplay deformity. Bertolotti (1928) used the term cubitolisthesis, meaning separation of the ulna from the radius. In the literature, one also meets with such terms as manus varus, manus valgus, manus furca, adolescent clubhand, carpal dysmorphosis, carpal kyphosis, carpoficiosis, radius brevior, radius parvus, radiovolar bayonet deformity, and dyschondrosteosis.

Zeitlin (1930) and many other authors used the term Madelung's disease. Burrows (1937) suggested calling the condition Madelung's syndrome. Anton et al (1938) did not think the deformity in question was a syndrome, and they also objected to the eponymic designation. They said that Madelung had already given his name to a disease characterized by a diffuse deposit of fatty tissue on the upper part of the back, shoulder, and neck. Anton et al argued against naming a disease or deformity after an author. Notwithstanding, Madelung deformity remains the most popular name for the progressive curvature of the distal radius due to a disturbance in its distal growth center. As Burrows put it, the terminology has all the faults of eponymous nomenclature, but a better name has yet to be devised.

OCCURRENCES

Anton et al (1938) listed 171 authenticated cases of Madelung deformity. Heredity features in nearly one-third of the reported cases, and transmission of the trait appears to follow the autosomal dominant pattern. The anomaly is four times as common in females as in males, and is twice as often bilateral as unilateral. In bilateral cases, the deformity is usually symmetrical, though one side might have become symptomatic earlier than the other. In unilateral cases, the right side seems to be involved slightly more often than the left, and the bones of the affected forearm — the radius in particular — are shorter than those of the unaffected side. Most authors claim that in bilateral cases the forearm bones are shorter than those in normal individuals of the same age.

Out of 171 cases of Madelung deformity tabulated by Anton et al (1938), in only six was the distal radius bent backwards; in addition, the head of the ulna had assumed a volar position. In the great majority of reported cases, the terminal radius is bent in the volar direction and the ulnar head maintains a dorsal stance. In both unreversed and reversed varieties, the terminal radius inclines in the ulnar direction. Normally, the distal portion of the radius is convex on its dorsal aspect and concave on its volar side; it is also convex along its radial border and concave on its ulnar margin. The distal part of the radius tends to incline in the volar and ulnar direction. In the unreversed variety of Madelung deformity, volar and ulnar inclination of the distal radius is accentuated.

BASIC DISTURBANCE

In Madelung deformity, the ulnar border of the shaft of the radius is much shorter than its radial margin. This discrepancy can only be accounted for by a disturbance in the distal growth cartilage plate. The ulnar sector of this plate is either absent or underdeveloped and fails to contribute to the growth of the corresponding border of the radial shaft. Continued deposition of bone by the unaffected radial and dorsal parts of the growth plate causes the corresponding sides of the radius to gain in length and to outstrip the borders where growth has been arrested. Since it is blocked by the carpus ahead, the fast-growing, newly formed soft bone bends toward the area where growth has been arrested—in the ulnar and volar directions. The curvature of the radius lies close to the wrist joint; it implicates and is in turn implicated by the changes which take place in various structures.

DISTAL EPIPHYSIS OF THE RADIUS

The appearance of the ossific core of the distal radial epiphysis is subject to considerable variation. It is known to become roentgenographically manifest in girls as early as the eleventh month after birth but may not be seen in hand films of boys until the end of the second year. In roentgenographs taken by dorsopalmar exposure at this early stage, the distal radial epiphysis has the appearance of a rounded seed. At the age of six, the epiphysis begins to flatten out. At eight, the ossific core extends radially to form the styloid process, which is ossified around the age of 10. At this age the ulnar half of the epiphysis is still narrower than the radial portion. From now until maturity—between the ages of 13 and 15 in females and two to three years later in males—the ulnar half of the epiphysis gains an increment of proximodistal depth but remains much thinner than the radial sector. The volar portion of the epiphysis is also thinner than the dorsal half.

In Madelung deformity, the ulnar and volar sectors of the distal radial epiphysis are reduced to flattened-out slivers and may not even be in evidence. It is perhaps for this reason that some authors—Rocher (1937) and his followers—have considered hemiatrophy of the distal radial epiphysis to be the basis of Madelung deformity. It may be significant that the ulnar half of the distal radial epiphysis is not ossified until after the age of seven. It is after this age that Madelung deformity is usually detected (Figs. 22–1 to 22–5).

RADIOCARPAL JOINT

At the elbow, the articular surface of the radial head, though dimpled in the center, lies in a horizontal plane, forming a small plateau. Measured respectively from the volar and dorsal rims of this plateau to the corresponding margins of the distal articular end, the dorsal border of the radius is slightly longer than the volar margin. As a result, the plane of the carpal articular facet of the radius tilts in the volar direction about 5 degrees. Measured from the ulnar and radial rims

(Text continued on page 759.)

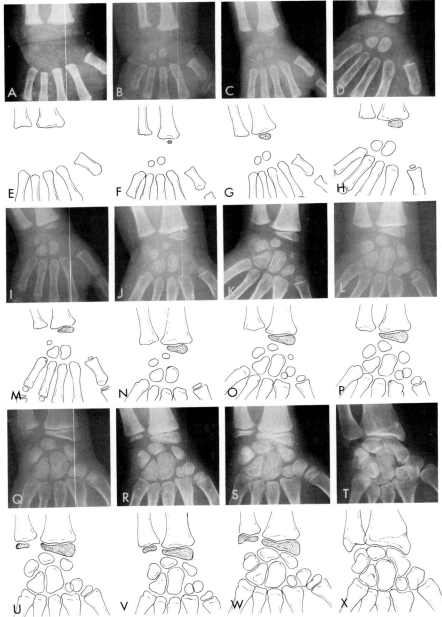

Figure 22–1 Distal epiphyses of radius and ulna in girls. *A*, Dorsovolar roentgenograph of a newborn girl. *B*, Ten-month-old girl: a small dot becomes visible in the center of the radial epiphysis. *C*, Fourteen-month-old: the ossific core assumes an ovoid shape with transversely disposed long axis. *D*, Fourteen-month-old: bony nucleus has elongated toward radial border. *E, F, G,* and *H* illustrate the roentgenograph above each. *I*, Two-and-a-half year old: the nucleus sprouts a beak which points toward the ulnar border while its radial sector thickens and expands in the opposite direction. *J*, Three-year-and-two-month-old: the nucleus has assumed the shape of a wedge with a radial base; as a whole it is closer to the radial border. *K*, Four-year-and-seven-month-old: the nucleus has extended in both the radial and ulnar direction. *L*, Six-year-old: the nucleus has reached the radial and ulnar borders of the metaphysis. *M, N, O,* and *P* illustrate the roentgenograph above each. *Q*, Six-and-a-half-year-old: the ulnar epiphysis has appeared. *R*, Eight-year-old: the radial border of the radial epiphysis begins to bulge beyond the corresponding margin of the metaphysis. *S*, Twelve-year-old: both styloids have developed. *T*, Fifteen-year-old: both epiphyses are matured, fused with metaphyses. *U, V, W,* and *X* illustrate the roentgenograph above each.

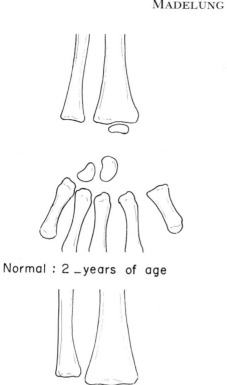

Normal : 2 _ years of age

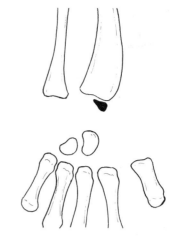

Madelung : 2 _ years of age

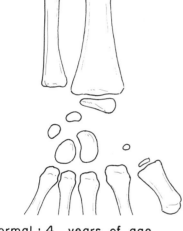

Normal : 4 _ years of age

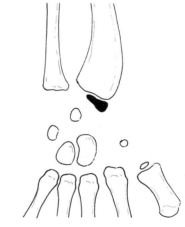

Madelung : 4 _ years of age

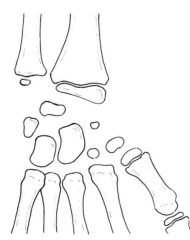

Normal : 6 _ years of age

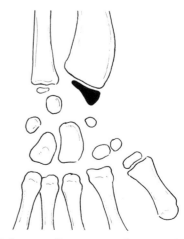

Madelung : 6 _ years of age

Figure 22-2 Configuration of the carpal epiphysis of the radius in Madelung deformity contrasted with that in normal individuals between the ages of two and six.

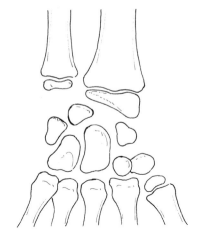

Normal : 8 _ years of age

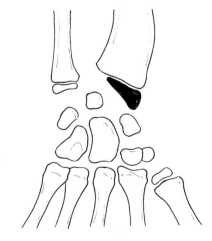

Madelung : 8 _ years of age

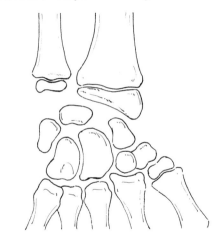

Normal : 10 _ years of age

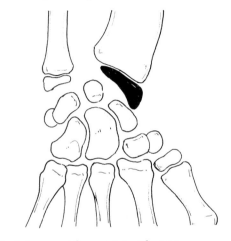

Madelung : 10 _ years of age

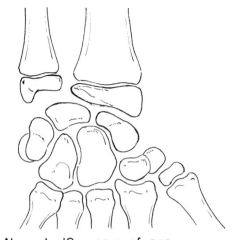

Normal : 12 _ years of age

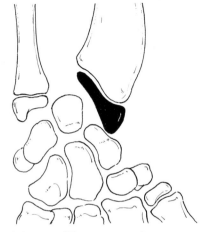

Madelung : 12 _ years of age

Figure 22–3 Configuration of the carpal epiphysis of the radius in Madelung deformity contrasted with that of normal individuals between the ages of eight and twelve.

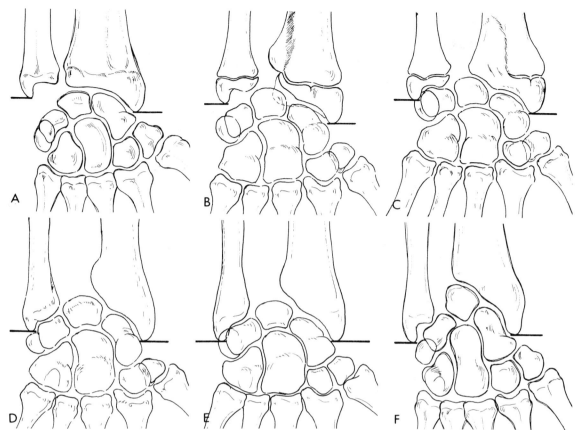

Figure 22–4 Sketches of dorsovolar roentgenographs. *A,* Normal wrist. *B,* Separation of distal radius and ulna and attenuated ulnar segment of radial epiphysis. *C,* Precociously fused ulnar sector of radial epiphysis. *D,* Ulnar styloid approaching the level of radial styloid. *E,* Both styloids reaching the same joint distally. *F,* Ulnar styloid reaching a point further distal than the radial styloid and carpal bones assuming the configuration of a pyramid.

of the capital plateau to the corresponding points of the distal articular surface, the radius is considerably longer on the radial than on the ulnar side. Accordingly, the plane of its distal articular facet is inclined in the ulnar direction to almost 15 degrees. The carpal articular facet of the radius is divided by a faint anteroposterior ridge into two concavities. The smaller of these lies on the radial sector and the larger on the ulnar; the former articulates with the scaphoid, and the latter with the lunate bone. The triangular fibrocartilaginous disc spans the gap between the radial rim and the styloid process of the ulna. The radial portion of the triangular disc articulates with the lunate, and its ulnar half with the triquetrum.

In the usual unreversed form of Madelung deformity, because of the great discrepancy between the lengths of the dorsal and volar borders of the radius and the forward bent of its distal portion, the plane of the carpal articular facet of the radius becomes greatly antiverted — it may incline in the volar direction to as much as 60 degrees. For similar reasons, the plane of the articular surface takes an exaggerated turn toward the ulna and inclines in that direction to about 80 degrees or more. The ridge separating the fossa lodging the lunate from that occupied by the scaphoid is effaced. The carpal articular surface of the

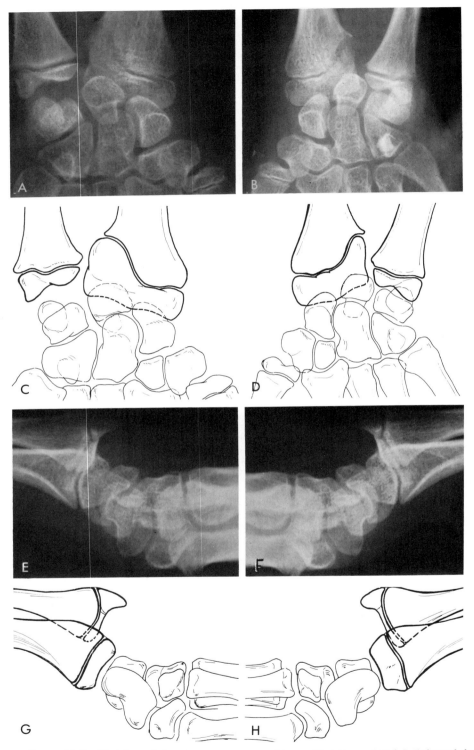

Figure 22–5 Madelung deformity: roentgenographic manifestations. *A* and *B*, Enlarged dorsopalmar roentgenographs of the right and left wrists of a 12-year-old girl. *C* and *D*, Sketches illustrating the same. *E* and *F*, Enlarged lateral roentgenographs of the right and left wrists. *G* and *H*, Sketches illustrating the same.

radius becomes continuous with the ulnar border of the distal radius, which normally bears a concave notch to house the head of the ulna. In Madelung deformity, this notch is also effaced.

It was Kirmisson (1902)—not Bennecke (1904) as stated by Anton et al (1938)—who first introduced the concept of the pyramidation of carpal bones in Madelung deformity. Normally, the carpal bones of the proximal row are arranged in an arc and present a convex dome toward the radius and the triangular ligament. In Madelung deformity, this dome becomes peaked, at the apex of which the lunate bone is seated. The carpal bones are pushed toward the palm. The lunate and triquetrum lose contact with the triangular fibrocartilage and shift volarward, while the fibrocartilage remains in its dorsal position. In addition, the carpal bones are pushed toward the ulnar border of the wrist. The hand follows suit—it is displaced volarward in an ulnar direction.

THE HEAD OF THE ULNA

The epiphysis of the distal end or the head of the ulna becomes roentgenographically manifest around the age of six, and its styloid process begins to ossify three years later. The capital epiphysis of the ulna matures at the same time as the distal epiphysis of the radius—between the ages of 13 and 15 in females and two to three years later in males. Normally, the head of the ulna is lodged in the fossa on the ulnar aspect of the distal radius. In Madelung deformity, the distal end of the radius is bent in the volar direction, away from the head of the ulna, giving the impression that the latter is dislocated. Actually, the head of the ulna remains in situ and continues to grow forward. It is the distal end of the radius which has changed position. Normally, the tip of the radial styloid extends about 1 cm. further distal than the ulnar styloid. In Madelung deformity, the tips of the two styloids may lie on the same horizontal line or the ulnar styloid may reach a point further distal than the radial styloid. This assessment is made on dorsopalmar roentgenographs.

REVERSED MADELUNG (Madelung Inversé)

Only seven cases of reversed variety of Madelung deformity have heretofore been recorded. Kirmisson (1902) reported one case; Stetton (1909), two cases; Peckham and Hammond (1909), one case; Gaudier (1909), one case; Burrows (1937), one case; and Bossaert (1960), one case. In reversed Madelung deformity the distal radius presents a volar instead of dorsal convexity, the carpal articular surface of the radius is retroverted, and the ulna has assumed a relative palmar position.

ASSOCIATIONS

Coexistence of Madelung deformity with the following anomalies has been recorded: short femur and ulnar ray defect of the opposite arm—by Hoffmann

(1900); cervical ribs—by Kajon (1934); scoliosis—by Duplay (1885), Ardouin (1902), Kirmisson (1902), Gevaert (1902), Bennecke (1904), Lenormant (1907), Siegrist (1908), and Brinsmade (1908); sacralization of the fifth lumbar vertebra—by Kuhn (1933) and Ingber (1934); spina bifida occulta—by Vianna (1931) and Kuhn (1933); absence of the head of the humerus—by Rocher (1934); cubitus valgus—by Roget (1899), Bennecke (1904), Schulze (1905), Volkmann (1905), Putti (1906), and Franke (1908); dislocation of the radial head and radiohumeral separation—by Thompson and Kalayjian (1939) and Negré et al (1948); osteitis fibrosa cystica of the distal radius—by Björkroth (1932); coalescence of carpal bones—by Alexander and Johnson (1941) and Travaglini (1962); short fingers—by Bergmann (1888), Melchior (1912), and Bertolotti (1913); bilateral dislocation of the hips—by Schulze (1905); laxity of the knee ligaments—by Gangolphe (1899); genu varum—by Solberg (1906); genu valgum—by Gevaert (1902) and Franke (1908); bowing of the tibia—by Brinsmade (1908), Stokes (1910), Mathieu and Joseph (1922), Brown (1923), Beder (1935), and Chierici (1936); pes planus—by Volkmann (1905), Solberg (1906), and Siegrist (1908); short stature—by Solberg (1906), Franke (1908), and Fazio (1930); multiple exostoses—by Franke (1908), Curtillet (1912), and Dimitriu (1934); exostosis of fibular head—by Corcos et al (1951); and loss of conductive hearing—by Nassif and Harboyan (1970).

Stetten (1909) recognized the association of Madelung deformity with various congenital anomalies, especially with multiple exostosis. Deformities of the wrist simulating Madelung are known to occur in mucopolysaccharidosis of the Hurler and Morquio variety, in multiple enchondromatosis, and in Turner's gonadal dysgenesis. Anton et al (1938) stated that if patients with Madelung deformity were subjected to general roentgenographic survey, "numerous other osteochondritic anomalies would have been discovered."

IDENTIFICATION WITH DYSCHONDROSTEOSIS

It has lately become fashionable to consider Madelung deformity as a local manifestation of the systemic disorder known as dyschondrosteosis, also called Léri-Weill disease. Dyschondrosteosis is a variant of mesomelic dwarfism described originally by Léri and associates (1929–1931). Almost nothing was written about it for two decades. Kaplan et al (1951) revived the discussion on the subject. Lamy and Maroteaux (1960) spoke of *formes frustes*, which they suspected might easily be confused with Madelung deformity. Their suspicion was confirmed. Langer (1965), Herdman et al (1966), and Aegerter and Kirkpatrick (1968) went so far as to identify dyschondrosteosis with Madelung deformity.

As pointed out by Berdon et al (1965), it is perhaps more correct to say that Madelung deformity of the wrist is only one of the features of dyschondrosteosis; however, it may be the sole feature of *formes frustes*. Felman and Kirkpatrick (1969) thought it fallacious to maintain that all patients with radiographic manifestations of Madelung deformity have dyschondrosteosis. They pointed out that patients with dyschondrosteosis have marked shortening of the tibia relative to the femur. In dyschondrosteosis, the proximal radius is thick and bowed, presenting an accentuated convexity in the radial direction; the radial head tends to tilt in the dorsal direction and may even subluxate. In Madelung deformity, the proximal radius is unaffected (Figs. 22–6 and 22–7).

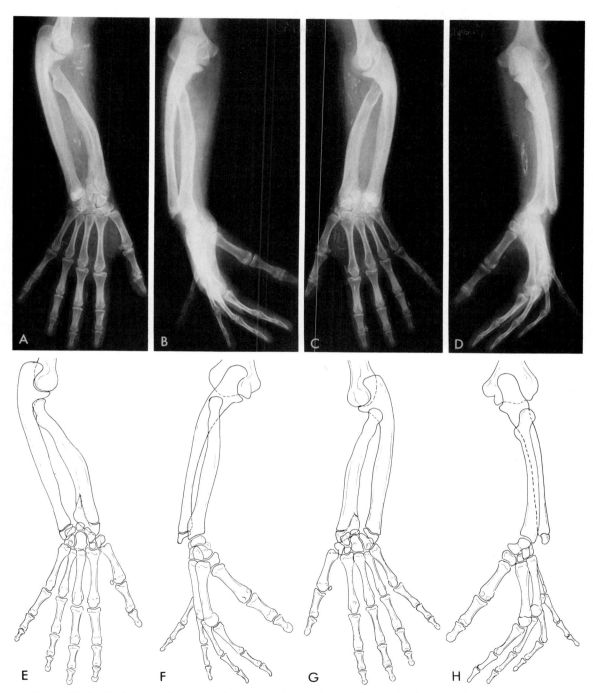

Figure 22–6 Madelung deformity probably secondary to dyschondrosteosis. *A*, Dorsopalmar roentgenograph of the right forearm, wrist, and hand of a 16-year-old girl, four feet two inches in height and with bowed tibias. *B*, Lateral roentgenograph of the same. *C* and *D*, Similar roentgenographs of the left forearm, wrist, and hand. *E*, *F*, *G*, and *H* illustrate the roentgenograph above each.

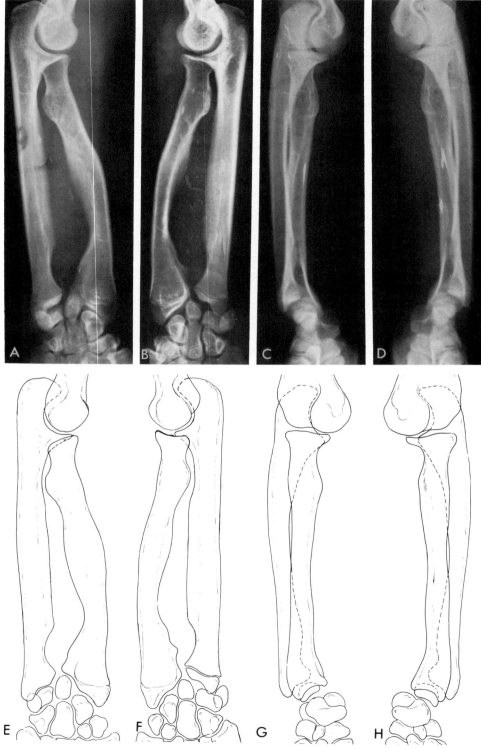

Figure 22–7 Madelung deformity probably due to dyschondrosteosis. *A* and *B*, Dorsovolar roentgenographs of the forearms of a 13-year-old girl: both radii are thin and curved at the midshaft and expanded at each end. *C* and *D* lateral roentgenographs of the right and left forearms. *E*, *F*, *G*, and *H* illustrate the roentgenograph above each.

DIAGNOSIS

Madelung deformity is characterized by an insidious onset of pain in one wrist, then the other, and progressive development of malformation. The patient is usually a girl between the ages of 6 and 13; she is moderately short in stature, presents none of the tell-tale signs of rickets, and gives no history of having incurred a previous injury or infection. Pseudo-Madelung deformity is not an uncommon aftermath of osteomyelitis of the distal radius with involvement of physis and growth arrest. Pseudo-Madelung deformity is also seen in cases of multiple enchondromatoses and multiple exostoses (Fig. 22–8).

The first roentgenographic study of Madelung deformity was conducted by Jagot (1897). Three decades later, Dannenberg et al (1939) listed 12 diagnostic criteria revealed by roentgenographs. The following are perhaps the most constant, hence reliable, signs of the usual unreversed variety of Madelung deformity: (1) increased dorsal and radial convexity of the distal radius, (2) exaggerated palmar and ulnar tilt of the distal articular surface of the radius, (3) pyramiding of carpal bone, (4) wide interosseous space, and (5) a relatively dorsal position assumed by the ulnar head. In reversed Madelung deformity, (1) the distal radius presents a volar, instead of dorsal, convexity, (2) the plane of the distal articular surface of the radius is retroverted, and (3) the carpus has shifted in the dorsal direction, giving the impression that the head of the ulna has dislocated in the volar direction.

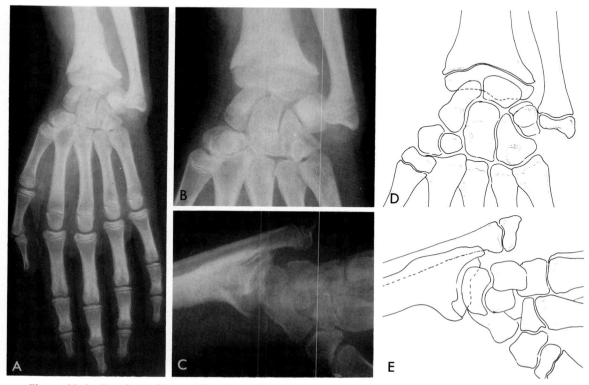

Figure 22–8 Pseudo-Madelung deformity. *A*, Dorsopalmar view of the wrist and hand of a 14-year-old boy who suffered arrest of growth at the distal growth plate of the radius due to osteomyelitis. *B*, Enlarged dorsovolar roentgenograph of the wrist. *C*, Lateral roentgenograph of the same. *D* and *E* illustrate the roentgenograph next to each.

FUNCTIONAL DISTURBANCE AND DISCOMFORT

In children, the hand normally extends at the wrist to about 80 degrees and flexes to 90 degrees; it radially deviates around 15 degrees and in the ulnar direction about 35 degrees. In the common variety of Madelung deformity, extension and radial deviation at the wrist are diminished to varying degrees, while flexion and ulnar deflection are increased. Depending upon the extent to which the interosseous space is widened, and upon the wedged incarceration of the carpus between the separated forearm bones, pronation and supination are also affected. As a rule, supination is definitely diminished, while pronation is only slightly impaired. Functionally, reversed Madelung deformity differs from the usual variety only in one respect: extension of the hand at the wrist is increased, while flexion is diminished.

Madelung deformity develops insidiously. It pursues a progressive course and reaches its zenith at about the time of closure of the distal radial epiphysis. During the progressive phase, it is usually accompanied by pain, which subsides when the deformity becomes stabilized. The pain may return in the future owing to friction by incongruous articular surfaces and to degenerative joint changes. The intensity of pain varies from patient to patient, as does the degree of deformity or disability. The distal radius is not curved in every case of Madelung deformity. Not uncommonly, the only objective finding is the exaggerated ulnar inclination of the distal articular end of the radius. A patient with mild deformity may complain of more severe pain than one who shows marked curvature of the distal radius. The treatment of Madelung deformity is directed primarily toward alleviation of pain and the restoration of functions lost as a result of the malposition of the hand.

TREATMENT

Madelung (1878) advised his patients to avoid forced extension of the wrist and to wear leather bracelets. Retentive and corrective appliances of diverse designs had their period of popularity until Stetten (1909), and after him Stokes (1910), pronounced them "useless." What these authors meant was that casts or splints neither improve the deformity nor check its progress. Stetten conceded that "sparing of the extremity" (meaning rest) would relieve the pain. Night splints are still recommended for this purpose.

Very few patients with Madelung deformity require surgical interference. For more obvious malformations the following procedures have been recommended, alone or in combination: cuff resection of the distal ulna, shortening of the ulna, resection of the ulnar head, osteotomy of the distal radius, epiphysiodesis of the distal ulna, epiphysiodesis of the radial sector of the distal radius, and bone-block operation, which was described by Bazy and Galtier (1935) and revived more recently by Barcat (1959). In this last procedure, in order to avoid interference with pronation and supination, a sufficient gap is created between the resected end of the proximal ulnar fragment and the head portion which is attached to the radius. If the curvature of the distal radius is marked, it is corrected at a later date by osteotomy.

The bone-block operation, together with cuff resection of the distal ulna,

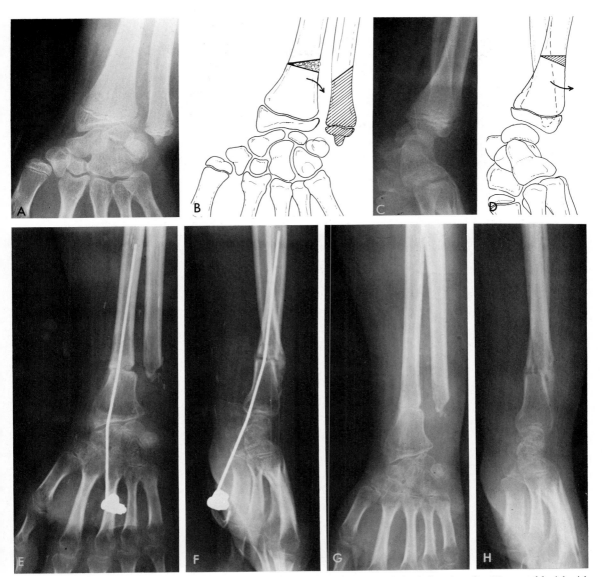

Figure 22–9 Madelung deformity. *A*, Dorsopalmar roentgenograph of the left wrist of a 12-year-old girl with moderate deformity but persistent pain over the distal radioulnar joint. *B*, Sketch illustrating the site of open wedge osteotomy of the distal radius and the segment of distal ulna to be resected: chips of bone obtained from the distal ulna were packed into the open wedge created in the distal radius. *C*, Lateral roentgenograph of the wrist. *D*, Sketch illustrating closed-wedge osteotomy of the distal radius. *E* and *F* show fixation of fragments of the osteotomized radius with an intramedullary K-wire. As will be shown in Figure 22–11, the split half of the extensor carpi ulnaris was utilized to reconstruct an ulnar collateral ligament. *G* and *H*, Dorsopalmar and lateral roentgenographs after removal of K-wire and union of the fragments of the osteotomized distal radius.

shortening of the ulna, and epiphysiodesis of one or both forearm bones, must be relegated to the category of meddlesome procedures. For moderate deformities of the wrist with pain over the distal radioulnar junction, all one has to do is resect the head of the ulna. In order to obviate ulnar drift of the carpus, the author threads the split half of the extensor carpi ulnaris tendon through a tunnel in the distal end of the remaining ulna and sutures it to the other half of the tendon. It should be pointed out that in more advanced deformities this tendon lies on the volar, instead of the dorsal, aspect of the ulnar head.

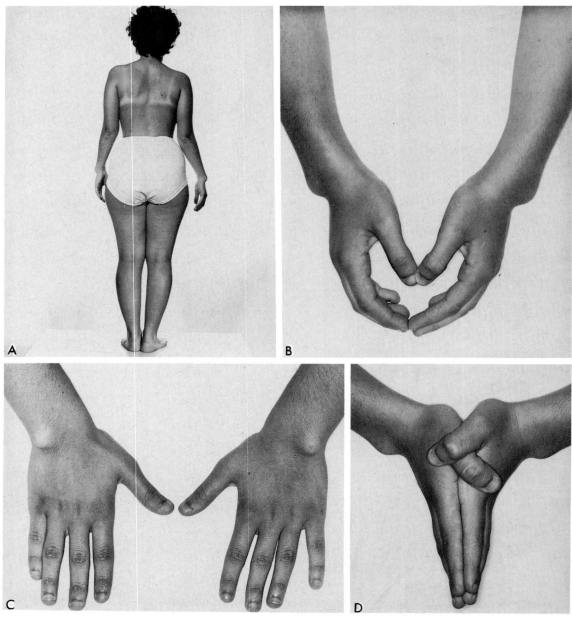

Figure 22–10 Madelung deformity. *A*, Dorsal view of a 12-year-old girl who measured four feet six inches in height. *B*, Radial view of the wrists and forearms. *C*, Dorsal view of the same. *D*, Radial view, bringing the prominent ulnar heads into greater relief.

The plane of resection of the distal ulna is oblique. It begins at a point about 3 cm. proximal to the distal articular surface on the radiodorsal aspect of the shaft and slants ulnarward; the dorsal and radial sector of the ulnar head, including the epiphysis, is resected. When the curvature of the terminal radius is marked, this should be corrected by osteotomy. The author prefers open-wedge osteotomy from the ulnar aspect of the distal radius; into this wedge is inserted a triangular piece of bone fashioned from the resected distal end of the ulna. The

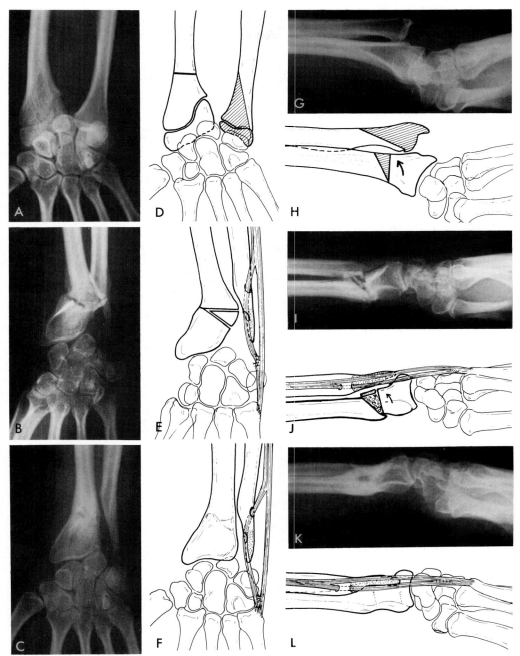

Figure 22-11 *A,* Preoperative dorsopalmar roentgenograph of the left wrist of the 12-year-old girl featured in Figures 22-9 and 22-10. *B,* Roentgenograph soon after open-wedge osteotomy of the distal radius and excision of the ulnar head. *C,* Roentgenograph a year after surgery. *D,* Sketch showing the site of osteotomy of the distal radius and the segment of the distal ulna to be resected. *E,* A triangular piece of bone is inserted into the opened wedge of the distal radius; the split half of the extensor carpi ulnaris tendon is threaded through the remaining fragment of the distal ulna and sutured to the main stem of the tendon. *F,* The same after healing of the osteomized radius. *G,* Preoperative lateral roentgenograph of the same wrist. *H,* Sketch illustrating the same. *I,* Roentgenograph showing the line of excision of the ulnar head. *J,* Sketch illustrating *E* in side view. *K,* Lateral roentgenograph after union of the osteotomized distal radius showing correction of volar tilt of its distal articular surface. *L* represents *F* as seen from the ulnar aspect.

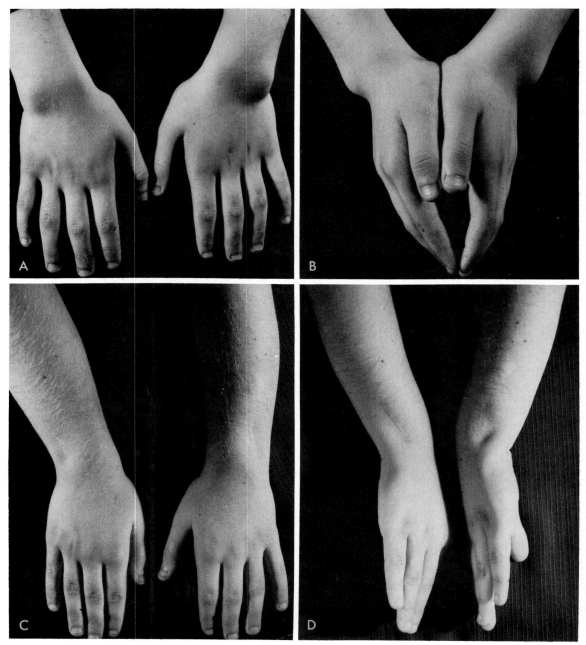

Figure 22–12 Results. *A*, Preoperative dorsal view of the wrists and hands of the 12-year-old girl featured in Figure 22–11. *B*, Preoperative radial view. *C*, Postoperative dorsal view. *D*, Postoperative ulnar view.

volar tilt of the distal radius is corrected by removing enough bone from the dorsal aspect of the proximal fragment and pushing the distal fragment in the dorsal direction; the fragments are immobilized by means of a heavy intramedullary K wire (Kirschner wire) and plaster cast. Old inveterate cases accompanied by painful arthritis are best treated by fusion of the radiocarpal joint. A sufficiently long segment of the distal ulna is resected to permit unhampered pronation and supination of the hand (Figs. 22–10 to 22–12).

SUMMARY

Madelung deformity is a congenital disorder which becomes manifest during late childhood or adolescence. It is four times more common in girls than in boys and twice as often bilateral as unilateral. It is a genetic disorder, being transmitted as an autosomal dominant trait. The affected individual is moderately short in stature. The carpal extremity of the radius constitutes the primary seat of the disturbance. In the more common unreversed variety, the ulnar and volar half of the distal radial physis fails to contribute its share of growth. As a consequence, the carpal end of the radius curves in the volar direction and toward the ulnar border of the wrist. The carpal articular surface of the radius slants in the volar and ulnar direction to a degree greater than normal; the carpus, and with it the hand, shift volarward while the ulna remains in its wonted position. Most cases of Madelung deformity do not need any treatment. Surgery is indicated when the wrist is painful or deformity is marked. The best results are obtained by excision of an inch or more of the carpal end of the ulna and corrective osteotomy of the distal radius.

References

Abadie, J.: De la luxation progressive du poignet chez l'adolescent. *Rev. d'Orthop.*, (n.s.), *4*:481–510, Pl. XIII, SIV, 1903.

Abadie, J.: Sur le mécanisme des luxations du poignet. *Bull. Soc. Anat.* (Paris), *6*:274–275, 1904.

Adams, R.: Wrist, abnormal conditions of. Congenital dislocations. In Todd, R. B., (ed.): *Cyclopedia of Anatomy and Physiology*. London, Longman, Brown, Green, Longmans & Roberts, Vol. IV, Part II, pp. 1508–1513, 1854.

Adams, R.: Wrist, abnormal conditions of. Congenital dislocations. In Todd, R. B., (ed.): *Cyclopedia of*

Aegerter, E., and Kirkpatrick, J. A.: *Orthopedic Diseases*. Third edition. Philadelphia, W. B. Saunders, pp. 205–206, 1968.

Albertin: Radius curvus. *Bull. Soc. Chir.* (Lyon), *8*:115–120, 1905.

Albertin, and Leclerc: Radius curvus. *Rev. Chir.*, *31*:551–552, 1905.

Alexander, H. H., and Johnson, G. H.: Dyschondroplasia of the distal radial epiphysis (Madelung's deformity) with fusion of the semilunar and triangular bones. *Am. J. Surg.*, *53*:349–351, 1941.

Amaral, B.: Doenca de Madelung. *Cir. Aparato Locomot.*, *2*:332–335, 1945.

Anton, J. I., Reitz, G. B., and Spiegel, M. B.: Madelung's deformity. *Ann. Surg.*, *108*:411–439, 1938.

Anzilotti, G.: Supra una deformita del polso tipo Madelung. *Arch. Ortop.*, *28*:537–549, 1911.

Ardouin, P.: Un cas de luxation congénitale incomplète du poignet. *Rev. d'Orthop.*, *3*:351–353, pl. XIII, 1902.

Aschoff, H.: Beitrag zur Enstehung der Madelung'schen Deformitat, ihere übergangsformen und zu ihrer nichtoperativen Behandlung. *Z. Orthop.*, *99*:465–473, 1965.

Barcat, J.: L'opération de Bazy-Gartier dans la maladie de Madelung. *Mém. Acad. Chir.* (Paris), *76*:337–339, 1950.

Barcat, J.: La maladie de Madelung et son traitément. *J. Chir.*, *77*:212–225, 1959.

Barsoum, S.: Madelung's deformity. *Lancet*, *2*:428, 1935.

Barthés, L. C.: *De la Luxation Progressive du Poignet chez l'Adolescent et chez l'Adulte*. Thèse. Paris, Imp. Faculté Méd., 1904.

Bauer, K. H., and Bode, W.: Madelungsche Deformität des Handgelenkes. *In* Abel, W., et al., (eds.): *Erbiologie und Erbpathologie Korperlicher Zustande und Funktionen*. Berlin, Springer, pp. 168–170, 1940.

Bazy, L., and Galtier, M.: Traitément sanglant de la luxation isolée de l'extrémité inférieure du cubitus en avant. *J. Chir.*, *45*:868–876, 1935.

Bazzano, H. C., and Carnelli, J. L.: Enfermidad de Madelung. *Arch. Pediatr. Uruguay*, *9*:73–86, 1938.

Becker, P. E.: Ein weiterer Fall von Dyschondrosteose (Leri-Weill). *Humangenetik*, *1*:563–570, 1965.

Beder, W. L., and Heimismann, J. I.: Zur Genese der Madelung'schen Deformität. *Fortschr. Röntgenstr.*, *52*:595–601, 1935.

Bégin, L. J.: Articulation radio-carpien. *Dictionaire de Science Médicale*. Paris, Vol. 13, pp. 491–498, 1825. Also in *Dictionaire Abrégé des Sciences Medicales*, Vol. 13, p. 493, 1841.

Bennecke: Ueber einen Fall von progressiver luxation des Handgelenkes. *Verh. Dtsch. Ges. Chir.*, *33*:131–135, 1904.

Bennett, W. H.: A case of spontaneous displacement forward of both wrists. *Tr. Clin. Soc.* (London), *25*:265–267, 1892.

Berdon, W. E., Grossman, H., and Baker, D. H.: Dyschondrostéose (Leri-Weill syndrome). Congenital short forearms, Madelung-type of wrist deformities and moderate dwarfism. *Radiology*, *85*:678–680, 1965.

Berg, P.: Die *Madelung'sche* Deformität des Handgelenkes. (Carpus valgus). *Arch. Orth. Unfallchir.*, *12*:325–338, 1913.

Bergan, F.: Madelungs deformitet, Familiaer optredon, tre sostre. *Norsk Mag. Laeg.*, *15*:2403–2406, 1942.

Bergmann, V.: Subluxation beider Hände. *Dtsch. Med. Wochenschr.*, *14*:861, 1888.

Bertolotti, M.: Nanism familiale par aplasie chondrale systématisée. Mésomelie et brachymélie metapodiale symétrique. *Presse Méd.*, 21st year, *1*:165–170, 1913.

Bertolotti, O.: La malattia di Madelung o cubitolistesi posteriore. *La Medicina Pratica*, *13*:95–99, 1928.

Binet, A., and Mutel, M.: Le radius curvus. *Rev. Chir.*, *48*:567–584, 1913.

Björkroth, T.: An extraordinary case of deformity of the wrist (symptomatic form of Madelung's deformity). *Acta Orthop. Scand.*, *2*:242–252, 1932.

Bode, O.: Demonstration eines Falles von Spontanluxation der Hand. *Berl. Klin. Wochenschr.*, *28*:900, 1891.

Bode, O.: Ein Beitrag zur Aetiologie und Casuistik der Spontanluxation der Hand. *Berl. Klin. Wochenschr.*, *28*:1128–1130, 1891.

Bossaert, P.: Un cas de maladie de Madelung "inverse" traité chirurgicalement. *Acta. Chir. Belg.*, *59*:649–653, 1960.

Brandes, M.: Zur Madelungs'chen Deformität der Handgelenkes. *Z. Orthop. Chir.*, *28*:392–414, 1911.

Brandes, M.: Zur Madelungs'chen Deformität der Handgelenkes. Ein Nachtrag. *Z. Orthop. Chir.*, *42*:20–38, 1922.

Brinsmade, W. R.: Madelung's deformity of the hands. *Ann. Surg.*, *47*:794–795, 1908.

Broca, A.: Radius curvus. *La Tribune Méd.*, (Paris), *3*:759–760, 1905.

Broca, A.: *Chirurgie Infantile*. Paris, G. Steinheil, pp. 210–214, 1914.

Brown, G. M.: Report of a case of Madelung's deformity. *Med. Clin. N. Am.*, *6*:1313–1318, 1923.

Bsteth, O.: Radiusfraktur bei Madelung'sher Deformität. *Zentralbl. Chir.*, *58*:1955–1957, 1931.

Burckhardt, H.: Spontane Luxationen und Subluxationen im Handgelenk. *Beitr. Klin. Chir.*, *88*:403–422, 1914.

Burnier, R., and Néveux, A.: Luxation bilatérale et symmetrique de l'extremité inférieure du cubitus en arrière avec radius curvus (Maladie de Dupuytren-Madelung et ses variétés). *Arch. Gen. Chir.*, *3*:805–817, 1909.

Burrows, H. J.: An operation for the correction of Madelung's deformity and similar conditions. *Proc. R. Soc. Med. London* (Sect. on Orthopedics), *30*:565–572, 1937.

Busch, W.: *Lehrbuch der Chirurgie*. Berlin, J. Springer, Vol. 2, p. 111, 1864.

Cabeca, C.: Sub-luxacao espontanea do punho; carpus curvus. *Rev. Portug. Med. Cir. Pratica*, *6*:51–58, 1899.

Cantagrel, A.: *Contribution à l'Étude de la Dyschondroséose;* à propos d'un cas familial. Thèse. Paris, No. 293, 1951.

Cantas, M.: Contribution a l'étude de la pathogénie de la déformation de Madelung ou radius curvus: sur un cas de maladie de Madelung ou radius curvus d'origine tuberculeuse. *Lyon Chir.*, *10*:434–469, 1913.

Canton, J.: Un cas de dyschondroplasie radio-cubitale inférieure avec hemiatrophie epiphysaire radiale. *Rev. d'Orthop.*, *22*:58–61, 1935.

Canton, J.: A propos de la maladie de Madelung. *Rev. d'Orthop.*, *27*:322–325, 1941.

Carrido-Lestache, J.: Un caso de enfermidad de Madelung. *La Pediatr. Espan.*, *14*:138–143, 1925.

Catterina, A.: Contributo allo studio della malattia di Madelung. *Chir. Organi. Mov.*, *10*:517–532, 1926.

Chastinent, de G., and Colombier: Deux cas de radius curvus. *Bull. Mém. Soc. Anat.* (Paris), *17*:370–376, 1920. See also *Presse Méd.*, *42*:418, 1920.

Chierici, R.: Madelung e pseudo-Madelung. *Quaderni Radiol.*, 7:3–24, 1936.

Chrysospathes: Zwei Fälle von gegenleicher Madelung's Deformität. Zugleich ein Beitrage zur Aetiologie derselben. *Arch. Orthop. Unfallchir.*, *11*:328–338, 1912.

Ciaccia, S.: Lussazione isolata, volare, dell'ulna, nell articulazione radio-ulnare inferior. *Arch. Ital. Chir.*, *8*:641–657, 1924.

Claiborne, E. M., and Kautz, F. G.: Madelung's deformity with report of a case. *Radiology*, *27*:594–599, 1936.

Clutton, N. H.: On adolescent or late rickets. *Lancet*, *2*:1268–1271; fig. 3, 1906.

Cnopf: Uber Madelung's spontane Subluxation des Handgelenks nach vorn. *Festschrift fur Hofrat.* Goschel, Tubingen, 1902; abstracted in *Zentral. Chir.*, *30*:574–575, 1903.

Cocchi, U.: Madelung's deformity. *In* Schinz, H. R., Baensch, E., Friedl, E., and Uehlinger, E., (eds.): *Roentgen-Diagnostics.* Translated by J. T. Case. New York, Grune and Stratton, Vol. I (Part I), pp. 789–792, 1951.

Codet-Boisse, P.: Deformation symétrique de deux poignets de type Dupuytren-Madelung. *Rev. d'Orthop.*, *2*:35–45, 1911.

Corcos, A., Mokkadem, S., Stam'rad, M., and Abitbol, S.: Un cas familial de maladie de Madelung. *Arch. Fr Pédiatr.*, *8*:313–315, 1951.

Cserey-Pechany, A.: Beitrag zur Aetiology und Therapie der Madelung'schen Krankheit. *Zentralbl. Chir.*, *57*:774–777, 1930.

Curtillot, J.: Quatre cas d'exostoses ostéogenique multiples héréditaires et familiales. *Rev. d'Orthop.*, *3*:193–206, 1912.

Dalbera, M.: *La Loi d'Ollier.* Son application en pathologie notamment dan la maladie de Madelung et l'hemimélie partielle. Thèse. Paris, M. Vigne, pp. 1–55, 1927.

Dannenberg, M., Anton, J. I., and Spiegel, M. B.: Madelung's deformity: consideration of its roentgenological diagnostic criteria. *Am. J. Roentgenol.*, *42*:671–676, 1939.

Darrach, W.: Habitual forward dislocation of the head of the ulna. *Ann. Surg.*, *57*:928–930, 1913.

Darrach, W.: Derangements of the inferior radio-ulnar articulation. *In Livre Jubilaire offert au docteur Albin Lambotte par ses amis et ses élèves.* Bruxelles, Vromant and Co., pp. 147–153, 1936.

Davoigneau, and Lehmann, R.: Trois cas de maladie de Madelung. *Presse Méd.*, *31*:955, 1923.

De-Bernardi, R.: Contributo radiologico allo studio delle deformita di Madelung. *Radiol. Medica*, *12*:392–398, 1925.

Dee: Spontaneous luxation of wrists—Madelung deformity. *Med. J. South Afr.*, *16*:158–159, 1921.

Define, B.: Sobre un cas de deformidade di Madelung. *Ann Paulistas Med. Cir.*, *15*:237–245, 1924.

Dekeyser, A.: Subluxation spontanée du poignet; subluxation de Madelung. *J. Med. Bruxelles, 6*:593–597, 1901.

Delbet, P.: Carpus curvus. *In Leçons de Clinique Chirurgicale Faites a l'Hôtel-Dieu.* Paris, G. Steinheil, pp. 161–190, 1899.

Delitala, F.: Sulla malattia Madelung. *Clinica Chir.*, *31*:1256, 1928. See also *Riforma Med.*, *44*:1498, 1928.

Delitala, F., and DeGennaro, R.: *Trattato di Tecnica Orthopedica e Traumatologica.* Milano, F. Vallardi, pp. 192–193, 1950.

Denucé, and Rabère: Subluxation progressive des poignets. Maladie de Madelung. *J. Med. Bordeaux*, No. 4, pp. 58–59, 1908.

Depouz, L.: *Contribution a l'Étude de la Maladie de Madelung*. Thèse, Lausanne, 1938.

Destot, E.: *Traumatismes de Poignet et Rayons-x*. Paris, Masson Cie, pp. 136–140, 1923.

Destot, E.: *Injuries of the Wrist, a Radiological Study*. New York, P. B. Hoeber, pp. 137–141, 1926.

D'Ettore, A.: La displasia radio-ulnare tipo Madelung. *Radiol Med.* (Torino), 49:540–552, 1963.

Digby, K. H.: The measurement of diaphyseal growth in proximal and distal directions. *J. Anat. Physiol.*, 50:187–188, 1916.

Dimitriu, V.: Un cas rare de maladie de Madelung. *J. Radiol. Electrol.*, 18:535–536, 1934.

Dodinval, P., and Collard, M.: Un cas isolé de dyschondrostéose. *Humangenetik*, 6:557–562, 1965.

Duplay, S.: De l'ostéotomie linéaire du radius pour remédier au difformités du poignet soit spontanées, soit traumatiques. *Arch. Gen. Med.*, 15:385–395, 1885.

Duplay, S.: Un cas de rachitism tardif der poignets. *Gaz. Hop.*, 64:1397–1398, 1891.

Dupuytren: *Leçons Orale de Clinique Chirurgicale Faites a l'Hôtel-Dieu de Paris*. Paris, F. Baillière, Vol. 4, pp. 197, 209–210, 1834.

Earl, G.: Madelung's deformity. *Journal-Lancet*, 36:229–232, 1916.

Ellsworth, H. A.: Inheritance of carpal displacement. *J. Hered.*, 18:132–133; fig. 8, 1927.

Elmslie, R. C.: Madelung's deformity of left wrist. *Proc. R. Soc. Med. London* (Sect. Surgery, Subsect. Orthopedics), 15:82, 1922.

Erlacher, P.: Gabelhand bei kongenitaler lues. Beitrage zur Enstichung der Madelung'schen Deformität. *Arch. Klin. Chir.*, 123:776–789, 1923.

Estor, E.: De la subluxation congénitale du poignet. *Rev. Chir.*, 36:145–168, 317–348, 1907.

Ewald, P.: Madelungsche Deformität als Symptom und als Krankheit sui Generis. *Z. Orthop. Chir.*, 23:470–497, 1900.

Ewald, P.: Zur Aetiologie der Madelung'schen Deformität. *Arch. Klin. Chir.*, 84:1099–1111, 1907.

Fazio, L.: Sulla radiodistrofia del Madelung. *Arch. Ortop.*, 44:551–565, 1930.

Felix, J.: *Étude sur la subluxation spontanée du Poignet en Avant*. Thèse. Lyon, Imp. Nouvelle, pp. 5–80, pl. 1–11, 1884.

Felix, W.: Beitrag zur Kasuistik der Madelungschen Deformität. *Z. Orthop. Chir.*, 49:563–568, 1928.

Felman, A. H., and Kirkpatrick, J. A., Jr.: Madelung's deformity: Observation in 17 patients. *Radiology*, 93:1037–1042, 1969.

Felman, A. H., and Kirkpatrick, J. A.: Dyschondrosteose. Mesomelic dwarfism of Léri and Weill. *Am. J. Dis. Child.*, 120:329–331, 1970.

Féré, C.: Note sur les deformités de développement du cubitus et de la clavicule. *Rev. Chir.*, 16:398–409, 1896.

Fick, R., and Pahl, J.: Über einen Fall von doppelseitiger Madelung'schen Fehlform der Handgelenkes mit Berucksichtigung seiner Mechanik. *Arch. Klin. Chir.*, 163:499–518, 1931.

Finzi, N. S.: The cause of Madelung's deformity. *The International Congress of Medicine*. 17th. London, Discussion and Proceedings, Section 7, Part 2, Orthopedics, pp. 339–344, 1913.

Finzi, N. S.: Quelques belles épreuves de radiographies de la difformité de Madelung. *Presse Méd.*, 21:727, 1913.

Foschini, D.: Contributo alla patogenesi della deformita di Madelung. *G. Clin. Med.*, 8:510–513, 1927.

Fournier, A., Pauli, A., Cousin, J., Cecile, J. P., Régnier, G., and Cuvelier, J.: Dyschondrostéose de Léri-Weill. *Pediatrie*, 26:291–303, 1971.

Franke: Zur Anatomie der Madelungschen Deformität der Hand. *Dtsch. Z. Chir.*, 92:156–180; Taf. v.; figs. 2–5, 1908.

Frassi, G.: Considerazioni su aspetii anatomico-radiografici della displasie del polso e dell avanbraccio tipo Madelung. *Arch. Ortop.*, 74:80–91, 1961.

Frere, J. M.: Madelung's deformity (case report). *South. Med. J.*, 35:168–171, 1942.

Froelich, M.: Radius curvus ou maladie de Madelung. *Rev. Med. l'Est.*, 1:586–587, 1922.

Fromme, A.: Madelungsche Handdeformität. *Ergeb. Chir. Orthop.*, 14:148–149, 1922.

Gadrat, J., and Marques, P.: Exostoses ostéogéniques multiples et main de Madelung. *J. Radiol. Electrol.*, 19:72–78, 1935.

Gaillot, G. H.: *Contribution a l'Étude du Radius Curvus*. Thèse. Lille, Imp. Centrale du Nord, pp. 5–115, 1907.

Gallardo, L. S.: Estudio de la anatomia y patogenia de un caso de deformidad de Madelung. *Rev. Med.* (Barcelona), 4:251–274, 1925.

Galliard, L., and Levy, F.: Micromélie avec malformation symétrique des radius. *Bull. Soc. Méd. Hop.* (Paris), 21:1103–1106, 1904.

Gangolphe: Déformation singulière du poignet inexactment dénommee subluxation spontanée. *Bull. Soc. Chir.* (Lyon), 2:117–123, 1899.

Gangolphe: Malformation congénitale du poignet, *Lyon Méd.*, 90:451, 1899.

Garrido-Lestache, J.: Un caso de enfermidad de Madelung. *La Pediatr. Espan.*, 14:138–143, 1925.

Gasne, E.: Déformation rachitiques tardives du poignet: Subluxation de Madelung et radius curvus. *Rev. d'Orthop.*, (2 s.), 7:153–170, 241–260, 1906.

Gasne, E.: La maladie de Madelung. *Rev. d'Orthop.*, 2:435–476, 493–513, 1911.

Gatto, I.: Contributo alla genetica delle deformita di Madelung. *Acta Genet. Med. Gem.*, 4:205–216, 1955.

Gaudier, H.: Déformation rachitique symétrique des deux poignets par radius curvus. *Rev. d'Orthop.,* (2 s.), *10*:263–266, 1909.

Gaugele, K.: Gibt es eine genuine Madelung'sche Handgelenks Deformität? *Z. Orthop. Chir., 24*:462–479, 1909.

Gaugele, K.: Madelung'sche Handgelenksdeformität. *Arch. Klin. Chir., 88*:1058–1075, 1909.

Gazzotti, L.: Contributo al trattamento delle deformita di Madelung mediante l'osteotomia lineare obliqua del radio. *Atti S.L.O.T., 21*:77–78, 1930.

Gazzotti, L.: Contributo al trattamento della deformita di Madelung. *Chir. Organi. Mov. 16*:263–273, 1931.

Gazzotti, L.: Deformita schléltriche da chondrodystrofia. *Boll. Soc. Med. Chir.* (Reggiana), *6*:84–90, 1933.

Gellis, S. S., and Feingold, M.: Picture of the month – Dyschondrosteosis (Léri-Weill syndrome, Léri's pleonosteosis). *Am. J. Dis. Child., 122*:429–430, 1971.

Geraud, Verger, and Pepet: Un cas de maladie de Madelung. *Presse Méd., 59*:377–378, 1951.

Gery, de Chastenet, and Colombier: Deux cas de radius curvus. *Bull. Mém. Soc. Anat.* (Paris), *17*:370–376, 1920.

Gevaert, G.: Un cas de subluxation de poignet de Madelung. *Rev. d'Orthop.,* (2 s.), *3*:335–343, 1902.

Ghormley, R. K., and Pollock, G. A.: Osteochondrodystrophy of the inferior radial epiphysis (Madelung's deformity). *Proc. Staff Meet. Mayo Clin., 14*:759–763, 1939.

Gickler, H.: Wachstumsstorung der Radiusepiphyse und Madelungsche Deformität. *Arch. Orthop. Unfallchir., 33*:312–318, 1933.

Ginliani, K.: Zur Therapie der habituellen Subluxation und veralteten Luxation im distalen Radio-ulnar-Gelenk. *Z. Orthop., 92*:626–629, 1960.

Giordano, G., and Palmieri, C. A.: A proposito della deformita di Madelung: le epifisiti et le metafisiti *Boll. Sci. Mediche, 110*:54–57, 1938.

Girardet, P.: Un cas de dyschondroplasie déformante du radius ou maladie de Madelung chez une fille de 8 ans. *Helvet. Pediatr. Acta, 13*:75–80, 1958.

Goetz, A. G., and Fatheree, T. J.: Madelung's deformity. *U.S. Naval Med. Bull., 44*:148–151, 1945.

Gogdet-Boise, P.: Déformation symétrique de deux poignets du Dupuytren-Madelung. *Rev. d'Orthop.,* (3 s.), *5*:305, 1923.

Grebe, H.: Madelungsche Deformität. *In* Becker, P. B., (ed.): *Humangenetik.* Stuttgart, G. Thieme, Vol. 2, p. 218, 1964.

Greig, D. M.: Congenital distal dislocation of the ulna. *Edinburgh Med. J., 31*:373–391, 1924.

Guépin, A.: Laxité congénitale de l'articulation radiocubitale inférieure et subluxation consecutive de la tête du cubitus en arriè. *C. R. Hebd. Soc. Biol., 4*:627–631, 1892.

Guéry, A.: Un cas de luxation progressive du poignet (subluxation spontanée de Madelung). *Rev. d'Orthop., 9*:277–282, 1898.

Guye: Observation d'un cas de maladie de Dupuytren-Madelung bilatérale. *Rev. Med. Suisse Romande, 39*:191–192, 1919.

Henry, A., and Thorborn, M. J.: Madelung's deformity: a clinical and cytogenic study. *J. Bone Joint Surg., 49B*:66–73, 1967.

Herdman, R. C., Langer, L. O., and Good, R. A.: Dyschondrosteosis. The most common cause of Madelung's deformity. *J. Pediatr., 88*:432–441, 1966.

Hoffmann, P.: A case of congenital dislocation of the wrist. *Trans. Am. Orthop. Assoc., 13*:96–97, 1900.

Hohmann, G.: *Hand und Arm.* Munchen, J. F. Bergmann, pp. 163–169, 1949.

Holenstein, P., and Buchs, P.: Die Madelungsche Deformität: Ausdruck einer Dyschondrosteose. *Z. Orthop. Chir., 102*:585–594, 1967.

Homuth, O.: Die Madelung'sche Deformität in ihrer Beziehung zur Rachitis. *Beitr. Klin. Chir., 74*:562–584, 1911.

Hopf, A.: Die Madelung'sche Deformität der Handgelenkes. *In* Hohmann, G., MacKenbroch, M., and Lindemann, K., (eds.): Stuttgart, G. Thieme, Vol. 3, pp. 480–484, 1959.

Horwitz, T.: An anatomic and roentgenologic study of the wrist joint. Observations on a case of recurrent radiocarpal dislocation complicating Madelung's deformity and its surgical correction. *Surgery, 7*:773–783, 1940.

Hucherson, D. C.: The Darrach operation for lower radio-ulnar derangement. *Am. J. Surg., 53*:237–241, 1941.

Hulten, O.: Über anatomische Variationen der Handgelenksknochen. *Acta Radiol., 9*:157–168; Tab. IX-XII, 1928.

Humphry, G. M.: *A Treatise on the Human Skeleton* (including the joints). Cambridge, Macmillan & Co., pp. 383–398, 1858.

Hutchinson, J.: Some general remarks on the series of cases and on the employment of names. *Arch. Surg., 9*:26–27, 1898.

Ianni, R.: Radius curvus (Deformita de Madelung-Duplay). *Ann. Ital. Chir., 3*:40–61, 1924.

Ingber, E.: Un caso tipico di deformita di Madelung bilaterale e concomitante reperto radiologico di sacralizzazione genuina ed asintomatica del Ve metamero lombare. *Quaderni Radiol., 5*:251–257, 1934.

Jacoulet: Un cas de maladie Dupuytren-Madelung. *Rev. d'Orthop., 1*:35–42, 1910.

Jagot: Sur un vice héréditaire de conformation des deux poignets. *Arch. Med. Angers, 1*:159–170, 1897.

Jantzen, P. M.: Madelung'sche Deformität bei Zwillingen. *Z. Orthop.*, 89:121–124, 1957.

Jean, A.: Double luxation congénitale, complète du cubitus et incomplète du radius sur les os du carpe. *Bull. Soc. Anat.* (Paris), 10:398–400, 1875.

Jeune, M., and Larbre, F.: Un cas dyschondrostéose. *Pédiatrie*, 9:58–61, 1954.

Jones, S. F.: Bilateral congenital dislocation of the lower end of the ulna. *Am. Orthop. Assoc.*, 10:199–217, 1912.

Josa, L.: A csuklo Madelung-fele deformitasanak egy esete. *Orvosi Hetilap.*, 70:1321–1324, 1926.

Joüon, R.: Déformation de l'avant-bras par arrête développement de l'extrémité inférieure du cubitus, de cause inconnue. *Rev. d'Orthop.*, 6:81–84, 1905.

Kajon, V. C.: Madelung'sche Deformität Kombiniert mit Halsrippen. *Wien Med. Wochenschr.*, 84:460–462, 1934.

Kaplan, M., Guy, E., and Cantegrel, A.: Dyschondrostéose familiale. *Presse Méd.*, 59:1723–1725, 1951.

Kieffer, C. F.: Congenital dislocation of both ulnae at the wrists. *Ann. Surg.*, 38:119–120, 1903.

Kirmisson, E.: *Les Difformités Acquisés de l'Appareil Locomoteur Pendant l'Enfance et l'Adolescence.* Paris, Masson et Cie, pp. 363–375, 1902.

Kirsch, J., and Valetas: Maladie de Madelung et dyschondroplasie. *J. Radiol. Electrol.*, 31:625–628, 1950.

Kirschmair, H.: Angeborene Fehlbildungen und Anomalien. 3. Dyschondrosteose (Léri-Weill Syndrom): mit über einen weiteren Fall. *Med. Monatsschr.*, 16:174–175, 1962.

Kollicker, T.: Die Dupuytren'sche und Madelung'sche Deformität der Handgelenkes. *In* Joachimsthal, (ed.): *Handbuch der Chirurgie.* Vol. II, pp. 34–36, 1907.

Koptis, E.: Ein seltene Form der Unterarmverbiegung. *Z. Orthop.*, 69:402–410, 1939.

Kuhn, E.: *Contribution a l'Étude de la Maladie de Madelung.* Thèse. Paris, Imp. Studio, pp. 13–45, 1933.

Lamy, M., and Biennenfeld, C.: La dyschondrosteose. *Analecta Genetica* (Roma), pp. 153–164, 1954.

Lamy, M., and Maroteaux, P.: *Les Chondrodysplasie Génotypique.* Paris, Expansion Scientifique Française, pp. 33–39, 1960.

Landivar, A. F., Iparraguirre, and Cesar, A. L.: Radius curvus bilateral de comienzo tario. *Bol. Trab. Soc.* (Buenos Aires), 20:1160–1168, 1936.

Lange, M.: *Orthopädisch-Chirurgische Operationslehre.* Munchen, J. F. Bergmann, pp. 365–366, 1951.

Langer, L. O.: Dyschondrosteosis, a hereditable bone dysplasia with characteristic roentgenographic features. *Am. J. Roentgenol.*, 95:178–188, 1965.

Laurence, J.: La maladie de Dupuytren-Madelung. *Rev. Gen. Clin. Therap. J. Practiciens*, 37:75, 1923.

Leclerc: Radius curvus. *Bull. Soc. Chir.* (Lyon), 8:115–120, 1905.

Leni, E.: Sul morbo di Madelung. *R. Ass. Previd. Soc.*, 26:25–33, 1939.

Lenormant, C. H.: Un nouveau cas de radius curvus. *Rev. d'Orthop.*, (2 s.), 8:1–10, 1907.

Léri, A., and Weill, J.: Une affection congénitale et symétrique du développement osseux: la dyschondrostéose. *Bull. Mém. Soc. Méd. Hôp. Paris*, 53:1491–1494, 1929.

Léri, A., Flandin, C., and Arnaudet: La dyschondrostéose: présentation d'un nouveau cas. *Bull. Mém. Soc. Méd. Hôp. Paris*, 54:385–388, 1930.

Léri, A., Layant, F., and Weill, J.: La dyschondrostéose: variété nouvelle de nanism. *Presse Méd.*, 39:262–264, 1931.

Leriche, R.: Sur un cas de maladie de Madelung bilatérale par lesion du cartilage de conjugation radial. *Rev. d'Orthop.*, (2 s.), 10:495–500, 1909.

Levy, R.: Ueber Madelung'sche Hangelenksdeformität. *Berl. Klin. Wochenschr.*, 452:2213–2216, 1908.

Levyn, N. L.: Madelung's deformity. *Radiology*, 3:145–149, 1924.

Llado, A. C., and Gallardo, L. S.: Estudio de la anatomia y patogenia de un caso de deformidad de Madelung. *Rev. Med.* (Barcelona), 4:251–474, 1935.

Lombard, P., and Natter, S.: Impuissance ostéogénique et perturbations encephalographiques dans un cas de maladie de Madelung. *Rev. Chir. Orthop.*, 39:161–170, 1953.

Lowman, C. L.: The use of fascia lata in the repair of disability at the wrist. *J. Bone Joint Surg.*, 12:400–402, 1930.

Macciocchi, B.: Rilievi genetici sulla dismorfosi di Madelung. *Minerva Ortop.*, 7:266–269, 1956.

MacLennan, A.: Report of a case of Madelung's deformity. *Br. Med. J.*, 2:759–760, 1909.

Madelung, V.: Die spontane Subluxation der Hand nach vorne. *Arch. Klin. Chir.*, 23:395–412; Taf. V; fig. 3–8, 1878. Also in *Verhandl. Dtsch. Ges. Chir.*, 7:259–276, 1878.

Magnus, G.: Ueber Madelungsche Deformität. *Med. Klin. Berl.*, 8:2069–2070, 1912.

Malgaigne, J. F.: *Traité des Fractures et des Luxations.* Paris, J. B. Baillière. Vol. 2. pp. 711–713, 1855.

Maroteaux, P., and Lamy, M.: La dyschondrostéose. *Sém. Hôp. Paris*, 35:3460–3470, 1959.

Marsan, F.: Sur un noveau cas de maladie de Madelung. *Arch. Gen. Chir.*, 2:472–482, 1908

Marsan, F.: La maladie de Madelung (radius curvus). *Gaz. Hôp.* (Paris), 81:1671–1679, 1909.

Marti, T.: De la maladie de Madelung-Dupuytren. *Rev. Med. Suisse Romande*, 60:31–50, 1940.

Masmonteil, F.: A propos de la pathogénie de la maladie de Madelung (radius brevior). *Gaz. Hôp.*, (Paris), 93:101–103, 1920.

Masmonteil, F.: Toujours a propos de la pathogénie de la maladie de Madelung. *Lyon Chir.*, 18:351–355, 1921.

Masmonteil, F., and Leuret, J.: Deux cas de maladie de Madelung, dont l'un compliqué tardivement de rupture spontanée des tendons extenseurs des trois derniers doigts. *Soc. Chir.* (Paris), 37:26–30, 1946.

Mathieu, C., and Joseph, V.: A propos d'un cas de maladie de Dupuytren Madelung bilatérale. *Rev. Méd. l'Est, 1*:691–701, 1922; also, Radius curvus bilatérale. *Rev. Méd. l'Est, 1*:586, 1922.

Mau, H.: Dysostotische Minusvarianten der Elle und Speiche (Abortive Madelungsche Deformität-Subluxation der Elle-Lunatummaladie). *Z. Orthop. Chir., 89*:17–29, 1958.

Mauclaire, P.: Trois observations de subluxation progressive du poignet avec alterations du cartilage conjugal dans deux cas. *Bull. Mém. Soc. Chir.* (Paris), *42*:344–346, 1916.

Mauclaire, P., and Labadie-Lagrave: Un cas de maladie de Madelung. *Bull. Mém. Soc. Chir.* (Paris), *35*:695–696, 1909.

Mazzini, O. F.: Enfermidad der Madelung. *Semana Med.* (Buenos Aires), *32*:626–639, 1925.

Melchior, E.: Ueber die Kombination von symmetrischer Madelungscher Handgelenksdeformität mit doppelseitiger metakarpaler Brachydaktylie. *Z. Orthop. Clin., 30*:532–537, 1912.

Melchior, E.: Die Madelung'sche Deformität des Handgelenkes. *Ergeb. Chir. Orthop., 6*:649–680, 1913.

Merlini, A.: La deformita di Madelung. *Chir. Organi. Mov., 9*:245–268, 1925.

Milch, H.: Cuff resection of the ulna for malunited colles fracture. *J. Bone Joint Surg., 23*:311–313, 1941.

Milch, H.: Short radius. *Arch. Surg., 59*:856–869, 1949.

Monastero, G., and Mandala, L.: Contributo alla genetica della deformita di Madelung. *Minerva Ortop., 3*:103–106, 1958.

Monticelli, G.: Osservazioni sulle displasia del polso tipo deformita di Madelung. *Ortop. Tram. App. Mot., 18*:167–183, 1950.

Monticelli, G.: Sulle deformita de polso tipo pseudo-Madelung e sui distacchi epiphisari del radio. *Ort. Traum. App. Mot., 18*:265–280, 1950.

Moore, B. H.: Radius curvus (Madelung's wrist). *J. Bone Joint Surg., 6*:568–574, 1924.

Muller, W.: Madelung'schen Deformität des Handgelenkes. *Zentralbl. Chir., 34*:1333–1334, 1907.

Narakas, A.: Die Dyschondrosteose. *Schweiz. Med. Wochenschr., 95*:609, 1965.

Nassif, R., and Harboyan, G.: Madelung's deformity with conductive hearing loss. *Arch. Otolaryngol., 91*:175–178, 1970.

Natvig, R.: Madelungs haanddeformitet. *Tdskrft. Laegef., 25*:553–555, 1905.

Negré, A., Villat, M., and Kaydel, P.: A propos de la maladie de Madelung. *J. Radiol. Electrol., 30*:472–473, 1948.

Negri, L., and Zappoli, S.: Sul trathamento del morbo di Madelung. *Chir. Organi. Mov., 47*:50–61, 1959.

Nelaton, Ch.; Luxations radio-carpiens. *In* Duplay and Reclus, (eds.): *Traité de Chirurgie.* Vol. 3, pp. 121–125, 1897.

Niccolini, G., and Andreini, G.: Osservazione sopra tre casi di malattia di Madelung. *Atti S.I.O.T., 40*:277–282, 1955.

Nissen, R.: Verfahren bei Madelungscher Deformität. Die Operationen an der oberen Extremität. *In* Bier, Braun, and Kummell, (eds.): *Chirurgische Operationslehre.* Leipzig, J. A. Barth, Vol. 5, pp. 180–184, 1933.

Nove-Josserand, G.: La maladie du Dupuytren-Madelung. *Seventeenth International Congress of Medicine,* London. Part I, Orthop., pp. 206–208, 1913.

Nove-Josserand, G.: Radius curvus (subluxation progressive du poignet. *In* Denuce and Nove-Josserand, G., (eds.): *La Pratique de Maladies des Enfants.* Denuce; G. Nove-Josserand. Paris, J. B. Baillière et Fils, pp. 95–96, fig. 37, 1913.

Painter, C. F.: Congenital dislocation of the carpus. *In* Bryan and Buck, (eds.): *American Practice of Surgery.* Vol. 4, pp. 742–746, 1908.

Palazzi, G.: Contributo alla cura operatoria della deformita di Madelung. *Clin. Chir., 17*:804–815, 1909.

Palmieri, G. G.: A proposita delle dismorfosi di Madelung. *Arch. Ital. Chir., 53*:392–497, 1938.

Palmieri, G. G.: Ulterior contributi alla interpretazione patogenetica della dismorfosi di Madelung. *Boll. It. Sci. Med., 3*:157–165, 1939.

Palmieri, G. G.: Un caso di "pseudo-Madelung." *Boll. Sci. Med.* (Bologna), *112*:424–429, 1940.

Paltrinieri, M.: Sulla deformita di Madelung. *Boll. Sci. Med.* (Bologna), *110*:32–39, 1938.

Parkes, W. R.: Madelung's deformity of wrist. *Illinois Med. J., 27*:286–288, 1915.

Paulsen, K.: Über die Madelungsche Deformität der Hand. *Arch. Klin. Chir., 75*:506, 1905.

Paus, B.: Madelung's deformity. Its etiology and pathogenesis. *Acta Orthop. Scand., 21*:249–258, 1951.

Peckham, F. E.: Report of a case of congenital deformity of the wrist joints. *Am. J. Orthop. Surg., 4*:388–389, 1907.

Peckham, F. E., and Hammond, R.: Madelung's deformity. *Boston Med. Surg. J., 160*:448; figs. 4, 5, 1909.

Pedrazzi, C.: Deformità di Madelung famigliare. *Radiol. Medica, 14*:125–132, 1927.

Pels-Leusden: Madelung'sche Deformität der Hand. *Zentralbl. Chir., 1*:190–191, 1907.

Pels-Leusden: Madelung'sche Deformität der Hand. Freir Vereingung der Chirurgen Berlins. *Z. Chir., 34*:190, 1907.

Pels-Leusden: Ueber die Madelung'sche Deformität der Hand. *Dtsch. Med. Wochenschr., 33*:372–374, 1907.

Perricone, F.: Sulla cura della deformita di Madelung. *Chir. Organi. Mov., 34*:291–294, 1950.

Perthies: Madelung, Otto Wilhelm. *Arch. Klin. Chir., 143*:1–7, 1926.

Phemister, D. B.: Operative arrestment of longitudinal growth of bones in the treatment of deformities. *J. Bone Joint Surg.*, *15*:1–15, 1933.

Pilatte, R. E.: *Contribution a l'Étude du Radius curvus.* Thèse. Paris, A. Maloine et Fils, pp. 9–84, 1919.

Pilatte, R.: Sur la pathogénie du radius curvus. *Rev. d'Orthop.*, 8:223–224, 1921.

Pinais, D., and Heimann, W. G.: Mesomelic dwarfism (dyschondrosteosis of Léri and Weill). *J.A.M.A.*, *193*:1056–1057, 1965.

Piollet: Un cas de radius curvus. *Bull. Soc. Chir.* (Lyon), *107*:274–277, 1906.

Poncet, A., and Leriche, R.: La maladie de Madelung. Ses modalités, sa pathogénie. *Gaz. Hôp.*, 82:187–191, 1909.

Ponte, A.: Osteotomia ad incastro del radio come trattamento di "pseudo-Madelung." *Arch. Putti*, *14*:387–395, 1961.

Pooley, J. H.: Congenital dislocation of the wrists. *Am. Practitioner*, *21*:216–220, 1880.

Poucel: Carpus Séance de la Société de Chirurgie de Marseille, November, 1929. *Presse Méd.*, *38*:24, 1929.

Poulsen, K.: Om den Madelung'sche Deformität af Handen. *Hospitalstid.* (Kopenhagen), *12*:817–838, 1904.

Poulsen, K.: Ueber die Madelung'sche Deformität der hand. *Arch. Klin. Chir.*, *75*:506–532, 1905.

Putti, V.: Le deformita di Madelung. *Arch. Int. Chir.*, *3*:64–98, 1906.

Putti, V.: Sulla deformità di Madelung. *Arch. Ortop.*, *25*:469, 1908.

Putti, V.: Sur la malformation de Madelung. *Rev. d'Orthop.*, *10*:207–220, 1909.

Quadrone, C.: Contribution a l'étude de la maladie de Madelung (subluxation spontanée du poignet). *N. Iconog. Salp.*, *24*:71–80, 1911.

Racansky, F.: La deformidad de Madelung. *Seplek. Cesk.*, *66*:1190–1197, 1927.

Redard, P.: Sur une déformation rare du poignet. *Arch. Gen. Med.*, *30*:651–667, 1892.

Redard, P.: Difformité congénitale rare des avant-bras, synostoses radio-cubitales. Radius curvus. *Rev. d'Orthop.*, *9*:113–119; Pl. V, 1908.

Reich: Die Madelung'sche Handgelenksdefosmität als Erbkrankheit *Zentralbl. Chir.*, *54*:1015–1016, 1927.

Reinhard, W. E.: Die Madelungsche Deformität des Handgelenkes und ihre Grundlagen. *Dtsch. Med. Runsch.* (Mainz), *3*:153–159, 1949.

Robinson, R.: De la carpocyphose. (Anatomie normale et pathologique de l'articulation radio-cubitale inférieure.) *C. R. Acad. Sci.* (Paris), *147*:1412–1413, 1908. See also *Gaz. Hôp.*, *81*:1781, 1908.

Robinson, R., and Jacoulet, F.: La luxation congénitale de l'extrémite inférieure du cubitus. *Arch. Gén. Chir.*, *3*:1–30, 1909.

Rocher, H. L.: A propos de notre septième observation de maladie de Madelung: Dyschondroplasie radio-cubitale inférieure par hemiatrophie epiphysaire radiale interne. *J. Med. Bordeaux*, *114*:513–518, 1937.

Rocher, H. L.: Maladie de Madelung, radius curvus. *In* Ombredanne, L., and Mathieu, P.: *Traite de Chirurgie Orthopédique.* Paris, Masson et Cie, Vol. 3, pp. 2485–2500, 1937.

Rocher, H. L.: Dyschondroplasie de l'epiphyse radial inférieure ou maladie de Madelung. *Presse Méd.*, *49*(2):717–718, 1941.

Rocher, H. L.: Maladie de Madelung, quelques considérations a propos de deux nouvelles observations. *Rev. Rheum.*, *11*:213–217, 1942.

Rocher, H. L., and Canton, J.: Pathogénie de la difformité de Madelung. *Arch. Franco-Belges Chir.*, *35*:98–102, 1935.

Rocher, H. L., and Rocher, C.: La maladie de Madelung, Dyschondroplasie radio-cubitale inférieure conditionée essentiellement par l'héimatrophie épiphysaire radiale. *Chir. Organi. Mov.*, *20*:20–30, 1934.

Rocher, H. L., and Roudil, G.: Dysmorphose congenitale bilatérale des poignets par hemiatrophie epiphysaire radiale. *Presse Méd.*, *38*:1089–1090, 1930.

Roederer, C.: Un cas de maladie de Madelung larvée. *Bull. Mém. Soc. Chir.* (Paris), *20*:235–237, 1928.

Roget, E.: *Étude sur le Radius Curvus.* These. Lyon, Imp. P. Legendre Cie, pp. 5–56, pl. 1–2, 1899.

Rosenfeld, L.: *Lehrbuch der Orthopädie.* Jena, G. Fischer, pp. 650–652, 1914.

Roudil, G., Drevon, and Mourgues: Dysmorphose congénitale bilatérale des poignets (Maladie de Madelung). *J. Radiol. Electrol.*, *20*:241–245, 1936.

Salisachs, L. G.: Contribucion al estudio de la deformidad de Madelung. *Rev. Med.* (Barcelona), *20*:105–137, 1933.

Sauer, F.: Die Madelung'sche Deformität des Handgelenkes. *Beitr. Klin. Chir.*, *48*:179–203; Taf. VIII, 1906.

Scharizer, E.: Zur Behandlung der Madelung'schen Deformität. *Z. Orthop.*, *87*:209–214, 1956.

Schinz, H. R.: Verebrung und Knochenban. *Schweiz Med. Wochenschr.*, *5*:1151–1156, 1924.

Schnek, F.: Federne dorsalluxation de elle Konsulenradius Madelung'sche Deformität. *Z. Ortop. Chir.*, *52*:101–110, 1930.

Schnek, F.: Die operative Besserung der echten und der sogenannten symptomatischen Madelungschen Deformität. *Z. Orthop. Chir.*, *53*:101–110, 1931.

Schulze, H.: Ein Fall von spontaner Subluxation der Hand nach un ten (Dupuytren-Madelungscher Subluxation). *Münch. Med. Wochenschr.*, *52*(2):1441–1443, 1905.

Scoutetten: Des luxation du poignet. *Bull. Acad. R. Med.*, *5*:796–804, 1841.

Siegmund, E.: Isolierte volare Luxation der Ulnaköpfchens. *Zentralbl. Chir.*, 55:1742–1745, 1928.

Siegrist, V. H.: Über manus valga oder sogenannte Madelungsche Deformität des Handgelenkes. *Dtsch. Z. Chir.*, 91:524–586; Taf. XII, 1908.

Sloane, D.: Madelung's deformity in sisters. *Am. J. Surg.*, 60:272–276, 1943.

Smith, E. W.: Compendium on shortness of stature. *J. Pediatr.*, 70:501–519, 1967.

Smith, R.: *Treatise on Fractures in the Vicinity of Joints and Congenital Dislocations.* Dublin, Hodges and Smith, pp. 236–265, 1847.

Solberg, M.: To tielfaulder af Madelung haandderformitat. *Tdschrf. Norske. Laegefr.*, 26:195–196, 1906.

Sorrel: Radius curvus opere, *Presse Méd.*, 33:189–190, 1925.

Spitzy: Die Madelungsche Deformität. *Verh. Dtsch. Orthop. Ges.*, 25:88–103, 1931.

Springer, C.: Zur Kenntnis der "Madelungschen Deformität" der Handgelenkes. *Z. Orthop. Chir.*, 29:216–244, 1911.

Springer, C.: Zur Operation der Madelung'schen Deformität: Korrektur der Gabelhand durch Osteotomie und Supination (Depronation). *Z. Orthop. Chir.*, 33:590–601, 1913.

Stehr, L.: Die ulnar-volare Bajonetthand als typische Fehlbildung bei Chondrodysplasien. *Fortschr. Röntgenstr.*, 57:587–604, 1938.

Steinhauser, J., and Merhof, G.: Röntgenstudien an Handgelenken zur Minusvariante der Elle (Hulten). *Z. Orthop.*, 107:11–24; Abb 4a–4d, 1969.

Stetten, W. de: Zur Frage der sog. "Madelung'schen Deformität" des Handgelenkes, mit besonderer Rücksicht auf eine umgekehrte Form derselben. *Zentralbl. Chir.*, 35:949–952, 1908.

Stetten, W. de: Idiopathic progressive curvature of the radius or so-called Madelung's deformity of the wrist (carpus varus and carpus valgus). *Surg. Gynecol. Obstet.*, 8:4–31, 1909.

Stieda, A.: Verein fur vessentschaftliche Heilkund in Konigsberg. *Dtsch. Med. Wochenschr.*, 31:989–990, 1907.

Stokes, A. C.: Spontaneous forward dislocation of wrist-joint (Madelung's deformity). *Ann. Surg.*, 52:229–238, 1910.

Tancredi, G.: Sulla deformita de Madelung (Contributo alla curo chirurgica). *Bull. Atti. Reale Acad.* (Roma), 57:153–158, 1931.

Taylor, H. L.: Progressive curvature of the radius (Madelung's deformity) corrected by osteotomy. *Med. Rec.*, 12:752–755, 1912.

Thiel, H. V., and Berquet, K. H.: Zwillingsheobachtung bei familiarer Dyschondrosteose. (Ein Beitrag zur Kenntnis des Morbus Léri-Weill). *Arch. Unfallchir.*, 65:182–188, 1968.

Thompson, C. F., and Kalayjian, B.: Madelung's deformity and associated deformity at elbow. *Surg. Gynecol. Obstet.*, 69:221–230, 1939.

Tillier, R.: Sur la pathogénie du "radius curvus." *Lyon Chir.*, 17:739–743, 1920.

Tollas, H.: Zur Ätiologie der Madelungschen Knochenkrankung an der Hand eines selbstbeobachteten Fälles. *Arch. Krankheilkd.*, 82:112–144, 1927.

Tomesku, I.: Ein Fälle einer atypischen Madelungschen Handgelenks-deformität. *Fortschr. Röntgenstr.*, 36:627–629, 1927.

Travaglini, F.: La cura chirurgica della deformità di Madelung. *Arch. Putti*, 16:409–421, 1962.

Trillmich, F.: Beitrag zur Madelung'schen deformität. *Z. Orthop. Chir.*, 31:69–80, 1913.

Vianna, B.: Doenca de Madelung. *Folla. Med.*, 12:241–251, 1931.

Vidal, C. A.: Sub-luxacao de Madelung-Duplay (carpur curvus). *Lisboa Med.*, 6:219–239, 1929.

Vigyazogy: Madelung's deformity of the hand (Hungarian). *Orvesi Hetilap.* (Budapest), 47:450–474, 1913.

Volkmann, Th.: *Ueber Madelung'sche Subluxation der Hand nach Vorne.* Inaug.-Diss. Leipzig, Druck von Bruno Georgi, pp. 5–30, 1905.

Vulpius, O., and Stoffel, A.: *Orthopädische Operationslehre.* Stuttgart, F. Enke, pp. 348–350, 1913.

Walther, C.: Décoloration de l'epiphyse inférieure du radius. *Rev. d'Orthop.*, 6:385–390, 1905.

Weill, J.: Les maladies osseuses constitutionelles VI. Une chondrodysteophic genetique. La dyschondrosteose. *Rev. Rheum.*, 32:133–139, 1965.

Werthemann, A.: *Die Entwicklungs-storungen der Extremiäten.* Berlin, Springer, pp. 274–276, 1952.

Wéry: Deux cas de maladie de Madelung. *Bruxelle Med.*, 2:45–46, 1921.

Weyers, H.: Die radio-ulnare Luxation oder Madelungsche Deformität, maladie de Madelung-Dupuytren, radio-ulnar Bajonethand. *In* Diethelm, L., (ed.): *Rontgendiagnostik der Skeleter Krankungen.* Berlin, Springer, Band V, Teil 3, pp. 430–431, 1968.

Whitman, R.: *A Treatise on Orthopedic Surgery.* Eighth edition. Philadelphia, Lea & Febiger, pp. 529–530, 1927.

Wright, L. T., and Kaufman, J.: Unusual type of Madelung-like deformity. *Am. J. Surg.*, 34:365–368, 1936.

Young, J. K.: *Manual and Atlas of Orthopedic Surgery.* Philadelphia, P. Blakiston Sons & Co., pp. 883–903, 1906.

Zeitlin, A.: Morbus Madelung oder Madelung'sche Deformität. *Zentralbl. Chir.*, 57:929–932, 1930.

Chapter Twenty-Three

RADIAL RAY DEFECT

The radius serves as the main support of the hand. When this bone is totally absent or is deficient in its distal portion, the hand inclines toward the radial border of the forearm and bends in the volar direction. The resulting radiopalmar deformity is called clubhand. The term radial clubhand is often used to distinguish this deformity from similar postural anomalies associated with spastic states, lower motor neuron lesions, arthrogryposis, craniocarpotarsal dystrophy, and various contractural conditions seen at birth. Bunnell and Dehne (1955) introduced the designation *clinarthrosis,* and Farmer and Laurin (1958) qualified this term with the adjective *radial.* Pardini (1968) indicated his preference for the term radial dysplasia. Dysplasia is an equivocal term meaning abnormal development, either over- or underdevelopment. Defects of the radial ray belong to the latter category; in many instances, it is not even a question of underdevelopment but of complete absence. O'Rahilly (1946, 1951) called this defect radial hemimelia, a term which most authors seem to prefer. In the present book, the terms radial hemimelia and radial ray defect are used interchangeably.

The radial ray consists of one solid bone, the radius, and a segmented portion composed of the scaphoid, the trapezium, the first metacarpal, and the two phalanges of the thumb. All these bones are absent in total terminal defect of the radial ray. In partial terminal deficiency, the first metacarpal and the two phalanges of the thumb, and sometimes varying portions of the distal radius, may be missing. When the radius is absent in part or as a whole but the skeletal elements of the pollical ray—the first metacarpal and the two phalanges of the thumb—persist, the defect is qualified as being proximal intercalary. In distal intercalary defect, the first metacarpal is missing in part or as a whole and occasionally the epiphysis of the proximal phalanx is absent. The radial carpal ossicles—the scaphoid and the trapezium—may be missing in partial terminal deficiency as well as in either proximal or distal intercalary defect. Isolated absences of the radial styloid and of the scaphoid or trapezium are classed with intercalary radial ray defect.

Davaine (1850) stated that absence of the radius entails absence of the thumb and its metacarpal. From this it was inferred that skeletal deficiencies of the thumb were invariably associated with defects of the corresponding radius.

During the ensuing decade, Dolbeau (1864) reported a case with rudimentary thumb and well-formed radius. Gruber's (1865) patient presented the opposite picture: suppressed radius and five digits, one of which was considered to be a thumb. Woodward (1869) reported a newborn infant with absent thumb on one side and floating pollex on the other. Parker's (1882) patient had bilateral absence of the radius; on the right side there were "five fingers and five metacarpal bones, but... no thumb." Horrocks (1889) reported a case of "arrested growth of the lower end of radius"; the accompanying photograph showed a radially deviated hand with a well-formed thumb and four fingers.

Ehrhardt (1890) cited five cases from the literature and added one of his own, of what he called ectromely of the thumb and its metacarpal; in none of these was the radius affected. Cases of absent thumb with intact radius have since been reported by Picqué and Poix (1896), Joachimsthal (1895), Mouchet (1904), and numerous recent authors. It is now generally recognized that in radial ray defect, the thumb may be present while the radius is absent or underdeveloped; conversely, the radius may remain while the thumb is missing. In distal intercalary deficiency, the first metacarpal is absent or stunted and the proximal

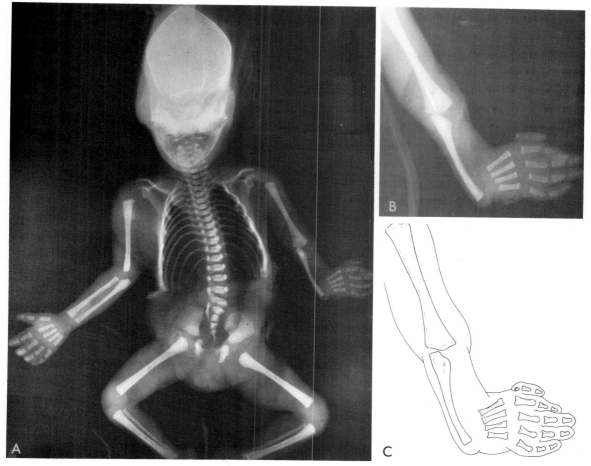

Figure 23–1   Unilateral intercalary defect of the radial ray. *A,* Anteroposterior roentgenograph of a stillborn fetus with absence of the left radius and proximal portion of the left first metacarpal, associated with dysplasia of the left acetabulum. *B,* Enlarged roentgenograph of the left upper limb. *C,* Sketch illustrating the same.

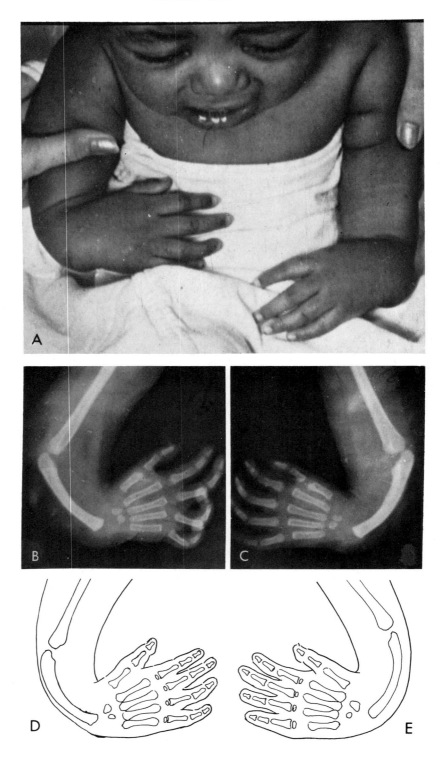

Figure 23–2   Bilateral intercalary defect of the radial ray. *A*, Frontal view of the upper limbs of a seven-month-old boy. *B*, Roentgenograph of the right upper extremity: the radius is missing but the skeletal components of the pollical ray are present. *C*, Roentgenograph of the left upper limb, showing the same defect as the right one. *D* and *E* illustrate the roentgenograph above each.

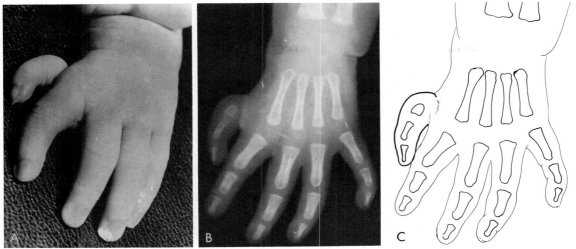

Figure 23–3 Intercalary defect of the pollical ray: floating thumb. *A*, Dorsopalmar view of the left hand of a three-month-old boy. *B*, Dorsopalmar roentgenograph. *C*, Sketch illustrating the same.

phalanx of the thumb is reduced in size. The last two segments of the thumb are attached to the side of the hand by a pedicle which contains nerves and vessels but seldom a tendon and only rarely a bone; the thumb dangles limply and is incapable of voluntary action—it is nonfunctional, useless.

The intercalary defect of the pollical ray just described was called *pouce flottant* by Dolbeau (1864). This term or its English equivalent, floating thumb, has become entrenched in the literature. Cases of distal intercalary defect do not always conform to the classic pattern of *pouce flottant*. In some instances the thumb is merely reduced in size and possesses extensor and flexor tendons, more commonly the former. Its metacarpal is slender and caught in the common bondage of a deep transverse ligament; the thumb cannot be fully abducted or circumducted nor made to press effectively against the fingers (Figs. 23–1 to 23–13).

(Text continued on page 791.)

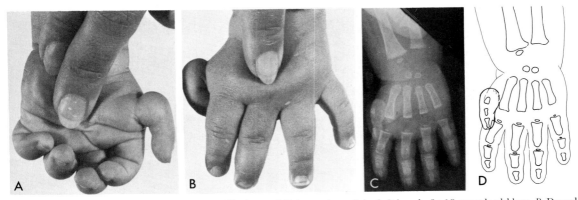

Figure 23–4 Intercalary defect of the pollical ray. *A*, Palmar view of the left hand of a 19-month-old boy. *B*, Dorsal view. *C*, Dorsopalmar roentgenograph: the first metacarpal is represented by a small ossicle; the phalanges of the thumb are puny slivers. *D*, Sketch illustrating the same.

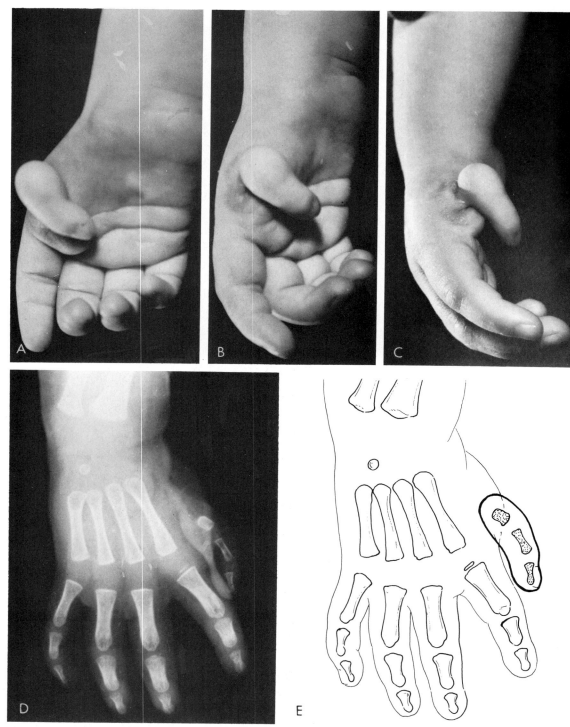

Figure 23–5   Intercalary defect of the pollical ray. *A*, *B*, and *C*, The right hand of a three-month-old girl with floating thumb. *D*, Dorsopalmar roentgenograph of the right hand: the proximal portion of the first metacarpal is missing. *E*, Sketch illustrating the same.

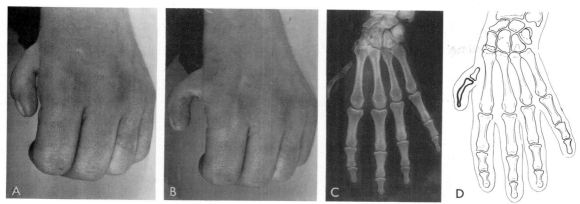

Figure 23–6 Intercalary defect of the pollical ray with functioning long abductor of the thumb. *A*, Dorsal view of the left hand of a 30-year-old man with hypoplastic thumb. *B*, The same, with the thumb partly abducted. *C*, Dorso-palmar roentgenograph of the left hand: the trapezium and the proximal portion of the first metacarpal are missing. *D*, Sketch illustrating the same.

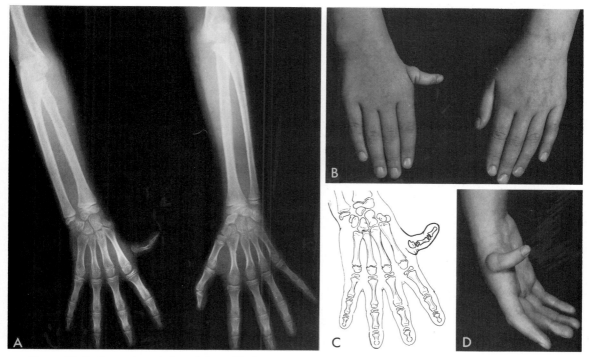

Figure 23–7 Intercalary defect of the pollical ray. *A*, Dorsovolar roentgenograph of the forearms and hands of a 10-year-old girl with absent right scaphoid and absence of the proximal portion of the first metacarpal of the right hand; the right radius is present but it is shorter than the left radius; the right ulna is likewise shorter than the left ulna. *B*, Dorsal view of the hands. *C*, Sketch illustrating the skeletal components of the right hand. *D*, Radial view of the right hand.

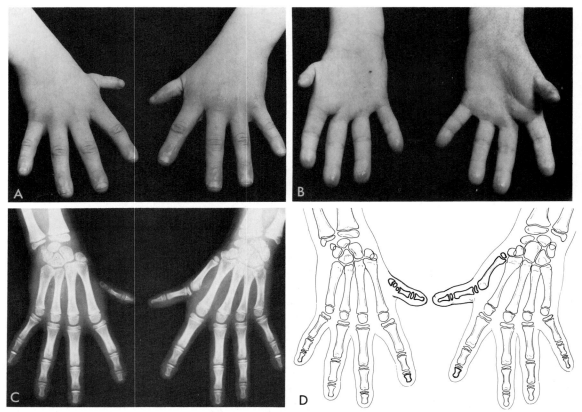

Figure 23–8 Intercalary defect of the pollical ray associated with hypoplastic adducted thumb on the opposite side. *A*, Dorsal view of the hands of a 12-year-old girl. *B*, Palmar view. *C*, Dorsopalmar roentgenograph: the scaphoid bone and the proximal portion of the first metacarpal are missing on the right side and the epiphyses of the ungual phalanges of the middle and little fingers are dense. On the left side, the scaphoid is hypoplastic, the first metacarpal is thin and adducted; in the left hand, the condensation affects the epiphyses of the ungual phalanges of the index and little fingers. *D* illustrates *C*.

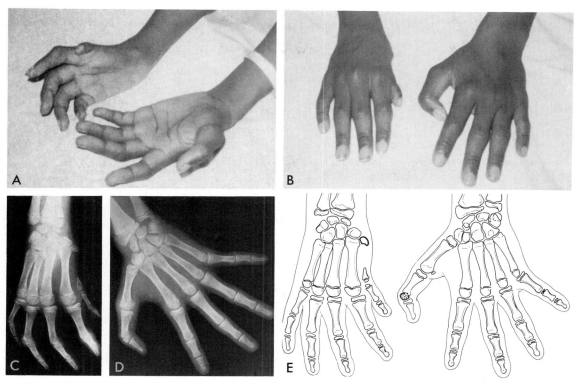

Figure 23–9 Intercalary defect of the right pollical ray associated with opposable triphalangeal thumb of the left hand. *A,* Palmar view of the hands of an 11-year-old boy. *B,* Dorsal view. *C,* Dorsopalmar roentgenograph: the right ulna extends as far distal as the right radius, which lacks a styloid process; the right scaphoid is diminutive and the right trapezium is missing, as is most of the shaft of the first metacarpal, whose remaining proximal and distal ends are rudimentary, as are the two phalanges of the thumb. *D,* Dorsopalmar roentgenograph of the left hand: the left thumb has a wedge-shaped middle phalanx. *E,* Sketch illustrating *C* and *D.*

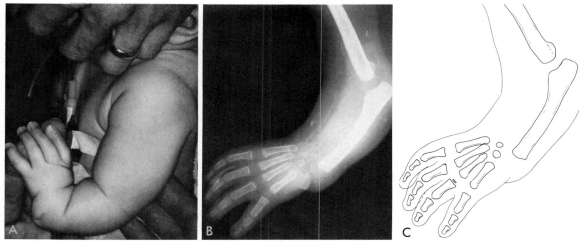

Figure 23–10 Total terminal longitudinal defect of the radial ray. *A,* Lateral view of the left upper limb of an 18-month-old boy with absent radius and missing pollical ray: note the dimple on the ulnar aspect of the wrist. *B,* Roentgenograph of the same. *C,* Sketch illustrating the roentgenograph.

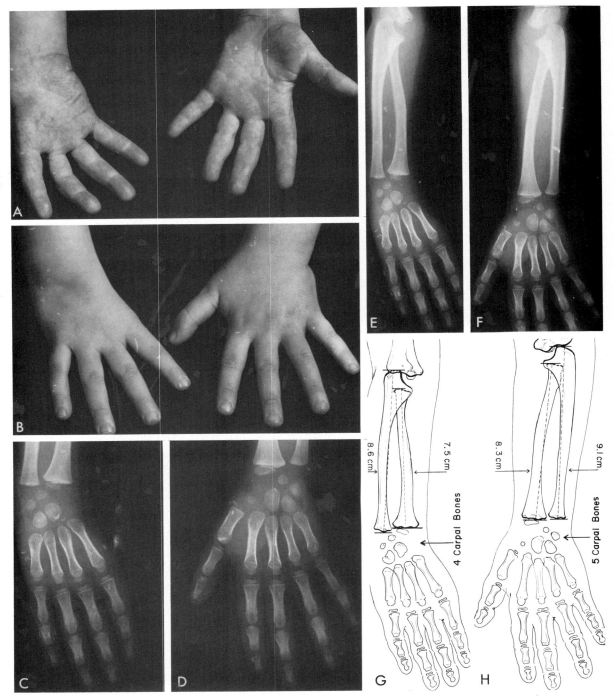

Figure 23–11   Partial terminal longitudinal defect of the radial ray. *A*, Palmar view of the hands of a five-year-old girl with absent right thumb. *B*, Dorsal view. *C* and *D*, Dorsopalmar roentgenograph of the right and left wrists and hands. *E* and *F*, Dorsovolar roentgenographs of right and left forearms and wrists: the right radial shaft is shorter than the right ulnar shaft; it is shorter than the left radius and has a smaller carpal epiphysis; the right wrist has four carpal bones; the left has five. *G* and *H*, Composite illustrative sketches of the right and left forearms and hands.

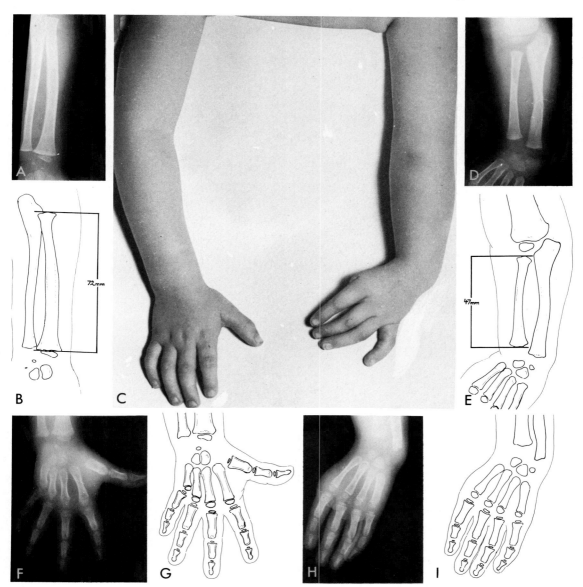

Figure 23–12 Distal terminal longitudinal defect of the radial ray. *A*, Dorsovolar roentgenograph of the right forearm of a four-year-old boy. *B*, Sketch illustrating the same. *C*, Dorsal view of both upper limbs: the left upper limb is shorter; the left hand lacks a thumb and tilts in the radial direction. *D*, Dorsovolar roentgenograph of the left forearm: both radius and ulna — but especially the former — are shorter on this side and the distal epiphysis of the radius is not evident. *E*, Sketch illustrating the same. *F*, Dorsopalmar roentgenograph of the right hand: the fifth metacarpal is dwarfed. *G*, Sketch illustrating the same. *H*, Dorsopalmar roentgenograph of the left hand: the pollical ray is completely absent. *I*, Sketch illustrating the same.

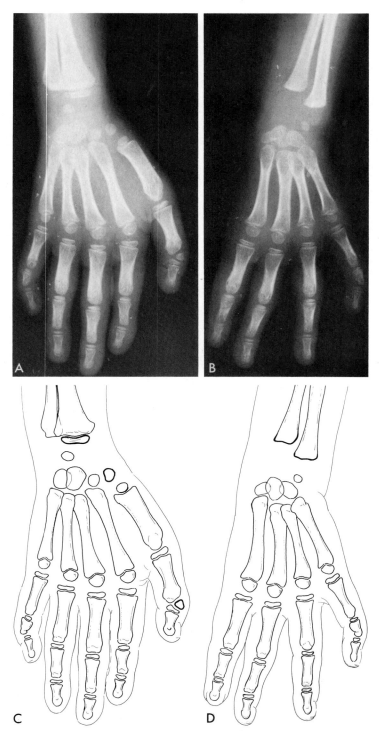

Figure 23–13   Partial terminal longitudinal defect of the radial ray associated with opposable triphalangeal thumb of the opposite hand. *A*, Dorsopalmar roentgenograph of the right wrist and hand of a six-year-old boy with a triangular ossicle wedged between the proximal and distal phalanges of the thumb. *B*, Dorsopalmar roentgenograph of the left wrist and hand: the radial epiphysis is not evident. *C* and *D* illustrate the roentgenograph above each.

OCCURRENCE

Since Petit (1733) recorded the autopsy findings of a newborn infant with bilateral radial ray defect, numerous cases of this anomaly have been reported and a number of collective reviews published. Hoffa (1890) cited 39 cases; Schmid (1893), 55; Kummel (1895), 67; Antonelli (1905), 114; Lewin (1917), 200; Kato (1924), 253; and Riordan (1955), 274 cases. Birch-Jensen (1949) described 73 cases which seem to have escaped Riordan's attention. Heikel (1959) reviewed 180 cases, some of which were not included in Kato's list, and added 47 more. "Between 1959 and December 1966, 97 more cases may be added," Pardini (1968) wrote; he reviewed 39 others, which brought the total number of reported cases to 639. Pardini's bibliography is comparatively meager. Radial ray defect is much more common than his report indicates.

"The frequency at birth of radial defect is one in about 55,000," Birch-Jensen (1949) wrote. Radial ray defects are more commonly unilateral than bilateral, involving the right side more frequently than the left and occurring more often in males than in females.

THEORIES OF ORIGIN

Three concepts feature prominently in the discussion of the origin of radial ray defect: (1) it is caused by amniotic adhesions or compression, (2) it is another example of reversion to an ancestral form, and (3) it is the outcome of focal deficiency or necrosis. Numerous criticisms have been leveled against the first concept. Perhaps the most damaging argument is that radial ray defect is occasionally seen in successive members of a genealogical tree, that it is often bilateral, and that it pursues a distinct morphological pattern which cannot be expected to have been reproduced time after time by haphazard mechanical influences. Not uncommonly, radial ray deficiency is accompanied by a defective interventricular septum, which is well protected from external pressure.

The concept of atavism — "the history of the individual represents the history of the species" or "ontogeny recapitulates phylogeny" — is implicit in Gegenbaur's (1876) archipterygial theory. Gegenbaur advanced the view that the skeletal components of the vertebrate limb evolved from the fin rays of the dipnoan fish, the upper limb being developed from a main stem and four secondary rays. Herschel (1878) subscribed to this view and regarded the defect of the radial ray as an expression of atavism. He contended that the bones of this ray tend to disappear progressively in distoproximal sequence and that the absence of the radius with intact thumb — what is now called intercalary defect — was an example of side-to-side fusion of the forearm bones. Riordan (1955) pointed out that this theory failed to explain the abnormalities which are often associated with radial ray defect.

Huxley and De Beer (1934) advanced the view that the limbfield is polarized along the anteroposterior axis and that the pre-axial border, destined to form the radius and the thumb, inevitably arises "from the anterior portion of the limb-disc," even if the latter is grafted in areas of abnormal orientation. O'Rahilly (1946) coupled this concept of polarization of the limbfield with Streeter's (1930) theory of focal necrosis.

O'Rahilly maintained that radial ray defects occur in the area of focal deficiency "where congneital or hereditary malconstitution of the germ-plasm results in imperfect histogenesis." When focal necrosis affects the polarized limb-field prior to the occurrence of regional differentiation, the involved ray suffers varying degrees of deficiency—the entire ray may be absent, or it may have lost one of its segments. "Hemimelic pattern," O'Rahilly (1951) wrote in a later communication, "is dependent on a successive longitudinal development of embryonic vertebrate limb. . . . In particular the radius, scaphoid, trapezium, first metacarpal and the thumb form a radial ray in the sense that they display a close ontogenic interdependence."

ENDOGENOUS AND EXOGENOUS INFLUENCES

Most radial ray defects are sporadic. Heredity features in about 10 per cent of reported cases. Goldenberg's (1948) patients were identical twins: "Each child presented bilateral clubhand with complete bilateral absence of the radius and the thumb." None of the known members of the family revealed any evidence of congenital deformity. Familial nonsyndromatic absences of the radius or the thumb, or both, have been transmitted as autosomal dominant phenotypes. Defects of the radial ray occurring in association with congenital heart disease (Holt-Oram atriodigital dysplasia, Lewis upper limb cardiovascular disease) are transmitted as autosomal dominant phenotypes, while those accompanying blood dyscrasias (Fanconi's anemia, thrombocytopenia) pursue autosomal recessive modes of inheritance. Radial ray defect seen in connection with cervical rib (Funston syndrome) and cervical vertebral anomalies (Klippel-Feil syndrome) are also inherited as autosomal dominant phenotypes. The inheritance of a radial ray defect seen in association with craniosynostosis is recessive, while that occurring with acrofacial dysostosis is dominant.

Syphilis has long been blamed as an exogenous cause of radial ray defect. Petersen (1880) treated a 31-year-old man with ozena syphilitica and absent radial diaphysis. Cuff (1896) described another man with congenital syphilis and defective radii. Thalidomide has replaced syphylis as the chief prompter of exogenous radial ray defect.

ANATOMY

Since many children with radial ray defect are stillborn or die soon after birth, there is a plethora of autopsy material. Prior to the advent of radiography, a number of detailed anatomical studies were published. The first roentgenograph of radial ray defect was published by Taylor (1897). Structural aberrations recorded since are legion. Only surgically significant data will be surveyed here.

At the shoulder, the head of the humerus may sag or subluxate owing to atrophy of the deltoid muscle. Distally, the capitulum and the radial epicondyle are defective. Flexion and extension at the elbow are usually normal. In total absence of the radius, pronation and supination are nil. The radius may be missing completely or partially, and absences of midshaft and proximal portions have been reported, but these are extremely rare. In most partial absences, only the distal half or more of the radius is missing; occasionally, the distal epiphysis or the radial styloid alone is absent.

The ulna conforms to the canon enunciated long ago by Ollier (1867): "Where there are two parallel bones and one of them is missing, the one which is present tends to curve. . . . " In radial ray defect, the ulna is curved, short, and thick. When the hand is held in pronated position—as it usually is in radial ray defect—the concavity of the ulna is directed toward the midline of the body. The carpal end or the head of the ulna is dislocated in the opposite direction—away from the midline of the body. The ulnar styloid is prominent. The triangular fibrocartilage joining the distal ends of the radius and ulna is absent. There is no synovial cavity between the subluxated ulnar head and the carpus.

The ulna gains most of its length—as does the radius when present—from its distal growth center. Normally, the carpal epiphysis of the ulna appears during the sixth year of postnatal life and unites with the shaft between the ages of 14 and 16. Epiphyses need functional stimulus to develop properly. When the radius is absent, the hand shifts away from the carpal epiphysis of the ulna and cannot impart to it any stimulus for development. The growth potential of the ulna is reduced considerably; the ulna, and with it the forearm of the affected limb, remains short.

The carpal scaphoid and trapezium are usually absent or undeveloped. Rarely, the lunate bone is missing. The first metacarpal is absent in total terminal defect of the radial ray and in intercalary and terminal defects of the pollical component. In 7 out of 10 cases of total absence of the radius, the thumb is said to be absent; the thumb is actually totally absent in about half and is vestigial in one-fifth of the reported cases. Of the four lesser digits, the index finger seems to be involved most. Forbes (1938) presented autopsy findings of a fetus with absence of all the skeletal elements of the radial ray. In addition, the second phalanx of the index finger and the trapezoid were missing. In radial ray defect, the index finger may be flexed, fused with its immediate ulnar neighbor, or may present an anomalous—usually triangular—middle phalanx; occasionally, the finger lacks muscular control.

A great deal has been written about the muscles, nerves, and vessels in radial ray defect. As is to be expected, muscles originating from the radial epicondyle of the humerus, the radius, and the adjoining interosseous membrane of the forearm exhibit some abnormalities, such as confluence and anomalous insertions, but mainly absences. When the thumb is wanting, the muscles acting on it are absent, and not infrequently the extensor indicis proprius is also missing. In a number of dissected specimens, all the extrinsic tendons of the index finger failed to reach their usual points of insertion.

The radial artery is often reported as being absent or attenuated. The hand as a whole has adequate blood supply. The digits which are present—including the pedunculated pollex—are well supplied by sensory enervations. The radial nerve sometimes terminates at about the level of the elbow. Ulnar and median nerves are intact. Of particular surgical importance is the fact that the median nerve assumes a superficial position because of the absence of overlying muscles.

Many authors have described a fibrous chord, which is said to act as a bowstring, between the proximal forearm and the carpus. Some consider this band to represent the missing radius; others insist that it is nothing more than a muscle or tendon which has undergone fibrous degeneration. It is generally agreed that this chord serves as a tether which perpetuates, or even aggravates, the deformity of both the forearm and the wrist; it counteracts attempts to bring the hand up from a displaced, deviated position to place it in line with the ulna.

CONTRALATERAL LIMB

Defects of the radial ray are more commonly unilateral than bilateral. Rarely, in bilateral cases, the deficiency is symmetrical. The pollical ray may be missing or have an intercalary defect on one side while the opposite hand possesses a triphalangeal thumb. In some instances, one pollical ray is adducted and has short and thin skeletal components, while the corresponding trajectory of the opposite hand manifests an intercalary or terminal longitudinal defect.

REGIONAL ASSOCIATIONS

Occasionally in connection with defects of the pollical ray, the index finger has a triangular middle phalanx with a broad ulnar base which causes the distal segment to tilt radially. Rarely, the last two ulnar metacarpals are confluent and the corresponding digits incline toward each other, simulating the configuration of a parenthesis. Side-to-side fusion of the ulnar metacarpal bones is also known to occur, and one or more fingers may be missing. In most cases, the lesser digits remain unaffected, each finger retaining its normal axial alignment, its cylindrical contour, and its full quota of bones.

As has been noted, the radius and the thumb are absent in ulnar dimelia or mirror hand. In phocomelia, the radius and the ulna are absent or dwarfed. In radioulnar synostosis, the radius is present, but has affected a union with the ulna. Extreme examples of radioulnar coalescence have been reported by Evans et al (1950) and by Margolis and Hasson (1955). Proximal radioulnar synostosis is not an uncommon accompaniment of partial terminal radial ray defect. Less commonly, absence of the pollical ray is associated with dislocation of the radial head. Curiously, dislocations of the radial head are more often seen in cases in which the metacarpals or the phalanges of the last ulnar digital rays have affected side-to-side union.

REMOTE AND RARE ASSOCIATIONS

Meckel (1826) described a patient with bilateral absence of both radius and thumb, a diminutive index finger on one side, absence of a lung, and a cystic kidney. Larcher (1868) said that in 1827 he had run across three cases of congenital absence of the radius accompanied by absence of homolateral lung lobes. In the case reported by Chalaiditi (1914), a defective right lung was associated with an intercalary deficiency of the pollical ray. These reports seem to have escaped the attention of Riordan (1955), who said that an association of radial ray and aplasia or collapse of the lung had not previously been mentioned in the literature.

Defects of the radial ray have also been reported in association with absence of the fibula by Krichler (1940); with anencephalia by Hann (1921); with atresia of the anus by Tunte (1968); with atresia of the common bile duct by Angelescu et al (1964); with contralateral facial paralysis by Essen-Möller (1929); with cerebellar meningocele by Gonnet (1908); with dorsal kyphosis and dextrocardia by Middleton (1898); with malformed auricle and facial palsy by Hartofilakidis-Garofalidis (1971); with nonrotation of the intestine by Grant (1930); with scoliosis by Feutelais (1930) and Makley and Heiple (1970); with tracheoesophageal fistula and esophageal atresia by Kirkpatrick et al (1965), and with word-deafness by Malewski (1903). Defects of the radial ray are also known to occur in a number of well-defined syndromes. Contracture of the joints is a common feature of chondrodystrophia calcificans congenita. Hewitt and van Bochove (1971) described a child with this type of short-limbed dwarfism whose radius was inordinately short, causing the hand to be deflected in the radial direction. Nager and de Reynier (1948) presented an 18-year-old girl with mandibulofacial dysostosis and absent thumbs; Becker's (1961) patient — an eight-day-old boy — with mandibulofacial dysostosis had bilateral absence of the thumb.

CARDIOMELIC COMPLEXES

Holt-Oram atriodigital dysplasia, also called heart and hand syndrome I, has been taken up in Chapter Ten, since its most common melic manifestation is nonopposable triphalangeal thumb. Occasionally, the pollical portion of the radial ray is missing. In two families described by Holmes (1965), congenital heart disease was associated with three types of thumb abnormality characterized, respectively, as fingerlike, vestigial, and absent. Cascos (1967) described a mother and her four children with electrocardiographic changes. The mother had hypoplastic triphalangeal thumb on the right hand and a malformed index finger; the youngest daughter had no thumb on the left hand, and on the right hand there were two triphalangeal thumbs which were webbed together. Rybak et al (1971) reported three siblings with radial ray defect. The trait was transmitted through three generations. There were nine affected members. Partial deletion of the long arm of a B-group chromosome was found in two siblings.

Melic malformations of the heart and hand syndrome II is also called Lewis upper limb–cardiovascular syndrome. Kuhn and associates (1963) described a family, the affected members of which presented the following abnormalties: primary pulmonary hypertension, congenital heart disease, and skeletal defects ranging from homolateral hypoplasia of the thumb to complete aplasia of the radial ray. In an occasional case there was hypoplasia of the humerus or dibrachial phocomelia with hypoplasia of the shoulder girdle. The basic deficiency involved predominantly the radial projection of the upper extremities. The defect was more pronounced on the left side than on the right. The middle phalanx of the little finger was short on both sides.

Lewis et al (1965) presented a pedigree in which 18 members in three generations were affected with a variety of cardiac anomalies, including the following: atrial septal defect, ventricular septal defect, anomalous coronary artery, retroesophageal subclavian artery, and transposition of the great vessels. The ensuing anomalies of the upper limb were listed: absent or hypoplastic thumb; soft-tissue syndactyly between the thumb and index finger; shortened radius and ulna; dwarfed clavicle; small, deformed scapula; flattened humeral head; absent pectoralis major muscle; various carpal bone defects; and, in two patients, phocomelia (Figs. 23–14 and 23–15).

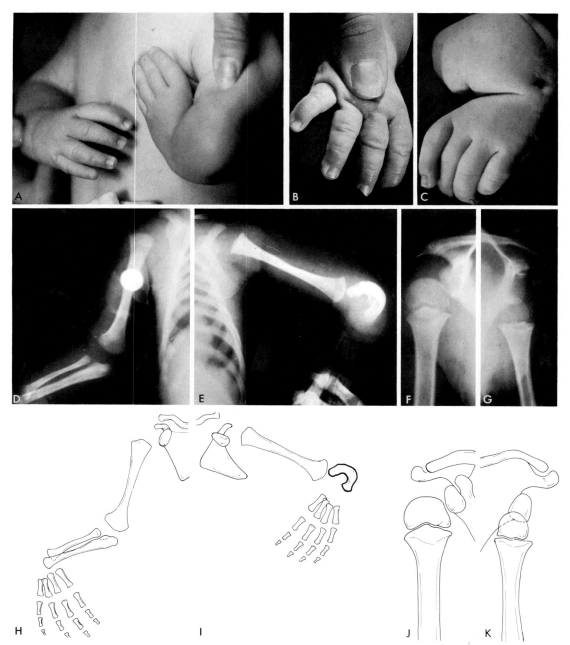

Figure 23–14 Cardiomelic complex. *A*, Dorsal view of the upper limbs of a three-month-old boy with absent right pollical ray, total terminal defect of the radial ray, semicircular ulna, dislocated left shoulder, and patent ductus arteriosus. *B*, Dorsal view of the right hand. *C*, Dorsal view of the left upper limb: note the dimple over the elbow. *D*, Anteroposterior roentgenograph of the right upper limb: the radius is shorter than the ulna. *E*, Anteroposterior view of the left upper limb: the radius is absent, the ulna is curved, and the glenoid of the scapula is tilted up. *F*, Roentgenograph of the right shoulder taken at the age of 10 years: the humeral head is subluxated downward. *G*, Roentgenograph of the left shoulder taken at the age of 10: the humeral head is definitely dislocated. In *H* and *I*, an attempt has been made to sketch the skeletal components of the right and left upper limbs at the age of three months. *J* and *K* illustrate the roentgenograph above each.

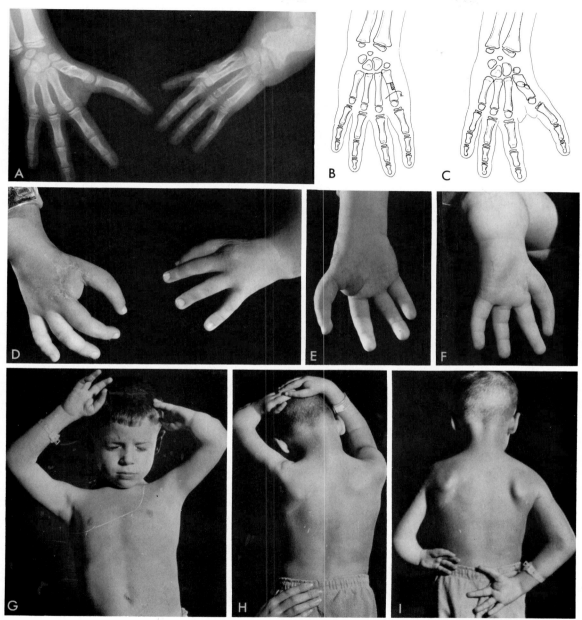

Figure 23–15 *A*, Dorsopalmar roentgenograph of the three-month-old boy featured in Figure 23–14: this roentgenograph was taken at the age of eight years—after pollicization of the right index finger. The left index was subsequently pollicized but lacked flexor and opponens muscles, which are being replenished by tendon transfer. *B* and *C* illustrate abbreviation, abduction, and rotation osteotomy of the right index metacarpal. *D*, Dorsal view of the hands after pollicization of the index fingers. *E* and *F*, Palmar view of the same. *G*, *H*, and *I* show limitation of shoulder movements of the shorter left upper limb with dislocated humeral head.

CHROMOSOMAL ABERRATIONS

Voorhess et al (1964) described a young girl who, in addition to the characteristic findings of trisomy 18 syndrome, had an absent radius and a rudimentary thumb. Zellweger's (1965) patient, a white female, had unequal arms. The fingers of her right hand were flexed, and the right thumb was relatively small; there was also a simian palmar crease. Her left forearm was very short. The thumb on this side consisted of a small soft-tissue appendix attached to the hand by a thin bridge of skin; the left four ulnar digits were kept flexed.

Sparkes et al (1967) described three cases of bilateral aplasia of the thumb; a karyotype was interpreted as showing a ring D_2 chromosome. Juberg and associates (1969) reported a female infant with ring D chromosome and multiple congenital malformations. Among the latter were included bilateral absence of the pollical ray, bilateral fusion of the metacarpals of the ring and little fingers, and absence of the middle phalanx of the little finger of both hands. Dellaire (1969) presented a young girl whose karyotype revealed a ring B chromosome. There was complete absence of the thumb on the right side. On the left side there was a slight hypoplasia of the radius. The thumb on the left hand was hypoplastic, with a rudimentary first metacarpal.

CRANIOSYNOSTOSIS AND RADIAL RAY DEFECT

This complex consists of oxycephaly and absent radius. Baller (1950) presented a female patient whose parents were third cousins. Gerold (1959) reported a brother and a sister, aged 16 years and 2 days, respectively. Each sibling had tower skull, aplasia of the radius, and slight hypoplasia of the ulna. This trait is transmitted as an autosomal recessive.

FUNSTON'S SYNDROME

Funston (1932) described a mother and daughter with bilateral cervical ribs and radial ray defects: "The mother had a bilateral absence of the radius with clubhand deformity and rudimentary thumbs. The daughter had an exactly similar deformity of the right hand. The left hand . . . had no thumb and there was synostosis between the radius and ulna just distal to the elbow joint. . . . Roentgenograms revealed well developed cervical ribs in both mother and daughter." Funston reported three other unrelated individuals with cervical rib and radial ray defect. It is perhaps significant to note that radial ray defect is seen in association with Klippel-Feil syndrome.

HEMATOMELIC COMPLEXES

Fanconi (1927) and many others have described a severe form of congenital anemia associated with hypoplasia or aplasia of bone marrow, generalized purpura, brown patchy pigmentation of the skin, dwarfism, microcephaly, mental retardation, malformations of the heart and kidneys, and a wide spectrum of skeletal anomalies, the most striking of which is some degree of radial ray defect. The distal segmented portion of the radial ray—the thumb and its metacarpal—is affected more often than the proximal solitary segment or the radius. Aplasia or hypoplasia of the thumb appears to be the most common melic anomaly seen in cases of Fanconi's pancytopenia—it is three times as frequent as total or partial absence of the radius. Only occasionally both the thumb and the radius are reported as having been absent in the same case. Numerical reduction of the carpal bones has been noted in two-thirds of reported cases of this type of hematomelic complex, which is transmitted as an autosomal recessive phenotype.

In recent years, a number of communications have appeared concerning congenital amegakaryocytic thrombocytopenia and bilateral defect of the radius. The syndrome is variously referred to as radius-platelet hypoplasia (RPH) or thrombocytopenia–absent radius (TAR) syndrome. The melic malformation consists of bilateral absence of the radius. The thumb and the fingers are present. TAR is distinguished from Fanconi's syndrome by the absence of cutaneous pigmentation and microcephaly, and by the presence of a high white cell count; the bone marrow biopsy shows absent or abnormal megakaryocytes with normal myeloid and erythroid precursors.

KLIPPEL-FEIL SYNDROME

Francais and Egger (1906) described a woman with short stiff neck and total longitudinal defect of the right radial ray. In their original communication, Klippel and Feil (1912) emphasized the following features of the syndrome which bears their hyphenated names: limitation of movements of the head; low implantation of the hairline at the nape; and a short neck, giving the impression that the head is directly connected with the trunk. The basic disturbance consists of the anomalous segmentation of the thoracocervical vertebral column—two or more vertebrae are wedged or fused together. Most recorded cases have been sporadic. Instances of Klippel-Feil syndrome occurring in several members of the same family were reported by Clemmesen (1936) and Jarcho and Levin (1938). The inheritance of this trait appears to be autosomal dominant with variable expression.

Ingelrans and Piquet (1928) presented a case of Klippel-Feil syndrome with the following associated anomalies: absence of the auditory canal and short left forearm with absent radius, underdeveloped radial carpal bones, and floating thumb. Houdart et al (1961) reported a case with total longitudingal defect of the radial ray. Temtamy (1966) spoke of a patient who had bilateral thumb hypoplasia. Luppis and Bachiocco (1969) featured the photograph and radiograph of a boy with unilateral total terminal radial ray defect. Klippel-Feil anomaly is also known to occur in patients suffering from congenital heart disease and Fanconi pancytopenia, which are not uncommon accompaniments of radial ray defect.

OCULO-AURICULO-VERTEBRAL DYSPLASIA

This complex consists of the following microphthalmia; diminutive external ears, at times without patent meatus; bilateral sessile or pedunculated nodules on the face, just in front of the auricle; fusion of two or more cervical vertebrae; and malformations of the hand and forearm. In a boy reported by Gorlin and Pindborg (1964), the radius on both sides was comparatively short and the hand deviated in a radial direction, the first metacarpal of the left thumb was rudimentary, and the little fingers had cube-shaped middle phalanges. Hypoplasia of the thumb seems to be the most significant upper limb anomaly occurring in connection with oculo-aruiculo-vertebral dysplasia.

OROMELIC COMPLEXES

In Birch-Jensen's (1949) survey of harelip and cleft palate, there were five cases of radial ray defect. In one, the radius was completely absent; in the others, there were varying degrees of defects affecting the distal portions of the radii. Gorlin and Pindborg (1964) featured the photograph of a brother and sister with cleft lip-palate and popliteal pterygium. The brother had hypoplastic thumbs and fingernails; the sister had no thumbs. These authors considered cleft lip-palate to be far more frequent in persons with deficiencies of the upper extremity than in the normal population, and absence of the radius was regarded as the most common associated melic anomaly. Immeyer (1967) reported more than a dozen cases of thalidomide embryopathy with radial ray defect and cleft lip-palate.

TEGUMENTARY COMPLEX

Thomson (1936) reported a female infant with congenital poikiloderma. She had bilateral partial terminal radial ray defect: "The metacarpals and phalanges of the thumbs were completely absent, whilst both ulnae and radii were rudimentary, the latter particularly so, with curvature of the ulna." The association of poikiloderma congenita and absent radius was also noted by Castel et al (1967).

THALIDOMIDE EMBRYOPATHY

In about 80 per cent of reported cases of thalidomide embryopathy, the upper limb is affected, involving most often the components of the radial — the radius, the carpal scaphoid, trapezium, the first metacarpal and the phalanges of the thumb. Radial ray deficiencies range from mild hypoplasia or attenuation of the thumb to total terminal absence (Fig. 23–16).

PROGNOSIS AND PRECAUTION

Children with radial ray defect were given a very poor prognosis by nineteenth century authors — Voigt (1863) and Krönig (1894) among many others.

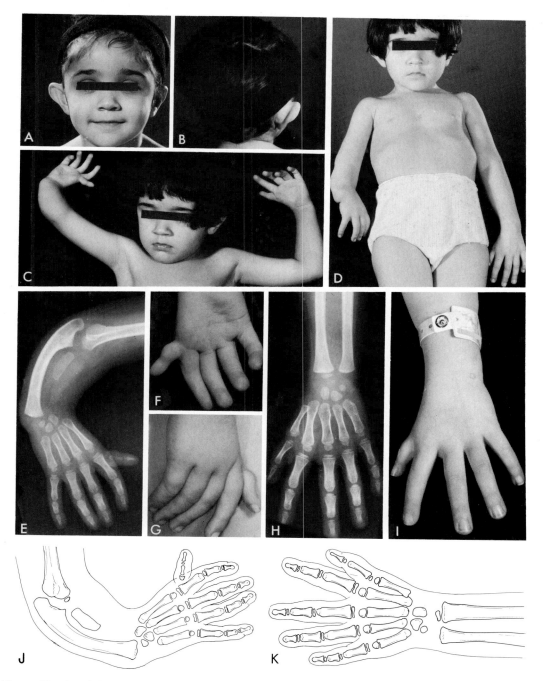

Figure 23–16 Thalidomide embryopathy—bilateral, asymmetrical, multiple abnormalities of the upper limbs and auricles. *A,* Frontal view of the head of the four-year-old girl featured in Figure 2–11: note the forward inclination of the right auricle. *B,* Dorsal view of the same. *C,* Volar view of the upper limbs. *D,* Dorsal view of the same: the right upper limb is considerably shorter. *E,* Roentgenograph of the right forearm and hand: there is an intercalary defect involving the distal portion of the radius and the proximal part of the first metacarpal. *F* and *G,* Palmar and dorsal views of the right hand with distally placed floating thumb. *H,* Dorsovolar roentgenograph of the left distal forearm, wrist, and hand: there are four carpal bones in this hand as compared to three on the right side; the first metacarpal is thin and is snugged close to its ulnar neighbor. *I,* Dorsal view of the left hand: the thumb is distally placed; the first webspace is narrow. *J* and *K* illustrate *E* and *H,* respectively.

Antonelli (1905) was astonished to see a 27-year-old patient with radial ray defect still alive. In Kato's (1924) list of 253 cases, there was a preponderance of children "either prematurely born or under one year of age." Birch-Jensen (1949) also augured a grave prognosis and drew attention to the fact that more than about 25 per cent of patients with radial ray defect have congenital heart disease, "which greatly aggravates prognosis." Birch-Jensen did not specify the nature of the heart disease, but most authors seem to lean toward the diagnosis of defective ventricular septum, which is now amenable to surgical treatment. There is as yet no published statistics concerning the concurrence of radial ray defects and blood dyscrasias. From the available reports, one might say that this combination occurs in about 5 per cent of the cases.

Before the surgeon subjects a patient with radial ray defect to surgery, he should have the condition of the heart appraised and the blood studied. Fanconi s anemia constitutes a definite contraindication to surgery. Thrombocytopenia should be brought under control prior to operative interference. The surgeon should heed the advice given by hematologists and cardiologists as to when, if at all, he should operate on a child with radial ray defect. Rarely are children with radial ray defect mentally deranged; those that are should not be subjected to surgery. Operations accomplish very little if the muscles acting on the digits either are absent or have lost their contractility. In the absence of the thumb, pollicization of the index finger should be avoided when this digit has insufficient muscular control. Subcutaneous tenotomy to release contracted structures on the radial side of the wrist belongs to the medieval age of surgery. Taut structures should be exposed by an adequate incision and examined. In doing this, the surgeon should be aware of the superficial position of the median nerve. No tendon belonging to a contractile muscle is ever severed.

TREATMENT

Conditioned by his training and experience, the surgeon tends to be a regionalist. His aim is to procure a hand which will perceive and prehend — feel and grasp — effectively. In varying degrees, radial ray defects present the following regional problems: short limb, curved forearm, and a hand which is flexed at the wrist, pronated, and radially deflected. Depending upon the extent of musculoskeletal deficiency, the following functional disturbances may be present: inability to pronate and supinate the forearm, inability to dorsiflex the hand at the wrist or pull it in an ulnar direction, inadequate prehension of the hand, and weak grip.

To a degree, the deformities of the forearm and wrist can be corrected by surgery and the hand may be brought in line with the ulna. Surgery will also improve the prehensile function of the hand. When the curvature of the forearm is straightened, the limb gains an increment of length, but it remains diminutive, dwarfed. Shortness of the limb is, on the whole, intractable. The best that a surgeon can hope for is to avoid interfering with the already reduced growth potential of the ulna, the only remaining forearm bone — to be more specific, with its distal growth plate. Since this plate lies close to the seat of deformity in the wrist, where surgical efforts are most effective, the surgeon should exercise special precaution not to damage it.

At the turn of the century, no less an authority than Lovett (1901) recommended amputation of the hand for situations "where the radius is deficient and deformity severe." Amputation has no place in the treatment of radial ray defect. Lovett, as others in his time, formed such sweeping conclusions on the basis of the analogy between clubfoot due to a defective tibia and clubhand associated with radial ray defect. A patient with severe discrepancy in leg length cannot walk without elevated footwear. One with a short arm can use his hand if it is properly positioned.

The name clubhand was tagged onto radial ray defect by way of the simplistic analogy with clubfoot; it was thought that therapeutic measures which had proved beneficial for the latter would also help the former. Sayre (1892) described a patient afflicted with what would now be categorized as longitudinal radial ray defect: "the hand being destitute of the thumb and the lower two-thirds of the radius having suffered complete arrest of development." Sayre manipulated the deformed parts. As he brought the hand to a certain point of extension, it became "snowy white." Sayre realized that he had "completely arrested the circulation." He returned the hand to partial flexion and maintained what little correction he had obtained by a plaster of paris cast. Ten days later, Sayre made another attempt at manipulative correction and found that "the tissues were less contracted and still further extension could be made without obstructing circulation."

Osteotomy for the correction of the curvature of the ulnar shaft appears to have been first performed by Hoffa (1890). It is not indicated whether Sayre (1894) had read Hoffa's article when a case of radial ray defect came under his care and he "did an osteotomy of the ulna to correct the curve." After the osteotomized fragments had united firmly, Sayre applied traction with adhesive plaster, hoping to elongate the contracted structures on the radial side of the forearm and the wrist. At the end of three weeks, he made an incision over the wrist and severed all ligamentous attachments of the distal ulna but was unable to bring the hand in line with this bone. Sayre removed the ulnar styloid, excised from the carpus two bones which seemed to block reduction of the subluxated wrist, and into the cavity thus created, he slotted the trimmed end of the ulna. Sayre considered partial carpectomy preferable to "the extensive division of tendons and muscles which would have been required to permit the carpus to be pulled down to the extremity of the ulna."

Six decades later, Speed and Knight (1956) detailed a similar technique which they ascribed to Campbell: "A cavity is excavated in the midline of the dorsum of the carpus, and the distal end of the ulna is countersunk into this slot and fixed by removable criss-cross threaded wires." Skerik and Flatt (1969) thought early soft-tissue correction followed by implantation of the ulna into the carpus provided the best possible functional status for the growing child. These authors recommend surgical squaring of the distal ulna and insertion of this end of the bone into a slot created in the carpus and aligned with the third metacarpal; they felt that careful trimming of the cartilage of the distal ulna with a sharp scalpel and central transfixation with Kirschner wire would not disturb epiphyseal growth. Sayres (1894) original operation and later modifications tend to stabilize the wrist by fusion.

Sayre (1894) set down the following principles, which are still valid today: (1) preliminary measures—periodic manipulations, stretching, traction, corrective casts, and splints—should be initiated as early as possible after birth, before

fixed contractures get a chance to become established; (2) in order not to embar-
rass the circulation, correction of palmar flexion and radial deviation of the hand
at the wrist must be attained in steps, gradually; (3) the curvature of the ulna is
corrected by osteotomy; (4) tenotomy and section of muscles should be
avoided — these structures may be given a relative increase in length by the
removal of the blocking carpal bones; and (5) the hand must be brought in line
with the ulna and stabilized at the wrist. Sayre left out one basic item: substitution of the index finger for the missing thumb to enhance the prehensile function of the hand.

The story of the surgical treatment of radial ray defect during the next
three-quarters of a century consists of descriptions of many operations and
reports of successful short-term results. Some procedures, like Sayre's, have survived in modified form; in many instances, the modification has been so artful as
to convince the novice, and also the naive modifier himself, that the method
described is original. Many of the earlier operations have been relegated to
limbo.

The graveyard of discarded procedures — documented by book after book
and article after article — includes Romano's (1894) trapezoid osteotomy of the
distal ulnar shaft, Thomson's (1889–1890) cuneiform osteotomy of the proximal
segment of the same bone, McCurdy's (1896) transportation of the ulnar
diaphysis to the radial side of its epiphysis, Antonelli's (1905) reconstruction of
the missing radius by the split half of the ulna, Küttner's (1917) transplant of the
distal end of a monkey's radius, and Ryerson's (1924) operation.

Bardenheuer's (1894) inverted Y operation may be regarded as the champion chameleon of procedures used in the treatment of radial ray defect; it has
reappeared time and again under deceptively different guises. In the original
version of this operation, the distal end of the ulna was split longitudinally, the
two halves were pried apart, and the carpus was pushed up between them and
transfixed with an ivory peg. Tubby (1911) secured the diverging limbs of the
split distal ulna to the carpus with silkworm gut. Axhausen (1919) extended the
radial limb of the split ulna to the proximal shaft by using an osteoperiosteal
tibial graft as a connecting bridge.

Albee (1921) simulated Bardenheuer's inverted Y operation; with the aid of
a tibial graft, he established an oblique bridge between the midportion of the
ulna and the radial carpal bones. Davidson and Horwitz (1962) reported a failure with the bone-graft reconstructive operation advocated by Albee, and they
revived Bardenheuer's original procedure with a slight modification: they
resected a block of bone from the distal end of the ulna and inserted this piece
into the diverging limbs of the inverted Y. Peabody (1947) used a keystone-
shaped iliac graft for the same purpose, transfixing it to the limbs of the ulna and
carpal bones with threaded wires. Farmer and Laurin (1958) also favored iliac
graft.

Define (1966, 1970) has recently recommended the following modification
of Bardenheuer's bifurcation procedure: the distal end of the ulna is dissected
subperiosteally; with the periosteal tube in situ, the denuded segment of the
ulnar metaphysis bearing the adjoining epiphysis is osteotomized and transposed toward the radial border of the carpus. The periosteal tube with its normal connections is said to eventually form a segment of new bone, assuming,
with the transposed distal ulna, an inverted Y. As pointed out by Pulvertaft
(1969), the bone strut which forms in the periosteal sleeve is static and cannot
keep pace with the growing ulna.

The ultimate aim of Bardenheuer's operation and many of its modifications was the stabilization of the wrist by fusion. Albee (1928) boasted that five years after surgery his patient had joined "a tennis tournament in which she was one of the semifinalists." Davidson and Horwitz (1962) reported that their patient, a year after they had operated, showed clinical and roentgenographic evidence of "fusion of the wrist, with excellent and apparently permanent correction of the deformity." Their patient was 10 and Albee's 12 years of age at the time of surgery. After the age of 12, the growth potential of the lone ulna is practically nil and arthrodesing operations are justifiable — but not in children under this age.

Bardenheuer's bifurcation operation underwent further modifications. Instead of using a tibial bone graft to provide the carpus with a radial buttress as Albee had done, Starr (1945) utilized the proximal segment of the fibula. He reversed the direction of this graft by turning its epiphyseal end toward the carpus. Individual modifications of this operation were introduced by Bintcliffe (1954), Riordan (1955), Entin and Petrie (1957), Heikel (1959), and Entin (1964). It was hoped that an epiphysis-bearing fibular transplant would keep pace with the longitudinal growth of the ulna and would stabilize the wrist without stiffening it. These expectations have not materialized. In due course, the transplanted fibular fragment receded away from the carpus and took on the appearance of an icicle hanging from the midshaft of the ulna. The deformity of the wrist recurred. As pointed out by Heikel, the lower extremity from which the fibular graft had been obtained manifested growth and functional disturbances; the remaining segment of the fibula angled toward the tibia, which caused instability at the ankle and eversion of the foot.

The dilemma of the surgeon undertaking the care of a growing child with radial ray defect is obvious: he must avoid procedures which might curtail the already reduced growth potential of the distal ulna; yet, knowing that function is the greatest stimulus to growth, he must place the parts in position to function properly and to supply adequate stimulus for growth. This means placing the hand in line with the ulna and maintaining this alignment continuously, which entails immobilization of the parts. As is well known, prolonged immobilization retards the growth of the immobilized parts. The surgeon must compromise and resort to those measures that are least harmful.

The treatment must be initiated early, immediately after birth. The parts are manipulated periodically and a circular cast is applied to preserve what little correction is obtained. After two weeks, the cast is removed. The contracted structures are stretched at intervals during the day, and a gutter splint is worn at night. An alternative method is that proposed by Entin and Petrie (1957). These authors recommend the use of a light elastic splint to maintain the alignment of the hand with the forearm and advise that it be worn "for a minimum of 12 hours a day, until 6 to 8 years of age." Dynamic splints of various sorts have also been recommended.

Splints and casts are useless if the hand cannot be placed in line with the ulna. When contracted tissues on the radial and volar aspect of the wrist fail to yield to more conservative measures, an incision is made over the ulnar epicondyle of the humerus; the origins of the flexor tendons are released and allowed to shift to a distal point in the proximal forearm. The volar aspect of the wrist is explored, and the "tethering" fibrous chord is severed. No tendon needs to be cut or lengthened by Z-plasty. Skeletal traction is applied with the aid of a Kirschner wire passed through the central metacarpal bones. Roentgenographic

(*Text continued on page 811.*)

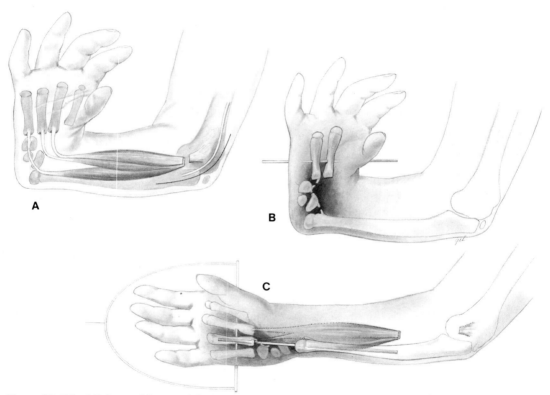

Figure 23–17 *A*, Release of flexor origin from the medial condyle of the humerus. *B*, Transmetacarpal K-wire for skeletal traction. *C*, Shows longitudinal K-wire holding the fourth metacarpal in line with the ulna.

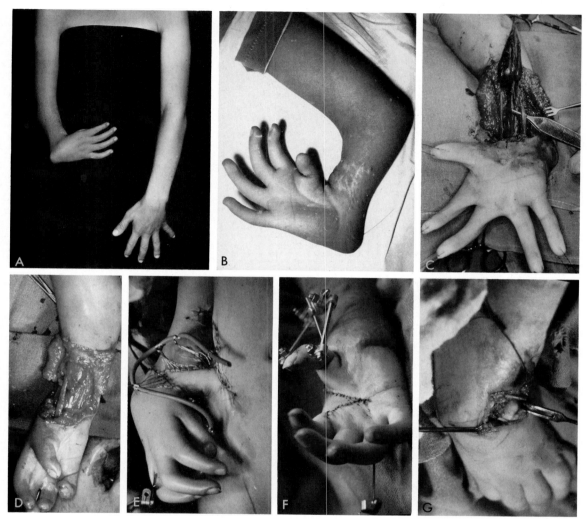

Figure 23-18 Absent radius with volar and radial deflection of the hand which had been subjected to Z-plasty of the skin on the palmar aspect of the wrist and angulation osteotomy of the distal ulna without any improvement. Subsequently, this limb was treated by replacement of tendon-bound scar in front of the wrist with a distant flap, Z-plasty of the first webspace, release of flexor tendons from the medial condyle of the humerus, carpectomy, and corrective osteotomy of the distal ulna. *A,* The upper limbs of an eight-year-old boy with absent right radius. *B,* Volar view of the right upper limb. *C,* Exposure of the taut structures after excision of the scar in front of the wrist: the flexor carpi radialis was tenotomized and reflected. *D,* Defect left after excision of the scar: the common origin of the flexors was released from the medial condyle; the wrist was straightened and held in the corrected position with the aid of a K-wire. *E,* Surfacing the raw area with a distant flap. *F,* Z-plasty to widen the first webspace, the thumb being held in extreme abduction with the aid of K-wire and external fixation apparatus. *G,* Carpectomy, which was carried out at the same time as osteotomy of the distal ulna (shown in Figure 23–19).

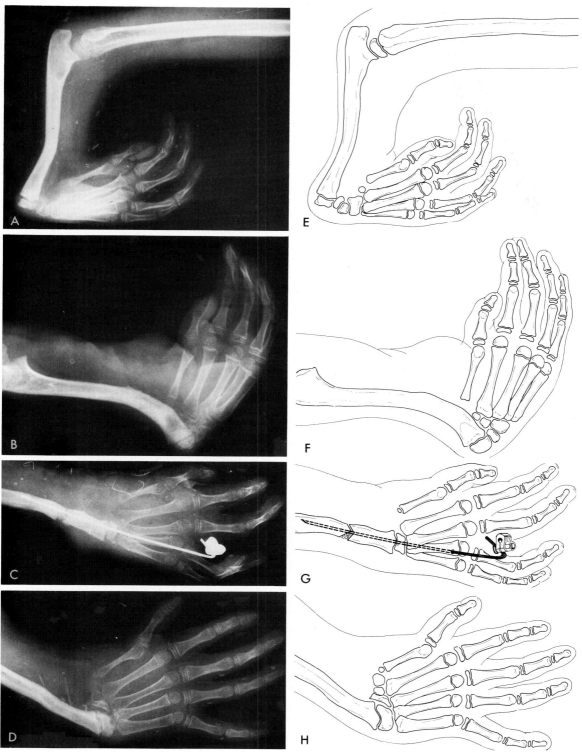

Figure 23–19 Corrective osteotomy of the distal radius and carpectomy. *A*, Roentgenograph of the right upper limb of the eight-year-old boy featured in Figure 23–18; this boy had a previous osteotomy of the distal ulna elsewhere. *B*, The same after the second osteotomy, which failed to bring the hand into a dorsal position. *C*, Roentgenograph after carpectomy, corrective osteotomy, and fixation of fragments with a K-wire. *D*, The same after healing of surgical fracture and removal of K-wire. *E*, *F*, *G*, and *H* illustrate the roentgenograph next to each.

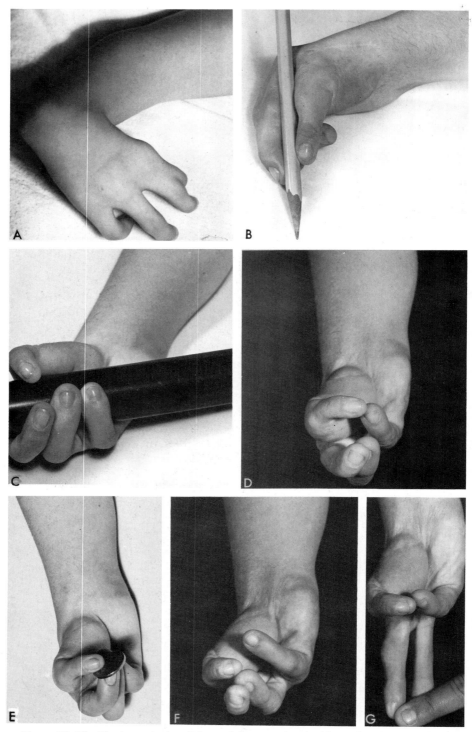

Figure 23–20 Total terminal radial ray defect associated with syndactyly of the index and middle fingers—treated by separation of the index from the middle finger, deepening and widening of the commissure between the two, carpectomy, two attempts at osteotomy of the distal ulna, and finally, fusion of the wrist. *A*, Preoperative view of the right forearm and the hand of a 13-year-old girl. *B, C, D, E, F,* and *G*, Postoperative results.

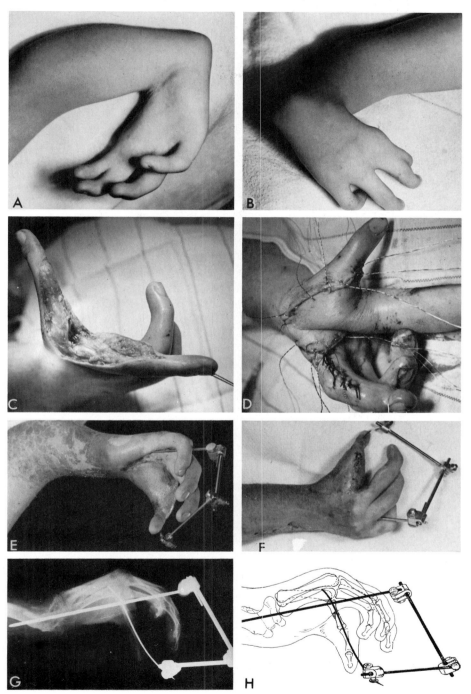

Figure 23–21 Separation of the webbed index and middle fingers; two-stage pollicization of the index finger and osteotomy of the distal ulna. *A*, Volar view of the right forearm and hand of the 13-year-old girl featured in Figure 23–20. *B*, Dorsal view. *C*, Separation of the webbed digits and deepening and widening of the commissure between them. *D*, Distant flap covering the deepened and widened commissure. *E*, Ulnar view after osteotomy of the ulna and abduction-angulation–clockwise rotation osteotomy of the index metacarpal. *F*, Radial view of the same. *G*, Lateral roentgenograph showing the transfixation wires and the external fixation apparatus. *H*, Sketch illustrating the same.

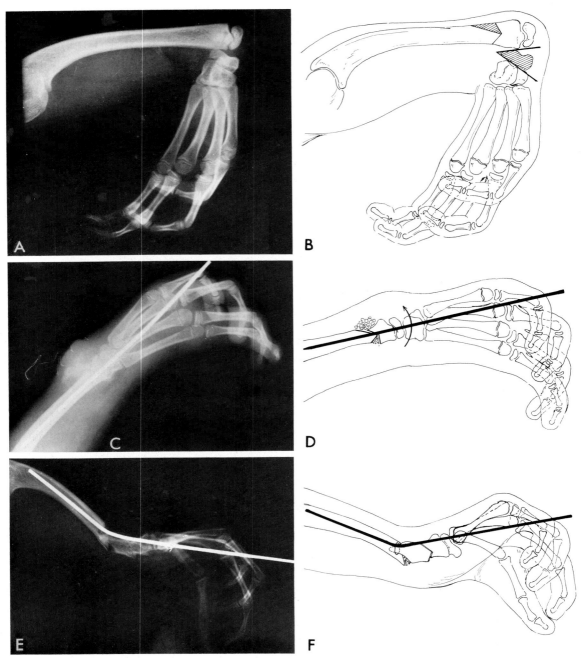

Figure 23–22 Carpectomy and two successive osteotomies of the distal ulna. *A*, Preoperative ulnar roentgenograph of the right forearm and hand of the 13-year-old girl featured in Figures 23–20 and 23–21. *B*, Sketch illustrating the osteotomy of the distal ulna and wedge resection of the proximal row of carpal bones. *C*, Roentgenograph after fixation of osteotomized fragments by K-wire. *D*, Sketch illustrating the same. *E*, Roentgenograph after second osteotomy of the distal ulna. *F*, Sketch illustrating the same.

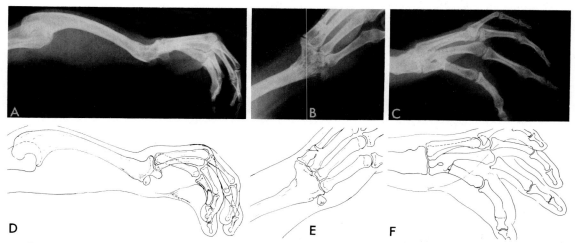

Figure 23–23 Fusion of the wrist. *A, B,* and *C,* Roentgenographs of the right forearm and hand of the 13-year-old girl featured in Figures 23–20 to 23–22, following surgical fusion of the right wrist. *D, E,* and *F* illustrate the roentgenograph above each.

studies are made. When the carpus seems to have come to a point distal to the ulnar styloid, the wrist is opened through a dorsal incision. The radial and volar ligaments are then cut; these structures should be severed from their attachment to the carpus, but their connection to the ulnar epiphysis must be preserved because they convey nutrient vessels to the latter. A Kirschner wire is passed longitudinally through the center of the ulnar epiphysis and allowed to come out the convex side of its shaft. The hand is brought in line with the ulna, and the Kirschner wire is drilled back in retrograde fashion into one of the central metacarpal bones.

To facilitate its removal in the future, the proximal protruding end of the Kirschner wire is cut about 1 cm. from the ulnar cortex. The time when this wire should be removed depends upon the age of the patient and the necessity for further surgery. In intractable deformities—usually in older children—one may have to remove two or more bones from the proximal row of carpals before the hand can be brought in line with the ulna. Residual deformities of the wrist may be corrected by osteotomy of the ulna at a point slightly proximal to the growth cartilage plate. Osteotomy at this level may be repeated until the hand is brought to functional position—10 to 15 degrees of dorsiflexion and midway between pronation and supination. Curvature of the proximal ulna is corrected by single or double osteotomy. At about the age of 12 years, the wrist may be fused if the deformity seems to be recurring. In thumbless hands, the index finger is pollicized (Figs. 23–17 to 23–24).

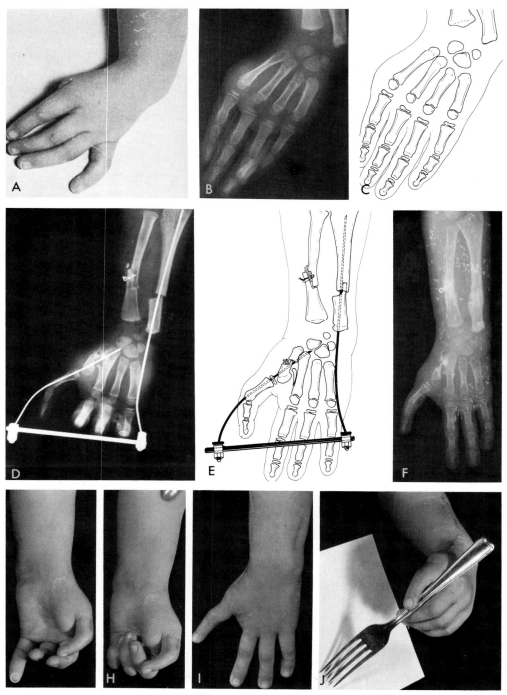

Figure 23–24 Distal terminal longitudinal ray defect treated by corrective osteotomy of the forearm bones and pollicization of the index finger. *A*, Dorsal view of the left hand of a four-year-old boy. *B*, Preoperative dorsopalmar roentgenograph of the left hand. *C*, Sketch illustrating the same. This child was operated on at the age of five: the distal radial epiphysis was still missing and the ulna had extended further distally and needed to be shortened. *D*, Dorsovolar roentgenograph of the forearm and hand after corrective osteotomy of the forearm bones and pollicization of the index finger. *E*, Sketch illustrating the same. *F*, Postoperative dorsovolar roentgenograph: surgical fractures of the forearm bones healed; fractured shortened first metacarpal resolved into nonunion. Notwithstanding, the transposed index functioned as a thumb. *G, H, I,* and *J,* Results.

SUMMARY

The radius supports the hand at the wrist. When this bone is absent, the wrist is unstable and becomes the main seat of distortion. The unsupported hand is acutely flexed at the wrist and turns sharply toward the radial border of the forearm, almost touching it; the ulna is thick, short, and bowed—its distal end is dislocated dorsally and ulnarward. Depending upon the length of the remaining radial segment, pronation and supination are limited or nil. The scaphoid and the trapezium are usually absent; the first metacarpal is often missing, and the second may possess an additional epiphysis at its proximal end. The thumb is frequently absent. With the exception of the index finger—which may have an anomalous middle phalanx, causing its distal segment to incline radially—the lesser digits are unaffected.

Symmetrical deficiencies of the radial ray are not uncommon. Absence of the radius and the distal elements of the radial ray are often associated with anomalies of the heart, blood, and viscera; they also occur in connection with thalidomide embryopathy. In the young, clubbing of the hand should be corrected by manipulation and splintage. At a propitious time, the carpus is then surgically explored, and the hand is placed in line with the ulna; this correction is maintained by an intramedullary Kirschner wire. This procedure may later be supplemented by release of the flexor origin from the ulnar condyle of the humerus, osteotomy of the curved ulna, carpectomy, and fusion of the wrist. In cases of defective radius with absent thumb, the index finger is pollicized—the technique of which will be described in Chapter Twenty-four.

References

Alamartine, H.: Main bote bilatérale, avec absence congénitale du radius. *Rev. d'Orthop.*, (2 s.), *3*:425–429, 1907.

Albee, F. H.: *Bone Graft Surgery.* Philadelphia, W. B. Saunders Co., pp. 373–392; figs. 300–310, 1915.

Albee, F. H.: *Orthopedic and Reconstruction Surgery.* Philadelphia, W. B. Saunders Co., pp. 903–916, 1921.

Albee, F. H.: Formation of radius congenitally absent; condition seven years after implantation of bone graft. *Ann. Surg.*, *87*:105–110, 1928.

Albrecht, R.: Beitrag zum Vorkommen der Unterarmmissbildungen. *Z. Orthop.*, *103*:478–485, 1967.

Alonzo, P.: Di tre casi d'emimelia dell avanbraccio. *Reforma Med.*, *41*:487–489, 1925.

Althoff, H., and Dagenhardt, K. H.: Kongenitale hypoplastische Thrombopenie mit Missbildungen. *Mschr. Kinderheilkd.*, *105*:40, 1957.

Ammon, F. A.: *Die angeborenen Chirurgischer Krankheiten des Menschen.* Berlin, F. A. Herbig, pp. 101–102, Tab. XXXIII, figs. 2–4, 1842.

Angelescu, V., et al.: Note on a case of congenital atrasia of the common bile duct and congenitale absence of both radii in a child with concomitant cytomogalic inclusion disease. (In Rumanian.) *Rev. Medicochir. Iasi.*, *68*:171–175, 1964.

Antonelli, I.: Ein Fall von kongenitalem bilateralem Radiusdefekt. *Z. Orthop. Chir.*, *14*:213–232, 1905.

Apert, E., and Morisetti: Absence congénitale bilatérale du radius et doigts radiaux (ectromélie longitudinal radiale bilatérale). *N. Iconog. Salp.*, *21*:412–420, 1908.

Axhausen, G.: Zur operativen Behandlung von Klumphand und Knickfuss bei bestehendem Knochendefekt (Radius-resp. Fibuladefekt). *Arch. Klin. Chir.*, *111*:621–643, 1919.

Ballantyne, J. W.: *Manual of Antenatal Pathology and Hygiene, The Embryo.* Edinburgh, W. Green & Sons, Vol. II, pp. 583–584, 1904.

Baller, F.: Radiusplasie und Inzucht. *Z. Menschl. Vererb. Konstitutionslehre, 29*:782–790, 1950.

Bardeleben, v.: Ein operierter Fall von beiderseits fehlendem Radius. *Dtsch. Med. Wochenschr.*, *25*:221–222, 1899.

Bardenheuer, B.: Vorstellung von 4 Patienten, an welchen die totale Hüftgelenkresection mit totaler Pfannenresection ausgefuhrt worden war. *Verh. Dtsch. Ges. Chir.*, 23rd Congress, Section I, *23*:85–87, 1894.

Bayrakci, C., and Walsh, J. R.: Amegakaryocytic thrombocytopenia and bilateral absence of the radii. *Postgrad. Med.*, *33*:401–405, 1963.

Beaudoing, A., Butin, L. P., Pont, J., Hadjian, A. J., and Bachelot, C.: Un cas de thrombocytopénie hypoplastique amégacaryocitaire congenitale avec malformations squelettiques et viscérales. *Pediatrie, 23*:111–116, 1968.

Becker, K.: Ueber die angeborene Unterkieferhypoplasie (Mikrogeni) und ihre Beziehungen zu anderen Korpmissbildungen. *Thesis*, Kinderklinsk Munster i. Lv. 1954, quoted by P. J. Waardenburg. *In* Waardenburg, P. J., Franceschetti, A., and Klein, D., (eds.): *Gentics and Ophthalmology.* Netherlands, Royal Van Gorum Publishers Assn., Vol. I, pp. 387–388, 1961.

Bell, A. D., Mold, J. W., Oliver, R. A. M., and Shaw, S.: Study of transfused platelets in a case of congenital hypoplastic thrombocytopenia. *Br. Med. J.*, *2*:692–695, fig. 2, 1956.

Belloni, G.: Contributo allo studio dell assenze e malformazioni ossee congenite degle arti. *Arch. Ortop.*, *45*:305–343, 1929.

Benazzi, R. B., and Berquist, E.: Congenital hypoplasia along the radial ray. *Am. J. Roentgenol.*, *110*:572–576, 1970.

Bergerhoff, W.: Kongenitaler doppelseitiger Radiusdefekt. *Fortschr. Röntgenstr.*, *36*:376–377, 1927.

Bertwistle, A. P.: Congenital absence of radius. *Br. Med. J.*, *1*:325–326, 1923.

Bilbrey, G. L.: Isolated congenital familial thumb deformities. *N. Engl. J. Med.*, *274*:1057–1060, 1966.

Bintcliffe, E.: Congenital club hand. *J. Bone Joint Surg.*, *36B*:154, 1954.

Birch-Jensen, A.: *Congenital Deformities of the Upper Extremities.* Translated from the Danish by E. Aagesen. Commission, Andelsbogtrykkereit i Odense and det Danske Forlag, pp. 18–22, 74–88, 143, 192–204, Proposit. 106, 133, 135, 155, and 162. pp. 134–140, 193, 197, 198, 202, 1949.

Birch-Jensen, A.: Two rare cases of congenital absence of forearm and aplasia of radius. *Ann. Eugenics, 17*:89–91, 1952.

Birnbacher, G.: *Drei Beobachtungen über Verkummerung der Oberen Extremitäten.* Inaug.-Diss. Konigsberg, P. Kreiss, pp. 1–29, 1891.

Blackett, A. E.: Congenital absence of radius with other abnormalities. *Radiology, 14*:70–71, 1930.

Blauth, W.: Der hypoplastische daumen. *Arch. Orthop. Unfallchir.*, *62*:225–246, 1967.

Blauth, W.: Erfehrungen in der operativen Behandlung von Klumphanden. *Verh. Dtsch. Orthop. Ges. 54 Kongress, 103*:439–445, 1967.

Blauth, W.: Zur Morphologie und Therapie der radialen Klumphand. *Arch. Orthop. Unfallchir.*, *65*:97–123, 1969.

Blencke, A.: Ein weiterer Beitrag zur Sogem. Klumphand. *Z. Orthop. Chir.*, *13*:654–657, 1904.

Blockey, N. J.: Observations of the fate of fibular transplants for congenital absence of the radius. *J. Bone Joint Surg.*, *49B*:762, 1967.

Boinet, E.: Ectromélie longitudinale externe de l'avant-bras et de la main gauche. *C. R. Soc. Biol.*, *66*:883–885, 1909.

Bora, F. W., Jr., Nicholson, J. T., and Cheema, H. M.: Radial meromelia. The deformity and its treatment. *J. Bone Joint Surg.*, *52A*:966–979, 1970.

Borok, J. G.: Bilateral congenital absence of the radius. *Centr. Afr. J. Med.*, *4*:524–525, 1958.

Botreau-Roussel: Léger degré de main bote causée par l'absence congénitale des deux scaphoides. *Bull. Soc. Anat. Paris*, (6 s.), *19*:33–35, 1922.

Bouvier: Anatomische Untersuchung einer Klumphand. *Jb. Kinderkrank.*, *40*:295–307, 1863.

Bouvier: Main bote. *In Dict. Encyc. Sc. Med.* Paris, (2 s.), Vol. 4, pp. 162–191, 1871.

Branciforti, S.: Il trattamento della mano torta congenita. *Chir. Organi. Mov.*, *37*:475–486, 1952.

Broca, A.: *Chirurgie Infantile.* Paris, G. Steinheil, pp. 686–687, 1914.

Broman, I.: *Normale und Abnorme Entwicklung des Menschen.* Wiesbaden, J. F. Bergmann, pp. 229; fig. 194, 1911.

Bruckova, Z., and Cihak, R.: Clinical and anatomical remarks concerning the surgical treatment of congenital manus vara. (In Czech.) *Acta Chir. Orthop. Traum. Cech.*, *23*:219–223, 1955.

Bruno: Demonstration eines Falles von Doppelseitiger Klumphand. Radius- und Daumendefekt und Syndaktylie. *Munch. Med. Wochenschr.*, *53*:724, 1905.

Buchbinder, H.: Ein Beitrag zur Kasuistik des kongenitalem Radiusdefekt. Festschr dem hochverehuten Freunde und Lehrer Benno Schmidt zur Frier der Vollendung seines siebenzigsten Lebensjahres. 80 Leipzig, pp. 47–57, 1896.

Bülow-Hansen, V.: Et tilfaelde af Kongenital komplet radiusdefekt opereret efter Bardenheuer's methode. *Norsk Mag. Laegev.*, *6*:956–960, 1908.

Bunnell, S., and Dehne, E.: Z-plasty for clinarthrosis of the wrist. *Plast. Reconstr. Surg.*, *16*:169–173, 1955.

Burckhardt, L.: *Beitrage zur Diagnostik und Therapie congenitalen Knochendefect an Vorderarm und Unterschenkel.* Inaug.-Diss. Leipzig, B. G. Teubner, pp. 22–29, 1890.

Calo, A.: Cardiopatie congenite e malformazioni degli arti. *Cuore Circulazione*, *37*:303–313, 1953.

Canepa, G., and Sanguinetti, C.: Deformita congenita della mano. *Arch. Chir. Ortop. Med.*, *24*:109–146, 1959.

Carrol, R. E.: Use of the fibula for reconstruction in congenital absence of the radius. *J. Bone Joint Surg.*, *48A*:1012, 1966.

Cascos, A. S.: Holt-Oram syndrome. *Acta Paediatr. Scand.*, *56*:313–317, 1967.

Cassimos, C., and Zammos, L.: Congenital hypoplastic anemia associated with multiple developmental defects (Fanconi's syndrome). *Am. J. Dis. Child.*, *84*:347–350, 1952.

Castel, Y., Masse, R., Roch, J., and Mollaret, J.: Sur un cas de poikilodérmie congénitale de Thomson. *L'Ouest Méd.*, *20*:890–896, 1967.

Catterall, R. C. F.: Congenital deformity of wrists (complete absence of both radii). *Proc. R. Soc. Med. London* (Sect. on Orthop.), *47*:600, 1949.

Catterall, R. C. F.: Congenital absence of the radius. *J. Bone Joint Surg.*, *38B*:777, 1956.

Chalaiditi, D.: Zur Diagnostik angeborener Lungenmissbildungen. *Fortschr. Röntgenstr.*, *15*:108–114; Taf. XII; figs. 3, 4, 1914.

Claassen, S. A., Becker, W. F., and Pratt, P. T.: Congenital thrombocytopenia with aplasia of the radii. *Nebraska Med. J.*, *49*:419–423, 1964.

Clarke, J.: A case of macrostomia with congenital club-hand (bilateral absence of the radius). *Report Soc. Study Dis. Child.*, *1*:100, 1901.

Clarke, J. J.: *Orthopedic Surgery: Textbook of the Pathology and Treatment of Deformities.* London, Cassell & Co., Ltd. pp. 215–219, 1899.

Clemmesen, V.: Congenital cervical synostosis (Klippel-Feil's syndrome). Four cases. *Acta Radiol.*, *17*:480–490, 1936.

Cocchi, U.: Aplasia of the radius. Hereditary diseases with bone changes. *In* Schinz, H. R., Baensch, W. E., Friedl, E., and Uehlinger, E., (eds.): *Roentgen-Diagnostics.* First American Edition based on fifth German edition. English translation arranged and edited by J. T. Case. New York, Grune & Stratton, Vol. I, Part I, pp. 786–789, 1951.

Corret, P.: *La main bote congénitale.* Paris, N. Maloin, pp. 1–78, 1926.

Coulon, H.: Main-bote avant l'apparence d'un pied. *Bull. Soc. Anat. Paris*, (2 s.), *10*:497, 1875.

Cowdell, R. H., Phizackerley, P. J. R., and Pyke, D. A.: Constitutional anemia (Fanconi's syndrome) and leukemia in two brothers. *Blood*, *10*:788–801, 1955.

Coyon, A., and Gasne: Malformation des membres superieurs. Absence de l'articulation du coude. Ectrodactylie du pouce. *Rev. d'Orthop.*, (3 s.), *5*:183–188, 1914.

Cranwell, D. J.: Ausencia congenita del radio. *Rev. Soc. Med. Argent.*, *11*:540–555, 1903.

Crespo, H., and de Medina, J. M.: Caso de ausencia congenita bilateral del radio. (Nota clinica.) *Progresos de la Clinica*, *44*:136–137, 1936.

Cuff, A.: Absence of radii. *Clin. Sketches, London*, *3*:41–42, 1896.

D'Abreu, A. R.: Congenital bilateral absence of the radius and the thumb. *Indian Med. Gaz.*, *65*:505–507, 1930.

D'Abreu, A. R.: Congenital bilateral absence of the radius and the thumb. *Indian Med. Gaz.*, *67*:266–267, 1932.

Dalbera, M.: *La Loi d'Ollier.* Thèse, Paris, M. Vigne, pp. 1–55, 1927.

Dannenberg, C.: Beitrag zur Frag der angeborenen Radiusdefekt. Heidelberg, pp. 1–32, 1926.

Davaine, C.: De l'absence congénitale du radius chez l'homme. *C. R. Soc. Biol.*, (1 s.), *2*:39–41, 1850.

Davidson, A. J., and Horwitz, T.: Congenital club-hand deformity associated with absence of radius: its surgical correction. *J. Bone Joint Surg.*, *21*:462–463, 1939.

Davidson, E. P.: Congenital hypoplasia of the carpal scaphoid bone. *J. Bone Joint Surg.*, *44B*:816–827, 1962.

Dawson, J.: Congenital pancytopenia associated with multiple congenital anomalies (Fanconi type). *Pediatrics*, *15*:325–333, 1955.

Define, D.: A aplicacao em cirurgia orthopedica do poder osteogenitio do periosteo na infancia. *Rev. Bras. Ortop.*, *1*:42–52; figs. 13–16, 1966.

Define, D.: Treatment of congenital radial club-hand. *Clin. Orthop.*, *73*:153–159, 1970.

Dellaire, L.: A ring B chromosome in a female with multiple skeletal abnormalities. *In* Bergsma, D., (ed.): *Birth Defects: Original Article Series.* New York, National Foundation — March of Dimes, Part V, Vol. V, No. 5, pp. 114–116, 1969.

Delorme, T. L.: Treatment of congenital absence of the radius by transepiphyseal fixation. *J. Bone Joint Surg.*, *51A*:117–129, 1969.

Denucé and Nové-Josserand, G.: *La Pratique des Maladies des Enfants.* Paris, J. B. Balliere et Fils, pp. 81–83; fig. 28. 1913.

Djorup, F.: Anatomisk Undersogelse af et Tilfaelde af dobbeltsidig Radiusdefekt. *Bibl. Laeger.*, *111*:395–451, 1919.

Dodson, E. O.: Hereditary absence of radius and thumb; a report of an additional family. *J. Hered.*, *47*:275–276, 1956.

Dolbeau: De la prothese dans les cas de malformation de la main; pouce flattant. *Bull. Gener. Therapie*, *64*:565–567, 1864.

Drinnenberg, A.: Klumphandbildung infolge angeborene Radiusdefekts und ihre Behandlung — Ein beitrag. *A. Orthop. Chir.*, *63*:297–307, 1935.

Dubin, W.: Schultergurtel und obere Extremitat. *In* Helner, H., Nissen, R., and Wasschulte, K., (eds.): *Lehrbuch der Chirurgie.* Stuttgart, G. Thieme, pp. 923–930; Abb. 464, 1962.

Ehrhardt, P.: Etude sur l'ectromelie du pouce et du premier métacarpien précédée de quelques considérations sur l'origine des anomalies dactyles. *Rev. d'Orthop.*, *1*:205–216, 1890.

Emery, J. L., Gordon, R. R., Rendle-Short, J., Varadi, S., and Warrack, A. J. N.: Congenital amegakaryocytic thrombocytopenia with congenital deformities and a leukemoid blood picture in the newborn. *Blood*, *12*:567–576, 1957.

Entin, M. A.: Reconstruction of congenital aplasia of radial component. *Surg. Clin. N. Am.*, *44*:1091–1105, 1964.

Entin, M. A., and Petrie, J. G.: Reconstruction of congenital absence of the radius. *In Trans. First Internat. Congress Plast. Surg.* Baltimore, Williams & Wilkins, pp. 448–452, 1957.

Erichsen: Congenital absence of the radius and its muscles. *Lancet*, *1*:605–606, 1858.

Essen-Möller, E.: Über angeborene Radiusdefekts. Ohrdefekte und Facialislahmungen anlasslich eines Falles von multiplen Missbildungen. *Z. menschl. Vererb. Konstitutionslehre*, *14*:52–70, 1929.

Estren, S., Suess, J. F., and Dameshek, W.: Congenital hypoplastic anemia associated with multiple developmental defects (Fanconi syndrome). *Blood*, *2*:85–93, 1947.

Evans, F. G., Alfaro, A., and Alfaro, S.: An unusual anomaly of the superior extremities in a Tarascan Indian girl. *Anat. Rec.*, *106*:37–47, 1950.

Eymer: Ein Fall von hereditärem kongenitalem Radiusdefekt. *Münch. Med. Wochenschr.*, *59*:502, 1912.

Faed, M., Stewart, A., and Keay, A. J.: Chromosome abnormalities in two cases with bilateral radial element defects. *J. Med. Genet.*, *6*:347, 1969.

Fanconi, G.: Familiäre infantile perniziösaartige Anämie (Perniziöses Blutbild und Konstitution). *Jb. Kinderheilkd.*, *117*:257–280, 1927.

Fanconi, G.: Familial constitutional panmyelocytopathy, Fanconi's anemia (F.A.) I. Clinical aspects. *Seminar Hemat.*, *4*:233–240, 1967.

Farmer, A. W., and Laurin, C. A.: Congenital absence of the radius. *Can. J. Surg.*, *1*:301–308, 1958.

Favel: Arrêt d'accroissement du radius. *Mem. C. R. Soc. Sci. Méd. Lyon*, *26*(2):266, 1887.

Feutelais, P.: Main bote radio-palmaire et scoliose congénitale. *Rev. d'Orthop.*, *17*:149–152; fig. 2, 1930.

Fisson, E.: *Absence Congénitale du Radius.* Thèse. Paris, No. 497, pp. 1–20, 1924.

Fletcher, J.: Malformations of the upper limb. *Proc. R. Soc. Med. London* (Sect. Plast. Surg.), *62*:55–56, 1969.

Florio, L.: La mano valga da assenza congenita del radio. *Arch. Putti*, *22*:406–421, 1963.

Follin: Main-bot palmaire. *Bull. Soc. Anat. Paris*, *26*:98–101, 1851.

Fontes, V.: Nota sobre un caso de hemimelia. *Arg. Anat. Anthropol.*, *13*:191–209; fig. 1–81, 1929–1930.

Forbes, G.: A case of congenital club-hand with a review of the aetiology of the condition. *Anat. Rec.*, *71*:181–199, 1938.

Francais, H., and Egger, M.: Agénésie totale du système radial. *N. Iconog. Salp.*, *19*:463–465, 1906.

Fritzsche, H.: Kausalitätsbiurteilung einer Lunatummalazie bei Daumenplasie ein seltene Beobachtung einer symmetrischen Tetradaktylie bei Mutter und Tochter. *Z. Unfallmed. Berufskr.*, *55*:84–89, 1962.

Funston, R. V.: The relation of congenital deformities of the hand to cervical ribs. *J.A.M.A.*, *98*:697–700, 1932.

Galliard, L., and Levy, F.: Micromelie avec malformation symetrique des radius. *Bull. Mem. Soc. Med. Hôp. Paris*, (3 s.), *21*:1103–1106, 1904.

Gardemin, H.: Zur Frühbehandlung der Radiusplasie. *Verh. Dtschr. Ges. 50 Kongress*, 97:422, 1963.

Gardemin, H.: Zur Frühoperation der angeborenen Radiusplasie. *Arch. Klin. Chir.*, *306*:183, 1964.

Garipuy: Un cas de main-bote par absence du radius. *Bull. Mem. Soc. Anat. Paris*, *82*:174–179, 1907.

Gayet, M. G.: La main bote héréditaire. *Gaz. Hôp.*, *74*:345–347, 1901.

Gegenbaur, C.: Zur Morphologie der gliedmassen der Wirbelthiere. *Morph. Jb.*, *2*:396–420, 1876.

Gellis, S. S., and Feingold, M.: Picture of the month. Fanconi's anemia (chronic pancytopenia with multiple congenital abnormalities.) *Am. J. Dis. Child.*, *113*:582–583, 1967.

Gerold, M.: Frakturheilung bei ein em seltenen Fall Kongenital er Anomalie der oberen Gliedmassen. *Zentralbl. Chir.*, *84*:831–834, 1959.

Glaesner, P.: Über angeborene Verbildungen Bereich der oberen Extremität. *Dtsch. Med. Wochenschr.*, *37*:2324–2326; figs. 1–7, 1911.

Goerlich, M.: Doppelseitiger kongenitaler Radiusdefekt. *Beitr. Klin. Chir.*, *59*:430–435, 1908.

Goerlich, M.: Erworbener linkseitiger partieller Radiusdefekt. *Beitr. Klin. Chir.*, *59*:435–439, 1908.

Goerlich, M.: Ueber einige Radiusmissbildungen. *Beitr. Klin. Chir.*, *59*:421–440, 1908.

Goldenberg, R. R.: Congenital bilateral complete absence of the radius in identical twins. *J. Bone Joint Surg.*, *30A*:1001–1003, 1948.

Goldstein, R.: Hypoplastic anemia with multiple congenital anomalies (Fanconi's syndrome). *Am. J. Dis. Child.*, *89*:618–622, 1955.

Gonnet: Absence congénitale du radius et meningocele cerebelleuse. *Bull. Soc. Obstet. Paris*, *11*:210–212, 1908.

Gorlin, R. J., and Pindborg, J. J.: *Syndromes of the Head and Neck*. New York, The Blakiston Division, McGraw-Hill Book Co., pp. 122–125, 427–431, 1964.

Grant, D. N. W.: Congenital absence of the radius and club hand. *Milit. Surg.*, *69*:578–621, 1931.

Grant, J. W. G.: Case of non-rotation of the intestine with congenital absence of radius. *Br. J. Surg.*, *18*:166–167, 1930.

Grebe, H.: Defekte der Radius. Klumphand Missbildung der Gliedmassen. *In* Becker, P. E., (ed.): *Humangenetik*. Stuttgart, G. Thieme, Vol. 2, pp. 213–215, 276, 1964.

Greenwood, H. H.: Reconstruction of the forearm for loss of radius. *Br. J. Surg.*, *20*:58, 1932.

Grisalli, M., and Samsone, G.: Constitutional infantile panmyelopathy with multiple malformations. *Helvet Beta Paediatr.*, *7*:299–308, 1952.

Grizaud, H.: Sur un cas de main bote congénitale bilatérale. *J. Radiol. Electrol.*, *16*:515–516, 1932.

Gross, H., Groh, C., and Weippl, G.: Kongenitale hypoplastische Thrombopenie mit Radiusaplasie, ein Syndrom multipler Abartungen. *Neue Osterr. Z. Kinderheilkd.*, *1*:574–582, 1956.

Gruber, W.: Ueber congenitalen Radiusmangel. *Arch. Pathol. Anat. Physiol.*, *32*:211–222, 1865.

Gruber, W.: Über congenitalen unvollstädigen Radiusmangel. *Arch. Pathol. Anat. Physiol.*, *40*:427–435; Tafel VII, 1867.

Guanti, G., Petrinelli, P., and Schettini, F.: Cytogenetical and clinical investigations in aplastic anemia (Fanconi's type). *Humangenetik*, *13*:222–223; fig. 2, 1971.

Guermonprez, F.: Absence congénitale du radius gauche avec développement rudimentaire du pouce et absence du premier metacarpien et l'éminence thenar. *Bull. Mem. Soc. Chir. Paris*, (n.s.), *10*:730–733, 1884.

Guerzoni, P. L.: Mano torte congenita e suo trattamento. *Atti S.E.R.T.O.T.*, *8*:913–920, 1963.

Hall, C. B., and Brooks, M. B.: Congenital skeletal deficiencies of the extremities. *J.A.M.A.*, *181*:590–599, 1962.

Hall, J. G. H., and Levin, J.: Congenital amegakaryocytic thrombocytopenia with bilateral absence of radius: radius-platelet hypoplasia or RPH. *In* Bergsma, D., (ed.): *Birth Defects: Original Article Series*. New York, National Foundation–March of Dimes. Vol. V, No. 3, pp. 190–195, 1969.

Hall, J. G., Levin, J., Kuhn, J. P., Ottenheimer, E. J., van Berkum, P., and McKusick, V. A.: Thrombocytopenia with absent radius (TAR). *Medicine*, *48*:411–439, 1969.

Hanley, T., and Conlon, P. C.: Congenital deformity of the carpus associated with maldevelopment of certain thenar muscles. *J. Bone Joint Surg.*, *39B*:458–462, 1957.

Hann, R. G.: Twin pregnancy with anencephalic foetus showing unilateral development and numerous deformities. *J. Obstet. Gynecol. Brit. Emp.*, *28*:311–313, fig. 2, 1921.

Harbeson, A. E.: Bilateral congenital absence of the radii. *Can. Am. Assoc. J.*, *36*:359–360, 1937.

Harris, L. C., and Osborn, W. P.: Congenital absence or hypoplasia of the radius with ventricular septal defect: ventriculoradial dysplasia. *J. Pediatr.*, *68*:265–272, 1966.

Hartofilakidis-Garofalidis, G., Matsoukas, J., Partazopoulos, T., and Giannikas, A.: Undescribed cranio-auriculo-radial syndrome. *Helv. Paediatr. Acta*, *26*:75–77, 1971.

Haudek, M.: Zur Aetiologie der angeborenen Klumphand ohne Defektbildung. *Z. Orthop. Chir.*, *16*:342–346, 1906.

Hay, F. W.: Das Bild der angeborenen Daumenhypoplasie. *Dtsch. Med. Wochenschr.*, *64*:1041–1042, 1938.

Heikel, H. V. A.: Aplasia and hypoplasia of the radius; studies on 64 cases and on epiphyseal transplantation in rabbits with the imitated defect. *Acta. Orthop. Scand.*, Supplement No. 39:1–155, 1959.

Hellmuth, K.: *Zur Casuistik der Missbildungen. Ein fall von congenitalem Vollstandigen Radiusdefect und von Dicephelus dibrachus tripus.* Inaug.-Diss. Erlangen, Druck der Universitaes, pp. 5–22, 1881.

Henzschel, O.: *Beitrag zur Casuistik des angeborenen Radiusdefektes.* Inaug.-Diss. Halle, Plotz'sche Buchdruckerei, pp. 5–38, 1872.

Herschel, W.: *Beitrag zur Casuistik und zur Theorie des congenitalen Radiusdefectes.* Inaug-Diss. Kiel, C. P. Mahr, pp. 5–35; fig. 1–2, 1878.

Herzog, A.: Angeborener Radiusdefekt mit Verbildung der Handwurzelknochen. *Fortschr. Röntgenstr., 34*:968–970, 1926.

Hewitt, H. L., and Van Bochove, M.: Chondrodystrophia calcificans congenita. *Radial. Clin. Biol., 40*:175–183; fig. 3, 1971.

Hill, L. L., Jr.: Congenital abnormalities—phocomelus and congenital absence of radius. *Surg. Gynecol. Obstet., 65*:475–479, 1937.

Hirotani, H., Yoshizumi, M., Tanaka, S., Otsuka, H., and Okamoto, S.: Congenital absence of the radius. (In Japanese.) *J. Jap. Orthop. Assoc., 38*:423–431, 1964.

Hodge, H. L.: Congenital absence of the radius. *Trans. Path. Soc. Philadelphia, 6*:4–6, 1877.

Hodgson, A. R.: Congenital retardation in development of the carpal navicular, first metacarpal and styloid process of the radius. *Br. J. Surg., 31*:95–96, 1943.

Hoffa, A.: Zur Statistik der Deformitäten. *Munch. Med. Wochenschr., 37*:237–240, 1890.

Holfelder, G.: Röntgenologische Studien uber das Wachstum der Arm von Dysmeliekindern. *Verh. Dtsch. Orthop. Ges. 31 Kongress, 100*:488–489, 1965.

Holmes, L. B.: Congenital heart disease and upper-extremity deformities: a report of two families. *N. Engl. J. Med., 272*:437–444, 1965.

Holt, M., and Oram, S.: Familial heart disease with skeletal malformations. *Br. Heart J., 22*:236–242, 1960.

Hopf, A.: Aplasie und hypoplasie der radius ("Radiusdefekt"). Die angeborenen Veränderungen des Unterarms und der Hand. *In* Hohmann, G., Hackenbroch, M., and Lindemann, K., (eds.): *Handbuch der Orthopädie.* Band III. *Spezielle Orthopädie obere Extremität.* Stuttgart, G. Thieme, pp. 426–428, 1959.

Horbeson, A. E.: Bilateral congenital absence of the radii. *Can. Med. Assoc. J., 36*:359–360, 1937.

Horrocks, W.: Arrested growth of lower end of radius. *Illustr. Med. News, 2*:200, 1889.

Houdart, R., Verley, K., and Mamo, H.: Malformations congénitales de la charnière crânio-rachidienne associées a des malformations de la face, de l'oeil, de l'omoplate et du membre supérieur. *Presse Méd., 69*:1127–1129, 1961.

Huisman, A.: Absence congénitale des deux radius. *J. Méd. Bruxelles, 10*:670–671, 1905.

Hutchinson, J.: Cases of congenital absence of the radius. (Dr. Niblett's case.) *Arch. Surg., 3*:299–304, 1891–1892.

Huxley, J. S., and De Beer, G. R.: *Elements of Experimental Embryology.* Cambridge, University Press, pp. 223–224, 1934.

Iketa, K., Yabe., Kato, T., Yamane, H., and Murakami, T.: The schema of the arteries in the defect of the radius. (In Japanese.) *Orthop. Surg., 19*:98–100, 1968.

Illyes, G.: Congenital defect of the radius. (In Hungarian.) *Orvosi Hetil.* Budapest 51:36, 1907.

Immeyer, F.: Lippen-Kiefer- Gaumenspalten bei thalidomideschadigten Kindern. *Acta Genet. Med. Gem., 16*:244–247, 1967.

Infante, C.: Un caso di assenza congenita del radio bilateral. *Atti Cong. Ital. Radiol. Med. 1913* (Pavia), 1:154, 1914.

Ingelrans, P., and Piquet, J.: Syndrome de Klippel-Feil accompagné de malformations multiples. *Rev. d'Orthop., 15*:297–307, 1928.

Jaboulay: Main bote par absence du radius. *Rev. Chir., 23*:447, 1901.

Jacobi: Case of uncommon congenital malformation of the arm (absent radius and thumb). *Am. J. Obstet., 8*:324, 1875.

Jacobsthal: Deformität der Vorderarmes bei erworbenem Radiusdefekt. *Dtsch. Z. Chir., 75*:554–568, 1904.

Jäger, M.: Ein funktionelle Klumphandschiene (Technische Mitteilung). *Z. Orthop. Chir., 103*:554–559, 1967.

Jäger, M., Refior, H. J., and Zenker, H.: Vergleichende Untersuchungen zur Frage der Fortenwicklungsstorung der Wirbelsaule bei Kingern mit Dysmelie-Syndrom und Kindern Peromelien. *Z. Orthop., 103*:283–308, 1967.

Jagot, L.: Absence congenitale du radius gauche et de la partie correspondante du massif osseux du carpe. *Arch. Med. Angers, 9*:161–167, 1905.

Jarcho, S., and Levin, P. M.: Hereditary malformation of the vertebral bodies. *Bull. Johns Hopkins Hosp., 62*:216–226, 1938.

Jeanne, A.: Main-bote congénitale (variété palmaire) par malformation des os du carpe et accompagnée d'une luxation congénitale du pouce. *Bull. Soc. Anat. Paris,* (5 s.), *11*:618–621, 1897.

Joachimsthal, G.: Über angeborene Anomalien der oberen Extremitäten. *Arch. Klin. Chir., 50*:495–506; Taf. II, 1895.

Johansson, S.: Ett fall av kongenitale defekt av radius och ulna. *Hygiea, 84*:81–84, 1922.

Juberg, R. C., Adams, M. S., Venema, W. J., and Hart, G.: Multiple congenital anomalies associated with Ring-D chromosome. *J. Med. Genet., 6*:314–321; fig. 3, 1969.

Judet, I.: Une technique chirurgicale du traitement de la main bote radiale, congénitale. *Rev. Chir. Orthop., 56*:277–278, 1970.

Juhl, J. H., Wesenberg, R. L., and Gwinn, J. L.: Roentgenographic findings in Fanconi's anemia. *Radiology, 89*:646–653, 1967.

Kaczander, J.: Über angeborenen Radiusmangel. *Arch. Pathol. Anat. Physiol., 71*:409–413; Taf. XV, 1877.

Kaganovich-Dvorkin, A. L.: Congenital absence of the radius with bilateral manus vara. (In Russian.) *Orthop. Traumatol., 12*:85, 1938.

Kashiwagi, D., Kataoka, D., Fujiwara, A., Kumon, H., Miyomoto, T., Fukita, H., and Miyake, M.: Surgical therapy of clubhand. *Orthop. Surg. Tokyo, 19*:100–102, 1968.

Kato, K.: Congenital absence of the radius. *J. Bone Joint Surg., 22*:589–626, 1924.

Kawamura, B., et al: Surgery of congenital clubhand. *Orthop. Surg. Tokyo, 8*:151–154, 1967.

Keiser, D. V.: Radius defekt. *In* Diethelm, L., (ed.): *Skeletanatomie (Röntgendiagnostik)*. Berlin, Springer, Band IV, Teil 2, pp. 203–204, 1968.

Kelikian, H., and Doumanian, A.: Congenital anomalies of the hand. *J. Bone Joint Surg., 39A*:1002–1019; 1249–1266, 1957.

Kindle, J.: Fünf Falle von angeborenen Defektbildungen an den Extremitäten. *Z. Heilkd., 28*:110–138, 1907.

Kirkpatrick, J. A., Wagner, M. L., and Pilling, G. P.: A complex of anomalies associated with tracheoesophageal fistula and esophageal atrasia. *Am. J. Roentgenol., 95*:208–211, 1965.

Kirmisson, E., and Longuet: Nouveau cas de main bote congénitale. *Rev. d'Orthop.*, (1 s.), *4*:59–64, 1893.

Kirmisson, E., and Sainton, R.: Note sur deux cas de main bote d'origine congénitale observés aux enfants-assistes. *Rev. d'Orthop.*, (1 s.), *3*:108–124, 1892.

Klaussner, F.: *Uber Missbildungen des Menschlichen Gliedmassen und ihre Entslehungsweise*. Wiesbaden, J. F. Bergmann, pp. 10–18, 1900.

Klippel, M., and Feil, A.: Anomalie de la colonne vertébrale par absence des vertèbres cervicales. Cage thoracique remontant jusqu'à la base du crâne. *Bull. Mem. Soc. Anat. 87*:185–188, 1912.

Klippel, M., and Feil, A.: Un cas d'absence des vertèbres cervicales avec cage thoracique remontant jusqu'à la base du crâne (cage thoracique cervicale). *N. Iconog. Salp., 25*:223–250, 1912.

Klippel, M., and Rabaud, E.: Sur une forme rare d'hémimélie radiale intercalaire. *N. Iconog. Salp., 16*:238–251, 1903.

Krevstovskey, V. V.: Arthrodesis between ulna and wrist in absence of lowest part of radius. (In Russian.) *Novy Khir. Arkhiv., 40*:445–449, 1938.

Krichler, U.: Über die Variationsbreite der kongenitalen Fibula und Radiusplasien. *Z. Mensch. Vererb. Konstitutionslehre, 24*:480–505, 1940.

Krönig: Vorstellung eines neugeborenen Kindes bei beiderseitigne Radiusdefekt. *Cbl. Gynakol., 18*:171–172, 1894.

Krückmeyer, K.: *Talipomanus, ein Beitrage zur Kenntnis des sog. cong. Radiusdefektes*. Dissertation. Gottingen, F. Pieper, pp. 3–31, 1938.

Kuhn, E. Schaaf, J., and Wagner, A.: Primary pulmonary hypertension, congenital heart disease and skeletal anomalies in three generations. *Japanese Heart J., 4*:205–223, 1963.

Kummel, W.: *Die Missbildungen der Extremitäten durch Defekt, Verwachsung und Ueberzahl*. Cassel, Th. G. Fischer & Co., Section E, Vol. II, pp. 1–11, 33–38, 1895.

Küttner, H.: Die Transplantation aus dem Afen und ihre Dauererfolge. *Munch. Med. Wochenschr., 64*:1449–1452, 1917.

Lackey, W. N.: Unusual congenital deformities of the upper extremities; absence of the radii with oligodactylia. *J.A.M.A., 93*:113–114, 1929.

Lange, M.: Erbbiologie der angeborenen Korperfehler. *Z. Orthop. Chir., 63*:73–99, Abb. 24, 1935.

Langlands, F. H.: Case of arrested development in the lower end of the radius. *Intercolon. Med. J. Melbourne, Australia, 104*:1 plate, 1900.

Larcher, J. F.: *Études Physiologiques et Médicales sur Quelques Lois de l'Organisme*. Paris, P. Asselin, pp. 221–223, 1868.

Layral, V., and Péju, G.: Absence congénitale totale du radius et malformation carpiennes multiples. *Prov. Méd., 20*:628, 1907.

Ledru: Main-bote radiale double congénitale, avec absence complète du radius des deux côtés. *Bull. Soc. Anat., Paris, 30*:269–277, 1855.

Legal: Angeborene Klumphände und angeborene Schulterverrenkung. *Zentralbl. Chir., 57*:534–535, 1930.

LeGendre, E. Q.: Observation de main bote. *Gaz. Med.*, (3s.), *14*:298, 1859. Also in *C. R. Soc. Biol., 11*:24–25, 1859.

Lehle, A.: Zur Kasuistik des kongenitalen Radiusdefektes. *Dtsch. Milit. Arztl. Z. Berlin, 41*:928–931, 1912.

Leloire, H.: Malformation congénitale de l'avant-bras et de la main. *Le Progrès Med., 7*:536–588, 1879. Also *Bull. Soc. Anat. Paris*, (4 s.), *4*:65–72, 1879.

Leprince, H.: *Contribution a l'Étude de la Main-bote Congénitale*. Thèse. Paris, Vigot Frères, pp. 5–70, 1900.

Lestache, G.: Un caso de ausencia congénita bilateral y completa del radio y de todos los huesos del carpo. *Pediatr. Espan.,* 7:91–94; figs. 1 and 2, 1918.

Letuelle, M.: Vice de conformation du membre supérieur droit; absence du radius, arrêt de développement du pouce et de la portion correspondante des régions carpienne et metacarpienne. *Bull. Soc. Anat. Paris,* (3 s.), *10*:309–316, 1875.

Lewin, P.: Congenital absence or defects of bones of the extremities. *Am. J. Roentgenol.,* (n.s.), *4*:431–448, 1917.

Lewis, K. B., Bruce, R. A., Baum, B., and Motulsky, A. G.: The upper limb–cardiovascular syndrome. An autosomal dominant effect on embryogenesis. *J.A.M.A., 193*:1080–1086, 1965.

Lexer, E.: *Die Freien Transplantationen.* Stuttgart, F. Enke, pp. 146–190; fig. 118; 174–179, 1924.

Leyral, V., and Peju, G.: Absence congénitale totale du radius et malformations carpiennes multiples. *Prov. Méd., 20*:628, 1907.

Lingabue, P.: Mano torta congenita e suo trattamento. *Arch. Ortop., 30*:712–730, 1913.

Loebell, A.: *Über Congenitalen Radiusdefekt.* Inaug.-Diss. Geissen, Munchow'sch Hof- und Universitats-Druckerei (O. Kindt.), pp. 6–34, 1906.

Lopez, E. H.: Anatomia pathologica de la mano zamba congenita por ausencia de radio. *Prog. Clinica,* Madrid, 37:583–590, 1929.

Lorenz, A.: Ein Fall von doppelseitigem angeborenem Defekt der Radius. *Wien Med. Wochenschr., 63*:1052–1058, 1913.

Lotsch, F.: Ein Fall von rechtesseitigem Radiusdefekt und linksseitiger daumenloser Klumphand. *Dtsch. Z. Chir., 82*:530–541, 1906.

Lovett, R. W.: Club-hand. *In* Park, R., (ed.): *A Treatise on Surgery.* Third edition. New York, Lea Brothers & Col., Vol. II, pp. 1280–1281, 1901.

Löwry, E.: Multiplen Missbildungen bei einer Zwillings-Fruehgeburt. *Wien. Med. Wochenschr., 71*:2019–2020, 1921.

Lugones, C., and Puglisi, A.: Ausencia congenita del radio. *Rev. Espec. Asoc. Med. Argent., 4*:300–308, 1929.

Lundholm, G.: Congenital manus vara. *Acta Orthop. Scand., 29*:207–216, 1960.

Luppis, F., and Bachiocco, R.: La mano torta congenita. *Chir. Organi. Mov., 58*:134–150, 1969.

Lynch, M. J., Sherman, L., and Elliot, F. G.: Fanconi's anemia (aplastic anemia with congenital abnormalities). *Can. Med. J., 71*:273–276, 1954.

Magalhaes, A. F. de: Mao radio-palmar, dupla congenita. *Brasil Med., 32*:25, 1918.

Magni, L.: Di alcune mon commumi malformazioni congenite degli arti. *Chir. Organi. Mov., 16*:185–206, Case No. III, 1931.

Makley, J. T., and Heiple, K. G.: Scoliosis associated with congenital deficiencies of the upper extremity. *J. Bone Joint Surg., 52A*:279–287, figs. 1-A, 2-A, 2-B, 1970.

Malewski, B.: Complete bilateral absence of the radius, combined with word deafness. (In Polish.) *Medicynia, Warsawa, 21*:235–240, 1903.

Margolis, E., and Hasson, E.: Hereditary malformations of the upper extremities in three generations. *J. Hered., 46*:254–262, 1955.

Martin, R., and Munier, J. P.: Sur un cas de malformations congénitales héréditaires des membres superieurs. *Soc. Pediatr. Paris, 11*:631–636, 1954.

Martmer, E. E.: Talipomanus: A report of three cases in one family. *Am. J. Dis. Child., 34*:384–387, 1927.

Massabuau, Guibal, A., and Marican: Absence congénitale du radius. *Bull. Soc. Sci. Méd. Bio. Montpellier, 4*:304, 1922–1923.

Massumi, R. A., and Nutter, B. O.: A syndrome of familial defects of heart and upper extremities (Holt-Oram syndrome). *Circulation, 34*:65, 1966.

Mastandrea, F.: Considerazioni patogenetiche e cliniche sulla mano torta congenita. *Ort. Traum. App. Mot., 23*:669–684, 1955.

Mathews, D.: Congenital abnormalities of the thumb. *Proc. R. Soc. Med. London* (Sect. Plast. Surg.), 62:53–54, 1969.

Mathews, W. P.: A Case of congenital absence of the radius and bones of the thumb. *Med. Reg. Richmond, 1*:29, 1 pl. 1897.

Matzen, P. F., and Fleissner, H. K.: Congenital malformation of the limbs. In: *Orthopedic Roentgen Atlas.* New York: Grune and Stratton Inc. pp. 387–474; figs. 589a, 589b, 600b, 1970.

McCurdy, S. L.: Congenital absence of radii, with operation. *Ann. Surg., 23*:44–47, 1896. Also: *Trans. Amer. Orthop. Assoc., 8*:8–14, 1895. Also *Boston Med. Surg. J., 133*:446, 1895.

McDonald, R., and Goldschmidt, B.: Pancytopenia with congenital defects (Fanconi's anemia). *Arch. Dis. Child., 35*:367–372, 1960.

Meckel, J. F.: Beschriebung einer merkwurdigne Missgeburt. *Arch. Anat. Physiol., 1*:36–43, 1826.

Metcalfe, J.: Congenital malformation of both hands and forearms. *Arch. Radiol. Electrol., 20*:18–20, 1915.

Michelson, J.: Ein Fall vontotalem Defekt der Radius. *Z. Orthop. Chir., 12*:445–452, 1904.

Middleton, G. S.: A case of congenital absence of the left radius and of the left thumb, malformation of the ulna, spinal curvature and complete displacement of the heart to the right. *Trans. Med. Chir. Soc.* (Glasgow), 2:156–160, 1897–1898. See also *Glasgow Med. J., 1*:244–248, 1898.

Milch, H.: Short radius. *Arch. Surg., 59*:856–869, 1949.

Miller, O. R.: Congenital absence of the radius. *Internat. J. Surg. N. Y.*, *38*:186–190, 1925.

Miller, R. C., and Phalen, G. S.: The repair of defects of the radius with fibular bone grafts. *J. Bone Joint Surg.*, *29*:629–636, 1947.

Milne, J. A.: Congenital absence of radii. *Br. Med. J.*, *2*:821, 1915.

Minagi, H., and Steinbach, H. L.: Roentgen appearance of anomalies associated with hypoplastic anemias of childhood. Fanconi's anemia and congenital hypoplastic anemia (erythrogenesis imperfecta). *Am. J. Roentgenol.*, *97*:100–109, 1966.

Mohanta, K. D., and Praharaj, K. C.: Hemimelia. *Indian Pediatr.*, *5*:277–279, 1968.

Mouchet, A.: Ectromelie du pouce du premier metacarpien avec persistance du radius. *Bull. Soc. Anat. Paris*, (6 s.), 6:29–30, 1904.

Mourad, A.: A case of club-hand. *Lancet*, 2:1222, 1922.

Mukarji, M.: A case of club hands. *Br. J. Radiol.*, (n.s.), *4*:507–508, 1931.

Muller, W.: Verschiedenen Fehlbildunstendenzen an Vorderarm. *Arch. Orthop. Unfallchir.*, *39*:541–557, 1939.

Muscatello, G.: Rer la cura operativa nella mancanza congenita del radio. *Arch. Ortop.*, *23*:366–371, 1906.

Mutel: Un cas de main bote radiale congenitals. *Rev. d'Orthop.*, (3 s.), *5*:119–128, 1914.

Myers, B.: Absence of both thumbs, with other deformities of the upper extremities in an infant. *Proc. R. Soc. Med.* (Sec. Dis. Child.), *16*:72, 1923.

Nager, F. R., and Reynier, J. P. de: Das Gehörorgan bei den angeborenen Kopfmissbildungen. *Pract. Oto-Rhino-Laryng.* (Basel), *10*(2):1–128, 1948.

Nicolas, R.: Contribution a l'étude de l'absence congénitale du radius. Thèse. Paris, pp. 1–72, 1835.

Nigst, P. F.: Radiusdefekte. *Schwiez. Med. Wochenschr.*, *57*:12–13, 1927.

Nilsson, L. R.: Chronic pancytopenia with multiple congenital anomalies. (Fanconi's anemia.) *Acta Paediatr.*, *49*:518–529, 1960.

Nilsson, L. R., and Lundholm, G.: Congenital thrombocytopenia associated with aplasia of the radius. *Acta Paediatr., Scand.*, *49*:291–296, 1960.

Oidtmann, A.: Resultaat der operatieve behandeling van een totaal radius-defect. *Ned. T. Geneesk.*, *61*:2172–2174, 1917.

Ollier, L.: *Traité Expérimentale et Clinique de la Régénération des Os et de la Production Artificielle du Rissu Osseux.* Paris, Victor Masson et Fils, Vol. II, pp. 202–211, 1867.

O'Rahilly, R.: Radial hemimelia and the functional anatomy of the carpus. *J. Anat.*, *80*:179–183, 1946.

O'Rahilly, R.: An analysis of cases of radial hemimelia. *Arch. Pathol.*, *44*:28–33, 1947.

O'Rahilly, R.: Morphological patterns in limb deficiencies and duplications. *Am. J. Anat.*, *89*:135–194, 1951.

Otto, A. W.: *Museum Anatomico-pathologicum Vrastislaviense.* Vratistaviae, F. Hibt, pp. 139–140, No. 235, Taf. XVII, figs. 1 et 2, No. 236, Taf XVI, figs. 11 et 12, 1841.

Pagliani, F., and Perazzo, G.: Osservazioni sopra un caso di mano torta da mancanza congenita del radio. *Boll. Sci. Med.* (Bologna), *106*:243–266, 1934.

Parahy, G.: Une technique chirurgicale de la main bote. *Paris Chir.*, *24*:27–32, 1932.

Pardini, A. G.: Radial dysplasia. *Clin. Orthop.*, *57*:153–177, 1968.

Parisel, F.: Absence congenitale et bilatérale du radius. *Bruxelles Méd.*, *27*:1176–1177, 1947.

Parisio, B.: L'assenza congenita bilaterale del radio. Nota casistica. *Folia Hered. Pathol.*, *4*:53–64, Tav. I, II, 1954.

Park, R.: Congenital defect of the forearm, absence of the radius. Clubhand and plastic operation. *Phila. Med. J.*, *8*:993, 1901. Also *Trans. Am. Orthop. Assoc.*, *14*:144–146, 1901.

Parker, R. W.: Congenital absence of radius from each arm, with defective carpus and hand. *Trans. Pathol. Soc. London*, *33*:236–239, 1882.

Pasquali: Un bambino mencanto di ambedue le ossa del radio. *Boll. Acad. Med Roma*, *6*:6, 1880.

Patel, and Charton: Hémimélie de quatre membres. *Lyon Chir.*, *32*:96–98, 1935.

Pavlos, M., and Petridis, A.: Un cas de main bote en valgus congénitale des deux côté chez un nouveau-ne debile, absence bilatérale du pouce; absence du radius du côté gauche. *Lyon Med.*, *132*:756–757, 1926.

Peabody, C. W.: Congenital absence of the radius. Orthopedic Correspondence Club Letter, 1947. (Cited by Speed and Knight, 1956).

Pereira, M. J. de F., and Pires de Lima, J. A.: As anomalias dos membros ilha de S. Miguel (Acores). *Arq. Anat. Anthropol.*, *13*:35–66, 1930.

Petersen, O.: Partieller Radiusmangel bei einem syphilitischen Manne. *St. Petersburg Med. Wochenschr.*, *5*:383–385, 1880.

Petit, J. L.: *Histoire de l'Académie Royale des Sciences, 1733.* Paris, Imprimérie Royale, pp. 1–21, 1733.

Petridis, P. A.: Un cas de main bote en valgus congénitale de deux côtés chez un nouveau-né debile. Absence bilatérale du pouce. Absence du radius du côté gauche. *Lyon Méd.*, *137*:756–757, 1936.

Picqué, L., and Poix, G.: Ectromélie du pouce et du premier métacarpien avec persistance du radius. *Bull. Soc. Anat. Paris*, *10*:226–229, 1896.

Poncet: Main bote radiale bilatérale par absence congénitale de radius. *Lyon Méd.*, *108*:17–18, 1907.

Pooley, J. H.: Malformation of the extremities, etc. *Illustrated Med. Surg.*, pp. 163–166, 1883.

Prokopova, L. V., and Pirigov, N. J.: The treatment of congenital clubhand in children. (In Russian.) *Klin. Khir. Odessa, 1*:27–31, 1963.

Pulvertaft, R. G.: Congenital radial clubhand. *J. Bone Joint Surg., 49B*:587, 1967.

Pulvertaft, R. G.: Aplasia and hypoplasia of the radius. *The Hand, 1*:60–62, 1969.

Püschel, E.: *Missbildungen der Gliedmassen Stuttgart,* F. K. Schattaus Verlag, pp. 122–138, 1970.

Rabinowitz, J. G., Moseley, J. E., Mitty, H. A., and Hirschhorn, K.: Trisomy 18A, esophageal atresia, anomalies of the radius and congenital hypoplastic thrombocytopenia. *Radiology, 89*:488–491, 1967.

Redard, P.: Surgical treatment of congenital clubhand. *Trans. Am. Orthop. Assoc., 15*:363–369, 1901.

Redard, P.: Du traitement chirurgicale de la main bote congénitale. *Rev. d'Orthop.,* (2 s.), *4*:247–252, 1903.

Reedy, J. J., and Bodner, L. M.: Dominant inheritance of radial hemimelia. *J. Hered., 44*:254–256, 1953.

Regnault, F.: Méchanisme de production de la main-bote congénitale. *Bull. Soc. Anat. Paris,* (6 s.), *2*:1051, 1900.

Reicz, O.: Congenital defect of the radius on both sides. (In Hungarian.) *Gyogyaszat. Budapest, 44*:226–227, 1904.

Reinhold, J. D. L., Neumark, E., Leightwood, R., and Carter, C. O.: Familial hypoplastic anemia with congenital abnormalities (Fanconi's syndrome). *Blood, 7*:915–926, 1952.

Reschke, K.: Zur operativen Behandlung der erworbenen Klumphand. *Dtsch. Z. Chir., 51*:458–562, 1931.

Rettig, H., and van Bommel, G.: Zur Behandlung schwerer Gliedmassenmissbildungen. *Orthop. Klin. Univ. Giessen, 36*:1731–1735, 1963.

Rincheval: Ein neues Operationsverfahren zur Behandlung congenitaler Defecte eines Unterarm- und Unterschenkelknochens. *Arch. Klin. Chir., 48*:802–810, 1894. Also *Verh. Dtsch. Ges Chir.,* 23 Kongress. Berlin, August Hirschwald, pp. 452–460, 1894. See review in *Ann. Surg., 21*:238–239, 1895.

Riordan, D. C.: Congenital absence of the radius. *J. Bone Joint Surg., 37A*:1129–1141, 1955.

Riordan, D. C.: Congenital absence of the radius. A fifteen year follow-up *J. Bone Joint Surg., 45A*:1783, 1963.

Rivarola, R. A.: Ausencia congenita de radio, mano bot y ectrodactilia. *Semana Med., 20*:757–762, 1913.

Robert, A.: *Des Vices Congenitaux de Conformation des Articulations.* Thèse. Paris, G. Baillière, pp. 100–104, 1851.

Robson, W. M., and Odgers, N. B.: Complete congenital absence of both radii in a boy, aged 6 years. *Proc. R. Soc. Med.* (Sect. Dis. Child.), *6*:203, 1913.

Rocher, H. L.: Main bote congénitale et main bote paralytique. *Rev. d'Orthop.,* (3 s.), *12*:633–695, 1925.

Rocher, H. L.: Double main bote radiale congénitale compliquée dans un cas de luxation du coude, dans l'autre de luxation de l'épaule. *J. Med. Bordeaux, 112*:880–882, 1935.

Roederer, C.: Absence congénitale de la lignée radiale. Main composée d'un seul doigt. *Bull. Soc. Pediatr. Paris, 24*:147, 1926.

Roederer, C., and Bouvaist, M.: Un cas d'absence congénitale du radius. *Rev. d'Orthop.,* (3 s.), *5*:129–134, 1914.

Roger, H., and Houel, M.: Note sur un example de double main-bot congénitale avec absence du radius, observée sur un enfant a terme. *Union Méd. Paris, 5*:562–563, 1851.

Romano, C.: Grave mano torta congenita. Reddrizzamento merce osteotomia segmentaria trapezoidale del cubito e tenotomia del muscolo grande palmare. *Arch. Ortop., 11*:80–93, 1894.

Rombeau, M.: Main-bot radiale. Absence du pouce. *Bull. Soc. Anat. Paris, 27*:414–421, 1852.

Roschke, E.: *Ein Fall von doppelseitigem Radius-Defect.* Inaug.-Diss. München, R. Muller & Steinicke, pp. 1–18, 1912.

Roullet, J., and Picault, C.: A propos d'un cas de greffe de l'extrémité supérieure de perone a l'avant-bras pour absence congénitale du radius. *Ann. Chir. Infantile, 6*:321–327, 1965.

Rouvillois, H.: Traitement de la main bote radiale invétérée. *Bull. Acad. Med. Paris,* (3 s.), *92*:1094–1097, 1924.

Rubin, S. L.: A case of congenital amegakaryocytic thrombocytopenia with leukemoid blood and picture of congenital deformities. *Arch. Pediatr., 76*:251–252, 1959.

Rybak, M., Kozlowski, K., Klechzkowska, A., Lewandowska, J., Skolowski, J., Soltysik-Wilk, E.: Holt-Oram syndrome associated with ectromelia and chromosomial aberrations *Am. J. Dis. Child., 121*:490–495, 1971.

Rybka, F. J., and Paletta, F. X.: Anomalies associated with congenital deformities of the thumb. *Plast. Reconstr. Surg., 46*:572–576, 1970.

Ryerson, E. W.: Cited by Kato, 1924, p. 593.

Ryoeppy, S., and Sulamaa, M.: Congenital defects of long bones of the extremities. *Duidecim* (Helsinki), *79*:56–68, 1963.

Savornin, A.: *Contribution à l'Étude de l'Absence Congenitale du Radius (Main bote).* Thèse. Lyon, P. Légendre, pp. 1–64, 1899.

Sayre, L. A.: *Lectures on Orthopedic Surgery and Diseases of the Joints*. Second edition. New York, D. Appleton & Co., pp. 161–163, 1892.

Sayre, R. H.: A contribution to the study of club-hand. *Trans. Am. Orthop. Assoc.*, 6:208–216, 1894.

Schaeffer, J., Parsons, J., and Nachamofsky, L. H.: Some observations on the anatomy of the upper extremities of an infant with complete bilateral absence of the radius. *Anat. Rec.*, 8:1–14, 1914.

Schekter, L.: Ectromélie radiale unilatérale heredo-syphilis probable. *Gaz. Hôp. Civ. Milit.*, 106:913–919, 1933.

Schiefel, H.: Korrekturschienen fur Klump- und Fallhand bei Dysmelie-Schaden. *Orthop. Technik*, 16:161–164, 1964.

Schmid, O.: Über eine bisher nicht beobachtete Form von partiellem Radiusdefekt. *Z. Orthop. Chir.*, 2:59–94, 1893.

Schnelle, A.: *Ueber angeborenen Defect von Radius und Ulna*. Inaug.-Diss. Gottingen, Univ. Buchdruckerei, pp. 1–16, 1875.

Schönenberg, H.: Missbildungen der Extremitäten. Basel (Schweiz.), New York, *Bibliotheca Paediatrica*, Fasc., 80, pp. 19–31, 1962.

Schönenberg, H.: Die Differentialdiagnose der radialen Defektbildungen. *Paediatr. Prax*, 7:455–467, 1968.

Schönenberg, H., and Scheidhauer, F.: Beidseitige radiale Hemimelie mit Megakaryocytopenie Ein neues Missbildungssyndrom. *Z. Kinderheilkd.*, 97:240–263, 1966.

Secord, E. R.: Bilateral congenital absence of the radius. *Ann. Surg.*, 61:381, 1915.

Shattock, S. G.: Congenital absence of the radius *Br. Med. J.*, 1:741, 1882.

Shattock, S. G.: On four specimens of congenital absence of the radius. *Trans. Pathol. Soc. London*, 33:240–246, 1882.

Shaw, S., and Oliver, R. A. M.: Congenital hypoplastic thrombocytopenia with skeletal deformities in siblings. *Blood*, 14:374–377, 1959.

Silver, H. K., Blair, W. C., and Kemp, C. H.: Fanconi syndrome. Multiple congenital anomalies with hypoplastic anemia. *Am. J. Dis. Child.*, 83:14–25, 1952.

Silvester, H. R.: A contribution to the science of teratology. (Trans.) *Medico-Chir.*, 41:73–111, 1858.

Simcha, A.: Congenital heart disease in radial clubbed hand syndrome. *Arch. Dis. Child.*, 46:345–349, 1970.

Simonini, A.: Sopra un caso di assenza congenita del radio. *Clin. Pediatr. Modena*, 1:175–181, 1919.

Skerik, S., and Flatt, A.: The anatomy of congenital radial dysplasia. *Clin. Orthop.*, 66:125–143, 1969.

Slingenberg, B.: Missbildungen von Extremitäten. *Arch. Pathol. Anat. Physiol.*, 193:1–92; Taf. V, VI, 1908.

Smith, R. J.: The radial club hand. *Bull. Hosp. Joint Dis.*, 25:85–93, 1964.

Sparkes, R. S., Carrel, R. E., and Wright, S. W.: Absent thumb with a ring D_2 chromosome. *Am. J. Hum. Genet.*, 19:644, 1967.

Spears, L. P.: Bilateral congenital absence of the radius. *Kentucky Med. J.*, 21:407–408, 1923.

Speed, J. S., and Knight, R. A.: Absence of the radius and ulna. Congenital clubhand deformity. *In Campbell's Operative Orthopedics*. St. Louis, C. V. Mosby Co., Vol. 2, pp. 2042–2047, 1956.

Spitzky: Zeigt einen Knaben, der mit angeborener Klumphand. *Munch. Med. Wochenschr.*, 60:2596, 1913.

Spitzy: Klumphand. *Verh. Dtsch. Orthop. Ges.*, 25:83–88, 1931.

Stamm, C.: Erworbener partieller Radiusdefekt bei einem hereditar luetischen Säuglinge. *Fortsch. Röntgenstr.*, 12:237–238; Taf. XV; fig. 6–7, 1908.

Starke, H., Schimke, R. N., and Dunn, M.: Upper limb cardiovascular syndrome. A family study. *Am. J. Cardiol.*, 19:588–592, 1965.

Starr, D. E.: Congenital absence of the radius: a method of surgical correction. *J. Bone Joint Surg.*, 27:572–577, 1945.

Stecher, R. T.: Identical twins discordant for intraventricular septal defect and absent radius and thumb. *Am J. Hum. Genet.*, 8:218–223, 1956.

Steindler, A.: Congenital malformations and deformities of the hand. *Am. J. Orthop. Surg.*, 2:639–668, 1920.

Steinsleger, M.: Mano bot congenita, *Rev. Med. Rosario*, 11:247–252, 1921.

Stiles, K. A., and Dougan, P.: A pedigree of malformed upper extremities showing variable dominance *J. Hered.*, 31:65–72, 1940.

Stöer, W. F. H.: Die Extremitätenmissbildungen und ihre Beziehungen zum Bauplan der Extremität. *Z. Anat. Entwicklung*, 108:136–160, 1938.

Stöer, W. F. H.: Über der Zusammentroffen von Hasencharte mit ernsten Extremitätenmissbildungen. *Der Erbarzt*, 7:101–104, 1939.

Stoffel, A., and Stempel, E.: Anatomische studien über Klumphand. *Z. Orthop. Chir.*, 23:1–157, 1909.

Stouffs: Mains-botes resultant de l'absence congénitale du radius (radiographie). *Bull. Soc. Belge Gynecol. Obstet.*, 10:124, 1899–1902.

Stracker, O. A.: Die Marknagelung in der Orthopädie. *Z. Orthop.*, 79:74–92; figs. 9–10, 1950.

Streeter, G. L.: Focal deficiencies in fetal tissues and their relation to intra-uterine amputation. Carnegie Inst. of Washington, Publication No. 414, 22:1–44, 1930.

Stricker: Doppelseitiger angeborener Defect des Radius und des Daumens. *Arch. Pathol. Physiol.*, 31:529–530, 1864.

Stubenrauch, V.: Ein Fall von congenitalem Defect des rachten Radius. *Sitzungsb. Arztl. Ver München (1897)*, 7:27, 1898.

Swaagmann, P. H.: Doppelseitiger angeborener Defect des Radius und des Daumens. *Arch. Pathol. Anat. Physiol.*, 33:228–231, 1865.

Takada, S.: Ein Fall von angeborenen beiderseitigen Fehlen des Radius (Japanese text.) *Z. Med. Ges. Tokyo*, 12:973–977, 1898.

Taylor, A. E.: A case of congenital absence of both radii. *Internat. Med. Mag. Phila.*, 5:89, 1896–1897.

Taylor, H. L.: Congenital absence of the radius. *Trans. Am. Orthop. Assoc.*, 10:170–175, 1897.

Temtamy, S. A.: *Genetic Factors in Hand Malformations.* Ph.D. Thesis. Baltimore, Johns Hopkins University, pp. 33–44; 110–152, 1966.

Thomson, C. E.: A case of club-hand treated by operation. *Trans. Am. Orthop. Assoc.*, 9:165–170, 1896.

Thomson, J.: Case of almost entire congenital absence of the radius on both sides. *Trans. Edinburgh Obstet. Soc.*, 15:56, 1889–1890.

Thomson, M. S. A.: Poikiloderma congénitale. *Br. J. Dermatol.*, 48:221–234, 1936.

Tognetti, G. P., Giaretta, V., and Cugola, L.: Interventi per il recupero funzionale in un caso di emimelia con mano valga. *Chir. Trivienta*, 9:699–710, 1969.

Töntz, O., Keller, H., and Cottier, H.: Beitrag zum Syndrom der kongenitalen Megakaryocytopenie mit Radiusaplasie. *Helvet. Paediatr. Acta*, 15(Supplement 9):1–26, 1960.

Torday, F.: Angeborener, beiderseitiger Ulna- und Radiusdefekt. *Pest. Med. Chir. Presse Budapest*, 45:482, 1909.

Tschmarke: Zwei seltene Tormen angeborener Missbildung. *Z. Orthop. Chir.*, 8:368–378; fig. 3, 1900.

Tubby, A. H.: Double congenital club-hand of the radio-palmar variety, with absence of the radius on both sides. *Proc. R. Soc. Med.* (Sect. Dis. Child.), 4:164, 1911.

Tunte, W.: A new polydactyly/imperforate-anus/vertebral-anomalies syndrome. *Lancet*, 2:1081–1082, 1968.

Tyrie, C. C. B.: Three cases of congenital absence of the whole or part of a bone. *J. Anat. Physiol.*, 28:411–413, 1894.

Van Haelst, A.: Main-bote par absence congénitale du radius. *Bull. Soc. Méd. Grand.*, 74:177–180, 1907.

Veit, G.: Über familiäres Vorkommen von Oligodaktylie. *Z. menschl. Vererb. Konstitutionslehre,* 23:620–635, 1939.

Virchow, R.: Ein neurer Fall ovon Halskiemenfistel. *Arch. Pathol. Anat. Physiol.*, 32:518–524, 1865.

Vogt, P.: *Die Chirurgischen Krankheiten der Oberen Extremitäten.* Stuttgart, F. Enke, pp. 1–292, 1881.

Voigt, L.: Beitrag zur Kasuistik des congenitalen Radiusdefectes. *Arch. Heilknd.*, 4:27–42, 1863.

Voller, A.: *Zum Problem der angeborenen Radiusdefektes mit Klumphand deformitat.* Inaug.-Diss. Augsburg, Univ. Munchen. pp. 5–35, 1957.

Voorhess, M. L., Aspilaga, M. H., and Gardner, L. T.: Trisomy 18 syndrome with absent radius, varus deformity of the hand and rudimentary thumb. *J. Pediatr.*, 65:130–133, 1964.

Wakeley, C. B. G.: A case of congenital absence of the radius in a woman aged 38. *J. Anat.*, 65:506–508, 1930–1931.

Warfield: Congenital absence of radius. *Bull. Johns Hopkins Hosp.*, 3:42, 1892.

Watermann, H.: Zur Frage der operativen Behandlung bei angeborehem Radiusdefekt. *Zentralbl. Chir.*, 57:1464–1467, 1930.

Wilbert, H. G., and Henkel, H. L.: *Klinik und Pathologie der Dysmelie.* Die Fehlbildungen an den oberen Extremitäten bei der Thalidomid-Embryopathie. Berlin, Springer Verlag, pp. 1–143. 1969.

Williams, P.: Congenital absence of the radius. *J. Bone Joint Surg.*, 49B:392, 1967.

Windle, B. C. A.: Note on a specimen of congenital suppression of the thumbs and dislocation of the wrists. *Anat. Anz.*, 3:63–65, 1888.

Woodward, W.: Case of congenital deformity of the hands. *Buffalo Med. Surg. J.*, 8:170–171, 1869.

Zellweger, H., Huff, D. S., and Abbo, G.: Phocomelia and trisomy E. *Acta Genet. Med.*, 14:164–173, 1965.

Zengerly, C.: *Beitrag zur Lehre der Klumphand.* Inaug.-Diss. Dresden, Albanus'sche Buchdruckerei, pp. 1–40, 1894.

Zetterquist, P.: The syndrome of familial atrial septal defect, heart arrythmia and hand malformation (Holt-Oram) in mother and son. *Acta Paediatr.*, 52:115–122, 1963.

Zinner, M.: Operative treatment of manus vara and manus valga. *J. Bone Joint Surg.*, 36B:690, 1954.

Chapter Twenty-Four

RESTORATION OF PREHENSILE FUNCTION

It is often stated that in the absence of the thumb, the hand loses 50 per cent of its utility. This assessment is arbitrary; it merely emphasizes the importance of the thumb in the prehensile function of the hand. Palmar surface to palmar surface opposition of two digits is a prerequisite for effective prehension. Because of its rotated position, its relative shortness, its power, and its ability to move in many directions, the thumb plays a major role in prehension. When too long and unrotated, as in the nonopposable variety of triphalangism, and when oversized and overstuffed, as in macrodactyly, the thumb fails to swing into apposition and press its tip against the palmar surface of one of the fingers. Pulp-to-pulp opposition is also hampered when the movements of the thumb are curtailed because of a missing muscle, blocked tendon, and fixed contractures. Prehension is drastically disturbed when the pollical ray is defective in its skeletal components.

Congenital deficiencies of the thumb occurring in connection with radial ray defect, acral absences, and split hand simulate deficiencies caused by injury during postnatal life. Many of the surgical methods originally designed for acquired deformities of the thumb are equally applicable to congenital defects of this most important digit. One must also consider the fact that a thumb without another part to press against is practically useless. For a hand with congenital absence of four ulnar digits, reconstruction of an oppositional strut or platform for the solitary pollex also comes under the category of restoration of prehension.

The primary aim of surgical interference in the deficiencies described is to convert the disabled hand into a prehensile organ. Ideally, the reconstructed thumb should be of such length and stance as would enable it to play its part efficiently in the prehensile action of the hand. It must have strength, mobility, and sensation; if possible, it must also simulate the appearance of the member it is intended to represent. As in mutilations caused by trauma, ideal conditions are seldom attained by surgical attempts, but what little is accomplished is often gratifying.

The degree of initial deficiency determines the range of improvement to be hoped for. The type of surgical procedure to be undertaken depends upon the nature of the defect. In historical sequence, four major operative methods have been developed: (1) deepening of the first interdigital cleft, (2) transfer of digits from the same hand, (3) composite bone and skin graft, (4) transfer of digits from the opposite hand, and (5) toe-to-hand transplants.

DEEPENING OF THE INTERDIGITAL COMMISSURE (Phalangization of Metacarpal; Clefting)

Huguier (1873, 1874), who pioneered reconstructive surgery of the thumb, advised surgeons to marshal their ingenuity and supplant the missing thumb or augment the length of what little basal segment may have survived. In cases of absent phalanges, Huguier thought that the metacarpal of the thumb could be given a relative gain in length and a measure of oppositional function when "individualized." Huguier accomplished this by creating a cleft between the first and second metacarpal bones. He deepened the first webspace by stripping the distal fibers of the first dorsal interosseous muscle from the metacarpal of the thumb; he also sectioned the transverse adductor about 1 cm. from its origin on the third metacarpal. Huguier's description of this operation was incorporated in a monograph extending over 70 pages; it was devoted solely to the thumb and was published piecemeal in a now extinct periodical. For this reason perhaps it has remained obscure and unread.

Lyle (1914–1923) was the first American surgeon to perform Huguier's operation. He described the technique in some detail and discussed the historical development of the operation. There are some indications that Bunnell (1931) obtained his information about Huguier and some other European surgeons from Lyle. In both Bunnell's and Lyle's articles, the same reference is made to Morestin's condemnation of the toe-to-thumb transplant, the difference being that Bunnell misspelled Morestin's name, converting it to Moreston. Both Lyle and Bunnell committed the same error about the date of Lauenstein's (1888) description of the rotary osteotomy of marginal metacarpal bones. Lauenstein described this operation in 1888 and not in 1880 as stated by Lyle and Bunnell.

Bunnell's (1931) article containing the following paragraph: "the index and long fingers together with a part or the whole of the metacarpal have been transplanted to the stump of the metacarpal of the thumb or to the trapezium, but without conservation of all nerves, tendons and muscles (Perthes; Verrall, two cases in 1919, no joining of tendons and nerves; Dunlop; in 1923, used pedicle skin from abdomen to the cleft; Huguier.)"

This paragraph reappeared verbatim in the second and with slight variation in the successive editions of Bunnell's book. It has been reproduced by other authors and given various interpretations. One implication is that, together with other surgeons mentioned, Huguier conducted his operation "without conservation of all nerves. . . ." Huguier could not have been more explicit about avoiding injury to the digital nerves. He insisted that in deepening the first intermetacarpal space, utmost care should be exercised to avoid injuring the collateral vessels and nerves. Huguier emphasized the importance of what is now called stereognosis.

In placing Huguier's name after Dunlop's, Bunnell also conveyed the impression that Huguier utilized pedicled skin graft to surface the surgically deepened cleft. This idea is expressed in a number of recent publications. "In 1923 Dunlop used an abdominal pedicle flap for the cleft, as did Huguier," Flynn and Burden (1962) wrote. In the fourth and fifth editions of Bunnell's book, revised by Boyes (1964, 1970) the following echo resounded: "In 1923 Dunlop used a pedicle from the abdomen for the digits as did Huguier." In Huguier's monograph, no mention is made of pedicled skin graft.

There is also some confusion as to when Huguier performed his operation. Tierny and Iselin (1937) gave 1868 as the date of Huguier's operation. Peacock (1966) wrote: "The operation of phalangization of the first metacarpal has been accepted universally as a satisfactory method of restoring prehensile function since it was first described by Huguier in 1825." Huguier performed his first operation in 1852; his second, in 1854. His description of it appeared posthumously in 1874.

Huguier's operation has had numerous modifications. In these variations, one or more of the following procedures are utilized: reattachment of surgically severed intrinsic muscles; extension of extrinsic muscle power to the new pollex; surfacing of the deepened cleft with Z-plasty or free skin or pedicled graft; excision of nonfunctioning second metacarpal; and—when the thumb and its metacarpal are absent and the phalanges of the index finger are missing—displacement of the second metacarpal in the radial direction and connection with the trapezium. Phalangized metacarpal has also been accorded absolute gain in length by Z-osteotomy or by composite skin and bone graft.

Huguier's operation owes its success to the mobility of the first metacarpal bone. Next in mobility comes the fifth and then the fourth metacarpals. The second and third metacarpals are immovable. Each ulnar metacarpal bone gains an increment of motion when it is freed from the common bondage of the deep transverse ligament and when the interosseous fibers binding its proximal extremity are severed. Resection of the basal, nonepiphyseal ends of the three central metacarpals enhances the movement of these bones. Sometimes one of these immovable metacarpals and the corresponding functionless finger need to be sacrificed.

TRANSFER OF DIGITS FROM THE SAME HAND

Guermonprez (1884, 1887) alone and Guermonprez with Derode (1889) ran through the entire gamut of digital transfer from one part of the hand to another. He particularized the transposition of the index finger—with its nerves, blood vessels, and tendons—to the location of the missing thumb: Guermonprez rightly deserves the accolade of being considered the originator of pollicization of the ulnar digits, in particular the index finger.

The forefinger, Guermonprez wrote, should be separated from its immediate ulnar neighbor and set at an angle to the latter; it should also be rotated until its palmar surface assumes a position opposite the main axis of the hand as represented by the middle finger. Guermonprez was emphatic about safeguarding the nerves, vessels, and tendons of the transposed digit. In an extensive monograph entitled "Functional Restoration of the Thumb," Hanotte (1888) described in detail Guermonprez's method of transferring the forefinger. Hanotte illustrated the main steps of this procedure with excellent drawings. According to these illustrations and the accompanying text, Guermonprez resected sizable segments from the bones entering into the metacarpophalangeal joint of the index finger; he shortened the pollicized digit but did not think it necessary to take in the slack of the tendons.

Guermonprez ranks with Huguier in having been least read and most often misconstrued. "Guermonprez de Lille did pollicization of the index finger without preserving the nerves or tendons," Bowe (1954) wrote. Guermonprez practiced in the city of Lille, France, and did not have the titular annexation "de Lille' attached to his name.

Bunnell (1958) bypassed Guermonprez and many others when he claimed to have first performed pollicization on April 10, 1929, and recorded it in 1931. In the fourth edition of Bunnell's book, revised by Boyes (1964), one is again reminded that Bunnell's "was the first reconstructed thumb which furnished both movement and normal sensation, including stereognosis."

Bunnell's (1931) patient had lost his thumb and its metacarpal; the index finger had been amputated through the proximal phalanx. Bunnell disarticulated the proximal end of the second metacarpal from the trapezoid and placed it in line with the trapezium to form "a new joint." He then excised 3 inches of the extensor carpi radialis tendon and passed it through drill holes in the trapezium and the translocated metacarpal "so as to encircle the joint and stabilize it against dislocating." It has since been discovered that fusion of the transferred metacarpal with the trapezium procures a more stable oppositional digit.

After studying the illustrations incorporated in Bunnell's article, one is left with the impression that only a small fragment of the proximal phalanx of the index finger had survived and this piece was bent and buried under the skin of the palm. The skin over this area is enervated by the palmar branch of the median nerve and not by the volar digital nerve as Bunnell indicated. His operation comes closer to phalangization of the second metacarpal than to pollicization of the index finger.

In his first communication on pollicization of the index finger, the author (1946) of this book stressed the importance of preserving the vessels and the nerves of the transported digit. This precaution was not new then. It is not new now. What appears new today is the sophisticated verbiage with which the descriptions of pollicization are garnished. Embellishment with resounding epithets does not alter an established surgical procedure or principle. Even to suggest that earlier surgeons did not consciously conserve the nerves, the vessels, and the tendons of the transferred digit is to deny them elemental intelligence.

In addition to Huguier (1873) and Guermonprez (1884), this condemned coterie includes such perceptive surgeons as Noesske, Tonnini, Perthes, and Moutier. Noesske (1920) was very careful in isolating the neurovascular bundle of the transplanted digit. Tonnini (1920) was explicit about replacing the thumb with an intact, unharmed index finger. He meticulously dissected the digital nerves and vessels in order to ensure, as he put it, the circulation and the sensibility of the transferred finger—"besogne badare di rispattare i collaterali vesali e nervosi che assicurano al ditto transporto la circulazione e la sensibilita." The patient presented by Perthes (1921) could move the transferred digit at both carpometacarpal and metacarpophalangeal joints and the sensation of the new thumb was normal throughout—"Das Gefühl ist an dem künstlichen Daumen überall normal." Moutier (1922) was adamant about respecting the integrity of the vessels and nerves of the transposed digit—"les vaisseaux et nerfs auront été soigneusement respectés au cours de ces manoeuvres," he wrote. No recent author has described the technique of isolating and preserving the neurovascular bundle of the pollicized index in as great detail as did Tonnini.

In congenital absence of the thumb, the index finger is fully equipped with nerves, blood vessels and, in most cases, with its full quota of tendons. Compared to the thumb, the index finger has one advantage and one disadvantage. Because of its extra joint and intrinsic muscles—the interossei and especially the lumbricals—the transposed index finger can effect more skillful movements. Yet, it is not as powerful as the thumb; what is gained in agility is lost in power. However, that power is irrevocably lost when the thumb is missing. It is often argued that in pollicization the hand loses a normal finger. There is very little the index finger can do that its immediate ulnar neighbor—which is stronger—cannot do. No transferred lesser digit can fully reproduce the strength and mobility of the thumb. When shortened and placed in opposition, the index finger becomes as nearly physiological a substitute for the missing thumb as can be expected.

Besides the index finger, the middle, ring, and little fingers have also been transferred as substitutes for absent thumbs. Machol (1919), Jepson (1925), Hilgenfeldt (1950), Boron and Fabre (1952), Gebauer and Ihl (1955), and May (1958) pollicized the middle finger. Schmiedt (1918), Müller (1920), Oudard (1922), Bocca et al (1959), Candiollo and Rinaldi (1960), and Butler (1964) utilized the ring finger. Letac (1952) and Kelleher (1958, 1964) used the little finger. There may be an exceptional circumstance for pollicizing one of these digits. In some cases of radial ray defect, not only the thumb but also the index finger is missing, necessitating pollicization of the middle finger. Some children with split hand have only a ring and a little finger which are usually webbed together; in such a case, the ring finger is separated from its ulnar neighbor and pollicized.

The further a finger is from the radial border of the hand, the more difficult and hazardous is its pollicization and the less propitious is the outcome. The ungual phalanges of the fingers flex less and less independently as one passes from the second to the fifth digit. The index finger is comparatively independent in its action; it is, moreover, closer to where the missing thumb should have been. Its pollicization is beset with less difficulty or hazard and yields more propitious results.

In congenital acral absences or transverse terminal defects and in longitudinal deficiencies of the pollical ray seen in connection with split hand, the radial carpal bones are unaffected, and in many instances a sizable portion of the first metacarpal bone remains. The transferred digit may be anchored to either one of these bones. In longitudinal absences of the thumb belonging to the category of radial ray defect, the first metacarpal, the trapezium, and the scaphoid are often absent. In a case of congenital absence of the pollical ray, Zancolli (1960) claimed to have successfully fixed the index metacarpal to the carpal bones. He did not specify which carpal bone or bones. From the drawing included in his article, one would suspect that he utilized either the trapezium or the trapezoid for anchorage. Even if present, these bones are mostly cartilaginous in children. The bony nucleus of the trapezium may not appear until the age of five, and that of the trapezoid is usually delayed another year.

Edgerton et al (1965) also asserted that in pollicizing the index finger for congenital absence of the pollical ray they had connected the second metacarpal with the carpal bones. In their drawing, the distal segment of the second metacarpal was shown slotted into the scaphoid bone. The ossific core of the scaphoid also appears late—often not before the age of six, even in normal children; it is frequently absent in terminal longitudinal defects of the radial ray.

In a child with congenital absence of the thumb belonging to the category of radial ray defect, one does not actually transfer the index finger but changes its position by osteotomy of its metacarpal. There is considerable discrepancy between the length of the normal thumb and that of the index finger. The thumb stems from a short metacarpal. It possesses two phalanges and one interphalangeal joint. The metacarpal of the index finger is longer, and this digit possesses three phalanges and two interphlalangeal joints. The index finger has an extra phalanx and one additional interphalangeal joint, as compared to the thumb.

It is now generally agreed that the pollicized index finger should be shortened. A sizable segment of bone is resected from the midshaft of the index metacarpal and the capital fragment is recessed toward the basal piece. Recession of the digit results in a soft-tissue bulge at the volar base of the pollicized index. This bulge is desirable, since it simulates the thenar eminence, which is absent in most skeletal deficiencies of the thumb belonging to the category of radial ray defect.

When the transferred digit is shortened, its tendons become lax. It is not necessary to take in the slack of these tendons; they soon readjust themselves. To provide the pollicized index finger with motor power of the opponents, Riordan (1955) transferred the sublimis tendon of the ring finger. For the same purpose, Zancolli (1960) transferred the origin of the first interosseous muscle to the proximal phalanx of the pollicized index finger. In his article entitled "Congenital absence of functioning thumb," Matthews (1960) wrote: "The first dorsal interosseous muscle, which is always well developed, is divided at its attachment around the metacarpophalangeal joint and allowed to fall back around the metacarpal stump to simulate the thenar eminence, together with the small thenar muscle mass which is often present." Littler (1964) advised shifting the insertion of the first dorsal interosseous muscle to the extensor communis tendon of the transferred index finger so that it might simulate the control of "an adductor pollicis brevis."

In congenital absence of a functioning thumb, the first interosseous is rarely well developed. The main belly of this muscle originates from the metacarpal of the thumb. In congenital deficiencies of the pollical ray, the first metacarpal, and with it the first dorsal interosseous muscle, is missing or vestigial. Adduction and opponens actions of the pollicized index finger are executed effectively by the coordinated efforts of the following muscles: second dorsal interosseous, first volar interosseous, first lumbrical, and extrinsic flexors. Abduction is controlled by the long extensor muscles.

In an earlier communication, the author (1957) of this book wrote: "Through a small incision over the dorsum of the wrist, the dorsal carpal ligament is slit and the extensor tendon is extricated from the wound and shifted to the lateral side of the radius, where it is held by a sling fashioned from part of the tendinous insertion of the brachioradialis." The author now agrees with Littler (1964), who states that in congenital absence of the thumb, rerouting of the extensor mechanism is not required. When the transferred digit is adequately rotated, the extensor communis and indicis proprius act as abductors and extensors.

Osteotomy of the metacarpal should permit axial rotation, abduction, and a measure of palmar angulation of the distal fragment, as well as shortening of the bone as a whole. The establishment of a bony bridge between bases of the index metacarpal and the metacarpal of its immediate ulnar neighbor, as has been advocated by Bowe (1954), virtually amounts to extra-articular fusion of the carpometacarpal articulation: elimination of this joint nullifies the rotary action of the transferred digit. Suturing the bones with flexible wire, or even stabilizing them with a removable intramedullary wire, is permissible. But firm, unyielding internal fixation of the osteotomized fragments should be avoided. Occasionally, at the termination of the reconstructive work—when the tourniquet is released—the rotated, abducted, and angulated digit will remain bloodless. It then becomes expedient to return the transferred digit to a moderate position and, in the course of the next few days, gradually attain the desired correction.

An ever-recurrent controversy concerns the question of whether the pollicization of the index finger should be performed in a single or two-stage procedure—more correctly, whether the web between the transferred index finger and the middle finger should be reconstructed with a local or distant skin flap. Historically, the one-stage operation antedates the two-stage method in which a distant flap is utilized to reconstruct a web between the transferred digit and its immediate ulnar neighbor. In the single-stage procedure, the operating time is prolonged, but the recovery period is curtailed by six weeks.

Contrary to the statement frequently recorded in the literature, children graciously tolerate the inconvenience of having the hand sutured to the abdominal flap. The short span of six weeks necessary to transfer a distant flap is not as important for a child as it is for a wage-earning adult. It is also argued that when pollicization is performed with flaps lifted from the hand itself, scarring of the abdomen is avoided. However, when local flaps are used, the hand—which is seen more often than the abdomen—is scarred more extensively; as the child grows, some of these scars contract and cause secondary deformities.

Pollicization of the index finger with the aid of local flaps has several other disadvantages. The reconstructed web between the transferred index finger and the middle finger is seldom as broad and yielding as that procured by a generous piece of pliable skin from a distant source. When the web is reconstructed with a local flap, the new thumb has limited range of abduction and it often appears spindly, as if sprouting from a split palm. Perhaps more significant is the fact that local flaps necessitate the use of incisions on the dorsum and radial border of the index metacarpal—the area which gives passage to the main venous channel draining the transferred digit.

Volar digital arteries are not accompanied by venae comitantes; the volar digital neurovascular bundles do not contain any longitudinally disposed veins. Both superficial and deep sets of volar digital veins exist as crisscrossing channels. Sizable vessels emanating from this network take the shortest course to the dorsum and empty into the veins in the back of the digit. As in other digits, the dorsal veins of the index finger are plexiform over the last two phalanges.

Proximal to the first interphalangeal joint, the dorsal venous plexus splits into two distinct vessels which diverge to encircle the knuckle of the metacarpophalangeal joint. These two veins converge over the neck of the index metacarpal to form a single vessel which slants toward the radial border of the thumbless hand and eventually empties into the cephalic vein. In children, the veins in the back of the hand are not as large and profusely intercommunicating as in adults; the longitudinal veins running along the dorsal aspect of the index metacarpal are smaller in caliber and have fewer anastomotic outlets than the axially disposed veins overlying the more ulnar metacarpal bones. When the index finger is transferred onto its volar neurovascular pedicle, it has to depend upon a single, or at the most two, dorsal metacarpal veins for adequate drainage. Incisions used for lifting local flaps invariably cross these veins, which may be injured and consequently become thrombosed. This hazard is obviated when no flaps are developed from skin on the dorsal and radial aspects of the index metacarpal.

Notwithstanding these arguments, one must consider the circumstances of the case and decide whether pollicization should be conducted with the aid of local or distant flaps. The training and experience of the surgeon also counts. If a surgeon has utilized one method repeatedly and obtained satisfactory long-range results, there is no reason why he should change it and adopt one that enjoys a current vogue. One could cite numerous examples of operative procedures which became fashionable at one time, were relegated to limbo or replaced, and later were revived again. Currently, the single-stage pollicization of the index finger—first performed by Guermonprez (1884) almost a century ago—is in vogue. The author of these lines is not convinced that it yields better results than the two-stage procedure. Heroic surgery is not necessarily better surgery; it is often more hazardous (Fig. 24–1).

Pollicization of the index finger with the aid of a distant flap is accomplished in two separate sessions. The first session is devoted to deepening the commissure between the index and middle fingers and to covering the deepened cleft with a distant flap. The hand is elevated. A tourniquet is applied. The hand is returned to the operating table and placed flat on its back. Number 000 silk threads are passed through the tips of the index and middle fingers for the purpose of holding these digits extended and apart during surgery.

The incision starts in the midpalm, at a point in line with the interdigital commissure between the index and middle fingers; it runs distally, bisecting the web between these two digits. It is deepened, and the interlacing fibers of the palmar aponeurosis are cut. The common arterial trunk—which bifurcates into digital branches for the adjacent sides of the index and middle fingers—is identified. The digital artery going to the radial side of the middle finger is isolated, doubly ligated, and cut between the two ligatures. The digital nerves split from their common trunk more proximally and they are left unmolested. The common digital nerve need not be slit longitudinally to the base of the palm, as was recommended by Bunnell (1931) and many others after him. The deep transverse metacarpal ligament which binds the adjacent metacarpal heads together is severed.

The hand is pronated. From the apex of the interdigital commissure, the incision is continued dorsally into the groove between the metacarpals of the index and the middle fingers. The incision is directed longitudinally toward the wrist until it reaches a joint just distal to the carpometacarpal junction. The two binding structures are severed through the dorsal incision. These structures include: the junctura tendinum, which connects the common extensor of the index to that of the middle finger, and the interosseous fibers, which bind the bases of the two radial metacarpal bones of the thumbless hand. The bases of these bones are pried apart and the interval between them is packed with a small plug of oxycel gauze or a piece of silicone rubber sheet in order to keep the interosseous fibers from reuniting.

The cleft between the metacarpals of the index and middle fingers is now deepened toward the carpus—along the space between the volar interosseous of

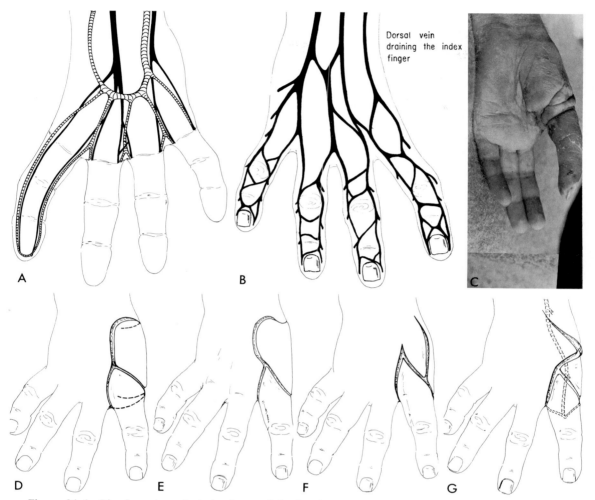

Figure 24–1 Blood supply to the index finger of the thumbless hand. *A*, Diagram showing the arterial supply of the right index finger as seen from the palmar aspect: this digit, like all others, has an artery on each side which pursues a straight course and is not accompanied by venae comitantes. *B*, Diagram showing the venous supply as seen on the dorsal aspect. The index finger is drained by a smaller straight vein in the back of the hand; this vein is often injured in raising flaps of skin from the area in the back of the index metacarpal. *C*, Palmar view of the left hand, showing a congested, dark index finger which had been pollicized by the single-stage method. *D, E, F,* and *G:* All the incisions commonly utilized for single-stage pollicization of the index threaten the dorsal metacarpal vein draining this digit.

the index finger and the dorsal interosseous on the radial side of the middle finger. The volar interosseous of the index finger arises from a single head on the second metacarpal. The dorsal interosseous on the radial side of the middle finger is bicipital: it arises from two heads on the adjacent surfaces of the metacarpals of the index and middle fingers. Unless its attachment to the index metacarpal is released, the second dorsal interosseous muscle will not permit this bone to be abducted radially. With the stripping of this muscle, the index finger is now abducted as far as possible. The constrictor is released. Hemostasis is secured.

A partially tubed flap is raised from the contralateral upper quadrant of the abdominal wall. The skin edges of the proximal portion of the dorsal incision on the hand are approximated and sutured together. The remainder of the surgically deepended cleft is surfaced with the detached end of the pedicled flap. The latter is secured to the hand with interrupted stitches, using No. 34 stainless steel wire for suture material. When tied together, the wire sutures often become buried in the skin and their removal at a later date causes considerable difficulty. The threads of each wire suture should be twisted together; three weeks later, they are untwisted, cut on one side, and removed. At the time when the wound is closed, the threads of the wire suture are twisted for a distance of 1 inch and tied over a comparatively stiff rubber catheter. This maneuver serves a dual purpose: it keeps the index and middle fingers apart and prevents the ends of the wire suture from turning toward the skin and sticking into it. Postoperatively, the arm is bound to the torso with a Velpeau bandage, which is discarded after a week.

During the second session—usually after six weeks—the skin graft is weaned from the abdomen. In cases of bilateral absence of the thumb, the detached end of the pedicled skin is utilized for pollicization of the opposite index finger. Ordinarily, the newly detached end of the graft is used to even up the irregularities around the base of the shortened index finger and to pad the thenar area.

The hand is again elevated and a tourniquet is applied. The hand is then placed palm up on the operating table while the proximal portion of the previous palmar incision is retrenched and extended up to the base of the index metacarpal. The shaft of this bone is isolated and a segment—the size of which depends upon the age of the individual and the degree of shortening desired—is resected from the midshaft. A window is created on the radiopalmar aspect of the basal fragment of the index metacarpal, and the spiked proximal end of the distal fragment is inserted into it. The two fragments are secured with a flexible wire suture. The resected metacarpal segment is split and used as an onlay graft. The surgical wound is closed. A wire is passed transversely through the proximal phalanx of the transferred index finger, and another wire is passed across the basal phalanx of the middle finger. The index finger is abducted, tilted in the volar direction, and rotated until its pulp assumes a position opposite the palmar surface of the middle finger. The protruding ends of the wires are connected with the bars of the external fixation apparatus.

The tourniquet is released. The circulation of the transferred digit is checked. Fluffed gauze dressings are packed between the fingers and all around the hand and forearm, to be followed by a mildly compressive elastic bandage. The external fixation apparatus is removed when the metacarpal fragment of the transferred digit has effected a firm union, which usually occurs in about six weeks. A great deal has been written about the need for postoperative physiotherapy and reeducation of muscles. Children very quickly learn to use their properly transferred and positioned index fingers as thumbs, and they learn faster if the opposite hand is immobilized—encased in an occlusive bandage or a firm, fingerless glove.

Pollicization of the index finger in congenital absence of the thumb was frowned upon at one time, but this attitude has changed recently. It is now generally agreed that a child born without a thumb should have his index finger pollicized. The treatment of intercalary defects of the pollical ray or floating thumb remains controversial. As often happens, the description of an irrational operation may creep into the literature; this becomes copied, modified, and refined ad absurdum; it takes years to discard such a procedure, especially when its originator is an affluent surgeon.

(Text continued on page 850.)

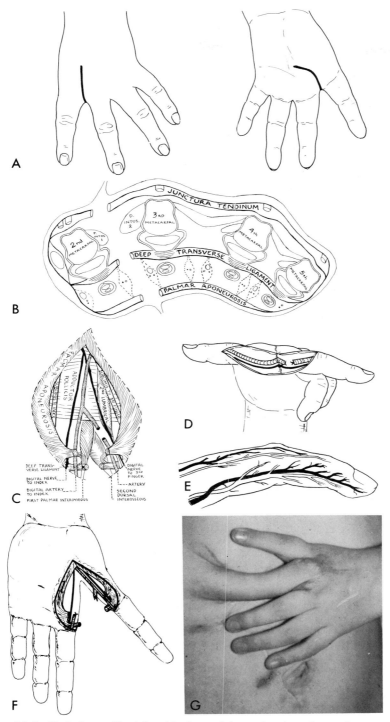

Figure 24–2 Technique utilized for widening and deepening the webspace between the index and middle fingers and surfacing the raw area with the aid of a distant flap. *A*, Dorsal and palmar incision on a four-fingered left hand. *B*, Three tethering bands are cut: the junctura tendinum which connects the extensors of the index and middle fingers, the deep transverse metacarpal ligament, and the transverse fibers of palmar aponeurosis. *C, D, E,* and *F* show that the digital artery on the radial aspect of the middle finger has been doubly ligated and severed between the ligatures. *G*, Surfacing the widened and deepened commissure with a distant flap.

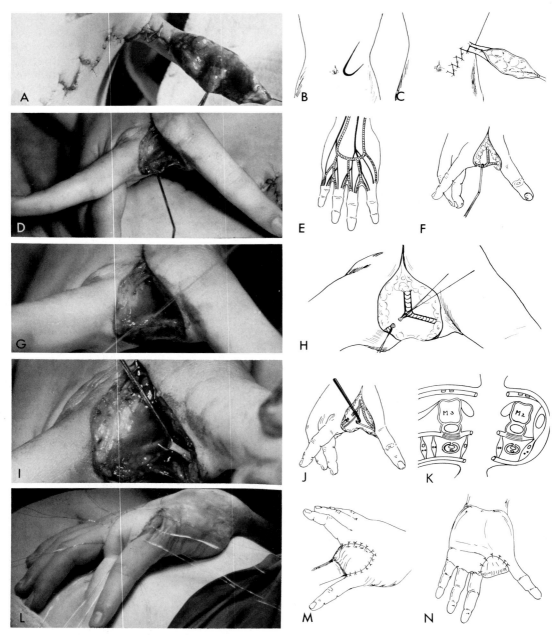

Figure 24–3 Technique utilized for widening and deepening the webspace between the index and middle fingers and covering the raw surface with the aid of a distant flap. *A*, Stem-petal flap raised from the right upper quadrant of the abdomen. *B* and *C*, Sketches illustrating elevation of the stem-petal. *D*, Isolation of the digital artery going along the radial aspect of the left middle finger. *E*, Sketch showing digital arteries as they split away from palmar vessels. *F* illustrates isolation of the digital artery of the middle finger which, as shown in *G*, is doubly ligated and, as shown in *H*, severed between the two ligatures. *I*, Isolation of the digital nerve on the ulnar aspect of the index finger. *J*, Sketch illustrating the same. *K*, Sketch illustrating fascial bands to be severed in deepening the commissure between the index and middle fingers, namely the junctura tendinum on the dorsal aspect, the deep transverse metacarpal ligament, and the transverse fibers of palmaris fascia on the palmar aspect. *L*, Covering the cleft between the index and middle fingers with the distant flap. *M*, Illustrates the same. *N*, Illustrates suturing the weaned portion of the flap to the palm.

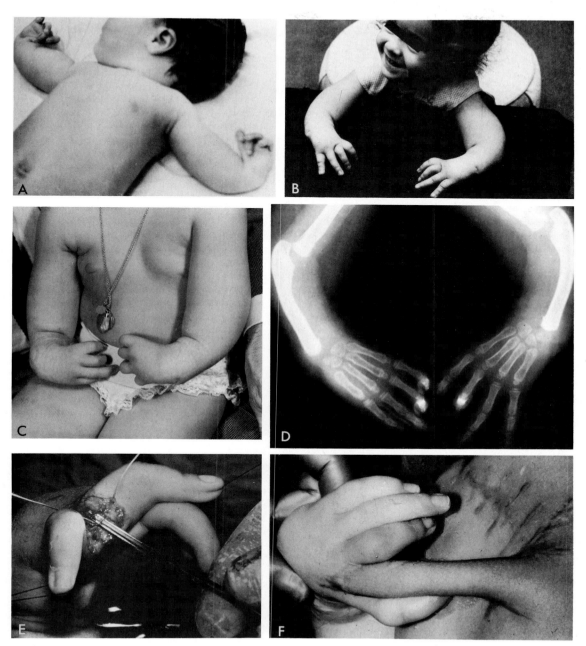

Figure 24–4 Pollicization of both index fingers. *A*, Volar view of the upper limbs of a newborn girl with total terminal longitudinal radial ray defect due to thalidomide embryopathy. *B* and *C*, Dorsal views of the upper limbs taken at the ages of 2 and 3 years, respectively. *D*, Dorsovolar roentgenograph of the forearms and hands taken at the age of three. *E* shows the deepened commissure between the left index and middle fingers and isolation of the digital artery going to the radial aspect of the middle finger, which is to be doubly ligated and severed between the ligatures. *F*, Surfacing the deepened and widened webspace with a distant flap.

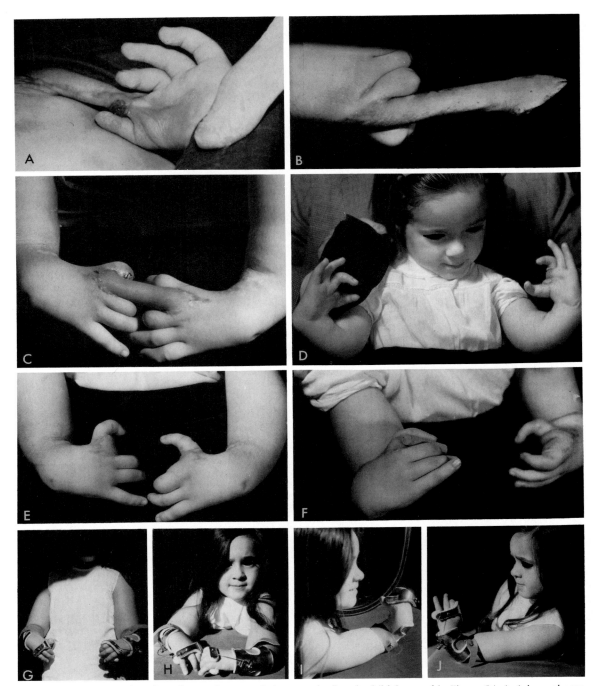

Figure 24–5   Continuation of procedures carried out on the female child featured in Figure 24–4. *A* shows the underaspect of the tubed flap attached to the left hand. *B*, This flap was weaned from the donor site six weeks after it was attached to the left hand. *C*, The free end of the tubed flap was then utilized to surface the surgically deepened and widened webspace between the right index and middle fingers. After another six weeks, it was sectioned in the middle and the halves were utilized to reconstruct the thenar bulge on each hand. *D, E,* and *F*, Results. *G, H, I,* and *J* show the splints which are worn periodically to counteract the progressive radial deflection of the hands. The splints will be used until the parents consent to more definitive treatment.

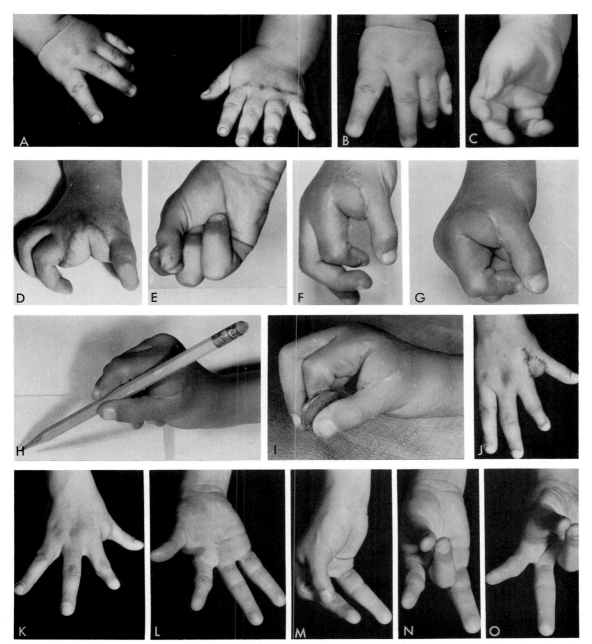

Figure 24-6   Adduction contracture of the thumb in a hand with four digits, one of which — the one next to the thumb — has a squat eccentric middle phalanx with a broad ulnar side and narrow radial border, causing the distal segment to tilt toward the thumb. This child was treated by (1) release of the thumb metacarpal from the bondage of the deep transverse ligament, (2) widening of the first webspace with the aid of a distant flap, and (3) open wedge osteotomy of the dwarfed middle phalanx of what was taken to be the index finger. *A*, Dorsal view of the hands of a seven-month-old boy with a thumb and three fingers on the right hand. *B*, Dorsal view of the right hand — enlarged. *C*, Palmar view of the same. *D*, Dorsal view of the right hand after widening the webspace between the two radial digits and osteotomy of the middle phalanx of the index finger. *E*, *F*, *G*, *H*, and *I*, Early postoperative results. *J*, Interdigital web was defatted five years after surgery. *K*, *L*, *M*, *N*, and *O*, Late results.

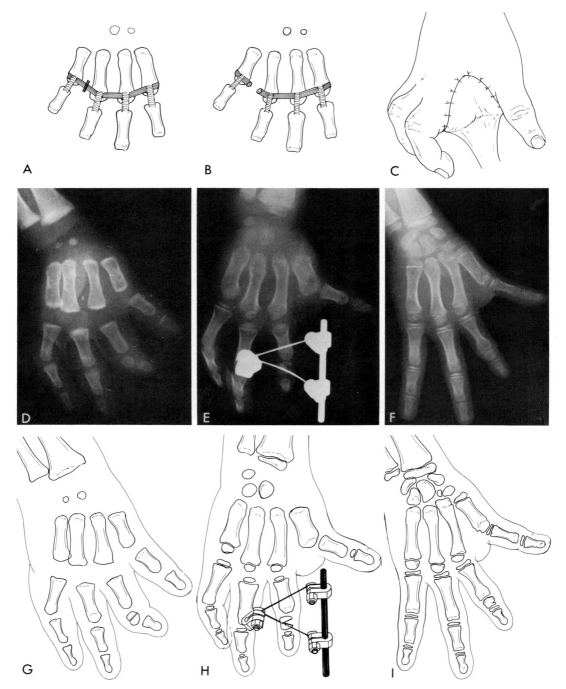

Figure 24–7 Procedures utilized for the seven-month-old boy featured in Figure 24–6. *A*, Sketch showing the deep volar transverse ligament on the palmar aspect of the right hand which had extended to the metacarpal of the thumb. *B*, Release of the thumb metacarpal from the common bondage of the deep volar metacarpal ligament. *C*, Widening the webspace and surfacing it with the aid of a distant flap. *D*, Preoperative dorsopalmar roentgenograph of the right hand: the middle phalanx of the second digit (index finger) is squat and eccentric. *E*, Roentgenograph showing open-wedge osteotomy of the middle phalanx of the index finger. *F*, Dorsopalmar roentgenograph of the right hand taken at the age of eight—five years after open-wedge osteotomy of the middle phalanx of the index finger. *G*, *H*, and *I* illustrate the roentgenograph above each.

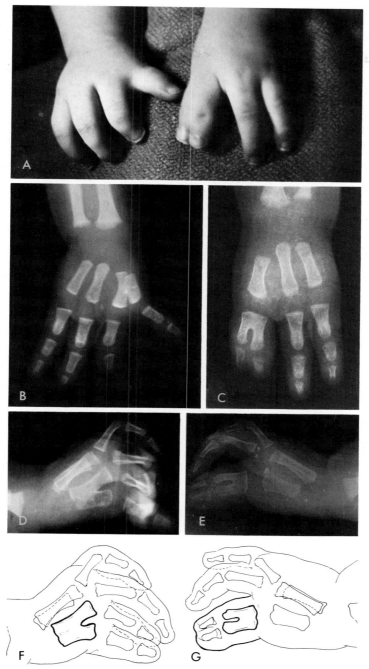

Figure 24–8 Bizarre form of bilateral oligodactyly in which the radialmost digit of each hand was shifted away from its neighbor and made to assume opposition by appropriate adjustment of a distant flap, one end of which was utilized to establish a broad webspace on the left side first; seven weeks later, the weaned end of the tubed graft was utilized similarly for the right hand. *A*, Dorsal view of the hands of a two-month-old boy. *B*, Dorsopalmar roentgenograph of the right hand: there are four digits; the two radial metacarpals have affected partial side-to-side union, and each of the corresponding digits possesses two phalanges. *C*, Dorsopalmar roentgenograph of the left hand: there are three metacarpals and four digits: each of the two radial digits possesses two phalanges; the bases of the proximal phalanges of these two radial digits have coalesced. *D* and *E*, Oblique roentgenograph of the right and left hands. *F* and *G* illustrate the roentgenograph above each.

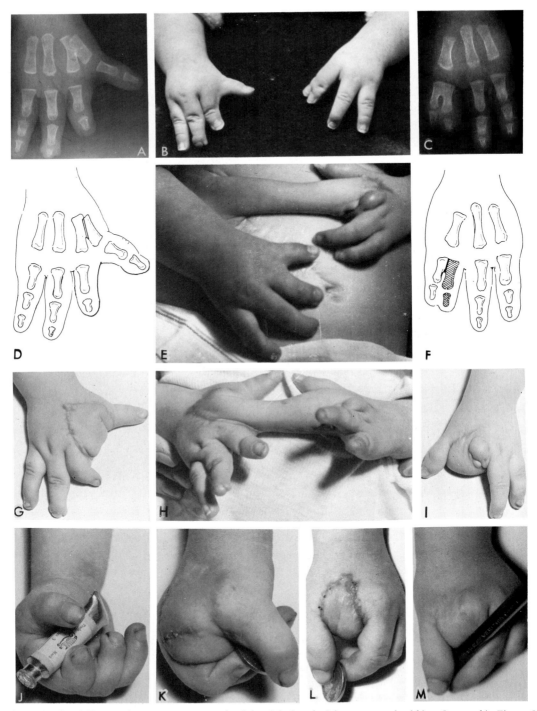

Figure 24–9   *A*, Dorsopalmar roentgenograph of the right hand of the two-month-old boy featured in Figure 24–8. *B*, Dorsal view of both hands. *C*, Dorsopalmar roentgenograph of the left hand. *D*, Sketch illustrating the line of surgical separation of the two fused metacarpals of the right hand. *E*, Attachment of the abdominal tube to the left hand. *F*, Sketch illustrating the resected phalanges of the left hand. *G*, Dorsal view showing the widened and deepened web of the right hand. *H*, Tube attached to both hands. *I*, Widened web of the left hand. *J*, *K*, *L*, and *M*, Opposition of the right and left hands after the final surgery.

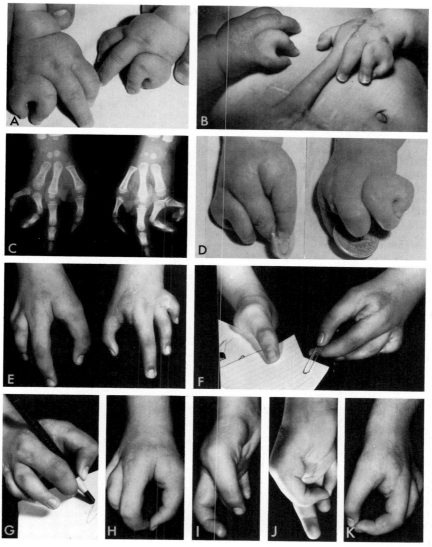

Figure 24–10 Pollicization of what were taken to be index fingers of an infant with bilateral absence of the thumb, three metacarpals in each hand, and two ulnar digits stemming from a single metacarpal and simulating parentheses. As shown in Fig. 27–2, this child subsequently developed radioulnar synostosis on the right and dislocation of the radial head on the left side. *A*, Dorsal view of the hands of a six-week-old girl. *B*, Distant tubed flap attached to the widened and deepened commissure between the left index and middle fingers; six weeks later the other end of the tube was weaned from the abdomen and attached to the deepened and widened webspace between the right index and middle fingers. After seven weeks the tube was divided and the halves were utilized to build a thenar bulge for each hand. *C*, Dorsopalmar roentgenograph of the right and the left hands taken at the age of 18 months, about 16 months after pollicization of the index fingers: the proximal phalanges of the last two ulnar digits of the left hand share one continuous epiphysis. *D*, Postoperative dorsal view of the hands, with the index and middle fingers of each hand holding a coin. The proximal phalanges of the last two ulnar digits were osteotomized to straighten the curvature of the fingers. *E*, Dorsal view of the hands at the age of 12 years. *F*, *G*, *H*, *I*, *J*, and *K*, Functional propensity at 16 years of age. It is to be noted that pollicization of the index finger was accomplished in this six-week-old infant by simply widening and deepening the commissure between this digit and its immediate ulnar neighbor — without abduction-rotation osteotomy of the index metacarpal — thus demonstrating that the earlier the operation is performed on a child the simpler is the surgical procedure.

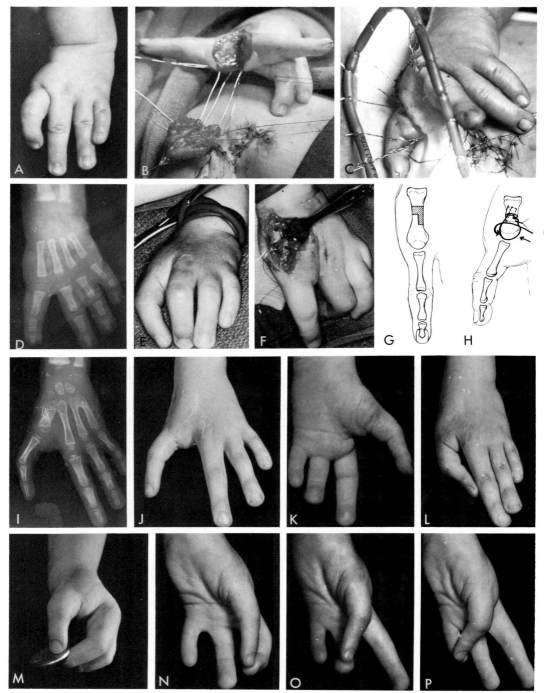

Figure 24–11　Pollicization of the left index finger. *A,* Dorsal view of the left hand of a six-week-old girl with absent thumb. *B,* The webspace of the two radial digits has been deepened and an abdominal flap is being sutured to surface the raw area. *C,* Surfaced web. *D,* Preoperative dorsopalmar roentgenograph of the left hand. *E,* Catheter used as a tourniquet for the next step of surgery which consisted of abbreviation-angulation-counterclockwise rotation osteotomy of the index metacarpal as shown in *F, G,* and *H. I,* Dorsopalmar roentgenograph of the hand two years after surgery: the bases of the last two ulnar metacarpals have coalesced; this patient had dislocation of the ipsilateral radial head. *J, K, L, M, N, O,* and *P,* Results.

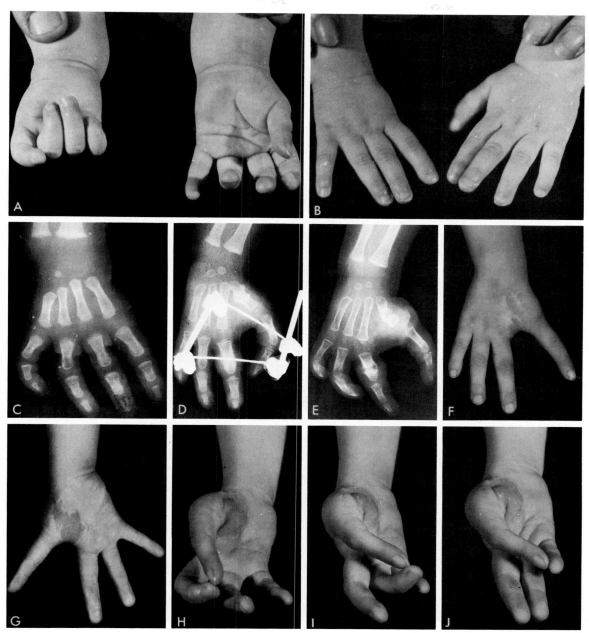

Figure 24–12 Pollicization of the right index finger. *A*, Palmar view of the hands of a three-month-old girl with absent right thumb. *B*, Dorsal view. *C*, Preoperative dorsopalmar roentgenograph of the right hand. *D*, The same, following establishment of a wide commissure between the right index and middle fingers and osteotomy of the index metacarpal—shortening it and abducting and rotating the distal fragment clockwise and maintaining opposition by fixation apparatus. *E*, Roentgenograph after osteosynthesis of metacarpal fragments and removal of fixation apparatus. *F*, *G*, *H*, *I*, and *J*, Results.

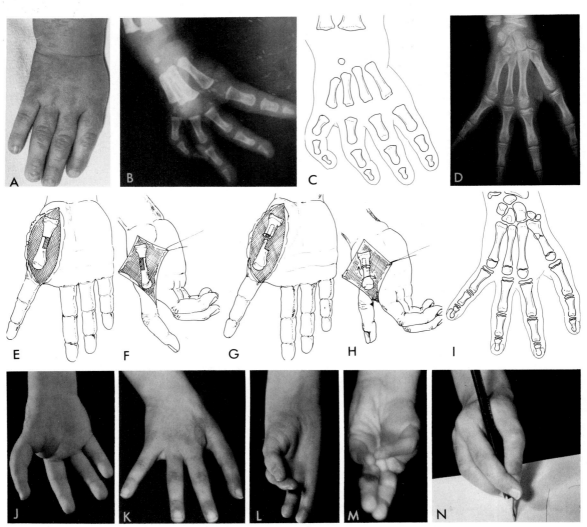

Figure 24–13   Pollicization of the right index finger. *A*, Dorsal view of the right hand of a four-month-old boy. *B*, Oblique roentgenograph of the right hand. *C*, Sketch illustrating preoperative dorsopalmar roentgenograph of the right hand. *D*, Postoperative dorsopalmar roentgenograph taken at the age of seven years—six years after shortening and rotary osteotomy of the index metacarpal: note the absence of the carpal scaphoid; osteotomized fragment of the metacarpal have been secured by a stainless steel wire suture. *E*, *F*, *G*, and *H* illustrate various steps for reduction of the length and rotary osteotomy of the index metacarpal. *I* illustrates the roentgenograph above it. *J*, *K*, *L*, *M*, and *N*, Functional results.

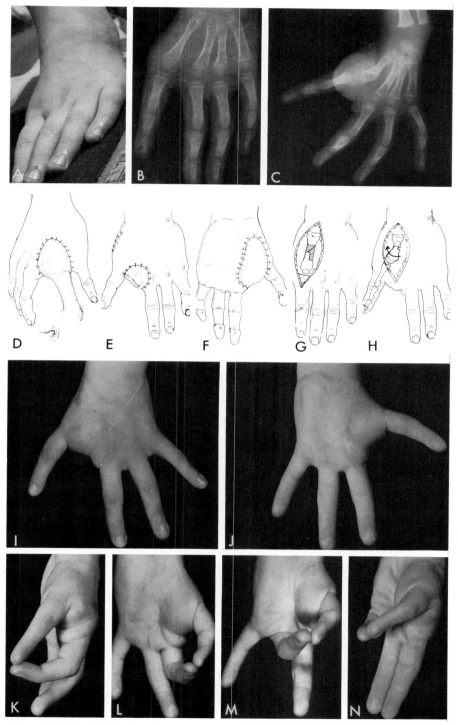

Figure 24–14 Pollicization of the left index finger and building up a thenar eminence. *A*, Dorsal view of the left hand of a 14-month-old girl. *B*, Preoperative dorsopalmar roentgenograph. *C*, Roentgenograph following abbreviation osteotomy of the index metacarpal and abduction, angulation, and counterclockwise rotation of the distal fragment. *D, E*, and *F* illustrate utilization of distant flap for widening the webspace between the pollicized index finger and its ulnar neighbor and for reconstructing a thenar eminence. *G* and *H* illustrate abbreviation-rotation osteotomy of the index metacarpal. *I, J, K, L, M*, and *N*, Results.

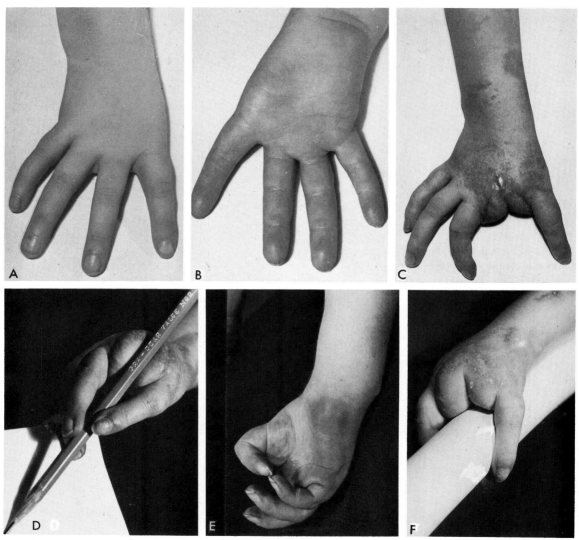

Figure 24–15   Pollicization of the right index finger. *A*, Dorsal view of the right hand of a three-year-old girl born with unilateral absent thumb. *B*, Palmar view. *C*, Dorsal view after widening and deepening of the webspace between the index and middle fingers. *D, E,* and *F,* Results after osteotomy of the index metacarpal, shown in Figure 24–16.

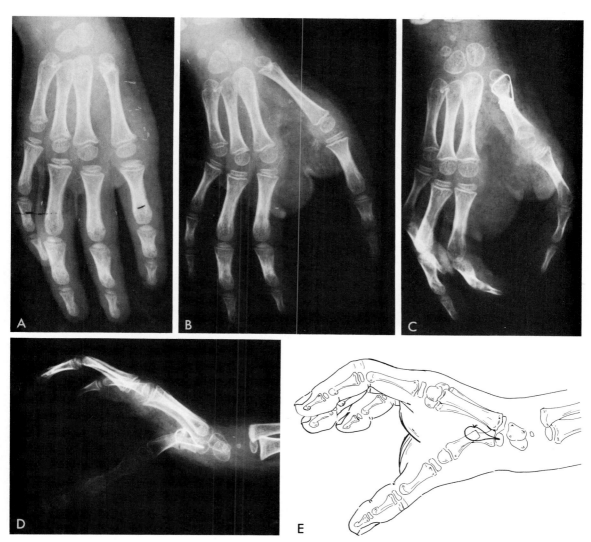

Figure 24–16   Abduction-angulation-clockwise rotation osteotomy of the index metacarpal and arrest of growth from its proximal physis. *A*, Dorsopalmar roentgenograph of the right hand of the three-year-old girl featured in Figure 24–15. *B*, The same, after the commissure between the index and middle fingers had been deepened and widened and the index metacarpal had been shifted in the radial direction. *C*, Dorsopalmar roentgenograph taken after arrest of its proximal physis, osteotomy of its shaft, and abduction, angulation, and clockwise rotation of the distal fragment. *D*, Lateral roentgenograph. *E*, Sketch illustrating the same.

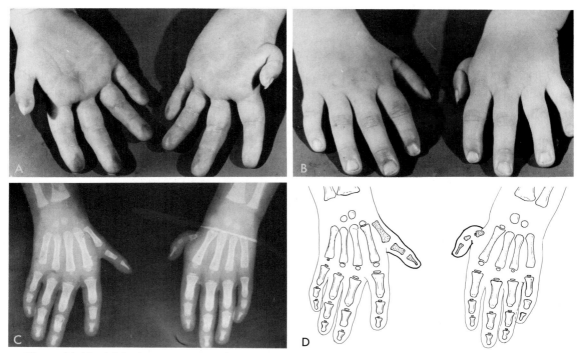

Figure 24–17   Adduction contracture of attenuated right thumb associated with intercalary defect of the pollical ray of the opposite hand. *A*, Palmar view of the hands of an 11-month-old boy. *B*, Dorsal view. *C*, Dorsopalmar roentgenograph of the right and left hands: the bones of the right pollical ray are present, but they are short and thin; the proximal portion of the left first metacarpal is missing. The remaining distal part is puny, as are the phalanges of the left thumb. *D*, Sketch illustrating the same.

     Roswell Park (1901) operated on a four-year-old female child with absent radius and missing first metacarpal bone. Park "made an incision over the location of the first metacarpal bone and transplanted therein a piece of bone about 1 inch long and ⅛ inch in diameter, taken from the humerus of a still live rabbit for this purpose." The article states that the surgical wound closed "without drainage ' and the subsequent course of the case was "uneventful." The little girl went home to Saginaw, which was such a distance from Buffalo, New York, where Park practiced, that he could not examine her in person, but "the accounts of the case sent by the family are exceedingly encouraging."

     During the ensuing decades, homogeneous bone grafts—from tibia, iliac crest, rib, metatarsals, and pedal phalanges—were utilized to establish a bridge of bone between the phalanges of the floating thumb and the second metacarpal or the surviving radial carpal bone. Prior to the insertion of the bone graft, it was necessary to create room for it; distant skin flaps were transferred from elsewhere in order to broaden the base of the rudimentary thumb; it was also necessary to shift the attachment of the vestigial thumb to a more proximal and palmar location. The entire undertaking required numerous sessions, extending over months, even years, and the results were anything but encouraging. Pollicization of the index yields far better functional and cosmetic results.

     For congenital deficiencies of the pollical ray in which the first metacarpal is attenuated, unrotated, and adducted but possesses funtioning extensors and

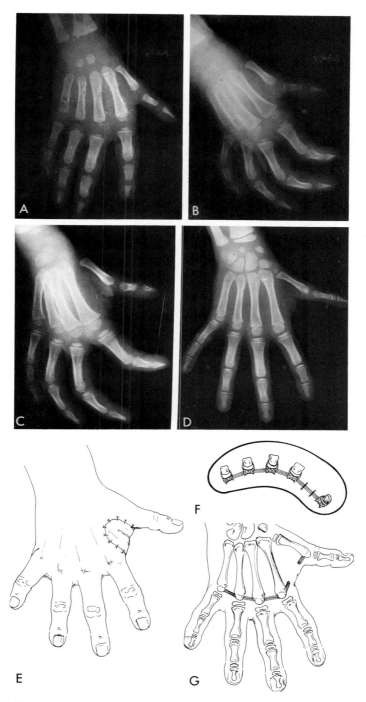

Figure 24–18 Management of the right hand of the 11-month-old boy featured in Figure 24–17. *A*, Preoperative dorsopalmar roentgenograph of the right thumb: the first metacarpal is short and thin and is held close to the second metacarpal—it is adducted. *B*, Oblique roentgenograph with the thumb actively abducted, an action which takes place not at the carpometacarpal junction but at the metacarpophalangeal joint. *C*, Oblique roentgenograph four years after severance of the deep transverse metacarpal ligament and widening of the first webspace. *D*, Dorsopalmar roentgenograph six years after surgery. *E*, Sketch illustrating the widened first webspace and the surfacing of it with the aid of a distant flap. *F* and *G* illustrate the severance of the segment of the deep transverse metacarpal ligament in the first intermetacarpal space.

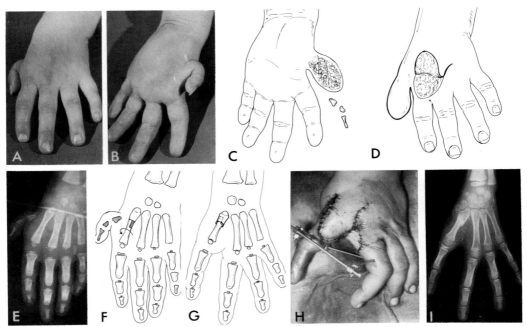

Figure 24–19   Management of the left hand of the 11-month-old boy featured in Figures 24–17 and 24–18. *A,* Dorsal view of the left hand. *B,* Palmar view. *C,* Sketch illustrating evacuation of the bony content of the floating thumb, saving the skin, which was utilized to establish a broader webspace between the index and middle fingers. *D,* Lifting an additional flap from the dorsum of the hand. *E,* Dorsopalmar roentgenograph of the left hand. *F,* Sketch illustrating the same. *G,* Sketch illustrating shortening and abduction-rotation of the index metacarpal. *H,* Immediate postoperative dorsal view of the hand with index and middle fingers being held in opposition with the aid of K-wire and external fixation apparatus. *I,* Dorsopalmar roentgenograph of the hand six years after surgery.

flexors, the following procedures—alone and in combination, depending upon the demands of the case—may be utilized: widening of the first webspace by Z-plasty; detachment of fibrous bands—particularly, the extension of the deep transverse ligament to the pollical ray; and osteotomy of the first metacarpal followed by abduction, axial rotation, and volar angulation of the distal fragment.

There are two other congenital anomalies for which pollicization of a lesser digit is indicated: in the unopposable variety of triphalangeal thumb, or five-fingered hand, and in ulnar dimelia or mirror hand. Pollicization of the first radial digit of a five-fingered hand is carried out along the lines already described for index finger transfer: a web is reconstructed between the first and second radial digits; the metacarpal of the first digit is osteotomized and shortened; and the finger is axially rotated, abducted, and tilted in the volar direction.

In mirror image deformity, there may be six, seven, or even eight fingers. When there are six fingers, the second radial digit is deleted; when there are seven fingers, the second and third radial fingers are sacrificed. In both instances, the eliminated digit is filleted, and the extra skin thus made available is utilized to reconstruct a thenar web; the first radial digit is shortened and placed in apposition. When there are eight fingers, the second, third, and fourth radial digits are deleted, and the first member is migrated in the ulnar direction and pollicized (Figs. 24–2 to 24–22).

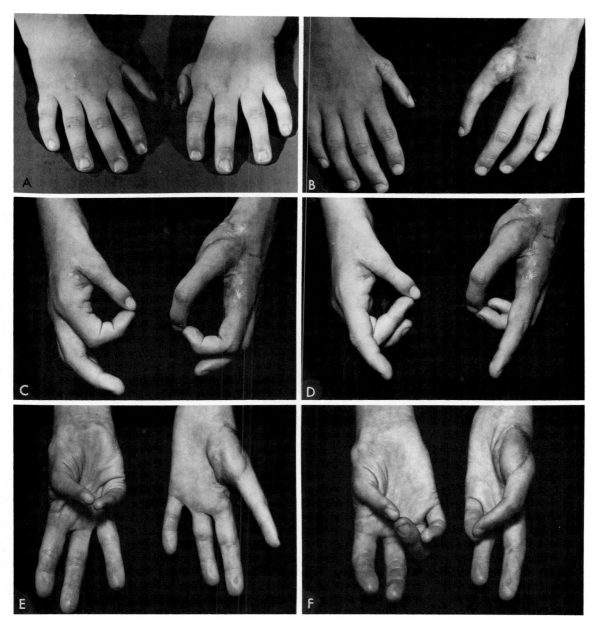

Figure 24–20 Results of the treatment of the bilateral thumb defect featured in Figures 24–17 to 24–19. *A*, Preoperative dorsal view of the hands at the age of eleven months. *B*, Postoperative dorsal view at the age of seven years. *C, D, E*, and *F*, Final functional and cosmetic results – the webspace between the pollicized left index finger and the middle finger was less resilient than the deepened and widened commissure of the right hand which was surfaced with the aid of a distant flap. The left hand, which was subjected to one-stage pollicization, is extensively scarred.

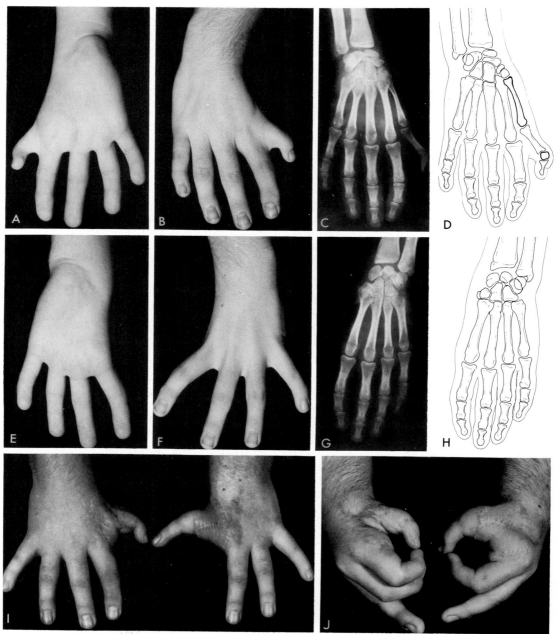

Figure 24–21 Hypoplastic nonopposable triphalangeal thumb of the right hand and absent pollical ray of the left hand. This patient also had bilateral radioulnar synostosis (Fig. 29–18). The hypoplastic thumb was treated by (1) deepening of the first commissure which involved freeing the metacarpal and the proximal phalanx of the thumb from the bondage of the deep transverse metacarpal ligament and tenotomy of the adductor transversus, and (2) abduction-rotation osteotomy of the first metacarpal; the left index finger was pollicized by two-stage procedure. *A,* Palmar view of the right hand of a 13-year-old girl: note the distally placed diminutive thumb. *B,* Dorsal view. *C,* Dorsopalmar roentgenograph: the radial styloid is missing; the lunate and triquetrum have coalesced; the scaphoid has wedged itself between the lunate and capitate, and the trapezoid lies between the scaphoid and trapezium; the first metacarpal is long and thin, and there is a squat, square, middle phalanx between the proximal and distal phalanges of the thumb. *D,* Sketch illustrating the same. *E,* Palmar view of the left hand. *F,* Dorsal view. *G,* Dorsopalmar roentgenograph: the radial styloid is absent; the scaphoid and trapezium are undersized, and the pollical ray is absent. *H,* Sketch illustrating the same. *I* and *J,* Results.

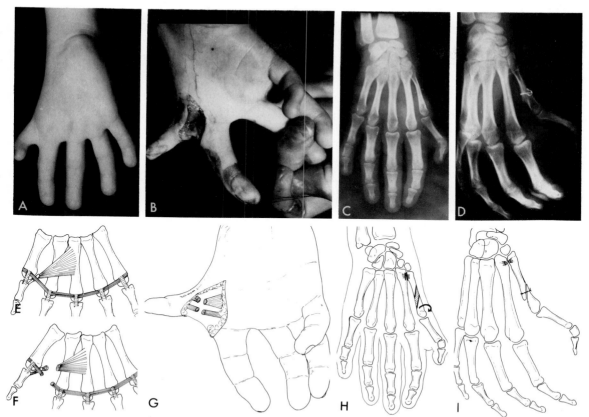

Figure 24–22 Procedures utilized for the treatment of the right hand of the 13-year-old girl featured in Figure 24–21. *A*, Palmar view of the right hand. *B*, Incision exposing a thick fibrous band—interpreted as the extension of the deep transverse volar metacarpal ligament—tethering the distally placed diminutive thumb and the tendon of the adductor transversus pollicis. *C*, Preoperative dorsopalmar roentgenograph of the right hand, showing a thin and long first metacarpal which lies close to its ulnar neighbor; its proximal end is overlapped by the corresponding extremity of the second metacarpal and its shaft bows in the ulnar direction, bringing its head closer to that of the second metacarpal. *D*, Postoperative dorsopalmar roentgenograph: the proximal extremity of the first metacarpal has been freed from the corresponding extremity of the second metacarpal by severing the interosseous ligament, and its shaft has been subjected to abduction and clockwise rotation. *E*, Sketch showing the insertion of the adductor transversus and extension of the deep transverse metacarpal ligament to the first metacarpal. *F* and *G* shows tenotomy of the adductor transversus and sectioning of the segment of the deep transverse ligament in the first webspace which was subsequently surfaced by a distant flap. *H* and *I* show the abduction-rotation osteotomy of the first metacarpal shaft.

COMPOSITE BONE AND SKIN GRAFT

In 1896, Nicoladoni (1897, 1900) fashioned a flap of skin from the chest wall into a tube and connected its free end to the stump of the thumb. After weaning it from the donor site, Nicoladoni stiffened the cylinder attached to the hand with a bone graft. During ensuing decades, what became known as the autoplastic method of digital reconstruction underwent numerous modifications. A more recent modification is that proposed by McGregor and Simonetta (1964). Their method consists of simultaneous transfer of skin and bone and provision of sensation by neurovascular island transfer from the ulnar pulp of the ring finger. When there is only a single solitary digit—as seen in some cases of split hand or ulnar ray defect—reconstruction of an oppositional post with composite skin and bone is definitely indicated. Obviously, in such a case one does not consider dissecting out a neurovascular island flap from the only remaining digit and transferring it to the reconstructed post. The latter rmains insensitive for as long as six to twelve months, during which it is protected by a celluloid encasement. Sensations of light touch and pinprick begin to appear during this period. Stereognosis never appears. Unless anchored to a mobile metacarpal or carpal bone, such a post, moreover, lacks movement.

TRANSFER OF A DIGIT FROM THE OPPOSITE HAND

Joyce (1918, 1928) and Oudard (1922) utilized the ring finger of the contralateral hand to reconstruct a thumb. Joyce reconstructed two thumbs by this method. Oudard added another one. All three patients had lost their thumbs because of trauma. This procedure does not seem to have been attempted for congenital defects of the thumb.

TOE-TO-HAND TRANSPLANTS

Nicoladoni (1900) pioneered this procedure: he transferred the second toe to take the place of the missing thumb. The first hallux-to-pollex transfer appears to have first been performed by Krause (1906). The operation has since been carried out by Esser (1917), Clarkson (1950–1966), and Freeman (1956, 1964) for acquired defects of the hand; and by Reid (1960) and Davis (1964) for congenital deficiencies. Buncke et al (1966) performed this procedure on a rhesus monkey. Davis (1964) singled out four main objections which had been leveled against this method and contributed to its unpopularity: (1) the intolerable position entailed during the period of attachment of the hand to the foot; (2) the precarious circulation of the transferred toe and the failure of anastomosed tendons to function; (3) failure to suture the nerves to procure adequate stereognosis; (4) trophic disorders of the transplanted digit. During the period of immobilization of the hand and foot—which necessitates enclosure of the torso and leg in a plaster cast—the patient is forced to sit on his buttocks most of the time. Clarkson spoke of a patient who had developed sciatic palsy as a result of protracted sedentary posture. Buncke et al—who carried out the enitre procedure on a rhesus monkey, performing "micro-miniature vascular anastomosis," with the aid of a binocular operating microscope and ultrafine sutures, needles and instruments—wrote: "The potentialities of tissue transplantation by these techniques are most challenging, and have wide application in the field of experimental and clinical reconstructive surgery." One may ask: challenging at whose expense? A child is not an inarticulate monkey. The child subjected to this operation, moreover, loses a big toe, which is not a dispensable appendage.

SUMMARY

When only the thumb is missing, this author's preference continues to be pollicization of the index finger. This operation is also preferred for the treatment of *pouce flottant,* the unopposable type of triphalangeal thumb, for mirror hand or ulnar dimelia, and in absence of the thumb seen in connection with split hand. In partial absences of the digit, the author deepens the interdigital commissure. In some instances, he also turns the dorsal skin in the palmar direction and surfaces the skin defect thus created with a pedicled flap, later fashioning distal digital pouches and inserting into each a piece of bone, usually the proximal phalanx of one of the lesser toes. When only two marginal digital rays remain, the cleft between them is deepened, and the metacarpal bones are subjected to rotary osteotomy. These digits are often webbed, and the repair of the syndactyly precedes rotation osteotomy of the metacarpals. In terminal absences of the three central fingers, the little finger is migrated in the radial direction closer to the thumb. In a monodactylous hand, often seen in split hand and in longitudinal defect of the radial ray, one is justified in reconstructing an oppositional post by composite skin and bone graft.

References

Adam, R.: *La Restauration du Mouvement d'Opposition du Pouce.* Thèse. Paris, Librairie Marcel Vigne, pp. 1–113, 1941.

Aguirre, S. C., and Oberlander, H.: Sobre reconstruccion total del pulgar. *Prensa Med. Argentina, 43:*2360–2364, 1956.

Albee, F. H.: Synthetic transplantation of tissues to form new finger. *Ann. Surg., 69:*379–383, 1919.

Allende, B. T., and Wilson, J. N.: Chirurgie reconstructive du pouce possibilités offertes par l'utilisation des doigts voisins blessés. À propos des observations. *Rev. Chir. Orthop. Rep. App. Mot.* (Paris), 54:715–728, 1968.

Almasanu, S.: Phalangisation du premier metacarpien. Resultats. Presentation du malade. *Rev. Chir., 74:*807–809, 1934.

Anglade, J. J.: *Contribution au Traitement Chirurgical des Pertes du Pouce par Blessure de Guerre.* Thèse, Paris, Imprimérie R. Foulon, pp. 1–80, 1958.

Apetrosyan, K. A.: Plastic reconstruction of fingers by means of transplantation of toes. (In Russian.) *Ortop. Travm., 13:*74–78, 1939.

Arana, G. B.: Phalangization of the first metacarpal. *Surg. Gynecol. Obstet., 40:*859–862, 1925.

Ardao, H.: La pulgarizacion del dedo indice. *Bol. Soc. Cir. Uruguay, 18:*78–79, 1947.

Arlt, B.: Daumenplastik. *Wien. Klin. Wochenschr., 30:*15–16, 1917.

Balico, G.: Falangizzazione del primo metacarpo. Da un caso curato con successo. *Chir. Plast., 5:*128–130, 1939.

Baron, R., and Fabre, A.: Technique de reconstruction du pouce. *Presse Méd., 60:*1597, 1952.

Barsky, A. J.: Restoration of the thumb by transplantation, plastic repair, and prosthesis. *Surgery, 23:*227–247, 1948.

Bartolini, G.: La reconstruccione del pollice: translazione di un dito secondo, Helgenfeldt. *Clinica Ortop., 12:*6–16, 1960.

Baxter, H., Entin, M., Drummond, J., and Sullivan, D.: Reconstruction of digits of deformed hands. *Can. Med. Assoc. J., 61:*401–405, 1949.

Beardsley, J. M., and Zechino, V.: Reconstruction of the thumb. *Am. J. Surg., 71:*825–827, 1946.

Beck, C., and Beck, W. C.: Plastic reconstruction of fingers by transplantation of the toes. *Surg. Clin. N. Am., 14:*763–767, 1934.

Benton, S. G.: Reconstruction of the thumb. *Am. J. Surg., 83:*347–351, 1952.

Berson, M. I.: Reconstruction of index finger with nail transplantation. *Surgery, 27:*594–599, 1950.

Bianchi, C.: Considerazioni su 53 casi di falangizzazione del l'metacarpo. *Clinica Ortop., 3:*45–54, 1951.

Blair, V. P., and Byars, L. T.: Toe to finger transplant. *Ann. Surg., 112:*287–290, 1940.

Blake, H. E.: Notes on the reconstruction of the thumb. *Br. J. Plast. Surg., 1:*119–122, 1948–1949.

Blauth, W.: Der hypoplastische Daumen. *Arch. Orthop. Unfallchir., 62:*225–246, 1967.

Blauth, W.: Indikation und Technik des "Zeigefinger-Daumens" bei Daumenplasie. *Handchirurgie, 1:*28–33, 1969.

Bocca, M., Fongo, A., and Rinaldi, F.: Pollicizzazione del quatro dito. *Boll. Soc. Piedm. Chir., 29:*499–500, 1959.

Boehler, J.: Primäre wiederherstellende Eingriffe bei schwersten Handverletzungen. *Arch. Klin. Chir.,292:*158–162, 1959.

Bolté, R.: Pollicisation du premier métacarpien. *J. Hôtel-Dieu Montreal, 7:*359–365, 1938.

Bonnet, P., and Carcassone, F.: Restauration anatomique du pouce par la greffe de l'index de la même main, mutilé et perdu au point de vue fonctionnel. Résultat éloigné. *Lyon Chir., 28:*247–248, 1931.

Bonnet, P., and Carcasssone, F.: Restauration du pouce par la greffe d'un doigt fonctionnellement lésé de la main traumatisée. *Lyon Chir., 28:*529–540, 1931.

Bonnet, P., and Carcassonne, F.: La phalangisation du premier métacarpien. Sa technique, ses indications, ses résultats. *Rev. Chir., 50:*341–355, 1931.

Bonvallet, J. M.: Allongement du pouce par le procédé de Gillies. *Ann. Chir. Plast., 5:*297–299, 1960.

Bonzon: Absence congénitale du pouce droit. Essai de restauration fonctionnelle. *Scalpel, 86:*799–803, 1933.

Boron, R., and Fabre, A.: Technique de reconstruction du pouce. *Presse Méd., 60:*1597–1598, 1952.

Bowe, J. J.: Transposition of the index finger for congenital absence of the thumb and thenar eminence. *Plast. Reconstr. Surg., 13:*474–480, 1954.

Bowe, J. J.: Thumb construction by index transposition. *Plast. Reconstr. Surg., 32:*414–424, 1963.

Boyes, J. H.: Reconstruction of the thumb. *In Bunnell's Surgery of the Hand.* Fourth edition. Revised by Joseph J. Boyes. Philadelphia, J. B. Lippincott Co., pp. 535–560, 1964. See also the Fifth edition, p. 506, 1970.

Broadbent, T. R., and Wollf, R. M.: The reconstruction with contiguous skin-bone pedicle graft: a case report. *Plast. Reconstr. Surg., 26:*494–499, 1960.

Brunelli, G.: La chirurgia riparatrice nei gravi infortuni della mano in rapporto al lavoro ed all machine modern e la sua attuazione "d'urgenza." *Arch. Ortop., 73:*545–551, 1960.

Brunelli, G.: Le varie possibilita di riconstruzione del pollice. *Arch. Ortop., 75:*94–104, 1962.

Buchen, A. C.: The neurovascular island flap in reconstruction of the thumb. *The Hand, 1*:19–20, 1969.

Buck-Gramcko, D.: Daumenersatz dem zweiten Mittelhandknochen bei Verlust des ersten und zweiten Fingers. *Arch. Klin. Chir., 306*:153–157, 1963.

Buck-Gramcko, D.: Operative Behandlung eines Spiegelbild. Beformität der Hand. *Ann. Chir. Plast., 9*:180–183, 1964.

Buck-Gramcko, D.: Daumenrekonstruktion bei Aplasie und Hypoplasie. *Klin. Med. (Wien), 21*:325–329, 1966.

Buck-Gramcko, D.: Daumenrekonstruktion bei traumatischem Verlust und Aplasia. *Münch. Med. Wochenschr., 108*:1252, 1966.

Buck-Gramcko, D.: Indikation und Tecknik der Daumenbildung bei Aplasia und Hypoplasie. *Chir. Plast. Reconstr., 5*:46, 1968.

Buck-Gramcko, D.: Operativer Daumenerstaz bei Aplasie und Hypoplasie. *Verh. Dtsch. Orthop. Ges., 55*:417–421, 1968.

Buck-Gramcko, D.: Pollicisation de l'index en cas d'aplasie et d'hypoplasie du pouce. Methodes et résultats. *Rev. Chir. Orthop. Rep. App. Mot., 57*:35–48, 1971.

Buck-Gramcko, D.: Pollicization of the index finger. Method and results in aplasia and hypoplasia of the thumb. *J. Bone Joint Surg., 53A*:1065–1067, 1971.

Buncke, H. J., Jr., Buncke, C. M., and Schulz, W. P.: Immediate Nicoladoni procedure in the Rhesus monkey, or hallux-to-hand transplantation, utilizing microminiature mascular anastomoses. *Br. J. Plast. Surg., 19*:332–337, 1966.

Bunnell, S.: Physiological reconstruction of a thumb after total loss. *Surg. Gynecol. Obstet., 52*:245–248, 1931.

Bunnell, S.: Digit transfer by neurovascular pedicle. *J. Bone Joint Surg., 34*:772–774, 1952.

Bunnell, S.: Reconstruction of the thumb. *Am. J. Surg., 95*:168–172, 1958.

Butler, R., Jr.: Ring-finger pollicization with transplantation of nail bed and matrix on a volar flap. *J. Bone Joint Surg., 46*:1069–1076, 1964.

Buzello, A.: Umstellungsplastik des Zeigefingers bei Verlust des ganzen Daumens. *Zbl. Chir., 63*:2945–2952, 1936.

Byars, L. T.: Toe to finger transplant. *Plast. Reconstr. Surg., 9*:274–275, 1952.

Cabarro, P.: Reconstruction of hand with transposition of a finger. *Plast. Reconstr. Surg., 13*:462–473, 1954.

Candiollo, L., and Rinaldi, F.: Indagini anatomiche sulla vascolarizzazione arteriosa del IV dito della mano translato sul primo metacarpo (IV dito "pollicizzato"). *G. Acad. Med. Torino, 123*:82–87, 1960.

Cannon, B., Graham, W. C., and Brown, J. B.: Restoration of grasping function following loss of five digits. *Surgery, 25*:420–423, 1949.

Carcasonne, F.: *Contribution à l'étude des Restaurations Anatomiques et Functionelles du Pouce dans les Traumatism.* Thèse. Lyon, Bosc. Riou, Imprimeurs, pp. 1–412, 1930.

Chauvenet, M. A.: Autoplastie de la main par lambeaux digitaux. *Bordeaux Chir., 1*:18–25, 1935.

Chu, H., Wang, T., Kung, F., and Hou, C.: Reconstruction of the thumb. *Acta Chir. Plast.* (Praha), *2*:197–206, 1960.

Cipollino, O.: La intermetacarpolisi. *Policliuico (Soz. Chir.), 28*:138–139, 1921.

Clarkson, R.: Treatment of congenital adactyly by pedo-carpal transference. *Proc. R. Soc. Med.* (Clinical section), *43*:905, 1950.

Clarkson, P.: Reconstruction of hand digits by two transfers. *J. Bone Joint Surg., 37*:270–276, 1955.

Clarkson, P.: On making thumbs. *Plast. Reconstr. Surg., 29*:325–331, 1962.

Clarkson, P.: Toe-hand transfers. *In* Flynn, J. Edward: *Hand Surgery.* Baltimore, Williams & Wilkins Co., pp. 583–596, 1966.

Clerico-Rogozzi, I.: Tecnica per la reconstruzione del pollice a mezzo di lembo cutaneo tubolato e di trapianto osseo. *Minerva Ortop., 6*:285–288, 1955.

Cobbett, J. R.: Free digital transfer. Report of a case of transfer of a great toe to replace an amputated thumb. *J. Bone Joint Surg., 51B*:677–679, 1969.

Colson, P., and Honot, R.: Chirurgie reparatrice du pouce, greffe articulaire. *Lyon Chir., 42*:721–724, 1947.

Colson, P., Gangolphe, M., and Honot, R.: Pollicisation d'un index. Pollicisation d'un moignon d'index. *Lyon Chir., 60*:768–771, 1964.

Cotta, H., and Jäger, M.: Die operative Behandlung der angeborenen Daumenfehlbildung einschliesslich der Daumenplasie. *Arch. Orthop. Unfallchir., 62*:339–358, 1967.

Cuthbert, J. B.: Pollicisation of the index finger. *Br. J. Plast. Surg., 1*:56–59, 1949.

Dabrowski, T.: Behavior of the grafts taken from the ribs in reconstructed finger. *Plast. Reconstr. Surg., 36*:218–226, 1965.

d'Aubigne, R. M., Tubiano, R., and Ramadier, J. O.: *Reconstruction du pouce. Mém. Acad. Chir., 76*: 901–904, 1950. Also in *Rev. d'Orthop., 38*:456–475, 1952.

Davis, J. E.: Toe-to-hand transfers (pedochyrodactyloplasty). *Plast. Reconstr. Surg., 33*:422–436, 1964.

Dega: La plastique du pouce d'après la méthode de Wierzejewski et ses résultats éloignés. *Rev. d'Orthop.,* (3 s.), *13*:497–501, 1926.

Dehne, E.: Operativer Ersatz des Daumens. *Der Chirurg., 23*:566–567, 1952.

D'Este, S.: Su la pollicizzazione del 1° metacarpale dupo la perdita total del pollice correspondente. *La Med. Internaz., 50*:224–236, 1942.

Dial, D. E.: Reconstruction of thumb after traumatic amputation. *J. Bone Joint Surg.*, (n.s.), *21*:98–100, 1939.

Dunlop, J.: The use of the index finger for the thumb: some interesting points in hand surgery. *J. Bone Joint Surg., 21*:99–103, 1923.

Duval, P.: Malade ayant subi une autoplastie complète du pouce avec son métacarpien par le procédé de M. G. Warren-Pierce. *Bull. Mém. Soc. Chir.* (Paris), *55*:882, 1929.

Edgerton, M. T., Snyder, G. B., and Webb, W. L.: Surgical treatment of congenital thumb deformities (including psychological impact of correction). *J. Bone Joint Surg., 47*:1453–1474, 1965.

Eiselsberg, F. V.: Ersatz des Zeigefingers durch die zweite Zehe. *Arch. Klin. Chir., 61*:988–997, 1900.

Esser, J. F. S.: Operativer Ersatz der Mittelhand nebst 4 Fingern. *Beitr. Klin. Chir., 108*:244–248, 1917.

Esser, J. F. S., and Ranschburg, P.: Reconstruction of a hand and four fingers by transplantation of the middle part of the foot and four toes. *Ann. Surg., 3*:655–659, 1940.

Ferrari, R. C.: Plástica reconstructiva de los dedos por el método italiano. *Sem. Méd., 2*:1104–1105, 1933.

Flynn, J. E., and Burden, C. N.: Reconstruction of the thumb. *Arch. Surg., 85*:56–60, 1962.

Francois, M. J., and Frezieres, H.: Reconstitution du pouce par lambeau cylindrique et greffe osseuse. *Ann. Chir. Plast., 3*:9–14, 1958.

Freeman, B. S.: Reconstruction of the thumb by toe transfer. *Plast. Reconstr. Surg., 17*:393–398, 1956.

Freeman, B. S.: Toe-hand transplantation: indications, technic, complications and end results. *Trans. Third Internat. Congress Plast. Surg.*, pp. 954–962, 1964.

Froste, N.: Tvo handskador behandlade med phalangisation. *Svensk. Lakart., 30*:337–341, 1933.

Gabarro, P.: Reconstruction of a hand, with transposition of a finger. *Plast. Reconstr. Surg., 13*:462–473, 1954.

Gabriel, E.: Der Daumenersatz aus dem Zeigefinger. *Münch. Med. Wochenschr., 832*:1391–1393, 1936.

Gebauer, T.: Reparacion plastica del pulgar transplante del dedo medio. *Arch. Soc. Chir. Chile, 5*:270–272, 1953.

Gebauer, T., and Ihl, W.: Reparacion del pulgar por transplante de un dedo de la misma mano. *Rev. Orthop. Traumat. Lat. Amer., 1*:28–44, 1955.

Gillies, S. H.: Autograft of amputated digit: a suggested operation. *Lancet, 1*:1002–1003, 1940.

Gillies, S. H., and Reid, D. A. C.: Autograft of amputated digit. *Br. J. Plast. Surg., 7*:338–342, 1955.

Gioia, T.: La Falangizacion del Primer Metacarpiano. *Semana Med., 1*:490–497, 1943.

Goebel, W. : Ersatz von Finger- und Zehenphalangen. *Münch. Med. Wochenschr.*, No. 7, *60*:356–357, 1913.

Gonzales, R., and Ulloa, M.: Digital reconstruction. *Plast. Reconstr. Surg., 22*:309–314, 1958.

Gordon, S.: Autograft of amputated thumb. *Lancet, 2*:823, 1944.

Gosset, J.: La pollicisation de l'index (technique chirurgicale). *J. Chir., 65*:403–411, 1949.

Gosset, J.: Technique de Jean Gosset. *In Traité de Technique Chirurgicale.* Zème ódid. par B. Fey, p. Mocquet S. Oberlin, et J. Quenu. Paris: Masson. édit. T. 1, pp. 630–634, 1955.

Gossett, J., and Sells, M.: Technique, indication et résultat de la pollicisation du zéme doigts. *Ann. Chir., 18*:1005–1014, 1964.

Graham, W. C., Brown, J., and Cannon, B.: Elongation and digitization of first metacarpal for restoration of function of hand. *Arch. Surg., 61*:17–22, 1950.

Greeley, P. W.: Reconstruction of the thumb. *Ann. Surg., 124*:60–70, 1946.

Grégoire, R.: Restauration du pouce par greffe du gros orteil. *Paris Méd., 11*:164–166, 1921.

Grundt, B.: Methods of re-establishing amputated fingers. *Trans. First Internat. Soc. Plast. Surg.*, pp. 444–452, 1957.

Guellemin, G., Barry, P., and Feit, R.: Pollicisation de l'index (à propos d'un cas pratique d'urgence). *Lyon Chir., 50*:626–629, 1955.

Gueullette, R.: Étude critique des procédés de restauration du pouce. *J. Chir., 36*:1–23, 1930.

Guermonprez, F.: Sur le prognositc des mutilations de la main. *Bull. Soc. Chir. Paris*, (n.s.), *10*:363–378, 1884.

Guermonprez, F.: *Notes sur quelques Résections et Restaurations du Pouce.* Paris, P. Asselin, pp. 1–53, 1887.

Guermonprez, F., and Derode: *Note sur les Indications de la Restauration du Pouce.* Toulouse, Imprimérie Pinel, pp. 1–10, 1889. Also in *Rev. Méd. Toulouse, 23*:231–236, 1889.

Guignard, J. M. J.: *La Reconstitution du Pouce par Pollicisation.* Thèse. Paris, Librairie Arnette, pp. 1–42, 1954.

Haas, S. L.: Plastic restoration for loss of all fingers of both hands. *Am. J. Surg., 36*:720–723, 1937.

Hallberg, K.: Ersatz des Daumens durch die Grosszehe. *Hygiea. Stockh., 90*:452–456, 1928.

Hanotte, G.: *Restauration Fonctionelle du Pouce.* Thèse. Lille, Imprimérie L. Daniel, pp. 3–109, 1888.

Harrison, S. H.: Restoration of muscle balance in pollicization. *Plast. Reconstr. Surg., 34*:236–240, 1964.

Harrison, S. H.: Pollicization in cases of radial club hand. *Br. J. Plast. Surg. 23*:192–200, 1970.

Harrison, S. H.: Pollicization in children. *The Hand, 3*:204–210, 1971.

Hayd, F. W.: Das Bild der angeborenen Daumenhypoplasie. *Dtsch. Med. Wochenschr., 64*:1041–1042, 1938.

Hilgenfeldt, O.: *Operativer Daumenersatz und Beseitigung von Greifstörungen bei Fingerverlusten.* Stuttgart, Enke V., pp. 1–144, 1950.

Hoffman, S., Seifert, R., and Simon, B. E.: Experimental and clinical experiences in epiphyseal transplantation. *J. Plast. Reconstr. Surg., 50*:58–65, figs. 5–9, 1972.

Hoffmann, E.: Daumenersatz. *Dtsch. Med. Wochenschr., 45*:839, 1919.

Hörhammer, C.: Beitrag zur plastischen Operation des Daumenersatzes. *Münch. Med. Wochenschr., 62*:1681–1684, 1915.

Hueck, H.: Ein Fall von Daumenersatz durch einen unbrauchbaren Finger. *Dtsch. Z. Chir., 153*:321–330, 1920.

Huffstadt, A. J. C., and Bom, A. W.: Verdere Ervaringen met de Pollicistie Operatie. *Ned. T. Geneesk., 113*:65–68, 1969.

Hughes, N. C., and Moore, F. T.: A preliminary report on the use of a local flap and peg bone graft for lengthening a short thumb. *Br. J. Plast. Surg., 3*:34–39, 1951.

Huguier, P. C.: Considérations anatomiques et physiologiques sur le rôle du pouce et sur la chirurgie de cet organe. *Arch. Gén. Méd., 2*:404–421; 567–580; 692–707, 1873. Also in *1*:54–82, 1874.

Irwin, C. E.: Transplants to the thumb to restore function of opposition. End results. *South Med. J., 35*:257–262, 1942.

Iselin, M., and Murat, J.: Restauration du pouce par pollicisation du deuxième métacarpien. *Presse Méd., 45*:1099–1102, 1937.

Iselin, M., and Schaffarz, R.: Zum Problem der Chirurgie der Mittelhand: Die Metacarpalhand. *Z. Dtsch. Chir., 299*:88–95, 1961–62.

Jeffrey, C. C.: A case of pollicization of the index finger. *J. Bone Joint Surg., 39*:120–123, 1957.

Jepson, P. N.: Transformation of the middle finger into a thumb. *Minn. Med., 8*:552–553, 1925.

Johnson, H. A.: Formation of a functional thumb post with sensation in phocomelia. *J. Bone Joint Surg., 49A*:327–332, 1967.

Joyce, J. L.: A new operation for the substitution of a thumb. *Br. J. Surg., 5*:499–504, 1918.

Joyce, J. L.: The results of a new operation for the substitution of a thumb. *Br. J. Surg., 16*:362–369, 1928.

Kallio, K. E.: Sur les opérations plastiques due pouce. *Acta Chir. Scand., 93*:231–253, 1946.

Kaplan, I.: Primary pollicization of injured index finger following crush injury. *Plast. Reconstr. Surg., 37*:531–535, 1966.

Kaplan, I., and Plaschkes, J.: One-stage pollicization of little finger. *Br. J. Plast. Surg., 13*:272–276, 1961.

Karewski, F.: Zur Funktionierung des verkrüppelten Daumens. *Dtsch. Z. Chir., 153*:423–425, 1920.

Karfik, V.: Cartilage as a substitute for the finger skeleton. *Trans. Second Internat. Congress Plast. Surg.,* pp. 234–235, 1960.

Kazakewitch, J.: Reconstruction of the thumb by Nicoladini's method. (In Russian.) *Kirurgija, 7*:69–74, 1940.

Kelikian, H.: The crippled hand. *In American Academy of Orthopaedic Surgeons Instructional Course Lectures.* J. W. Edwards, Ann Arbor, Michigan, Vol. XIV, pp. 163–182, 1957.

Kelikian, H., and Bintcliffe, E. W.: Functional restoration of the thumb. Pollicization of the index. *Surg. Gynecol. Obstet., 83*:807–814, 1946.

Kelikian, H., and Daumanian, A.: Congenital anomalies of the hand Part. II. *J. Bone Joint Surg., 39A*:1249–1266, 1957.

Kelikian, H., and Daumanian, A. A.: Skin grafts in hand surgery. *Clin. Orthop., 9*:205–226, 1957.

Kelikian, H., and Daumanian, A.: Some problems of hand surgery. *Surg. Clin. N. Am., 37*:1–15, 1957.

Kelleher, J. C., and Sullivan, J. G.: Thumb reconstruction by fifth digit transposition. *Plast. Reconstr. Surg., 21*:470–478, 1958.

Kelleher, J. C., and Sullivan, J. G.: Thumb reconstruction by fifth digit transposition. *Trans. Third Internat. Congress Plast. Surg.,* pp. 968–975, 1964.

Kelly, A. P., Jr.: Subtotal reconstruction of the thumb. *A.M.A. Arch. Surg., 78*:583–585, 1959.

Kessler, I.: Five-fingered hand: one-stage pollicization of radial finger. *Israel J. Med. Sci., 6*:280–283, 1970.

Klapp, R.: Ueber einige kleinere plastische Operationen an Fingern und Hand. *Dtsch. Z. Chir., 118*:479–482, 1912.

Kleinschmidt, O.: Zum Ersatz des Daumens durch die zweite Zehe. *Arch. Klin. Chir., 164*:809–811, 1931.

Klemm, P.: Plastische Operationen an den Händen. *Arch. Klin. Chir., 96*:181–194, 1911.

Köster, K. H.: Plastische Operationen bei Verlust des Daumens. *Acta Orthop. Scand., 9*:115–131, 1938.

Kraft, F.: Ueber Ersatz von Fingern durch Zehentransplantation. (Dactyloplastik). *Wien. Klin. Wochenschr., 19*:1443–1447, 1906.

Kraft, R.: Daumenplastik bei vollständigem Fingerverlust. *Dtsch. Z. Chir., 226*:426–430, 1930.

Krause, F.: Ersatz des Daumens aus der grossen Zehe. *Klin. Wochenschr., 34*:1527–1528, 1906.

Kuhn, H.: Reconstruction du pouce par "lambeau de Hilgenfeldt." *Ann. Chir. Plast., 6*:259–268, 1961.

Kuslik, M. I.: Transplantation of a toe according to the method of Nicoladoni. *Arch. Surg., 32*:123–130, 1936.

Labunskaya, O. V.: Transplantation of toes for fingers. *Ann. Surg., 102*:1–4, 1935.

Lambret, O.: Résultat éloigné d'une transplantation du gros orteil en remplacement du pouce. *Bull. Soc. Chir.* (Paris), *46*:689–695, 1920.

Lambrinudi, C.: Plastic operation for congenital absence of thumb. *Proc. R. Soc. Med.,* (Sec. Orthopedics), *31*:181–183, 1938.

Landivar, A.: Falangizacion del primer metacarpino. Operacion de Wiezerjewsky y Dega. *Bol. Soc. Cir.* (Buenos Aires), *23*:637–645, 1939.

Larry, R.: Résultat éloigné d'une disarticulation des doigts de milieu et de leurs métacarpiens (pince de homard). *Lyon Chir., 38*:77, 1943.

Lassar, G. N.: Reconstruction of a digit following loss of all fingers with preservation of the thumb. *J. Bone Joint Surg., 41A*:519–523, 1959.

Lauenstein, C.: Ein neuer Vorschlag, auf operativem Wege die Brauchbarkeit der daumenlosen Hand zu verbessern: *Dtsch. Med. Wochenschr., 14*:612–613, 1888.

LeMer, A., Foray, J., and Penot, B.: Pollicisation du médius pour néo-pouce gauche chez un enfant amputé de l'avant-bras droit, selon la technique de Boron et Fabre. *Lyon Chir., 61*:394–397, 1965.

Lenormant, C.: Le traitement des mutilations des doigts et en particulier du pouce par les autoplasties et transplantations. *Presse Méd., 28*:223–227, 1920.

Letac, R.: Reconstruction du pouce detruit par pollicisation de l'annulaire ou du 5e doigt. *Mem. Acad. Chir., 78*:262–264, 1952.

Letac, R.: Pollicization of the ring finger. *J. Internat. Coll. Surg., 22*:649–655, 1954.

Lewin, M. L.: Partial reconstruction of thumb in a one-stage operation. *J. Bone Joint Surg., 35*:573–576, 1953.

Lewin, M. L.: Sensory island flap in osteoplastic reconstruction of the thumb. *Am. J. Surg., 109*:227–229, 1965.

Littler, J. W.: Subtotal reconstruction of the thumb. *Plast. Reconstr. Surg., 10*:215–226, 1952.

Littler, J. W.: The neurovascular pedicle method of digital transposition for reconstruction of the thumb. *Plast. Reconstr. Surg., 12*:303–319, 1953.

Littler, J. W.: Neurovascular skin island transfer in reconstructive hand surgery. *Trans. Second Internat. Congress Plast. Surg.,* pp. 175–178, 1960.

Littler, J. W.: Principles of reconstructive surgery of the hand. *In* Converse, J. M., (ed.): *Reconstructive Plastic Surgery.* Philadelphia, W. B. Saunders Co., Vol. IV, pp. 1612–1673, 1964.

Littler, J. W.: *Current Practice in Orthopedic Surgery.* St. Louis, C. V. Mosby Co., Vol. 3, pp. 157–172, 1966.

Luksch, L.: Ueber eine neue Methode zum Ersatz des verlorenen Daumens. *Verh. Dtsch. Ges. Chir., 32*:221–223, 1903.

Lyle, H. H. M.: The formation of a new thumb by Klapp's method. *Ann. Surg., 59*:767, 1914.

Lyle, H. H. M.: Deformity of hand — formation of a new thumb from the stump of the first metacarpal. *Ann. Surg., 74*:121, 1921.

Lyle, H. H. M.: The formation of a new thumb from the first metacarpus. *Ann. Surg., 76*:121–127, 1922.

Lyle, H. H. M.: The disabilities of the hand and their physiological treatment. *Ann. Surg., 78*:816–845, 1923.

Machol: Beitrag zur Daumenplastik. *Beitr. Klin. Chir., 114*:181–188, 1919.

Maltz, M.: Reconstruction of thumb: a new technic. *Am. J. Surg., 58*:429–433, 1942.

Manasse, P.: Vorstellung eines Falles mit Daumenersatz und Fingerauswechselung. *Klin. Wochenschr., 56*:717–718, 1919.

Marcer, E.: Pollicizzazione dell'indice e del secondo metacarpo. *Minerva Ortop., 2*:42–48, 1951.

Matev, I.: Angeborene Daumenlosigkeit. *Z. Orthop., 102*:166–169, 1966.

Matev, I. B.: Thumb reconstruction after amputation at the metacarpophalangeal joint by bone-lengthening. *J. Bone Joint Surg., 52A*:957–965, 1970.

Matthews, D.: Congenital absence of functioning thumb. *Plast. Reconstr. Surg., 26*:487–493, 1960. See also *Arch Klin. Chir., 299*:95–99, 1961–1962.

Matthews, D.: Congenital abnormalities of the thumb. *Proc. R. Soc. Med.* (Sect. Plast. Surg.), *62*:53–55, 1969.

May, H.: *Reconstructive and Reparative Surgery.* Second edition. Philadelphia, F. A. Davis Co., pp. 784–828, 1958.

McGregor, I. A., and Simonetta, C.: Reconstruction of the thumb by composite bone-skin flap. *Br. J. Plast. Surg., 17*:37–48, 1964.

McLaughlin, C. R.: Reconstruction du pouce par la méthode de Gillies. *Ann. Chir. Plast., 3*:15, 1958.

Meyer, A. W.: Ueber Fingerplastik. *Münch. Med. Wochenschr., 59*:2506, 1912.

Meyer, H.: Der plastische Ersatz des Daumens. *Beitr. Klin. Chir., 119*:286–400, 1920.

Meyer-Wildisen, R.: Differenzierungsplastik bei Daumenverlust. *Helv. Med. Acta, 6*:872–873, 1940.

Michon, J.: Le pouce sans doigts. *Chirurgie, 96*:433–438, 1970.

Micotti, R.: Neofalangizzazione del pollice amputato allo sua base. *Arch. Ortop., 41*:481–492, 1925.

Mikhail, I. K.: Reconstruction of the amputated thumb. *A.M.A. Arch. Surg., 76*:372–378, 1958.

Mirabaha, M.: Pollicization of the middle finger. *J. Int. Coll. Surg., 43*:522–528, 1965.

Mocci, A., and Massara, F. S.: Sul trattamento chirurgico di una rara deformita congenita della mano. *Ortop. Traum. App. Mot., 30*:227–233, 1962.

Moore, F. T.: The technique of pollicization of the index finger. *Br. J. Plast. Surg., 1*:60–68, 1948–1949.

Morandi, G.: Indicazioni e risultati della riconstruzione chirurgica del pollice. *Chir. Organi. Mov., 30*:41–51, 1946.

Moutier, G.: Les procédés operatoires de restauration du pouce. *J. Chir., 19*:225–244, 1922.

Müller, G. M.: Construction of a palmar post. *Br. J. Plast. Surg., 3*:47–49, 1950.

Müller, W.: Anatomische Studien zur Frage des Daumenersatzes. *Beitr. Klin. Chir., 120*:595–598, 1920.

Murat, J.: *Restauration du Pouce per Pollicisation.* Thèse. Paris, Vigot Frères, pp. 1–101, 1936.

Murray, A. R.: Reconstructive surgery of the hand with special reference to digital transplantation. *Br. J. Surg., 34*:131–140, 1946.

Müsham, R.: Ueber Ersatz des Daumens durch die grosse Zehe. *Berl. Klin. Wochenschr., 44*:1045–1047, 1918.

Müsham, R.: Fingerplastik. *Zentralbl. Chir., 53*:585–588, 1926.

Muskat: Gewinnung eines Daumenersatzes ohne Operation. *Arch. Orthop. Unfallchir., 16*:255–259, 1919.

Nasta, R., Balcu, St., and Vladescu, V.: Un cas de falangisare al primului metacarpien. *Rev. Chir.* (Bucharest), *37*:234–237, 1934.

Nemethi, E.: Reconstruction of the distal part of the thumb after traumatic amputation. *J. Bone Joint Surg., 42A*:375–391, 1960.

Neuhaueser, H.: Ein neues Operationsverfahren zum Ersatz von Fingerverlusten. *Berl. Klin. Wochenschr.,* No. *18*:1287–1290, 1916.

Neuhof, H.: Transplantation of toe for missing finger. *Ann. Surg., 112*:291–293, 1940.

Nicoladoni, C.: Daumenplastik. *Wien. Klin. Wochenschr., 10*:663–665, 1897.

Nicoladoni, C.: Daumenplastik und organischer Ersatz der Fingerspitze (Anticheiroplastik und Daktyloplastik). *Arch. Klin. Chir., 69*:695–703, 1900.

Noesske, K.: Chirurgische Demonstrationen, zum Teil neue Operationsmethoden. *Münch. Med. Wochenschr., 58*:1157–1158, 1911.

Noesske, K.: Ueber Ersatz des Metakarpus samt verlorenen Daumens durch operative Umstellung des Zeigefingers. *Münch. Med. Wochenschr., 67*:465–466, 1920.

Novickij, S.: Total transplantation of a toe to take the place of a thumb. (In Russian.) *Vestnik. Chir., 57*:352–361, 1939.

Nuzzi, O.: Ricostruzione dell pollice mediante falangizzazione del 1° metacarpo. *Ann. Ital. Chir., 2*:957–963, 1923.

Oberlin, S.: Reconstitution du pouce. *Traite Technique Chirurgicale.* Paris, Masson et Cie, Tome 1, pp. 626–648, 1955.

Oehlecker, F.: Aus dem Gebiete der Knochen- und Gelenktransplantation. *Bruns. Beitr. Chir., 162*:135–181, 1922.

Oehlecker, F.: Aus dem Gebeite der Knochen- und Gelenktransplantation. *Bruns. Beitr. Chir., 162*:135–181, 1922.

Oehlecker, F.: Endergebnis der Ueberpflanzung der grossen Zehe als Daumenersatz. *Arch. Klin. Chir., 189*:674–680, 1937.

Ombrédanne, L.: Constitution autoplastique d'un pouce prenant au moyen du leur métacarpien. *Bull. Soc. Chir. Paris, 46*:158–161, 1920.

Oudard: Greffes des doigts par transplantation. *Rev. d'Orthop.,* (3 s.), *9*:413–427, 1922.

Pachner, E.: Autoplastiche del pollice. *Arch. Ortop., 48*:817–828, 1932.

Palmstierna, K.: En tumplastik. *Nord. Med., 1*:243–244, 1939.

Parin, B. V.: Reconstruction of the thumb. (In Russian): Trudy Molotovsk. *Gas. Med. Inst., 21*:125–142, 1942.

Parisel, C.: Deux cas d'atrophie congénitale due pouce. Essai de reconstitution par greffe osseuse. *Bull. Soc. Belge d'Orthop., 6*:231–233, 1934.

Park, R.: Congenital defect of forearm, absence of radius, clubhand and plastic operation. *Trans. Am. Orthop. Assoc., 14*:144–146, 1901. See also *Philad. Med. J., 8*:993, 1901.

Peacock, E. E., Jr.: Reconstruction of the thumb. *In* Flynn, J. Edward, (ed.): *Hand Surgery.* Baltimore, Williams and Wilkins Co., pp. 561–582, 1966.

Perthes, G.: Plastischer Ersatz des verlorenen Daumens. *Münch. Med. Wochenschr.,* No. *4*:113, 1919.

Perthes, G.: Ueber Daumenplastik. *Zentralbl. Chir., 48*:669–670, 1921.

Perthes, G.: Ueber plastischen Daumenersatz insbesondere bei Verlust des ganzen Daumenstrahles. *Arch. Orthop. Unfallchir., 19*:199–214, 1921.

Perthes, G., and Jungling, O.: Ueber Ergänzungsprothesen bei Versteifung sämtlicher Finger. *Münch. Med. Wochenschr., 64*:1221–1222, 1917.

Petersen, N.: Plastic reconstruction of the thumb. *S. Afr. Med. J., 17*:137–138, 1943.

Petit, L. H.: Eclatement de la main gauche. Arrachement de tous les doigts, sauf le cinquième. Reconstitution d'une pince utile par greffe du gros orteil droit a la place du pouce. *Bull. Soc. Chir. Paris, 47*:725–729, 1921.

Pierce, G. W.: Reconstruction of thumb after loss. *Surg. Gynecol. Obstet., 45*:825–826, 1927.

Pierce, G. W., and O'Connor, G. B.: Pedicle flap patterns for hand reconstruction. *Surg. Gynecol. Obstet., 65*:523–527, 1937.

Pieri, G.: Ricostruzione del pollice del moncone della falange basale. *Chir. Organi. Mov., 3*:325–331, 1919.

Pieri, G.: Contrivuto alla recostruzione plastica del pollice. *Chir. Organi. Mov., 11*:89–93, 1926.

Pierre, M., Carcassonne, M., and Guasconi, H.: Reconstruction du pouce par la méthode autoplastique. *J. Chir., 68*:449–460, 1952.

Piotet, G.: Remarques sur la reconstruction du pouce et de la main. *Helv. Chir. Acta, 25*:345–349, 1958.

Polonsky, B.: Reconstruction of missing thumb. *S. Afr. Med. J., 23*:812–814, 1958.

Porzelt, W.: Erfolgreiche Daumenplastik aus der Grosszehe der Gegenseite, 4-½ Jahre nach missaglücktem Transplantations-versuch. *Arch. Klin. Chir., 135*:340–355, 1925.

Porzelt, W.: Daumenersatz aus dem verstümmelten Zeigefinger unter Erhaltung der Trennungsfalte zum Mittelfinger. *Der. Chirurg., 5*:61–65, 1933.

Prpìc, I.: Reconstruction of the thumb immediately after injury. *Br. J. Plast. Surg., 17*:46–52, 1964.

Rank, B. K., and Wakefield, A. R.: Reconstruction of opposition digits for mutilated hands. *Aust. N. Z. J. Surg., 17*:172–188, 1947–1948.

Reghini, A.: Pollicizzazione dell'indice in primo tempo per grave trauma. *Chir. Organi. Mov., 33*:294–296, 1949.

Reid, D. A. C.: Reconstruction of the thumb. *J. Bone Joint Surg., 42B*:444–465, 1960.

Reid, D. A. C.: Pollicization—an appraisal. *The Hand, 1*:27–31, 1969.

Rettig, H.: Zur operativen Behandlung angeborener Daumenfehlbildungen und ihrez Funktionsstörungen. *Arch. Orthop. Unfallchir., 60*:132–137, 1966.

Rettig, H. G., Mans, G., and Seibel, E.: Ein Beitrag zur Funktionsbeurteilung und Funktionsverbesserung von Daumenmissbildungen. *Arch. Orthop. Unfallchir., 60*:132–137, 1966.

Riedel: Niloladoni'sche Daumenplastik. *Berl. Klin. Wochenschr., 55*(1):559, 1918.

Righni, A.: Pollicizzazione dell'indice in primo tempo per grave trauma della mano. *Chir. Organi Mov., 33*:294–296, 1949.

Rinaldo, M.: Neofalangizzazione del pollice amputato alla sua base. *Arch. Ortop., 41*:481–492, 1925.

Riordan, D. C.: Congenital absence of the radius. *J. Bone Joint Surg., 37A*:1129–1141, 1955.

Ritzmann, W.: Primäre Daumenersatzplastik. *Chirurgie, 23*:315–317, 1952.

Rogova, K. F.: Phalangization of first metacaral bone. (In Russian.) *Chirurgija, 11*:150–151, 1939.

Roullet, J., Hoirclerc, J. A., and Landreau, F. R.: De la pollicisation. *Lyon Chir., 67*:114–121, 1971.

Roux, F.: *Contribution a l'Étude de la Reconstitution Ostéoplastique du Pouce d'Emblée en Traumatologie.* Thèse. Paris, Imprimérie R. Foulon, pp. 13–58, 1959.

Salamanca, D. F. E., Jr., and Lopez, D. R.: Cirurgia plastica y reparadora del pulgar. *Rev. Lat. Am. Cir. Plast., 6*:287–338, 1962.

Sandblom, P.: Tumplastik genom falangisation av metacarpal. I. *Nord. Med., 40*:2403–2410, 1948.

Schepelmann, E.: Plastischer Ersatz bei Totaldefekt des rechten Daumens. *Z. Orthop. Chir., 34*:174–181, 1914.

Schepelmann, E.: Weitere Erfahrungen ueber Fingerplastik. *Z. Orthop. Chir., 35*:827–850, 1916.

Schepelmann, E.: Das spätere Schicksal einer Daumenplastik. *Z. Orthop. Chir., 39*:181–200, 1920.

Schmiedt, W.: Beitrag zur Daumenplastik. *Dtsch. Z. Chir., 145*:420–423, 1918.

Schosserer, W.: Ueber primäre Plastiken bei Hand- und Fingerverletzungen. *Dtsch. Z. Chir., 233*:434–440, 1931.

Schroeder, W. E., and Plummer, S. C.: Congenital absence of metacarpal bone and part of the first phalanx of the thumb. *Chicago Med. Recorder, 11*:187–188, 1896.

Seiffert, K.: Hand- und Fingerplastiken. *Arch. Orthop. Unfallchir., 28*:370–375, 1920.

Sels, M.: *Les Méthodes Actuelles de Reconstitution du Pouce Amputé.* Thèse, Paris, Editions A. G. E. M. P., 1963.

Shaw, M. H., and Wilson, I. S. Pl: An early pollicization. *Br. J. Plast. Surg., 3*:214–215, 1950.

Shirokov, B. A.: Phalangization of the first metacarpal bone in plastic restoration of thumb. (In Russian.) *Khirurgjia, 7*:115–122, 1939.

Smith, R. J.: Surgery of thumb reconstruction. *Bull. Hosp. Joint Dis., 26*:56–58, 1965.

Soiland, H.: Lengthening a finger with the "on the top" method. *Acta Chir. Scand., 122*:184–186, 1961.

Spencer, W. G.: Plastic operations of the thumb. *In* Milford, H., (ed.): *Medical Science Abstracts and Reviews.* London, Oxford University Press, Vol. III, pp. 29–35, 1920–1921.

Spitzy, H.: Einen Daumen Operativ. *Berl. Klin. Wochenschr., 55*:363, 1918.

Stefani, A. E., and Kelly, A. P., Jr.: Reconstruction of the thumb: a one-stage procedure. *Br. J. Plast. Surg., 15*:289–292, 1962.

Szlazak, J.: Total reconstruction of the thumb. *Plast. Reconstr. Surg., 8*:67–70, 1951.

Takazawa, H., et al.: 3 cases of pollicization by Littler method. (In Japanese.) *Orthop. Surg. Tokyo, 18*:401–402, 1967.

Tanzer, R. C., and Littler, J. W.: Reconstruction of the thumb by transposition of an adjacent thumb. *Plast. Reconstr. Surg., 3*:533–547, 1948.

Tierny, A., and Iselin, M.: Restauration d'un pouce detruit par pollicization de l'index. *Mém. Acad. Chir., 63*:1007–1012, 1937.

Tonnini, L.: Ricerche sull'anatomofisiologia del pollice e dell'indice in riguardo ad un metodo di sostituzione del pollice. *Chir. Organi. Mov., 4*:213–238, 1920.

Tubiana, R., and Duparc, J.: Un procédé nouveau de reconstruction d'un pouce sensible. *Mém. Acad. Chir., 86*:264, 1960.

Uselac, O.: Reconstruction of the thumb: another possibility. *Br. J. Plast. Surg., 23*:85–89, 1970.

Verdan, C.: Hautplastiken bei der Wiederherstellungschirurgie der verletzten Hand—Indikation und Technik. *Arch. Klin. Chir., 299*:69–82, 1961–1962.

Verdan, C.: The reconstruction of the thumb. *Surg. Clin. N. Am., 48*:1033–1062, 1968.

Verdan, C., Tubiana, R., Harrison, S., and Littler, W.: Reconstruction of the thumb. (Panel discussion.) *Trans. Third Internat. Congress Plast. Surg.,* pp. 25–27, 1964.

Verrall, P. J.: Three cases of reconstruction of the thumb. *Br. Med. J., 2*:775, 1919.

Vogt, P.: *Die chirurgischen Krankheiten der oberen Extremitäten.* Stuttgart, Verlag von Ferdinand Enke, pp. 354–358, fig. 225, 1881.

White, W. F.: Pollicization for the missing thumb, traumatic and congenital. *The Hand, 1*:23–26, 1969.

White, W. F.: Fundamental priorities in pollicization. *J. Bone Joint Surg., 52B*:438–443, 1970.

Wierzejewski, I.: Daumenstumpfbildung. *Münch. Med. Wochenschr., 66*:19–20, 1919.

Wilflingseder, P.: Ein neues Verfahren zur Daumenplastik. *Arch. Orthop. Unfallchir., 45*:617–623, 1953.

Wilson, J. S. P., and Braithwaite, F.: The autografting of an amputated thumb. *Trans. Third Internat. Congress Plast. Surg.,* pp. 1012–1017, 1964.

Wittek, A.: Erfolgreicher Daumenersatz. *Der. Chirurg., 13*:577–581, 1941.

Young, F.: Transplantation of toes for fingers. *Surgery, 20*:117–123, 1946.

Zancolli, E.: Transplantation of the index finger in congenital absence of the thumb. *J. Bone Joint Surg., 42A*:658–660, 1960.

Zarotti, F.: Pollicizzazione dell'indice, resorse vasculari. Atti dell XLVII Congresso della *Soc. Ital. Ortop. Trauma., 47*:410–415, 1962.

Zoltan, J.: Su alouni problemi della chirurgia ricostruttiva della mano lesa. *Minerva Chir., 16*:1453–1467, 1961.

Zrubecky, G.: Zur Wiederherstellung der Sensibilität an der Kuppe eines aus Bauchhaut gebildeten, gefühllosen Daumens. *Zentralbl. Chir., 85*:1671–1679, 1960.

Zrubecky, G.: Aesthetische Gesichtspunkte der Chirurgie der Fingerendglieder. *Z. Dtsch. Chir., 299*:105, 1961–1962.

Zrubecky, G.: Operativer Daumenersatz an beiden Händen. *Z. Dtsch. Chir., 299*:142–144, 1961–1962.

Zrubecky, G.: Traitement operatoire dell'ectrodactylie du pouce. *Ann. Chir. Plast., 9*:187–190, 1964.

Zsulyevich, I.: Ein Fall von plastischem Daumenersatz. *Der. Chirurg., 10*:433–435, 1938.

Chapter Twenty-Five

DEFECTS OF THE ULNAR RAY

In longitudinal absence of the ulnar ray, any or all of the following elements may be missing: the ulna, the ulnar digits and their metacarpals, and the intervening carpal bones. When the ulna is entirely absent or deficient in its distal extremity, the hand deviates in the ulnar direction; this deformity is referred to as ulnar clubhand or manus valga. As in the case of radial ray defect, ulnar hemimelia can be intercalary or terminal. Terminal longitudinal defect of the ulnar ray may be total or partial. In total terminal deficiency, all the skeletal components of the ulnar ray from the elbow to the tip of the little finger, and sometimes including the next two or three digits, are missing. Partial deficiencies of the ulnar ray are qualified as being proximal or distal. In proximal deficiency, the ulna is missing in part or entirely; in distal defect, the ulnar digital rays are absent. The intervening carpal ossicles may be missing in either proximal or distal partial terminal deficiency. Occasionally, in partial distal terminal deficiency, the carpal end of the ulna or its styloid is also missing. Absence of the ulnar styloid alone is classed with intercalary defects (Figs. 25–1 and 25–2).

The ulna serves as the main skeletal element of the forearm at the elbow. It supports the elbow in the same manner that the radius supports the wrist. In defects of the ulnar ray, the elbow bears the brunt of distortion; deformities at the wrist are minimal. At the elbow, the proximal end of the radius is often fused with the humerus or is dislocated. The radius is short. The hand tilts in the ulnar direction and is slightly flexed. This deformity is not as conspicuous as the radiopalmar deflection of the hand seen in connection with defects of the radial ray. In the hand there is an increasing tendency for the digital rays to fail as one passes from the radial to the ulnar aspect. The surviving digits exhibit degrees of stunting, syndactyly, or symphalangism. Defects of the ulnar ray are only occasionally bilateral; they are seldom symmetrical. Absence of the ulna is more often incomplete. Bilateral defects of the ulna and short upper limbs are often confused with phocomelia (Fig. 25–3).

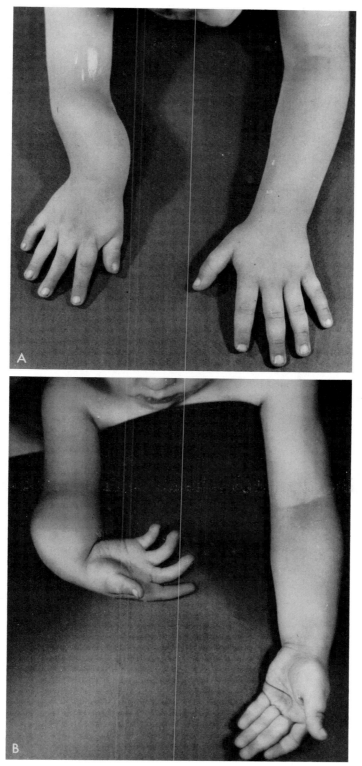

Figure 25–1 Shortness of the limb and posture of the hand in ulnar ray defect. *A*, Dorsal view of the upper limbs. *B*, Volar view.

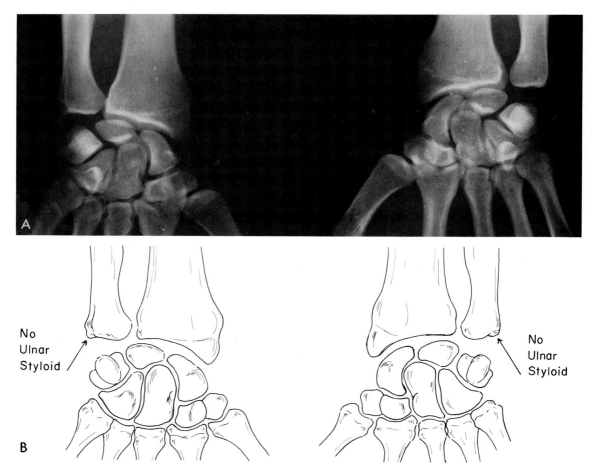

Figure 25-2   Intercalary defect of the ulnar ray: bilateral absence of the ulnar styloid. *A*, Dorsopalmar roentgenograph of the right and left wrists of an adult man. *B*, Sketch illustrating the same.

OCCURRENCE

Priestley (1856) described a neonate whose right ulna was entirely absent, and the hand had only a thumb and an index finger. Priestley contrasted this deformity with another type of ectrodactyly in which "the force directing or giving rise to malformation, seems to have acted in a transverse direction, lopping off the fingers and shortening the limb in some portion of its length." In the case Priestley himself presented, "the amputation seems to have been longitudinal, parallel to the axis, depriving the limb not only of its three inner fingers, but, at the same time, of the inner half of the hand, with the ulna and its dependencies in the arm as far as the elbow." This perceptive clinician anticipated his more recent colleagues by almost 100 years in making a distinction between longitudinal and transverse deficiencies or hemimelias.

Defects of the ulnar ray are not as common as those of the radial trajectory. Prior to the advent of roentgenography, Kümmel (1895) could collect only 13 cases of ulnar deficiency from the literature as compared to 69 absences of the radial component. Rabaud and Hovelacque (1924) cited only 72 deficiencies of

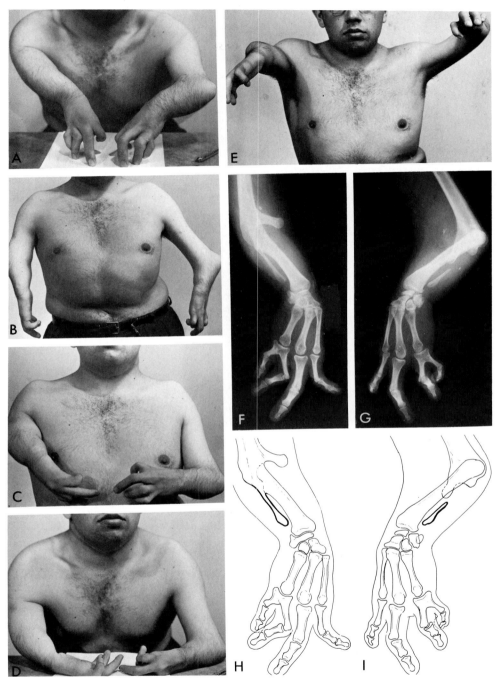

Figure 25–3 Bilateral ulnar ray defect simulating phocomelia. *A, B, C, D,* and *E,* The upper limbs of the 15-year-old boy shown in Figure 5–8 with bilateral ulnar ray defect simulating phocomelia and often qualified with the adjective phocomeloid. *F,* Dorsovolar roentgenograph of the right upper limb: there is complete radiohumeral ankylosis; the ulna has the appearance of a stalactite hanging from the humerus; both the proximal and distal rows of carpal bones are coalesced. *G,* Dorsovolar roentgenograph of the left upper limb: on this side there is no radiohumeral ankylosis; the radial head is dislocated and the ulna is seen as a detached sliver; there are four discrete carpal bones. *H* and *I* illustrate the roentgenograph above each.

the ulna as against 268 cases of radial ray defect. Birch-Jensen (1949) gave the statistic of radial ray defect as 1 in about 31,000 births and ulnar deficiency as 1 in 100,000 births.

TYPES

Kümmel (1895) distinguished three main classes of ulnar ray defect. In the first group he placed cases of normal radiohumeral articulation; the second group comprised cases of radiohumeral ankylosis; and the third group included those with dislocation of the radial head. Lausecker (1954) considered five categories: (1) deficiency of ulnar digital rays, (2) the same deficiency plus absence of the distal portion or even of the entire ulna, (3) defect in the midshaft of the na, (4) absence of the ulna or ulnar digital ray, or both, associated with bilateral malformation of the radial digital rays, and (5) deficiency of the ulna associated with defects of the long bones of the lower extremity, particularly with the fibula.

HEREDITY

Most reported cases of ulnar ray defect have been sporadic. Roberts (1886) described a 73-year-old man whose right ulna was absent along with the second to fifth digital rays and the intervening carpal bones — the pisiform, triquetrum, and hamate. On the left side, the ulna was present, but the middle, ring, and little fingers, with their metacarpals, were absent. One of the proband's sisters was said to have had a similarly deformed hand, as did the child of another sister. The inheritance in this instance is obviously autosomal dominant, but it is questionable whether Robert's case should be classified as isolated ulnar ray defect or as ulnar ray defect occurring in association with split hand complex. The deficiency of the ulna occurring in connection with split hand complex and multiple exostoses is inherited as an autosomal dominant trait; defects of the ulna seen in achondrogenesis and de Lange syndrome are considered to be recessive. Weyer's oligodactyly syndrome is sporadic. Some of the reported cases of mesomelic dwarfism of the ulna-fibula type seem to have been transmitted as dominant and others as recessive phenotypes. Hereditary cases of ulnar ray defect are far less common than those of the radial ray, which are rare enough.

EXOGENOUS INFLUENCES

In numerous reports concerning thalidomide embryopathy, one finds no mention of a defective ulna independent of an absent radius. The present author has seen one case — a boy with ulnar ray defect — which might possibly be ascribed to his mother's ingestion of thalidomide in early pregnancy.

Another boy with bilateral absence of the fourth and fifth digits had unrotated nonopposable thumbs, and the second and third digits of one hand were webbed. His mother wrote: "I had missed just one menstrual period but had slight spotting at about the time the period was due. Since I am the worrying type, I went to see an obstetrician.... He...told me to keep a record of my morning temperature.... It was while I was keeping this record that I caught a cold and one of the temperatures recorded was 104°.... The first missing period was due about January 15, 1965, and I would place this cold in time about the first week in February.... Tommy was born September 4, 1965, about two weeks before the predicted birth date. I don't remember how long the spotting went on—perhaps as long as a month. The obstetrician gave me pills to help me hold onto the pregnancy." The name of the "pills" was not revealed. Another mother, whose daughter was born with ulnar ray defect and absence of the sternocostal head of the ipsilateral pectoralis major muscle, reported that she had taken some pills for nervousness early in pregnancy (Fig. 25–4).

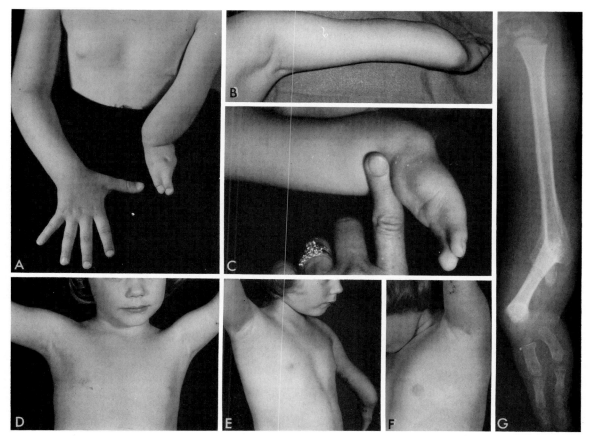

Figure 25–4 Unilateral defect of the ulnar ray associated with absence of the sternocostal head of the ipsilateral pectoralis major muscle. *A*, Dorsal view of both upper limbs of a four-year-old girl whose mother claimed to have taken some "pills" early in pregnancy. *B*, Radial view of the left upper limb. *C*, Volar view of the same. *D*, Frontal view showing sagging left nipple and absence of anterior axillary fold. *E*, Right axilla. *F*, Left axilla. *G*, Roentgenograph of the left upper limb, showing fusion of the radius and the remnant of the ulna with the humerus and two radial digits which are webbed together.

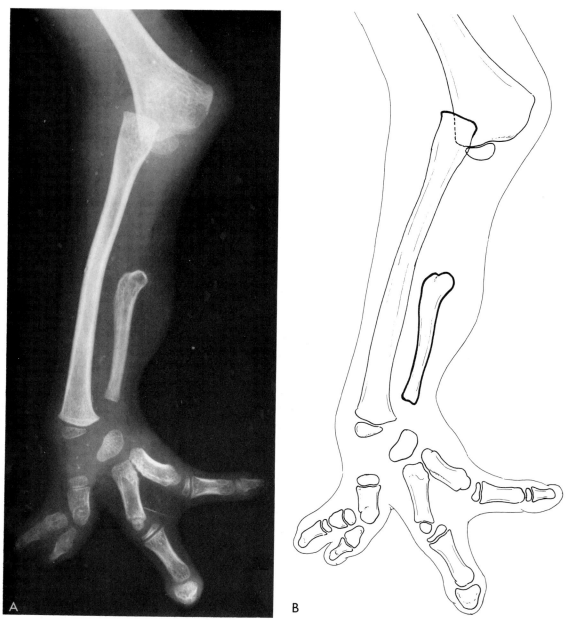

Figure 25–5   Dwarfed ulna with dislocated radial head and sundry malformations of the digits. *A*, Dorsovolar roentgenograph of the left elbow, forearm, wrist, and hand of a two-year-old child: the head of the radius is dislocated at the elbow; the ulna is diminutive but appears to possess an olecranon process which is far away from the elbow; at the wrist, the capitate and hamate bones are fused. The thumb is bifurcate; what appear to be ring and little fingers have two phalanges each. *B*, Sketch illustrating the same.

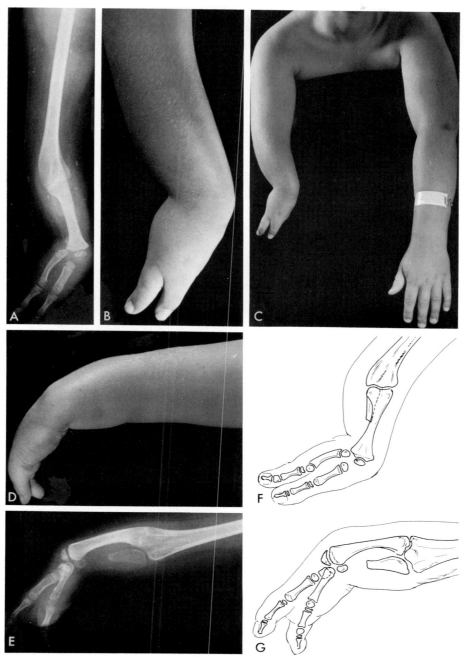

Figure 25–6 Partial terminal ulnar ray defect. *A*, Dorsovolar roentgenograph of the right upper limb of a seven-year-old boy. *B*, Dorsal view of the right forearm and hand. *C*, Dorsal view of both upper limbs. *D*, Radial view of the right forearm and hand. *E*, Roentgenograph of the same. *F* and *G*, Sketches illustrating the skeletal contents of right forearm and hand.

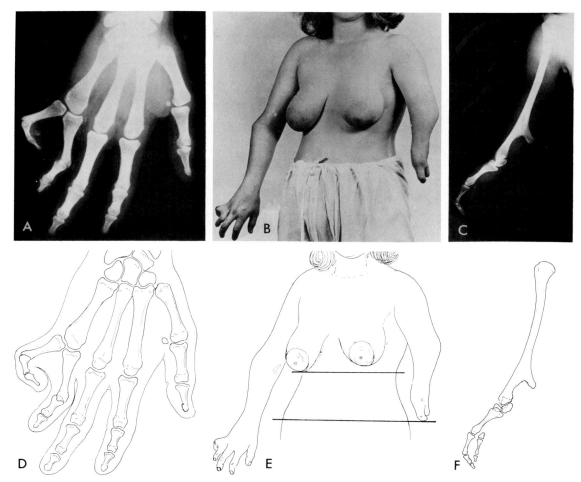

Figure 25–7   Bilateral asymmetrical defect of the ulnar ray. *A*, Dorsopalmar roentgenograph of the right hand of a 16-year-old girl with absent right fifth metacarpal, fusion of the left radius and humerus, and bidactylic left hand, one of the digits of which, probably the fifth, lacks metacarpal foundation. *B*, Frontal view of the torso and dorsal view of the upper limbs. *C*, Roentgenograph of the left upper limb: the humerus has fused with a dwarfed radius; there are two digits, one of which lacks a metacarpal. *D* and *F* illustrate the roentgenograph above each. *E* illustrates the photograph above it.

REGIONAL ASSOCIATIONS

Defects of the ulnar ray have a greater tendency to be accompanied by regional than by remote abnormalities. Absent sternocostal head of the ipsilateral pectoralis major muscle, ankylosis of the elbow, dislocation of the radial head, Madelung deformity, split hand, brachydactyly, symphalangism, syndactyly, and oligodactyly constitute the main regional accompaniments of ulnar ray defect. When it serves — which it preferentially does — as the seat of exostoses or enchondromatoses, the ulna is usually dwarfed and the longer radius dislocates at the elbow. Dislocation of the radial head is the most common regional accompaniment of defective ulna and ulnar oligodactyly (Figs. 25–5 to 25–13).

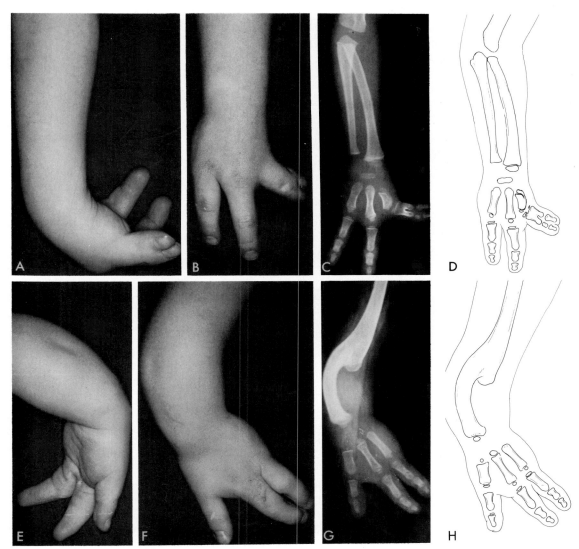

Figure 25–8 Ulnar ray defect. *A*, Radial view of the right forearm and hand of a two-year-old boy. *B*, Dorsal view. *C*, Dorsovolar roentgenograph: there is one carpal bone representing the coalesced hamate and capitate; two ulnar digital rays are missing; the first metacarpal is thick, probably caused by the confluence of the first and second metacarpals; the thumb is bifid—its radial component has two and its ulnar component three phalanges and the proximal ends of the basal phalanges are fused. *D*, Sketch illustrating the same. *E*, Ulnar view of the left forearm and hand. *F*, Dorsal view: the two ulnar digits had been webbed; they were surgically separated. *G*, Dorsovolar roentgenograph: there is radiohumeral coalescence; there is no ulna and no visible carpal bone as yet; two ulnar digital rays are missing and the second metacarpal has an epiphysis at each end. *H*, Sketch illustrating the same.

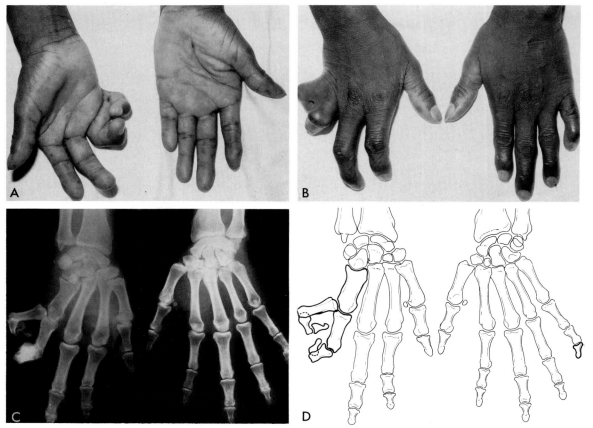

Figure 25–9   Intercalary defect of the left ulnar ray, with absent pisiform, missing or fused fifth metacarpal, camptodactyly of the ring and little fingers, and clinocamptodactyly of the right little finger. *A*, Palmar view of the hands of an adult man. *B*, Dorsal view. *C*, Dorsopalmar roentgenograph of the hands. *D*, Sketch illustrating the same.

REMOTE ASSOCIATIONS

Ulnar ray defect is not associated with as many distant malformations as is radial ray deficiency. Göller (1698) described a seven-month fetus with bilateral absence of the ulna and absence of four ulnar digits of each hand, leaving only the thumbs; in the lower extremities, both fibulas and all fibular toes were absent. Gessner's (1894) patient with ulnar ray defect had diaphragmatic hernia and uterus unicornis. In the case reported by Collins (1895), one fibula was missing and there were an imperforate anus, clubfoot deformity, and defective penis. Watt (1917) described a seven-month fetus with bilateral absence of the ulna, monodactylism, and diaphragmatic hernia. Kajon's (1921) patient with bilateral defect of the ulna had a bifid thumb on the right side. Ke Ping Jen (1937) noted the association of ulnar ray deficiency and defective tibia. Kozlowski's (1965) case of defective ulna had bilateral calcaneocuboid coalescence. Mackley and Heiple (1970) reported a patient with ulnar ray defect and scoliosis. Deficiencies of the ulna have also been recorded in connection with a few syndromes (Fig. 25–14).

(Text continued on page 882.)

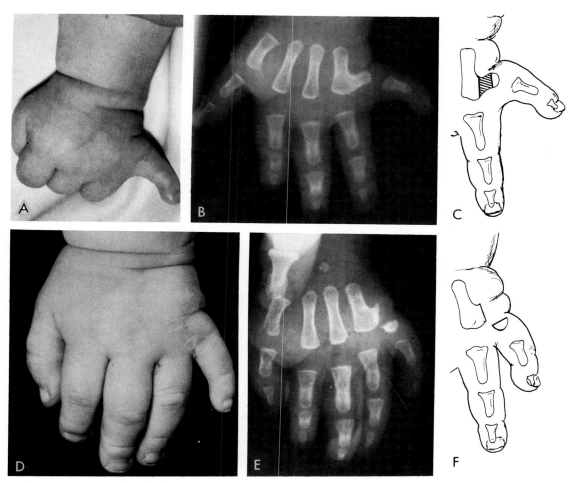

Figure 25–10   Distal intercalary defect of the ulnar ray, with absence of the proximal portion of the fifth metacarpal and fusion of the distal half with the fourth metacarpal. *A*, Dorsal view of the left hand of a newborn infant. *B*, Dorsopalmar roentgenograph of the left hand. *C*, Sketch illustrating the segment of bone removed to correct the ulnar angulation of the fifth digit. *D*, Postoperative dorsal view of the hand. *E*, Postoperative dorsopalmar roentgenograph. *F*, Sketch illustrating corrected stance of the little finger.

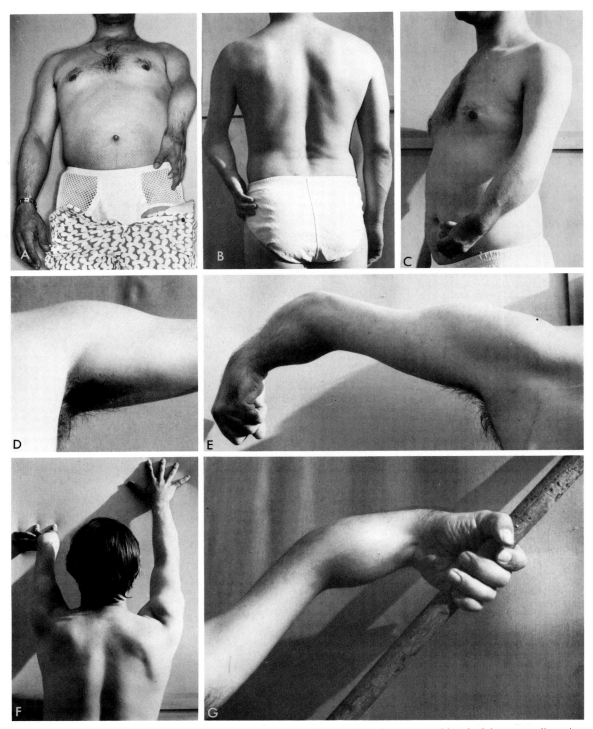

Figure 25–11   Ulnar ray defect associated with absence of the ipsilateral sternocostal head of the pectoralis major; ankylosis of the elbow; hypoplastic lunate, triquetrum, and hamate; and triangular middle phalanx with a broad ulnar base of the index finger, causing the ungual segment to tilt toward the thumb. *A, B, C,* and *F,* An adult man with a short, malformed left upper limb. *D,* Right axilla. *E,* Left axilla: the anterior axillary fold is absent. *G,* The functional propensity of the left hand.

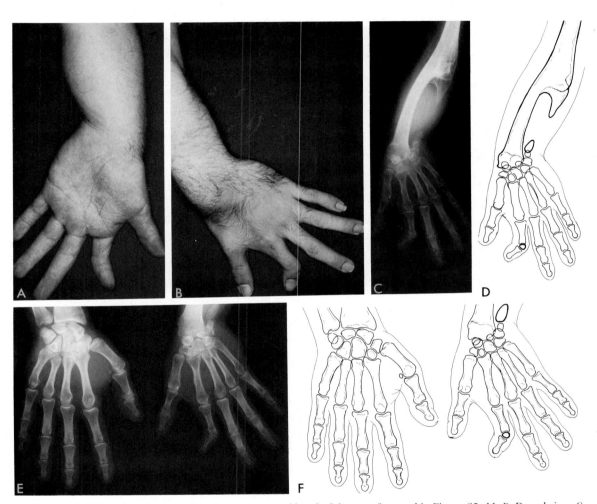

Figure 25–12 *A*, Palmar view of the left forearm and hand of the man featured in Figure 25–11. *B*, Dorsal view. *C*, Dorsovolar roentgenograph: the humerus is fused with the radius and the proximal remnant of the ulna; the ulnar shaft is missing; the distal end of the ulna is present in segments. *D*, Sketch illustrating the same. *E*, Dorsopalmar roentgenograph of the right and left hands: the left carpal lunate, triquetrum, and hamate are diminutive; the middle phalanx of the left index finger is represented by a small triangular ossicle, causing the ungual segment to tilt in the radial direction. *F*, Sketch illustrating the same.

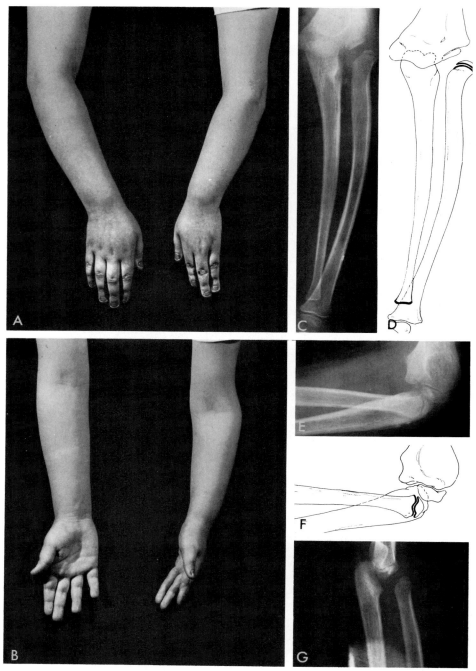

Figure 25–13 Partial terminal longitudinal defect of the ulnar ray accompanied by dislocation of the radial head. *A*, Dorsal view of both forearms and hands of a seven-year-old girl with missing left little finger. *B*, Palmar view of the right forearm and hand and radial view of the left forearm and hand, which failed to supinate fully. *C*, Dorsovolar roentgenograph of the left elbow and forearm: the ulna has no distal epiphysis and is short; the head of the radius is dislocated at the elbow. *D*, Sketch illustrating the same. *E*, Lateral roentgenograph of the left elbow, showing posterior dislocation of the radial head. *F*, Sketch illustrating the same. *G*, Dorsovolar roentgenograph of the left elbow following skeletal traction via the shaft of the radius: this procedure failed to bring the distal head of the radius down and exaggerated the separation between it and the proximal ulna.

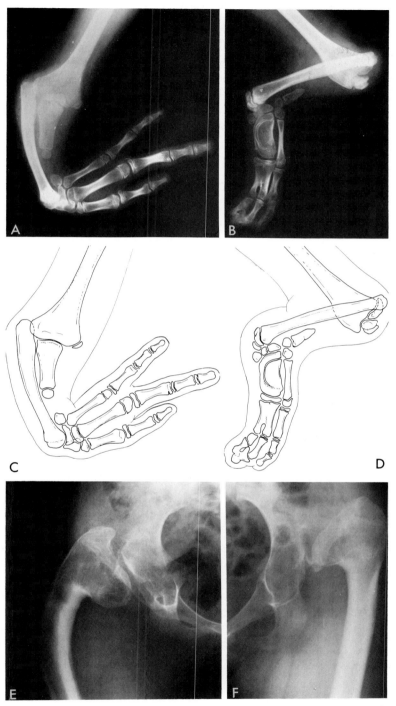

Figure 25–14 Bilateral ulnar ray defect associated with bilateral dislocation of the hip and micrognathia. *A,* Anteroposterior roentgenograph of the right forearm and hand of a 12-year-old girl with partial terminal longitudinal defect of the ulnar ray, including the distal portion of the ulna and the two ulnar digital rays: the radius is dislocated at the elbow. *B,* Anteroposterior roentgenograph of the left forearm and hand: here the proximal portion of the ulna is missing and the hand has three digital rays, two of which have effected almost total side-to-side bony union. *C* and *D* illustrate the roentgenograph above each. *E,* Anteroposterior roentgenograph of the right hip. *F,* Anteroposterior roentgenograph of the left hip.

DE LANGE DEGENERATION

This complex consists of primordial dwarfism, microcephaly and brachycephaly, retardation of psychomotor development, muscular hypertrophy, leonine features (characteristic facies with hypertrichosis) raucous voice, and malformations predominantly of the upper extremities. Among the latter are included stunted first metacarpal, hypoplastic middle phalanx of the little finger, monodactylic hands, and absence of forearm bones, usually the ulna.

MESOMELIC DWARFISM OF HYPERPLASTIC ULNA, FIBULA, MANDIBLE TYPE (Ophthalmomandibulomelic Dysplasia; Boomerang Bone Disease; Ulnafibular Dysplasia)

Absence of the fibula is the most common distant skeletal anomaly associated with defective ulnar ray. Guerin-Valmale and Jeanbrau (1899) dissected an infant with congenital dislocation of the elbow and ulnar deviation of the hand; the ulna was considerably shorter than the radius, and the index finger was dwarfed. Bertolotti (1913) described a variety of mesomelic dwarfism with symmetrical hypoplasia of the ulna, the metacarpals, and the middle phalanx of the little finger. The three central metatarsals were short, and the head of the fibula extended to a point about 2 cm. below the level of the tibial plateau.

Comparable anomalies have been reported by the following authors: Brailsford (1935), Helweg-Larsen and Morch (1950), Böök (1950), Grebe (1955), Blockey and Lawrie (1963), Reeves (1966), Cholmeley (1966), Reinhardt and Pfeiffer (1967), and Langer (1967). In all the reported cases, hypoplasia of the fibula alone, ulna alone, or of the ulna and fibula together appears to be the most constant feature. As in most conditions involving a disproportionately short ulna, the head of the radius is dislocated at the elbow, its shaft is curved, and its carpal articular surface simulates the obliquity seen in Madelung's deformity. The hand is deviated in the ulnar direction. Helweg-Larsen and Morch described the hand as being trident. Böök considered the configuration of the hand "intermediate between normal and isodactylic." Grebe's patients had small carpal bones, short metacarpals, and trapezoid middle phalanges of the index fingers, with radial deviation of the terminal segments. The two siblings reported by Blockey and Lawrie had "fixed flexion-deformity of the fingers and thumbs." The infant reported by Reeves had "clawing of the fingers and absence of the intrinsic muscles of the thumb."

Brailsford (1935) and Böök (1950) both made it clear that the parents of their patients were short in stature and had short fingers. Böök and Reinhardt and Pfeiffer (1967) considered the transmission of the trait in the cases they reported to be dominant. The inheritance in Grebe's cases — a brother and sister from a first-cousin marriage — was obviously recessive.

SICKLE CELL ANEMIA

Van Der Sar (1947) presented a patient with the following associated anomalies: cervical rib, hypoplastic second and third right ribs and underdeveloped right chest wall, congenital aplasia of the right ulna with absence of the right fourth and fifth digital rays, and sickle cell anemia.

WEYERS' OLIGODACTYLY SYNDROME

Weyers (1957) reported two sporadic cases with the following findings: congenital abnormality of the kidney and spleen; reduced sternal segments and hypoplasia of the acromial end of the clavicle; and, in one case, cleft palate and hypoplastic maxilla, bilateral absence of the ulna, and diminished number of digits. One child had only two digits on the right hand and a single pinlike finger on the left side; the other child had two digits on each hand.

TREATMENT

The functional disturbance in ulnar ray defect depends upon the following factors: (1) radiohumeral fusion and the angle at which these two bones are united, (2) dislocation of the proximal end of the radius, (3) the size of the surviving segment of the ulna, (4) the number of digits destroyed, and (5) syndactylism of those digits that are present.

Radiohumeral ankylosis is not an uncommon accompaniment of ulnar ray defect, and arthroplasty of the elbow has been recommended in order to secure mobility. It is questionable whether arthroplasty in such cases will yield an actively mobile yet stable joint. In defects of the ulnar component, as in deficiencies of the radial ray, the muscles connected to the missing bone are absent, fused, or fibrotic. In bilateral cases, when both elbows are fixed in extension, one arm should be given functionally useful angle by osteotomy.

The dislocated proximal end of the radius may have to be resected, especially if the radial head impinges on the skin or has pushed its way through it. Goddu (1930) reported a woman with absent distal ulna, unstable wrist and elbow, and absence of all three ulnar digits. The radius was long and curved, and the radial head had bypassed the level of the elbow joint and reached a point above the humeral condyles. Goddu sawed off the proximal radius at a point which would allow the distal part to articulate with the lower end of the humerus. He reversed the direction of the resected segment and connected it with the remnant of the ulna; he then reinforced the elbow and the wrist with fascial slings. After a year the patient wrote: "My elbow which was formerly loose. . .is now firm. . . . The previously long curved bone of my forearm is now straight. . . . The previous absence of support of my forearm is now perfectly adjusted."

Lane (1898–1899) reported a three-year-old girl with a defect in the midshaft of the ulna—the distal end failed to reach the corpus. Lane spanned the gap between the two fragments of ulna with a graft obtained from the femur of a rabbit. The deformity was said to have been corrected successfully. Rabbit bone has since been supplanted by autogenous bone graft. Bone graft is also used to extend the moderately short proximal ulna towards the wrist. In a patient with a large "osteochondroma in the distal half of the ulna with luxation of the radial head, after resection of the tumerous bone," Vitale (1952) utilized the

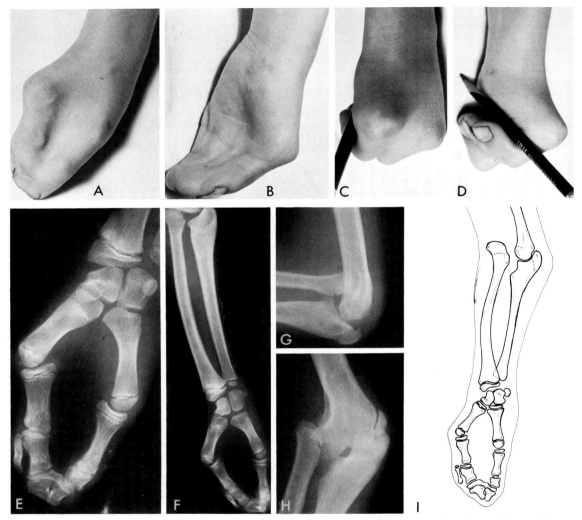

Figure 25–15 Ulnar ray defect of the right upper limb associated with central adactylia, webbing of the two marginal digits of the opposite hand, and bilateral dislocation of the radial head. *A*, Dorsal view of the left hand of an eight-year-old boy with distal terminal defect of the contralateral ulnar ray: this hand had only two marginal digital rays and they were webbed. *B*, Palmar view of the left hand. *C* and *D* show the functional propensity of this hand: this boy could wield a pencil or a tool effectively and was a good baseball catcher. It was felt that surgery would not improve and might in fact vitiate the function of this hand—it was left alone. *E*, Dorsopalmar roentgenograph of the left carpus and hand. *F*, Dorsopalmar roentgenograph of the hand and forearm showing dislocation of the radial head. *G* and *H*, Roentgenographs showing anterior dislocation of the right radial head. *I*, Composite sketch illustrating the skeletal contents of the left forearm and hand.

principle of surgical radioulnar synostosis recommended by Groves (1921). Vitale resected the proximal radius 1½ inches above the level of the lower end of the ulna. The pointed distal end of the ulna was then driven into the medullary cavity of the remaining radius.

In one case that came under this author's care, the distal portion of the ulna and the four ulnar digital rays were missing—only the thumb and a vestigial ulnar metacarpal, possibly the fifth, remained. The proximal end of the radius was dislocated about 4 cm. past the level of the elbow. Skeletal traction was

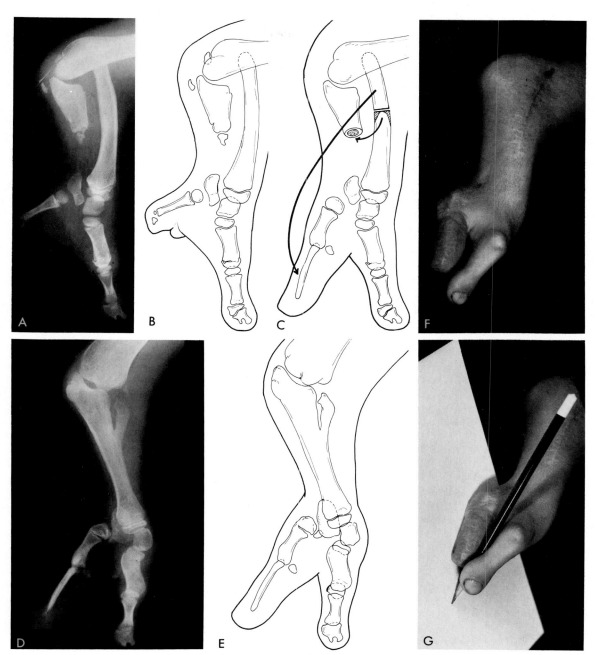

Figure 25–16 *A*, Preoperative dorsovolar roentgenograph of the right forearm and hand of the eight-year-old boy featured in Figure 25–15: the distal portion of the right ulna is missing; there are three carpal bones—two sizable and one small; there is one ulnar metacarpal, at the distal end of which are seen two small pieces of bone; the thumb is present but has a bifid ungual phalanx. *B*, Sketch illustrating the same. *C*, Sketch illustrating the surgical procedure: a pedicled tube was transferred from the abdomen to the ulnar border of the hand; a bony stem was fashioned out of the proximal portion of the radius and inserted into the pedicled tube; the proximal end of the distal fragment of the radius was osteosynthesized with the remnant of the ulna; and the site of apposition was reinforced with inlay graft. *D*, Postoperative roentgenograph: the union of the bone in the transferred tube and the ulnar metacarpal was delayed, but union eventually occurred; the forearm bones united; some of the strayed bone grafts formed a radial projection. *E*, Sketch illustrating the same. *F* and *G*, Postoperative results.

applied to mobilize the radius and bring it into a more distal position. A segment of the proximal radius was then resected, and the excised bone was utilized for reconstruction of a composite oppositional post for the thumb. The remaining distal portion of the radius was connected with the surviving proximal ulna. In several other cases, the author has carried out corrective osteotomy of the radius, repair of syndactyly, and rotation osteotomy of the metacarpals to enable the surviving digits to effect a pulp-to-pulp pinch (Figs. 25–15 and 25–16).

SUMMARY

The ulna serves as the main skeletal element of the forearm at the elbow. In defects of the ulna, the hand deviates in the ulnar direction, but the elbow bears the brunt of distortion and functional derangement. When the ulna is disproportionately dwarfed, the radius dislocates at the elbow. The defects of the ulna are less frequent than those of the radius; they have a greater tendency to be accompanied by regional abnormalities and have fewer syndromic associations. Total absence of the ulna is comparatively uncommon. When the proximal extremity of the ulna is present, surgical radioulnar osteosynthesis procures the best functional result.

References

Abadie, J.: Contribution à l'étude d'une "malformation curieuse du membre supérieur." *Rev. d'Orthop.* (2 s.), *9*:317–319, 1908.

Abadie, J., and Gagnière: Hemimélie portant sur la tige cubitale. *Bull. Mém. Soc. Anat.* (Paris), *78*:436–439, 1903.

Agayeff, G.: Rare congenital anomalous development of the humerus and both wrists. (In Russian.) *Vrach. Gaz. St. Petersburg, 12*:155–157, 1905.

Ballantyne, J. W.: *Manual of Antenatal Patho-Hygiene. The Embryo.* Edinburgh, W. Green & Sons, Vol. 2, pp. 584–585, 1904.

Bankart, A. S. B.: Congenital absence of the ulna. *Proc. R. Soc. Med. London.* (Sect. Surgery: sub-sect. orthopedics), *13*:211–212, 1919–1921.

Barrot, M.: Un cas complex d'absence partielle du cubitus. *Rev. d'Orthop., 12*:367–369, 1925.

Bertolotti, M.: Nanism familial par aplasia chondrale systematisée. Mésomélie et brachymelie métapodiale symétrique. *Presse Méd., 1*:165–170, 1913.

Birch-Jensen, A.: *Congenital Deformities of the Upper Extremities.* Odense, Andelsbogtrykkereit and Det Danske Forlag, pp. 20–21; 89–94; 143; 205–207, 1949.

Birnbacher, G.: *Drei Beobachtungen ueber Verkuemmerung der oberen Extremitaeten.* Koenigsberg, R. Leopold, pp. 5–29, 1891.

Blockey, N. J., and Lawrie, R. J.: An unusual symmetrical distal limb deformity in siblings. *J. Bone Joint Surg., 45B*:745–747, 1963.

Böök, J. A.: A clinical and genetical study of disturbed skeletal growth (chondrohypoplasia). *Hereditas, 36*:161–180, 1950.

Bordet, M.: Vices de conformation du membre thoracique supérieur gauche (le cubitus manqué dans sa partie moyenne). *Bull. Soc. Anat. Paris,* (1 s.), *11*:82–91, 1836.

Bosch, O. V.: Mano zamba por ausencia parciale del cubito. *Cir. Ap. Locomot., 2*:284–287, 1945.

Brailsford, J. F.: Dystrophies of the skeleton. *Br. J. Radiol., 8*:533–569, 1935.

Brodhurst, B. E.: Cases of intrauterine fracture (case 2 is about defective ulna). *Medico-Chir. Trans., 43*:115–126, 1860.

Broman, I.: *Normale und abnormale Entwicklung des Menschen.* Wiesbaden, J. F. Bergmann, pp. 229–230; fig. 195, 1911.

Brown, E.: An isolated human case of malformed upper extremity and thorax. *J. Hered., 34*:284–288, 1943.

Budin: Mains bote, variété cubito-palmaire. *Bull. Soc. Anat. Paris,* (2 s.), *17*:597–599, 1874.

Cange, A.: Déformations singulières et symétriques des avant-bras et des mains. *N. Iconog. Salp., 17*:283–288; Pl. XLI, 1903.

Castro, A. (de): Sur quelques cas hemimélie. *N. Iconog. Salp., 28*:292–296, 1916.

Cholmeley, J. A.: See Reeves, 1966.

Cleret, F., and Bienvenue, F.: Un cas d'ectrodactylie avec malformations du coude et luxation congénitale du radius droit. *Rev. d'Orthop., 1*:455–458; figs. 1 and 2, 1910.

Collins, R. G.: Report of a case of club-hand and foot. *Chicago Clin. Rev., 4*:11–14, 1895.

Delchef, J.: Greffes osseuses libres dans un cas d'agénésis cubitale, un cas d'agénésis radial, un cas d'agénésis peroniere bilateral. *Rev. d'Orthop. Chir. l'App. Mot., 35*:99–102, 1949.

Denninger, H. S.: Multiple anomalies. *Med. Radiog. Photog., 24*:86–87; fig. 23, 1948.

Deville, A.: Absence d'une grande partie du cubitus droit, luxation de l'extrémité supérieure du radius. Fractures et luxations congénitales. *Bull. Soc. Anat. Paris, 24*:153–162, 1849.

Feil, A.: Absence congénitale du cubitus et ectrodactylie. *Bull. Soc. Anat.* (Paris), (6 s.), *20*:572–577, 1923.

Genee, E.: Une forme extensive de dysostose mandibulo-faciale, *J. Génét. Hum., 17*:45–52; figs. 3 and 7, 1969.

Gessner: Ein Kind mehrfacher Missbildungen. (Defekt der Ulna am rechten Arme.) *Cbl. Gynek., 18*:824, 1894.

Goddu, L. A. O.: Reconstruction of elbow and bone graft of rudimentary ulna. *N. Engl. J. Med., 202*:1142–1144, 1930.

Göller, D. G. C.: Abortus humani monstros: hist. anat. Misc. Acad. Nat. curios. *Norimb decuria, 2*:ii, 311–318, 1698.

Gorgerot, M.: Ectrodactylie (absence of fifth digit and fusion of lunate with trignetrum). *Bull. Mém. Soc. Anat., 7*:300, 1905.

Grebe, H.: *Chondrodysplasia.* Rome, Inst. Greg. Mendel, pp. 300–303, 1955.

Grimaud, J. B. R.: *Variations Familiales Associées* (Hémimélie cubitale partielle, exostoses-ostéogéniques syndactylie). Thèse. Paris, Éditions Médicales, pp. 1–47, 1926.

Grimault, L., and Epirtalbags, A.: Absence congénitale bilaterale du cubitus. *Bull. Mém. Soc. Anat.* (Paris), *93*:738–743, 1923.

Groves, E. W. H.: *On Modern Methods of Treating Fracture.* Second edition. Bristol, J. Wright & Sons, pp. 313–323; figs. 247–249, 1921.

Gruca, A.: Un cas de main bote cubito-palmaire congénitale avec subluxation de phalanges. *Rev. d'Orthop., 14*:407–412, 1927.

Guerin-Valmale, C., and Jeanbrau, E.: Dissection d'une main-bote congénitale pure avec luxation congénitale du coude. *Bull. Soc. Anat. Paris,* (6 s.), *1*:911–915, 1899.

Guerin-Valmale, C., and Jeanbrau, E.: Etude d'un cas de main bote cubitale pure. *Montpellier Méd.*, 8:385–393, 1899.

Handlich, R.: Eine vierfingerige rechte Hand als kongenitale Missbildung. *Arch. Pathol. Anat. Physiol.*, 174:392–401, 1903.

Helweg-Larsen, H. F., and Morch, E. T.: Chondrodistrofi hos to soskende med. normale foraeldes. *Nordisk Med.*, 43:180–182, 1950.

Hoffmann, L.: Missbildungen der oberen Extremität. *Fortschr. Röntgenstr.*, 17:301–305, Taf. XXXIII, fig. 2, 1911.

Huet, E., and Infroit, C.: Description d'un ectromélie hémimélie, avec quelques considérations sur l'hémimélie. *N. Iconog. Salp.*, 14:128–148, 1901.

Jones, H. W., and Roberts, R. E.: A rare type of congenital club hand. *J. Anat.*, 60:146–147, fig. 2, 1926.

Jones, M. V.: Oligodactyly. *J. Bone Joint Surg.*, 34B:752–754; fig. 1–3, 1957.

Joüon, E.: Déformation de l'avant-bras par arrêt de développement de l'extrémité inférieure du cubitus, de cause inconnue. *Rev. d'Orthop.*, (2 s.), 6:80–84; Pl. II-IV, 1905.

Kachkachiff, A. B.: Absence of ulna. (In Russian.) *Russk. Vrach. St. Peterburg*, 3:325, 1904.

Kajon, C.: Angeborener doppelseitiger Ulna Defekt und Pollex bifudus dexter. *Z. Orthop. Chir.*, 41:526–528, 1921.

Keiser, D. V.: Ulnadefekt. *In* Diethelm, L., (ed.): *Skeletanatomie (Roentgendiagnostik).* Berlin, Springer, Band IV, Teil 2, pp. 205–206, 1968.

Ke Ping Jen: Der angeborene Defekt des ulnaren Strahls und angeborene Defekt der Tibia. *Arch. Orthop. Unfallchir.*, 37:42–47, 1937.

Kirmisson, E.: Malformation curieuse de membre supérieure gauche (absence de l'articulation du coude; développement incomplète du cubitus: ectrodactylie). *Rev. d'Orthop.*, (2 s.), 9:141–144, 1908.

Klaussner, F.: *Gliedmassen und ihre Entstehungslehre.* Wiesbaden, F. Bergmann, pp. 19–21; fall 6–7; figs. 3–4, 1900.

Klippel, M., Francois-Dainville, and Feil, A.: L'absence congénitale du cubitus. Un nouveau cas. *Paris Méd.*, 55:107–109, 1925.

Knapp, R. E.: Ulnar dorsal talipomanus. *Radiog. Clin. Photog.*, 18:25–26, 1942.

Kozlowski, K.: Hypoplasie bilatérale congénitale du cubitus et synostose bilatéral calcanco-cuboide chez une fillette. *Ann. Radiol.*, 8:389–392, 1965.

Kuh, R.: Der angeborene Defekt der Ulna. *Z. Orthop. Chir.*, 41:437–441, 1921.

Kümmel, W.: Ulnadefekt. *In* Die *Missbildungen der Extremitäten durch Defekt, Verwachsung und Uberzahl.* Bibliotheca Medica, Section E, Vol. III. Kassel, Th. G. Fischer, pp. 11–12, 38–40, 1895.

Lane, W. A.: Two cases of deficiency of the shaft of the ulna treated successfully by the insertion of a rabbit's femur. *Trans. Clin. Soc. London*, 32:44–45, pl. II, 1898–1899.

Langer, L. O., Jr.: Mesomelic dwarfism of hypoplastic ulna, fibula, mandible type. *Radiology*, 89:654–660, 1967.

Laurin, C. A., and Farmer, A. W.: Congenital absence of ulna. *Can. J. Surg.*, 2:204–207, 1959.

Lausecker, H.: Der angeborene Defekt der Ulna. *Arch. Pathol. Anat. Physiol.*, 325:211–226, 1954.

Letoire, H.: Malformation congénitale de l'avant bras et de la main. *Bull. Soc. Anat. Paris*, (4 s.), 4:65–72, 1879.

Liu, S. H.: A case of congenital partial absence of the right ulna and associated deformities. *Chinese Med. J.*, 47:1052–1055, Pl. I-II, 1933.

Loeweneck: Ein Beitrag zum kongenitalen Ulnadefekt. *Zentralbl. Chir.*, 50:3254–3255, 1927.

Longuet, and Peraire: Malformation congénitale du cubitus avec synostoses congénitales. *Bull. Mém. Soc. Anat. Paris*, (6 s.), 3:147–148, 1901.

Maas, O.: Angeborener linksseitiger Ulnadefekt. *Berl. Klin. Wochenschr.*, 1:234–236, 1917.

Mackley, J. T., and Heiple, K. G.: Scoliosis associated with congenital deficiencies of the upper extremity. *J. Bone Joint Surg.*, 52A:279–286, figs. 2A and 2B, 1970.

Manzinilla, M. A.: Atrophie congénitale de la partie inférieure du cubitus. *Ann. Anat. Pathol.*, 16:1031–1041, 1939–1940.

Metcalfe, J.: Congenital malformation of both hands and forearms. *Arch. Radiol. Electrol.*, 20:18, Pl. 3, 1915.

Motta, A.: Su di un caso di lussazione anteriore del capitello del radio da ipoplasia congenita dell'ulna. *La Clinica Ortopedica*, 12:480–485, 1960.

Mouchet, A.: Un cas d'hémimélie avec radiographie. *Bull. Soc. Anat.*, (6 s.), 1:937–942, 1899.

Mouchet, A.: Un ectromélien hémimélie par absence du cubitus. *J. Belge Chir.*, 10:655, 1901.

Mouchet, A.: Absence partielle du cubitus gauche. *Rev. d'Orthop.*, 29:96–98, 1943.

Mouchet, A., and Pakowski: Deux cas d'absence du cubitus (une absence totale et une absence partielle). *Rev. d'Orthop.*, (3 s.), 10:147–153, 1923.

Müller, W.: *Die angeborenen Fehlbildungen der menschlichen Hand.* Leipzig, G. Thieme, pp. 69–71, 1937.

Neumann: Ein Fall von angeborenem Ulnadefekt. *Berl. Klin. Wochenschr.*, 53:1376–1377, 1916.

Nicholson, J. T., and Qualis, D. M.: Early evaluation of musculoskeletal lesions by the pediatricians. *Pediatr. Clin. N. Am.*, 6:1190–1196; fig. 108, 1959.

Nigit, P. E.: Ulnadefekte. *Schweiz. Med. Wochenschr.*, 57:13–14, 1927.

Orel, H.: Kleine Beitraege zur Vererbungswissenschaft, IV. *Mitteilung Konstitutionslehre, 14*:347–355, 1929.

Pagenstecher, F.: Beitraege zu den Extremitätenmissbildungen. Defekte an der oberen Extremität. *Dtsch. Z. Chir., 50*:427–435, 1899.

Pardini, A. G.: Congenital absence of the ulna. *J. Iowa Med. Soc., 57*:1106–1112, 1967.

Patterson, F. D.: Congenital defect in the ulna. *Ann. Surg., 48*:296–299, 1908.

Pillay, V. K.: Ophthalmo-mandibulo-melic dysplasia. A hereditary syndrome. *J. Bone Joint Surg., 46A*:858–862, 1964.

Pingel, P., and Rompe, G.: Einteilungsprinzipien der Dysmelie, dargestellt am Beispiel der ulnaren Ektromelie. *Z. Orthop. Grenzgbt., 109*:137–144, 1971.

Pircard: Deux cas interessants de malformations congénitales des membres supérieures. *Rev. d'Orthop.*, (3 s.), *11*:145–149, 1924.

Pircard: Hémimélie cubitale; absence presque complète du cubitus droit. *Rev. d'Orthop.*, (3 s.), *12*:269–272, 1925.

Piulachs, M.: Absence congénitale partielle du cubitus, fracture de l'extrémité inférieure du radius. *Rev. d'Orthop., 26*:672–676, 1939–1940.

Poulalion, S. M. A.: Note sur un cas d'ectrodactyly congénitale avec absence total du métacarpien correspondant (ectromélie de l'auriculaire et du cinquieme metacarpien du côte gauche). *Arch. Gen. Med.*, (7 s.), *2*:548–563, 1891.

Priestley, W. O.: A dissection of a curious malformation of the forearm. *Med. Times Gaz., 15*:489–490, 1856.

Pringle, J. H.: Notes of a case of congenital absence of both ulnae. *J. Anat. Physiol., 27*:239–244, 1893.

Rabaud, E., and Hovelacque, A.: Absence congénitale du cubitus, du radius, du tibia et du péroné (ectromélie longitudinale-intercalaire-hémisegmentaire). *Rev. d'Orthop.*, (3 s.), *11*:21–38, 1924.

Reeves, B.: Boomerang bone disease: bilateral dysplasia of ulna and fibula. *Proc. R. Soc. Med. London* (Sect. Orthopedics), *59*:711–712, 1966.

Reichart, A.: Über eine eigentuemliche typische Deformierung des Griffelfortsatzes der ulna. *Münch. Med. Wochenschr., 60*:1146–1147, 1913.

Reimann-Hunziker, G.: Über den angeborenen Ulnadefekt. *Z. Orthop., 73*:160–164, 1942.

Reinhardt, K., and Pfeiffer, R. A.: Ulno-fibulare Dysplasie. Eine autosomal-dominant vererbte Mikromesomelie, ahnlich dem Nievergeltsyndrom. *Fortschr. Röntgenstr., 107*:379–391, 1967.

Reinike: *Zur Kenntnis des kongenitalen Ulnadefekts.* Inaug. Diss. Berlin, G. Schade, pp. 1–30, 2 pl. 80, 1912.

Riedinger: Über Gelenkmissbildungen. *Verh. Dtsch. Berl. Ges. Chir. Berlin.* 18th Congress. Berlin, A. Hirschwald, pp. 76–80, 1889.

Rigal: Main bote par insuffisance de longueur du cubitus, d'origine indeterminée. Allongement du cubitus par greffe osseuse. Résultat excellent. *Lyon Chir., 19*:606–609, 1922.

Roberts, A. S.: A case of deformity of the forearm and hands, with an unusual history of hereditary congenital deficiency. *Ann. Surg., 3*:135–139, 1886.

Roome, N. W.: Bone defect of ulna treated by bone graft. *Can. M.A.J., 34*:64–65, 1936.

Roth, B.: Case of arrested growth of right ulna by exostosis near styloid process and continued growth of radius bending round lower end of ulna. *Trans. Clin. Soc. London 21*:283–284, 1888.

Roth, P. B.: A case of congenital defect of the ulna. *Lancet, 1*:1457–1458, 1914.

Roth, P. B.: Congenital defect of the left ulna. *Proc. R. Soc. Med. London.* (Sect. Dis. Child.), *9*:81–83, 1916.

Rothschild, H. de: Main bote cubitopalmaire avec absence complète du cubitus; absence de l'annulaire, de l'auriculaire et de la region hypothénar. Syndactylie de l'index et du médius. *Bull. Soc. Obstet.* (Paris), *6*:114–115, 1903.

Rübsamen, W.: Beitrag zur Kasuistik des kongenitalen Ulnadefekts. *Münch. Med. Wochenschr., 42*:2284, 1912.

Schenck, E.: Ueber zwei Falle von typischer Extremitäten-Missbildung. (Ulnadefekt, Fibuladefekt.) *Frankfurter Z. Pathol., 1*:544–562, 1907.

Schnell, A.: *Über angeborenen Defekt von Radius und Ulna.* Inaug. Diss. Göttingen, Univ. Buchdruckerei, pp. 5–23, 1875.

Schoenenberg, H.: Ulnadefekte. *In Über Missbildungen der Extremitäten.* Bibliotheca Paediatrica. Fasc. 80. Basel, S. Karger, pp. 31–33, 1962.

Schwarzbach, W.: Über angeborenen Defekt der Tibia und Ulna. *Z. Chir. Mech. Orthop., 6*:345–370, 1912.

Senftleben, H.: Notiz über eine angeborene Luxation des Radius mit Defekt des mittleren Teils der Ulna. *Arch. Pathol. Anat. Physiol., 55*:303–304, 1869.

Shertzer, J. H., Bickel, W. H., and Stubbins, S. G.: Congenital pseudarthrosis of the ulna. *Minn. Med., 52*:1061–1066, 1969.

Southwood, A. R.: Partial absence of the ulna and associated structures. *J. Anat., 61*:346–351, 1927.

Spinner, M., Freundlich, B. L., and Abeler, E. D.: Management of moderate longitudinal arrest of development of the ulna. *Clin. Orthop., 69*:199–202, 1970.

Steffal: Ein Fall von seltener Missbildung. *Oesterr. Jahrb. Paediatrik*, Bd. II, p. 33, 1875.

Straub, L. R.: Congenital absence of the ulna. *Am. J. Surg., 109*:300–305, 1965.

Strecker, C.: Eine angeborene vierfingerige rechte. Hand. *Arch. Pathol. Anat. Physiol.*, *127*:181–187, figs. 1 & 2, 1892.

Stricker, G.: Grossartiger Defekt an beiden Vorderarmen und Händen einer Neugeborenen. Arch. *Pathol. Anat. Physiol.*, *72*:144, 1878.

Thorndike, A.: Some notes on malformations. *Am. J. Orthop. Surg.*, *7*:311–318, 1910.

Van Der Sar, A.: Over aageboren afwijkingen aan den onderarm. *Ned. T. Geneesk.*, *91*:313–315; figs. 4 and 5, 1947.

Vitale, C. C.: Reconstructive surgery for defects in the shaft of the ulna in children. *J. Bone Joint Surg.*, *34*:804–810, 1952.

Vulpius, O.: Knochenplastik zur Beseitigung der manus vara. *Z. Orthop. Chir.*, *17*:287–292, figs. 1 & 2, 1906.

Wagenseil, F.: Über einen angeborenen doppelseitigen Ulnadefekt. *Anat. Anz.*, *52*:439–447, 1919–1920.

Watt, J. C.: Anatomy of seven month foetus exhibiting bilateral absence of ulna accompanied by monodactyly (and also diaphragmatic hernia). *Am. J. Anat.*, *22*:385–427, 1917.

Wernscheid, H.: Ein Beitrag zur Entstehungsmoeglichkeit des kongenitalen Defektes der Ulna. *Med. Klin. Berl.*, *19*:11578, 1923.

Werthemann, A.: *Handbuch der speziellen pathologischen Anatomie und Histologie.* Berlin, Springer Verlag, Vol. IX, Section VI, pp. 86–89, 1952.

Weyers, H.: Das Oligodaktylie-Syndrom des Menschen und seine Parallel-mutation bei der Hausmaus. *Ann. Paediatr.*, *189*:351–370, 1957.

Wierzejewski, I.: Über den kongenitalen Ulnadefekt. *Z. Orthop. Chir.*, *27*:101–131, 1910.

Willard, de F.: Deformities, congenital multiple—arms and legs—femurs deficient. *Trans. Am. Orthop. Assoc.*, *13*:305–312, 1900.

Yudt, I. M.: Rare congenital anomaly of development. (In Russian.) *Vrach. Gaz. St. Peterburg*, *10*:392, 1903.

Chapter Twenty-Six

PHOCOMELIA

Saint-Hilaire (1836) compounded the designation phocomelia from the Greek *phoke* meaning seal and *melos* which means limb. The classic phocomelus is an individual whose hands and feet sprout directly from the trunk, simulating the flippers of a seal. It is implied that two intermediary segments are missing in each upper and lower limb—the arm and the forearm in the upper, and the thigh and the leg in the lower extremity. In phocomelia, one or two digits may be missing, though some functioning terminal element is always present. Johnson (1967) wrote an article about a case in which there was "absence of elements distal to the carpal bones of the left hand except for useless nubbins of digits with tiny deformed nails." This was obviously a case of acral defect or transverse terminal deficiency (also called intrauterine amputation) with rudimentary digits. Yet Johnson reported it as one of phocomelia and the editors of a highly esteemed journal allowed this bit of semantic abuse to be printed.

Alice Vance was a mulatto born in Texas but living in Berlin. She had short forearms—her radius and ulna measured about 6 cm. in length. Her lower legs contained rudimentary tibias, the fibulas were absent, and her body was covered with hair. When on all fours, she resembled a bear, hence her nickname bearwoman—*Das Barenweib*. She was often exhibited in sideshows. Alice Vance's mother was "similarly formed," but her sister and her own offspring were unaffected. Hers might have been a case of mesomelic dwarfism with hypoplastic ulna-fibula. However, more than one nineteenth century German author erroneously reported her case to be one of hereditary phocomelia.

PHOCOMELUS AND PHOCOMELOID

The phocomelus with involvement of both upper and lower limbs is a dwarf whose limbs lack root and midsegments. Roentgenographic studies of a newborn phocomelus may not show any vestige of intermediary bones, but x-rays taken in later years will reveal a rudiment or two. In the literature, there are a number of cases reported as phocomelia in which the intermediary segments of the limb are not absent but are drastically reduced in length. These subjects, called phocomeloids, constitute the majority of reported cases in the literature.

891

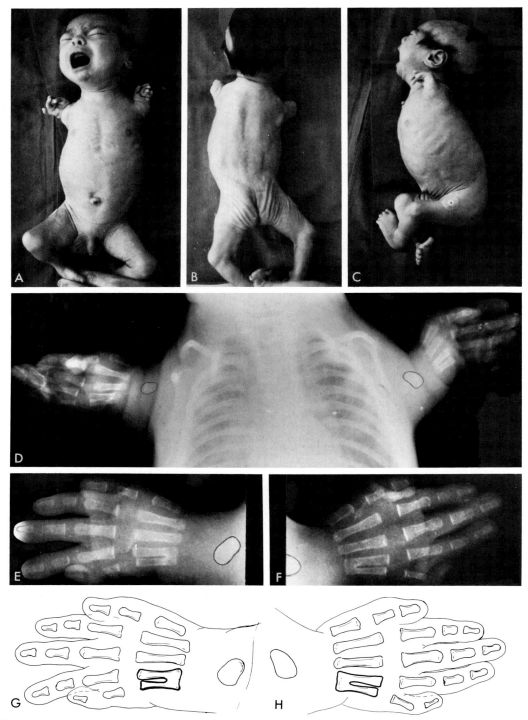

Figure 26–1   Phocomelia. *A*, Frontal view of a newborn boy with upper limb phocomelia and varus feet. *B*, Dorsal view. *C*, Side view. *D*, Anteroposterior roentgenograph of the torso and upper limbs: on each side there is an oblong piece of bone between the shoulder girdle and the hand. *E*, Roentgenograph of the right hand: there are five digital rays; the fourth and fifth metacarpal bases are coalesced; each marginal digit has two phalanges. *F*, Roentgenograph of the left hand showing the same anomalies as the right hand. *G* and *H* illustrate the roentgenograph above each.

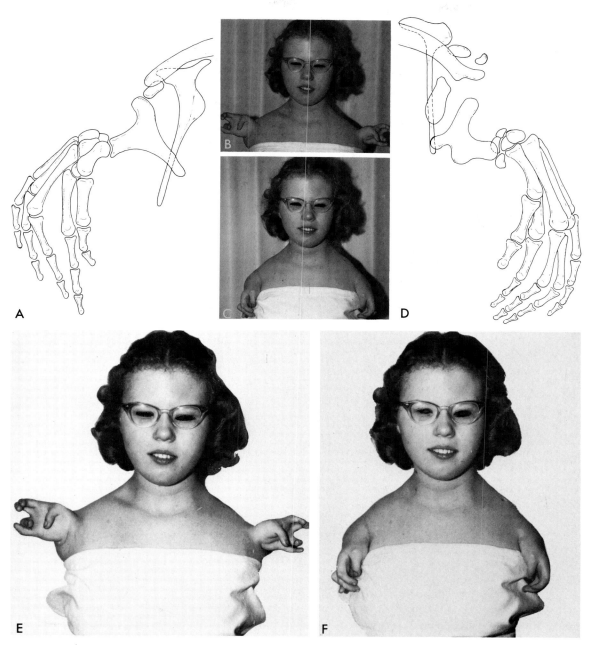

Figure 26–2 Phocomelia. *A*, Tracing from the roentgenograph of the right upper extremity of a 15-year-old girl born in 1941, long before the manufacture and marketing of thalidomide. *B* and *C*, Frontal views of the patient. *D*, Tracing from the roentgenograph of the left upper extremity. *E* and *F* represent *B* and *C*, respectively: the background has been retouched and the figures have been enlarged.

Phocomelia is classified with intercalary defects in which, by definition, the middle part is deficient and parts proximal and distal are present but not necessarily normal. In many reported cases of phocomelia, parts proximal and distal to the affected area show detectable deficiencies. In the upper extremity, the clavicle, the scapula, and occasionally the homolateral ribs are malformed; distally, one or more digits, usually the thumb, may be missing. Of the intermediary elements between the hand and the shoulder, the humerus seems to survive most often or undergoes the least degree of abbreviation in length; the radius and ulna are affected most frequently and severely, the carpal bones may be missing or are coalesced, and the thumb is usually absent, especially in thalidomide-induced phocomelia (Figs. 26–1 and 26–2).

SOME EARLIER REPORTED CASES

Sheldrake (1740) described a newborn whose "arms were without the elbow joint" and consisted only of "two bones"; this infant had "no legs or thighs, but had two feet joined into the lower part of the body." Dumeril (1800), Saint-Hilaire (1836), Guinard (1893), Gould and Pyle (1897), Ballantyne (1904), Socin (1917), O'Brien and Mustard (1921), Wepler (1937), and Hill (1937) all speak of a notorious phocomeloid variously named Marc Catozze, Marco Catozzo, or Marc Cazotte, and nicknamed Pepin. This character is described as being "quite intellectual . . . quite a clever man." He traveled through Europe on foot or horseback and spoke four languages. Pepin was exhibited before the public and was celebrated for his dexterity. He performed nearly all necessary actions and exhibited skillfulness in his movements. Pepin died in Paris around 1800 at the age of 62. His body was carefully dissected by Dumeril, whose findings were published by Socin. Pepin had well-formed hands and feet. Each hand was connected with the corresponding scapula by a short tubular bone, probably a remnant of the humerus. Each leg contained a very short bone which was interpreted as being the tibia; he had no scrotum but "was credited for his ability to perform coitus."

INHERITANCE

In a family reported by Kutzenok (1929), the father and his brother had partial absence of the radius and the son and daughter had phocomelia. The variable expression is also exemplified in the pedigree described by Stiles and Dougan (1940). In this family, a father and his son were definite phocomeloids with "fin-like arms." Altogether 26 relatives had malformed upper extremities; some members had deformed fingers only, others had malformed wrists as well, and in a few the entire upper limb was affected. In an occasional case, the radius and ulna were partially fused. It is possible that these dominantly inherited cases belong to the category of Holt-Oram syndrome.

O'Brien and Mustard (1921) reported a phocomeloid whose father and mother were double first cousins. The mother was 19 when she married. "She bore eight children, five normal and three monstrous." One stillborn infant was "anatomically exactly" like the propositus. Freire-Maia et al (1959) described a family in which consanguinity was a definite factor. There were four cases of phocomelia involving the upper extremities. The data suggested "the action of an autosomal recessive gene with variable expression." This family came from a low social stratum, from a rural community in southern Brazil, where such a disfiguring anomaly is said to have no effect on the frequency of marriage or reproduction; in a more sophisticated society the same anomaly would deter partners from selecting each other, Freire-Maia and associates argued.

SPORADIC CASES

The argument offered by Freire-Maia et al would in part account for the comparative scarcity of hereditary phocomeloids and the relatively greater number of sporadic cases reported in the literature. The phocomeloid infant reported by Sheldrake (1790) was sporadic, as was Pepin, the phocomeloid described by Dumeril (1800) and many others. In the literature, one also finds reports by the following authors: Barton (1740), Cole (1868), Rodenstein (1875), Chason (1879), Van Der Hoeven (1884), Santex (1886), Morgan (1888), Hirst (1889), Tyrie and Baxter (1894), Gittings (1898), Virchow (1898), Orgler (1900), Joachimsthal (1900), Klaussner (1900), Ballantyne (1904), Kindl (1907), Falk (1908), Skillern (1912), Stiell (1916), Socin (1917), Carey (1919), Homi (1920), McConnell (1922), Schurig (1922), Feller (1922), Perkins (1922), Nigst (1927), Hill (1937), Wepler (1937), Schwanke (1938), Brown (1943), Birch-Jensen (1949), and Potter (1952). Birch-Jensen (1949), who reviewed some of these earlier cases, said that the deformity was unilateral in about half of the cases; when bilateral, the involvement was asymmetrical. Quite frequently, both upper and lower extremities were involved. Birch-Jensen estimated that combined radioulnar defect occurred once in about 75,000 births.

ASSOCIATIONS

Pepin (Marc Catozze) had no scrotum. In some phocomeloids, the carpal bones were missing; in others, these ossicles had coalesced. The thumb and the index finger seem to be the most common digits missing, and the remaining members were usually flexed, weak, and, in Kutzenok's (1929) case, webbed. Carey (1919) noted "the rudimentary development of the related muscles." Hill's (1937) patient had adducted thumbs which could not be voluntarily abducted. In many cases, the bones of the pectoral girdle were hypoplastic. Some subjects had bilateral involvement, and in others all four limbs were affected. Makley and Heiple (1970) reported a patient with phocomelia of both upper limbs and scoliosis. Phocomelia is also known to occur in a number of syndromes.

CARDIOMELIC COMPLEX

Birch-Jensen (1949) noted the association of phocomelia and congenital heart disease. He did not specify the nature of the heart disease except to say that the five-year-old girl he described had an enlarged heart and systolic prolongation and had been liable to cyanosis since birth. Murdock (1969) reported a male infant with bilateral upper limb phocomelia and with "at least two ventricular septal defects." The child's mother had absent left thumb, triphalangeal fingerlike right thumb, and atrial septal defect; the grandmother possessed a nonopposable small left thumb and had "marked cardiac enlargement, with contour characteristics of atrial septal defect." The mother's and grandmother's defects were interpreted as those of Holt-Oram syndrome, discussed in Chapter Ten.

CHONDRODYSTROPHIA CALCIFICANS CONGENITA (CCC)

This complex was discussed in Chapter Seventeen. It is a form of mesomelic dwarfism with radiographic evidence of calcific densities in cartilaginous epiphyses and contracture of joints, including those of the hand and forearm. Moselkilde (1968) presented a patient with CCC and short flipperlike arms, resembling a phocomelus.

CHROMOSOMAL ABERRATIONS
(E-trisomic Phocomelia)

Kajii et al (1964) reported a male infant who died soon after birth. The following findings were recorded: "phocomelia of the left arm, an absence of the left diaphragm and exophthalmos, in addition to typical features of 17–18 trisomy."

The female infant with 17–18 trisomy described by Zellweger et al (1965) also died soon after birth. Her right arm, particularly the right forearm, was longer than the left. The fingers of the right hand were in flexed position. The right thumb was relatively small. The left upper limb consisted of a slightly shortened root segment and a very short forearm; the thumb on this side was represented by a small mass of soft tissue with a narrow pedicle, and the fingers were flexed. Both palms possessed four finger lines.

HEMATOMELIC COMPLEX
(Thrombocytopenic Phocomelia)

Radius platelet hypoplasia (RPH) or thrombocytopenia–absent radius (TAR) syndrome was taken up in Chapter Twenty-Three. A characteristic feature of this complex is absence of the radius with a pentadactylic hand. In thrombocytopenic phocomelia, the hand likewise has five digits; this is in contrast to thalidomide-induced phocomelia, in which at least the thumb is missing. Dignan et al (1967) described five patients with phocomelia of the upper extremities and associated blood cell abnormalities. These patients have "five-fingered hands," absent radii and ulnae, and hypoplastic thrombocytopenia which was most profound in the early months of life and tended to improve with age. Each patient also had episodes of myeloid-leukemoid reactions. Two of the subjects were siblings. Hall et al (1969) reviewed 40 examples of TAR, 27 of which had been reported in the literature. Among the 13 new cases, there was a female whose "right arm was very short." In another female patient belonging to this group, the "right arm was very short; the hand appeared to arise from the shoulder."

OROMELIC COMPLEX (Robert's Syndrome)

Roberts (1919) presented an infant whose parents were first cousins. The child had double cleft of the lip and palate, protrusion of the intermaxillary portion of the upper jaw, and imperfect development of the bones of the extremities. The bones of the legs were almost absent and those of the arms were hypoplastic. There were two other affected sibs in this family. One was a "monstrosity"; the other was born with deformities almost identical to those of the propositus and died shortly after birth.

One of the sibs with phocomelia described by O'Brien and Mustard (1921) had harelip. Stroer (1939) reported a patient with analogous malformations. The parents of this proband were also first cousins. Brown's (1943) patient had minor abnormalities of the ribs, misshapen clavicles, and scapulas, vestigial humerus, completely absent ulnae and rudimentary radii, carpal coalescence, and two absent digits on each hand. One of the relatives had cleft palate and another had mental deficiency. The propositus was unable to abduct his arms at the shoulders, supinate the vestigial forearm and carry his hands in the ulnar direction, nor extend his fingers. The trait is considered to be an autosomal recessive.

THALIDOMIDE-INDUCED PHOCOMELIA

Thalidomide was synthesized in West Germany in 1954 and dispensed as a sedative during the following six or seven years. The incidence of phocomelia in West Germany and in many other countries where the drug was marketed under various names took on an unprecedented upsurge. According to Zellweger et al (1965), prior to the synthesis of thalidomide, the incidence of phocomelia was estimated "to be between one in 22,000 and one in 70,000 live births. It rose to one to three in 1,000 live births in areas where thalidomide and related drugs were used. After the withdrawal of the drug, the incidence of phocomelia fell again, yet the malformation did not disappear. Thus thalidomide cannot be the only cause of phocomelia. A number of etiological factors were listed which can be grouped in three main categories: hereditary, cytogenic and environmental causes." Perhaps it is safe to say that thalidomide is the most common cause of what Lenz (1964) called "atypical" phocomelia.

Lenz (1964) spoke of classic phocomelia, which is taken to refer to cases which had been reported prior to the introduction of thalidomide, and stated that most patients with classic phocomelia had five digits, but that in thalidomide-induced phocomelia usually at least one thumb was absent, and that only a small minority of phocomelia patients born before the introduction of thalidomide were similar to the thalidomide-induced variant. The latter was usually associated with one or more of the following anomalies: "capillary hemangioma of the upper lip and the nose, anotia and internal malformations such as aplasia of the gallbladder and appendix, uterus duplex and atresia of the duodenum." Lenz pointed to the comparative scarcity of these associated defects in classic phocomelia, which is true.

It is not true, however, as stated by Lenz, that "most classical cases of phocomelia had five fingers." In many cases of phocomelia reported prior to the thalidomide epidemic, the thumb was missing. To support this statement, one need only mention the cases cited by Morgan (1888), Klaussner (1900), Skillern (1912), Steill (1916), O'Brien and Mustard (1921), McConnell (1922), Schurig (1922), Kutzenok (1929), Schwanke (1938), Brown (1943), Birch-Jensen (1949), and Freire-Maia et al (1959). It is possible that some of the cases of phocomelia reported prior to the introduction of thalidomide were caused by a drug or drugs with an analogous embryotoxic effect.

TREATMENT

"In bilateral phocomelia," Swanson (1965) wrote, "the problem for the patients is that they cannot get the hand into the desired position in space because of the absence of the proximal extremity. In order for the hand to be placed in the desired position, a great deal of trunk activity is necessary. The patient will frequently bend the trunk down to get the hands in a position to function. Frequently these patients have some deformity in the lower limbs so that good foot prehension is not possible. The chief problems of patients with bilateral phocomelia are toilet activity and feeding. There is also cosmetic concern about the fact that the extremities are short and the trunk positioning required in eating in public is usually embarrassing. Frequently the phocomelic extremity can be used to control the terminal device or the elbow lock of a nonconventional prosthesis. The problem in designing these prostheses for patients with phocomelia is to keep them from being so complex that the patient will reject them because of their gadgetry."

SUMMARY

Phocomelia of the upper limb is characterized by the stunting of the upper arm and the forearm. These segments are seldom completely absent. Heredity features in a few cases. Most reported cases have been sporadic. It is possible that some of the so-called classic cases reported in the literature were caused by exogenous agents—drugs with embryotoxicity analogous to that of thalidomide—and others might have accompanied undetected blood dyscrasias and congenital heart disease. In drug-induced phocomelia, the thumb and the adjacent digit or adjacent two digits are usually absent. In thrombocytopenic phocomelia, the thumb and the four ulnar digits are present. In Robert's syndrome, phocomelia is associated with cleft lip-palate. Patients with E-trisomic phocomelia have not survived. Very little can be said about the treatment of phocomelia.

References

Appelt, H., Gerken, H., and Lenz, W.: Tetraphokomelie mit Lippen-Kiefer-Daumenspalte und Clitorishypertrophie: ein syndrom. *Paediatr. Paedol., 2*:119–124, 1966.

Ballantyne, J. W.: *Manual of Antenatal Pathology and Hygiene. The Embryo.* Edinburgh, W. Green & Sons, pp. 580–582, 1904.

Barton: On congential malformation of the left upper extremity. *Dublin Quart. J. Med. Sci.,* (2 s.), *38*:446–448, 1864.

Birch-Jensen, A.: *Congenital Deformities of the Upper Extremities.* Translated by E. Aagensen: Commission Andelsbogtrykkeriet; Odense and det danske Forlag. pp. 94–101, 207. Prop. 190. figs. 104, 105, and 106, 1949.

Bitny-Schliacto, F. A.: Beitrag zu den Missbildungen der oberen Extremitäten. *Arch. Orthop. Unfallchir., 24*:597–609, 1927.

Blakeslee, B., and Hoston, L.: *The Limb-Deficient Child.* Berkeley, University of California Press, pp. 153–171, 1963.

Blauth, W., and Willert, H. G.: Klinik und Therapie ektromeler Missbildungen der unteren Extremität. *Arch. Orthop. Unfallchir., 55*:521–570, figs. 1, 4, 14a, 17, 18, 1963.

Boerner, E.: *Anatomische Untersuchung eines Kindes mit Phokomelie.* Inaug.-Diss. Marburg, Universität Buchdruckerei (R. Freiderich), pp. 1–28, 1887.

Brandt, W.: Experimental production of atrophied and partly deficient limbs (phocomelias) in the axolotl embryo. *J. Exp. Biol., 20*:117–119, pl. 5, 1944.

Broman, I.: *Normal und abnormer Entwicklung des Menschen.* Wiesbaden, J. F. Bergmann, pp. 228–231; figs. 188–190, 1911.

Brown, E.: An isolated human case of malformed upper extremities and thorax. *J. Hered., 34*:284–288, 1943.

Carey, E.J.: Teratological studies: on a phocomelus with a special reference to the extremities. *Anat. Rec., 16*:45–70, 1919.

Charon, M.: D'un monstre éctromélien se rapprochant de phocomélien. *J. Med. Pharmacol., 19*:187–191, 1879.

Charon, and Stoquart: Note sur l'absence congénitale de l'humerus observée chez un enfant de six ans. *J. Med. Chir. Pharmacol.* (Bruxelles), *68*:13–17, 1879. See also report by E. Houzein *J. Méd. Bruxelles, 68*:110–111, 1879.

Chauvin, E.: *Précis de Teratologie,* Paris, Masson et Cie, pp. 87–88, 1920.

Cole, G. C.: Case of malformation of both upper extremities; living specimen. *Trans. Pathol. Soc.* (London), *20*:417–418, 1869.

Coodin, F. j., Uchida, I. A., and Murphy, C. H.: Phocomelia. Report of three cases. *Can. Med. Assoc. J., 87*(2):735–739, 1962.

Daffner, F.: Über einen Fall von angeborener Missbildung der Gliedmassen. *Münch. Med. Wochenschr., 25*:782, 1898.

Danlos, Apert, and Flandin: Micromélie congénitale limités aux deux humerus. *N. Iconog. Salp., 22*:682–688, 1909.

Degenhardt, K. H., and Geipel, G.: Zur Aetiologie und Phänogenese phokomeler Entwicklunsstörungen. *Z. Menschl. Vereb. Konstitutionslehre, 31*:1–53, 1952.

Dignan, P. St. J., Mauer, A. M., and Frantz, C.: Phocomelia with congenital hypostatic thrombocytopenia and myeloid leukemoid reactions. *J. Pediatr., 70*:561–573, 1967.

Dumeril: Venetian appele Marc Catozze. *Bull. Soc. Philomatique.* Tom III, p. 122, An Xi, 1800. Cited by Saint Hillaire (1836), Falk (1907), Socin (1917), and many others.

Dunn, P. M., Fischer, A. M., and Kohler, H. G.: Phocomelia. *Am. J. Obstet. Gynecol., 64*:348–355, 1962.

Evans, F. G., Alfaro, A., and Alfaro, S.: An unusual anomaly of the superior extremities in a Tarascan Indian girl. *Anat. Rec., 106*:37–47, 1950.

Falk, E.: Eine seltene menschiche Missbildung und ihre Bedeutung für die Entwicklungsgeschichte. *Arch. Pathol. Anat. Physiol., 192*:544–564, Taf. XIV, 1908.

Feller, A.: Missbildung der beiden oberen Extremitäten (linksseitige Phokomelie). *Wein. Klin. Wochenschr., 35*:707–708, 1922.

Forster, A.: *Die Missbildungen des Menschen.* Jena, F. Mauke, p. 64; Taf. XI, figs. 6 and 7, 1865.

Freire-Maia, A., Quelce-Salgado, A., and Koehler, R. A.: Hereditary bone aplasias and hypoplasias of the upper extremities. *Acta Genet., 9*:33–40, 1959.

Gittings, J. C.: Congenital absence of the humerus. *Arch. Pediatr., 15*:927–928, 1898.

Gould, G. M., and Pyle, W. L.: *Anomalies and Curiosities in Medicine.* Philadelphia, W. B. Saunders Co., pp. 263–264, fig. 106, 1897.

Grandmaire, A. E.: *Essai de la Teratologie Humaine. Une Famille de Phocomédiens.* Thèse. Bordeaux, Imp. du Midi–P. Cassigol, pp. 13–42, 1897.

Grebe, H.: Phokomelie. *In* Becker, P. E., (ed.): *Humangenetik.* Stuttgart, G. Thieme, Vol. 2, pp. 226–229, 1964.

Grillo, R. A.: Über einen Fall von Phokomelie. *Dtsch. Med. Wochenschr., 62*:1332–1336, 1936.

Gruber G. B.: *Die Morphologie der Missbildungen des Menschen und der Tiere.* Jena, G. Fischer, 3T, 17 Lief., 1 Abt, 7 Kap., 1 Halfte, pp. 300–328, 1937.

Guinard, L.: *Précis de Teratologie. Anomalies et Monstrosites chez l'Homme et chez les Animaux.* Paris, J. B. Ballière et fils, pp. 346–358, 1893.

Hall, G.: A case of phocomelia of the upper limbs. *Med. J. Aust., 1*:450–499, 1963.

Hall, J. G., Levin, J., Kuhn, J. P., Ottenheimer, E. J., Peter van Beskum, K. A., and McKusick, V. A.: Thrombocytopenia with absent radius. *Medicine, 48*:411–439, 1969.

Hamburger, V.: Monsters in nature. *Ciba Symposia, 9*:666–683, 1947.

Herrmann, J., Feingold, M., Tuffli, G. A., and Opitz, J. M.: A familial dysmorphic syndrome of limb deformities, characteristic facial appearance and associated anomalies: the 'pseudo-thalidomide" or "SC-syndrome." *In* Bergsma, D., (ed.): *Birth Defect Original Article Series.* New York: National Foundation-March of Dimes, Vol. V, No. 3:81–89, 1969.

Hill, L. L., Jr.: Congenital abnormalities—phocomelus and congenital absence of radius. *Surg. Gynecol. Obstet, 65*:475–479, 1937.

Hirsch, W.: Phocomelia. *J. Int. Coll. Surg., 39*:238–251, 1963.

Hirst, B. C.: A phocomelic monster. (Dr. A. H. Dag's case). *University Med. Mag.* (Philadelphia), *2*:374–375, 1889.

Hoeven, L. Van Der: Over phocomele. *Ned. T. Geneesk., 20*:13–19, 1884.

Holbron, P.: Un cas de phocomélie et hémimélie. *N. Iconog. Salp., 16*:123–128, 1903.

Homi, C.: A case of phocomelus. *Lancet, 2*:128, 1920.

Joachimsthal, G.: *Die angeborenen Verbildungen der oberen Extremitäten.* Hamburg, L. Gräfe & Sillem, pp. 9–10; figs. 8 and 10; Taf. II, fig. 1, 1900.

Joachimsthal, G.: *Die angeborenen Verbildungen der unteren Extremitäten.* Hamberg, L. Gräfe & Sillem, pp. 22–23, 1902.

Johansson, S.: Ein Fall kongenitalen Defekts von Radius und Ulna. *Z. Orthop. Chir., 42*:1–3, 1922.

Johansson, S.: Ett fall av kongenital defekt av radius och ulna. *Hygiea, 84*:81–84, 1922.

Johnson, H. A.: Formation of a functional thumb post with sensation in phocomelia. *J. Bone Joint Surg., 49A*:327–332, 1967.

Kahn, A. A.: Phocomelia in three Ugandan Children. *Br. Med. J., 2*:1326–1327, 1962.

Kajii, T., Oikawa, K., Itakuro, K., and Ohsawa, T.: A probable 17–18 trisomy syndrome with phoco-melia, exomphalos, and agenesis of hemidiaphragm. *Arch. Dis. Child., 39*:519–522, 1964.

Kaul, A.: *Uber eine besondere Form der Phokomelie.* Inaug.-Diss. Würzburg, P. Scheiner's Buchdruckerei, pp. 5–27, 1899.

Kenny, S.: Phocomelia—three cases. *Br. J. Radiol., 35*:462–467, 1962.

Kindl, J.: Phokomelie beider oberen Extremitäten. *Z. Heilkd. Chir., 28*:122–127, 1907.

Klaussner, F.: *Über Missbildungen der Menschlichen Gliedmassen.* Wiesbaden, J. F. Bergmann, pp. 67–77, figs. 38–40, 1900.

Krueger, R.: *Die Phokomelie und ihre Uebergänge.* Eine Zusammenstellung sämtlicher veröffentlichten Fälle. Berlin, A. Hirschwald, pp. 1–117, 1906.

Kutzenok, B.: Ein Fall von angeborener familiärer Missbildung der oberen Extremitäten. *Arch. Orthop. Unfallchir., 27*:246–259, 1929.

Lafusco, F., and Buffa, V.: Su di un caso di focomelia probablimente secondario a virosi influenzale materna. *Pediatria* (Naples), *70*:954–961; figs. 1–4, 1962.

Lamb, D. W., MacHaughtan, K. M., and Fragiadakis, E. G.: Phocomelia of the upper limb. *Hand, 3*:200–203, 1971.

Lange, M.: *Erbbiologie der angeborenen Körperfehler,* Stuttgart, F. Enke, pp. 79–80, Abb. 27, 1935.

Leloire, H.: Malformation congénitale de l'avant bras et de la main. *Bull. Soc. Anat. Paris,* (4 s.), *4*:65–72, 1879.

Lenz, W.: Kinkliche Missbildungen nach Medikament-Einnahme während der Gravität? *Dtsch. Med. Wochenschr., 86*:2555–2556, 1961.

Lenz, W.: *Congenital Malformations.* New York, The International Medical Congress Ltd., pp. 263–276, 1964.

MacDougall, J.: Foetal monstrosity (phoco-melus). *Trans. Edinburgh Obstet. Soc., 4*:50–52, 1878.

Makley, J. T., and Heiple, K. G.: Scoliosis associated with congenital deficiencies of the upper extremity. *J. Bone Joint Surg., 52A*:279–287; fig. 3A, 1970.

Margolis, E., and Hasson, E.: Herediatry malformations of the upper extremities in three generations. *J. Hered., 46*:255, 1956.

Martin, R., and Munier, J.-P.: Sur un cas de malformations congénitales et héréditaires de membres supérieures. *Arch. Fr. Pediatr., 11*:631–636, 1954.

McConnell, G.: A case of congenital absence of both forearms simulating phocomelus. *Int. Assoc. Med. Mus. J. Tech. Month. Bull., 8*:156–159, 1922.

Megelheier, P. S. de: Un cas de raccourcissement considérable du bras du coté gauche dû ä un arrêt de croissance de humerus correspondant. *Rev. Chir. Paris, 18*:422–447, 1898.

Morgan, J. H.: Arrested development of right upper extremity. *Lancet, 2*:1237, 1888.

Moselkilde, E.: Chondroangeopathia calcarea seu punctata. *In* Diethelm, L, (ed.): *Roentgen. Diagnostik der Skeletterkrankungen.* Berlin, Springer Verlag, Band V, Teil 3, pp. 49–67; figs. 2 and 3, 1968.

Murdock, J. L.: Holt-Oram syndrome: digital and heart anomalies in three generations. *In* Bergsma, D., (ed.): *Birth Defects Original Article Series.* New York: National Foundation-March of Dimes, Vol. V, no. 3:187–189, 1969.

Nigst, P. F.: Die Phokomelie. *Schweiz. Med. Wochenschr., 8*:53, 1927.

O'Brien, H. R., and Mustard, H. S.: An adult living case of total phocomelia. *J.A.M.A.*, 77:1964–1967, 1921.

Oikawa, K., Kochen, J. A., Schorr, J. B., and Hirschhorn, K.: Trisomy 17 syndrome with phocomelia due to complete and partial chromosomal trisomy. *J. Pediatr.*, 63:715, 1963.

Orgler: Demonstration der Radiogramme eines Falles von Phokomelie. *Dtsch. Med. Wochenschr.*, 26:293, 1900.

Patten, B. M.: *Human Embryology.* New York, Blakiston Co., pp. 121–122; fig. 1270, 1946.

Perkins, C. W.: X-ray demonstration of rudimentary development of both arms, with lacking elbow joints. *Med. Rec.*, 101:436, 1922.

Potter, E. L.: *Pathology of the Fetus and the Newborn.* Chicago, Year Book Medical Publishers Inc., pp. 184–185; fig. 521, 1952.

Puschel, E.: *Missbildungen der Gliedmassem.* Stuttgart, F. K. Schattauer, pp. 95–121, 1970.

Roberts, J. B.: A child with double cleft of lip and palate, protrusion of the intermaxiallary protion of the upper jaw and imperfect development of the bones of the four extremities. *Ann. Surg.*, 70:252, 1919.

Rodenstein, L. A.: A case of arrest of development of both upper extremities (Dr. G. W. Snow's case). *Am. J. Obstet.*, 8:663–664, 1875–1876.

Saint-Hilaire, J. G.: *Histoire Générale et Particuliére des Anomalies de l'Organisation chez l'Homme et les Animaux.* Paris, J. B. Ballière, Vol. II, pp. 208–213, 1836.

Sayli, B. S., Asmaz, A., and Yemisc, B.: Consanguinity, aspirin and phocomelia. *Lancet,* 1:876, 1966.

Schonenberg, H.: *Missbildungen der Extremitäten.* Bibliotheca Paediatrica. Fasc. 80, Basel, S. Karger., pp. 40–47, 1962.

Schurig, H.: Über einen Fall symmetrischer Missbildung beider oberen Extremitäten (Phocomelie) nebst einigen Bemerkungen zur Atiologie. *Morph. Jahrb.*, 51:231–257, 1922.

Schwanke, D.: Beitrag zur Kenntnis über Missbildungen der oberen Extremität. *Z. Anat.*, 108:719–725, Abb. 1–3, 1938.

Sentex, L.: Phocomélie accompagnée d'éctrodactylie. *J. Méd. Bordeaux,* 16:53–54, 1886.

Sheldrake, T.: A monstrous child born of a woman under sentence of transportation. *Philosophical Tr.*, 41:341–343, 1740.

Skillern, P. G.: A child with rudimentary left upper extremity (perobrachium). *Ann. Surg.*, 55:421–422; figs. 1 and 2, 1912.

Socin, H.: La morphologie de la phocomélie. *Arch. Méd. Ex. Anat. Pathol.*, 28:485–532, 1917.

Steill, W. F.: A rare congenital malformation. *Lancet,* 2:1015–1016, 1916.

Stiles, K. A., and Dougan, P.: A pedigree of malformed upper extremities. *J. Hered.*, 31:65–72, 1940.

Stroer, W. F. H.: Über das Zusammentreffen von Hasenscharte mit ernsten Extremitätenmiss-bildungen. *Erbarzt.*, 7:101–104, 1939.

Sulamaa, M.: Upper extremity phocomelia: a contribution to its operative treatment. *Clin. Pediatr.*, 2:251–257, 1963.

Swanson, A. B.: Phocomelia and congenital limb malformations reconstruction and prosthetic replacement. *Am. J. Surg.*, 109:294–299, 1965.

Thapar, R. K., Grewal, H. S., and Kalra, K.: Phocomelia with radioulnar synostosis. Report of a case with review of the literature. *Indian J. Pediatr.*, 33:85–87, 1966.

Tiberghein, L.: Notes sur un cas de phocomélie. *Ann. Méd. Chir.* (Bruxelles), 4:45–50, 1893.

Tyrie, C. C., and Haigh, J. W.: Report of a case of phocomelus. *Teratologia,* 1:89–95, Pl. I–VIII, 1894.

Unterricher, L.: Beiträge zur Kenntnis der angeborenen Anomalie der Extremitäten. *Z. Konstitutionslehre,* 18:317–338, 1934.

Virchow: Die Phocomelen und das Bärenweib. *Z. Ethnologie* (Berlin), 11:55–61, 1898.

Wallenstein, F.: Ein Fall von angeborenem totalem Defekt der beiden oberen Extremitäten (Abrachus) und partiellem Defekt der unteren Extremitäten (Phokomelie nach Virchow). *Berl. Klin. Wochenschr.*, 18:390, 1899.

Weidenbach, A.: Total phocomelie. *Z. Gynäkol.*, 81:2048–2052, 1956.

Weil, S.: Die Phokomelie. *In* Hohmann, G., Hackenbrach, M., and Lindemann, K., (eds.): *Handbuch der Orthopädie.* Stuttgart, G. Thieme, Band 3, pp. 6–8, 1959.

Wepler, W. V.: Die sogenannte Phokomelie. *Dtsch. Med. Wochenschr.*, 62:1302–1305, 1937.

Werthemann, A.: *Die Entwicklungsstörungen der Extremitäten.* Berlin, Springer, pp. 113–119, 1952.

Wiedemann, H. R.: Hinweis auf eine derzeitige Häufung hypo- und aplastischer Fehlbildungen der Gliedmassen. *Med. Welt.*, 37:1863–1866, 1961.

Willert, G. G., and Henkel, H. L.: *Klinik und Pathologie der Dysmelie.* Die Fehlbildungen an den oberen Extremitäten bei der Thalidomide-Embryopathie. Berlin, Springer, pp. 43–45, 1969.

Zellweger, H., Huff, D. S., and Abbo, G.: Phocomelia and trisomy E. *Acta Genet. Med.* (Rome), 14:164–172, 1965.

Chapter Twenty-Seven

DISLOCATION OF THE RADIAL HEAD

Bizarre forms of congenital dislocation of the elbow have been reported by a number of authors. McGavin (1913) described a newborn infant whose roentgenographs showed "transposition of the heads of the radius and ulna; the radius articulating with the trochlea and the ulna with the capitellum." Mead and Martin (1963) presented a mother and three children with aplasia of the trochlea and humeroulnar dislocation. The radial head remained in articulation with the capitulum, but the ulna, with its sigmoid notch, was displaced in the ulnar direction and proximally, there being a diastasis between the radius and ulna. Congenital dislocation of the radial head is far more common, is a more definite entity, and is based upon fairly constant structural alterations often referred to as radiocapitellar dysplasia.

OCCURRENCE

Prior to the introduction of radiography—and in fact for many years after—congenital dislocation of the radial head and proximal radioulnar synostosis were confused and even identified with one another. Radioulnar synostosis was considered to be a form of subluxation and was included in most collective reviews of congenital dislocation of the radial head. Bonnenberg (1893) reviewed 30 cases of what he considered to be congenital dislocation of the radial head. Blodgett (1906) cited 51 cases and stated that in one-third of these there was "bone fusion of the upper parts of the radius and ulna." Even some of the other cases which he reported as having no osseous union would now be considered to be examples of incipient radioulnar synostosis. Bergtold's case—number 47 in Blodgett's list—is one example. Bergtold's (1891) patient, an eight-year-old boy, had "complete and perfect" flexion and extension at the elbow, but pronation and supination of the forearm were "entirely wanting." On forced rotation of the forearm, what was considered to be the radial head moved slightly. On the basis of this finding, Bergtold concluded that there was interlocking but "no co-

902

alescence of radius and ulna." It is now known that in some cases of radioulnar synostosis the bony bridge does not mature until the age of 10 or 12 years, and slight movement of the radial head can be elicited passively.

The number of cases reviewed by Blodgett, but not his name, appeared in Lovett's (1909) article in Keen's *Surgery*. "In searching through several textbooks, we found that Keen gave the best description and stated that 51 cases had been reported up to 1907," Mauck and Butterworth (1940) wrote. The search must have been very cursory. These authors did not mention Lovett's name nor the fact that 17 out of 51 reported congenital dislocations of the radial head were cases of proximal radioulnar synostosis. White (1942–1943) described a case of dislocation of the radial head without synostosis; he also reviewed 21 other cases, 11 of which belonged to McFarland (1936). Caravias (1957) could find only 25 cases recorded in all the literature, and among the four cases he added to White's list, he included roentgenographs of a case shown by Watson-Jones (1941).

If a roentgenograph deserves a place in tabulations of congenital dislocation of the radial head, cases which have been subjected to careful clinical study and confirmed by dissection have more justification to be accorded their niche. In most later tabulations — by Almquist et al (1969) and others — continental authors who have reported numerous authenticated cases of congenital dislocation of the radial head are not mentioned. As with many other congenital defects, this anomaly is far more prevalent than statistics indicate.

BASIC CHANGE

Robert Smith (1852), who was mentioned in Chapter Eighteen, studied a number of patients with congenital dislocation of the radial head and dissected their elbows after their deaths. Smith recorded the following findings in each: a relatively small, underdeveloped forearm; shrunken hypoplastic or completely absent humeral capitulum; partially defective trochlea; prominent ulnar epicondyle; absent lesser sigmoid cavity on the radial aspect of the proximal ulna; short ulna or one which does not quite reach the carpus distally; comparatively long radius which bypasses the level of the elbow joint; undersized radial head bearing a domed, instead of dimpled, proximal articular plateau; and grooving of the distal humerus at the point of impingement of the dislocated radial head. Smith likened the last change to the false acetabulum formed on the side of the ilium in congenital dislocation of the hip. The excavation, he said, might be located in the back, front, or radial aspect of the distal humerus, depending upon whether the head of the radius had become displaced backward, forward, or to the radial side. Regardless of the direction of the displacement of the radial head, the capitulum of the humerus was found defective.

Over 100 years after Robert Smith's communication, Caravias (1957) pronounced the failure of growth of the humeral capitulum as the primary defect in congenital dislocation of the radial head and considered the altered configuration of the latter to be "a secondary deformity." As had Smith, Caravias singled out the underdeveloped capitulum as the most reliable sign of congenital dislocation of the radial head (Fig. 27–1).

Spinner and Kaplan (1970) described what they called quadrate ligament of the elbow. This structure emanates from the radial aspect of the proximal ulna and connects with the neck of the radius just distal to the articular margin. The

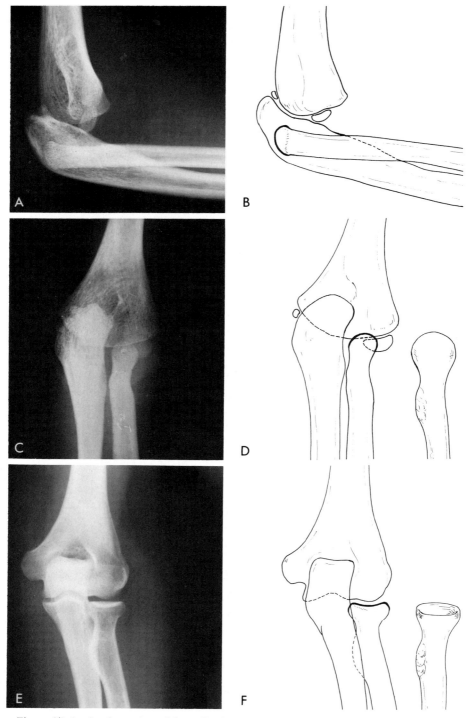

Figure 27–1 Configuration of the radial head in congenital dislocation. *A*, Lateral roentgenograph of the right elbow of an adolescent with posterior dislocation of the radial head. *B*, Sketch illustrating the same. *C*, Dorsovolar roentgenograph: the radial head is dome-shaped; the neck is thin. *D*, Sketch illustrating the same. *E*, Dorsovolar roentgenograph of the right elbow of a normal young adult: the radial head presents a dimpled, or concave, superior articular surface and has a broader neck. *F*, Sketch illustrating the same.

ligament has an anterior and posterior border, the former being denser and stronger. In full supination of the forearm, the thicker anterior fibers of the quadrate ligament are said to stabilize the radioulnar joint. Laxity or tear of this portion of the ligament is said to be responsible for "pulled elbows" and traumatic dislocations of the radial head. "In addition, one may question whether some congenital dislocations of the radial head in childhood are not the end result of an accidental dislocation of the newborn which was not recognized. In support of this speculation a 30 per cent incidence of dislocations of the radial head (anterior and posterior) in cases of Erb's palsy is reported by Aitken (1952)," Spinner and Kaplan wrote. The speculation remains farfetched, since in many cases of congenital dislocation of the radial head there are other prenatally determined anomalies; some cases, moreover, have hereditary antecedents and are associated with anomalies of other parts.

CAUSAL RELATIONS

Ambard (1901) reported a patient with congenital dislocation of both radial heads; he considered hereditary syphilis to be the cause, since the patient presented such telltale stigmata as collapsed nasal bridge and keratitis. In the course of his discussion of Power's (1903) paper on congenital dislocation of the radius, Bottomley (1903) reported two cases belonging to F. J. Cotton of Boston City Hospital. Both patients were said to have congenital syphilis of the elbow. One patient had unilateral involvement; the other, bilateral. Guilleminet and Leclerc (1937) reported three cases of bilateral congenital dislocation of the radial head. All three belonged to the same family and had the characteristic features of hereditary syphilis—"facies d'heredo-syphilitique." Mauck and Butterworth (1940) described a 40-year-old man who had never been able to flex his elbow beyond a right angle. Diagnosis of bilateral congenital dislocation of the radius was made. The Wasserman reaction of both blood and spinal fluid was positive. It is perhaps significant that since the introduction of penicillin, syphilis is not mentioned in discussions of congenital dislocation of the radial head.

Gunn and Pillay (1964) described a mother and daughter, and another girl. The three belonged to a tribe of Tamils residing in Malaya. All three had dislocated radial heads. The Tamils, it is said, often marry their cousins. On the basis of the prevalence of consanguineous marriage in the small community from which the affected individuals came, Gunn and Pillay considered the transmission of the trait to be probably recessive. Dislocation of the radial head is inherited as a dominant phenotype when it occurs in connection with such complexes as multiple exostosis, nail-patella syndrome, and antecubital pterygium.

DELAYED RECOGNITION

Congenital dislocation of the radial head is often overlooked until pain and dysfunction following injury invite attention. Leisbrink's (1879) patient was an 18-year-old boy who sought advice after he injured his left arm. The radial head was found to be dislocated anteriorly, and the ulna was fractured. The fracture of the ulna was reduced, but the radial head remained dislocated and could not be reduced. On further inquiry, it was discovered that the patient had had a deformed elbow since the age of 3. Mouchet and d'Allaines (1928) reported a 14-year-old boy who was not aware of the fact that he had anything the matter with his elbow until he injured it. McFarland (1936) related the story of another boy who had sustained a fracture of the ulna for which he had been treated by a general practitioner. The parents of this boy complained of a persistent lump in front of the elbow which interfered with function. "I was able to establish that this radius had been dislocated before the accident, and was in fact a congenital dislocation," McFarland wrote. Rose (1938) spoke of a patient who had injured his right elbow in an unsuccessful attempt to grasp the handrail of a quickly moving omnibus. Rose reduced what was diagnosed as traumatic dislocation of the radial head. Immediately afterward, the dislocation recurred. The opposite elbow was examined. It presented an exaggerated carrying angle or cubitus valgus, and the extension at the elbow was curtailed; roentgenographic examination revealed bilateral dislocation of the radial head. Magee (1947) saw a 27-year-old man soon after he had injured his left elbow by being thrown from a motorcycle. Roentgenographic examination of both the injured and uninjured elbows showed bilateral dislocation of the radial head; the latter was "rounded" and had lost its "cup-shaped articular surface."

RECURRENT OR HABITUAL DISLOCATION

In all reported cases of congenital dislocation of the radial head, there are only three which are incriminated as being recurrent or habitual. The first of these was reported by Heelis (1886). His patient was a "loose-jointed" boy with bilateral dislocation of the radial head; the left head stayed in its dislocated locus and, when reduced, it slipped out of place on slight pronation of the forearm; the right head was partially dislocated. Bindman's (1945) patient was a young girl. While attempting to loosen a button on the left shoulder with her right hand she suddenly felt a pain in the right elbow and noticed that a lump appeared in front of the elbow. The dislocation, which was anterior, could be reduced by simple thumb pressure, but it recurred when the forearm was supinated and the elbow extended beyond 90 degrees. Roentgenographs revealed a shallow, poorly developed radial head, which made Bindman suspect congenital origin of the condition. This suspicion was strengthened by the absence of any history of trauma. Wahren (1945) reported the third case, calling it habitual luxation of the capitulum radii.

QUESTION OF DISLOCATION BY ELONGATION

Transient subluxation of the radial head often occurs in young children. Since the presumed displacement happens following traction of the hand or forearm, the designation dislocation by elongation is applied to this condition. In France, the condition is often referred to as Goyand's (1842) injury. In America, the condition is called pulled elbow. "Its features," Stimson (1888) wrote, "are well marked: a young child generally less than three-years-old, is lifted or pulled by the hand, it cries out with pain, and refuses to use the limb, which hangs motionless by the side, somewhat flexed at the elbow, and more or less pronated. A careful examination fails to discover marked changes in anatomical relations of the bones at the elbow or wrist; passive motion at both joints is free but painful, except supination which is resisted; often during the manipulation made in the examination or on forced supination, a slight click is heard, and the child is at once able to use the limb freely without pain."

Van Arsdale (1889) cited 100 consecutive cases of transient subluxation of the radial head. He reviewed the literature on this subject extensively and conceded that the anatomical lesion underlying subluxation of the radial head in children had not yet been established. It is not established, even now. Congenital defects of the orbicular ligament, of the joint capsule, or even of the radial head have been incriminated—conjecturally. The facts that this variety of subluxation is preceded by injury and that it is easily reduced, and stays reduced, point to its being acquired rather than congenital.

REGIONAL ASSOCIATIONS

It is a general rule that when one of two parallel bones, such as the radius or ulna, is short, the other tends to outstrip its mate and push its smaller extremity out of the joint where it is least resisted. Digby (1916) estimated that the radius obtains 75 per cent of its growth in length from its distal epiphyseal plate; the radius grows mostly in the direction of its nutrient vessels—toward the elbow. The carpal extremity of the radius is massive; it affords anchorage and is anchored in turn by such muscles as the brachioradialis and pronator quadratus and by a number of stout ligaments; it has, moreover a broad buttress ahead and is not likely to dislocate. No muscle or ligament connects with and tethers the head of the radius, which is small and is covered with cartilage on the top and around, making it slippery and prone to dislocate. The radial head has a comparatively small bone, the capitulum of the humerus, standing in its way; this ossicle serves as an obstacle only when the elbow is in extension. In flexion—which is the usual position of the elbow in the fetus—the head of the radius has no bony block in its path and may easily slip past the humeral capitulum, especially when the latter is hypoplastic or completely absent. An ulna with adequate length would normally counteract this tendency. A short ulna fails to exert any restraining action and permits the radius to push its growth in the direction of its nutrient artery, proximally; at the elbow, the hypoplastic capitulum of the humerus fails to provide an effective obstruction and permits the head of the radius to slip behind or in front.

Dislocation of the radial head is a common accompaniment of absent or short ulna. Guérin-Valmale and Jeanbreau (1899) noted the association of what they called pure congenital club hand and congenital luxation of the elbow—"main-bote congénital pure avec luxation congénitale de coude." Zorn (1967–1968) recorded the association of congenital dislocation of the radial head and Sprengel's deformity. The head of the radius is dislocated in some cases of absent pollical ray and side-to-side fusion of the ulnar metacarpals or phalanges. Dislocation of the radial head is more often seen in association with oligodactyly, especially in ulnar oligodactyly (Figs. 27–2 to 27–9).

(Text continued on page 912.)

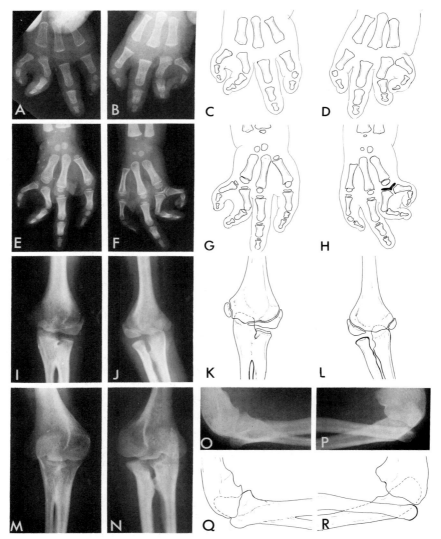

Figure 27–2 Dislocation of the radial head associated with side-to-side fusion of the epiphyses of the proximal phalanges of the ipsilateral two ulnar digits and proximal radioulnar synostosis of the opposite limb—in an infant with bilateral absence of the thumb, three metacarpals in each hand, and two ulnar digits stemming from a single metacarpal and simulating parentheses. *A* and *B*, Dorsopalmar roentgenographs of the right and left hands of the six-week-old girl featured in Figure 24–10: note that the proximal ends of the basal phalanges of the last two ulnar digits are closer. *C* and *D* illustrate roentgenographs of the right and left hands, respectively. *E* and *F*, Dorsopalmar roentgenographs of the right and left hands taken at the age of 18 months—about 16 months after pollicization of the index fingers: the distal epiphysis of the radius and the two carpal bones are smaller on the left side; the proximal phalanges of the two last ulnar digits share a single continuous epiphysis. *G* and *H* illustrate roentgenographs of the right and left hands, respectively, at the age of 18 months. *I* and *J*, Dorsovolar roentgenographs taken at the age of nine years: the proximal ends of the right radius and ulna have affected solid bony union; the left radial head lacks an epiphysis—it is thinner and domed and tilts away from the olecranon process of the ulna. *K* and *L* illustrate the roentgenographs of the right and left elbow, respectively, at the age of nine years. *M* and *N*, Dorsopalmar roentgenographs of the right and left elbows, taken at the age of 16 years. *O* and *P*, Lateral roentgenographs of the right and left elbows, taken at the same age: the head of the left radius is dislocated posteriorly. *Q* and *R* illustrate the roentgenograph above each. Curiously, the radial head is dislocated on the side of the confluent epiphyses of the proximal phalanges of the last two ulnar digits and radioulnar synostosis affects the opposite limb in which there is no fusion of distal elements.

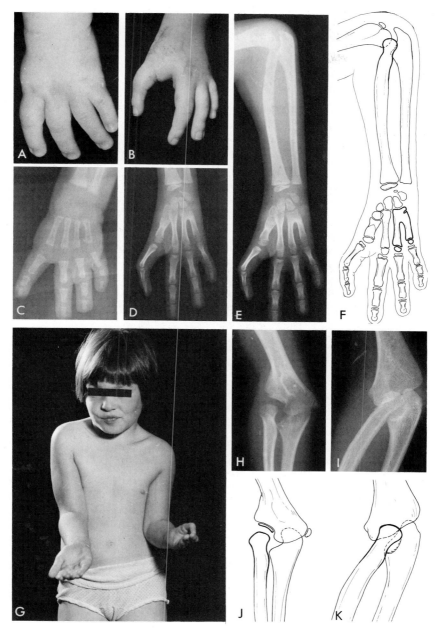

Figure 27–3 Dislocation of the radial head in radial oligodactyly: *A*, Preoperative dorsal view of the left hand of the six-week-old girl featured in Figure 24–11. *B*, Same after pollicization of the index finger. *C*, Dorsopalmar roentgenograph of the left hand taken at the age of six weeks. *D*, The same at the age of five years. *E*, Dorsovolar roentgenograph of the left elbow, forearm, and wrist taken at the age of five years: the head of the radius is dislocated anteriorly and the bases of the last two ulnar metacarpals have affected bony union. *F*, Sketch illustrating the same. *G*, Photograph taken at the age of eight years, showing diminished supination of the left forearm and hand. *H*, Dorsovolar roentgenograph of the left elbow: the capitulum humeri is dysplastic and the head of the radius presents a dome-shaped articular surface — these two features are characteristic of congenital dislocation of the radial head. *I*, Lateral roentgenograph of the left elbow showing anterior dislocation of the radial head. *J* and *K* illustrate the roentgenograph above each. In this subject, as in the one featured in Figure 27–4 with ulnar oligodactyly, dislocation of the radial head has occurred on the side where two elements of the ulnar digital rays have affected side-to-side bony union.

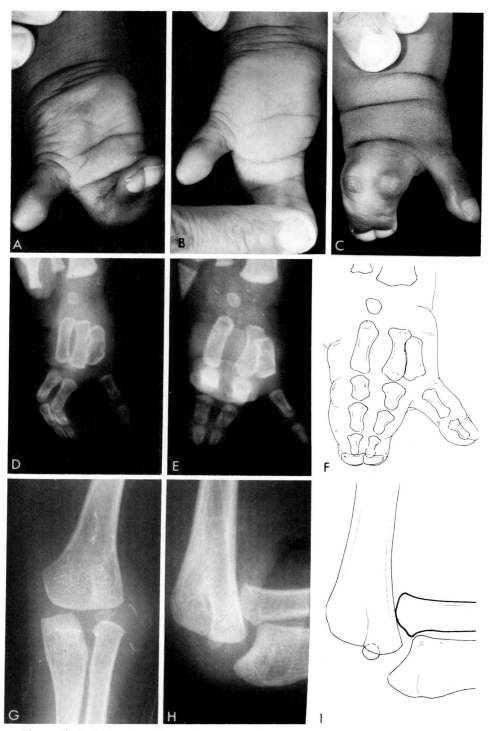

Figure 27–4   Dislocation of the radial head associated with ulnar oligodactyly, fenestrated fusion of the first two metacarpals, and syndactyly of the second and third digits. *A, B,* and *C,* Views of the right hand of a four-month-old boy. *D,* Oblique roentgenograph of the hand. *E,* Dorsopalmar roentgenograph. *F,* Sketch illustrating the same. *G,* Dorsovolar roentgenograph of the right elbow. *H,* Lateral roentgenograph. *I,* Sketch illustrating the same.

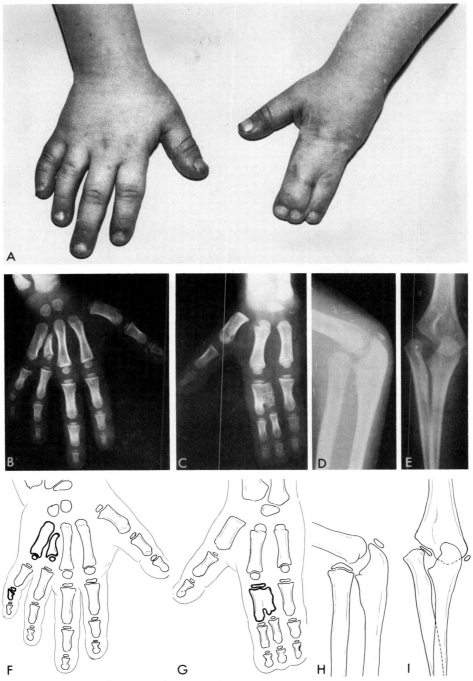

Figure 27–5 Dislocation of the radial head associated with ulnar oligodactyly and intercalary defect of the metacarpals. *A*, Dorsal view of the hands of a two-year-old boy. *B*, Dorsopalmar roentgenograph of the right hand: the fourth metacarpal is defective proximally. *C*, Dorsopalmar roentgenograph of the left hand: the distal radial epiphysis is not in evidence; there is only one carpal bone; the third metacarpal is missing; the proximal phalanges of the index and middle fingers are united by bone; the three fingers are webbed; and the fifth digital ray is absent. *D*, Lateral roentgenograph of the left elbow: the head of the radius is dislocated anteriorly. *E*, Dorsopalmar roentgenograph of the left elbow: the radial head is dislocated upwards. *F*, *G*, *H* and *I* illustrate the roentgenograph above each.

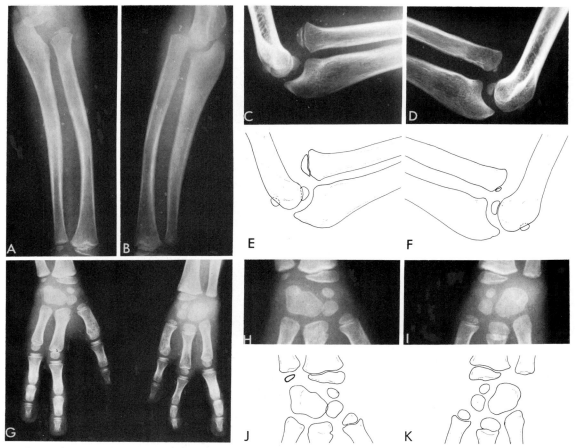

Figure 27–6   Bilateral anterior dislocation of the radial head associated with ulnar oligodactyly and disharmonious development of the epiphyses of the radius and ulna and carpal bones. *A*, Dorsovolar roentgenograph of the right forearm of an eight-year-old boy with bilateral ulnar oligodactyly. *B*, The same of the left forearm. *C*, Lateral roentgenograph of the right elbow, showing a sizeable radial epiphysis. *D*, Lateral roentgenograph of the left elbow with a barely discernible radial epiphysis. *E* and *F* illustrate the roentgenograph above each. *G*, Dorsopalmar roentgenograph of the wrists and hands: the distal epiphysis of the left ulna is not visible as yet. *H*, Roentgenograph of the right wrist. *I*, Roentgenograph of the left wrist. *J* and *K* illustrate the roentgenograph above each.

Senftleben (1869) described a patient with congenitally dwarfed ulna and dislocation of the radial head. The accompanying illustration showed an overexpansion of the proximal ulna, probably due to regional enchondromatosis or exostosis. Numerous instances of dislocation of the radial head have been reported in multiple exostoses of the ulna, which leaves this bone short; the combination was described by Hagen (1891), and the syndrome bears his name. For analogous reasons, the radial head is dislocated in multiple enchondromatosis—with or without hemangiomas. Dislocation of the radial head is often seen in mucopolysaccharidosis. There are a number of other complexes in which the radial head is dislocated. Some of these syndromes are discussed in alphabetical order in the following paragraphs (Figs. 27–10 and 27–11).

(Text continued on page 918.)

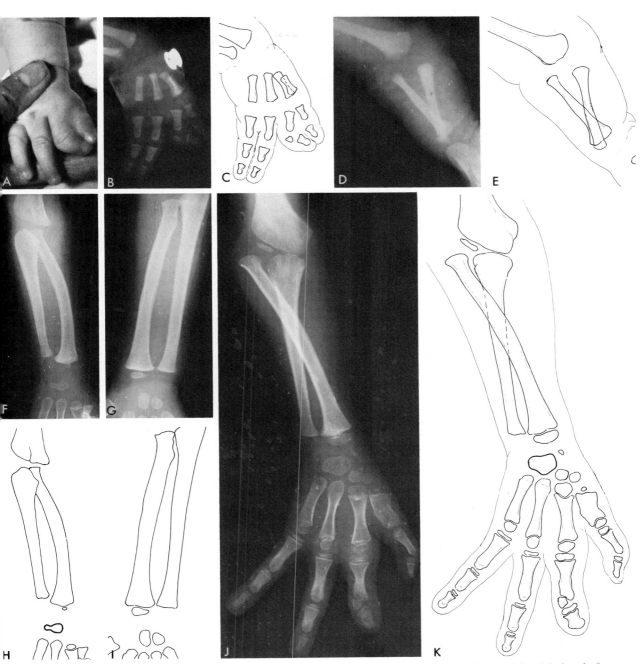

Figure 27–7   Dislocation of the radial head associated with ulnar oligodactyly. *A,* Dorsal view of the right hand of a three-month-old boy (see Figure 12–24) with syndactyly of the thumb and index finger and absence of an ulnar digit. *B,* Dorsopalmar roentgenograph of the right hand: the index finger has an eccentric triangular middle phalanx. *C,* Sketch illustrating the same. *D,* Anteroposterior roentgenograph of the right forearm. *E,* Sketch illustrating the same. *F,* Dorsovolar roentgenograph of the right forearm in prone position taken at the age of 2 contrasted with the left forearm *G:* on the right side, the radius and ulna are shorter and thinner; the distal epiphysis of the radius is puny; the capitate and hamate are fused. *H* and *I* illustrate the roentgenograph above each. *J,* Anteroposterior roentgenograph of the right forearm and hand taken at the age of 5 after correction of syndactyly, angulation osteotomy of the proximal phalanx of the index finger, and abduction-rotation osteotomy of the pollical metacarpal. *K,* Sketch illustrating the same.

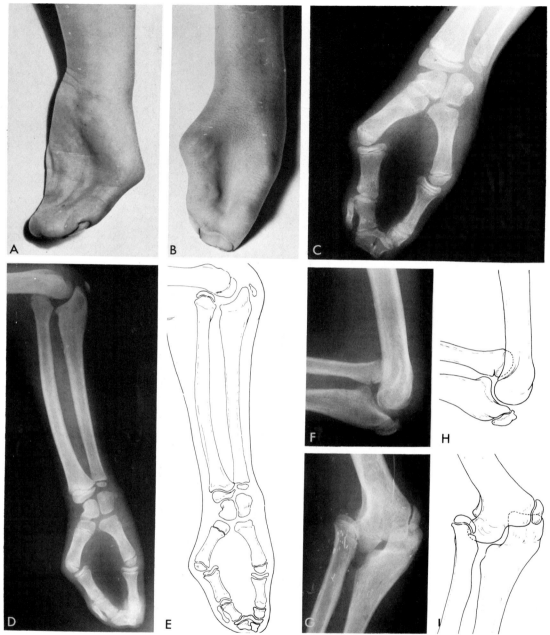

Figure 27–8   Dislocation of the radial head in central oligodactyly and webbing of the two remaining marginal digits. *A*, Palmar view of the left hand of the eight-year-old boy featured in Figures 25–15 and 25–16. *B*, Dorsal view. *C*, Dorsopalmar roentgenograph of the left wrist and hand. *D*, Dorsovolar roentgenograph of the left elbow, forearm, wrist, and hand: the head of the radius is dislocated anteriorly; there are two massive carpal bones at the wrist and a small ossicle on the ulnar aspect of one; the radial metacarpal has an epiphysis at each end; the ulnar metacarpal has a distal epiphysis but bears a notch at its proximal extremity, suggesting a pseudoepiphysis at this end. Each digital ray possesses two phalanges; a longitudinally disposed sliver of bone lies on the radial aspect of the distal phalanx of the radial digit; a transversely disposed undulating flat piece of bone unites the tips of the two digital rays; ahead of this bridge of bone lie two rudimentary ungual phalanges. *E*, Sketch illustrating the same. *F*, Lateral roentgenograph of the left elbow taken at the age of eight years. *G*, Oblique roentgenograph taken a year later. *H* and *I* illustrate the roentgenograph next to each.

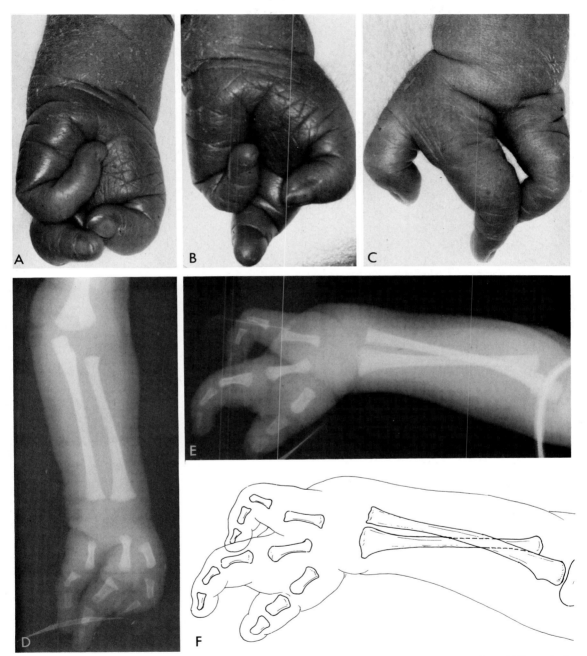

Figure 27–9 Dislocation of the radial head associated with two missing central digits—the middle and ring fingers?—and congenital heart disease which was diagnosed as pseudotruncus and for which the infant was subjected to a Waterstone procedure. *A*, *B*, and *C*, Views of the left hand of a one-day-old boy. *D*, Anteroposterior roentgenograph of the left elbow, forearm, and hand, showing only one biphalangeal and two triphalangeal digits. *E*, Oblique roentgenograph of the same, showing posterior dislocation of the left radial head. *F*, Sketch illustrating the roentgenograph above it.

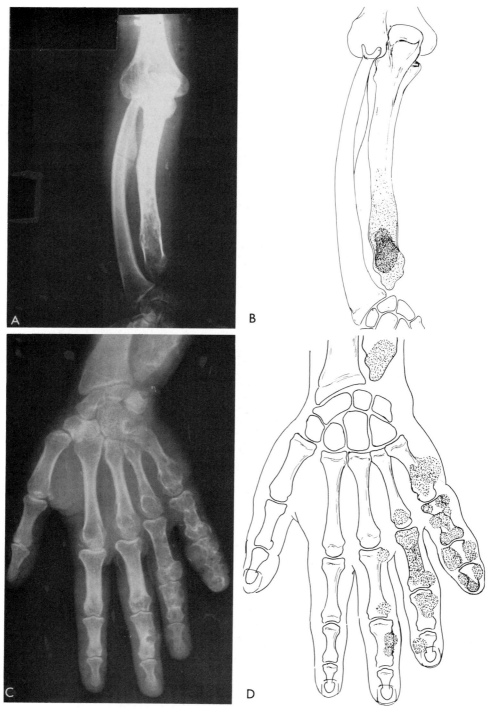

Figure 27–10   Multiple enchondromatosis without hemangioma—Ollier's disease. *A*, Dorsovolar roentgenograph of the left forearm of the 24-year-old woman featured in Figures 20–5 to 20–7: the head of the radius is hypoplastic—it is dislocated upward and backward; the ulna is short and its distal shaft is bulbous and bears intraosseous translucent areas. *B*, Sketch illustrating the same. *C*, Dorsopalmar roentgenograph of the hand: the two ulnar metacarpals are short and the three ulnar digital rays, but especially the ring and middle fingers and their metacarpals, are affected most. *D*, Sketch illustrating the same.

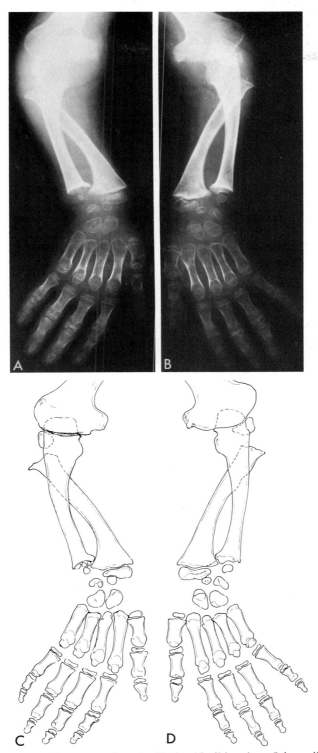

Figure 27–11 Morquio's mucopolysaccharidosis with dislocation of the radial heads. *A*, Dorsovolar roentgenograph of the right forearm and hand of a seven-year-old child: trapezium, trapezoid, and scaphoid bones have not yet appeared. *B*, Roentgenograph of the left forearm and hand. *C* and *D* illustrate the roentgenograph above each.

ACRO-OSTEOLYSIS CONGENITA

This complex was discussed in Chapter Eight. In the case reported by Hajdu and Kauntze (1948), the roentgenograph of the right elbow showed aplasia of the capitulum humeri and dislocation of the radial head.

ANTECUBITAL PTERYGIUM

Congenital web formation in front of the elbow joint is comparatively uncommon. Shun-Shin (1954) described eight affected individuals in three generations of one family. Roentgenographs of the elbows revealed bilateral posterior subluxation of the radial head and "maldevelopment of the radioulnar joint." Cockshott and Omololu (1958) described a female infant with restrained extension of both elbows. Her father's elbow likewise could not be extended farther than a right angle. The proband had posterior dislocation of both radial heads. The subjects reported by Shun-Shin were natives of the very small isolated town of Rodriquez, 300 miles east of Mauritius. Cockshott's and Omololu's patients—father and daughter—resided in Nigeria. Presumably all these affected individuals were dark-skinned. It may be of some interest to note in this connection that Jacklin (1964) reported six persons—four females and two males—affected by ocular pterygium in three generations of the same family, also Negroes. Pterygium antecubiti is transmitted as an autosomal dominant phenotype (Figs. 27–12 and 27–13).

AURICULO-OSTEODYSPLASIA

Beals (1967) described the pedigrees of two families in which the affected members manifested the following characteristics: peculiarly shaped external ear, with an elongated lobe and posteriorly placed lobule; dysplasia of the radiocapitellar joint, with or without dislocation of the radial head; and short stature. In some instances, there was also dysplasia of the hips, and the superior medial angle of the scapula was prominent. Dysplasia of the radial head was the most constant feature of the symptom complex. The trait is regarded as an autosomal dominant.

BIRD-HEADED DWARFISM

Seckel (1960) gave the following characteristics of this complex: extremely short stature, small head and small brain, mental retardation short of true idiocy, beaklike protrusion of the central face, receding chin, and frequent association with multiple congenital malformations. Among the latter he included anterior dislocation of the radial head.

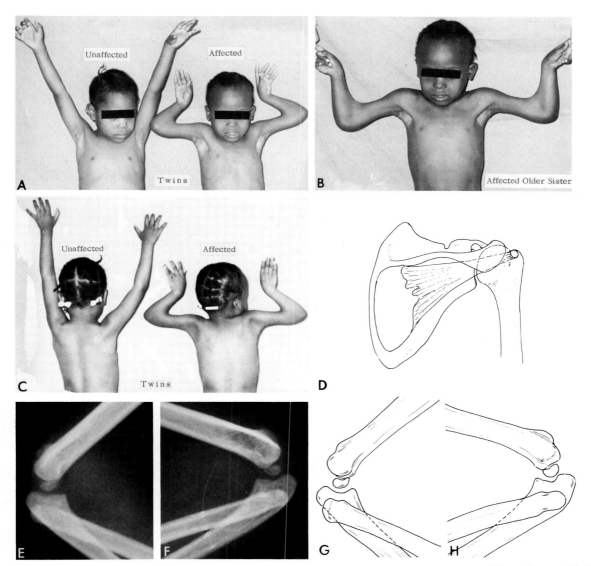

Figure 27–12 Antecubital pterygium. *A,* Frontal view of twin sisters, one of whom has bilateral antecubital pterygium and cannot extend the forearms at the elbows or the upper arms at the shoulders. *B,* An older sister with less marked bilateral pterygium antecubiti: note that this child also has limited extension at both the elbows and the shoulders. The mother of these three girls reported that their father, living in the South, also had webbing of the elbows. *C,* Dorsal view of the twins: the twin without pterygium antecubiti had atrophy of the left infraspinatus muscle; the twin with antecubital pterygium had a vestigial infraspinatus on the right side and a completely absent muscle on the left side. *D,* Sketch showing the hypoplastic left infraspinatus muscle. *E* and *F,* Lateral roentgenographs of the right and left elbows of the twin with antecubital pterygium: note bilateral posterior dislocation of the radial heads as illustrated in sketches *G* and *H.* The older sister, shown in *B,* also had bilateral dislocation of the radial head (see Fig. 27–13).

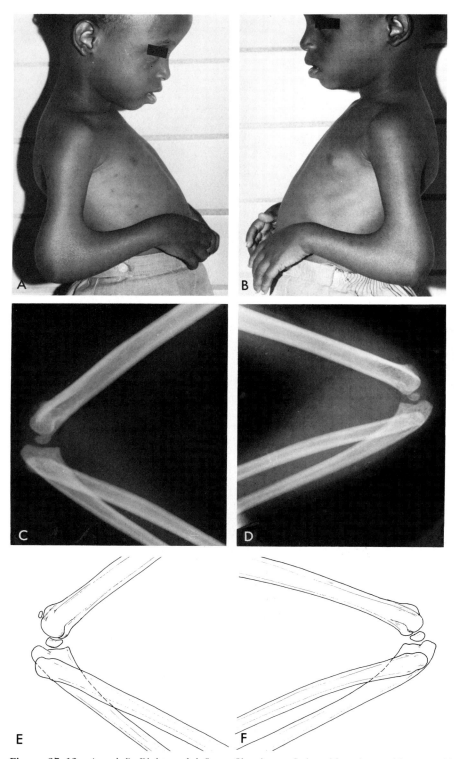

Figure 27–13   *A* and *B*, Right and left profile views of the older sister with antecubital pterygium featured in Figure 27–12. *C* and *D*, Lateral view roentgenographs of the right and left elbows, showing posterior dislocation of the radial heads. *E* and *F* illustrate the roentgenograph above each.

CHROMOSOMAL ABERRATIONS

Almquist et al (1969) reported a 12-year-old boy with atrophic testicles, tall stature, chromosome pattern XXXY or XXXXY, and bilateral elbow deformities which had been present since birth. In the right elbow there was radioulnar synostosis; in the left, anterior dislocation of the radial head. Walker and Borgaonkar (1969) presented a male child whose karyotype contained three extra XY chromosomes; roentgenographs showed delayed maturation of the epiphyses. The head of the right radius was displaced in the radial direction.

CRANIO-CARPOTARSAL DYSTROPHY

This complex was taken up in Chapter Seventeen. Walker (1969) described a black woman with what he called whistling-face and windmill-vane syndrome; roentgenograph of the right elbow showed posterior dislocation of the radial head.

CRANIOSYNOSTOSIS

Pillay (1964) reported two cases of acrocephalosyndactyly with bilateral dislocation of the radial head.

DE LANGE DWARFISM

Zweymüller (1957) presented a De Lange dwarf with bilateral dislocation of the radial head. Jervis and Stimson (1963) described five patients and in all of them the elbows could not be completely extended. In four cases of their series, "posterior dislocation of the head of the radius was present." Hypoplasia and dislocation of the radial head were present in four other cases reported by Lee and Kenny (1967). Gerald and Umansky (1967) also reported cases of de Lange dwarfism with dislocation of the radial head.

DETENBECK-ABRAMS SYNDROME

Detenbeck and Abrams (1970) reported a 15-day-old Negro infant with the following abnormalities: short limbs, syndactyly of the thumb and index finger, fusion of the first two and last two metacarpals, absent middle phalanx of the little finger, and anterior dislocation of the radial head. The anomalies were bilateral and symmetrical. There were no hereditary antecedents with similar malformations.

EHLERS-DANLOS SYNDROME

Key (1927) wrote an article entitled "Hypermobility of joints as a sex-linked hereditary characteristic." One patient he reported had habitual dislocation of the elbow. One of five patients with Ehlers-Danlos complex—laxity of skin, fragility of small vessels, parchment-thin scars, and hyperextensibility of joints—reported by Hass and Hass (1958) had bilateral dislocation of the radial head. Almquist et al (1969) spoke of a patient who had habitual dislocation.

FAMILIAL RADIOULNAR OR TIBIOFIBULAR SYNOSTOSIS

Almquist et al (1969) reported an eight-year-old boy with posterior dislocation of the left radial head and proximal radioulnar synostosis on the right side. He also had bilateral synostosis of the tibia and fibula. "All men in the kindred for eight generations had bone deformities of their arms and legs; in the last three generations these deformities were synostosis of the tibia and fibula, and radius and ulna."

JÄGER-REFIOR SYNDROME

Jäger and Refior (1968) reported a case which bore some resemblance to Rubinstein-Taybi syndrome as well as to otopalatodigital syndrome but in some respects differed from both. The propositus was mentally retarded and had hypertelorism and general skeletal dysplasia, with stub thumb, clubbing of the ungual phalanges, and subluxation of the radial head.

KÖNIG'S DISEASE

An hereditary form of osteochondritis dissecans is said to occur only in males. Almquist et al (1969) reported a 12-year-old boy with osteochondral defects of the right and left femoral medial condyles and the right capitulum. He had a posterior dislocation of the left radial head.

LARSEN'S SYNDROME

Larsen et al (1950) reported six sporadic cases featuring the following abnormalities: flattened facies, with prominent forehead, depressed nasal bridge, and wide-spaced eyes; bilateral dislocation of the elbows, hips, and knees; equinovarus or equinovalgus of the feet; supernumerary carpal ossicles; cylindrical fingers which do not taper normally, short metacarpals, and stub thumb; and, occasionally, cleft palate and failure of spinal segmentation. In the elbow,

(Text continued on page 926.)

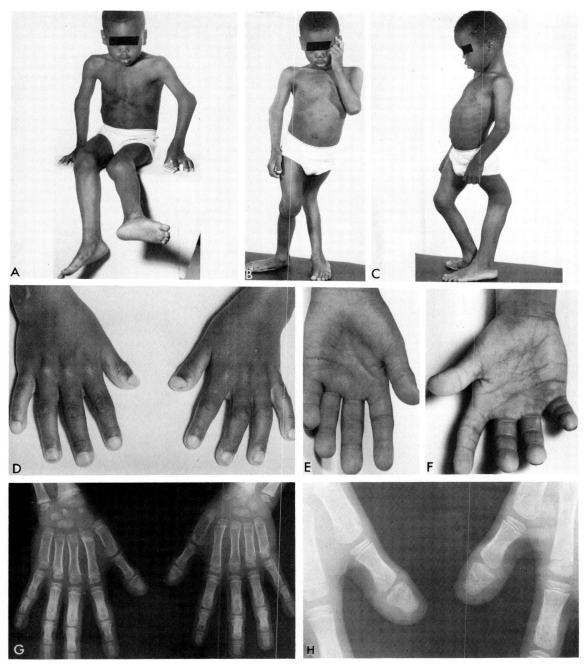

Figure 27–14   Larsen's syndrome. *A, B,* and *C,* A four-year-old boy (see also Figure 8–9) with multiple deformities, mainly dislocations of the knees and elbows. *D,* Dorsal view of the hands, showing stub thumbs. *E,* Palmar view of the right hand. *F,* The same of the left hand. *G,* Dorsopalmar roentgenograph of the wrists and hands, showing precocious appearance of the ulnar epiphyses; appearance of the scaphoid before the trapezium on both sides; and accessory ossicles—one near the right and two around the left lunate bones. *H,* Dorsopalmar roentgenograph of the thumbs, showing precocious closure of the epiphyses of the ungual phalanges.

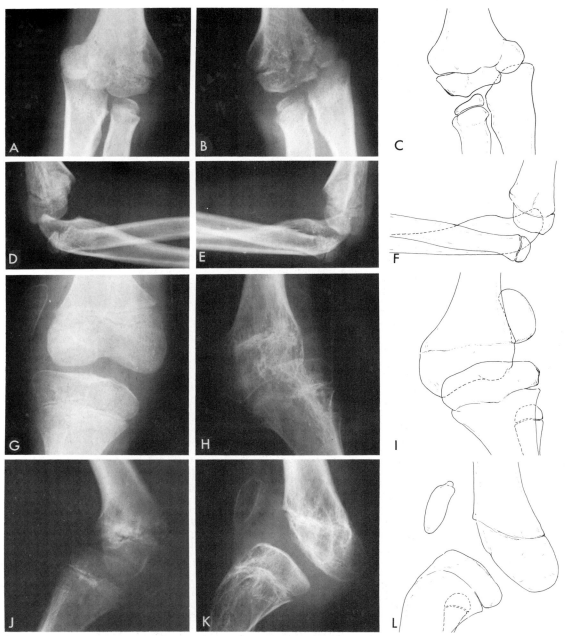

Figure 27–15   *A,* Dorsovolar roentgenograph of the right elbow of the boy featured in Figure 27–14 taken at the age of 9. *B,* The same of the left elbow. *C,* Sketch illustrating *B. D* and *E,* Lateral roentgenographs of the right and left elbows, respectively, showing bilateral dislocation of the radial heads. *F,* Sketch illustrating *E. G,* Anteroposterior roentgenograph of the right knee, showing laterally dislocated patella and slight valgus deformity. *H,* The same of the left knee, showing severe valgus deformity. *I,* Sketch illustrating *H. J,* Lateral roentgenograph of the left knee, showing posterior subluxation of the tibia. *K,* Lateral roentgenograph of the left knee, showing anterior dislocation of the tibia. *L,* Sketch illustrating *K.*

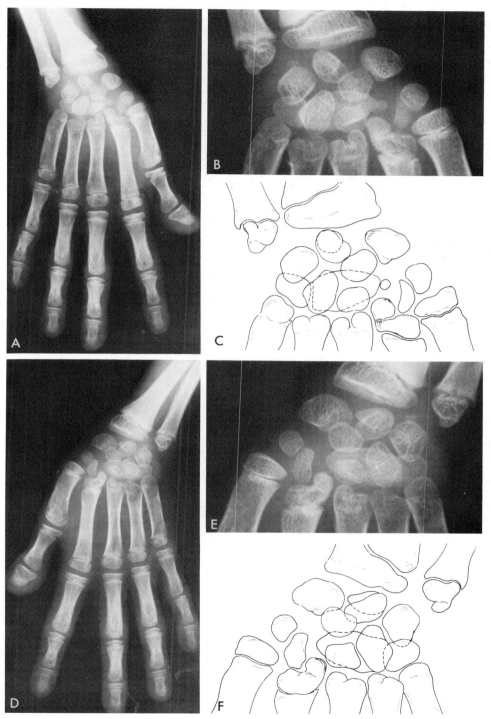

Figure 27–16 *A*, Dorsopalmar roentgenograph of the right wrist and hand of the boy featured in Figures 27–14 and 27–15 taken at the age of nine years. *B*, Enlarged roentgenograph of the right wrist, showing supernumerary—13—carpal bones and accessory epiphyses at the proximal ends of the ulnar metacarpals. *C*, Sketch illustrating the same. *D*, Dorsopalmar roentgenograph of the left hand. *E*, Enlarged roentgenograph of the left wrist. *F*, Sketch illustrating the same.

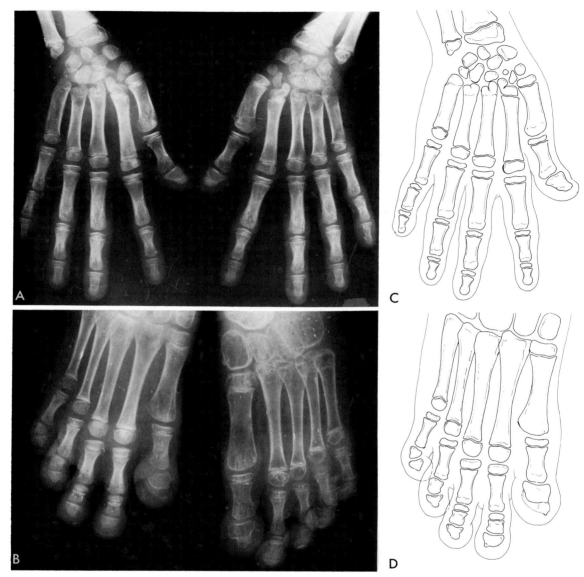

Figure 27–17   *A*, Dorsopalmar roentgenograph of the hands of the boy featured in Figures 27–14 to 27–16. *B*, Dorsoplantar roentgenograph of the forefeet: the right great toe is short. *C*, Sketch illustrating the roentgenograph of the right hand. *D*, Sketch illustrating the roentgenograph of the right forefoot.

the radial heads are dislocated mainly; at the knee, the tibias are displaced forward. Steel and Kohl (1972) described three siblings with multiple dislocations; all three had delayed coalescence of centers of ossification of the calcaneus. Two out of three had multiple anomalous ossification of the calcaneous. Bilateral dislocation of the radial head was noted in two children. Latta et al (1971) drew attention to a juxtacalcaneal accessory bone which they considered to be specific for Larsen's syndrome. This ossicle was not present in the author's case. The most characteristic feature of Larsen's syndrome is anterior dislocation of the tibias. The radial heads are dislocated posteriorly (Figs. 27–14 to 27–17).

MULTIPLE EPIPHYSEAL DYSPLASIA

This condition, already discussed in Chapter Nine, is a genetically determined, disseminated disorder affecting mainly the appendicular skeleton. The ossification of the epiphyses is retarded and patchy, paving the way for precocious osteoarthritis. Waugh (1952) reported three sisters with dysplasia epiphysealis multiplex and noted the occurrence of dislocated radial head.

MULTIPLE SKELETAL MALFORMATIONS WITH PECULIAR FACIES

Gordon et al (1948) reported a 13-year-old girl with hypertelorism, epicanthic folds, broad nose, receding chin, Klippel-Feil type of brevicollis, asymmetrical thorax, genu valgus, lunotriquetral fusion of both wrists, and bilateral anterior dislocation of the radial head. She was the seventh child in a family with no other malformed member.

NAIL-PATELLA SYNDROME (NPS)

This complex has been described in part in Chapter Seven. NPS is a fully penetrant autosomal dominant phenotype linked with the ABO blood group. It affects both ectrodermal and mesodermal derivations; among the former are included the nails and the nervous system and among the latter, the skeleton and kidneys. The nervous system and the kidneys are affected only occasionally. The nails and the skeleton are involved constantly. The main skeletal manifestations of NPS are the following: iliac horns, absence or hypoplasia of the patellae, bilateral hypoplasia of the capitulum humeri, and hypoplasia or dislocation of both radial heads. The capitulum of the humerus is hypoplastic and flat; the head of the radius is diminutive and dislocated posteriorly. In old cases, owing to unwanted friction, the radial head may become mushroomed and appear enlarged. Radiocapitellar dysplasia or dislocation of the radial head has been noted in the pedigrees described by the following authors: Servier (1872), Pye-Smith (1883), Judet and Touchard (1903), Roskoschny (1905), Sieber (1924), Stocks (1925), Trauner and Rieger (1925), Österreicher (1930), Turner (1933), Aschner (1934), Lester (1936), Montant and Eggermann (1937), Sever (1938), Passarge (1940), Senturia and Senturia (1944), Montagard (1945), Rondil-Pernix (1945), Gordon et al (1948), Mino et al (1948), Brixey (1950), Hawkins and Smith (1950), Mosebech (1951), Roeckerath (1951), Wildervanck (1951), Lunardo (1959), Saunders (1961), Zimmerman (1961), Elliott et al (1962), Duncan and Souter (1963), Gibbs et al (1964), Beaumont (1965), Pillay (1965), Maini and Mittal (1966), Palacios (1967), Seyss (1970), and perhaps some others (Fig. 27–18).

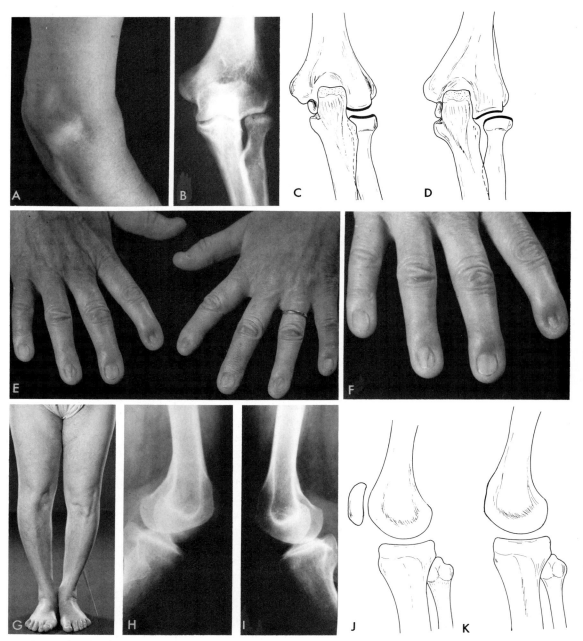

Figure 27–18   Nail-patella syndrome. *A,* Lateral view of the right elbow of an adult woman (see Figure 7–7) whose father was similarly affected. *B,* Dorsovolar roentgenograph of the same, showing dysplasia of the capitulum humeri and dome-shaped radially displaced head of the radius. *C,* Sketch of a dorsovolar roentgenograph of a normal elbow. *D,* Sketch illustrating *B. E,* Dorsal view of the hands, showing dystrophic nails. *F,* Dorsal view (enlarged) of right lesser digits, showing that nail dystrophy is less marked on middle and little fingers. *G,* Photograph showing bowlegs due to bilateral tibia vara. *H* and *I,* Lateral roentgenographs of the right and left knees, showing bilateral absence of the patella. *J,* Sketch of a lateral roentgenograph of a normal left knee. *K,* Sketch illustrating *I.*

NIEVERGELT SYNDROME (Nievergelt-Pearlman Syndrome)

Synostotic states—symphalangism, carpal and tarsal coalescence, and radioulnar synostosis—are more characteristic of Nievergelt (1944) syndrome than dislocation. The complex will be described in greater detail in Chapter Twenty-Eight. Pearlman et al (1964) described a mother and daughter with Nievergelt syndrome and dislocation of the radial head. In the case reported by Dubois (1970), there was "dysplasia of the elbows."

OCULOMELIC COMPLEXES

Ophthalmo-mandibulo-melic dysplasia described by Pillay (1964) consists of corneal clouding, fusion of the temporomandibular joints, absent coronoid process of the mandible and obtuse mandibular angles, aplasia of the distal ulna, dysplasia of the humeral capitulum, and dislocation of the radial head. There were flexion contractures of the middle, ring, and little fingers. This syndrome might be a variant of mesomelic dwarfism of the hypoplastic ulna, fibula, and mandible type. Pillay reported a father and son with this complex. The trait is regarded as an autosomal dominant.

Mietens and Weber (1966) described six sibling offspring of unaffected parents who were second cousins. Each affected child was mentally retarded, had corneal opacity, nystagmus, strabismus, a small pinched nose, flexion contracture of the elbows, dislocation of the head of the radius, abnormally short forearm bones, and clinodactyly. The syndrome is listed with the autosomal recessive phenotypes.

OROMELIC COMPLEX

A male infant reported by Juberg and Hayward (1969) had bilateral cleft of the lip; hypoplastic columella nasi and associated deformity of the external nares; broad nasal bridge; hypoplasia and distal positioning of the thumbs, which were stiff and unopposable; limitation of motion of his elbow joints; and, on the left side, anterior dislocation of the radial head.

OTOPALATODIGITAL SYNDROME (Taybi Syndrome; OPD)

This complex, already described in Chapter Eight, consists of conductive deafness, dwarfism, cleft palate, and pleiotropic skeletal dysplasia. Among manifestations of the latter, Dudding et al (1967) included hypoplasia of the proximal radius with posterior dislocation of the radial head. Langer (1967) reported two patients with gross dislocation of the radial head. Curtis and Fisher (1970) described a seven-and-one-half-year-old boy with left club foot, a cleft palate, bilateral tibiofemoral subluxation, broadened nasal base, broad thumbs and great toes, and "bilateral dislocated elbow."

RUBINSTEIN-TAYBI SYNDROME

Rohlfing et al (1971) presented a 26-year-old mentally retarded white man whose mother had had rubella during the first trimester of pregnancy. The proband had broad thumbs and big toes, "lateral displacement of the patella bilaterally," and "bilateral posterior dislocation of the radial heads."

SILVER-RUSSELL SYNDROME

This complex has been taken up in Chapter Twenty. It consists of intrauterine dwarfism, asymmetry between the two halves of the body, elevated urinary gonadotropins, precocious sexual maturation, and retarded skeletal development. Almquist et al (1969) reported a five-year-old girl with short stature and "left hemihypertrophy." She had bilateral posterior dislocation of the radial head.

DIAGNOSTIC CRITERIA

One or more of the following findings are mentioned in the literature as proof of the fact that the dislocation of the radial head is prenatal and congenital: (1) discovery of dislocation prior to occurrence of injury—in infancy, (2) absence of paralysis of the arm muscles, (3) involvement of the contralateral elbow, (4) concurrence of other congenital anomalies, (5) occurrence in other members of the family or ancestry, (6) greater mobility of congenitally dislocated radius as compared to traumatic dislocation, (7) irreducibility except by surgery and, on very rare occasions, by manipulation, (8) radiographic evidence of an undersized radial head with a dome-shaped top and thin elongated neck, but above all (9) an underdeveloped capitulum of the humerus. A defective humeral capitulum is considered to be the most reliable radiological sign of congenital dislocation of the radial head.

DISABILITY

In congenital dislocation of the radial head, flexion and extension at the elbow is impeded. When the head of the radius is displaced anteriorly, flexion at the elbow is checked; when it is dislocated posteriorly, extension is blocked. Pronation and supination of the forearm are affected only slightly; in anterior dislocation, supination is limited and in posterior dislocation pronation is curtailed.

TREATMENT

Many cases of congenital dislocation of the radial head do not cause any great inconvenience and are, therefore, left alone. McFarland (1936) saw 11 patients with the anomaly. In six, the function of the elbow was unimpaired. The remaining five "suffered from continual or intermittent blocking of flexion. "In such a case," McFarland wrote, "it is a simple matter to excise the head of the radius. . . . I am opposed to attempting to replace the head. For successful reduction, the child must be very young, preliminary traction must be employed, and at operation an orbicular ligament must be formed." In a case of anterior dislocation of both radial heads, Brennan (1963) surgically reduced the displaced bones and held them in place by a newly reconstructed annular ligament.

Hagen (1891) and Bonnenberg (1893) practiced excision of the radial head. In adults, this operation is now regarded as a legitimate procedure for cases of congenital dislocation causing pain or functional disturbance. Resection of the radial head is avoided in growing children because it aggravates the already existing exaggerated carrying angle—the cubitus valgus.

SUMMARY

Prior to the advent of roentgenography in 1896, congenital dislocation of the radial head was confused with proximal radioulnar synostosis and one notes the persistence of this confusion even now. In many recent communications, one also encounters the ever recurring cliché which, in effect, states that congenital dislocation of the radial head is a rare anomaly. This is not true. In addition to numerous isolated cases reported in the literature, congenital dislocation of the radial head is known to occur in association with many regional and remote disorders. Most cases do not require any treatment. In growing children, open reduction is feasible provided that the operation is preceded by a period of direct skeletal traction of the radius. During surgery, an attempt is made to reconstruct some semblance of an orbicular ligament. In adults, the best result is obtained by excision of the dislocated radial head.

References

Abbott, F. C.: Hereditary congenital dislocations of the radius. *Trans. Path. Soc.* (London), *43*:129–139, 1892.

Abbott, F. C.: Congenital dislocation of the radius. *Lancet, 1*:800, 1892.

Adams, R.: Case of congenital malformation of the elbow joint; the head of the radius dislocated laterally and upwards, above the outer condyle of the humerus. *Dublin J. Med. Sci., 17*:504–505, 1840.

Aimes, Adengue, and Hutin: Luxation congénitale bilatérale de l'extrémité superidéure du radius avec synostose des os de l'avant-bras. *Rev. d'Orthop., 6*:69–74, 1919.

Aitken, J.: Deformity of the elbow joint as a sequel to Erb's obstetrical paralysis. *J. Bone Joint. Surg., 34B*:352–365, 1952.

Albanese, A.: Contributo allo studio della lussazione congenita del radio. *Arch. Orthop., 45*:455–486, 1929.

Albertini, B.: Sulla lussazione isolata anteriore del capitello del radio. *Arch. Chir. Orthop. Med., 17*:376–379, 1952.

Allen, W.: On the anatomical changes induced at the elbow by luxation backwards of the head of the radius in early life. *Glasgow Med. J., 14*:44–50, 1880.

Almquist, E. A., Gordon, L. H., and Blue, A. J.: Congenital dislocation of the head of the radius. *J. Bone Joint Surg., 51A*:1118–1127, 1969.

Ambard: Double luxation congénitale du radius en haut et en arrière chez un malade soupçonné de syphilis héréditaire. *Rev. d'Orthop.,* (2 s.), *2*:173–176, P. VI, 1901.

Andreini, G.: La lussazione congenita della testa del radio. Contributo clinico e critico allo studio della patogenesi e della anatomia patologica della deformita. *Arch. Ortop., 31*:704–788, 1914.

Appraillé, G.: *Malformations Congénitales de l'Extremite Superieure du Radius.* Thèse. Paris, G. Steinheil, pp. 7–46, 1901.

Aschner, B.: A typical hereditary syndrome: dystrophy of the nails, congenital defect of the head of the radius. *J.A.M.A., 102*:2017–2020, 1934.

Barettoni, M.: Lussazione congenita bilaterale del radio ecc. *Rass. Prev. Social.,* Anno XVI, No. 1, pp. 12–23, 1914.

Barret, M.: Un cas de maladie de Bassel-Hagen. Exostosis multiples. Malformation du cubitus et luxation du radius en haut avec perforation des teguments. *Bull. Mem. Acad. Chir. Paris, 62*:232–236, 1936.

Barros, M.: *Contribution a l'Etude des Luxations de l'Extremité Superieure du Radius.* Genéve, H. Georg, pp. 1–120, 1886.

Bassel. See Hagen (1891).

Beals, R. K.: Auriculo-osteodysplasia. A syndrome of multiple osseous dysplasia ear anomaly and short stature. *J. Bone Joint Surg., 49A*:1541–1550, 1967.

Beaumont, F. de: L'onycho-ostéodysplasie. *J. Génét. Hum., 14*:93–131, 1965.

Bélot, and Chaperon: Double luxation congénitale du radius en haut et en arrière. *Soc. Radiol.* (Paris), p. 246, 1910. See Review in *Z. Orthop. Chir., 27*:565, 1910.

Belot, J., Lepennetier, F., and Pelizza, J.: Radiodiagnostique de quelques altérations osseuses de l'articulation du coude. *J. Radiol. Electrol., 12*:457–500, 1928.

Berger: Luxation congénitale bilaterale de l'extrémité supérieure du radius. *Bull. Soc. Chir. Paris, 20*:219–220, 1894.

Bergtold, W. J.: A case of symmetrical congenital dislocation of the head of each radius. *Ann. Surg., 14*:370–373, 1891.

Bernard, E.: *Des Luxations Congénitales de la Tête de Radius.* Thèse. Lille, C. Dunbar & Cie, 11–138, 1908.

Bertini, S., and De Pasquale, F. M.: La lussazione congenita del capitelo radiale. (Contributo clinico.) *Clin. Ortop., 12*:70–78, 1960.

Bindman, E.: Congenital recurrent dislocation of the head of radius. *Br. Med. J., 2*:254, 1945.

Blodgett, W. E.: Congenital luxations of the head of radius. Report of two cases. Analysis of fifty-one cases. Summary. Certain other considerations. Conclusions. *Am. J. Orthop. Surg., 3*:253–270, 1906.

Bonnenberg, T.: Die Luxatio capituli radii congenita (angeborene Verrenkung des Radiuskoepfchens). *Orthop. Chir., 2*:376–409, 1893.

Bottomley, J. T.: Discussion following Powers (1903) paper. *J.A.M.A., 41*:168, 1903.

Bouvier: Luxation double de l'éxtrémité supérieure du radius. *Bull. Soc. Chir. Paris, 2*:471–475, 1861.

Braine, J.: Luxation congénitale bilaterale du radius en arrière. *Bull. Soc. Anat. Paris, 17*:475–480, 1920.

Brennan, J. J.: Annular ligament construction for congenital anterior dislocation of both radial heads. *Clin. Orthop., 29*:205–209, 1963.

Brindeau, A.: Luxation congénitale du radius. *Bull. Soc. Obstet. Paris, 11*:140–141, 1908.

Brixey, A. M., Jr., and Burke, R. M.: Arthro-onychodysplasia. Hereditary syndrome involving deformity on head of radius, absence of patellae, posterior iliac spurs, dystrophy of finger nails. *Am. J. Med., 8*:738–744, 1950.

Burman, M. S.: Paradoxical crossing of the radius in anteromedial dislocation of the head of the radius to give supination contracture of the forearm. *Am. J. Roentgenol., 70*:422–424, 1953.

Bussati, P. F.: Un caso di lussazione congenita tardiva della testa del radio. *Arch. Ortop., 44*:366–387, 1928.

Cafati, A., and Morelli, E.: La lussazione congenita del capitello radiale (presentazione di 6 casi). *Arch. Ortop., 73*:662–670, 1960.

Camplani, M.: Un caso di lussazione della testa del radio. *Radiol. Med., 16*:1093–1100, 1929.

Camurati, C.: Un caso di Lussazione anteriore congenita del radio. *Clinica Ortop., 3*:65–70, 1951.

Caravias, D. E.: Some observations on congenital dislocation of the head of the radius. *J. Bone Joint Surg., 39B*:86–90, 1957.

Carling, W. R., and Ross, J. P.: *British Surgical Practice*. St. Louis, C. V. Mosby, Vol. 3, pp. 185–186, 1948.

Catterina, A.: Sulla lussazione congenital del capitello del radio. *Chir. Organi. Mov., 19*:480–487, 1934.

Charlet, A.: *Luxation Congénitale Total du Coude*. Thèse. Paris, Impremerie Industrielle, pp. 11–47, 1937.

Chassaignac: Double luxation des deux radius. *Bull. Soc. Chir. Paris, 5*:400–402, 1855.

Chlumsky, V.: Über Subluxation des Radiusköpfchen bei Kindern. *Z. Orthop. Chir., 29*:213–215, 1911.

Christopher, F.: Radial exostosis complicating anterior dislocation of the elbow. *J. Bone Joint Surg., 14*:949–952, 1932.

Chryssafis, M.: Un cas de luxation congénitale bilatérale de la tête du radius en avant. *Rev. d'Orthop., (3 s.), 9*:549–952, 1932.

Cleret, F., and Bienvenue, F.: Un cas d'ecrodactylie avec malformation du coude et luxation congénital du radius droit. *Rev. d'Orthop., (3 s.), 1*:455–458, 1910.

Cockshott, W. P., and Omololu, A.: Familial congenital posterior dislocation of both radial heads. *J. Bone Joint Surg., 40B*:483–486, 1958.

Condict, W. L.: Bilateral congenital dislocation of the radius. *Ann. Surg., 71*:798–799, 1920.

Cotton, F. J.: See Powers (1903).

Cozzolino, A.: Sulla lussazione congenita del capitello radiale. *Arch. Ortop., 73*:313–321, 1960.

Curtillet, J., and Lombard, P.: Double genu recurvatum congénitale bilatérale, luxation congénitale bilatérale, luxation congénitale de coudes. Traitément de genu recurvatum par le procède de Wolf. *Rev. d'Orthop., (3 s.), 3*:289–298, 1912.

Curtis, B. H., and Fischer, R. L.: Heritable congenital tibiofemoral subluxation. *J. Bone Joint Surg., 52A*:1104–1114, fig. 9a, case 5, 1970.

Cushing, H. W.: Subluxation of the radial head in children. *Boston Med. Surg. J., 114*:77–80, 1886.

DeRuggero-Romanini: Sulla lussazione congenita del capitello radiale. *Ortop. Traum. App. Mot., 27*:317–325, 1959.

Detenback, L. C., and Abrams, R. C.: Congenital symmetrical limb deformities. *Am. J. Dis. Child., 120*:354–355, 1970.

Detzel, H.: Zur Behandlung der angeborenen Radius-Köpfchen-Luxation. *Arch. Orthop. Unfallchir., 45*:536–542, 1953.

Diebel, H. W.: Congenital luxation of the head of the radius. *Trans. Luzerne Co. Med. Soc.* (Wilkesbarre), *15*:25, 1907.

Digby, K. H.: The measurement of diaphysial growth in proximal and distal directions. *J. Anat. Physic., 50*:187–188, 1916.

Dreifuss, A.: Uber die isolierte Luxation des Capitulum Radii nach vorn *Z. Orthop. Chir., 17*:257–265, 1906.

Dubois, H. J.: Nievergelt-Pearlman syndrome. Synostosis of feet and hands with dysplasia of elbow. *J. Bone Joint Surg., 52B*:325–329, 1970.

Dudding, B. A., Gorlin, R. J., and Langer, L. O.: The oto-palato-digital syndrome. A new symptom-complex consisting of deafness, dwarfism, cleft palate, characteristic facies, and a generalized bone dysplasia. *Am. J. Dis. Child., 113*:214–221, fig. 8, 1967.

Duncan, J. G., and Souter, W. A.: Heriditary onycho-osteodysplasia. The nail-patella syndrome. *J. Bone Joint Surg., 45B*:242–258, 1963.

Elliott, G. B.: A study of a child presenting multiple deformities, with presentation of specimens. *Tr.. Am. Orthop. Assoc., 12*:282–294, 1899.

Elliott, K. A., Elliott, G. B., and Kindrachuk, W. H.: The "radial subluxation–fingernail defect–absent patella" syndrome: observations on its nature. *Am. J. Roentgenol., 87*:1067–1074, 1962.

England, J. P. S.: Congenital dislocation of the head of the radius. *British Association Meeting*, September 24–26, 1964.

Evans, E. L.: Case of congenital dislocation of right radius. *Proc. Roy. Soc. Med.* (Sect. Orthopedics), *17*:16, 1923–1924.

Exarhou, E. J., and Antoniou, N. K.: Congenital dislocation of the head of the radius. *Acta. Orthop. Scand., 41*:551–556, 1970.

Fairbank, H. A. T.: Dyschondroplasia synonyms—Ollier's disease, multiple enchondromata. *J. Bone Joint Surg., 30B*:689–708, fig. 35, 1948.

Farfan, C. R.: Lussazione congenita bilateral del radio. *Acad. Peru Cir., 17*:209–210, 1964.

Feil, A.: Luxation congénitale et allongement symétrique des deux radius au niveau de coude. *Bull. Soc. Anat. Paris*, (6 s.), *3*:147–151, 1921.

Feil, A.: Malformation symétrique de deux radius. *Presse Méd., 29*:661–662, 1921.

Févre, M.: Luxation de la tête radiale par racourcissement du cubitus dans la maladie exostotique. *Rev. Chir. Orthop. Rep. App. Mot., 54*:67–72, 1968.

Fox, K. W., and Griffin, L. L.: Congenital dislocation of the radial head. *Clin. Orthop., 18*:234–243, 1960.

Fusari, A.: Lussazione congenita bilaterale del capitello del radio. *Ortop. Traum. App. Mot., 1*:13–22, 1929.

Galeazzi, R.: Contributo alla cura chirurgica della lussazione anteriore congenita del radio. *Arch. Ortop., 24*:323–342, 1907.

Gardner, J.: On an undescribed displacement of the bones of the forearm in children. *London Med. Gaz., 20*:878–879, 1837.

Gaudier, and Bernard: Double luxation congénitale du radius. *Echo Med. Nord* (Lille) *10*:501, 1906.

Gerald, B., Umansky, R.: Cornelia de Lange syndrome: roentgenographic findings. *Am. J. Roentgenol., 100*:96–100, 1967.

Gibbs, R. C., Berczeller, P. H., and Hyman, A. B.: Nail-patella-elbow syndrome. *Arch. Dermatol. Syph., 89*:196–199, 1964.

Goerlich, M.: Rechtseitige kongenitale Radiusluxation nach hinten und aussen. *Beitr. Klin. Chir. 59*:427–430, 1908.

Gordon, E., Shechter, N., and Perlman, A. W.: Multiple congenital malformations of the skeletal system. A case report. *Am. J. Roentgenol., 59*:533–538, fig. 4, 1948.

Goyrand: Quelques mots sur la luxation incomplète de l'extrémité supérieure du radius commune chez les enfants en bas age. *Ann. Chir. Fr. Etrang., 5*:129, 1842.

Grewal, N.: Bilateral congenital dislocation of the head of the radius with brachydactyly in British Guiana—case report. *W. Indian Med. J., 15*:147–149, 1966.

Grimault, L., and Epitalbra, A.: Un cas d'absence congénital bilateral du cubitus. *Bull. Mem. Soc. Anat. Paris,* (6 s.), *20*:738–743, 1923.

Guerin, J.: Recherches sur les luxations congénitales, exposées dans les conférences cliniques du 29 Janvier et du 3 Fevrier 1841, a l'hôpital des enfants (sic) malades. *Gaz. Medicale 9*:97–105, 1841.

Guérin-Valmale, and Jeanbreau: Dissection d'une main bote cubitale pure avec luxation congenitale du coude. *Bull. Soc. Anat. Paris,* (6 s.) *1*:911–915, 1899.

Guilleminet, M., and Leclerc, G.: Luxation congénitale héréditaire des coudes et des hauches. *Lyon Chir., 34*:207–210, 1937.

Guilleminet, M., and Leclerc, G.: Trois cas de luxation congénitale bilatérale des coudes. *Rev. d'Orthop., 24*:596–605, 1937.

Gunn, D. R., and Pillay, V. K.: Congenital posterior dislocation of the head of the radius. *Clin. Orthop., 34*:108–113, 1964.

Hagen, F. B.: Üeber angeborene und pathologische Luxationen des Radius Köpfchen. *In* Ueber Knochen- und Gelenkanomalien, insbesondere bei partiellem Riesenwuchs und bei multiplen cartilaginären Exostosen. *Arch. Klin. Chir., 41*:420–466, Tafel V, VI, VII, 1891.

Hajdu, N., and Kauntze, R.: Cranio-skeletal dysplasia. *Br. J. Radiol., 21*:42–48, 1948.

Hass, J., and Hass, R.: Arthrochalasis multiplex congenita. Congenita. Congenital flaccidity of the joints. *J. Bone Joint Surg., 40A*:663–674, 1958.

Hawkins, C. F., and Smith, O. E.: Renal dysplasia in a family with multiple hereditary abnormalities including iliac horns. *Lancet, 1*:803–808, 1950.

Heelis, R.: A case of congenital dislocation of radius. *Lancet, 2*:249, 1886.

Herskowitz: Ein Fall angeborener beiderseitiger Luxation des Radius. *Wien. Med. Press, 24*:217–221, 1888.

Hertel, E., Stotz, S., Jacobi, H. M., and Murken, J. D.: Zur Diagnose Arthrogryposis multiplex congenita. *Arch. Orthop. Unfallchir., 67*:114–134; Abb. 8, 1969.

Herzog, A.: Missbildung im Ellbogengelenk. Eine unbekannte Anomalie. *Fortschr. Röntgenstr., 36*:407–409, 1927.

Hipp, H., and Hahle, K.: Luxation im proximalen Radio-Ulnargelenk. *Roentgenpraxis, 9*:120, 1937.

Horsch, K.: Beitrag zur isolierten angeborenen Radiuskoepfchen-Luxation. *Zentralbl. Chir., 61*:993–995, 1934.

Hussein, K.: Multiple congenital dislocations. *J. Bone Joint Surg., 20*:488–489; fig. 2., 1938.

Jacklin, N.: Familial predisposition to pterygium formation. *Am. J. Ophthalmol., 57*:481–482, 1964.

Jäger, M., and Refior, H. J.: Knochendysplasie-Syndrom. *Z. Orthop., 105*:196–208; Abb. 7, 1968.

Japiot, and Fouilloud-Buyat: Luxation congenitale du coude. Radiographie. *Lyon Med., 131*:435, 1923.

Jaulin, and Limousi: Luxation congénitale bilaterale de la tête du radius. *J. Radiol. Electrol., 14*:27–29, 1930.

Jervis, G. A., and Stimson, C. W.: De Lange syndrome. The "Amsterdam type" of mental defect with congenital malformation. *J. Pediatr., 63*:634–645, 1963.

Jones, T. T.: Notes on a case of multiple exostoses. *Br. Med. J., 1*:709–710, 1878.

Joppich, J.: *Beitrag zur Kenntnis der angeborenen Luxation des Capitalune radii.* Inaug. Diss., Greifswald, J. Abel, pp. 5–36, figs. 1–3, 1888.

Juberg, R. C., and Hayward, J. R.: A new familial syndrome of oral, cranial and digital anomalies. *J. Pediatr.*, *74*:755–762, 1969.

Judet, H., and Touchard: Luxation congénitale de la rotule coincident avec une double luxation en arrière de la tête du radius. *Bull. Soc. Pédiatr.*, *5*:197–198, 1903.

Keith, A.: Studies on the anatomical changes which accompany certain growth-disorders of the human body. *J. Anat.*, *54*:2–31, 1920.

Kelikian, H., and Clayton, I.: A method of repair of radial head dislocations. *Quart. Bull., Northwestern Univ. Med. School, Chicago*, *29/4*:365–367, 1955.

Key, J. A.: Hypermobility of joints as a sex-linked hereditary characteristic. *J.A.M.A.*, *88*:1710–1712, 1927.

Kienböck, R.: Das Ellbogengelenk bei chondraler Dysplasie des Skeletts mit multiplen Exostosen. A. Luxation des Radiuskoepfchens. *Fortschr. Röntgenstr.*, *15*:104–108; Tafel XI; figs. 8–11, 1910.

Kieser, W.: Die sogenannte Flughaut beim Menschen. *Z. Konstitutionslehre*, *23*:594–619, 1939.

Kirch, J.: La maladie exostosant de Bassel-Hagen et le problem de la croissance de l'os en longeur. *J. Radiol. Electrol.*, *32*:386–387, 1951.

Knish, J. T.: Congenital dislocation of the radial head. (In Russian.) *Orthop. Traum.*, *9*:48–51, 1965.

Komparda, J.: Congenital dislocation of the head of the radius. (In Czech.) *Acta. Chir. Orhop. Traum. Cech.*, *34*:347–351, 1967.

Kraus, A.: Un nuovo caso di lussazione congenita del capitello del radio. *Policlinico (Sez. Prat.)*, *29*:8–10, 1922.

Kunne, B.: Die Kombination der "angeborenen" Luxation des Radiusköpfchens mit der Littleschen Krankheit. *Z. Orthop. Chir.*, *31*:138–154, 1913.

Lange, M.: *Erb-biologie der angeborenen Korperfehler*. Stuttgart, F. Enke, pp. 1–143, 1935.

Langer, L. O., Jr.: The roentgenographic features of oto-palato-digital (OPD) syndrome. *Am. J. Roentgenol.*, *100*:63–70, fig. 5, 1967.

Larsen, L. J., Schottstaedt, E. R., and Bost, F. C.: Multiple congenital dislocations associated with characteristic facial abnormality. *J. Pediat.*, *37*:574–581, 1950.

Lasserre, C., and Saft, G.: Luxation congénitale bilatérale du radius en dehors. *Rev. Orthop. Chir. App. Mot.*, *20*:166–167, 1933.

Latta, R. J., Graham, C. B., Aase, J., Scham, S. M., and Smith, D. W.: Larsen's syndrome. A skeletal dysplasia with multiple joint dislocations and unusual facies. *J. Pediatr.*, *78*:291–298, 1971.

Lee, F. A., and Kenny, F. M.: Skeletal changes in the Cornelia De Lange syndrome. *Am. J. Radiol.*, *100*:27–38, 1967.

Le Gendre, E. Q.: Observation de luxation de l'extrémité supérieure du radius en dehors et en arrière. *C. R. Soc. Biol.*, *11*:31–33, 1859.

Leisbrink, H.: Case reported by C. Hueter. *Dtsch. Z. Chir.*, *11*:173–176, 1879.

Lester, A. M.: A familial dyschondroplasia associated with anonychia and other deformities. *Lancet*, *2*:1519–1521, 1936.

Lievre, C. A.: Contributó allo studio della lussazione congenita dell'epifisi prossimale del radio. *Minerva Ortop.*, *9*:112, 1958.

Lovett, R. W.: Dislocation of the head of the radius. *In* Keen, W. W., (ed.): *Surgery: Its Principles and Practice*. Philadelphia, W. B. Saunders Co., Vol. 2, pp. 541–542, 1909.

Lowy, M.: Angeborene Radius Luxation mit Synostose der beiden Unterarmknochen. *Mitteil S. Ges. Innere Mediz. Kinderheilkd. Wien. Ig.*, *20*:187–188, 1921.

Ludloff, K.: Die Subluxation radii und die Bewegunseinschränkungen im Ellenbogengelenk. *Z. Orthop. Chir.*, *25*:303–322, 1910.

Lunardo, C.: Rara sindrome malformativa articolare associata a ipotiroidismo e ad altre deformita. *Arch. Putti*, *11*:394–401, 1959.

Magee, R. K.: Bilateral congenital dislocation of radial head. *Lancet*, *1*:14, 519, 1947.

Maini, P. S., and Mittal, R. L.: Hereditary onycho-osteo-arthrodysplasia. *J. Bone Joint Surg.*, *48A*:924–930, 1966.

Maioli, M.: Sopra un caso raro di lussazione congenita del radio. *Chir. Organi. Mov.*, *30*:52–56, 1946.

Malgaingne, J. F.: *Traité des Fractures et des Luxations*. Paris, J. B. Bailliere, Tome II, pp. 680–681, 1855.

Mauck, H. P., and Butterworth, R. D.: Two cases of bilateral congenital dislocation of the head of the radius. *J.A.M.A.*, *114*:2542–2543, 1940.

McFarland, B.: Congenital dislocation of the head of the radius. *Br. J. Surg.*, *24*:41–49, 1936.

McFarland, B.: Congenital dislocation of the head of the radius. *In* Platt, H., (ed.): *Modern Trends in Orthopedics*. London, Butterworth & Co., p. 131, 1950.

McGavin, L. H.: Bilateral congenital displacement of the upper ends of the radius and ulna. *Proc. R. Soc. Med. London.* (Clin. Sect.), *6* (Part 1):25, 1913.

Mead, C. A., and Martin, M.: Aplasia of the trochlea—an original mutation. *J. Bone Joint Surg.*, *45A*:379–383, 1963.

Meijers: Luxatio congenita radii. *Ned. T. Geneesk.* *40*:946–950, 1904.

Meng. C. M.: Congenital dislocation of the radius. *Chinese Med. J.*, *57*:479–489, 1940.

Merlini, A.: La lussazione congenita del capitello del radio. *Arch. Ortop.*, *42*:97–126, 1926.

Meyer: Über multiple kongenitale Gelenkdeformitäten. *Z. Orthop. Chir.*, *22*:563–580, 1908.

Mietens, C., and Weber, H.: A syndrome characterized by corneal opacity, nystagmus, flexion contracture of the elbows, growth failure, and mental retardation. *J. Pediatr.,* 69:624–629, 1966.

Milch, H.: Dislocation of the head of the radius. Suggestion for a new operative procedure. *J. Bone Joint Surg.,* (n.s.), 10:89–93, 1928.

Mino, R. A., Mino, V. H., and Livingstone, R. F.: Osseous dysplasia and dystrophy of the nails. Review of the literature and report of a case. *Am. J. Roentgenol.,* 60:633–641, 1948.

Mitscherlich, A.: Ein Fall von angeborener Verbildung beider Ellenbogengelenke. *Arch. Klin. Chir.,* 6:218–222, 1865.

Montagard, F.: Un syndrome héréditaire rare d'anomalies de développement. La triade: absence congénitale de rotules – dysplasie articulaire des coudes – dystrophie des ongles (une observation personelle). *Presse Méd.,* 53:696–697, 1945.

Montant, R., and Eggermann, A.: Syndrome héréditaire caracterise par une hypoplasia des rotules, une malformation des radius et une hémi-atrophie de l'ongle du pouce. *Presse Méd.,* 45:770–772, 1937.

Mordeja, J.: Die angeborene Radiusluxation. *Arch. Orthop. Unfallchir.,* 48:474–493, 1956.

Mosebech, J.: Congenital malformation of the nails associated with deformities of the elbows and knees (monozygotic twins). *Acta. Genet. Statist. Med. Basel,* 2:312–317, 1951.

Mouchet, A., and d'Allaines, F.: Luxation congénitale en dehors et en arrière du radius gauche restée méconnue jusqu'à l'âge de 14 ans et révélée par un traumatisme. *Rev. d'Orthop.,* 15:43–49, 1928.

Muller, V.: Erfahrungen bei der luxation der Radiusköpfchen jugendlicher Gelenke. *Zentralb., Chir.,* 66:2319–2329, 1939.

Münter, O.: *Congénitale Luxation des Radiusköpfchens mit Vererbung* Würzburg, Druck der K. Universität, Druckerei von H. Sturtz, pp. 5–14, figs. 1–5, 1899.

Nievergelt, K.: Positiver Vaterschaftsnachweis auf Grund erbicher Missbildungen der Extremitäten. *Arch. Julius-Klaus Stift.,* 19:147–159, 1944.

Ollier: Da la dyschondroplasie. *Bull. Soc. Chir. Lyon,* 3:22–27, 1899–1900.

Osmond-Clarke, H.: Congeniatal dislocation of head of radius. *In* Carling, E. R., and Ross, J. P., (eds.): *British Practice of Surgery.* London, Butterworth & Co., Vol. 3, pp. 185–186, 1948.

Österreicher, W.: Gemeinsame Vererbung von Anonychie bzw. Onychatrophie, Patellardefekt und Luxatio radii. Dominantes Auftreten in 5 Generationen. *Z. Konstitutionslehre,* 15:465–476, 1930.

Oto, T., Kohoda, M., Suzuki, G., and Serizawa, Y.: Case of congenital anterior dislocation of the small head of the radius. (In Japanese.) *Orthop. Surg. Tokyo,* 17:740–743, 1966.

Pagenstecher, E.: Beitrag zu den Extremitätsmissbildungen II. Brachydaktylie – Pollex valgus – Luxation der Radius Köpfchen und Missbildung der Daumen u.s.w. *Dtsch. 2. Chir.,* 60:239–249, 1901.

Painter, C. F.: Congenital dislocation of the elbow. *In* Bryant, J. D., and Buck, A. H., (eds.): *American Practice of Surgery.* New York, William Wood & Co., Vol. 4, pp. 741–742, 1908.

Palacios, E.: Hereditary osteo-onycho-dysplasia. The nail-patella syndrome. *Am. J. Roentgenol.,* 101:842–850, 1967.

Passarge, E.: Familiäre aseptische Nekrose der Patella bei gleichzeitiger doppelseitiger Ellbogengelenkmissbildung. *Mschr. Unfallheilkd.,* 47:193–200, 1940.

Pastormerlo, P.: Un raro caso di lussazionne congenita bilaterale de la testa del radio. *Policlinico,* 54:659–660, 1947.

Pearlman, H. S., Edkin, R. E., and Warren, R. F.: Familial carpal synostosis with radial head subluxation (Hievergelt's syndrome). *J. Bone Joint Surg.,* 46A:585–592, 1964.

Pfeiffer, R.: Die angeborene Verrenkung des Speichenköpfchens als Teilerscheinung anderer kongenitaler Ellenbogengelenkmissbildungen. *Z. Menschl. Vererb. Konstitutionslehre,* 21:530–544, 1938.

Phillips, M. N., and Stark, K. F.: Bilateral congenital dislocation of the radial head. *Br. J. Clin. Pract.,* 19:35–37, 1965.

Phillips, S.: Congenital dislocation of radii. *Br. Med. J.,* 1:773–774, 1883.

Piccinini, G.: Sulla lussazione congenita del capitello del radio. *Arch. Putti,* 5:350–358, 1954.

Piccioli, G.: Lussazione congenita bilaterale del radio. *Arch. Ortop.,* 26:161–178, 1909.

Piccioli, G.: Contributo alla statistica delle lussazioni congenite posteriori del capitello radiale. *Arch. Ortop.,* 27:225–228, 1910.

Pièrre, J. R.: Anomalie congénitale des coudes. *Bull. Soc. Anat. Paris,* 93:255–257, 1923.

Pillay, V. K.: Congenital (developmental) abnormalities of the elbow joint. *Singapore Med. J.,* 4:142–146, 1963.

Pillay, V. K.: Acrocephalosyndactyly in Singapore. A study of five Chinese males. *J. Bone Joint Surg.,* 46B:94–101, 1964.

Pillay, V. K.: Ophthalmo-mandibulo-melic dysplasia, a hereditary syndrome. *J. Bone Joint Surg.,* 46A:858–862, 1964.

Pillay, V. K.: Onycho-osteodysplasia (nail-patella syndrome). Study of a Chinese family with this condition. *Ann. Hum. Genet.,* 28:301–307, Pl. 1–3, 1965.

Piulachs, P., and Tutor, R. N.: Luxation congenita de la extremidad superior del radio. *Cir. Aparato Locomotor,* 2:140–151, 1945.

Poli, A.: Contributo alla cura chirurgica della lussazione anteriore inveterata del radio. *Arch. Ortop.*, *68*:695–711, 1955.

Pollono, F., Toscano, G., and Cavalli, F.: Considerazioni sulla lussazione congenita del capitello del radio (presentazione di 5 casi). *Minerva Ortop.*, *18*:492–498, 1967.

Porter, F. T.: Congenital luxation of the head of the radius. *Proc. Path. Soc. Dublin*, (n.s.), *5*:258, 1874.

Powers, C. A.: Congenital dislocations of the radius. *J.A.M.A.*, *41*:165–168, 1903.

Preiser: Angeborene Gelenkmissbildungen. *Dtsch. Med. Wochenschr.*, *36*:1885, 1910. See also the review in *Am. J. Orthop. Surg.*, *8*:651, 1910.

Princeteau: Subluxation congénitale des deux extrémités supérieures des radius en haut et en avant. *J. Méd. Bordeaux*, *37*:474, 612, 1907.

Pye-Smith, R. J.: Dislocation backwards of the head of the left radius. *Lancet*, *2*:993–994, 1883.

Pye-Smith, R. J.: Notes on a family presenting in most of its members certain deformities about the joints of both limbs. *Med. Press Circular*, (n.s.), *34*:504–505, 1883.

Roeckerath, W.: Hereditaere Osteo-onycho-dysplasie. *Fortschr. Roentgstr.*, *75*:700–712, 1951.

Rohfling, B., Lewis, L., and Singleton, E. B.: Rubinstein-Taybi syndrome. *Am. J. Dis. Child.*, *121*:71–74, 1971.

Rondil-Perneix: Un cas de luxation congénitale des deux têtes radiales et deux rotules. *Rev. d'Orthop.*, *31*:69–73, 1945.

Rose, T.: Bilateral congenital dislocation of the head of the radius. *Med. J. Aust.*, *1*:741–742, 1938.

Roskoschny, F.: Ein Fall von angeborener, vererbter Verbildung beider Knie- und Ellenbogengelenke. *Dtsch. Z. Chir.*, *76*:569–580, 1905.

Rostad, H.: Congenital dislocation of the head of the radius. *Acta. Chir. Scand.*, *133*:75–77, 1967.

Rowland, S.: Report on the application of the new photography to medicine and surgery. *Br. Med. J.*, *1*:1059–1061, 1896.

Schoen, H.: Luxation der radius bei multiplen cartilaginaren Exostosen. *Röntgenpraxis*, *14*:276–277, 1942.

Schroeder, C. H.: Familiäre congenitale Luxation. *Z. Orthop. Chir.*, *57*:580–595, 1932.

Schroeder, G.: Osteo-Onycho-Dysplasia hereditaria (albuminurica). *Z. Menschl. Vererb. Konstitutionslehre*, *36*:42–73, 1961.

Schubert, J. J.: Dislocation of the radial head in the newborn infant. *J. Bone Joint Surg.*, *47A*:1019–1923, 1965.

Seckel, H. P. G.: *Bird-Headed Dwarfs.* Springfield, Illinois, Charles C Thomas, pp. 12 and 190, figs. 7c and 54b, 1960.

Senftleben, H.: Notiz ueber eine angeborene Luxation des Radius mit Defect des mittleren Theils der Ulna. *Arch. Pathol. Anat. Physiol.*, *4512*:303–304, Tafel XI, figs. 1 and 2, 1869.

Senturia, H. R., and Senturia, B. D.: Congenital absence of the patellae associated with arthrodysplasia of the elbows and dystrophy of the nails: a hereditary syndrome. *Amer. J. Roentgenol.*, *51*:352–358, 1944.

Servier: Note sur une cas de difformité congénitale des articulations de genou et des coudes. *Gaz. Hebdm. Med. Chir.*, *9*:214–215, 1872.

Sever, J. W.: Hereditary arthrodysplasia associated with dystrophy of the nails: report of a case. *N. Engl. J. Med.*, *219*:87–89, 1938.

Seyss, R.: Die Manifestation der Arthro-osteo-onycho-Dysplasie im Kindesalter. *Arch Kinderheilkd.*, *182*:82–87; Abb. 3, 4, 1970.

Squazzini-Viscontini, C.: Un caso di lussazione anteriore congenita della epifisi prossimale del radio. *Arch. Orthop.*, *72*:1331–1337, 1959.

Shun-Shin, M.: Congenital web formation. *J. Bone Joint Surg.*, *36B*:268–271, 1954.

Sieber, H.: Doppelseitige angeborene Luxation der Patella und des Radius-Köpfchens nach aussen. *Z. Orthop. Chir.*, *46*:555–561, 1924.

Silver, H. K.: Asymmetry, short stature, and variations in sexual development. *Am. J. Dis. Child.*, *107*:495–515, 1964.

Smith, R. W.: Congenital dislocation of the head of the radius forwards. *Dublin Quart. J. Med. Sciences*, (n.s.), *10*:213–216, 1850.

Smith, R. W.: Congenital luxations of the radius. *Dublin Quart. J. Med. Sciences*, (n.s.), *13*:208–210, 1852.

Sorrel, E.: À Propos de la luxation congénitale du radius et des troubles de croissance des os présentant des exostoses osteogéniques. *Bull. Mém. Soc. Nat. Chir.*, *58*:806–808, séance du 25 mai, 1932. Review in *Rev. d'Orthop.*, *20*:165–166, 1933.

Sorrel, E., and Parin: Luxation congénitale double du radius en dehors. *Bull. Soc. Anat. Paris*, *17*:488–492, 1920.

Soupault, R., and Portes: Luxations congénitales doubles des coudes et des hauches; anomalies congénitales de l'appareil routilien. *Bull. Soc. Anat. Paris*, *90*:101–105, 1920.

Spinner, M., and Kaplan, E. B.: Quadrate ligament of the elbow—its relation to the stability of the proximal radio-ulnar joint. *Acta. Orthop. Scand.*, *41*:632–647, 1970.

Spitzy: Die isolierte Luxation des Radius nach vorne. *Verh. Dtsch. Orthop. Ges.*, *25*:81–83, 1931.

Steel, H. H., and Kohl, E. J.: Multiple congenital dislocations associated with other skeletal anomalies. *J. Bone Joint Surg.*, *54A*:75–82, 1972.

Stimson, L. A.: *A Treatise on Dislocations*. Philadelphia, Lea Brothers & Co., pp. 106, 349–352, 1888.

Stocks, P.: Congenital dislocation of radius. Eugenic Laboratory Memoirs XXII. *In* Pearson, K., (ed.): *The Treasury of Human Inheritance*. New York, Cambridge University Press, pp. 139–140, 1925.

Stocks, P.: Hereditary disorders of bone development. *In* Pearson, K., (ed.): *The Treasury of Human Inheritance*. New York, Cambridge, University Press, Vol. III, Part I, pp. 7–48, 141–167, 1925.

Stone, C. A.: Subluxation of the head of the radius. Report of a case and anatomic experiments. *J.A.M.A.*, *67*:28–29, 1916.

Sury, K. V.: Beitrag zur Kenntnis der kongenitalen Radiusmissbildung mit Rücksicht auf die dadurch bedingte Erwerbseinbusse. *Korresp. Schweiz. Arzte.*, *39*:79–83, 1909.

Taybi, H.: Generalized skeletal dysplasia with multiple anomalies. *Am. J. Roentgenol.*, *88*:450–452; figs. 2 and 7B, 1962.

Thomas, L. C.: Radio-ulnar olisthy. *Eugenical News*, *11*:150–153, 1926.

Togenetti, G. P., Giaretta, V., and Cugola, L.: Interventi per il recupero funzionale in un case di emimelia con mano valga. *Chir. Trivienta*, *9*:699–710, 1969.

Trauner, R., and Rieger, H.: Eine Familie mit 6 Fällen von Luxation radii congenita mit übereinstimmenden Anomalien der Finger und Kniegelenke, sowie der Nagelbildung in 4 Generationen. *Arch. Klin. Chir.*, *137*:659–666, 1925.

Turner, J. W.: An hereditary arthrodysplasia associated with hereditary dystrophy of the nails. *J.A.M.A.*, *100*:882–884, 1933.

Uffreduzzi, O.: Sulla lussazione congenita et acquisita del capitello del radio. *Arch Ortop.*, *30*:658–687, 1913.

Valdueza, A. F.: The nail-patella syndrome: a report of three families. *J. Bone Joint Surg.*, *55B*:145–162, 1973.

Van Arsdale, W. W.: On subluxation of the head of the radius in children – with a resumé of one hundred consecutive cases. *Ann. Surg.*, *9*:401–423, 1889.

Van Hook, W.: Double congenital dislocation of the heads of the radii. *Ill. State Med. J.*, (n.s.), *5*:958, 1903–1904.

Wahren, H.: A case of habitual luxation of capitulum radii. *Acta. Chir. Scand.*, *92*:327–330, 1945.

Walker, B. A.: Whistling-face–windmill-vane hand syndrome (cranio-carpotarsal dystrophy; Freeman-Sheldon syndrome). *In Birth Defects, Original Article Series*. Editor: D. Bergsma. New York, National Foundation – March of Dimes, Vol. V, No. 2, pp. 228–230, 1969.

Walker, B. A., and Borgaonkar, D. S.: Quadruple-XY syndrome. *In* Bergsma, D., (ed.): *Birth Defects: Original Article Series*. New York, National Foundation – March of Dimes, Vol. V, No. 5, pp. 142–143, 1969.

Watson-Jones, R.: *Fractures and Other Bone and Joint Injuries*. Second edition. Baltimore, Williams & Wilkins Co., pp. 375–389, 1941.

Waugh, W.: Dysplasia epiphysialis multiplex in three sisters. *J. Bone Joint Surg.*, *34B*:82–87, 1952.

Weil, S.: Die angeborene Luxation des Radiusköpfchen (R.K.L.). *In* Hohmann, G., Hackenbroch, M., and Lindemann, K., (eds.): *Spezielle Orthopädie obere Extremität of Handbuch der Orthopädie*. Stuttgart, G. Thieme, Band 3, pp. 327–332, 1959.

White, J. R. A.: Congenital dislocation of the head of the radius. *Br. J. Surg.*, *30*:377–379, 1942–1943.

Wildervanck, L. S.: Hereditary congenital abnormalities of the elbows, knees and nails in five generations. *Acta Radiol.*, *33*:41–48, 1950.

Wildervanck, L. S.: Hereditary congenital anomalies of bones and nails in five generations: luxation of the capitulum radii, luxation or absence, respiratory hypoplasia of the patella, crooked little fingers and dystrophy or absence of the nails and abnormal lunulae. *Genetica*, *25*:1–28, 1951.

Windfeld, P.: On congenital and acquired luxations of the capitulum radii with discussion of some associated problems. *Acta. Orthop. Scand.*, *16*:126–141, 1946.

Zimmerman, C.: Iliac horns: a pathognomonic roentgen sign of familial onycho-osteodysplasia. *Am. J. Roentgen*, *86*:478–483, 1961.

Zorn, B.: Sprengelsche Deformität und angeborene Ellenbogensubluxation. *Z. Orthop.*, *104*:592–593, 1967–1968.

Zukschwerdt, L.: Doppelseitige kongenitale Radiusluxation nach hinten mit kongenitaler Hueftluxation. *Dtsch. Ztschr. Chir.*, *231*:45–48, 1931.

Zweymüller, E.: Neue Beobachtungen an einem Typus degenerativus Amstelodamensis. *Neue Öst. Z. Kinderheilkd.*, *2*:40–48, 1957.

Chapter Twenty-Eight

RADIOULNAR SYNOSTOSIS

The region of the elbow constitutes the most common site of congenital synostosis. Humeroradial ankylosis often occurs in cases of longitudinal defects of the ulnar ray. Bizarre forms of fusion of the humerus with either or both forearm bones have been reported by the following authors: Mitscherlich (1865), Kümmel (1895), Andérodias (1921), Michelsson (1922), Aitken (1928), Mouchet and Saint-Pierre (1931), Romanus (1933), Frostad (1940), Mouchet and DiMatteo (1942), Frankel (1944), Murphy and Hanson (1945), Storen (1946), Lambert (1947), Camera (1954), and Keutel et al (1970).

Romanus (1933) cited 24 cases of congenital fusion of the elbow and added one of his own. Frostad (1940) reported five additional cases which occurred in two unrelated families. Frostad thought it very strange that both families lived in the same locality and had almost daily intercourse, and that the abnormalities were precisely the same. This locality was identified by Storen (1946) as Sunmore, Norway. The two patients that Storen himself reported—a brother and sister—came from the same district and had deformities similar to those of Frostad's cases. One notes a preponderance of Scandinavian patients afflicted with this comparatively uncommon congenital anomaly. As was indicated in an earlier chapter, coalescence of carpal bones is more common in African races. Congenital fusion of the proximal radioulnar joint seems more prevalent in Jews from eastern European countries—Hungary, Roumania, Poland, and particularly Russia.

Congenital fusion of the distal ends of the radius and ulna is extremely rare. In a case of proximal radioulnar synostosis reported by Longuet and Peraire (1901), the tapered distal end of the ulna was snug against the adjacent portion of the radius and penetrated the proximal row of carpal bones. This came case was described again by Appraillé (1901), and Wilkie (1914) referred to it as an example of synostosis of the distal ends of the radius and ulna. Jemma (1935) reported an isolated case in which both the proximal and distal extremities of the forearm bones had coalesced. Müller (1939) described a similar case. Another case of distal radioulnar synostosis was featured by Hopf (1959). Harrison and

Wardle (1958) described an unusual outgrowth from the shaft of the radius which articulated with the concave tip of a similar projection jutting out from the ulna.

NOMENCLATURE

Nontraumatic fusion of the forearm bones has been variously referred to as congenital pronation, defective supination, ankylosis of the superior radioulnar joint, proximal radioulnar synostosis, or — because of the rarity of fusion of the distal parts of the forearm bones — simply radioulnar synostosis. Since the advent of radiography, the last designation has gained acceptance and is the one most commonly used at present. Andreini (1953) expressed dissatisfaction with this term, contending that it places far too great an emphasis on the osseous anomaly and does not take into account muscular defects and functional disturbances. Andreini proposed instead the designation "congenital dysplasia of the prono-supinatory complex." Redundancy in this coinage has precluded its adoption by other authors. A title need not denote every aspect of the subject to which it is applied, but should suggest the one that appears salient.

OCCURRENCE

Sandifort (1793) featured excellent lithographs illustrating proximal radioulnar synostosis. In the course of a postmortem examination, Lenoir (1827) discovered that the proximal ends of the forearm bones had consolidated. Prior to the advent of roentgenography, only 22 cases of radioulnar synostosis were recorded in the literature, 15 of which were autopsy specimens; only seven were living patients. After the introduction of roentgenography, almost as many cases were reported in each single decade: Rais (1907) cited 24 cases; Baisch (1913), 38; Wilkie (1914), 42; Thomas (1917), 46; and Greig (1925), 84. Of the last number, 47 were males and 32, females; in five individuals, the sex was not stated. The defect was bilateral in 59 cases; in unilateral cases, the left side was affected 16 times and the right side, nine times. Within one year, Blaine (1930) produced two papers: in one he gave 100 and in the other 200 as the total number of reported cases. Two years after Blaine, Fahlstrom (1932) collected 184 cases from the literature and added one of his own. Jeanty (1964) raised this number to 220. Albrecht (1967) stated that during the period between 1912 and 1967 a total of 124 patients with congenital malformations of the forearm had been seen in the Orthopedic Clinic in Munich, and of these only seven had radioulnar synostosis.

According to Hansen and Andersen (1970), in a period of ten years (1958 to 1968), 37 cases of congenital radioulnar synostosis had been diagnosed in various orthopedic departments in Denmark. Of these patients, 21 were males and 16 females; in 12, the right side was affected and in six, the left side. Nineteen patients had bilateral involvement, all of whom appeared to have inherited their defect from an affected father. It is to be remembered that only a small percentage of patients with radioulnar synostosis seek surgical advice, and not many surgeons report the cases they see. Radioulnar synostosis is far more common than reported (Fig. 28–1).

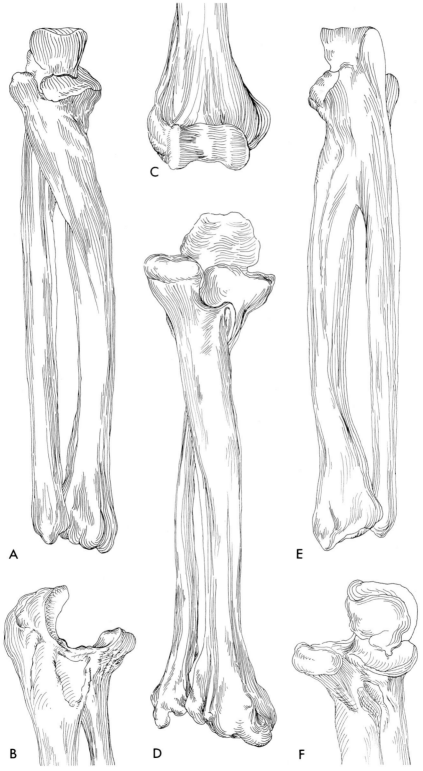

Figure 28–1 Sandifort's (1793) lithographs—redrawn.

THEORIES OF ORIGIN

A number of theories have been proposed to account for the origin of radioulnar synostosis. The proponents of the theory of mechanical interference glibly reason that the proximal ends of the forearm bones are compressed and molded together in utero by pressure from without. The ensuing facts argue against this contention: radioulnar synostosis presents a fairly uniform morphological pattern; it is often bilateral and symmetrical; in many instances, it is hereditary and members of the same family tree manifest other synostotic traits. The theory of mechanical interference fails to account for these and for many diversified, deep-seated abnormalities which are often associated with radioulnar synostosis and which recur generation after generation.

The concept of reversion to an ancestral type is often evoked in connection with radioulnar synostosis. Hamilton (1905), Davenport et al (1924), and Blaine (1930) drew attention to the fact that, in some animals, the radius and ulna are fixed proximally, permitting no rotary movement. Blaine regarded radioulnar synostosis as an atavistic throwback and pointed out that a similar development is found in the forelimb of the deer. The radius and ulna are separate in young deer, but they become fused in the mature animals. Hamilton said that in camels the radius and ulna are completely ankylosed. He leaned to the view that radioulnar synostosis presents "a partial return to one of the lower vertebral forms." Hamilton and Davenport et al advised looking to embryology for further interpretation.

EMBRYOLOGY

In the human embryo, the radius and ulna develop from the same block of condensed mesenchymal cells. At the fourth post-ovulatory week, the precartilaginous precursors of the radius and ulna are contiguous. During the fifth week, cartilage begins to form, creating two longitudinally disposed rods within the common mesenchymal block; these rods tend to diverge distally, but their proximal ends are continuous with one another. At this stage, the forearm and the handplate lie flat on the chest. In this semiprone position, the rod destined to form the radius crosses the precursor of the ulna, and its proximal end rolls toward what is to become the coronoid process. During the sixth week, the perichondrium, investing the cartilaginous radius and ulna, insulates their diverging distal extremities but provides a common envelope for their proximal ends, which lie close to each other. Within this common perichondrial encasement, an interzone of condensed mesenchymal cells separates the proximal end of the future radius from the corresponding extremity of the ulnar anlage.

At the seventh week, the cartilaginous precursor of each forearm bone has gained in girth and length, and the olecranon and coronoid processes of the ulna have become delineated. Interzonal mesenchyma between this part of the ulna and the radial head persists; there is as yet no suggestion of a proximal radioulnar joint. Articular space is formed by the dissolution of interzonal tissue. This process takes place toward the end of the second or the beginning of the third post-ovulatory month. It is presumed that some factor inhibits the interzonal mesenchyma from undergoing dissolution so that a joint space may be formed. Instead of degeneration, the interzonal mesenchyma undergoes chondrification; cartilage, in turn, becomes converted into bone, thus constituting synostosis. The embryonic position of the forearm in semi- or full pronation is perpetuated.

PROGRESS

Radioulnar synostosis is to be regarded as an anomaly of longitudinal segmentation. The proximal end of the radius is assimilated by the proximal ulna, or a bridge of bone connects its neck to the ulna. In the last instance, tethered as it is distally, the head of the radius grows away from the ulna and is said to be dislocated. Thus two varieties of radioulnar synostosis are distinguished—one with and the other without a head. The latter is called primary and the former secondary. This is one of the many arbitrary distinctions that lingers on in the literature. In headless or primary radioulnar synostosis—also called "pure" or type I—the bridge of bone is more extensive: it may measure 4 to 8 cm. in length. In the type of synostosis in which the head of the radius persists proximal to the point of osseous union—called "secondary," "modified," type II or, by earlier authors "dislocated"—the bridge of bone measures about 2 to 4 cm. in length. In many bilateral cases, the head is assimilated by the ulna on one side; on the other side, it bears on epiphysis and eventually the fully matured head angles away from the ulna. In an occasional case, there may be radiographically manifest translucent space in the center of the bony bridge. The aperture or fenestrum within the osseous bridge is ascribed to the incomplete dissolution of interzonal mesenchyma, representing a partly formed joint.

In some instances, for several years after birth, one may discern on radiographs a definite space between the proximal ends of the radius and ulna; in time, this space is effaced and an osseous bridge becomes established. These cases are considered analogous to the condition seen in young and old deer mentioned by Blaine (1930), where the tendency to synostosis is present at birth, but the lesion attains maturity only after a lapse of years. In the roentgenograph of synostotic subjects, one often sees the persistence of the negative shadow cast by the joint space, but pronation and supination of the forearm are nullified. It is conjectured that lack of rotary motion in these cases is due to the fibrous union of bones or the interlocking of the contiguous surfaces of the radius and ulna.

In girls, the carpal epiphysis of the radius may appear as early as the end of the first year after birth. In boys, it usually appears during the second postnatal year. The ossific center of the radial head becomes roentgenographically manifest between the sixth and seventh years after birth. The proximal physis of the radius contributes least to the growth in length of the main bone; the radius grows mostly from the distal end. In radioulnar synostosis, when the proximal end is fixed, continued growth from the carpal extremity causes the shaft of the radius to thicken and become bowed. It presents a convexity away from the ulna, the ulna is thin, and the interosseous space is widened (Figs. 28–2 to 28–7).

HEREDITY

Feidt (1917) considered it plausible that the delayed appearance of the proximal radial epiphysis plays a part in the production of radioulnar synostosis;
(*Text continued on page 949.*)

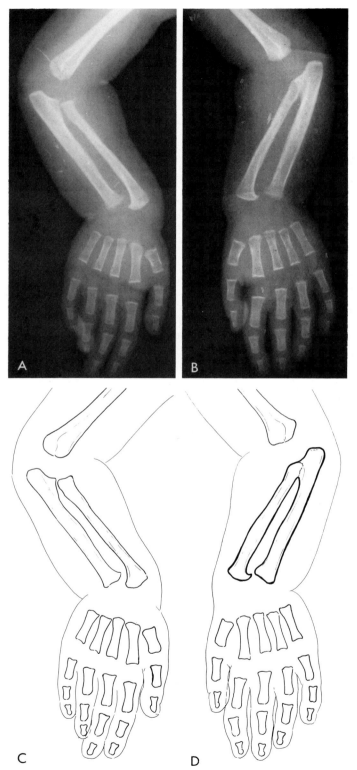

Figure 28–2 Unilateral radioulnar synostosis detected soon after birth. *A*, Dorsovolar roentgenograph of the right forearm and wrist of a neonate. *B*, The left forearm and wrist. There is already osseous union between the proximal ends of the radius and ulna. *C* and *D* illustrate the roentgenograph above each.

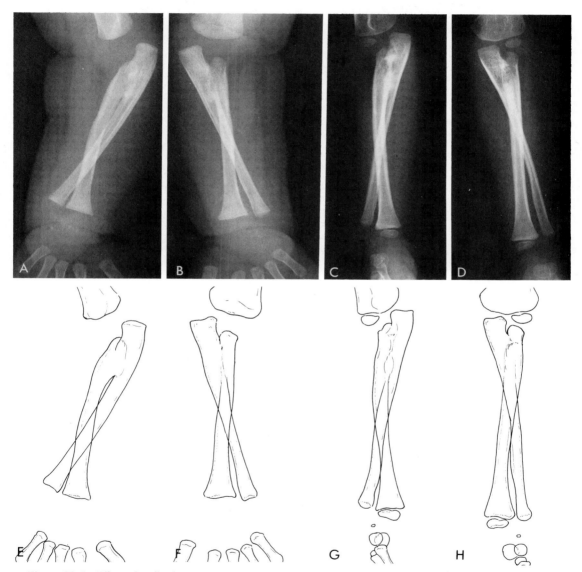

Figure 28–3 Bilateral radioulnar synostosis. *A*, Dorsovolar roentgenograph of the right forearm of a two-month-old boy. The radial head is assimilated. *B*, Dorsovolar roentgenograph of the left forearm: the radial head is free. *C* and *D*, Lateral roentgenographs of the right and left forearms taken at the age of 2. *E*, *F*, *G*, and *H* illustrate the roentgenograph above each.

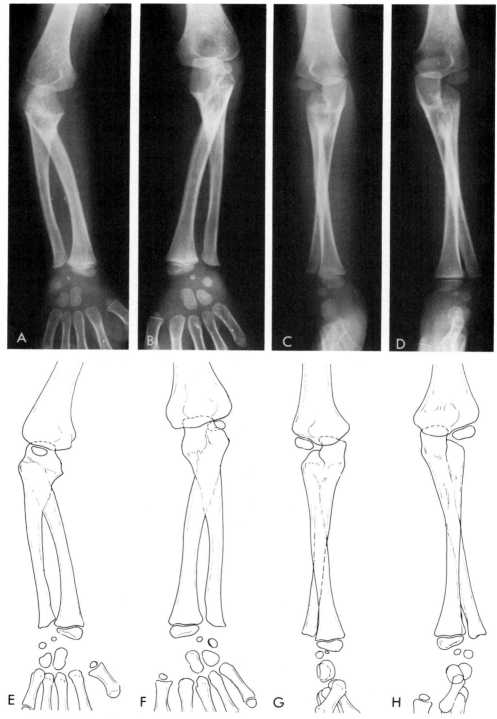

Figure 28–4   Bilateral radioulnar synostosis. *A*, Dorsovolar roentgenograph of the right forearm of a four-year-old boy. *B*, Dorsovolar roentgenograph of the left forearm. *C*, Lateral roentgenograph of the right forearm. *D*, Lateral roentgenograph of the left forearm. *E, F, G,* and *H* illustrate the roentgenograph above each.

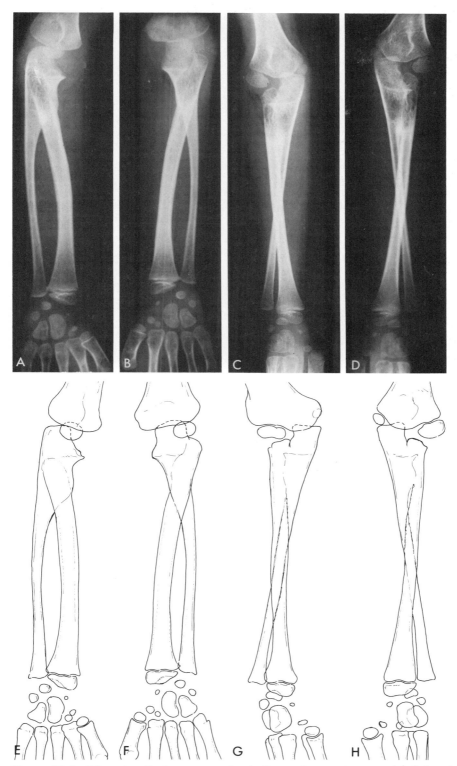

Figure 28–5 Bilateral radioulnar synostosis. *A*, Dorsovolar roentgenograph of the right forearm of a five-year-old boy *B*, Dorsovolar roentgenograph of the left forearm. *C*, Lateral roentgenograph of the right forearm. *D*, Lateral roentgenograph of the left forearm. *E*, *F*, *G*, and *H* illustrate the roentgenograph above each.

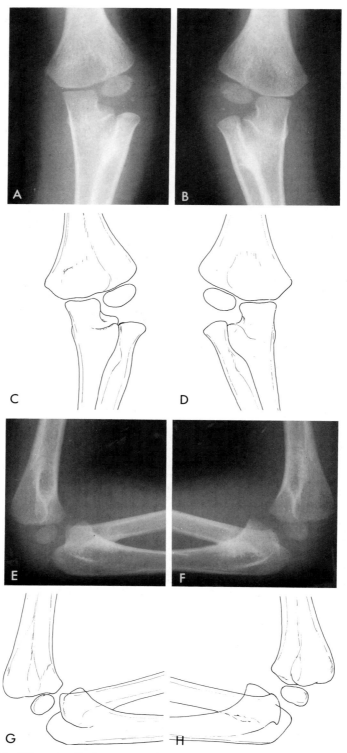

Figure 28–6 Bilateral radioulnar synostosis. *A* and *B*, Dorsovolar roentgenographs of the right and left elbows of a five-and-one-half-year-old boy. *C* and *D* illustrate the roentgenograph above each. *E* and *F*, Lateral roentgenographs of the right and left elbows. *G* and *H* illustrate the same.

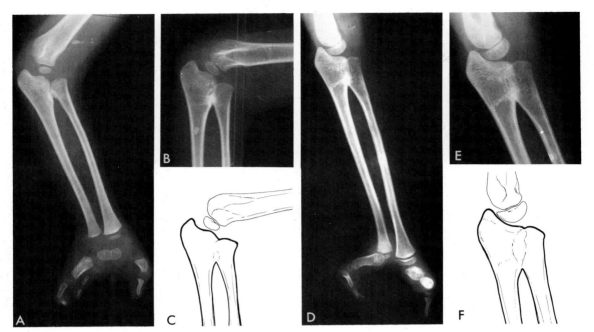

Figure 28–7   Insidious development of radioulnar synostosis. *A,* Dorsovolar roentgenograph of the right forearm and hand of a three-year-old boy with central adactylia, capitate-hamate fusion, and incipient radioulnar synostosis. *B,* Roentgenograph of the elbow a year later, showing osseous fusion of the two forearm bones. *C,* Sketch illustrating the same. *D,* Roentgenograph of the forearm and hand taken at the age of 11 — after clefting operation which consisted of removing the vestigial bones on the radial aspect of the ulnar digit and rotating and putting the coalesced carpal bones in line with the phalanges of what was taken to be a thumb without a metacarpal. *E,* Enlarged roentgenograph of the elbow, showing advanced radioulnar synostosis. *F,* Sketch illustrating the same.

he placed the primary onus on "some inhibitory influence" which presumably had been active during the prenatal period. Most authors seem to agree that the events leading to the final establishment of radioulnar synostosis are genetically determined.

Feidt reported two unrelated patients with radioulnar synostosis; in each report he inserted the following, "Nativity Russia." Kurlander's (1917) patient was born in Russia, and so were the two cases reported by Boorstein (1918). Davenport and associates (1924) traced the pedigree of 13 families, nine of which were Jews of eastern European extraction—mainly Russian. "Even in New York," they wrote, "this is an undue proportion of Jews." Mouchet and Leleu (1925) identified the patients reported by Boorstein and Kurlander as being Russian Jews; the patient they themselves reported was a Polish Jew.

Familial cases of radioulnar synostosis have been reported by Joachimsthal (1900), Blumenthal (1904), Roskoschyn (1905), Sury (1909), Ahreiner (1909), Dawson (1912), Adams (1912–1913), Martin-du Pan (1914), Feidt (1917), Beuchard (1921); Friedjung (1933), and many others. Davenport et al (1924) traced the pedigree of 13 families and, in part, concluded the following: that there are genotypical differences in various families with radioulnar synostosis and that there are diverse biotypes; that the trait may have been activated by one, two, or three genes; and that males are affected twice as frequently as females. In the same family the extent of bony fusion varies from member to member. Radioulnar synostosis is a dominant phenotype with variable expression.

REGIONAL ASSOCIATIONS

Defects of the hand associated with radioulnar synostosis usually involve the pre-axial components. The thumb may be missing, or it is at times diminutive. Occasionally, the first metacarpal is dwarfed and held adducted by being included in the common bondage of the deep transverse ligament. Coalescence of carpal bones and symphalangism have also been reported in cases of radioulnar synostosis. Abbott (1892) spoke of attenuated "supinator brevis" in a dissected arm with radioulnar synostosis. During surgical exploration, Dawson (1912) found the "supinator longus and pronator radii teres muscles much

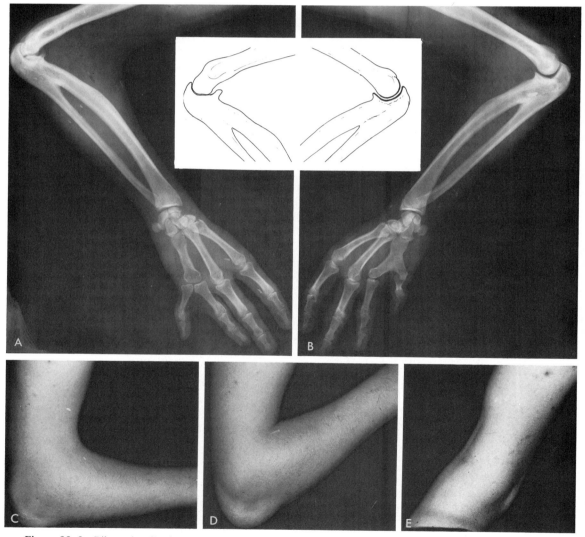

Figure 28–8 Bilateral radioulnar synostosis with limited extension at the right elbow and defective development of the carpal and manual bones. *A*, Dorsovolar roentgenograph of the right elbow, forearm, wrist, and hand of a 17-year-old boy with narrowing of the joint space of the elbow and osteoarthritic lipping of the proximal ulna as shown by the illustrative inset. *B*, Dorsovolar roentgenograph of the left elbow, forearm, wrist, and hand: as shown in illustrative sketch (inset), the elbow joint is unaffected on this side. *C* and *D*, Range of extension and flexion of the right elbow. *E*, Extension of the left elbow.

smaller and thinner than normal." Total absence of the supinator and contracture of the pronator teres and pronator quadratus have also been mentioned in the literature. Greig (1925) considered that soft tissue changes seen in connection with radioulnar synostosis were secondary to the skeletal anomaly (Figs. 28–8 and 28–9).

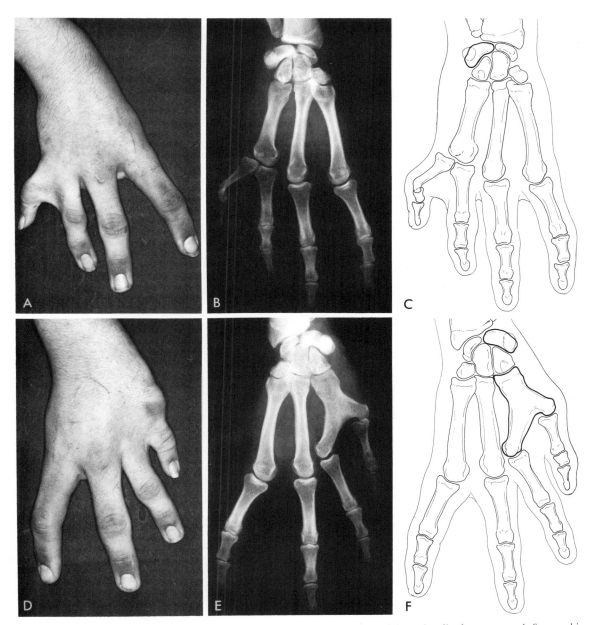

Figure 28–9 *A*, Dorsal view of the right hand of the 17-year-old boy with bilateral radioulnar synostosis featured in Figure 28–8. *B*, Dorsopalmar roentgenograph of the same: the lunate and triquetrum have coalesced; the scaphoid is flat and small; the trapezium is absent, as is the pollical ray; the last two ulnar digits stem from a common metacarpal and the middle phalanx of the little finger is squat. *C*, Sketch illustrating the same. *D*, Dorsal view of the left hand. *E*, Dorsopalmar roentgenograph of the same: the anomalies are similar to those of the right hand except for the configuration of the last ulnar metacarpal, which starts with a thick stem and bifurcates distally. *F*, Sketch illustrating the same.

Patients with radioulnar synostosis will at times present other skeletal abnormalities or have relatives with varied defects. Joachimsthal (1900) described a 12-year-old boy with radioulnar synostosis on the left side. The corresponding hand had no thumb; all the bones of the left arm were shorter and thinner than those on the right side. This patient's brother had a hypoplastic right thumb, and on the left side there was almost complete deficiency of the radial ray. What was left of the proximal radius had coalesced with the ulna. His two sisters and his mother had malformed fingers. In one of the families reported by Boorstein (1918), all members—four males and three females—had "club finger." Not the same finger was affected in all, but a "club finger" was invariably present and the male members had no hair over their cheek bones. In the pedigree featured in Chapter Eleven, mention was made of a teenage boy with radioulnar synostosis. His mother, maternal uncle, and three of his cousins from the mother's side had bilateral symphalangism of their little fingers. The male members were more severely affected—they had solid bony fusion of the proximal and middle phalanges. Roentgenographs of the hands of the females showed a joint space between the phalanges, and motion was drastically curtailed but not completely eliminated.

ASSOCIATED LOWER LIMB ANOMALIES

Roskoschyn's (1905) patient with radioulnar synostosis had bowed legs. Ahreiner's (1909) case showed a subluxated hip, and in the case reported by Evans (1921), bilateral radioulnar synostosis was associated with congenital dislocation of both hips. Grunfeld (1911) and many others have noted the association of clubfoot—usually due to coalescence of the tarsal bones—with radioulnar synostosis. Radioulnar synostosis is also known to occur in a number of established syndromes.

ACROFACIAL DYSOSTOSIS OF NAGER AND DE REYNIER

This complex, already described in Chapter Twenty-Three, consists of a short, small mandible, absent radius or thumb, and radioulnar synostosis. Nager and de Reynier (1948) presented an 18-year-old girl with mandibulofacial dysostosis, absent thumbs, an accessory finger on the left hand, and bilateral radioulnar synostosis. Becker's (1954) patient was an eight-day-old boy with bilateral absence of the thumbs and limited extension of the elbows. Marden et al (1964) presented a male infant whose father and mother were 42 and 41, respectively, at the time of his birth, thus suggesting dominant mutation.

CHROMOSOMAL ABERRATIONS

Davenport et al (1924) had surmised that at least in some families the gene responsible for radioulnar synostosis might be located on the Y chromosome.

Klinefelter and associates (1942) described nine patients with "gynecomastia, aspermatogenesis, without a-leydigism and increased excretion of follicle-stimulating hormone." One of these cases had bilateral radioulnar synostosis. Radioulnar synostosis has been reported with XXY, XXXY, XXXXY, XYY, and XXYY patterns. It is more likely to occur with the XXXXY pattern. Neu and Gardner (1969) estimated that radioulnar synostosis occurred in 42 per cent of cases with XXXXY pattern and in 3 per cent of individuals with XY/XXY constitution; they suspected the Y chromosome to be the carrier of genetic information. Cleveland et al (1969) expounded upon the existence of a close relationship between the extra Y chromosome and radioulnar synostosis—just as Davenport et al (1924) had surmised almost half a century earlier.

As was to be expected, all reported cases of abnormal sex chromosomes and radioulnar synostosis have been males. Bilateral radioulnar synostosis with XXXXY constitution was reported by the following authors: Fraser et al (1961), Barr and associates (1962), Fraccaro et al (1962), Atkins and Connelly (1963), Schade et al (1963), Scherz and Roeckel (1963), Turner et al (1963), Jancur (1964), Joseph et al (1964), and Jancur (1971). The case with the same sex chromosome constitution presented by Van Went et al (1965) had unilateral synostosis of the forearm bones. Anders et al (1960), Ferguson-Smith et al (1960), and Greenstein et al (1970) reported unilateral radioulnar synostosis with XXXY pattern. Robinson et al (1964) presented a case of unilateral radioulnar synostosis with XXYY pattern, and Cleveland et al (1970) reported two prepuberal boys with one-sided involvement of the forearm bones and XYY chromosomal constitutions; both of these boys manifested aggressive behavior. As will be shown in the next chapter, adult males with an extra Y chromosome tend to be antisocial and indulge in violent criminal acts.

CRANIOSYNOSTOSIS

Jewesbury (1920–1921) described a three-week-old infant who, in addition to acrocephaly and syndactyly, had proximal radioulnar synostosis.

FUNSTON'S CERVICAL RIB SYNDROME

Funston (1932) described a mother and daughter with bilateral cervical ribs and radial ray defects. He stated: "The mother had a bilateral absence of the radius with club hand deformity and rudimentary thumbs. The daughter had an exactly similar deformity of the right hand. The left hand. . .had no thumb and there was synostosis between the radius and ulna just distal to the elbow joint. . . . Roentgenograms revealed well-developed cervical ribs in both mother and daughter."

MANDIBULOFACIAL DYSOSTOSIS

Franceschetti and Klein (1949) presented a patient with radioulnar synostosis aplasia of the thumb and mandibulofacial dysostosis. Vitré (1971) described an eight-year-old girl with mandibulofacial dysostosis, radioulnar synostosis, aplasia of the right thumb, hypoplasia of the left thumb, bilateral dislocation of the hips, and excessive laxity of the knees.

MULTIPLE EXOSTOSES

Davenport et al (1924) reported a family in which some members had radioulnar synostosis and others had multiple exostoses. In another family reported, all affected members were short in stature, as are individuals with multiple exostoses. Davenport and his associates relegated congenital radioulnar synostosis to "the general rubric of dyschondroplasia," meaning multiple exostoses. They considered the tendency of bone formation to be inherited, and surmised about the localizing factors which caused the basic trend to become centralized on some particular bones. They also called attention to the fact that in both multiple exostoses and radioulnar synostosis, males are affected more commonly than females.

NIEVERGELT SYNDROME (Nievergelt-Pearlman Syndrome)

Nievergelt (1944) described a man with short forearms and short lower legs. This mesomelic dwarf had three male offspring by three different women. All three sons had short forearms and short lower legs. In each forearm, the radius and ulna were short and bulky; they had coalesced proximally. In only one instance was radioulnar synostosis absent; extension at the elbow and pronation and supination of the forearm were limited. In the lower leg, the tibia and fibula were short and rhomboidal in shape. The trait was regarded as an autosomal dominant. Radioulnar synostosis was also present in the cases reported by Solomen and Sulamma (1958) and Pearlman et al (1964).

DISABILITY

The most constant sign of radioulnar synostosis is the pronated or semipronated position of the forearm. The usual complaint by the patient is inability to supinate the forearm and hand. Pronation and supination materially enhance the functional usefulness of the hand; conversely, absence of these movements diminishes its usefulness. Muscles control these rotary movements, but it is the radius which rotates. In radioulnar synostosis, the muscles undergo atrophy of disuse and contracture because the radius resists rotation. Patients with radioulnar synostosis experience no difficulty in flexing and extending the forearm at the elbow.

The radius has been likened to the spoke of a wheel and is said to have acquired its name because of this resemblance. The radius functions more like an axle than a spoke; the hand serves as its rotating terminal. Unlike the arrangement between an ordinary axle and wheel, the connection between the

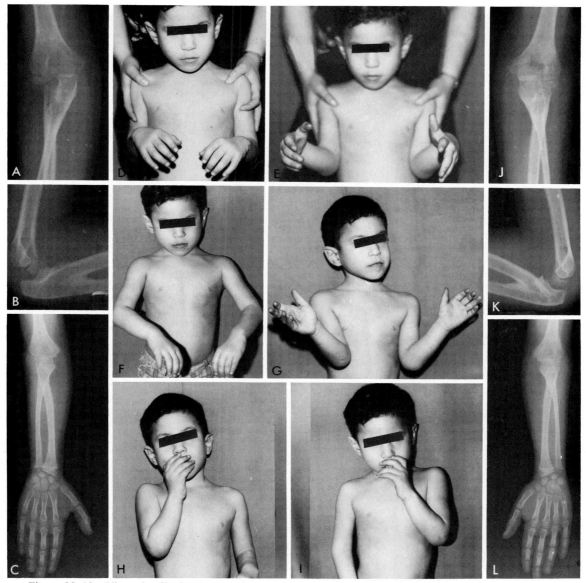

Figure 28–10   Bilateral radioulnar synostosis: compensatory movements at the shoulders and at the wrist. *A,* Dorsovolar roentgenograph of the right elbow. *B,* Lateral roentgenograph of the same. *C,* Dorsovolar roentgenograph of the right forearm and hand. *D* and *E,* Pronation and supination when compensatory movement at the shoulders is eliminated. *F* and *G,* Pronation and supination aided by compensatory movements of the shoulders and wrists. *H* and *I,* Palm-to-mouth opposition by the right and left hand. *J,* Dorsovolar roentgenograph of the left elbow. *K,* Lateral roentgenograph of the same. *L,* Dorsovolar roentgenograph of the left forearm and hand.

hand and forearm is not rigid. A movable joint, the wrist, links the two and adds considerably to the motion permitted at the proximal radioulnar joints. In long-standing cases of radioulnar synostosis, the wrist tends to be hypermobile and allows a greater degree of pronation and supination than when the radius is not fixed proximally. To a minimal degree, pronation and supination are augmented by the side-to-side rocking of the olecranon on the trochlea of the humerus. Most of the supplementary contribution to the rotary action of the ra-

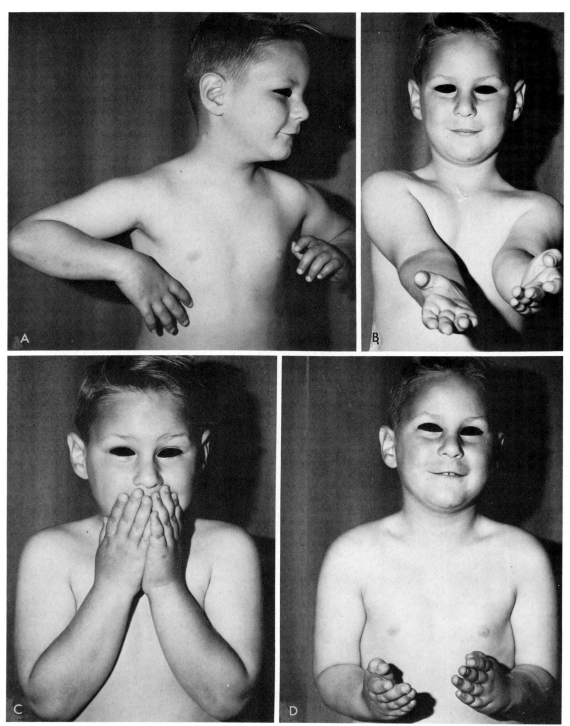

Figure 28–11   Movements at the shoulder and wrist compensating for lack of pronation and supination incident to radioulnar synostosis. *A*, Photograph of a boy with bilateral proximal radioulnar synostosis. He abducts his arms and flexes the wrists to simulate pronation of the forearms. *B*, Supination is simulated by adduction of the arms and extension of the wrists. *C*, Surgical interference is deemed unnecessary when the patient has developed sufficient hypermobility of the wrists to kiss his palm or when the forearm is frozen in midsupination as shown in *D*.

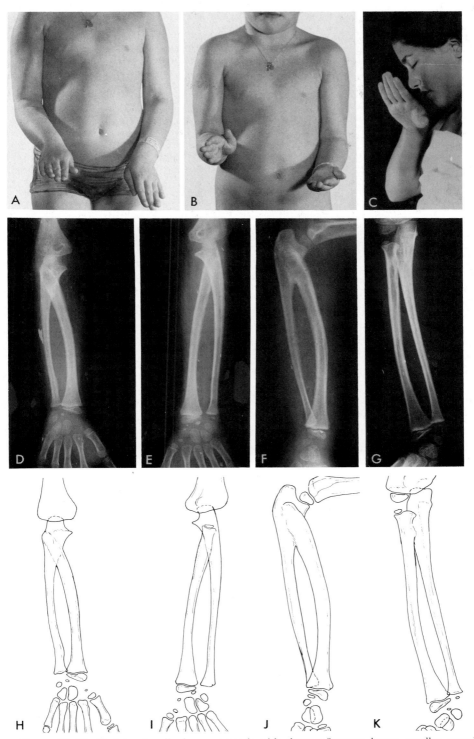

Figure 28–12 Unilateral radioulnar synostosis with shorter forearm bones, smaller carpal bones, and delayed appearance of the distal epiphysis of the ulna of the affected limb. *A*, Frontal view of a six-year-old girl with radioulnar synostosis of the right forearm. *B*, Failure to supinate the right forearm. *C*, Failure to kiss the right palm. *D*, Dorsovolar roentgenograph of the right forearm. *E*, Dorsovolar roentgenograph of the left forearm. *F*, Lateral roentgenograph of the right forearm. *G*, Semi-lateral roentgenograph of the left forearm. *H, I, J,* and *K* illustrate the roentgenograph above each.

dius is made by the shoulder joint. The radius may thus be regarded as the segment of a long caterpillared axle which begins to rotate at the shoulder and gains increments at the distal articulations, but mainly at the proximal radioulnar joint. When this articulation is rendered immobile, as in radioulnar synostosis, rotary movements of the other joints—in particular, the shoulder and the wrist—come into play and mimic pronation and supination. These compensatory movements are at best awkward and fatiguing.

In many instances, radioulnar synostosis is discovered accidentally. The parents of Hamilton's (1905) patient did not suspect that anything was wrong with their son. At school the teacher asked the boy to hold out his hand. The boy tried "but failed to perform the act of supination. The teacher grasped his hand and tried to forcibly supinate it but was unable to do so." Lunn's (1906) patient, a waitress, carried trays on the back of her hand. Painter's (1909) patient, a young girl, tired easily when learning to write. Dawson (1912) reported that if his patient made an effort to hold anything with the palm turned uppermost, an extremely awkward exposure of the deformity resulted, the elbow being pressed firmly to the side and the hand simulating a spiral twist. Wilkie's (1914) patient, a woman, "noticed the disability most when receiving change in a shop, as she could not take it into the palm of her hand, but required always to pick it up with the hand pronated." Feidt (1917) spoke of a housewife who complained that, when doing the wash, she experienced great difficulty in wringing the water out of clothes. When offered a coin, Chesser's (1919) patient, a boy, flexed the elbow-joint and turned the hand backwards to receive the coin in the palm of the hand.

Grossman (1928) stated that the disability in radioulnar synostosis, though a handicap, was by no means an insuperable one. Cohn's (1932) patient was a telegraph operator who later became a brakeman. The only awkwardness of movement that he experienced was in dealing cards or accepting coins. "In the latter instance, whenever possible," Cohn wrote, "he first puts his hand on a counter and then rotates his arm from the shoulder in order to obtain supination." Patients with fully pronated forearm and hand cannot button their shirts, tie their ties, feed themselves, carry on toilet duties, or turn a doorknob with ease and grace (Figs. 28–10 to 28–12).

TREATMENT

Only a small minority of patients with radioulnar synostosis require surgical interference. These are individuals with fully pronated forearm and hand who, even with compensatory movements of the shoulder and wrist, are sufficiently handicapped that they cannot earn a livelihood in the occupation of their choosing nor feed themselves. The surgeon tries to procure a measure of supinatory movement or, at least, to bring the hand into a functionally useful position, which is about midway between pronation and supination but slightly in favor of the latter. As noted by Gibson (1923), "full supination is certainly not an optimum position." An improved fixed position can be attained by rotary osteotomy of the radius and ulna. Procurement of active pronation and supination necessitates more complicated procedures.

Numerous attempts have been made to disconnect the two bones; muscle or metal sheet has been interposed between them, and the separated radial head has even been insulated by an appropriately shaped cap made of stainless steel.

The results have been disappointing. A favorite operation at one time was to resect a segment from the midshaft of the radius and establish a pseudarthrosis between the two fragments. Following this procedure, the proximal end of the distal fragment slanted toward the ulna and resulted in radial deviation of the hand.

In the course of his discussion of Bennett's (1924) paper on congenital synostosis of the radius and ulna, Prince made the following startling confession: "Some years ago," he said, "I had a very unfortunate experience with a young Italian girl on whom I performed a section of the radius with the removal of about one-half inch of the shaft. The condition was bilateral and the forearms were fixed in full pronation. At the time of the operation following the removal of the section of the radius, the forearm could be easily supinated, and accordingly it was put in this position and retained by means of a plaster of paris cast. The hand became quite swollen and cyanotic, and in spite of the fact that the cast was removed as soon as the seriousness of the condition was noted, gangrene of that portion of the arm supplied by the radial artery resulted. The thumb and most of the radius sloughed away and an ischemic paralysis resulted in the remaining fingers. It is my belief that the torsion correction occluded radial circulation, giving rise to the disastrous results."

In 1957, the author of this book described what he called a swivel operation for proximal radioulnar synostosis. This procedure is carried out in a single surgical session; it consists of three dovetailed steps: (1) insertion of the swivel, (2) tendon transplantation, and (3) resection of the distal ulna. In the procedure described originally, the author transferred either the flexor carpi ulnaris or flexor carpi radialis. He has since found it equally efficacious to transfer the extensor carpi ulnaris. The interposition of the swivel is preceded by resection of a commensurate segment of radial shaft just proximal to the insertion of the pronator teres. In cases of congenital radioulnar synostosis, since younger individuals tend to deposit new bone more generously, the author removes the periosteal sleeve with the resected segment of the radius and cauterizes the ends of the remaining bones. In growing children, he has osteotomized the distal shaft of the ulna instead of excising its carpal end. The author has found the years between 12 and 16 to be the optimum time of surgery for congenital radioulnar synostosis.

The segment of the radial shaft between the insertions of the supinator muscle and pronator teres is exposed through a longitudinal dorsoradial incision over the proximal forearm. The tendinous insertion of the pronator teres, which curls around the junction of the upper and middle thirds of the radius, is identified; the fibers of the supinator attached to the radius just proximal to this insertion are stripped, and appropriate segment of the radius is resected. The medullary cavity of the proximal fragment of the radius is reamed and gouged out in order that 2 inches of the central rod of the prosthesis may be inserted; the cavity of the distal fragment of the radius is similarly widened for an inch or a little more from the resected end. The soft tissues are retracted by wooden tongue depressors, and the ends of the remaining bones are cauterized to prevent overgrowth.

The swivel is made of stainless steel and consists of a cylinder-shaped body and a central rod. The cylinder should be slightly shorter than the piece of bone resected and about the same size in girth; there are depressions in the upper and lower surfaces; and there is a set-screw at the midsection. The cylinder is perforated from top to bottom in order that the central rod may be inserted, and the perforation is large enough so that the rod may glide easily. The central rod is three times the length of the cylinder and one-third its size in diameter. There is a small hole beneath the superior rim of the cylinder, and another through the upper portion of the central rod. A loop of suture wire is placed through these holes, and when this loop is tugged, the central rod glides down within the cylinder to the desired level, where it can be secured by tightening the set-screw.

Because of the synostosis, the proximal fragment of the radius is fixed; it cannot be moved. The central rod of the swivel is inserted into the cylinder until its distal end is flush with the lower rim; the extruding 2 inches of the rod is then inserted into the end of the proximal fragment. The cylinder is now aligned with the proximal end of the distal fragment, and by pulling the wire,

(Text continued on page 965.)

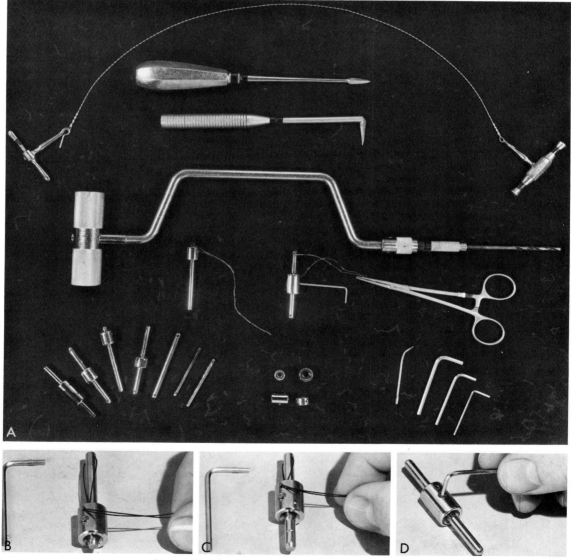

Figure 28–13   Armamentarium for swivel operation.

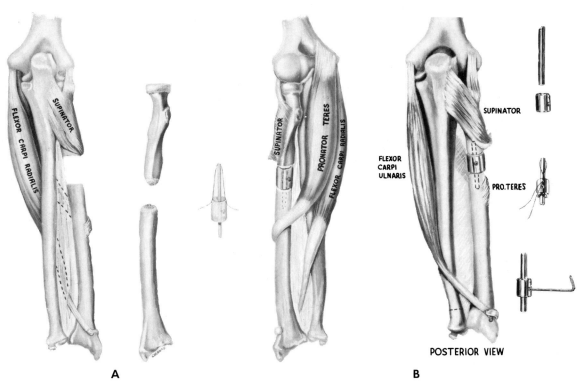

A **B**

Figure 28–14 Older technique of swivel operation. *A*, Drawing showing the insertion of a swivel in a forearm in which the flexor carpi radialis has been transplanted to serve as the supinator. *B*, Drawing of a forearm in which the flexor carpi ulnaris has been transplanted to serve as the supinator. The dotted line across the distal end of the ulna shows the level at which the resection is performed. In the newer technique shown in Figure 28–15 the distal ulna is resected obliquely and the split half of the extensor carpi ulnaris tendon is passed through the distal end of the remaining ulnar fragment and sutured to itself in order to establish a collateral ligament; the main body of the flexor carpi ulnaris is transplanted to serve as the supinator.

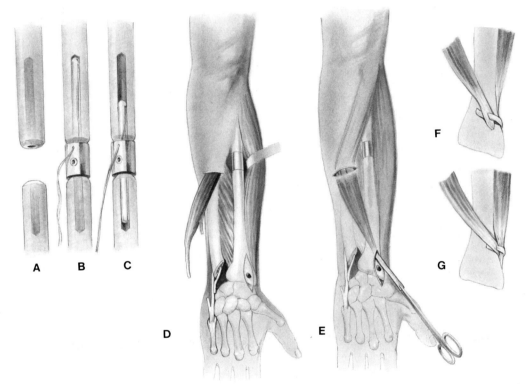

Figure 28–15 Newer technique for swivel operation. *A*, Segment of radius resected. *B*, The central rod of the swivel has been driven up into the proximal fragment of the radius. *C*, The rod is pulled down into the medullary cavity of the distal fragment. *D*, Split half of the extensor carpi ulnaris tendon is utilized to establish a collateral ligament: it is made to pass through the resected end of the distal ulna and sutured onto its main stem. *E*, Extensor carpi ulnaris is passed subcutaneously and its tendon is made to come out near the point of insertion of brachioradialis. *F*, After the closure of the carpal physis of the radius, the tendon of extensor carpi ulnaris is anchored to the radial border of the distal radius. *G*, In growing children it is moored to the tendinous insertion of brachioradialis.

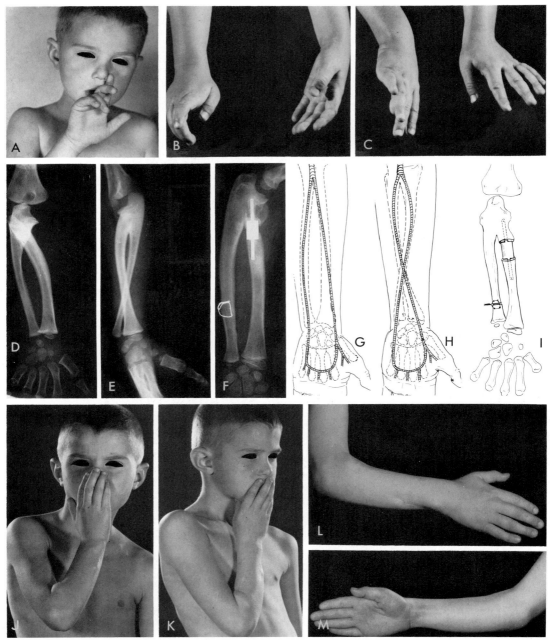

Figure 28–16   Swivel for proximal radioulnar synostosis. *A,* Frontal view of the six-year-old boy featured—with his mother who had symphalangism as did several members of her family—in Figure 11–7. Even with the aid of compensatory movements of the right shoulder and wrist, this boy could not supinate his right forearm and hand to feed himself. *B* and *C,* Attempts to pronate and supinate the hands. The right hand does not supinate. *D* and *E,* Preoperative dorsovolar and lateral roentgenographs of the right forearm. *F,* Postoperative dorsovolar roentgenograph. Surgery consisted of inserting the swivel, shortening the ulna, and transferring the extensor carpi ulnaris insertion into the tendon of the brachiradialis. During surgery, when the distal forearm and the hand were fully supinated, the digits remained white, bloodless; the limb was immobilized in a compromised position between pronation and supination. *G,* Sketch showing the position of the radial and ulnar arteries in a normal forearm or in one which had not remained in fixed pronation since birth or even before. *H* illustrates the course of the forearm arteries in the right forearm of this young boy. *I* illustrates *F.* *J, K, L,* and *M,* Results one year after surgery.

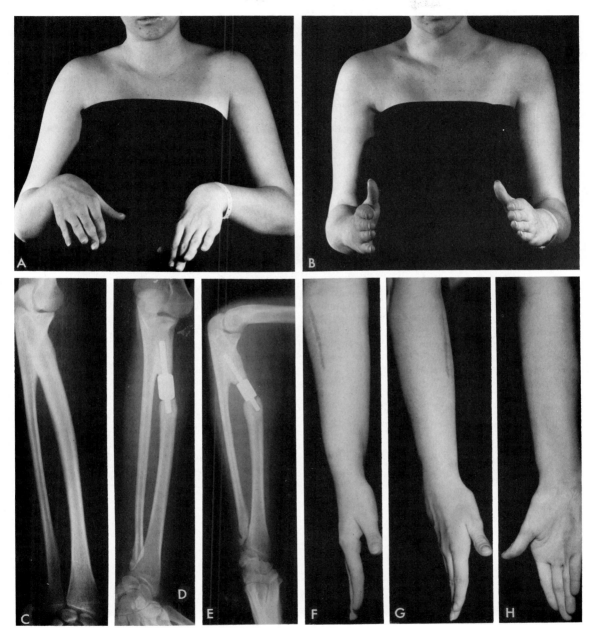

Figure 28–17   Swivel for proximal radioulnar synostosis. *A*, Photograph of a 16-year-old girl with bilateral radioulnar synostosis, more severe on the right side. The right forearm was fully pronated. *B*, Attempt at supination which is made possible by the hypermobility of the wrists. *C*, Preoperative dorsovolar roentgenograph of the right forearm. *D* and *E*, Postoperative roentgenographs: a segment of the radius distal to synostosis and proximal to the insertion of the pronator teres was resected and a stainless steel swivel inserted. The distal end of the ulna was obliquely resected. The extensor carpi radial was transferred to the radial border of the distal radius. *F*, *G*, and *H*, Functional results.

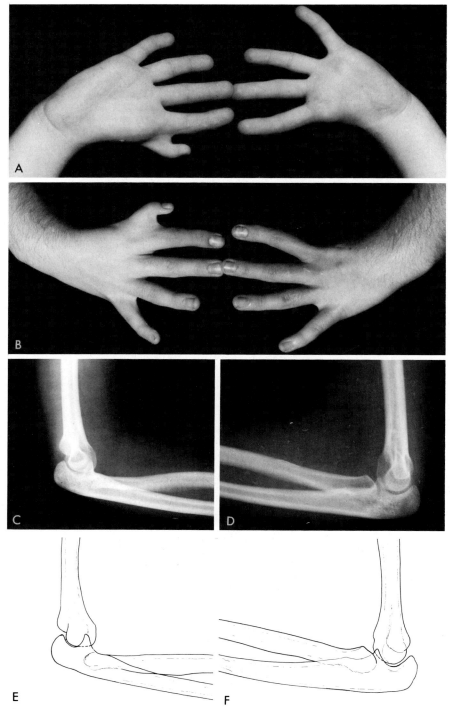

Figure 28–18   Bilateral radioulnar synostosis in a patient with nonopposable triphalangeal thumb of the right hand and absent left pollical ray. *A*, Palmar view of the hands of the 13-year-old girl featured in Figures 24–21 and 24–22. This patient could supinate her hands only by raising them above her head. *B*, Dorsal view. *C*, Lateral roentgenograph of the right elbow, showing that the radial head has been completely assimilated by the proximal ulna. *D*, Lateral roentgenograph of the left elbow. There is side-to-side coalescence of the proximal ends of the radius and ulna. *E* and *F* illustrate the roentgenograph above each.

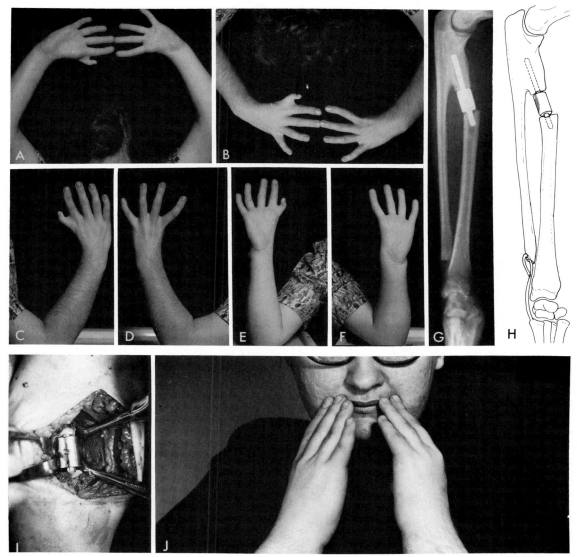

Figure 28–19 *A* and *B*, Palmar and dorsal views of the hands and forearms of the 13-year-old girl featured in Figure 28–18. These photographs were obtained with the patient lying face down and putting her hands above her head. *C, D, E,* and *F*, show pronation and supination by the action of the shoulders. *G,* Lateral roentgenograph of the right forearm after the insertion of a swivel, resection of the distal ulna and transfer of the extensor carpi ulnaris to the insertion of the brachioradialis. *H,* Sketch illustrating the same. The left forearm was similarly operated on. *I,* Swivel in the right forearm. *J,* Postoperatively, after bilateral swivel operation, this patient was able to touch her lips without abduction and external rotation of the arm at the shoulder and to feed herself.

which has been previously threaded through the holes in the upper rim of the cylinder and the proximal end of the central rod, an inch of the central rod is doweled into the distal fragment. The position of the central rod within the medullary cavities of the two radial fragments is ascertained by roentgenographs; each fragment should contain about 1 inch of the rod. When the rod is in this position, it is secured by tightening the set-screw with an Allen wrench.

In proximal radioulnar synostosis, the action of the supinator muscle is

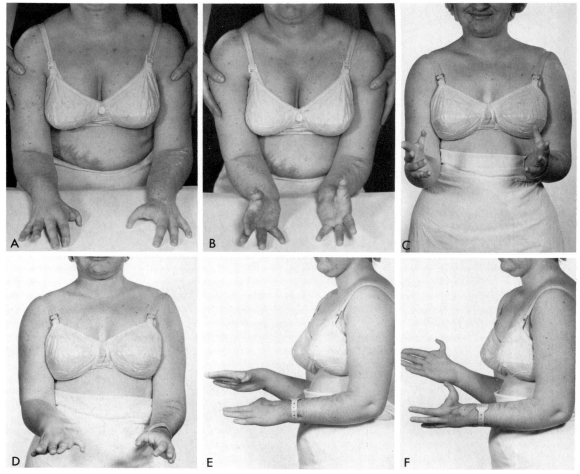

Figure 28–20   Late results. *A, B, C, D, E,* and *F* show pronation and supination of the forearms and hands of the girl featured in Figures 28–18 and 28–19 four years after surgery.

nullified. In order to counterbalance the pronator teres and to bring the hand into supination, the extensor carpi ulnaris is used, the insertion of this muscle being shifted to the distal end of the radius. In older subjects, the tendon of the extensor carpi ulnaris is moored to the radial border of the distal radius. In growing children, it is attached to the tendinous insertion of the brachioradialis. Resection of the distal end of the ulna may be accomplished through the incision used for the detachment of the original insertion of the extensor carpi ulnaris. The ulna is sectioned obliquely. An attempt is made to establish a collateral ligament by utilizing a split half of the extensor carpi ulnaris tendon which is threaded through a tunnel in the distal end of the remaining ulna and sutured to itself.

At the termination of reconstructive work, the hand is placed in semisupine position, the tourniquet is released, and the return of blood to the fingertips is observed. If those digits remain bloodless, the parts are returned to their original position, with the hope of improving this stance later on. Postoperatively, the arm is encased in a cast, immobilizing both the elbow and wrist. Ordinarily, the forearm is placed in a position of about 20 degrees of supination. In cases of precarious circulation, optimum supination is procured gradually by periodic changes of cast. The cast is removed after six weeks, at which time the attachment of the transplanted tendon to the distal end of the radius should be firm. Functional exercises are then initiated (Figs. 28–13 to 28–20).

SUMMARY

Radioulnar synostosis is an anomaly of longitudinal segmentation. It is genetically determined and is often associated with other synostotic states. It is more common in males than in females, and it is not an uncommon accompaniment in males with supernumerary X chromosomes or XYY constitution. Radioulnar synostosis appears to prevail in Jews of Eastern European extraction. Only occasionally does radioulnar synostosis cause sufficient disability to require surgical interference. When the hand is in fixed pronation and the patient is not able to kiss his own palm, it should be brought into a position of midsupination either by osteotomy of the forearm bones or by the swivel operation described by the author.

References

Abbott, F. C.: Hereditary congenital dislocations of the radius. *Path. Soc. London, 43*:129–139, 1892.

Accardi, V., and Catalano, V.: Le sinostosi radio-ulnari post-traumatiche. *Chir. Organi Mov., 34*:120–129, 1950.

Adams, J. E.: Congenital coalescence of radius and ulna. *Proc. R. Soc. Med. London* (Sect. Dis. Child.), 6:136–137, 1913.

Ahreiner, F.: Ein Fall von doppelseitiger kongenitaler Synostose der oberen Gelenkenden von Radius und Ulna. *Beitr. Klin. Chir., 65*:467–471; fig. 8, 1909.

Aimes, Hadengue, and Hutin: Luxation congénitale bilatérale de l'extrémité supérieure du radius, avec synostose des os de l'avant-bras. *Rev. d'Orthop.,* (3 s.), 69–74, 1918.

Aitken, D. M.: Case of bilateral radioulnar synostosis associated with bilateral congenital dislocation of hips. Discussion of E. L. Evans' presentation. *Proc. R. Soc. Med. London* (Sect. Surg. Subsect. Orthop.), *1*:165, 1928.

Albrecht, R.: Beitrag zum Vorkommen der Unterarmmissbildungen. *Z. Orthop., 103*:476–485; Abb. 13, 1967.

Algyogyi, H.: Ein seltener Fall von Missbildung einer Oberextremität Brachydaktylie, mit Pero- und Ektrodaktylie. *Fortschr. Röntgenstr., 16*:286–290; Taf. xxii; fig. 5, 1911–1912.

Andérodias: Un cas d'ankylose congenitale du coude. *Rev. d'Orthop.,* (3 s.), *8*:133–134, 1921.

Anders, V. G., Prader, A., Hauschtech, E., Scharer, K., Siebenmann, R. E., and Heller, R.: Multiples Sex-Chromatin und komplexes chromosomales Mosaik bei einem Knaben mit Idiotie und multiplen Missbildungen. *Helv. Paediatr. Acta, 15*:515–532; Abb. 3, 1960.

Andreini, G.: La sinostosi congenita radio-ulnare. *Arch. Putti, 3*:336–349, 1953.

Appraillé, G.: *Malformations Congénitales de l'Extrémite Supérieure du Radius.* Thèse. Paris, G. Steinheil, pp. 1–46, 1901.

Atkins, L., and Connelly, J. P.: XXXY sex chromosome abnormality. *Am. J. Dis. Child., 106*:514–519, 1963.

Baisch, B.: Die kongenitale radio-ulnare Synostose. *Z. Orthop. Chir., 31*:46–57, 1913.

Baldwin, C. H.: Fusion of the radio-ulnar joint. *J. Bone Joint Surg., 11*:345, 1929.

Barr, M. L.: The natural history of Klinefelter's syndrome. *Fertil. Steril., 17*:429–441, 1966.

Barr, M. L., Carr, D. H., Pozsonyi, J., Wilson, R. A., Dunn, H. G., Jacobson, T. S., Miller, J. R., Lewis, M., and Chown, B.: The XXXXY sex chromosome abnormality. *Can. Med. Assoc. J., 87*:891–901; fig. 8, 1962.

Bartsch, H.: Ein Fall von angeborener radio-ulnarer Synostose. *Arch. Orthop. Unfallchir., 24*:84–94, 1926.

Bauer, K. H., and Bode, W.: Die Aplasie des proximalen Radio-Ulnar-gelenkes (sog. radio-ulnare Synostose). *In* Abel, W., et al., (eds.): *Erbbiologie und Erbpathologie körperlicher Zustände und Funktionen.* Berlin, Springer, pp. 183–188, 1940.

Beck, W.: Beitrag zur radio-ulnaren Synostose. *Fortschr. Röntgenstr., 83*:734, 1955.

Becker, K.: Ueber die angeborene Unterkieferhypoplasie (Mikrogeni) und ihre Beziehungen zu anderen Korpmissbildungen. *Thesis* Kinderklinsk Munster i. Lv. 1954, quoted by P. J. Waardenburg. *In* Waardenburg, P. J., Franceschetti, A., and Klein, D., (eds.): *Genetics and Ophthalmology.* Vol. 1. Netherlands, Royal Van Gorum Publishers Assn., pp. 387–388, 1961.

Becker, V.: Zwei mit angeborenen Hemmungsmissbildungen der oberen Extremitäten behaftete Geschwister. *Schmidt's Jahrb. Ges. Med., 179*:13, 1878.

Bennett, C. B.: A case of congenital synostosis of radius and ulna. *Calif. West. Med., 22*:435–436, 1924.

Bertolucci, G.: Un caso di sinostosi radio-ulnare bilaterale congenita. *G. Med. Mil., 74*:474–477, 1926.

Beuchard, R.: De la synostose radio-cubitale supérieure primitive et héréditaire. (Étude clinique et radio-graphique de 2 cas). *Rev. Chir., 59*:629–647, 1921.

Biesalski, K.: Zur Kenntnis der angeborenen und erworbenen Supinationsbehinderung im Ellbogen. *Z. Orthop. Chir., 25*:205–218, 1910.

Billant, Dufour, and Thibonmery: Un cas d'ankylose congénital bilatéral du coude. *Bull. Soc. Franc. Electro-Radiol., 26*:238–240, 1938.

Binty-Schiliachto, F. A.: Beitrag zu den Missbildungen der oberen Extremitäten. *Arch. Orthop. Unfallchir., 24*:597–609, 1927.

Blaine, E. S.: Congenital radioulnar synostosis, with report of a case. *Am. J. Surg.,* (n.s.), *8*:429–434, 1930.

Blaine, E. S.: Radioulnar synostosis, with report of a case. *Ill. Med. J., 57*:166–169, 1930.

Blank: Synostosis radioulnaris. *Berl. Klin. Wochenschr., 49*:423, 1912.

Blumenthal, M.: Über hereditare, angeborene doppelseitige Supinationsstörung des Ellbogengelenkes. *Z. Orthop. Chir., 12*:181–194, 1904.

Boeckh, C. A.: Über kongenitale Synostose zwischen Radius und Ulna. *Dtsch. Z. Chir., 213*:225–230, 1928–1929.

Boorstein, S. W.: Bilateral congenital radioulnar synostosis. *Am. J. Surg., 32*:221–223, 1918.

Boppe, M.: La synostose congénitale radio-cubitale. *In* Ombrédanne, L., and Mathieu, P., (eds.): *Traité de Chirurgie Orthopédie.* Parisc Masson et Cie, Vol. 3, pp. 2384–2990, 1937.

Borden, E. D.: Congenital radioulnar synostosis: case. *Boll. Soc. Cir. Chile, 23*:219–222, 1945. Also in *Rev. Med. Chile, 75*:151–154, 1946.

Borrel: Un cas de synostose radio-cubitale. *Rev. Méd. Centre Quest., 7*:78–81, 1935.

Bossi, P.: Anchilosi radio-ulnare superiore congenita. *Arch. Ortop., 21*:25–34, 1905.

Brezmes, M. S.: Sinostosis radio-cubitale superior. *Folia Anat. Univ. Conimb., 17*:1–4, 1942.

Broca, A.: *Chirurgie Infantile*. Paris, G. Steinheil, pp. 667–668, 1914.

Bychowsky, C.: Ein Fall von angeborener Ellbogenankylose eines im Wachstum zurückgebliebenen und Missgebildeten. *Z. Orthop. Chir., 31*:480–496, 1913.

Calabro, F.: Su di in caso sinostosi radio ulnare congenita trattamento chirurgicamente. *Arch. Ortop., 72*:1246–1253, 1959.

Camera, R.: La anchilosi congenita di gomito. *Chir. Organi Mov., 41*:385–398, 1954.

Campanacci, M.: Transposizione dell'ostensore ulnare del carpo pro supinatori. *Chir. Organi Mov., 50*:167–172, 1961.

Canton, J.: Sur un cas de synostose congénitale des deux os de l'avant-bras. *Bordeaux Chir., 4*:449–452, 1933.

Capecchi, V., and Casini, E.: Luzzazione, sinostosi radio-ulnare congenita e displasia del complesso prono-supinatorio. *Arch. Ortop., 68*:24–49, 1955.

Card, R. Y., and Strachman, J.: Congenital ankylosis of the elbow. *J. Pediatr., 46*:81–85, 1955.

Cenani, A., and Lenz, W.: Totale Syndactylie und totale radioulnare Synostose bei swei Brüdern. *Z. Kinderheilkd., 101*:181–190, 1967.

Ceresole, F.: Due case di rare malformazione congenita dell'avambraccio (Sinostosi radio-cubitale). *Radiol. Med. Torino, 4*:73–76, 1917.

Chasin, A.: Synostosis radioulnaris superior congenita. (Zur Frage uber die Anatomie, die Pathogenese und die Behandlung dieser erbkrankung). *Z. Orthop. Chir., 56*:353–377, 1932.

Chesser, E. S.: Congenital synostosis. *Lancet, 1*:298, 1919.

Ciaccia, S.: Sulla sinostosi radio-ulnare congenita. *Chir. Organi Mov., 11*:513–529, 1926.

Clarke, J.: Congenital fusion of the upper end of the radius to the ulna. *Proc. R. Soc. Med. London*, (Sect. Surg. Subsect. Orthop.), *7*:120–121, 1914.

Cleveland, W. W., Arias, D., and Smith, G. F.: Radioulnar synostosis, behavioral disturbance and XYY chromosomes. *J. Pediatr., 74*:103–106, 1969.

Cocchi, U.: Radio-ulnar synostosis. Hereditary diseases with bone changes. *In* Schinz, H. R., Baensch, W. E., Friedl, E., and Uehlinger, E., (eds.): *Roentgen-Diagnostics*. First American edition based on fifth German edition. English translation by J. T. Case. New York, Grune & Stratton, Vol. I, Part I, pp. 786–789, 1951.

Cohen-Sohal, L.: Pronation congénital de coude. *Pédiatrie, 19*:106–107, 1963.

Cohn, B. N. E.: Congenital bilateral radio-ulnar synostosis, with report of case. *J. Bone Joint Surg., 14*:404–405, 1932.

Coode, C. D.: Congenital radio-ulnar synostosis; case report. *J. R. Nav. Med. Serv., 32*:166–168, 1946.

Coppa, E.: Su di una rara anomalia congenita isolata dello scheletro dell'avambraccio. *Arch. Radiol., 5*:553–557, 1929.

Cotterill, J. M.: Congenital deformity of both forearms. (Exhibition of patient.) *Tr. Med. Chir. Soc. Edinburgh, 12*:169, 1893.

Coudray, P.: Deux cas de synostose radio-cubitale supérieure bilatérale, d'origine congénitale. *Rev. d'Orthop.*, (3 s.), *6*:361–365, 1919.

Coyon, A., and Gasne: Malformation des membres supérieurs. Absence de l'articulation du coude. Éctrodactylie du pouce. *Rev. d'Orthop.*, (3 s.), *5*:185–188, 1914.

Cramer, K.: Über kongenitale Supinationsstörungen. *Z. Orthop. Chir., 20*:127–147, 1908.

Crasselt, C.: Zur operativen Behandlung der radio-ulnaren Synostose. *Z. Orthop., 96*:478–488, 1962.

Crespellani, C.: Un caso di sinostosi radio-ulnare superiore congenita. *G. Med. Mil., 74*:471–473, 1926.

Creyssel, J., Fischer, A. R., and Machenaud, A.: Synostose radiocubitale supérieure congénitale. À propos de trois case. *Lyon Chir., 66*:175–179; fig. 2, 1970.

Cross, A. R.: Congenital bilateral radio-ulnar synostosis. *Am. J. Dis. Child., 58*:1259–1260, 1939.

Cueto, A. B.: Malformaciones esqueleticas en la extremidades superiores del recien nacido (Un caso de sinostosis radio-cubitale y ausencia del primer metacarpo y dedo pulger izquiero, sinostosis del III, IV y V metacarpio y clinodactilia desviacion lateral—del pulger derecho. *Acta Pediatr. Espan., 22*:927–931, 1964.

Curtis, B. F.: Congenital ankylosis of radio-ulnar articulations. *N.Y. Med. J., 42*:319–320, 1885.

Davenport, C. B., Taylor, H. L., and Nelson, L. A.: Radio-ulnar synostosis. *Arch. Surg., 8*:705–762, 1924.

Davies, D. J.: Congenital radio-ulnar synostosis. *Br. Med. J., 2*:557–558, 1930.

Dawson, H. G. W.: A congenital deformity of the forearm and its operative treatment. *Br. Med. J., 2*:833–835, 1912.

Derveaux, W.: *Contribution à l'Étude de la Synostose Radio-cubitale Congénitale*. Thèse. Paris, A. Legrand, pp. 11–47, 1934.

Diaz, E.: Sinostosis radiocubital congenita. *Bol. Soc. Cir. Chile, 23*:219–222, 1945. Also in *Rev. Med. Chile, 74*:151–154, 1946.

Dietz, P. J. P.: Die radio-ulnare Synostose, eine seltene angeborene Missbildung der Ellbogengegend. *Fortschr. Röntgenstr., 16*:22–23; Taf. VI; fig. a, b, 1910.

Dietz, P. J. P.: Een Geval van aageboren vergroeiing tusschen radius en ulna. *Ned. T. Geneesk., 23*:254–257, 1910.

Donovan, R. E., and Etchevere, A. O.: Radio-ulnar synostosis: congenital case. *Bol. Trab. Soc. Cir. Buenos Aires, 19*:772–782, 1935.

Drenkhahn: Ein Fall von seltener Missbildung der Vorderarme. *Z. Orthop. Chir., 11*:598–599, 1903.

Drenkhahn: Seltene Missbildungen. *Dtsch. Milit. Z., 41*:48–55, Bild 6, 1912.

Dubois, M.: Luxation du radius en arrière avec soudure des os de l'avant-bras. *Bull. Soc. Anat. Paris, 27*:67–70, 1852.

Dubs, J.: Weiterer Beitrag zur Kenntnis der kongenitale radio-ulnaren Synostose. *Z. Orthop. Chir., 38*:509–514, 1918.

Dubs, J.: Zur Kenntnis der kongenitalen radio-ulnaren Synostose. *Z. Orthop. Chir., 38*:173–182, 1918.

Dun, R. C.: A case of congenital deformity of both forearms. *Rep. Soc. Study Dis. Child.* (London), *5*:198–200, 1905.

Eckinger, W.: Radio-ulnare Synostose am distalen und proximalen Ende mit verschiedensten Formen von Missbildungen. *Z. Orthop. Chir., 68*:297–300, 1938.

Edwards, J. G.: Congenital radio-ulnar synostosis. *Med. J. Aust., 1*:494, 1918.

Etchevere, A.: Sinostosis radiocubital superior. *Rev. Ortop. Traumat.* (Buenos Aires), *17*:293–295, 1948.

Evans, E. L.: Case of bilateral radio-ulnar synostosis associated with bilateral congenital dislocation of hips. *Proc. R. Soc. Med. London* (Sect. Surg. Subsect. Orthop.), *14*:165, 1921.

Fahlstrom, S.: Radio-ulnar synostosis: Historical review and case report. *J. Bone Joint Surg.*, (n.s.), *14*:395–405, 1932.

Fanghanel, M.: Ein Fall von angeborener Ankylose des Ellbogengelenkes. *Zentralbl. Gynäkol.. 77*:1993–1996, 1955.

Feidt, W. W.: Congenital radio-ulnar syntstosis. *Surg. Gynecol. Obstet., 24*:696–700, 1917.

Ferguson-Smith, M. A., Johnson, A., and Handmaker, S. D.: Primary amentia and micro-orchidism associated with XXY chromosome constitution. *Lancet, 2*:184–187, 1960.

Fraccaro, M., Klinger, H. P., and Schutt, W.: A male with XXXXY sex chromosomes. *Cytogenetics, 1*:52–64; fig. 4, 1962.

Franceschetti, A., and Klein, D.: The mandibulo-facial dysostosis. A new syndrome. *Acta Opthal., 27*:143–149; figs. 17, 18, 1949.

Frank, A.: Über humero-radial Synostose. *Beitr. Pathol. Anat., 99*:247–249, 1937.

Frankel, E.: Humero-radial synostosis. *Br. J. Surg., 31*:242–245, 1944.

Fraser, J.: *Surgery of Childhood.* New York, W. Wood & Co., Vol. 11, pp. 995–1000; figs. 494–497, 1926.

Fraser, J. H., Boyd, E., Lennox, B., and Dennison, W. M.: A case of XXXY Klinefelter's syndrome. *Lancet, 2*:1064–1067, 1961.

Freyer, B.: Ungewöhnliche Beobachtung doppelseitiger kongenitaler Synostosen zwischen Radius und Ulna sowie zwischen Os lunatum und Os triquetrum verbunden mit einer doppelseitigen abortiform der Madelungschen Deformität (Sog. Hulten-Plus-Variant) in der II Generation bei doppelseitigem pes quinns–varus in der I Generation. *Radiologie, 6*:253–355, 1966.

Friedjung, J. K.: Hereditäre radio-ulnare Synostose. *Med. Klin., 29*:1677–1678, 1933.

Frostad, H.: Congenital ankylosis of the elbow-joint. *Acta Orthop. Scand., 11*:296–306, 1940.

Funston, R. V.: The relation of congenital deformities of the hand to cervical rib. *J.A.M.A., 98*:697–700, 1932.

Gayral, and Bru: Une synostose radio-cubitale congénitale ou l'explication radiologique d'une vocation pik-pocket. *J. Radiol. Electrol., 31*:99–100, 1950.

Gene, E.: Une forme extensive de dysostose mandibulo-faciale. *J. Genet. Hum., 17*:45–52; fig. 7, 1969.

Gherlinzoni, G.: L'anchilosi congenita del gomito. *Chir. Organi Mov., 26*:162–166, 1940.

Gibson, A.: A critical consideration of congenital radio-ulnar synostosis with special reference to treatment. *J. Bone Joint Surg., 21*:299–304, 1923.

Giorgacopulo, D.: Di un caso di sinostosi radioulnare congenita. *Chir. Organi Mov., 8*:342–356, 1924.

Glaessner, P.: Angeborene Verwachsungen von Radius und Ulna. *Jb. Orthop. Berlin, 2*:34–35, 1911.

Görlich, M.: Kongenitale partielle Synostose von Radius und Ulna. In: Über einige Radiusmissbildungen. *Beitr. Klin. Chir., 59*:421–440, 1908.

Gourdon, J.: Deux cas de synostose radio-cubitale supérieure. *Bull. Mém. Soc. Méd. Chir.* (Bordeaux), pp. 451–455, 1924. Review in *Rev. d'Orthop.*, (3 s.), *12*:299–300, 1925.

Graczynski, J.: Evaluation of surgical results in radio-ulnar synostosis. (In Polish.) *Chir. Narzad Ruchu Ortop. Pol., 29*:531–536, 1964.

Grebe, H.: Synostosis radioulnaris congenita. *In* Becker, P. E., (ed.): *Humangenetik.* Stuttgart, G. Thieme, Vol. 2, pp. 217–218, 1964.

Greenstein, R. M., Harris, D. J., Luzzatt, L., and Cenn, H. M.: Cytogenic analysis of a boy with XXXY syndrome. Origin of the X chromosome. *Pediatrics, 45*:677–686, 1970.

Greig, D. M.: Two cases of congenital superior radio-ulnar synostosis. *Edinburgh Med. J.*, (n.s.), *18*:281–284, 1917.

Greig, D. M.: Observations on the bones in congenital proximal radioulnar synostosis. *Edinburgh Med. J.*, (3 s.), *32*:354–369, 1925.

Grossman, J.: Congenital radioulnar synostosis with a report of three cases. *Med. J. Rec.*, *127*:186–188, 1928.

Grunfeld, K.: Ein Fall von radio-ulnarer Synostose (kongenitale Missbildung der Ellbogengegend mit Supinationshemmung). *Gesell. Inn. Med. Kinderheilkd.* (Wien), *10*:97–99, 1911.

Hamilton, S.: A case of congenital synostosis of both upper radio-ulnar articulations. *Br. Med. J.*, *2*:1327–1328, 1905.

Hansen, O. H., and Andersen, N. O.: Congenital radio-ulnar synostosis. Report of 37 cases. *Acta Orthop. Scand.*, *41*:225–230, 1970.

Harrison, R. G., and Wardle, E. N.: An unusual malformation of the radius and ulna. *J. Bone Joint Surg.*, *40B*:82–93, 1958.

Hefter, H.: Die radioulnare Synostose. *Med. Klin.*, *26*:1184–1186, 1930.

Henry, H.: Synostose radio-cubitale congénitale et unilatérale. *Bull. Mém. Soc. Belge d'Orthop.*, *5*:92–93, 1933.

Hlawacek: Über einige Extremitätenmissbildungen. *Dtsch. Z. Chir.*, *43*:140–160, 1896.

Hohmann, G.: Supinationsbehinderung des Vorderarms. *Z. Orthop. Chir.*, *38*:670–675, 1918.

Hohmann, G.: *Hand und Arm.* Munchen, J. F. Bergmann, pp. 123–125, 1949.

Hohmann, G.: Beitrag zur radio-ulnaren Synostose. *Arch. Orthop. Unfallchir.*, *54*:523–525, 1962.

Hopf, A.: Distale Synostose zwischen Ulna und Radius bei Hypoplasie des Radius. Ausserdem bestehen Synostosen zwischen navicular und radius, Lunatum und Trigietrum der distalen Handwurzelknochenreihe. Doppelepiphysen der Metacarpale I, Brachymesophalangie 2 bis 5. *In* Hohmann, G., Hackenbroch, M., Lindemann, K., (eds.): *Spezielle Orthopädie obere Extremität of Handbuch der Orthopädie.* Stuttgart, G. Thieme, Band 3, p. 425, Abb. 2, 1959.

Hornung, R.: Ein Fall von angeborenem beiderseitigem Fehlen des Radiusköpfchens mit der Ulna. *München Med. Wochenschr.*, *62*:1216–1217, 1915.

Houston, S.: Roentgen findings in the XXXXY chromosome anomaly. *J. Can. Assoc. Radiol.*, *18*:258–267, 1967.

Hoxter: Discussionsbemerkung zu "Familiare Synostose von Radius und Ulna." *Zentralbl. Chir.*, *55*:2075, 1928.

Humphries, S. V.: Congenital proximal radio-ulnar synostosis. *S. Afr. Med. J.*, *15*:486, 1941.

Jancur, J.: Mentally defective males with XXXXY chromosome. *In* Oster, J., (ed.): *Proceedings of International Congress on the Scientific Study of Mental Retardation.* Copenhagen, Vol. I, p. 179, 1964.

Jancur, J.: Radioulnar synostosis. A common occurrence in sex chromosomal abnormalities. *Am. J. Dis. Child.*, *122*:10–11, 1971.

Jean: Pronation permanente congénitale par malformation de la tête radiale. Reported by A. Mouchet. *Bull. Soc. Chir. Paris*, *50*:1102–1105, 1924.

Jeanty, M.: La synostose radiocubitale congénitale. *Acta Orthop. Belg.*, *30*:294–302, 1964.

Jedlicka, R.: *Die topographische Anatomie des Ellbogenegelenkes.* Hamburg, Lucas Grafe & Sillom, pp. 1–15; Taf. I–VIII, 1900.

Jemma, G.: Sur un cas très rare de synostose radio-cubitale inférieure congénitale. *Rev. d'Orthop.*, (3 s.), *22*:41–52, 1935.

Jewesbury, R. C.: Synostosis of radius and ulna—congenital. *Proc. R. Soc. Med. London* (Sect. Dis. Child.), I-II: 27–35; fig. 3, 1920–1921.

Joachimsthal, G.: Die angeborenen Verbildungen der oberen Extremitäten. *Fortschr. Röntgenstr.*, *2*:1–40; Taf. I–Vii, 1900.

Joseph, M. C., Anders, J. M., and Taylor, A. L.: A boy with XXXXY sex chromosomes. *J. Med. Genet.*, *1*:95, 1964.

Kato, T., Tanaka, I, Ota, M., et al: Three cases of radio-ulnar synostosis. *Orthop. Surg.* (Tokyo), *21*:804–810, 1970.

Kaufamn, J.: A case of bilateral congenital fusion of the radius and ulna. *J.A.M.A.*, *73*:1842, 1919.

Keiser, D. V.: Synostosen der Unterarmknochen. *In* Diethelm, L., (ed.): *Skeletanatomie (Röntgendiagnostik).* Berlin, Springer, Band IV, Teil 2, pp. 209–211; fig. 16, 1968.

Kelikian, H., and Doumanian, A.: Swivel for proximal radio-ulnar synostosis. *J. Bone Joint Surg.*, *39A*:945–952, 1957.

Keutel, J., Kindermann, I, and Mockel, H.: Ein wahrscheinlich autosomal recessiv vererbte Skeletmisbildung mit Humeroradial-synostose. *Humangenetik*, *9*:43–53, 1970.

Kienbock, R.: Die radio-ulnare Synostose. *Fortschr. Röntgenstr.*, *15*:93–108, 1910.

Kirmani, S. R.: Congenital ankylosis of elbow. *J. Pakistani Med. Assoc.*, *17*:297–300, 1967.

Kiwull, J.: Kongenitale Difformität an der oberen Extremität. *Fortschr. Röntgenstr.*, *6*:185–187, 1902–1903.

Klapp: Synostose der Unterarmknochen beobachtet. *Dtsch. Med. Wochenschr.*, *39*(1): 918, 1913.

Klinefelter, A. F., Jr., Reifenstein, E. C., and Albright, F.: Syndrome characterized by gynecomastia, aspermatogenesis without aleydigism and increased excretion of follicle stimulating hormone. *J. Clin. Endocrinol.*, *2*:615–627, 1942.

Kopelewitz, J. C.: A case of congenital radio-ulnar synostosis. *J.A.M.A.*, *72*:21, 1919.

Kreglinger, G.: Ein Fall von hereditärer, kongenitaler doppelseitiger Synostose beider Vorderarmknochenen der proximalen Epiphyse. *Z. Orthop. Chir.*, *28*:66–95, 1911.

Kuh, R.: Über congenitale Vorderarmsynostose. *Med. Klin.* (Berlin), *17*:604–605, 1921.

Kümmel, W.: *Die Missbildungen der Extremitäten durch Defekt. Verwachsung und Überzahl.* Bibliotheca Medica, Section E, Vol. III. Cassel, Th. G. Fisher & Co., pp. 1–12, 33–40, 1895.

Kurlander, J. J.: Congenital radio-ulnar synostosis. (Letter to the editor.) *Surg. Gynecol. Obstet. 25*:472, 1917.

Lambert, L. A.: Congenital humeroradial synostosis with other synostotic anomalies. *J. Pediatr., 31*: 573–577, 1947.

Lejeune: Fusion complète des extrémités supérieures des radius avec les parties correspondantes des humerus observée chez un nouveau-né. *Bull. Med. Nord, Lille*, pp. 264–272, 1861. Also in *Gaz. Hôp. Paris, 34*:462, 1861.

Lenoir: Un avant-bras gauche rachitique, dont les deux os, entrecroisés comme dans la pronation. *Bull. Soc. Anat., 2*:95, 1827.

Lett, H.: A case of synostosis of the upper ends of the radius and ulna. *Rep. Soc. Dis. Child.* (London), *8*:17, 1908.

Lhermitte, J., and Beuchard: Sur un cas de synostose radio-cubital supérieur congénital et héréditaire. *Rev. Neurol.* (Paris), *28*:322–324, 1921.

Lhermitte, J., Nemours-Auguste, and Parturier: Synostose radio-cubitale supérieure associée à une double luxation congénitale des hanches acompagné d'alliérations osseuses considérable de basin. *Presse Méd., 39*(1):325, 1931.

Lieblein, V.: Zur Kasuistik und Äetiologie der angeborene Verwachsung der Vorderarmknochen in ihrem proximalen Abschnitte. *Z. Orthop. Chir., 24*:52–70, 1909.

Longuet, and Peraire: Malformation congénitale du cubitus avec synostoses congénitales. *Bull. Soc. Anat. Paris*, (6 s.), *3*:147–148, 1901.

Lowe, H. G.: Radio-ulnar fusion for defects in the forearm bones. *J. Bone Joint Surg., 45B*:351–359, 1963.

Löwy, M.: Angeborene Radiusluxation mit Synostose der beiden Unterarmknochen. *Wien Med. Wochenschr., 71*:2018, 1921.

Löwy, M.: Radiusluxation mit Synostose der beiden Unterarmknochen vor. *Mitthl. Ges. In. Med. Kinderheilkd., 20*:187–188, 1921.

Lüdin, M.: Üeber familiäre, kongenitale radioulnare Synostose. *Schweiz. Med. Wochenschr., 54*:300–302, 1924.

Lunn, J. R.: Congenital synostosis of radio-ulnar articulations. *Br. Med. J., 1*:499, 1906.

Maass, H.: Über mechanische Störungen des Knochenwachstums. *Arch. Pathol. Anat. Physiol., 163*: 185–208, 1901.

Maass, H.: Die kongenitale Vorderarmsynostose. *Dtsch. Med. Wochenschr., 39*:704–706; also p. 918, 1913.

Maass, H.: Zur Operation der kongenitalen Vorderarmsynostose. *Z. Orthop. Chir., 34*:116–123, 1914.

Maccauro, L., and Zorzi, C.: Sinostosi radioulnare congenita. *Chir. Organi Mov., 42*:365–379, 1955.

Madrange, C.: *La Synostose Radio-cubitale Congénitale.* Thèse. Paris, Le François, pp. 1–127, 1914.

Marden, P. H., Smith, D. W., and McDonald, M. J.: Congenital anomalies in the newborn infant, including minor variations. A study of 4412 babies by surface examination for anomalies and buccal smear for sex chromatin. *J. Pediatr., 64*:357–371, 1964.

Margolis, E., and Hasson, E.: Hereditary malformations of the upper extremities. *J. Hered., 46*:255–262, 1955.

Marie, G.: *La Synostose Congénitale Radiocubitale Supérieure.* Thèse. Paris, Les Presses Universitaires de France, pp. 7–16, 1924.

Marotta, U., and Zorzin, L.: Sinostosi radio-ulnare. Descrizione di un caso. *Nunt. Radiol., 33*:1539–1544, 1967.

Marques, P., Dunglas, J., and Cukierstjein, W.: Synostose bilatérale des extrémités proximales du radius et du cubitus. *J. Radiol. Electrol., 27*:458, 1946.

Martin-du Pan, C.: Trois cas de synostose radio-cubitale congénitale. *Rev. Méd. Suisse Rom., 34*:697–710, 1914.

Mastromarino, R.: La sinostosi congenita radio-ulnare proxximale. *Ortop. Traum. App. Mot., 25*:901–909, 1957.

McFarland, B.: Less common orthopedic congenital defects. *Med. Press* (London), *110*:80–81, 1924.

McFarland, B.: Congenital radio-ulnar synostosis. *Br. Med. J., 2*:664, 1930.

McFarland, B.: Synostosis of the radius and ulna. *In* Platt, H., (ed.): *Modern Trends in Orthopedics.* New York, P. B. Hosbera pp. 132–134, 1950.

Melchior, E.: Zur Kenntnis der kongenitalen Vorderarmsynostosen. *Berl. Klin. Wochenschr., 49*:1659–1662, 1912.

Meves, F.: Über die Synostosen der Handwurzelknochen. *Z. Orthop., 67*:17–20, 1937.

Michelsson, G.: Knochen, Muskeln, Nerven und Arterien einer oberen Extremität mit kongenitaler humero-radio-ulnarer Synostose. *Arch. Pathol. Anat. Physiol., 236*:117–145, 1922.

Mitscherlich, A.: Ein Fall von angeborener Verbildung beider Ellenbogengelenke. *Arch. Klin. Chir., 6*:218–222, 1965.

Morestin, H.: Fusion congénitale des os de l'avant-bras a leur partie supérieure. *Bull. Soc. Anat. Paris*, (6 s.), *6*:60–64 1904.

Morrison: Radio-ulnar synostosis. *Br. Med. J.*, 2:1337, 1892.

Mouchet, A.: Synostose radio-cubitale congenitale. *Bull. Soc. Pediatr. (Paris)*, 15:206–209, 1913.

Mouchet, A., and DiMatteo, J.: Ankylose congénitale et symétrique des coudes. *Rev. d'Orthop.*, 28:224–228, 1942.

Mouchet, A., and Leleu, A.: La synostose congénitale radiocubitale supérieure. *Rev. d'Orthop.*, (3 s.), 12:421–443, 1925.

Mouchet, A., and Saint-Pierre, L.: Ankylose congénitale héréditaire et symétrique des deux coudes. *Rev. d'Orthop.*, (3 s.), 18:210–220, 1931.

Müller, W.: Die verschiedenen Fehlbildungstendenzen am Vorderarm. *Arch. Orthop. Unfallchir.*, 139:541–557, 1939.

Mummery, P. L.: A rare congenital deformity of both radii. *In Reports of the Society for the Study of Diseases in Children.* London, J. & A. Churchill, Vol. 7, pp. 13–15, 1906–1907.

Murphy, H. S., and Hanson, C. G.: Congenital humeroradial synostosis. *J. Bone Joint Surg.*, (n.s.), 27:712–713, 1945.

Nager, F. R., and Reynier, J. P. de: Das Gehörorgan bei den angeborenen Kopfmissbildungen. *Pract. Oto-Rhino-Laryng.* (Basel), 10(2):1–128, 1948.

Négrié, and Barge: Un cas de synostose radio-cubitale supérieure congénitale bilatérale. *Rev. d'Orthop.* (3 s.), 22:678–682, 1935.

Negro, R. C., Soto, J. A., and Valcarcel, B.: Congenital bilateral superior radio-ulnar synostosis; case. *Arch. Pediatr. Uruguay*, 12:349–353, 1941.

Neu, R. L., and Gardner, L. T.: Abnormalities of the sex chromosomes. *In* Gardner, L. T. (ed.): *Endocrine and Genetic Disease of Childhood.* Philadelphia, W. B. Saunders Co., pp. 682–703, 1969.

Neustadt, E.: Synostosis radio-ulnaris congenita. *Arch. Orthop. Unfallchir.*, 31:250–254, 1932.

Nievergelt, K.: Positiver Vaterschaftsnachweis auf Grund erblicher Missbildungen der Extremitäten. *Arch. Julius-Klaus Stift.*, 19:197–212, 1944.

Nigrisoli, P.: Sulla sinostosi congenita radio-ulnare superiore. *Arch. Putti*, 14:111–123, 1961.

Nilsonne: Ist operative Lösung der kongenitalen radio-ulnaren Synostosen berechtigt? *Acta Chir. Scand.*, 72:225–235, 1932.

Ober, F. R.: Congenital synostosis of upper end of radius and ulna. *In* Bancroft, F. W., and Marble, H. C., (eds.): *Surgical Treatment of the Motor-Skeletal System.* Second edition. Philadelphia, J. B. Lippincott Co., Part I, pp. 10–13, 1951.

Oeynhausen, R. F.: Angeborene Synostosen (kongenitale Ankylose, angeborene Gelenkaplasie). *In* Schwalbe, E., and Gruber, G. B., (eds.): *Die Morphologie der Missbildungen des Menschen und der Tiere.* Jena, G. Fishcer, T. 3, 19 Lief., Abb. 1, 7, Kap. 2. Halfte:893–917.

Orel, H.: Klein-Beiträge zur Vererbungswissenschaft. IV Mitteilung (Radioulnarsynostose). *Z. Menschl. Vererb. Konstitutionslehre*, 14:347–354, 1928.

Osmond-Clarke, H.: Deformities. *In* Carling, Sir E. R., and Ross, J. P., (eds.): *British Surgical Practice.* London, Butterworth & Co., Ltd. Vol. 3, pp. 180–191, 1948.

Painter, C. F.: Congenital pronation of the forearms. *Am J. Orthop. Surg.*, 7:529–532, 1909.

Palagi, P.: Sulla sinostosi radio-ulnare superiore. *Arch. Ortop.*, 24:298–317, 1907.

Pare, J.: Een geval van synostosis radio-ulnaris duplex. *Ned. T. Geneesk.*, 91:97–99, 1947.

Pasquali, E.: L'indirizzo terapeutico in duo infrequenti malformazion: congenite. *Atti XXVII Congr. S.I.O.T.*, pp. 245–317, 1907.

Pearlman, H. S., Edkin, R. E., and Warren, R. F.: Familial tarsal and carpal synostosis with radial-head subluxation (Nievergelt's syndrome). *J. Bone Joint Surg.*, 46A:585–592, 1964.

Pellegrini, L.: Sinostosi radio-ulanre congenita ereditaria. *Clin. Ortop.*, 1:346–351, 1949.

Pepi, O.: Della sinostosi radio-cubitale superiore congenital. *Policlinico*, 34:205–218, 1927.

Petit, P., and Bedouelle, J.: Synostoses congénitales du membre supérieure. *Encyc. Médico-Chir.* App. Mot. Vol. 3:15202 E10, pp. 1–2, 1956.

Pforringer: Zur Kasuistik angeborener Verbildungen. *Fortschr. Röntgenstr.*, 12:181–183, 1908.

Pollnow, and Levy-Dron: Angeborene Verwachsung von Radius und Ulna (Synostosis radio-ulnaris). *Berl. Klin. Wochenschr.*, 48:427–429, 1911.

Preiser: Angeborene doppelseitige Supinationsstörung des Ellbogens. *München. Med. Wochenschr.*, 57:1035, 1910.

Rais, G.: La synostose congénitale radio-cubitale. *Rev. d'Orthop.*, (2 s.), 8:431–450; Pl. 23–24, 1907.

Redard, P.: Difformité congénitale rare des avant-bras. Synostoses radio-cubitales, radius curvus. *Rev. d'Orthop.*, (2 s.), 9:113–118, 1908.

Ricciardi, L.: Sinostosi radio ulnare congenita. *Minerva Ortop.*, 20:363–374, 1969.

Ricciardi, M.: Su di un caso di sinostosi, isolata, radio-ulnare inferiore. *Ortop. Traum. App. Mot.*, 12:194–206, 1940.

Ritter, U.: Breite angeborene Synostose zwischen Elle und Speiche. *Fortschr. Röntgenstr.*, 75:495, 1951.

Robinson, G. C., Miller, J. R., Dill, F. J., and Kamburoff, T.: Klinefelter's syndrome with XXYY sex chromosome complex. *J. Pediatr.*, 65:226–232, 1964.

Rocher, L.: Synostose congénitale radio-cubitale supérieure double. *J. Méd. Bordeaux*, 48:80, 1921.

Rodriguez, A. P., and Bejarno, E. B.: Congenital radioulnar synostosis. *Rev. Clin. Esp.*, 61:44–46, 1956.

Roederer, C.: Un cas de synostose radio-cubitale. *Bull. Mém. Soc. Chir.* (Paris), *20*:151, 1928.

Romanus, R.: Ein Fall von angeborener Ankylose im Ellbogenegelenk. *Acta Orthop. Scand.*, *4*:291–306, 1933.

Rosas, F. F., and Castiarena, R.: Sinostoses congenita radio-cubital superior. *El Dia Medico.20*:315–318, 1948.

Roskoschyn, F.: Ein Fall von angeborener, vererbter Verbildung beider Knie- und Ellenbogengelenke. *Dtsch. Z. Chir.*, *76*:569–580; Taf. IV u. V, 1905.

Salisachs, L. G.: Contribution al estudio de la sinostosis radio-cubital congenital. *Rev. Med. Barcelona*, *22*:295–314, 1934.

Sandifort, E.: Ancyloses radii and ulnae. *In Museum Anatomicum Academiae Lugduno-Batavae*. Lugduni, Batavorum, S. et J. Luchtmans, Academiae Typographos, Vol. 2, p. 104; Tab. CIII; figs. 1–6, 1793.

Schade, H., Schoeller, L., and Toeberg, G.: Ein Patient mit XXXXY chromosomen. *Med. Welt.*, *16*:869–872, 1963.

Schenck, S. G.: Unilateral radio-ulnar synostosis. *Am. J. Dis. Child.*, *53*:128–131, 1937.

Scherz, R. G., and Roeckel, I. E.: The XXXXY syndrome. *J. Pediatr.*, *63*:1093–1098, 1963.

Schilling, R.: Ein Fall von doppelseitiger Synostose des oberen Radius- und Ulnaendes. Inaug. Diss. Kiel, Otto Krohn, pp. 5–12, 1904.

Schlapfer, F.: Beitrag zur operativen Behandlung der Vorderarm-synostosen (Bruckencallus). *Dtsch. Z. Chir.*, *137*:225–243, 1916.

Schmidt, A.: Ein Beitrag zur kongenitalen radio-ulnaren Synostose. *Dtsch. Z. Chir.*, *205*:326–332, 1927.

Schulz, P. Die Radio-ulnaren Synostosen. *Beitr. Orthop. Trauma*, *9*:421–434, 1962.

Scott, C. I.: The triple-XY syndrome. *In* Bergsma, D., (ed.): *Birth Defects. Original Article Series*. New York, National Foundation—March of Dimes, Vol. V, No. 5, pp. 140–141, 1969.

Sever, J. W.: Congenital radio-ulnar synostosis. *Surg. Gynecol. Obstet.*, *29*:203–204, 1919.

Siegmund, E.: Angeborene radio-ulnare Synostose. *Orv. Hetil.*, *34*:968–970, 1928.

Singleton, E. B., Rosenberg, H. S., and Yang, S. J.: The radiographic manifestations of chromosomal abnormalities. *Radiol. Clin. N. Am.*, *2*:281–295, 1965.

Siwon, P.: Kongenital hereditäre, doppelseitige Ankylose der Ellenbogengelenke. *Dtsch. Z. Chir.*, *209*:338–349, 1928.

Solomen, K. A., and Sulamma, M.: Nievergelt syndrome and its treatment. A case report. *Ann. Chir. Gynecol. Fem.*, *47*:142–147, 1958.

Sonntag, E.: Ein Fall von kongenitaler radioulnarer Synostose. *Z. Orthop. Chir.*, *40*:195–204, 1921. Also in *Beitr. Klin. Chir.*, *127*:716–720, 1922.

Sorokin, F. F.: Zur Frage der Synostosis. Radio-ulnaris. *Acta Radiol.*, *17*:191–199, 1936.

Steindler, A.: *Orthopedic Operations*. Springfield, Illinois, Charles C Thomas, pp. 425–426, 1946.

Storen, H.: Two operated cases of ankylosis cubiti congenita. *Acta Chir. Scand.*, *94*:65–74, 1946.

Stretton, J. L.: Congenital synostosis of radio-ulnar articulations. *Br. Med. J.*, *2*:1519, 1905.

Sury, K. V.: Beitrag zur Kenntnis der kongenitalen Radiusmissbildung mit Rücksicht auf die dadurch bedingte Erwerbseinbusse. *Korrespbll. Schwiz. Aerzte.*, *39*:79–83, 1909.

Szczepanski, J.: A case of congenital synostosis of forearm bones. (In Polish.) *Wiad. Lek.*, *21*:1369–1371, 1968.

Thomas, G. F.: Congenital radio-ulnar synostosis. *Am. J. Roentgenol.*, *4*:571–573, 1917.

Turner, B., Den Dulk, G. M., and Watkins, G.: The XXXY syndrome. *Med. J. Aust.* *2*:715–716, 1963.

Van Went, J. J., Van Geldren, H. H., and Schaberg, A.: Het XXXY syndrome. *Nederl. T. Geneesk.*, *109*:1563–1569, 1965.

Vitré, J.-L.: Etude génétique et classification clinique de 154 cas de dysoslose mandibulo-faciale (syndrome de Franceschetti) avec description de leur associations malformatives. *J. Génét. Hum.*, *19*:17–100, 1971.

Vogeler, K.: Die radio-ulnare Synostose. *Arch. Klin. Chir.*, *136*:422–426, 1925.

Voluter, G., and Klein, D.: Syndrom von Rocher-Sheldon. Synostose radio-cubitale près de l'articulation. *J. Radiol. Electrol.*, *31*:9–21, 1950.

Voskresensky, G. P.: Congenital bilateral synostosis of forearm in child. (In Russians) *Vrach. Gaz.*, *32*:265–268, 1928.

Vulpius, O., and Stoffel, A.: *Orthopadische Operationslehre*. Stuttgart, F. Enke, pp. 348–350, 1913.

Waegner, A.: Beiderseitige kongenitale radio-ulnare Synostose. *Arch. Klin. Chir.*, *163*:116–121, 1931.

Wakeley, C. P. G.: Congenital synostosis of the radius and ulna. *Arch. Radiol. Electr. Ther.*, *26*:185–200, 1921.

Wandel: Familiare Synostose von Radius und Ulna. *Zentralbl. Chir.*, *55*:2074–2075, 1928.

Watterott, A.: *Congenitale Radio-ulnare Synostose*. Inaug. Diss. Bonn, Paulinus-Druckerei, pp. 3–19, 1932.

Weil, S.: Die radioulnare Synostose (R. u. S.) oder die Aplasie des proximalen Radioulnar-Gelenkes. *In* Hohmann, G., Hackenbrach, M., and Lindenmann, K., (eds.): *Spezielle Orthopädie obere Extremität of Handbuch der Orthopädie*. Stuttgart, G. Thieme, Band 3, pp. 336–340, 1959.

Werthemann, A.: *Handbuch der Speziellen Pathologischen Anatomie und Histologie.* Berlin, Springer, Vol. IX, Sect. VI, pp. 89–93, 1952.

Weyers, H.: Aplasie des oberen radio-ulnar-Gelenkes, radio-ulnarse Synostose, Synostose radio-ulnaris congenita. *In* Diethelm, L., (ed.): *Röntgendiagnostik der Skeleterkrankungen.* L. Diethelm. Berlin, Springer Verlag, Teil 3, pp. 423–425, 1968.

Wilkie, D. P. D.: Congenital radio-ulnar synostosis. *Br. J. Surg., 1*:366–375, 1914.

Willert, H. G., and Henkel, H. L.: *Klinik und der Pathologie der Dysmelie.* Berlin, Springer, pp. 19–24, 1968.

Zaleski, W. A., Houston, C. S., and Porsonyi, J.: The XXXXY chromosome anomaly. Report of three new cases and review of 30 cases from the literature. *Can. Med. Assoc. J., 94*:1143–1154, 1966.

Zollinger, H.: Das XXXY-Syndrom. Zwei neue Beobachtungen im Kleinkindsalter und eine Literaturübersicht. *Helv. Paediatr. Acta, 24*:589–599, 1969.

Zollner, W.: Luxationsfraktur in einem Ellenbogenegelenk bei Kongenit radio-ulnarer Synostose. *Mschr. Unfallheilkd., 52*:232–239, 1949.

Chapter Twenty-Nine

IMPACT AND
EXPECTATIONS

Johannsen (1911), who coined the word gene, recognized the tyranny of words. "Language," he said, "is not only our servant when we wish to express—or even conceal—our thoughts, but . . . may also be our master, over-powering us by means of notions attached to current words."

Words used today are preformed and hence prejudicial: they convey connotations assigned to them years back and reflect the ratiocination of another generation. The word *monstrosity,* which bears the stamp of condemnation, was in the past—as it is even now—often used in connection with congenital anomalies of the forearm and the hand. One may also ponder such an unobtrusive deviation as lefthandedness and the diverse deprecatory meanings attached to the adjective left.

Since ancient times the left hand has been considered inferior to the right in power, performance, and dignity. Hollis (1875) spoke of carved stone figures dating back 2200 years before Christ. In these carvings the right hand crossed the breast in an attitude of supplication, while the left hand hung limply down the side of the body. The warriors depicted in the ancient Assyrian bas re-liefs—as well as in engravings illustrating the epic of Ramayana found among rock-sculptures at Mundor and on a terra-cotta dish belonging to the Greek archaic period—held their weapons in their right hands.

One learns from the Bible that Joseph (Genesis 48:13–17) was displeased when he saw Israel place his right hand on Joseph's younger son Ephraim and his left hand on Manasseh who, being older, deserved to be touched by the "better" hand. Joseph removed Israel's right hand from Ephraim's head and placed it on Manasseh's, saying, "for this is the firstborn: put thy right hand upon his head." A later chapter in the Bible (Judges 3:12–15) states that Ehud, the killer of Eglon, was a left-handed Benjaminite; that is, he descended from the youngest of Jacob's twelve sons. Consequently, he was assigned to the lowest nich of the tribal totem. Characteristically, Ehud conducted his act of killing Eglon clumsily. After he stabbed Eglon he could not pull his dagger out of the latter's belly and the wound yielded not blood but excrement—"dirt."

Hollis (1875) introduced what he called "internal evidence of language" in denigrating left-handeness. He and many others after him have pointed out that in most languages the word *left* is used synonymously with the adjectives clumsy, inept, contrary, inverted, gauche, and sinister. "Even in English," Hollis wrote, "left means that which is 'leaved' idle when only one hand of the two is to be employed."

From the root *sinister* comes the sinistral, meaning left-handed. Milleniums have not significantly modified the prejudicial conceptions concerning sinistrals. In this presumably enlightened age, there are parents who try to convert their left-handed children to right-handedness. In a previous chapter of this book, mention was made of psychic and physiological disturbances which ensue from attempts to convert sinistrals into dextrals. Prejudice thus precipitates mishaps.

LORE

At one time, the lore of the forbidden fruit featured prominently in discussions of the causes of congenital anomalies of the hand. Kellie (1808) visited a woman and her two children. She had normal thumbs but each one of her fingers possessed a single phalanx and had no nail. With slight variation, the defect was present in the other members of her family and it had affected nine previous generations. The progenitor of the first generation was said to be a parson with a penchant for cultivating fruit trees. The parson's favorite apple tree had been barren for some time but at long last had produced "an uncommonly kind of fruit" which disappeared overnight. The parson "taxed the gardener with the theft." The gardener insinuated that perhaps the mistress of the house might be the culprit. "The parson's lady was then in a state of pregnancy. Her husband inquired softly whether her longing had tempted her, like our original mother, to take the strictly forbidden fruit." She pledged innocence. The gardener thought she had lied, "and with dreadful rashness wished, that if she was guilty, the child which she was with then might be born without fingers! Poor woman! She had taken the fruit; and thus became the grand-progenitor of a fingerless race unto now the tenth generation."

MacKinder (1857) described a woman and her newborn. Both had what appears to have been bilateral apical dystrophy of the fingers. In describing the transmission of this defect through six generations and characterizing the progenitor of the trait as "the soil which gave such vigorous root to the unfortunate weed," MacKinder related the following story as told by the infant's grandmother:

"The foolish patriarch of six generations had in his garden a tree which bore a single apple. For this he entertained the most profound respect, and forbade anyone to pluck it. In a weak and evil moment, beguiled by some unhallowed power, his spouse put forth her hand and stole the solitary prize. Mighty was the anger of her lord and master when he beheld the fruitless tree; and, in a language unselect, he cursed the thief, and prayed for so heinous an offense that the fingers which touched the apple might be chopped off. His wife, *enciente*, feared much, and in solitude poured out mournful regrets, but dared not confess the crime. Alas! time passed by; her hour of pain drew near; the fearful prayer, too truly, had been heard; a child was born but, sad to tell, the fingers which its father had wished to be amputated had strangely forgotten to grow. . . ."

Maternal impression as a cause of congenital anomalies of the hand is another recurrent theme. Horne (1838) reported that Mrs. Walsh of Gort, Ireland, had a supernumerary thumb and spawned a brood of babies with the same anomaly. Mrs. Walsh's mother assigned the cause of her daughter's unusual supply of digits to the fright she herself had received from a well-known man in Gort named "Tom with the two thumbs." Nothing is said about the circumstances under which this emotional perturbation occurred. The malformation described by Horne was hereditary and could have been caused only by a potently dominant gene—most likely that of "Tom with the two thumbs." Genes were unknown in 1838, and the explanation offered by Mrs. Walsh's mother seemed to satisfy everyone, including the contemporary medical men.

In the past, such anecdotes often appeared in respected medical journals. Modern and sophisticated as the contemporary medical writer may pretend to be, he cannot rid himself completely of the cant insidiously instilled in him by his predecessors, inasmuch as he still uses the words and thinks in the terms handed down to him by his forebears. He may change some of these words and invent newer phrases, but outdated meanings seep into current usage or leave corroding residues. The modern equivalent of the emotion which accrues from having been tempted by the forbidden fruit is guilt complex, and the anomalies which Horne and his generation considered to be caused by fright are now ascribed to hypoxia due to psychic trauma.

THEORIES

Frequently a prestigious author concocts a convincing answer to a moot question—as Darwin (1896) did with his theory of atavism in explaining polydactyly—and the unquestioning majority adopts his pronouncement as ultimate truth. Busey (1878) was an influential medical writer in his time; he ascribed all macrosomies to congenital occlusion of lymphatic channels and dilatation of lymph vessels. Hurley (1878) was impressed by Busey's theory and thought it supplied the most plausible explanation for nerve territory–oriented macrodactyly (NTOM). The theory of lymphatic stasis as the cause of congenital hypertrophies persisted until the third decade of the present century, when the onus was shifted to Recklinghausen's neurofibromatosis. This protean disorder appears to have replaced syphilis in supplying an explanation for many bizarre malformations. As shown in Chapter Eighteen,, multiple neurofibromatoses may cause enlargements of parts, but no authentic case of NTOM has been reported in connection with it. In the 1950s, NTOM appears to have been replaced in popularity by split hand deformity. Ribeiro (1954) reported a case of bilateral macrodactyly under the heading "Lobster claw hand."

Another theory which enjoyed a temporary vogue is that which bears the hyphenated names of Bonnevie and Ullrich. Ullrich (1930) described a six-year-old girl with webbed neck and muscular and mammary defects. He related her condition to congenital lymphangiectatic edema. Bonnevie (1934) advanced the view that certain congenital anomalies might be explained on the basis of pressure caused by wandering blebs of cerebrospinal fluid. Ullrich (1936) adopted this theory because it appeared to supply a plausible mechanism for the development of the pterygium colli and muscular and mammary defects he had described earlier. This constellation of anomalies became known as status Bonnevie-Ullrich or pterygolymphangiectasia. Rossi and Caflisch (1951) suggested that the general term pterygium syndrome be adopted to include the following subgroups: (1) status Ullrich bilateralis, (2) Nielson's dystrophia brevicollis congenita, (3) Turner's gonadal dysgenesis, (4) status Ullrich unilateralis, and (5) arthrogryposis multiplex congenitalis or pterygo-arthromyodysplasia. Gharib and Stickler (1959) endorsed this classification and reported a case of arthrogryposis, which they claimed "belonged in this ill-defined group of congenital malformations." Most investigators see no fundamental relationship among the various signs and symptoms lumped together under the nondescript designation pterygium syndrome.

PREFERRED BODY-IMAGE AND THE PLIGHT OF THE INDIVIDUAL WITH MALFORMED LIMBS

It is expected that, among other perfections, the newborn infant have a pair of perfect hands; that each hand be equipped with a thumb and four fingers, five agile and perceptive digits which respond with skill and alacrity to the demands made upon them; and that these digits appear attractive, or at least not repulsive.

Society sets a definite goal for each child. The child with a malformed limb, unlike the normal infant, begins life with a distinct disadvantage. While other children strive toward their goal with relative ease and speed, the physically handicapped youngster inches his way with much effort through a maze of obstacles. On his way to the arena of competition with others and even after he gets there, he may remain incarcerated behind what may seem an insurmountable rampart. Does the obstacle serve him as a challenge and evoke compensatory capabilities? It is said that when a projection of an amoeba is blocked, the amoeba puts forth another one. Does the child with a congenitally defective hand activate substitute extensions of insight or skill to accelerate his progress toward the goal? Carlisle (1814) described a hexadactylous family, a member of which, Zerah Colburn, the son of Abiah Colburn, born in Vermont, was brought to London because of his "extraordinary power in arithmetical computation from memory." There have been a number of physically handicapped artists, writers, lawyers, and physicians who have achieved fame and fortune. Contrary to the popular adage, exceptions do not establish a rule.

The more fortunate members of society cannot fully appreciate the difficulties encountered by a malformed individual and they often fail to recognize the duality of the problem faced by him. Following the standards of traditional mores, society distinguishes variations in physique and places values upon them; it accords lower values to those who fall short of its requirements and as a result, tends to alienate them.

SHIFTING SOCIAL ATTITUDES

In the literature on congenital anomalies of the hand and forearm, there is very little coordinated discussion of historical perspectives and practically no meaningful interpretation of the available data. The Weisman collection in New York and the anthropological museum in Mexico City contain many remnants of pre-Colombian sculpture showing malformed hands. According to Parrot (1878), ancient Egyptians worshipped an achondroplastic deity named Phtah. The Standing Maitreya Buddha (A.D. 550–808) from Pra Kon Chai—whose statue is now in the Kimbell Art Museum, Fort Worth, Texas—had duplicated forearms and hands. Perthies (1902) spoke of the image of another deity with cloven hands and feet in the temple of Nikko, Japan. Plutarch (A.D. 46–120) wrote that Artaxerxes I, who reigned over Persia between 465 and 425 B.C., was nicknamed "macrocheir" because he had a gigantic right hand. According to Gates (1946), the Sultan of Pontianak (Borneo) was hexadactylous and regarded his surplus digit as a mark of royal distinction. It would seem that in some communities polydactylism carried no social stigma. It was, in fact, looked upon as a sign of virtue.

Of all congenital abnormalities of the hand, polydactyly has perhaps the oldest and the longest history. Chaldeans are often mentioned in the Bible (Genesis 11:28, Daniel 1:4, and so forth). "In the days of ancient Chaldeans," Gould and Pyle (1897) wrote, "it was for those of royal birth specially that divinations relative to extra digits were cast. Among the ancients we also occasionally see illustrations emblematic of wisdom in an individual with many fingers or rather double hands, on each arm." In the Bible (II Samuel 21:20) one also reads: "And there was yet a battle in Gath, where was a man of great stature, that had on every hand six fingers, and on every foot six toes, four and twenty in number; and he also was born to the giant." Renan (1903) placed the date of the Gath encounter prior to 1000 B.C. On the authority of Archbishop Ussher Julia Bell (1930), 1019, B.C. has been assigned as the date of the battle of Gath.

Chuang Tzu, the Taoist philosopher who lived in China about 400 B.C., considered extra fingers to be functionally superflous and useless excrescences. A Chinese story transcribed by H. A. Giles (1909) describes the plight of Sally Sun who was enamored of a beautiful rich girl named A-pao. Sally Sun had six fingers. Before she would marry Sally Sun, A-pao insisted that he cut off his sixth finger. This he did, and he almost died from hemorrhage. Social stigma against supernumerary digits does not appear to have been adopted by Europeans until many years after Marco Polo's return from China near the end of the thirteenth century—almost 2000 years after Chuang Tzu.

Ancient Romans took their hexadactylism for granted, and even used Sedigitus as a surname. Members of the Scipian family are said to have been hexadactylous. This family gave Rome some of its best generals and rulers. Perhaps the most famous of these is Scipio Africanus the Elder (237–183 B.C.), who destroyed the combined armies of the Carthaginians and Numidians. He also defeated Hannibal in the battle of Zama thereby gaining the title "Conqueror of Hannibal." His son, Scipio Africanus the Younger (185–129 B.C.) is considered one of Rome's most skillful generals; he is said to have been highly cultured. "Some people," Pliny the Elder (A.D. 23–79) wrote, "have six fingers on each hand. It has come down to us that the two daughters of the patrician, Marcus Curiatus, were called Misses Six-Fingers and that Volcatius Sedigitus was distinguished in poetry."

According to Mauclaire (1901, 1913) Attila, "scourge of God, King of the Huns," who terrorized the known world during the first half of the fifth century, also had six fingers. Many French authors, including Morand (1773), Saint-Hilaire (1832), Tapie (1885), Mauclaire (1901) and Christiaenes et al (1963), have claimed that in his celebrated fresco of the *Last Supper*, Leonardo da Vinci painted one of the 12 apostles with six fingers. Bell (1930) said she had seen a copy of the picture and thought that the anomalous digit resulted from the "artist's oversight (or over-painting) rather than a reproduction of an anomaly in the original design." Miss Bell could not conceive of any purpose on the part of the artist for paying attention to so "small a detail."

Leonardo da Vinci started the *Last Supper* in 1494; he finished it four years later. The original painting has suffered much damage from vandalism and neglect and has been subjected to many restorations. The refectory wall of St. Maria delle Grazie in Milan continues to crack and lose chunks of plaster from year to year, and the colors in the painting have long since faded. Upon viewing Leonardo's mural in its present state, one can barely distinguish the faces of the apostles and will find it even more difficult to count their fingers.

It is quite possible that Morand (1773) saw a faithful facsmile of the original painting. There is no reason to question the testimony of Morand, who is explicit on this point. As for the "small detail" that concerned Miss Bell, many great works of art are produced by paying attention to the smallest of details. Such perceptive artists as Leonardo da Vinci and Michelangelo seldom overlooked significant details. Lawrence (1929) points out that in Michelangelo's Laocoon the oldest son, who wears a scared expression, indicating weakness, had three phalanges in his left thumb. Michelangelo also showed Guilano de Medici with a triphalangeal right thumb (Figs. 29–1 and 29–2).

According to Bruno (1959), Leonardo da Vinci often utilized such anomalies as clinodactyly, camptodactyly, and arachnodactyly in his paintings as indications of hidden traits. One wonders if, in the original version of the *Last Supper*, da Vinci placed the anomalous finger on Judas Iscariot's hand to suggest his treachery symbolically. It was not many years after the completion of the painting that Europeans came to regard extra digits as a sign of a scheming character.

Anne Boleyn's hexadactylism appears to have established a more definite precedence. Historians place Anne's birth around 1507, when Leonardo da Vinci was still alive and, by curious coincidence, when he began his painting *Virgin in the Lap of St. Ann*. Da Vinci showed this painting to his friend, Cardinal Louid of Aragon, who might have been related to Catherine of Aragon—Henry VIII's lawful wife—whom Anne Boleyn replaced with a tactical skill reminiscent of the strategies of Scipian generals. Anne became pregnant by King Henry long before she was legally married; her only child, Elizabeth, the future queen of England and Ireland, was illegitimate by any standard. After she became Henry's queen, Anne treated her adversaries with an insolence that could well match Attila's.

Anne's predecessor, Catherine, had proved herself an exemplary queen. She came of royal stock and professed the Catholic faith. Anne was a commoner. Catholic historians were hypercritical of Anne, since she had set a precedent for divorce and had caused a major rift between England and Rome. They perhaps magnified her defects. Protestant historians overlooked Anne's shortcomings. They even praised her. After all, she was the mother of the great queen, Elizabeth I. Even her adversaries conceded that she was "brave as a lion" and faced death at the gallows cheerfully. Time was needed for proper perspective.

Anne Boleyn's physical defects, previously hush-hushed by Protestant historians, finally found their way into medical literature—both French and English. Saint-Hilaire (1832) singled out three distinct imperfections: badly aligned teeth, a supernumerary breast, and six fingers on one hand. Samuel Cooper (1838) wrote: "Anne Boleyn . . . was cruelly punished by her husband, Henry VIII, for having hidden from him another vice of conformation, a supernumerary

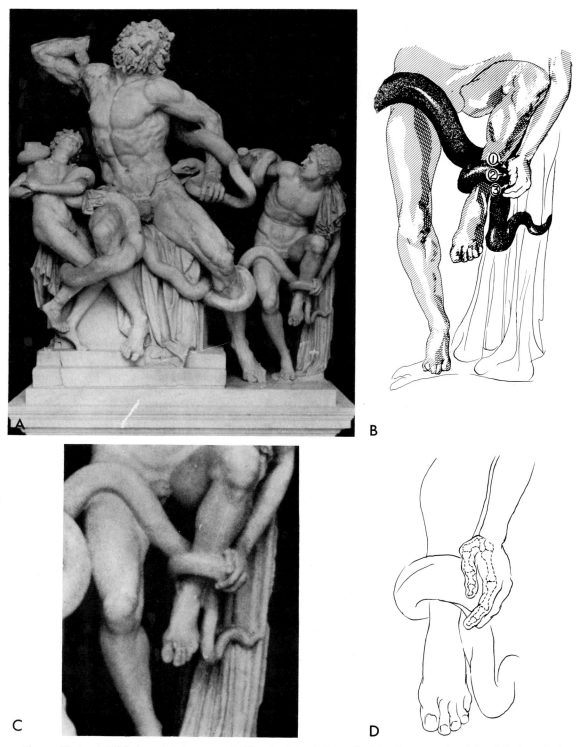

Figure 29–1 *A*, Michelangelo's Laocoon, *B*, Sketch of the left hand of the figure on the right. *C*, Enlarged photograph of the same left hand. *D*, Sketch illustrating the skeletal components of the left thumb and index finger.

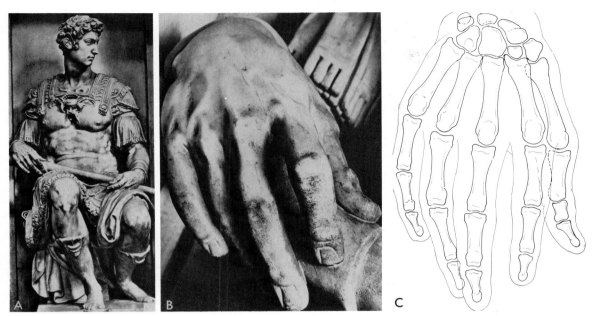

Figure 29–2 *A*, Michelangelo's Guilano de Medici. *B*, Enlarged photograph of the right hand, showing that the thumb extends beyond the second interphalangeal joint of the index finger. *C*, Sketch illustrating the skeletal components of the same hand.

breast." Oliver (1940) has recently described a recessive form of polydactyly in two female sibs, one of whom had a supernumerary nipple on her left breast. Anne might have suffered from a variation of this syndrome as, unlike Oliver's subjects, she was not mentally retarded.

Bell (1930) cast some doubt on the contention that Anne Boleyn was polydactylous and, moreover, had a supernumerary nipple, which had been repeatedly stated, particularly in French literature. Samuel Cooper was not French; he was an eminent surgeon in London, who compiled one of the best medical dictionaries in English. "Now the portraits of the beautiful queen show no defect," Bell argued naively. She might have known that no queen—and least of all, coquettish Anne—would permit an artist to demonstrate her defects. Anne is not known to have posed in the nude for any artist, which might have revealed her supernumerary breast. She also would not have shown the "sixth finger on her right hand," to an artist, and if she did, she would not have permitted him to include it in his portrait of her.

Almost all recent historians agree that Anne was an ambitious schemer and a conqueror of sorts in her own limited sphere. She was skillful in strategy and tactics just as Scipio the Elder was, and she could boast of culture and refinement like the younger Scipio. Anne was conversant about poetry and music; it is said that this was one of her principal attributes which attracted Henry. "Anne's worst enemies granted her one virtue, courage," Albert (1956) wrote. She was adventurous and cruel like Attila. One could also draw an analogy between Anne's cheerful attitude toward impending death and the hilarious recklessness with which Attila ended his own life.

Times change and standards of evaluation alter. What may have been regarded as the object of envy at one period, in one country, could well invite disdain at some other time, in another place. The modern era has rightly been dubbed the "age of conformity." The children of today wish to possess the same physical equipment as their peers. It is inevitable that, upon attaining a measure of self-awareness, the child with a discernible congenital anomaly will suffer some psychic trauma. This is not to say that such a child is destined to be backward or aggressive. Other factors enter into the picture.

SUBTERFUGE

As noted by Mattingly (1960), Anne Boleyn hid her hexadactylous hand "so well with gloves and the folds of her dress that many people never noticed it." Paget (1845) spoke of the governor of Luzon, Philippines, who kept his macrodactylic fingers within the breast of his coat "to avoid observation."

Malformed hands cannot be kept out of sight indefinitely. They are eventually seen and scrutinized. To dispose of "the stigma of congenitalism," Littler (1964) recommended altering a gestational defect by surgical intervention to make it appear as if it were the result of external trauma. Littler advised excision of rudimentary "functionless and bizarre" digital buds to make the limb simulate "a simple amputation stump" and thus become "relatively free from curious attention."

Rudimentary digits need not be subjected to surgical extirpation merely to divert attention. In cases of young girls and women with no hands, it is justifiable to prescribe a cosmetic glove. Friedmann (1968) points out that the cosmetic glove is expensive and, if stained, is likely to be discarded and thus will defeat the very purpose for which it was obtained. He advised wearing it only on special occasions. Boys do not seem to mind wearing prostheses which may appear unsightly but are functionally effective (Fig. 29–3).

EMOTIONAL ANCHORAGE AS AN AIM

In imaginative literature, one finds numerous references to malformed feet but only an occasional mention of congenitally maimed hands. In Willa Cather's (1918) *My Antonia,* Marek always "held up his hands to show . . . his fingers, which were webbed to the first knuckle, like a duck's foot . . . always trying to be agreeable . . . always coveting distinction." In Kafka's (1925) *The Trial,* Leni, the nurse, who had short, webbed fingers, zealously exhibits her malformed hand to her lover and hopes to replace her normally constituted rival. Leni had learned to live with her defect.

RELIGION

Faith enters into the picture with an apparent salutary effect. In answer to a questionnaire, one Catholic mother with a handless infant considered it a privilege that the Lord had selected her to care for a child who needed extra attention. Four Protestant pairs who had been proffered normal children for adop-

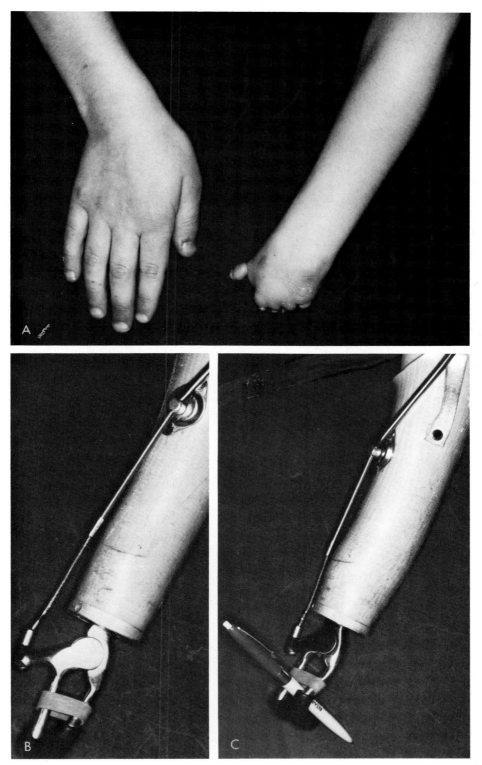

Figure 29–3 Prosthesis. *A*, Dorsal view of the hands of a left-handed boy with transverse terminal defect of the left hand who preferred a functionally useful prosthesis. *B*, Prosthesis. *C*, Wielding a pen.

tion chose infants with defective hands. One couple wrote: "We had a good marriage. We didn't 'need' a child for it to be a success, but we had something to offer a child . . . we had both placed the situation in the Lord's hands. If He wanted us to have a baby, we would have one. . . . We feel certain the Lord has been leading in this matter."

MARRIAGE AND PROCREATION

Individuals with widespread syndromic defects and repulsive appearance, such as those afflicted with acrocephalosyndactyly, may have difficulty in finding marital mates. Most subjects with isolated malformation of the hand and forearm seem to meet with no such hindrance. Murray (1863) described "a well-developed, healthy, active, and intelligent woman." These qualifications appear to have compensated for her defect, which consisted of ulnar dimelia or mirror hand. She was married and had a normal child. Brachydactylous women are compactly built and petite, and are preferentially selected by normal men. "They always pick us first," boasted a short-fingered female belonging to a pedigree recorded by Farabee (1905). In the fourth generation of this pedigree, 14 normal parents produced 28 offspring, an average of two per parent, while seven short-fingered parents claimed 33 children, an average of almost five offspring per parent. Farabee ascribed this discrepancy to the earlier marriage of brachydactylous individuals. "Abnormals all along the line have married earlier in life than normals," Farabee wrote, "so when the fifth generation is reached their families number ten, seven, five, etc., while normals in many cases have but one child." In Drinkwater's (1908) pedigree, six short-fingered females had 49 children, a little more than eight per female, while eight affected men had 39 offspring, an average of less than five children per parent. Drinkwater (1908) concluded that brachydactylous women were "clearly much more prolific than men."

BEHAVIOR

Gingras et al (1964) conducted behavioral studies on 41 patients with congenital limb anomalies and found no evidence of any major emotional disorder; a malformed individual's attitude toward his disability appeared to be definitely influenced by that of his parents as well as by the character of the emotional undertone in the total environment. These investigators considered the attitude of the parents, particularly of the mother, extremely important in the emotional development of the defective child. They advised counseling for the parents soon after the birth of a defective infant.

In a study of juvenile amputees, Spring and Epps (1968) encountered a wide spectrum of emotional problems, ranging from minor character disorders to inferiority complex and paranoia. These investigators also stressed the importance of parental attitude and of social acceptance in determining the child's psychomotor state; when these two factors were favorable the child learned to accept its deformity and attained emotional stability. Mental retardation accompanies a number of syndromic malformations of the hand and forearm; the affected individuals may manifest bizarre behavior but they rarely run afoul of the law.

In recent years a number of communications—by Jacob et al (1965), Price and Whatmore (1967), Court-Brown et al (1968), Cleveland et al (1969), Valentine (1969), and Fotheringham (1970)—appeared concerning the aggressive behavior and the criminal tendencies of males with XYY genotype, some of whom are known to have radioulnar synostosis. These investigators point out that affected individuals manifest criminal behavior after puberty. A prepubertal boy with XY/XYY mosaicism was described by Kajii et al (1968). This boy was tall and had a prognathic jaw. The thenar and hypothenar eminences of his hands were effaced; his thumbs and fingers were axially deviated. The span of his attention was short, and he had "hyperkinesis associated with learning difficulties." It is possible that this boy was too young—only 11 years old—to display aggressive, antisocial behavior.

PARENTAL ATTITUDE

Kerckringii's (1670) polydactylous dwarf was found drowned in a river—presumably thrown there by one of the parents. Quite likely this is not the first, nor the last, anomalous child to be discarded by the parents. It is not uncommon, especially in larger cities, to find malformed neonates left at the doors of homes for foundlings. Understandably, parents are shocked at the sight of their defective newborn. There follows a period of readjustment during which they undergo paroxysms of remorse, a sense of personal responsibility for the tragedy, and recrimination. Ultimately, most parents attain a realistic attitude and do what they can to improve the malformed child's condition.

ILLEGITIMACY

The medical literature contains numerous reports of illegitimate children with anomalous upper limbs. Victoire Barré was reported by Maygrier (1830) as having split hand complex. Victoire had two daughters with the same defect. She previously given birth to a son with split hand, but "the father of this boy was not. . . the father of the girls also." Snyder (1929) described a woman who was involved in a "set of critical matings"; she had seven normal children by a normal man whose family had never shown polydactylism and one illegitimate polydactylous child by a man who himself showed the same abnormality. Saethre (1931) spoke of a mother and her daughters with acrocephalosyndactyly: one of the daughters was illegitimate and, for some reason, was affected more severely than her half sister. The male progenitor of Nievergelt's (1944) syndrome had three affected sons by three different women. A male infant born to unmarried parents was described by Agazzi (1962). This child had rudimentary humeri on both sides, bilateral radioulnar synostosis, syndactyly of both ring fingers, and absence of both thumbs.

LEGAL COMPLICATIONS

An illicit relationship with legal complications was recorded by Mohr (1921). The affair concerned one Karen Hansen and her brachydactylous lover, Hans Olsen, who denied that he had fathered her brachydactylous son, Ole Kristian. Karen Hansen, as well as her mother, father, seven brothers and sisters, and her relatives, had normal hands. Roentgenographs of Hans Olsen's and Ole Kristina's hands showed an identical type of brachydactyly: the second row of phalanges of the middle, ring, and little fingers was dwarfed and the index finger had only two phalanges, the middle phalanx being entirely absent.

Hans Olsen himself was illegitimate. His mother, Anna Olsen, had an affair with a "traveling agent." The affair must have been fleeting and clandestine, since she could not remember the shape of his hands. She herself had normal hands. The case was further complicated by the fact that some other witnesses had to be examined, "who according to the opinion of the plaintiff may have had coition" with Karen Hansen. These men had normal hands. The sheriff, who said he knew almost everyone in the district, could not recall any man, other than Hans Olsen, with deformed hands.

Mohr, who served as an expert witness in this case, attested that Hans Olsen was Ole Kristian's father. The same verdict was passed by the court, and Hans Olsen "had to pay a sum in costs of proceedings to the State."

FUNCTIONAL PROPENSITY

Untreated giant fingers not only appear repulsive but, being oversized and overstuffed—too long and too thick—will not bend and effect pulp-to-pulp apposition with the other digits nor take part in the act of grasping. However, individuals with such extreme malformations as ulnar dimelia seem to have no functional impairment. The man with mirror hand reported by Jackson (1853) was a machinist. Jackson wrote: his "hand was not merely useful in the way of his business, but gave him some advantage . . . in playing upon the piano, upon which he was a performer." A man with no thumbs, stiff, flexed wrists, and almost no forearms was reported by Stiles and Dougan (1940) as having farmed 80 acres of land with little assistance.

In some forms of brachydactyly, dwarfed digits are stiff; they cannot be expected to perform as efficiently as fingers with flexible joints and normal length. In the pedigree of a brachydactylous family reported by Farabee (1905), the ladies complained that they could not reach a full octave and, hence, were not good piano players. Brachydactylous members of the pedigree studied by Drinkwater (1908) also complained of inability to play any musical instrument for which normal length of the fingers was requisite; the men had weaker and smaller grips, and the women could not do "netting." Most men and women in this family were engaged in occupations which made no demands upon manual dexterity; they were unskilled laborers and remained several scales below the social niche attained by their normal relatives.

Men with short fingers are usually short in stature. Individuals with Ellis-van Creveld chondroectodermal dysplasia are moderate dwarfs and have short middle and distal phalanges and comparatively long proximal ones. They cannot make a tight fist. The diastrophic dwarf with hitchhiker's thumb tends to wield a pen or a pencil with the index and middle fingers. People with pycnodysostosis also have short fingers. Many earlier authors—and more recently Rubin (1964) and Bergstrom (1969), among others—perpetuated the lore that Toulouse-Lautrec suffered from osteogenesis imperfecta, which is transmitted as a dominant phenotype. Toulouse-Lautrec was not a blue sclerotic; he did not suffer from numerous fractures; he always kept his hat on to hide his peculiarly contoured head; and he was the product of a consanguineous marriage. In a scholarly article, Maroteaux and Lamy (1965) concluded: "shortness of stature, moderate bone brittleness, the shortness of the hand, craniofacial deformity with absence of knitting of the fontanel, and autosomal recessive transmission, which are the main features of pycnodysostosis, are present in Toulouse-Lautrec's case. . . . This rare disease bequeathes us the artistic works of one of the greatest painters of our time." By implication, brachydactylic hands in pycnodysostosis are not disabling. Toulouse-Lautrec was the son of a rich man; he had all the opportunities to fully develop his particular talent; and he was self-employed. Short stature and short fingers do not preclude talent, but society can stifle latent talent. Toulouse-Lautrec lived in a society which placed a high value on art.

EMPLOYABILITY

A young woman who was operated upon for macrodactyly and since then has become an excellent stenographer, writes: "I don't want anybody's sympathy. I hate to think of myself as a handicapped person. It infuriates me to think that I can't get a job because everybody thinks I can't use my hands normally. Huh! I am a better worker than a lot of other people. Once I went to a place that hires only handicapped people. The agent did not try to find out how well I could type. He told me I should solicit sales by telephone since I am handicapped, and that was probably the only kind of work I would get. I walked out with a vow to myself that one day I"ll have a fine, normal job. It's frustrating when you know you can do something, but nobody realizes it."

What the malformed individual wants most is a gainful occupation commensurate with his ability. The last thing a disabled person needs is saccharine sympathy or cloying, sugar-coated pity. Employment agents and employers should be taught not to be swayed by cosmetic factors; they should learn to form judgments on the basis of functional capabilities of malformed individuals.

COUNSELING

Macrodactyly, acrosyndactyly, annular grooves, symbrachydactyly, and ulnar dimelia are not transmitted from one generation to another. Of the heritable hand or forearm malformations, type B brachydactyly (apical dystrophy), split hand complex, and radial ray defect associated with congenital heart disease, as well as syndromes accompanied by severe debility, mental retardation, or gross deformation, are considered sufficiently serious to warn the affected individual against procreation, but not necessarily against marriage. The same warning is accorded to consanguineous individuals, especially when either the man or the woman or both are known to be carriers of deleterious genes.

During the first three months of gestation, pregnant women should shun exposure to roentgen rays and viral infections and avoid ingestion of corticosteroids, anticoagulants, estrogens, and sedatives. Even daily use of nose drops and frequent exposure to insecticide sprays, as well as ingestion of contraceptive pills by women who are not aware of their incipient pregnancy, are said to invite "maximal fetal hazard." Sayli et al (1966) reported a case of phocomelia and considered aspirin to be one of the two causative factors, the other being parental consanguinity.

THE FUTURE

Tatum (1961), previously mentioned in Chapter One, spoke of the ultimate in biological engineering. He expressed the hope that, with increasing knowledge of the involved molecular chains of events, of the mechanism of gene mutation, of the finer details of DNA structure, and of the genetic code, it would be possible to restore an abnormal or potentially abnormal organism to normality, or to alter predictably and improve genes within the chromosomes of the living cell by a process of controlled and directed mutation. This, however, is only a hopeful projection.

SUMMARY

A malformed child soon realizes that he is different from others, and his sense of alienation can become aggravated or alleviated by those who surround him. The child, as well as his parents and society at large, must be indoctrinated to accept his defect. With more liberal legislation, better control of drugs, and enlightenment of the public, many congenital anomalies, especially exogenous ones, may in time be eliminated. A great deal also depends upon biological scientists and their ability to unravel the mysterious shrouds of the complex mechanism of being born normal. It is not beyond the ken of possibility that at some future date desirable elements will be introduced into the constituion of genetic material.

References

Agazzi, W.: Il problema delle malformazioni congenite negli illegittimi. *Minerva Nipiol, 12*:380–382, 1962.

Albert, H.: *The Divorce.* New York, Simon & Schuster, pp. 79–95, 1956.

Bagley, J. J.: *Henry VIII and His Times.* New York, Arco Publishing Co., Inc., pp. 59–61, 1963.

Bell, J.: Some new pedigrees of hereditary disease. A. Polydactylism and syndactylism. B. Blue scleroses and fragility of bone. *Ann. Eugen., 4*:41–49, 1930.

Bergstrom, W. H.: Hereditary and metabolic bone diseases. *In* Gardner, L. T., (ed.): *Endocrine and Genetic Diseases of Childhood.* Philadelphia, W. B. Saunders Co., pp. 738–756, in particular p. 754, 1969.

Bonnevie, K.: Embryological analysis of gene manifestation in Little and Bagg's abnormal mouse tribe. *J. Exp. Zool., 67*:443–520, 1934.

Bruno, G.: Malformazioni delle dita della mano nella patologia e nell'arte (aracnodactylia, klinodactylia, kamptodactylia). *Minerva Med., 50*:3685–3691, 1959.

Busey, S. C.: Congenital occlusion and dilatation of lymph channels. *Am. J. Obstet., 10*:223–253, 1877; *11*:65–115, 1878.

Carlisle, A.: An account of a family having hands and feet with supernumerary fingers and toes. *Phil. Trans. R. Soc., 104*:94–101, 1814.

Cather, W.: *My Antonia.* Sentry edition. Boston, Houghton Mifflin Co. The Riverside Press Cambridge, pp. 24, 77, 103, 1954. The original appeared in 1918.

Christiaenes, L., Laude, M., and Fontaines, G.: Les polydactylies à propos d'un cas familial. *Pédiatrie, 18*:790–814, 1963.

Chuang Tzu: *Chuang Tzu, Taoist Philosopher and Chinese Mystic.* Second revised edition. Translated from the Chinese by H. A. Giles. London, Ruskin House, pp. 92–96, 1961.

Cleveland, W. W., Arias, B., and Smith, G. F.: Radioulnar synostosis, behavioral disturbance and XXY chromosomes. *J. Pediatr., 75*:103–106, 1969.

Cooper, S.: *A Dictionary of Practical Surgery.* Sixth London edition. New York, Harper & Bros, Vol. 1, pp. 370–371, 1838.

Court-Brown, W. M., Price, W. H., and Jacobs, P. A.: The XXY male. *Br. Med. J., 4*:513, 1968.

Crouzon, O.: Étude de la main par H. Holbein. *N. Iconog. Salp., 21*:245–246; Pl. XXXVIII, 1908.

Darwin, C.: *The Variation of Animals and Plants under Domestication.* Third edition. New York, D. Appelton & Co., Vol. 1, pp. 457–460, 1896.

Drinkwater, H.: An account of a brachydactylous family. *Proc. R. Soc. Edinburgh, 28*:35–57, 1908.

Emery, A. E. H.: Genetic counseling. *Scot. Med. J., 14*:335–347, 1969.

Farabee, W. C.: Inheritance of digital malformation in man. *Am. Archeol. Ethnolog., 3*:69–76; tables V & VI; Pl. XXIII-XXVII, 1905.

Fotheringham, B. J.: XYY males in South Australia. *S. Australian Clin., 4*:265–266, 1970.

Fraser, F. C.: Genetic counseling and the physician. *Can. Med. Assoc., 99*:927–934, 1968.

Freire-Maia, N., and Freire-Maia, A.: Recurrence risks of bone aplasias and hypoplasias of the extremities. *Acta Genet.* (Basel), *17*:418–421, 1967.

Friedmann, L. W.: Rehabilitation of amputees. *In* Licht, S., and Kamenetz, H. L., (eds.): *Rehabilitation and Medicine.* Baltimore, Waverly Press, Inc., pp. 296–389, 1968.

Gates, R. R.: *Human Genetics.* New York, MacMillan Co., pp. 385–469, 1946.

Gharib, R., and Stickler, G.: Pterygium syndrome (Status Bonnevie-Ullrich). *J. Lancet, 79*:57–59, 1959.

Giles, H. A.: *Strange Stories from a Chinese Studio.* Second edition, revised. London, T. Werner Laurie, pp. 115–129, 1909.

Gingras, Q., Monçeau, M., Moreault, P., Dupuis, M., Hebert, B., and Corriveau, C.: Congenital anomalies of limbs. II. Psychological and educational aspect. *Can. Med. Assoc. J., 91*:115–119, 1964.

Gordon, H.: Genetic counseling: considerations for talking to parents and perspective parents. *J.A.M.A., 217*:1215–1225, 1971.

Gould, G. M., and Pyle, W. L.: *Anomalies and Curiosities of Medicine.* Philadelphia, W. B. Saunders Co., pp. 270–276, 1897.

Hollis: Lopsided generations. *J. Anat. Physiol., 9*:263–271, 1875.

Horne, A. G.: Hereditary malformations — supernumerary fingers. *Lancet, 1*:115, 1838.

Hurley, T. W.: Hypertrophy and elongation of the thumb, index and middle fingers of the right hand from congenital occlusion of lymph channels. *Am. Med. Bi-weekly, 9*:49–50, 1878.

Jackson, J. B.: Malformation in an adult subject, otherwise well formed, consisting of apparent fusion of two upper extremities. *Am. J. Med. Sci.,* (n.s.), *25*:91–93, 1853. See also *Descriptive Catalogue of the Warren Anatomical Museum, Harvard University.* Boston, A. Williams & Co., Entry 917; pp. 137–138, 1870.

Jacob, P. A., Brunton, M., Melville, M. M., Brittain, R. P., and McClement, M. F.: Aggressive behaviors, mental subnormality and the XYY male. *Nature, 208*:1351–1352, 1965.

Jaworska, M., and Popiolek, J.: Genetic counseling in lobster-claw anomaly: discussion of variability of genetic influence in different families. *Clin. Pediatr., 7*:396–399, 1968.

Johannsen, W.: The genotype conception of heredity. *Am. Naturalist, 45*:129–159, 1911.

Kafka, F.: *The Trial.* Translated from the German by W. & E. Muir. New York, Alfred A. Knopf, Definitive ed., pp. 132–139, 1957. The original German edition appeared in 1925.

Kajii, T., Neu, R. L., and Gardner, L. T.: XY/XYY mosaicism in a prebubertal boy with tall stature prognathism, and malformations of the hands. *Pediatrics, 41*:984–988, 1968.

Kallmann, F. J.: Psychiatric aspects of genetic counseling. *Am. J. Hum. Genet., 8*:96–101, 1956.

Kellie: Short fingers. Extract from a letter to M. L. from Dr. Kellie. *Edinburgh Med. Surg. J., 4*:252–253, 1808.

Kemp, T.: *Genetics and Disease.* Copenhagen, E. Munksgaard, pp. 190–242, 1951.

Kerckringii, T.: *Spicilegium Anatomicum.* Amsterdam, Angrae Firstii, pp. 51–53, 1670.

Lawrence, A. W.: *Classical Sculpture.* London, J. Cape, pp. 323–325, pl. 121, 1929.

Littler, J. W.: Principles of reconstructive surgery of the hand. *In* Converse, J. M., (ed.): *Reconstructive Plastic Surgery.* Philadelphia, W. B. Saunders Co., Vol. IV, pp. 1617–1673, 1964.

MacKinder, D.: Deficiency of fingers transmitted through six generations. *Br. Med. J., 2*:845–846, 1857.

MacLaurin, C.: The case of Anne Boleyn. *In Post Mortem Essays, Historical and Medical.* New York, George H. Doran & Co., pp. 13–33, 1922.

Maroteaux, P., and Lamy, M.: The malady of Toulouse-Lautrec. *J.A.M.A., 191*:715–717, 1965.

Mattingly, G.: *Catherine of Aragon.* New York, Vintage Books, pp. 234–235, 1960.

Matulsky, A. G., and Hecht, F.: Genetic prognosis and counseling. *Am. J. Obstet. Gynecol., 90*:1227–1241, 1964.

Mauclaire, P.: Chirurgie des membres. *In* LeDontu, A., and Delbot, P., (eds.): *Traité de Chirurgie.* Paris, J. B. Ballière et fils, pp. 77–111, 1901.

Mauclaire, P.: *Chirurgie Générale et Chirurgie Orthopédique des Membres.* Paris, J. B. Ballière et fils, pp. 77–111, 1913.

Maygrier: Remarkable case of hereditary monstrosity. *Lancet, 1*:791–792, 1830.

Mohr, O. L.: A case of hereditary brachyphalangy utilized as evidence in forensic medicine. *Hereditas, 2*:290–298, 1921.

Montgomery, D. W.: Mention made of the fingers by Rabelais. *Med. J. Rec., 120*:127–129, 1924.

Morand, M.: Recherches sur quelques conformations monstrueuses des doigts dans l'homme. *Histoire Acad. R. Sci.,* (Anne 1770), pp. 137–150, 1773.

Murphy, E. A.: The rationale of genetic counseling. *J. Pediatr. 72*:121–130, 1968.

Murray, J.: Case of a woman with three hands. *Med. Chir. Tr. 28*:29–31, 1863.

Nielson, H.: Dystrophis brevicollis congenita. *Hospitalstidende* (Kobenhaven), *77*:403–423, 1934.

Nievergelt, K.: Positiver Vaterschaftsnachweis auf Grund erblicher Missbildungen der Extremitäten. *Arch. Julius Klaus Stift, 19*:157–195, 1944.

Oliver, C. P.: Recessive polydactylism, associated with mental deficiency. *J. Hered., 31*:365–367, 1940.

Paget, J.: See Curling, T. B.: Case of remarkable hypertrophy of the fingers in a girl with a notice of some similar cases. *Med. Chir. Tr., 28*:337–339, 1845.

Parrot, J.: Sur la malformation achondroplastique et le Dieu Phtah. *Bull. Soc. Anthropol., 1*:296–308, 1878.

Perthies, G.: Über Spalthand. *Dtsch. Z., 63*:137–148, 1902.

Pliny: (A.D. 23–79): *Natural History.* Translated into English by H. Rackham. London, W. Heinemann Ltd, Vol. III, Book XI, p. 584–611, 1940.

Plutarch (A.D. 46–120): Artaxerxes and Aratus. *In Parallel Lives.* The Loeb Classical Library. Editors: E. Capps, T. E. Page, and W. H. B. Kouse. English Translation by B. Perrin from Souteurs (Teubuer 1873–1875) and Bekker (Tauchnitz 1855–1857) editions. London, W. Heinemann, Vol. XI, pp. 128–129, 1920.

Price, W. H., and Whatmore, P. B.: Behavior disorders and pattern of crime among males identified at a maximum security hospital. *Br. Med. J., 1*:533–536, 1967.

Renan, E.: *History of the People of Israel.* Boston, Little, Brown & Co., Vol. II, pp. 22–23, 1903.

Ribeiro, A. L.: "Lobster claw" hands. *Br. Med. J., 1*:1209, 1954.

Rossi, E., and Caflisch, A.: Le syndrome de pterygium. Status Bonnevie-Ullrich, dystrophia brevicolli congenita, syndrome de Turner et arthromyodysplasia congenita. *Helvet Paediatr. Acta, 6*:119–148, 1951.

Rossle, R.: Über Mythos und Pathologie. *Arch. Pathol. Anat. Physiol., 308*:519–539, 1932.

Roy, P. M.: *L'Enfant Malformé.* Paris, P. Lathielleux, pp. 115–123, 1963.

Rubin, P.: *Dynamic Classification of Bone Dysplasias.* Chicago, Year Book Medical Publishers, Inc., pp. 309–321, 1964.

Saethre, H.: Ein Beitrag zum Turmschadelproblem (pathogenese Erblickeit and Symptomatologic). *Dtsch. Z. Nervenheilkd., 119*:533–551, 1931.

Saint-Hilaire, I. G.: *Histoire Générale et Particulière des Anomalies.* Paris, J. B. Ballière, Vol. I, pp. 251–278, 671–702, 1832.

Sayli, B. S., Amaz, A., and Yemise, B.: Consanguinity, aspirin and phocomelia. *Lancet, 1*:876, 1966.

Schull, W. J.: Empirical risks in consanguineous marriages: sex ratio, malformation, and viability. *Am. J. Hum. Genet., 10*:294–343, 1958.

Schull, W. J.: Empirical risks in consanguineous marriages; sex ration, malformation, and viability.

Sedgwick, W.: On influence of sex in hereditary diseases. *Br. Foreign Med. Chir. Rev., 31*:445–479, 1863.

Snyder, L. H.: A recessive factor in polydactylism in man. Studies in human inheritance III. *J. Hered., 20*:73–77, 1929.

Spring, J. M., and Epps, C. H., Jr.: Juvenile amputee. Some observations and considerations. *Clin. Pediatr., 7*:76–79, 1968.

Stiles, K. A., and Dougan, P.: A pedigree of malformed upper extremities. *J. Hered., 31*:65–72, 1940.

Tapie: *De la Polydactylie.* Thèse. Paris, A. Parent, pp. 5–54, 1885.

Tatum, E. L.: Some molecular aspect of congential malformations. *In First International Conference on Congenital Malformations.* Philadelphia, J. B. Lippincott Co., pp. 381–388, 1961.

Tips, R., Smith, G. S., Lynch, H. T., and McNutt, C. W.: The whole family concept of clinical genetics. *Am. J. Dis. Child., 107*:67–76, 1964.

Tracy, E. J.: The mission of preventive medicine. *J.A.M.A., 165*:343–344, 1957.

Turner, H. H.: A syndrome of infantilism, congenital webbed neck and cubitus valgus. *Endocrinology, 23*:566–574, 1938.

Ullrich, O.: Über typische Kombinationsbilder multipler Abartungen, *Z. Kinderheilkd., 49*:271–276, 1930.

Ullrich, O.: Muskeldefekte und Beweglichkeitsstörungen im Gehirnervenbereich. *In* Bumke, O., and Foerster, O., (eds.): *Handbuch der Neurologie.* Berlin, J. Springer, Sechzehnter Band, pp. 142–181, 1936.

Ullrich, O.: Der Status Bonnevie-Ullrich im Rahmen und derer Dyscranio-Dysphalangie. *Ergebn. Inn. Kinderheilkd.,* (n.s.), *2*:413–446, 1951.

Valentine, G. H.: The YY chromosome complement. What does it mean? *Clin. Pediatr., 8*:350–355, 1969.

Yorke, P. C.: Anne Boleyn. *In The Encyclopaedia Britannica.* Eleventh edition. Cambridge, University Press, Vol. 4, pp. 159–161, 1910.

INDEX

Note: Page numbers in *italic* indicate illustrations.

Book Reviews

CONGENITAL DEFORMITIES OF THE HAND AND FOREARM. H. Kelikian. Philadelphia, W. B. Saunders, 1974. $35.00.

There is probably no area of surgical practice for which fewer rules or generalizations can be made than in the management of anomalies of the hand, for many defy easy description and would tax Solomon's judgment as to whether to attempt any reconstruction at all. Dr. Kelikian has rendered a signal service to the hand surgery community and the entire next generation of physicians by condensing a life's work in this area into an astonishingly well organized and readable text.

The chapter organization is excellent, with grouping by the general type of deformity and minimum use of obscure terminology in chapter headings. The bibliography is outstanding and will undoubtedly serve as the entry source for literature search in this area for many years. References are conveniently located at the end of each chapter.

The text is massively illustrated and indeed in many sections becomes solid illustrations with captions for pages at a time. The illustrations, including roentgenograms, photographs, and drawings, are of excellent quality and well coordinated with the text. This is not a primer for the beginning surgeon, but the descriptions and drawings of technique are adequate for a clear understanding of the corrections achieved or attempted in each case. Hundreds of case results are shown, and in a number of instances one seriously wonders if the improvement justified the extensive surgery and revisions required. One of the strengths of this presentation is that the illustrations will let one make many of these judgments for himself.

While no text fails to be superseded in time, I suspect that Dr. Kelikian has created an instant classic, that will be supplemented but not replaced for many years to come. It belongs in all hospital libraries and will be a necessity for any serious student of hand surgery.

Kingsbury G. Heiple, M.D.